The Principles and Practice of

MEDICINE

Twenty-Third Edition

D0080451

Edited by

John D. Stobo, MD
Professor of Medicine
Former Director, Department of Medicine
   The Johns Hopkins University School of Medicine
Chairman and Chief Executive Officer
   Johns Hopkins HealthCare

David B. Hellmann, MD
Associate Professor of Medicine
The Mary Betty Stevens Chair in Rheumatology
Executive Vice Chairman, Department of Medicine
   The Johns Hopkins University School of Medicine

Paul W. Ladenson, MD
John Eager Howard Professor of Medicine
Professor of Pathology
Joint Appointment in International Health
Director, Division of Endocrinology and Metabolism
   The Johns Hopkins University School of Medicine

Brent G. Petty, MD
Associate Professor of Medicine, Divisions of Clinical Pharmacology
   and Internal Medicine
   The Johns Hopkins University School of Medicine

Thomas A. Traill, FRCP
Associate Professor of Medicine
Director, E. Cowles Andrus Cardiac Clinic
   The Johns Hopkins University School of Medicine

APPLETON & LANGE
Stamford, Connecticut

Copyright © 1996 by Appleton & Lange
A Simon & Schuster Company

Copyright © 1988 by Appleton & Lange; © 1984, 1980, 1976, 1972, 1968 by Appleton-Century-Crofts

96 97 98 99 00 / 10 9 8 7 6 5 4 3 2 1

Prentice Hall International (UK) Limited, *London*
Prentice Hall of Australia Pty. Limited, *Sydney*
Prentice Hall Canada, Inc., *Toronto*
Prentice Hall Hispanoamericana, S.A., *Mexico*
Prentice Hall of India Private Limited, *New Delhi*
Prentice Hall of Japan, Inc., *Tokyo*
Simon & Schuster Asia Pte. Ltd., *Singapore*
Editora Prentice Hall do Brasil Ltda., *Rio de Janeiro*
Prentice Hall, Upper Saddle River, *New Jersey*

Library of Congress Catalog Card Number: 96-23756

Acquisitions Editor: Shelley Reinhardt
Managing Editor, Development: Gregory R. Huth
Production Editor: Christine Langan
Designer: Mary Skudlarek
Illustrator: Mollie Dunker
Cover illustration: *Composition* by Wassily Kandinsky

Printed in the United States of America

ISBN 0-8385-7963-9

9 780838 579633   90000

This volume is dedicated to all the students, physicians, and staff who have contributed to the success of Johns Hopkins Medicine.

Contents

Contributors

All titles without institutional listings are at The Johns Hopkins University and The Johns Hopkins Hospital.

Martin D. Abeloff, MD
Professor of Oncology and Medicine
Director, Oncology Center

Stephen C. Achuff, MD
David J. Carver Professor of Medicine
Director, Clinical Cardiology

N. Franklin Adkinson, Jr, MD
Professor of Medicine
Co-Director, Division of Allergy and Clinical Immunology

Richard F. Ambinder, MD, PhD
Associate Professor of Oncology and of Pharmacology and
   Molecular Sciences

Arnold E. Andersen, MD
Professor of Psychiatry
   University of Iowa College of Medicine
   Iowa City, Iowa

Wilmot C. Ball, Jr, MD
Associate Professor of Medicine
Joint Appointment in Environmental Health Sciences

Barbara J. Ballermann, MD
Associate Professor of Medicine

John G. Bartlett, MD
Stanhope Bayne-Jones Professor of Medicine
Joint Appointment in Epidemiology
Director, Division of Infectious Diseases

Kenneth L. Baughman, MD
Professor of Medicine
Director, Division of Cardiology

Theodore M. Bayless, MD
Professor of Medicine
Clinical Director, Meyerhoff Digestive Disease-
   Inflammatory Bowel Disease Center

William R. Bell, MD
Professor of Medicine, Radiology, and Nuclear Medicine
Edith Harris Lucas and Clara Lucas Lynn Professor of
   Hematology
Clinical Director, Division of Hematology

Bruce S. Bochner, MD
Associate Professor of Medicine

Charles B. Brendler, MD
Professor and Chief of Urology
   University of Chicago Hospitals–Pritzker School
   of Medicine
   Chicago, Illinois

Roy G. Brower, MD
Associate Professor of Medicine
Medical Director, Medical Intensive Care Unit

David W. Buchholz, MD
Associate Professor of Neurology
Director, Neurological Consultation Center

Gregory B. Bulkley, MD
Mark M. Ravitch Professor of Surgery

Christopher R. Burrow, MD
Assistant Professor of Medicine

James N. Campbell, MD
Professor of Neurosurgery
Director, Blaustein Pain Treatment Center

H. Ballentine Carter, MD
Associate Professor of Urology and Oncology

Richard E. Chaisson, MD
Associate Professor of Medicine
Joint Appointments in Epidemiology and International
   Health
Director, AIDS Service

Nisha Chibber Chandra, MD
Professor of Medicine
Director, Coronary Care Unit, Johns Hopkins Bayview
   Medical Center

Patricia Charache, MD
Professor of Pathology and Medicine

Samuel Charache, MD
Professor of Medicine and Pathology Emeritus

Augustine M. K. Choi, MD
Assistant Professor of Medicine

David S. Cooper, MD
Associate Professor of Medicine
Director, Thyroid Clinic
Director, Division of Endocrinology, Sinai Hospital of
   Baltimore

John L. Currie, MD
Professor and Chair, Department of Obstetrics
   and Gynecology
   Dartmouth Medical School
   Hanover, New Hampshire

Chi V. Dang, MD, PhD
Associate Professor of Medicine
Director, Division of Hematology

J. Raymond DePaulo, Jr, MD
Professor of Psychiatry
Director, Affective Disorders Section

Anna Mae Diehl, MD
Associate Professor of Medicine

Mark Donowitz, MD
Professor of Medicine
Paulson Professor of Gastroenterology
Director, Division of Gastroenterology

Henry E. Fessler, MD
Assistant Professor of Medicine

John H. Fetting, MD
Associate Professor of Oncology and Medicine
Co-Director, Johns Hopkins Breast Center

Robert S. Fisher, MD, PhD
Chief, Epilepsy Center and Neurophysiology
    Barrow Neurological Institute
    Phoenix, Arizona

Marshal F. Folstein, MD
Professor and Chairman, Psychiatry
    Tufts University School of Medicine
Psychiatrist-in-Chief
    New England Medical Center
    Boston, Massachusetts

Susan E. Folstein, MD
Professor of Psychiatry
    Tufts University School of Medicine
Director, Child and Adolescent Psychiatry
    New England Medical Center
    Boston, Massachusetts

Daniel E. Ford, MD, MPH
Associate Professor of Medicine
Joint Appointments in Epidemiology and in Health Policy
    and Management

Nicholas J. Fortuin, MD
Professor of Medicine

Angeliki Georgopoulos, MD
Associate Professor of Medicine
    University of Minnesota School of Medicine
Director, Lipid Clinic
    Veterans Affairs Medical Center
    Minneapolis, Minnesota

Francis M. Giardiello, MD
Associate Professor of Medicine
Director, Hereditary Colon Cancer and Polyposis Clinic

Luis F. Gimenez, MD
Assistant Professor of Medicine
Director, Renal Division, Good Samaritan Hospital,
    Baltimore
Director, Dialysis Unit, Good Samaritan Hospital

Sidney O. Gottlieb, MD
Associate Professor of Medicine

Diane E. Griffin, MD, PhD
Professor and Chair, Department of Molecular Microbiology
    and Immunology
Joint Appointments in Medicine and Neurology

John W. Griffin, MD
Professor of Neurology and Neuroscience

Stuart A. Grossman, MD
Associate Professor of Oncology, Medicine, and
    Neurosurgery
Director, Neuro-Oncology

Thomas Guarnieri, MD
Associate Professor of Medicine

Alan D. Guerci, MD
Associate Professor of Clinical Medicine
    College of Physicians and Surgeons
    of Columbia University
    New York, New York
Executive Vice President for Medical Affairs
Director of Research
    St. Francis Hospital
    Roslyn, New York

Stanley R. Hamilton, MD
Professor of Pathology and Oncology

Mary L. Harris, MD
Assistant Professor of Medicine

Katharine S. Harrison, MD
Attending Physician
Johns Hopkins University/Sinai Hospital Program in Internal
    Medicine, Sinai Hospital of Baltimore

David B. Hellmann, MD
Associate Professor of Medicine
The Mary Betty Stevens Chair in Rheumatology
Executive Vice Chairman, Department of Medicine

Thomas R. Hendrix, MD
Professor of Medicine
Director Emeritus, Division of Gastroenterology

H. Franklin Herlong, MD
Associate Professor of Medicine
Associate Dean for Student Affairs

Marc C. Hochberg, MD, MPH
Professor of Medicine and of Epidemiology and Preventive
    Medicine
Head, Division of Rheumatology and Clinical Immunology
    University of Maryland School of Medicine
    Baltimore, Maryland

Antoinette F. Hood, MD
Professor of Pathology and Dermatology
    Indiana University School of Medicine
    Indianapolis, Indiana

Janet E. Horn, MD
Associate Professor of Medicine

Richard L. Humphrey, MD
Associate Professor of Pathology, Oncology, Medicine, and
    Health Policy and Management
Director, Diagnostic Immunology Laboratory

David B. Jacoby, MD
Associate Professor of Medicine

Carol Johnson Johns, MD
Distinguished Service Associate Professor of Medicine
Eudowood Tuberculosis/Sarcoidosis Consultant and Review
  Physician

Constance J. Johnson, MD
Assistant Professor of Neurology
Director, Stroke Center, Johns Hopkins Bayview Medical
  Center

Richard J. Jones, MD
Associate Professor of Oncology

Anthony N. Kalloo, MD
Associate Professor of Medicine
Director, Gastrointestinal Endoscopy

Peter W. Kaplan, MB, FRCP
Associate Professor of Neurology
Chairman, Department of Neurology, Johns Hopkins
  Bayview Medical Center
Director, Clinical Electrophysiology, Johns Hopkins
  Bayview Medical Center

Michael G. Kauffman, MD, PhD
Division of Rheumatology
  Massachusetts General Hospital
  Harvard Medical School
  Boston, Massachusetts
Director, Medical Research
  Biogen, Inc.
  Cambridge, Massachusetts

M. John Kennedy, MB, FRCPI
Assistant Professor of Oncology

Thomas S. Kickler, MD
Associate Professor of Pathology and Medicine
Director, Diagnostic Hematology Laboratories

Michael J. Klag, MD, MPH
Associate Professor of Medicine
Joint Appointments in Epidemiology and in Health Policy
  and Management
Acting Director, Division of Internal Medicine

Freddy T. Kokke, MD
Fellow in Pediatric Gastroenterology
  Beatrix Children's Hospital
  Groningen, The Netherlands

Ralph W. Kuncl, MD, PhD
Associate Professor of Neurology

Paul W. Ladenson, MD
John Eager Howard Professor of Medicine
Professor of Pathology
Joint Appointment in International Health
Director, Division of Endocrinology and Metabolism

Howard M. Lederman, MD, PhD
Associate Professor of Pediatrics
Director, Immunodeficiency Clinic

Michael A. Levine, MD
Professor of Medicine and Pathology

Lawrence M. Lichtenstein, MD, PhD
Professor of Medicine
Director, Division of Allergy and Clinical Immunology

Mark C. Liu, MD
Associate Professor of Medicine

John J. Mann, MD
Associate Professor of Medicine

Simeon Margolis, MD, PhD
Professor of Medicine and Biological Chemistry

Justin C. McArthur, MB, BS, MPH
Associate Professor of Neurology
Joint Appointment in Epidemiology

Paul R. McHugh, MD
Henry Phipps Professor of Psychiatry
Director, Department of Psychiatry
Psychiatrist-in-Chief

Mack C. Mitchell, MD
Chairman, Department of Internal Medicine
  Carolinas Medical Center
  Charlotte, North Carolina

John F. Modlin, MD
Professor of Pediatrics and Medicine
  Dartmouth Medical School
  Hanover, New Hampshire
Director, Diagnostic Virology Laboratory
  Dartmouth-Hitchcock Medical Center
  Lebanon, New Hampshire

Thomas R. Moench, MD
Medical Director
  ReProtect, LLC
  Baltimore, Maryland

Alison Moliterno, MD
Fellow in Hematology

David R. Moller, MD
Assistant Professor of Medicine
Director, Sarcoidosis Clinic

Hamilton Moses III, MD
Professor of Neurology
  University of Virginia School of Medicine
  Charlottesville, Virginia

Patrick A. Murphy, MD, PhD
Professor of Medicine and of Molecular Biology and Genetics
Chief, Division of Infectious Diseases, Johns Hopkins
  Bayview Medical Center

Paul M. Ness, MD
Professor of Pathology and Medicine
Director, Division of Transfusion Medicine

Philip S. Norman, MD
Professor of Medicine

Jean L. Olson, MD
Professor of Clinical Pathology
  University of California, San Francisco
  San Francisco, California

David B. Pearse, MD
Assistant Professor of Medicine

Michelle Petri, MD, MPH
Associate Professor of Medicine

Brent G. Petty, MD
Associate Professor of Medicine

Jacqueline A. Pongracic, MD
Assistant Professor of Pediatrics and Medicine
  Northwestern University Medical School
Attending Physician
    Children's Memorial Hospital and Northwestern
    Memorial Hospital
    Chicago, Illinois

James K. Porterfield, MD
Assistant Professor of Medicine

Thomas J. Preziosi, MD
Associate Professor of Neurology

Reed Edwin Pyeritz, MD, PhD
Professor of Human Genetics, Medicine, and Pediatrics
Chair, Department of Human Genetics
Director, Institute for Medical Genetics
  Medical College of Pennsylvania and Hahnemann
  University
  Pittsburgh, Pennsylvania

Thomas C. Quinn, MD
Professor of Medicine

William J. Ravich, MD
Associate Professor of Medicine
Clinical Director, Division of Gastroenterology
Clinical Director, Johns Hopkins Swallowing Center

Stephen G. Reich, MD
Assistant Professor of Neurology
Director, Parkinson's Disease Center

Alan J. Romanoski, MD, MPH
Associate Professor of Psychiatry and Behavioral Sciences
Joint Appointment in Mental Hygiene
Director, World Health Organization Collaborating Centre
  for Methods of Assessment, Diagnosis and Classification
  in Psychiatry, Baltimore

Rebecca A. Roubenoff, RD, MPH (deceased)
Research Associate
  Tufts University School of Nutrition
  Boston, Massachusetts

Ronenn Roubenoff, MD, MHS
Assistant Professor of Medicine and Nutrition
  Tufts University
Scientist I
  USDA Human Nutrition Research Center
  Boston, Massachusetts

George H. Sack, Jr, MD, PhD
Associate Professor of Medicine, Pediatrics, and Biological
  Chemistry

R. Bradley Sack, MD, ScD
Professor of International Health
Joint Appointments in Immunology and Infectious Diseases,
  Medicine, and Molecular Biology and Genetics
Director, Travel Clinic

Roxan F. Saidi, MD
Fellow in Gastroenterology

Daniel G. Sapir, MD
Associate Professor of Medicine

Christopher D. Saudek, MD
Professor of Medicine
Director, Johns Hopkins Diabetes Center
Director, Clinical Research Center

Christine R. Schneyer, MD
Assistant Professor of Medicine
Associate Director, Division of Endocrinology,
  Sinai Hospital of Baltimore

Marvin M. Schuster, MD
Professor of Medicine
Joint Appointment in Psychiatry
Director, Division of Digestive Diseases, Johns Hopkins
  Bayview Medical Center

Alan R. Schwartz, MD
Associate Professor of Medicine

Eric J. Seifter, MD
Associate Professor of Medicine and Oncology

Stuart E. Selonick, MD
Assistant Professor of Medicine and Oncology

Keith T. Sivertson, MD
Medical Director
  LifeFlight
Emergency Physician
  Idaho Emergency Physicians
  Boise, Idaho

Philip L. Smith, MD
Professor of Medicine
Director, Sleep Disorders Clinic

Jerry L. Spivak, MD
Professor of Medicine and Oncology

Barney J. Stern, MD
Professor of Neurology
  Emory University School of Medicine
Chief of Clinical Services
  Section of Neurology
  The Emory Clinic
  Atlanta, Georgia

Mary Betty Stevens, MD (deceased)
Professor of Medicine

John D. Stobo, MD
Professor of Medicine
Former Director, Department of Medicine
Chairman and Chief Executive Officer, Johns Hopkins
  HealthCare

J. T. Sylvester, MD
David Marine Professor of Medicine
Associate Professor of Anesthesiology and Critical Care
 Medicine
Director, Division of Pulmonary and Critical Care Medicine

Mark L. Teitelbaum, MD
Associate Professor of Psychiatry and Medicine

Peter B. Terry, MD
Professor of Medicine
Joint Appointments in Anesthesiology and Critical Care
 Medicine and in Environmental Health Sciences

Patricia A. Thomas, MD
Assistant Professor of Medicine

Thomas A. Traill, FRCP
Associate Professor of Medicine
Director, E. Cowles Andrus Cardiac Clinic

Martin D. Valentine, MD
Professor of Medicine

Gary S. Wand, MD
Associate Professor of Medicine and Psychiatry
Director, Neuroendocrine Clinic

Alan J. Watson, MRCPI
Consultant Nephrologist
 St. Vincent's Hospital
 Dublin, Ireland

Alastair J. M. Watson, MD
Senior Lecturer in Medicine
Honorary Consultant Gastroenterologist
 Hope Hospital
 Salford, England

Gail G. Weinmann, MD
COPD/Environmental Lung Disease Scientific Research
 Group Leader
 National Heart, Lung, and Blood Institute
 Bethesda, Maryland

Andrew Whelton, MD
Professor of Medicine and Pharmacology
Executive Vice President for Planning
 Finch University of Health Sciences/
 The Chicago Medical School
 Chicago, Illinois

Paul K. Whelton, MD, MSc
Professor of Medicine and Epidemiology

Fredrick M. Wigley, MD
Associate Professor of Medicine
Director, Division of Rheumatology

Jerry A. Winkelstein, MD
Eudowood Professor of Pediatrics
Director, Division of Immunology, Department of Pediatrics

Robert A. Wise, MD
Associate Professor of Medicine
Instructor in Radiology (Nuclear Medicine)
Joint Appointment in Environmental Health Sciences
Director, Pulmonary Function Laboratories

Benjamin K. Yokel, MD
Dermatologist
 East Range Clinic
 Virginia, Minnesota

Carol M. Ziminski, MD
Assistant Professor of Medicine
Deputy Director, Johns Hopkins University Division of
 Rheumatology at Good Samaritan Hospital, Baltimore

Preface

This all-new edition of *The Principles and Practice of Medicine* returns to the book's roots as an introduction to clinical technique for medical students. The goal is to help students make the transition from the classroom to working with patients in the clinic and at the bedside.

The authors have approached their topics as they do on teaching rounds. They have kept the focus on the patient. Each chapter stresses why a condition is important, how patients present, and how to work through the differential diagnosis with the history, physical exam, and thoughtful use of diagnostic tests. The emphasis is on explanation and understanding rather than listing and memorizing. Since the book builds on previous instruction, the pathophysiology of each disorder is reviewed only in the context of the clinical manifestations that it explains. Management is covered in its broadest sense: caring for the patient before, during, and after diagnosis. We have minimized coverage of the specifics of treatment, particularly drug doses.

This book is not a medical encyclopedia. We have chosen not to cover every condition that students might encounter during their clerkships, nor do we discuss diseases that primarily affect children. Instead, the book offers a broad, clinically based perspective on how symptoms, syndromes, and diseases fit into the grand scheme of medicine, together with an overall appreciation for natural history, principles of management, and outcome.

We honor the memory of two authors who died during the preparation of this edition: Rebecca Roubenoff, RD, MPH, and Mary Betty Stevens, MD. Their colleagues remember with admiration their passionate devotion to Johns Hopkins Medicine and their many contributions to their own fields.

Acknowledgments

For special consultation on chapters, we thank Drs. John G. Bartlett, Duke E. Cameron, Jaquelyn F. Fleckenstein, Marc C. Hochberg, Paul D. Kessler, Michael A. Levine, Paul R. McHugh, Godfrey D. Pearlson, Michelle Petri, George H. Sack, Jr, Patricia B. Santora, Paul J. Scheel, Jerry L. Spivak, Frank M. Tamarin, and Carol M. Ziminski. We received valuable guidance from Susan L. Abrams, Frederick T. DeKuyper, Patricia L. Friend, Dr. Michael L. Gompertz, Dr. Mark C. Loury, Dr. Robert W. Massof, and Carol A. Sulak. We appreciate the knowledge and patience of the staffs of the William H. Welch Medical Library and the Drug Information Center of the Johns Hopkins Hospital Department of Pharmacy.

For photographs, we thank the American College of Rheumatology, the Franklin Square Hospital (Baltimore) Department of Medical Communications, and Drs. William S. Aronstein, Marie Bellantoni, Bernard A. Cohen, David M. Cook, Anne McB. Curtis, Pablo E. Dibos, Daniel Finkelstein, John A. Flynn, Abraham Genecin, Antoinette F. Hood, Bronwyn Jones, Peter O. Kwiterovich, Jr, Joao A.C. Lima, David H. Madoff, Anne M. Rompalo, Andrew P. Schachat, William W. Scott, Jr, Stuart E. Selonick, Eva F. Simmons-O'Brien, Jerold M. Wassel, Jane H. Wheeler, Paul S. Wheeler, S. Elizabeth Whitmore, Kirk J. Wojno, Randall V. Wong, Jonathan M. Zenilman, and Elias A. Zerhouni, as well as Marjorie Ewertz, RN, BSN, Catherine S. Sackett, RN, CANP, and Victoria E. Smith, MT(ASCP)SH. We thank the Pathology and Radiology Photography Departments of The Johns Hopkins University School of Medicine for preparation of photographs.

We thank all the authors' secretaries, and in particular our own secretaries, Kathleen D. Barnes, Barbara J. Benzing, Pamela S. Hill, Debra K. Kulle, Tambra E. Noethen, Barbara J. Pearce, Jennifer L. Raeke, Sandy VanFossen, Mary L. Williams, and Jo Ann L. Young.

We thank the past and present staff at Appleton & Lange, especially Al Averbach, Greg Huth, Alison Kelley, Christine Langan, Shelley Reinhardt, Bill Schmitt, Mary Skudlarek, and Marty Wonsiewicz.

Now we know why William Osler decided to finish his first edition of *The Principles and Practice of Medicine* before proposing marriage to Grace Revere Gross. We thank our families for their support and patience in seeing us through this project.

We thank Mollie Dunker, AMI, for illustrating this volume with such skill and creativity.

We particularly acknowledge our enormous gratitude to Edie Stern, our managing editor, whose scholarship permeates every aspect of this book and whose patience, persistence, and persuasion were essential to its successful completion.

The Editors

Introduction

The turn of the 20th century heralded a golden age of medicine. At the newly opened Johns Hopkins University School of Medicine, William Osler was first introducing American medical students to a European approach to medical training: Science became the foundation for the practice of medicine, to be taught concurrently in the classroom, laboratory, and clinic. Osler provided the impetus for changing medical training. Students no longer served an apprenticeship, but sought an understanding of the scientific basis of disease. It was during this revolution that Osler completed the first edition of *The Principles and Practice of Medicine.* This is not the occasion to recount the monumental influence that the first edition had on the transformation of medicine, nor to enumerate the extraordinary accomplishments of its author, but rather to convey the present editors' sense of how Osler's views continue to influence medicine.

Consider the state of American medicine when Osler published the first edition in 1892: He believed that beriberi was an infectious disease and that gout, diabetes mellitus, scurvy, and hemophilia were "constitutional" disorders—nonspecific indicators of disease in the same category as fever. Although Osler could not have predicted the directions that medicine would take over the next decades, throughout the first edition he etched some timeless principles that would hold true no matter how the practice of medicine or the knowledge of specific diseases might change. Among these principles:

- The patient is central to the learning of medicine. In Osler's words, "To study the phenomena of disease without books is to sail an uncharted sea, while to study books without patients is not to go to sea at all."

- Medicine is a calling. The physician should truly believe that the practice of medicine is a privilege to be embraced and cherished. The public trust bestowed on physicians requires constant attention to professional behavior and a commitment to the patient's well-being above one's own.

- Intellectual curiosity is essential. Only the curious physician can advance the health of patients as well as the science of medicine.

- The practice of medicine is an art as well as a science. Physicians' ability to help a patient depends not only on their knowledge but on how they use that knowledge.

- Physicians' most important tools are their eyes, hands, and ears. The basic skills in caring for patients require inspection, palpation, and, most important, listening.

We believe that adhering to these principles enables a physician to be effective, regardless of how medical practice changes. Indeed, through both its format and content, the current edition attempts to reinforce these principles.

We, too, are in a golden age of medicine. The 20th century witnessed an enormous accumulation of knowledge and its application to treat disease. In 1900, mean life expectancy in the United States was 45 years; by 1993, it was 75 years. The tools of molecular biology and recombinant DNA technology have facilitated great advances in our understanding of pathophysiology. At the turn of the 21st century, we will see these discoveries used not only to cure illness but to detect the potential for disease, prevent disease, and maintain health.

But this new knowledge will be applied in a new clinical framework. In the 20th century, a single physician treated the illness of a single patient; in the 21st, a health care team will address the needs of a population of patients. Indeed, the excitement of the next 100 years of health care will be to see how, for example, advances in molecular genetics can be used to prevent, diagnose, and treat disorders that affect large numbers of people. The focus must include addressing problems such as substance abuse and domestic violence, as well as managing resources to meet the health needs of both individuals and populations.

We believe that the principles that Osler etched in the first edition of *The Principles and Practice of Medicine* and that we have tried to reinforce in this edition are as relevant to the new as they were to the old framework of patient care. The primacy of the patient, medicine as a calling, and the importance of intellectual curiosity, the "art" of medicine, and physicians' basic tools—their eyes, hands, and ears—will be as fundamental to the medicine of the 21st century as they were to the 20th.

John D. Stobo, MD

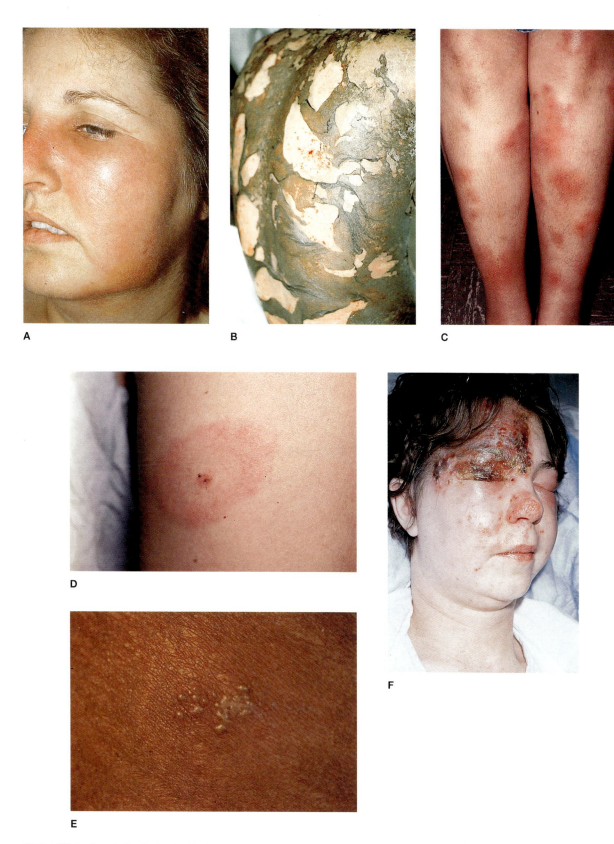

Color Plate 1. **A:** Erysipelas. **B:** Full-thickness loss of epidermis in toxic epidermal necrolysis. **C:** Tender reddish-brown nodules on the legs of a woman with erythema nodosum. **D:** Erythema migrans, the rash of Lyme disease. **E:** Clustered tense vesicles typical of herpesvirus infection. **F:** Herpes varicella zoster.

Panels A, B, C, E, F: Courtesy of Antoinette F. Hood, MD. D: Courtesy of S. Elizabeth Whitmore, MD.

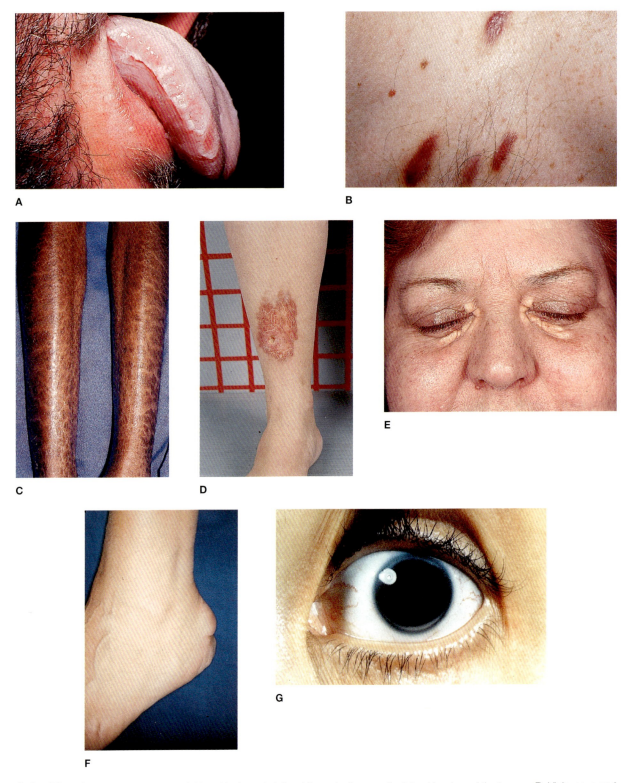

Color Plate 2. **A:** Oral hairy leukoplakia, with characteristic white projections on the lateral borders of the tongue. **B:** Violaceous and reddish-brown plaques of Kaposi's sarcoma in a patient with AIDS. **C:** Acquired ichthyosis in a patient with AIDS. **D:** Necrobiosis lipoidica diabeticorum. **E:** Xanthelasma in a patient with hypercholesterolemia. **F:** Achilles tendon xanthoma. **G:** Corneal arcus in a patient with hypercholesterolemia.

Panels A, B, C: Courtesy of Antoinette F. Hood, MD. D: Courtesy of Christopher D. Saudek, MD. E: Courtesy of Peter O. Kwiterovich, Jr, MD. F: Courtesy of Simeon Margolis, MD, PhD. G: Reproduced, with permission, from Haber C, Kwiterovich PO Jr: Dyslipoproteinemia and xanthomatosis. Pediatr Dermatol 1984;1:261. © 1984 Blackwell Scientific Publications, Inc.

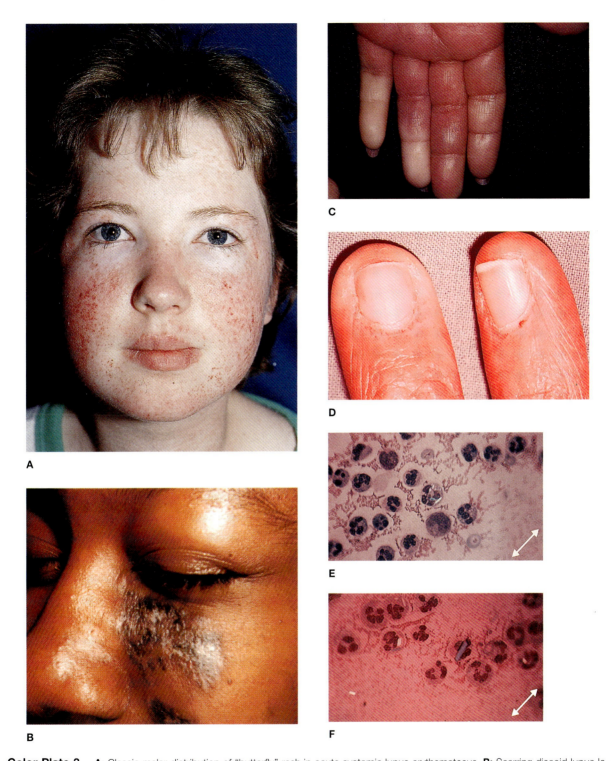

Color Plate 3.   **A:** Classic malar distribution of "butterfly" rash in acute systemic lupus erythematosus. **B:** Scarring discoid lupus lesion. **C:** Demarcated pallor in fingers during an attack of Raynaud's phenomenon. **D:** Dilated nailfold capillaries in Raynaud's phenomenon. Capillary abnormalities, seen just below the cuticle, can be subtle (left) or prominent (right). They usually indicate that the patient has Raynaud's secondary to another disorder. Gout **(E)** versus pseudogout **(F)** crystals that have been phagocytosed by polymorphonuclear leukocytes in the joint fluid during attacks. **E:** Needle-shaped monosodium urate crystals in gout. Under compensated polarized light, gout crystals lying parallel to the direction of the compensator look yellow and those lying perpendicular look blue. The arrow shows the direction of the compensator. **F:** Rhomboidal calcium pyrophosphate dihydrate (CPPD) crystals in pseudogout. In addition to their squatter shape, CPPD crystals differ from gout crystals under compensated polarized light: CPPD crystals parallel to the direction of the compensator look blue and those perpendicular look yellow.

Panel A: Courtesy of Antoinette F. Hood, MD. C: Courtesy of Fredrick M. Wigley, MD. D: Reprinted from the Clinical Slide Collection on the Rheumatic Diseases, © 1991. Used by permission of the American College of Rheumatology. E, F: Courtesy of Syntex Laboratories, Inc.

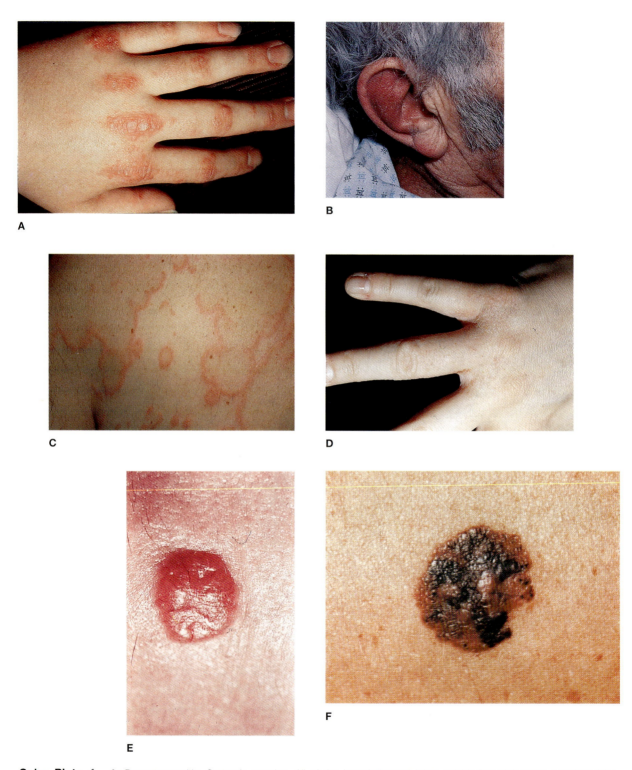

Color Plate 4. **A:** Dermatomyositis: Gottron's papules. All of the interphalangeal joints exhibit firm violaceous papulonodules. **B:** Prominent swelling and erythema of the ear in relapsing polychondritis. **C:** Small urticarial plaques and larger urticarial lesions with characteristic polycyclic and serpiginous borders. **D:** Linear vesiculation typical of a contact dermatitis. **E:** Nodular basal cell carcinoma with smooth surface and telangiectasia coursing over the superior border. **F:** Variegated color in a cutaneous melanoma.

Panel A: Courtesy of Eva F. Simmons-O'Brien, MD, and Bernard A. Cohen, MD. B, C, D, E: Courtesy of Antoinette F. Hood, MD.

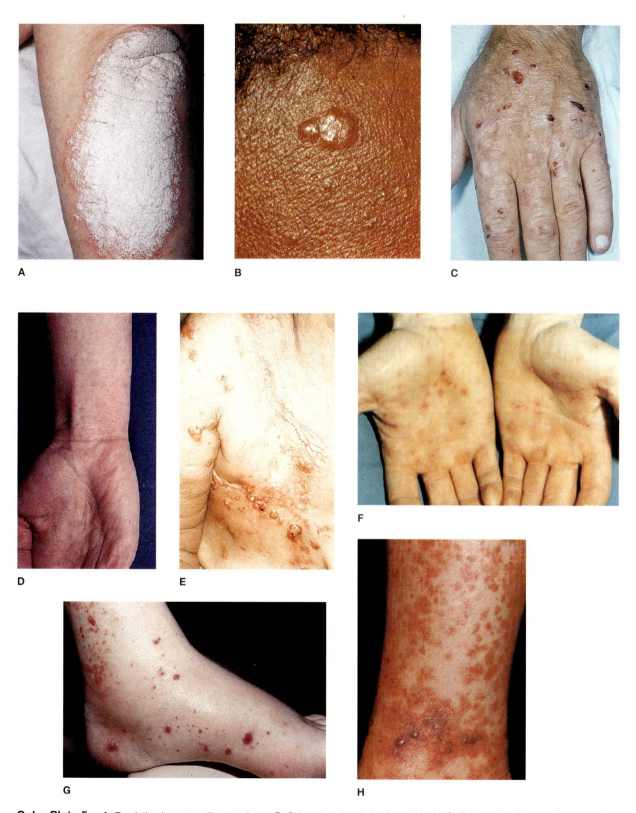

Color Plate 5. **A:** Psoriatic plaque on elbow and arm. **B:** Skin-colored nodule of sarcoidosis. **C:** Bullae, ulcerations, and scars on the hand of a patient with porphyria cutanea tarda. **D:** Blanchable erythematous morbilliform eruption characteristic of a drug reaction. **E:** Scattered nodules of metastatic breast carcinoma on the trunk and arm of a woman previously treated by radical mastectomy. **F:** Target lesions in erythema multiforme. **G:** Palpable purpuric lesions of leukocytoclastic vasculitis. **H:** Characteristic cutaneous features of vasculitis.

Panels A, C, D, E, G: Courtesy of Antoinette F. Hood, MD.

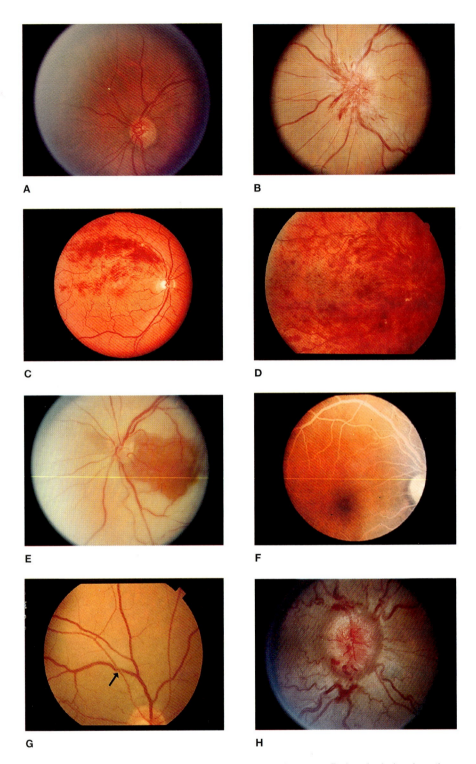

Color Plate 6. **A:** Arteriolar embolus following coronary artery bypass graft surgery. **B:** Anterior ischemic optic neuropathy. The disk is swollen, with dilated vessels and hemorrhage. **C:** Branch retinal vein occlusion. **D:** Central retinal vein occlusion with extensive intraretinal hemorrhage. **E:** Central retinal artery occlusion with diffuse ischemic whitening of the retina, sparing the macula (which is supplied by a separate cilio-retinal artery). **F:** Lipemia retinalis. **G:** Arteriovenous nicking in a patient with hypertensive retinopathy. **H:** Papilledema showing marked hyperemia and elevation of the optic disk, blurring at the disk margin, and superficial peripapillary hemorrhages.

Panel A: Courtesy of Andrew P. Schachat, MD. C: Reproduced, with permission, from Schachat AP, Cruess AF: *Diagnostic Diagrams: Ophthalmology.* © 1984, Williams & Wilkins. D: Courtesy of Daniel Finkelstein, MD. F: Courtesy of Simeon Margolis, MD, PhD. G: Courtesy of Randall V. Wong, MD.

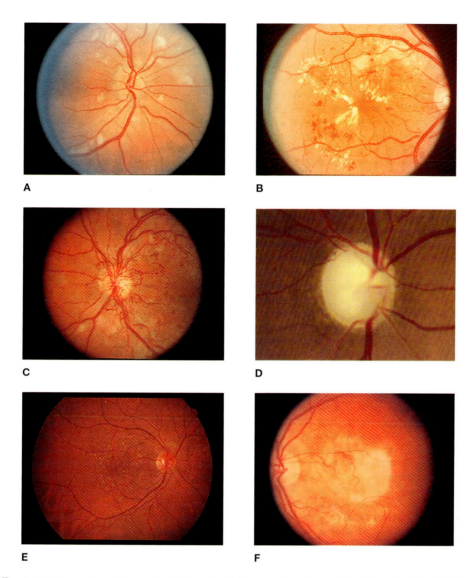

Color Plate 7. **A:** Cotton-wool spots in a patient with systemic lupus erythematosus. The picture is similar in diabetes mellitus and hypertension. **B:** Nonproliferative diabetic retinopathy with macular edema. **C:** Proliferative diabetic retinopathy characterized by optic disk neovascularization (NVD). **D:** Chronic (open angle) glaucoma with extensive cupping of the optic disk. **E:** Macular drusen in a patient with nonexudative age-related macular degeneration. **F:** Disciform scar in a patient with exudative age-related macular degeneration.

Panel A: Reproduced, with permission, from Jabs DA et al: Severe retinal vaso-occlusive disease in systemic lupus erythematosus. Arch Ophthalmol 1986;104;560. © 1986, American Medical Association. B, C, E, F: Courtesy of Andrew P. Schachat, MD.

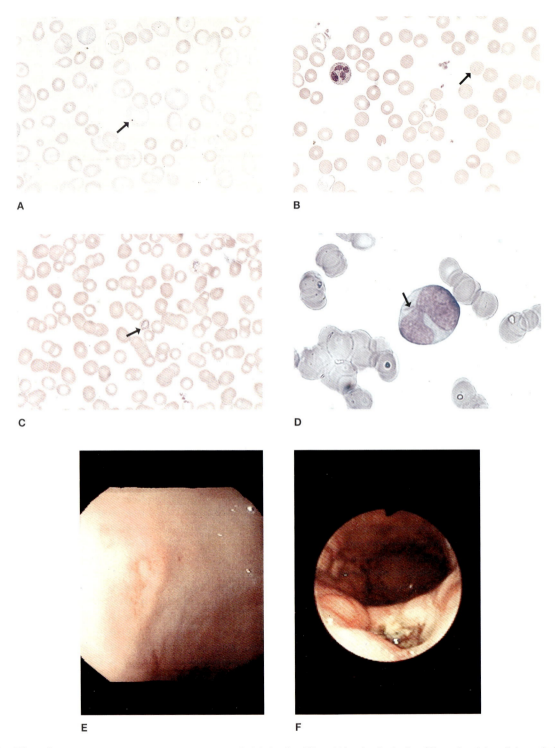

Color Plate 8. Peripheral blood smears showing Howell-Jolly bodies **(A)**, red blood cell stippling **(B)**, and an intracellular malaria parasite **(C)**. **D:** Auer rod in acute myelogenous leukemia. Endoscopic appearance of benign **(E)** and malignant **(F)** gastric ulcers.

Panels A, B, C: Courtesy of Victoria E. Smith, MT(ASCP)SH. D: Courtesy of Chi V. Dang, MD, PhD. E, F: Courtesy of Anthony N. Kalloo, MD.

Section 1

Cardiovascular Disease

Thomas A. Traill, FRCP, Section Editor

1.1

Approach to the Patient With Cardiovascular Disease

Thomas A. Traill, FRCP

The approach to patients with cardiovascular disease demands two kinds of expertise. One is "human," the other "physiological." When a patient complains of pain in the chest, whether in the outpatient clinic, the emergency room, or even by telephone, the physician has only the description of the pain, and any constitutional symptoms, from which to decide whether this is cardiac pain (angina) or pain from some other, usually less serious cause. There is no test that replaces the physician's skill in this setting—getting the diagnosis right depends solely on the ability to elicit and interpret the history. On the other hand, in a patient with a paroxysmal tachycardia, the choice of management depends on interpreting the electrocardiogram (ECG) and perhaps on electrophysiologic studies of the patient's cardiac conducting tissue, using intracardiac electrodes and multichannel recording apparatus. Here, understanding the physics of the disease is essential before choosing among medication, placing a catheter-guided lesion in the myocardium, or implanting an electrical device such as a pacemaker or an automatic defibrillator.

In cardiology, where physiologic changes occur mainly at a macroscopic level, the two kinds of interpretive skill, the human and the physical, generally overlap easily, and for many doctors the appeal of cardiology lies in the direct relation between the symptoms and signs of heart disease and the physiologic disturbances that underlie them.

THE HISTORY

Heart diseases make themselves known to patients through a limited repertoire of symptoms. Some reflect awareness of the heart, for example, palpitation or angina pectoris; others reflect awareness of altered circulatory function, for example, fatigue or breathlessness. Generally, symptoms of cardiovascular diseases are not specific

for the heart; chest pain, breathlessness, and fatigue all have noncardiac causes that are more common but less feared than heart diseases. It is the circumstances in which symptoms occur that signal their physiologic basis and allow the physician to identify them as cardiac. Thus, the astute history taker spends as much or more time learning about a patient's lifestyle and the effect of the symptoms on it as on the description of the feelings themselves. In doing this, it is important to obtain concrete details of a person's activities, rather than ask vague stock questions. It is no use asking those who live in the country how many blocks they can walk, or asking those with a small house how many stairs they can climb. It is better to ask about relevant activities—changing a flat tire, mowing grass, running a vacuum cleaner, doing laundry, going to the grocery store—and include leisure activities, such as dancing and swimming. Often people who can cope with walking do so by moderating their pace, and it may be helpful to know whether their family has to slow down for them or wait. People with more serious disability may have difficulty even with routine activities that we do not think of as exercise—dressing, bathing, or even brushing teeth.

The New York Heart Association scale was developed for describing effort tolerance of patients with angina pectoris in consistent and semiobjective terms (Table 1.1–1). Although it finds its main use in providing numeric data for stratifying patients in research projects, it is also helpful for clinicians when more than one person will be seeing a particular patient. The scale can be applied to patients with dyspnea caused by reduced heart function just as well as to those with angina.

Exploring the symptoms from the point of view of the patient's life and activities may also be the best way to obtain a sense of how acute or chronic the problem is. Sometimes patients with valvular heart disease believe that they have only recently begun to feel symptoms; yet it emerges

Table 1.1–1. New York Heart Association functional classification of patients with heart disease.

Class I	Patients with heart disease but no limitation of physical activity; no undue dyspnea, pain, or fatigue during ordinary activity
Class II	Patients with slight limitation of physical activity; symptoms only during the more strenuous grades of ordinary activity
Class III	Patients with marked limitation of physical activity; comfortable at rest, but symptoms with even mild degrees of ordinary activity
Class IV	Patients unable to carry on any physical activity without dyspnea or other cardiac symptoms; dyspnea at rest

that they have been curtailing their activities for years and are overdue for effective surgical treatment.

Often it becomes apparent during the history that a patient's symptoms are not caused by heart disease, and in some patients it is plain that there is no "organic" explanation at all. Physicians can be of great assistance to such patients provided that the doctor is not seen as dismissive, impatient, or patronizing. To be a credible source of reassurance, it is essential to listen carefully to complaints, however nonsensical they may sound; to spend time on the history, even when it is obvious from the outset that the heart is not the problem; and to be honest in trying to explain the real cause of the symptoms. Equivocation and overtesting are counterproductive, and so is spuriously attributing the complaints to disease in other systems. Authoritative reassurance, given in a sympathetic and unhurried fashion, is effective medicine and rewarding to provide.

THE CARDIAC EXAMINATION

The physical findings in heart disease, even more than the history, have their basis in very accessible pathophysiology; each finding, whether it is the jugular pressure in pericardial compression or the Austin Flint murmur in aortic regurgitation, is the direct effect of a disturbance in pressure or flow. For many doctors, auscultatory findings are the hardest to interpret. Yet all too often heart sounds and murmurs receive undue attention from the examiner at the expense of the more easily appreciated and basic information provided by the arterial and venous pulses and the character of the cardiac impulse.

It is important to develop a system early in one's career and stick to it; even though the new physician often has difficulty interpreting the findings correctly, only by doing things the same way for patient after patient will physical signs begin to become obvious. This system should always begin with the peripheral arterial pulses, including a check for symmetry, and progress via the jugular and arterial pulses in the neck to the precordial impulse and, finally, to cardiac auscultation. The chances of correctly detecting and interpreting a sound or murmur are

enormously enhanced by acquiring the information in this order.

A cardiologic examination includes more than just examining the heart and large vessels. It includes attention to whether the patient has lost weight, or whether the patient bears signs of any congenital or inherited syndrome, or hypercholesterolemia. The retinal arterioles should be checked for signs of hypertension and sclerosis of small arteries as well as for evidence of diabetes. The lungs should be examined for crackles, keeping in mind that the absence of rales does not rule out pulmonary venous congestion. Even though an assistant may have recorded the blood pressure, it is important for the physician to take it as well. If it is left to the end of the exam, the patient may be feeling more at ease than before, and the reading may be more representative of the true pressure.

Patients who have light-headedness, whose fluid balance is a concern, or who are taking blood-pressure–lowering drugs need lying and standing pressures taken to check for orthostatic hypotension. Patients in whom subclavian steal syndrome might be a cause of transient posterior cerebral circulation ischemia should have pressure taken in both arms to check for subclavian artery occlusion. Anyone who might need coronary bypass surgery should have both pressures taken as well, since the left internal mammary artery, a branch of the left subclavian, is often used as a bypass into the coronary circulation.

Physical findings are "physical"; they are never "wrong." But clinicians may misinterpret their significance. For example, patients with a pansystolic murmur caused by severe mitral regurgitation often have a diastolic murmur at the apex caused by excessive flow across the mitral valve during ventricular filling. This is not the murmur of mitral stenosis. The lesion would not be mistaken for mitral stenosis by an examiner who had recognized that the hyperkinetic left ventricular impulse implies an excessive volume load. Physical findings are also not always present when we need them; it is obvious that in a patient with angina pectoris, even that caused by very severe coronary disease, no abnormal signs may be found between attacks of pain. It is less obvious but also true that patients may have severe myocardial dysfunction and yet not have any detectable abnormality on examination. Often, therefore, even the most clinically skillful cardiologist requires various laboratory tests to arrive at an accurate diagnosis.

SPECIAL TESTS

The ECG, echocardiography, stress testing, cardiac catheterization, imaging techniques, and electrical studies all are physiologically based tests that can be essential to reach an accurate or complete assessment of a patient's heart disease. Like the physical signs, however, the information they provide has to be interpreted, and it is important not to be beguiled by the apparent "objectivity" of the results of special tests. The cardiology literature contains numerous warnings that technologic advances can diminish clinical expertise. Yet no field has demonstrated better than cardiology how the reverse can also be true. Thanks to objective studies of physiologic changes in patients we have learned the right interpretations of certain physical signs. One of the many examples of this can be found in the chapter on valvular heart disease: A low-frequency diastolic murmur heard in some patients with aortic regurgitation, first described by Flint in the last century, remained unexplained until the advent of echocardiography 100 years later. The murmur reflects closing of the mitral valve in mid-diastole caused by rapid rise in the left ventricular diastolic pressure. Until this was shown, the finding had been a curiosity, sought only by those eager to show off their knowledge of arcane cardiologic trivia. Now, by having a known physical significance, the murmur has become a valuable part of the clinical assessment of aortic regurgitation.

Electrocardiography

Clinical examination of a patient with suspected heart disease always includes an ECG. As a routine, the physician should check the rhythm and heart rate, the electrical axis of the heart in the frontal (coronal) plane, and look for evidence of ventricular enlargement, conduction disease, ischemic damage, and the most common finding, abnormalities in the ST segment and T wave. ST-segment and T-wave changes, although not specific, suggest that there may be some abnormality of the coronary circulation or the myocardium. A normal ECG does not exclude the possibility of heart disease, but it is uncommon for a patient to have a normal ECG after previous myocardial infarction, during ischemic pain, or with left ventricular hypertrophy. In patients admitted with unstable angina or acute myocardial infarction, ECGs are recorded serially every day or so, and these, in conjunction with the clinical course, give clues to whether further ischemic events are complicating the picture. Serial ECGs taken annually are also a way to detect the development of left ventricular hypertrophy in aortic valve disease and may thus provide a clue to when to recommend valve replacement.

In patients suspected of having episodic arrhythmias, it may not be possible to record an ECG during one of the spells. There are two ways around this. One is to make a continuous ECG recording, usually from two leads, using a small portable amplifier and tape recorder—this is referred to as a Holter monitor and can usually record for up to 3 days. For episodes that happen less frequently, the recommended approach is to use a so-called event recorder, which patients can activate to obtain a recording just when they have symptoms.

Stress Testing and Nuclear Cardiology

The role of treadmill stress testing for patients with coronary artery disease is discussed in Chapter 1.2. It should be noted that the treadmill, although a reliable means of quantifying the severity of ischemia, and contributing to our impression of a patient's level of risk, does not find much use as a means for diagnosis. There are two reasons for this. First, in patients whose suggestive symptoms, usually chest pain, are not caused by coronary disease, there is a high incidence of false-positive results. When the a priori expectation of coronary disease is not high, this limited specificity leads to a very low positive predictive value for the test. Second, in patients with unstable angina, caused by unpredictable reductions in coronary flow from thrombosis or spasm, stress testing has limited sensitivity. There is no particular reason that the events causing unstable pain should happen to be reproduced on the treadmill. Stress testing in patients with unstable angina may also be dangerous. Thus, the main uses of stress testing are in patients in whom the suspicion of coronary disease is strong, or certain, when the study can be used to assist in prognosis and risk stratification (Figure 1.1–1).

To improve its specificity, ECG stress testing can be combined with various imaging techniques. These include radionuclide myocardial perfusion scans using thallium or sestaMIBI, or, to follow left ventricular wall dynamics during exercise, echocardiography, or gated blood pool scanning. In patients for whom treadmill or bicycle exercise is impossible, there are ways to reveal inequalities in coronary perfusion pressure using vasodilators, in particular, dipyridamole, combined with perfusion scanning. Alternatively, the increase in heart rate and inotropic state caused by exercise can be mimicked by an infusion of dobutamine at incremental doses.

Chest X-Ray

Assessing the heart size is difficult at the bedside. Although a displaced point of maximal impulse is a sure guide, many patients have cardiomegaly that is not picked up by palpation, and cardiomegaly cannot be detected reliably by percussion. The chest x-ray is an excellent means of assessing overall heart size, and gives a useful impression of the state of the pulmonary vasculature. This is particularly valuable in patients with suspected pulmonary congestion, because not all patients with pulmonary venous hypertension have crackles, and in patients with congenital heart disease or other potential causes of pulmonary hypertension. Sometimes the x-ray is helpful for showing intracardiac or pericardial calcification. The echocardiogram is more sensitive for calcification of valves and the mitral anulus.

Computed Tomography

Computed tomographic (CT) scanning of the heart and great vessels is a useful way to sort out whether an enlarged cardiac silhouette is caused by enlargement of the heart or by a pericardial effusion. The study may also help to show up calcification in the pericardium and thus help with the difficult distinction between constriction of the pericardium and certain kinds of heart muscle disease. CT scanning is also of value for examining the dimensions of the aorta, and may occasionally be used to look for aortic

Rest

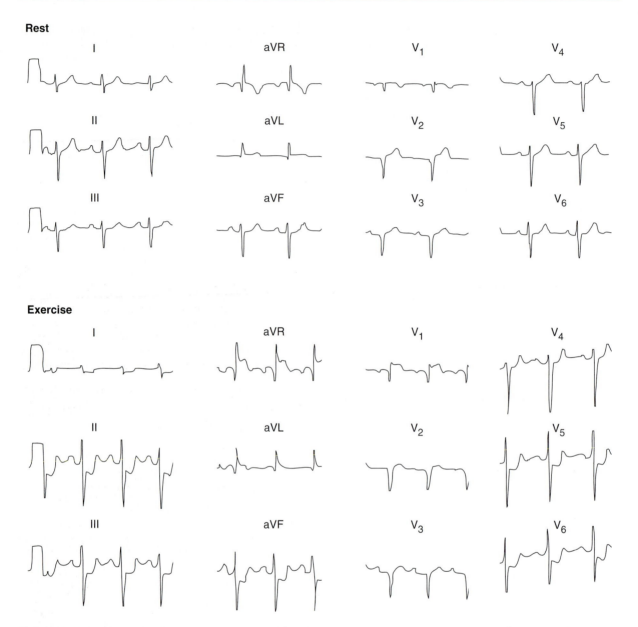

Figure 1.1–1. Positive treadmill stress test in a patient with coronary artery disease and angina pectoris. **Upper panel:** The resting tracing shows signs of a previous anterior myocardial infarction, with ST segments that are all isoelectric. **Lower panel:** During exercise, after 6 minutes the ECG shows pronounced ST-segment depression in leads II, aVF, III, V₅, and V₆. These changes, occurring at a heart rate of only 121 bpm, were accompanied by angina and a fall in blood pressure from 180/90 to 140/55. These measurements imply that the patient's coronary artery disease is life-threatening and that revascularization may be needed.

dissection. Magnetic resonance imaging and transesophageal echocardiography are both superior to CT for aortic imaging, however.

Echocardiography

By far the most valuable adjunct to clinical technique in cardiology is the echocardiogram. Ultrasound examination of the heart allows unambiguous measurement of

chamber size and function, inspection of the valves, measurement of wall thickness, and detection of additional functional abnormalities such as incoordinate wall movement, aneurysm development, and the effects of increased right heart pressures. Echocardiography can be performed along a single dimension (the M-mode) for the most accurate measurements of distance, or in two-dimensional tomographic slices, using videotape to record the heart's motion, and it can be combined with doppler ultrasound to provide quantitative information about the velocity and direction of blood flow. Usually, the echocardiogram is recorded by placing an ultrasound transducer on the patient's chest, but recordings also can be made from transesophageal echo probes, which give even clearer images, taken from behind the heart. Surprisingly, the discomfort and morbidity of passing an echo transducer part way down the esophagus are slight—patients receive topical anesthesia and need light, if any, sedation. The added clarity of the transesophageal echocardiogram is particularly useful when looking in the atria for mural thrombus, for example in patients with stroke. A view from behind may be essential in patients with mitral valve prostheses, which prevent a proper view from the front, or when valve or myocardial function has to be examined during the course of a cardiac surgery procedure.

By far the most common indication for echocardiography is to examine left ventricular function, either because of a clinical presentation that indicates left heart dysfunction, or because left ventricular function is relevant to assessing and planning treatment in a patient with valvular disease or an arrhythmia. Other indications are to assess the cause of an unexplained murmur, or the severity of valvular disease, to look for pericardial effusion, or to look for potential sources of systemic embolism, for example, in the young patient with unexplained stroke.

Cardiac Catheterization

Cardiac catheterization affords a method for measuring pressures, oxygen saturations and flow in any or all of the heart chambers, and for performing angiography—contrast radiography of the coronary arteries, ventricles, and great vessels. Hemodynamics is the measurement of flow and pressure, and the derived variables such as resistance, that describe the function of the heart and circulation. Early workers with these techniques in the 1950's may have imagined that such a powerful, accurate method would replace the more subjective clinical methods in cardiology. As the following chapters will bear out, this has not proved to be the case. The reasons are several. In coronary artery disease, pictures of the vessels convey only limited information about their potential for occlusion or about how rapidly their arteriosclerosis will progress. Information from the angiographic films has to be combined with the prognostic information provided by the clinical presentation and other tests of function, particularly the treadmill test, before good advice can be given about whether a patient's coronary arteries need to be repaired. Similarly, with valvular heart diseases, although catheterization and measurements of pressure and flow can give remarkably accurate estimates of orifice size, for example, in aortic or mitral stenosis, this is not enough information to determine whether valve surgery is needed. Patients may need an operation even when the measured reduction in the valve orifice is slight, and others can be managed without surgery even when there is a large measured volume of valvular regurgitation (Chapter 1.8). Indications for cardiac catheterization are discussed in Chapters 1.2 and 1.3.

Magnetic Resonance Imaging

Magnetic resonance imaging (MRI), especially when combined with ECG gating to "freeze" the heart's motion, provides valuable still pictures of cardiac and great vessel anatomy. Such images are particularly useful in sorting out structural details in patients with complex congenital malformations (Figure 1.1–2), and for examining the aorta when dissection or aneurysm are suspected (Chapter 1.4). Other indications include pericardial disease and cardiac masses. MRI can be used to create moving images, or to

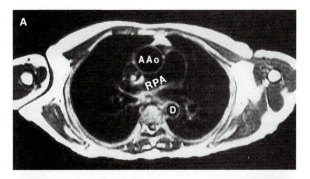

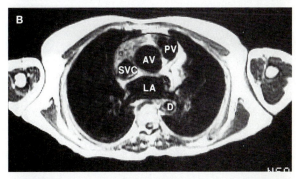

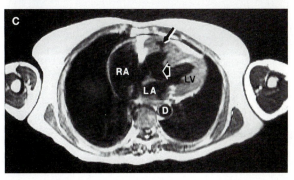

Figure 1.1–2. MRI scans showing tetralogy of Fallot. **A:** The right pulmonary artery (RPA), ascending aorta (AAo), and descending aorta (D). **B:** The left atrium (LA), aortic valve (AV), pulmonary valve (PV), and superior vena cava (SVC). **C:** The right atrium (RA), narrowed right ventricular infundibulum (thin arrow), ventricular septal defect (thick arrow), and left ventricle (LV). The mitral and tricuspid valves (not labeled) can also be identified.

follow blood flow, but when this sort of information is needed, echocardiography or contrast angiography is usually preferred.

SUMMARY

▶ The history should be taken with attention to specific details of patients' lifestyle and effort tolerance. Questions should relate to the real activities of their daily lives. The only way to get good at the cardiac exam is to be systematic and repetitive.

▶ The ECG is used to identify myocardial infarction, ventricular hypertrophy, and arrhythmias. Stress testing may be used to detect extent, severity, and threshold of ischemia, and thus help define prognosis, but is of limited specificity and sensitivity for diagnosis.

▶ Echocardiography and catheterization afford detailed views of disordered structure and function in patients with heart disease, yet prognosis and decision making are governed as much by the clinical situation as by any more objective measurements.

SUGGESTED READING

Cournand A: Recent observations on the dynamics of the pulmonary circulation. Bull NY Acad Med 1947;23:27.

Feigenbaum H: *Echocardiography*, 5th ed. Lea & Febiger, 1994.

Leatham A: *Auscultation of the Heart and Phonocardiography.* Churchill, 1970.

MacKenzie J: Introduction to: *Heart Disease and Pregnancy.* Hodder & Stoughton, 1921.

Wagner GS, Marriott HJL: *Marriott's Practical Electrocardiography*, 9th ed. Williams & Wilkins, 1994.

Angina Pectoris

Stephen C. Achuff, MD

Chest pain is one of the most common symptoms prompting patients to consult a physician. Most people are well aware that chest pain can signal a heart attack or cardiac death. Therefore, it is incumbent upon the physician to make an accurate diagnosis of cardiac or noncardiac pain and, whichever it is, to allay the patient's natural anxieties. Despite the impressive array of technology now available to evaluate and treat angina pectoris, the most basic encounter between patient and physician, the history, remains the keystone of diagnosis. Laboratory testing has an important—sometimes life-saving—place in the care of patients with angina, but when tests are done, on whom they are done, and why they are done are issues that require the physician's thoughtful consideration rather than reflex action.

PATHOPHYSIOLOGY

Angina pectoris is the symptom experienced during myocardial ischemia. As with other medical names for symptoms (eg, claudication, syncope), angina is not a "diagnosis." The physician using the term has interpreted the patient's symptom as cardiac pain, but must still identify its cause. By far the most common cause is coronary atherosclerosis, but the differential diagnosis of angina includes hypertrophic cardiomyopathy (Chapter 1.7), the secondary left ventricular hypertrophy that complicates aortic stenosis (Chapter 1.8), coronary spasm, and, much more rarely, vasculitis and congenital coronary artery anomalies.

Myocardial ischemia develops when oxygen supply is inadequate for demand. The balance can be tilted by a disproportionate drop in supply or increase in demand. Supply is determined primarily by coronary blood flow, the oxygen carrying capacity of blood, and the adequacy of ventilation in the lungs. Apart from such situations as profound anemia, hemoglobinopathy, and severe lung disease, the critical determinant of oxygen supply is coronary blood flow, and, as a corollary, patency of the coronary arteries.

The major factors affecting demand are heart rate, left ventricular wall tension, and the contractility of the myocardium. Myocardial oxygen demand is increased by tachycardia, high blood pressure, left ventricular hypertrophy or dilatation, and increased adrenergic tone, as with exercise or emotional upset. Since most of the factors that determine myocardial oxygen demand remain constant from moment to moment, the variable component of demand can be calculated as the heart rate multiplied by the mean systolic arterial pressure, the *rate-pressure product*.

The threshold for angina can be defined in terms of this rate-pressure product. For example, a patient might have angina reproduced during a treadmill exercise test, primarily because of a large increase in heart rate, or during isometric exercise (eg, hand grip exercise), mostly because of an increase in arterial pressure. Either way, pain is likely to begin at the same threshold of rate-pressure product. The physician can increase patients' exercise tolerance by lowering their baseline blood pressure with nitrates or their baseline heart rate with a β-blocker. However, the threshold of rate-pressure product for demand angina remains the same, because neither drug increases oxygen supply.

Most patients with angina have fixed atherosclerotic narrowings of ≥70% in at least one major coronary artery. These narrowings do not cause ischemia when patients are resting, but with exercise the demand for increased coronary blood flow cannot be met and ischemia develops. The pathophysiology of angina that results from temporary increases in myocardial oxygen demand can be called *demand angina*; the ischemia is precipitated by an increase in myocardial oxygen requirement and ceases promptly when the workload is reduced. An important feature of demand angina is that it is predictable, reproducible, and relatively stereotyped in its clinical manifestations in an individual patient. Roughly the same level of exercise under the same conditions produces the same symptoms. Angina that occurs with a fixed threshold of increased workload is called *stable angina*.

Common factors that may disrupt this stable pattern by increasing demand include the onset of hypertension, hyperthyroidism, and anemia. The major factors that disrupt stable angina by spontaneously reducing supply are coronary thrombosis and spasm. Thrombosis and spasm, usually triggered by plaque rupture, provoke chest pain that is unrelated to any change in myocardial workload and is as likely to occur at rest as with exertion. If a coronary artery remains occluded for longer than about 30 minutes, pain persists and the patient suffers a myocardial infarction. If occlusion is transient because spasm is relieved or a thrombus lyses spontaneously, the patient has spells of angina. This "supply-side" ischemia causes the syndrome of "unstable angina" (Chapter 1.3). Transient spasm of the coronary arteries can suddenly restrict blood flow in both diseased and angiographically normal coronary arteries. There is even credible evidence that spasm of intramyocardial arteries (microvascular angina) can cause ischemia. However, spasm is much less common than fixed atherosclerosis-mediated angina.

CLINICAL FEATURES

History

Angina is a symptom; recognizing angina starts and finishes with the history. The physician must take as much time as necessary to allow patients to tell their whole story in their own words. Patients respond to open-ended questions. For example, the physician might start by saying, "Describe the first time you had this pain," or "Describe your most recent episode" or "Describe your worst episode." Many patients do not describe their symptom as "pain." They may even correct the examiner by saying, "I don't have chest pain." This is because, as Heberden noted more than 200 years ago in the original description of angina, it has a deep, visceral, "strangling" quality. Patients tend to use words like "gripping," "pressure," and "tightness." Perhaps the most graphic expression of angina is Levine's sign: clenched teeth and a fist held firmly against the sternum. In contrast, when patients use terms like "sticking," "prickly," and "pinching," they are probably describing noncardiac symptoms.

Another important part of the history is location of the discomfort. Most patients with angina point to the sternum, although some perceive the focus to be up in the throat or down in the epigastrium. Anginal pain can radiate to other sites, sometimes without causing any chest symptoms whatsoever. Common sites of radiation are the jaw; one or both shoulders, arms, or wrists; and the back of the neck.

Stable (Demand) Angina: More important than the quality or location of discomfort is its relationship with exertion (increased myocardial oxygen demand). The physician should strongly suspect angina when patients—especially middle-aged and older people—describe almost any uncomfortable sensation above the waist that is provoked by physical activity and relieved by rest. People sometimes describe "a tired feeling in the chest," burning, or breathlessness. Any of these, if reliably brought on by physical effort and relieved by rest, may be angina.

Patients with demand angina learn that their discomfort worsens with continued exertion and that they must stop or slow down substantially to make their symptoms go away. Time of day, ambient temperature, and proximity to meals all can affect how much exertion is needed to provoke angina, but, in general, the circumstances that trigger discomfort in an individual person become stereotyped.

Response to nitroglycerin is also important in the diagnosis of angina, albeit less specific than might be expected. Sublingual nitroglycerin usually relieves angina within 1–2 minutes; the pain of esophageal spasm, which also responds to nitroglycerin, seldom abates before 10 minutes. Patients with angina may find that prophylactic nitroglycerin helps prevent pain in situations that would ordinarily provoke it, such as sexual intercourse or other aerobic activity.

Other Kinds of Angina: In addition to the classic angina of effort, there are several variations that may be harder to diagnose. Among these is angina that occurs exclusively at rest, in patients with normal exercise capacity. Prinzmetal termed this form "variant angina" in his original 1959 description. Now it is also called "vasospastic angina" because it is understood to be caused by coronary artery spasm—in atherosclerotic as well as angiographically normal arteries. Vasospastic angina is one form of unstable angina (Chapter 1.3).

Another presentation is known as "angina decubitus," implying that patients asleep in bed have symptoms that awaken them. The pathologic conditions usually are extensive coronary artery disease and poor left ventricular function; the left ventricular diastolic pressure is increased to a level at which it impairs subendocardial perfusion. When a patient lies down, and the diastolic pressure increases further, subendocardial blood flow falls and pain begins. This symptom is best thought of as evidence of left ventricular failure and is treated with measures that lower the left ventricular filling pressure (Chapter 1.5).

Still another presentation is known as "angina-equivalent." This is usually dyspnea or syncope, caused by transient myocardial ischemia; unless the patient also has chest discomfort, the physician may not think of angina. The critical factor here is that the pathophysiology of the dyspnea or syncope is transient myocardial ischemia, provoked, as with classic angina, by increased oxygen demand. The dyspnea may be caused by global ischemia and a resulting increased left ventricular diastolic pressure that leads to pulmonary venous congestion, or it may be caused by ischemia of a papillary muscle, leading to mitral regurgitation. Syncope as an angina-equivalent can also be attributed to severe global ischemia and a markedly reduced cardiac output, but more often the cause is an arrhythmia, either ventricular tachycardia or transient high-degree atrioventricular block.

The term *atypical angina* can be used to encompass all the foregoing unusual manifestations of myocardial ischemia. "Atypical chest pain" is sometimes used to describe symptoms that are difficult to interpret; it is a meaningless phrase and should be avoided.

Physical Examination

The physical examination of patients with suspected angina pectoris has three purposes: to detect conditions (eg, aortic stenosis) that may be causing the angina, to identify other diseases that may cause chest pain that mimics angina (see "Differential Diagnosis" below), and to look for other consequences of coronary artery disease, such as myocardial dysfunction, left ventricular aneurysm, and mitral regurgitation. If a patient happens to have a spell of angina during the exam, the physician may be able to hear third or fourth heart sounds that were not present in the asymptomatic state, or perhaps an apical systolic murmur of mitral regurgitation caused by transient papillary muscle dysfunction.

DIFFERENTIAL DIAGNOSIS

The physician can distinguish ischemic cardiac pain from other conditions using easily obtained (bedside) clinical information. The following differential diagnosis includes syndromes of episodic chest pain that can generally be diagnosed just with a detailed, unhurried history and physical exam. This discussion does not cover the pain of myocardial infarction (Chapter 1.3); although the differential diagnosis is similar, myocardial infarction causes a single episode of chest pain that often brings patients to an emergency room, where the focus may be less on bedside findings than on laboratory tests.

The first principle in sorting through the various causes of recurrent chest pain is to consider the host. What risk factors for coronary artery disease might increase the chance that an individual's chest pain is caused by myocardial ischemia? A 60-year-old diabetic male smoker with chest pain is far more likely to be having angina than a 40-year-old premenopausal woman who has never smoked and whose 75-year-old parents are alive and well. Another example is the busy, constantly stressed executive who develops chest pain at rest during times of worry or introspection, but has relief with exercise. Regardless of other traditional risk factors, the source of this person's symptoms is probably not cardiac. The astute physician seeks to understand the personality and lifestyle of patients with chest pain syndromes and inquires about cigarette smoking, diabetes, hypertension, cholesterol, and the cardiac histories of first-degree relatives. If treatment is to be comprehensive and effective, whatever the eventual diagnosis, the physician should also gain an empathic understanding of the impact that the symptoms are having on the patient's work, social, and family life.

After the host, the most important aspect of the history is the circumstances in which patients experience their symptoms. In contrast to people experiencing most of the noncardiac causes of chest pain, patients with angina can usually be specific in describing an activity that has elicited symptoms, and their accounts bespeak a vivid recollection of particular occasions. Patients with stable angina always show clear evidence of the increase in cardiac work, from some form of exertion or sometimes from emotional arousal.

Table 1.2–1 lists the most common causes of episodic chest pain and suggests features that distinguish them from typical angina pectoris. The most common conditions that cause difficulty in diagnosis are upper gastrointestinal and musculoskeletal disorders, with esophageal disease the most frequent source of confusion in middle-aged, "coronary-prone" patients. Gastroesophageal reflux of acidic stomach contents typically causes burning pain; begins after the patient eats, or drinks alcohol; and appears when the patient is recumbent. Reflux may be alleviated by antacids, sitting upright, and belching, and typically lasts longer than an episode of angina, even for 30 minutes or more. Esophageal spasm, a motility disorder that may or may not be triggered by reflux, more closely mimics angina in its quality, location, radiation, and relief with sublingual nitroglycerin. However, esophageal spasm is

Table 1.2–1. Differential diagnosis of episodic chest pain.

Condition	Location	Provocation	Relief	Duration
Typical angina	Retrosternal	Physical exertion	Rest	5–10 min
Esophageal reflux	Retrosternal	Recumbent position, large meal, alcohol	Antacids	20–60 min
Esophageal spasm	Retrosternal	Spontaneous; may relate to reflux, emotion	Nitroglycerin	5–30 min
Peptic ulcer	Epigastric	Lack of food	Food, antacids	Hours
Biliary colic	Right upper quadrant, right subscapular	Fatty foods	Time, analgesics	Hours
Cervical nerve root compression	Shoulders, arms, chest	Movement	Rest, analgesics	Minutes to hours
Arthritis or bursitis	Related to specific joint	Movement	Analgesics, nonsteroidal anti-inflammatory drugs	Minutes to hours
Pleuritis or pericarditis	Anywhere in chest	Respiration	Analgesics	Waxing, waning
Psychoneurosis	Retrosternal or left mammary	Anxiety, panic attack	Rest, sedation	5–10 min

not usually triggered by exercise, and it responds to nitrates much more slowly than angina does. Biliary tract and peptic ulcer disease can generally be differentiated from angina by the abdominal focus of the discomfort and by the association of symptoms with certain foods (or the lack of food) rather than with exercise.

Musculoskeletal or cervical spine pain may be mistaken for cardiac pain because of the shared nerve supply, precipitation by movement or exercise, and relief by rest. Acute inflammation or trauma in the shoulder bursa, costochondral cartilage, or cervical spine may cause pain that physicians can reproduce by palpating or moving the affected part, thus enabling them to distinguish these conditions from cardiac sources of pain. The pain of herpes zoster is continuous, and its cause is revealed after a day or so when the characteristic rash emerges (Chapter 8.11).

Occasionally, the pain of pericarditis or pleural irritation is episodic and becomes confused with angina. But it is usually easy to ferret out the underlying disorder, often a preceding viral illness, pneumonia, or pulmonary embolus. The characteristic friction rub should be readily apparent on auscultation of the chest.

Psychological causes of chest pain can be the most vexing to manage, not because the diagnosis is obscure but because treatment is difficult, poorly handled by most physicians, and often ineffective no matter how well-intended or directed. Anxiety disorders, sometimes mixed with depressive illness, panic attacks, and hyperventilation syndromes, can usually be detected by probing, thoughtful history taking and judicious, carefully explained use of laboratory tests. Unfortunately, even a normal coronary angiogram is insufficient to relieve some patients of their psychological symptoms.

Another type of disability is seen all too often in patients with mitral valve prolapse, a common and generally benign disorder (Chapter 1.8). Some of these patients have chest pain, palpitations, and dyspnea that they and their physician may attribute wrongly to their mitral valve prolapse. The cause of these symptoms is generally related to autonomic hyperreactivity, coupled with a degree of heightened cardiac awareness. The only serious medical consequence of these symptoms, apart from the burden of having "heart disease," is that the physician may prescribe inappropriate, ineffectual, and sometimes harmful medications.

LABORATORY EVALUATION

Noninvasive Testing

Initial evaluation of patients with chest pain should always include a 12-lead resting electrocardiogram (ECG). Even when the history and physical exam indicate a noncardiac source of the pain, patients and physicians are much reassured by a normal ECG. When the diagnosis of angina is secure, the ECG helps assess prognosis by documenting whether the patient has Q waves, ST-T wave abnormalities, left ventricular hypertrophy, or conduction defects. Echocardiography and radionuclide ventriculog-

raphy are noninvasive ways to get an objective assessment of left ventricular function. One or both of these tests may be desirable, for example, when the physician is considering giving a β-blocker and the physical exam suggests cardiomegaly. The echocardiogram can also be used to assess valve lesions when suspicious murmurs are heard on cardiac auscultation.

By far the most commonly used (and abused) noninvasive cardiac study is the stress test. Generally, the patient is connected to a modified 12-lead system and walks on a treadmill according to a standardized graded exercise protocol. The end points of the exercise are fatigue, chest discomfort, ischemic ECG changes, hypotension, and sustained arrhythmias. Ideally, patients with angina have their symptoms reproduced exactly, and the ECG shows concurrent ST-segment depressions. Patients with nonanginal chest pain have a normal ECG up to the "target" heart rate published in standard reference tables.

Unfortunately, stress testing is fraught with problems of sensitivity, specificity, over- and underinterpretation, and general misunderstanding of its usefulness and limitations by many physicians who order it for their patients. Furthermore, some doctors subject asymptomatic people to stress testing in an attempt to screen for coronary artery disease, thereby provoking unjustified anxiety and occasioning inappropriate additional tests and treatments.

The principal indication for stress testing is to assess prognosis in patients with known or strongly suspected angina—part of a larger process called *risk stratification*. Secondarily, stress testing may be used to sort out an equivocal diagnosis, such as to establish whether or not signs of myocardial ischemia accompany atypical symptoms such as the angina-equivalent syndromes (see "Other Kinds of Angina" above). Stress testing can also be part of the assessment of therapeutic efficacy, such as to demonstrate adequate protection against exercise-induced ischemia after initiating β-blocker treatment. Many patients need this documentation before they can be allowed to return to work, join a cardiac rehabilitation program, or begin an unsupervised vigorous exercise regimen.

Stress electrocardiography is unreliable in patients who have certain abnormalities of the resting ECG, in particular, left bundle branch block, Wolff-Parkinson-White syndrome, left ventricular hypertrophy with strain, or abnormal digitalis effect. When these abnormalities are seen on the resting ECG, stress thallium scintigraphy and stress radionuclide ventriculography have proved most valuable and reliable. These nuclear imaging techniques are also used sometimes to assess the likely significance of an abnormal stress ECG. In other patients, stress testing cannot be performed because of physical disabilities that preclude walking. These patients are tested with pharmacologic stressors, often combined with thallium scintigraphy or echocardiography. Dobutamine, adenosine, and dipyridamole all have been used as stressors to unmask ischemia.

Several findings on the routine treadmill exercise test predict high risk for morbidity and mortality from coronary artery disease in patients with angina and even in patients who are asymptomatic after myocardial infarction (Table 1.2–2). When patients who have already received a reasonable course of medical therapy are found to have one or more of these poor prognostic factors, the physician should recommend coronary angiography to determine whether revascularization is feasible. Patients without any of these factors have a good prognosis and should continue on drug therapy. Because coronary atherosclerosis progresses in fits and starts, it is not clear how often to repeat stress tests if the patient's symptoms remain stable. Once every 2–3 years seems reasonable.

Ambulatory electrocardiography (Holter monitoring) is another noninvasive way to correlate symptoms with ECG signs of ischemia. Unlike the artificial laboratory environment of treadmill or imaging tests, the monitor allows patients to go about their normal activities relatively unencumbered. If patients have spontaneous episodes of chest discomfort, atypical angina, or angina-equivalent symptoms, they mark those moments on the monitor tape with an electrical signal, so that the physician can examine the simultaneous multiple-lead ECG tracings. Holter monitoring is particularly useful for patients whose symptoms typically occur under peculiar circumstances or at times of day that cannot be duplicated in the laboratory. The monitor may be the only way to confirm vasospastic or Prinzmetal's angina. But the physician must use caution in interpreting asymptomatic ST-segment shifts (silent ischemia), especially when there is no corroborating evidence of coronary artery disease. The clinical significance of silent ischemia remains controversial.

Coronary Angiography

Cardiac catheterization is the only way to gain certain knowledge of coronary anatomy. But the value of this anatomic information is limited without an understanding of the functional or physiologic significance of obstructions. When physicians see a narrowed or occluded artery on angiography, they can only infer the dynamic process of ischemia. In this era of revascularization procedures, primarily coronary bypass surgery and balloon angioplasty, the natural tendency of physicians and patients alike is to "do something" once an obstructive lesion has been confirmed. Although revascularization is often appropriate for patients with ominous clinical presentations (see Table 1.2–2), numerous studies have proved the wisdom of more conservative management for most patients with angina.

Table 1.2–2. Treadmill exercise test findings that predict a poor prognosis.

Onset of ST depression at low level of exercise (<6 min exercise, heart rate <120/min)
ST-segment depression in multiple ECG leads
ST-segment depression >2 mm in one or more leads
Hypotension with ST-segment depression during exercise
≥10% drop in ejection fraction on stress radionuclide ventriculography
Reversible perfusion defects in more than one vascular region on stress thallium scintigraphy

Table 1.2–3. Indications for coronary angiography.

Intractable angina
Intolerance of medical therapy
Ominous stress test results
Prinzmetal's variant angina
Uncertain cause of chest pain
Possible angina equivalent
Definitive study because of occupation or lifestyle, or for reassurance

The fundamental indication for coronary angiography is the need to know the coronary anatomy, usually to determine whether revascularization is feasible (Table 1.2–3). Most patients who are referred for catheterization because of chest pain have already been diagnosed as having angina. Their physician believes that continued medical therapy may not be their best option, because of side effects or inadequate control of symptoms, or because noninvasive studies suggest that they have a coronary artery lesion for which surgery usually improves prognosis: left main or severe triple-vessel disease.

Admittedly, the widespread availability of balloon angioplasty has somewhat loosened the criteria for catheterization in recent years. Physicians feel that eliminating an obstructive coronary lesion is preferable to treating it medically and that eliminating the lesion without the risk, expense, and disability of open heart surgery is also preferable to bypass grafting. Unfortunately, current angioplasty techniques have enough limitations that this belief is based more on theory than on reality. Angioplasty thus far has proved to be more a delaying action than a true alternative to surgery. This is sometimes a perfectly legitimate argument. But angioplasty is an evolving technique, and its proper place in the treatment of coronary artery disease is yet to be determined.

Since it is desirable to establish a definite cause for chest pain, some patients appropriately undergo catheterization for strictly diagnostic purposes. There may be a compelling "need to know" the coronary anatomy, even when the likelihood of finding disease is low, such as in patients whose history and noninvasive studies are equivocal and who do not wish to take cardiac medications unless absolutely necessary, in patients who must know whether they have coronary disease because their occupation (eg, airline pilot) or lifestyle (eg, long-distance runner) entails unusual risk, and in patients who may have one of the atypical angina or angina-equivalent syndromes. For this last group of patients, the catheterization findings may necessitate radical changes in management.

TREATMENT

Upon establishing the diagnosis of angina, the physician must institute general measures such as risk factor modification and must decide among the three major treatment options: drugs, angioplasty, and bypass surgery. Some physicians believe that to make the correct choice they must send all patients for cardiac catheterization, the rationale being that this is the only way to diagnose left main or triple-vessel coronary artery disease, the lesions that require surgery. However, there is no evidence that universal catheterization for patients with angina improves their short-term or long-term outcome. A more reasonable approach is to recommend catheterization only when the clinical context or noninvasive test results suggest that revascularization will relieve symptoms or improve prognosis more reliably than medical treatment (Table 1.2–4).

General Measures

The ideal treatment for angina is one that causes regression of atherosclerotic plaques. With our current understanding of atherogenesis and with the ability of therapy to reduce known risk factors, this ideal is not as fanciful as it once seemed. Convincing studies document angiographic stabilization of coronary artery lesions and, in some patients, actual regression, with associated reductions in ischemic cardiac morbidity and mortality. It is essential, therefore, that physicians make every reasonable effort to convince patients with established coronary artery disease to eliminate or reduce all modifiable risk factors. Patients must be encouraged in the strongest terms possible to quit smoking, control hypertension, and lose weight by regular aerobic exercise and calorie restriction. Intensive diet modification and drug therapy to lower low-density lipoprotein (LDL) cholesterol or raise high-density lipoprotein (HDL) cholesterol levels are justifiable if they impose no undue hardship or hazard. In addition, unless they have a specific contraindication, all patients should regularly take low-dose aspirin.

Antianginal Medications

Everyone who has had angina should be counseled to take note of exactly what circumstances bring on symptoms. Patients should always have sublingual nitroglycerin available to relieve symptoms and, whenever feasible, to take prophylactically to prevent attacks. Other forms of nitroglycerin, mainly long-acting oral and cutaneous preparations, are not considered first-line therapy

but, taken in combination with other medications, may be appropriate for some patients who have refractory symptoms.

After sublingual nitroglycerin, the keystone to preventing angina is a β-blocker. This class of drugs reduces myocardial oxygen demand primarily by reducing heart rate and ventricular contractility, and secondarily by decreasing blood pressure, particularly during exercise. Once-a-day cardioselective β-blockers (eg, atenolol) are preferable to non-cardio-selective, multiple-daily-dose β-blockers (eg, propranolol), largely because the simpler regimen improves adherence. The cardioselective drugs can be given safely to most people with diabetes, and even to patients with bronchospastic lung disease. Peripheral vascular disease is not a contraindication to taking β-blockers.

For patients whose angina is inadequately controlled by nitrates and a β-blocker and for patients who cannot tolerate β-blockers because of side-effects or adverse reactions, the next line of therapy is a calcium channel blocker. Patients with normal left ventricular function benefit from verapamil, especially if they are susceptible to supraventricular arrhythmias or their heart is markedly hypertrophied. Patients who may have prominent vasospasm do better on nifedipine, amlopidine, or diltiazem, without or with at most a low-dose β-blocker. Vasospastic syndromes can be exacerbated by β-blockade, presumably because it leaves α-adrenergic activity relatively unopposed. Again, longer-acting or sustained-release calcium blockers improve adherence.

Patients who have both angina and heart failure require diuretics, plus digoxin if they are in atrial fibrillation, and probably long-acting nitrates to reduce preload. Since angina decubitus may be a manifestation of nocturnal heart failure, many patients can prevent it by taking a short-acting diuretic late in the afternoon and by putting on a nitroglycerin patch at bedtime. They should remove the patch in the morning, to prevent the development of nitrate tolerance.

Coronary Artery Bypass Graft Surgery

Patients who have disabling angina despite maximum tolerable doses of anti-ischemic drugs should undergo angiography to determine the potential for revascularization. The two goals of bypass surgery are to relieve symptoms and prolong survival. Among patients who have proximal obstructions but whose distal vessels are relatively healthy, more than 90% have angina relieved by surgery. Whether people live longer after surgery than after medical therapy is less certain. According to studies begun in the mid to late 1970's, the only patients whose lives were definitely lengthened were those with left main coronary artery disease or severe triple-vessel disease. However, it is possible that current surgical techniques—especially using the internal mammary artery for grafts, in addition to the saphenous veins—will improve long-term survival for everyone.

The role of balloon angioplasty may be clarified by current trials comparing it with bypass surgery in patients

Table 1.2–4. Indications for medical versus surgical therapy for angina pectoris.

Medical
Good response to therapy
Low risk indicated by stress test
Mild disease
Single-vessel disease
Inoperable disease
Poor general health

Surgical
Disabling symptoms
Intolerance of medications
Left main coronary artery disease
Triple-vessel disease, especially with left ventricular dysfunction

with multivessel disease. Also under investigation are adjuncts or alternatives to balloon angioplasty, such as atherectomy, laser angioplasty, and intracoronary stents.

SUMMARY

▶ Angina pectoris is not a disease, but a symptom caused by coronary artery blood supply not keeping up with myocardial oxygen demand.

▶ A careful history is generally sufficient to diagnose angina. Key questions address factors that provoke and relieve chest discomfort, location and quality of symptoms, and risk factors for coronary artery disease.

▶ Treadmill exercise testing is a valuable adjunct in assessing prognosis and is often the decisive factor in determining when patients need angiography to define the coronary anatomy.

▶ Goals of treatment are relieving symptoms, stabilizing coronary atherosclerosis, and improving prognosis. With current medical therapy, sometimes supplemented by coronary artery bypass surgery or angioplasty, most patients can achieve these goals.

SUGGESTED READING

Brown G et al: Regression of coronary artery disease as a result of intensive lipid-lowering therapy in men with high levels of apolipoprotein B. N Engl J Med 1990;323:1289.

Cameron A et al: Coronary bypass surgery with internal-thoracic-artery grafts: Effects on survival over a 15-year period. N Engl J Med 1996;334:216.

King SB et al: A randomized trial comparing coronary angioplasty with coronary bypass surgery. N Engl J Med 1994;331:1044.

McNeer JF et al: The role of the exercise test in the evaluation of patients for ischemic heart disease: Rationale, efficacy, and adverse effects. Circulation 1978;57:64.

Strauss WE, Parisi AF: Combined use of calcium-channel and beta-adrenergic blockers for the treatment of chronic stable angina. Ann Intern Med 1988;109:570.

Yusuf S et al: Effect of coronary artery bypass graft surgery on survival: Overview of 10-year results from randomised trials by the Coronary Artery Bypass Graft Surgery Triallists Collaboration. Lancet 1994;344:563.

Unstable Angina and Acute Myocardial Infarction

Alan D. Guerci, MD

Myocardial infarction (MI) is caused by coronary thrombosis and is usually signaled by the same kind of pain as angina pectoris, but more protracted and usually more severe. In the early 1960's, the mortality rate for patients admitted to the hospital with acute MI was more than 20%; now, although MI remains one of the most common causes of death in the middle-aged, the hospital mortality rate has been reduced to less than 10%. Some of this improvement stems from being able to reopen an occluded coronary artery with thrombolytic drugs. In a patient treated early enough, this may reduce the extent of myocardial necrosis. Even in those patients who are seen only when the damage is already done, we are better able to treat arrhythmias, repair mechanical catastrophes such as rupture of the mitral valve or ventricular septum, and prevent recurrent infarction by prompt attention to postinfarction angina.

Despite this increased expertise, and a heightened awareness among patients of the need for early treatment, there is probably an irreducible minimum of mortality from MI. Among hospital patients, this is related to simple pump failure, but a larger group die before they reach medical care, either from arrhythmias or immediate pump failure. The physician's role, therefore, is to recognize the presenting features of MI and then prevent further damage, treat the complications of myocardial necrosis, and take steps to prevent further coronary occlusions in the future. Many patients also need a period of rehabilitation to recover their former activity level and confidence.

Not all coronary occlusions cause infarction. Brief occlusions can be caused by temporary vasospasm, or when thrombosis is followed immediately by clot lysis. These brief interruptions in blood supply cause angina, described as "unstable angina," but without infarction. Whereas stable angina is caused by a temporary increase in oxygen demand (Chapter 1.2), unstable angina is caused by a temporary reduction in oxygen supply and is not precipitated by effort. The expression "unstable," or sometimes "preinfarction," angina, is accurate, since without treatment many patients with unstable, supply-side angina develop MI. For this reason and because in their initial phases unstable angina and MI may be indistinguishable, the two conditions are discussed together.

PATHOPHYSIOLOGY

The pathophysiologic events in unstable angina and MI occur at two levels. One is the coronary artery, where spasm and thrombosis are the products of an interplay between diseased endothelium and the blood. The other is the myocardium, where the site of infarction and the characteristics of ischemic muscle determine the mechanical consequences of a coronary occlusion.

Atherosclerosis, Platelets, and Thrombosis

Although many people think of coronary atherosclerosis as a continuous, gradual process that follows simple physical principles—"hardening of the arteries"—it is better imagined as the product of complex biologic interactions that proceed in an intermittent fashion. A coronary plaque has periods of intense biologic activity, during which it is at risk for complete occlusion, and periods during which it is biologically stable. Stability of a plaque has little to do with how much it narrows the artery; merely knowing the severity of a coronary stenosis is still a long way from knowing how likely it is at any moment to "heat up" and occlude.

Usually, the initiating event is rupture or fissuring of the plaque's endothelial surface. Exposure of tissue factors and collagen inside the plaque stimulates adhesion, aggregation, and activation of platelets, together with deposition of fibrin. In other cases, shear forces created by high velocity of flow through tight coronary stenoses, and turbulence distal to those stenoses, promote platelet aggregation and activation. In either case, potent vasoconstrictors released from platelets, such as thromboxane A_2 and serotonin, may induce coronary vasospasm. Spasm and fibrin deposition resulting from these processes may cause partial or complete interruption of coronary blood flow.

Although there is a spectrum of decreased coronary perfusion in both unstable angina and acute MI, transient and variable reductions of flow are more typical of unstable angina, whereas total vascular occlusion and cessation of antegrade flow are more typical of MI.

Pure spasm of coronary arteries accounts for perhaps 2% of infarctions, and an even smaller number are the result of embolism, congenital anomalies of the coronary circulation, and arteritis.

Coronary Artery Anatomy

The left coronary artery comprises the anterior descending artery, in the anterior interventricular groove, and the circumflex artery, in the atrioventricular groove. Both branches arise from a short common trunk, the left main coronary artery, which thus supplies blood to about 75% of the left ventricle (Figure 1.3–1). Infarction of more than 40% of the left ventricular myocardium is usually lethal, so that in the absence of extensive collateral supply from the right coronary artery, acute occlusion of the left main coronary artery is usually fatal.

The left anterior descending coronary artery is usually larger than the circumflex or right coronary artery. It supplies at least the anterior half of the septum and variable amounts of the anterolateral wall. Proximal occlusions of the anterior descending artery also carry a high mortality.

The left anterior descending artery perfuses the bundle of His and the initial portions of the right and left bundles as they traverse the proximal and anterior septum, so that in addition to pump failure, occlusions may cause intraventricular conduction disturbances and complete heart block.

The left circumflex coronary artery supplies the posterior wall of the left ventricle and some of the lateral and inferior walls. The circumflex artery is not usually a large vessel; severe pump failure from a circumflex occlusion is only likely in patients in whom the circumflex artery also perfuses most or all of the inferior wall (a "left dominant" circulation).

The right coronary artery supplies the right ventricle, inferior part of the septum, inferior wall, and posterolateral wall, and, in about 90% of persons, the atrioventricular (AV) node. As in the case of the circumflex artery, the right coronary artery usually perfuses a less than critical amount of left ventricular myocardium (20–25%), and right coronary occlusions do not ordinarily cause severe left ventricular dysfunction. More common complications of right coronary occlusions are AV heart block, papillary muscle dysfunction, and right ventricular dysfunction.

THE PATIENT WITH ACUTE CHEST PAIN

Patients with acute myocardial ischemia usually experience severe squeezing retrosternal pain. Radiation to the neck, jaw, or left arm is common; radiation to the right arm or back is somewhat less common. Just as in exertional angina, the character and distribution of pain are variable; some patients report pain only in the arms or

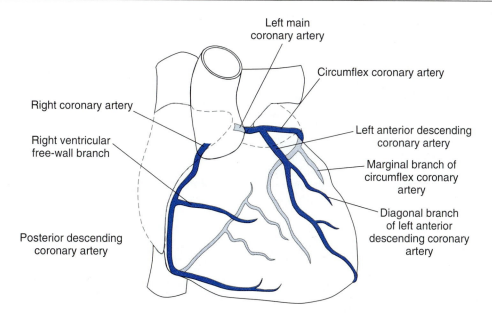

Figure 1.3–1. The coronary arteries.

confined to the upper part of the back. Others describe only dyspnea and "tightness"; hence, the common euphemism "chest discomfort." The pain of MI and that of unstable angina are the same; like the pain of chronic stable angina, they both represent cardiac pain. It is the pattern and clinical circumstances, not the description of pain, that separate these three syndromes.

Completely asymptomatic MIs are unusual, but unrecognized infarctions are not. Not all patients find the discomfort so intolerable as to require immediate medical attention. In some, the pain is epigastric and mistaken for indigestion. In others, the arm or neck discomfort overshadows the chest pain, and the cardiac origin is not obvious. Still other patients have symptoms of reduced cardiac output or a secondary increase in adrenergic tone, such as shortness of breath or some combination of malaise, weakness, and anxiety. Serial ECGs from longitudinal studies of large employee groups suggest that as many as 25% of patients with MI do not seek medical attention. At least another 25% die suddenly, from ventricular fibrillation or pump failure, before they reach a hospital.

Unstable Angina

Unstable angina is defined as ischemic myocardial pain occurring more frequently or at lower levels of physical exertion than during a previously stable period of exertional angina, or as episodes of ischemic myocardial pain occurring at rest without evidence of infarction. Some evidence also supports including any angina of new onset. Thus, the emphasis is on pain at rest or with minimal exertion, but the definition is broad and any change in the pattern of symptoms requires attention.

Prinzmetal's angina, sometimes called variant or vasospastic angina, is a syndrome characterized by episodes of chest pain at rest despite well-preserved exercise capacity. ST segments are characteristically elevated during an attack. This syndrome is caused by spasm of a coronary artery, often superimposed on atherosclerotic coronary disease.

Physical Examination

In acute MI, the physical examination has three purposes. The first is to identify the degree of circulatory embarrassment from the vital signs, the quality of the pulses, and any evidence of increased sympathetic activity, such as pallor, sweating, livedo, or goose bumps. The second is to help with the differential diagnosis; relevant signs include asymmetric or absent pulses in a patient with aortic dissection, crepitus over the thoracic inlet of a patient with ruptured esophagus, and a rub in a patient with pericarditis. The third is to evaluate the state of the heart itself. A fourth heart sound is common in acute MI and implies that the left ventricular diastolic pressure is elevated. Third sounds are less common and indicate severe myocardial dysfunction. Often when a patient has a third sound, the heart rate is high enough that the third and fourth sounds are superimposed, creating a "summation gallop."

The jugular venous pressure (JVP) is usually increased in inferior infarction, implying associated right ventricular dysfunction. Some patients with left coronary occlusions have a high JVP at the time of presentation because of intense vasoconstriction and relative increase in venous blood volume. A persistently high JVP in the patient with anterior infarction is a sign of seriously impaired heart function and is a worse sign than after right coronary occlusion. The structural disasters that may follow MI include mitral regurgitation and ventricular septal rupture, each of which causes a pansystolic murmur.

Electrocardiography

The electrocardiogram (ECG) is the most important test in the diagnosis of acute myocardial ischemia and infarction. There are two general patterns. When an epicardial artery is abruptly occluded, the resulting transmural ischemia is signaled by ST elevation, sometimes more than 5 mm (Figures 1.3–2 and 1.3–3). If the ischemia ceases, the ECG returns to normal, but if the ischemia lasts long enough to cause infarction, the ECG evolves in a characteristic way. Over the course of 3–12 hours, the R wave gradually loses amplitude, until eventually the affected ECG leads show characteristic Q waves. The ST segment gradually returns to baseline, at the same time that the T wave becomes inverted, beginning at its terminal portion. In a few patients, the ST segments remain permanently elevated. This corresponds to a true full-thickness scar and often accompanies aneurysm formation. ST-segment elevation and development of Q waves are usually signs of acute transmural ischemia and infarction. In other patients, acute ischemia causes ST depression, and MI may occur without changes in the QRS complex. This is termed non-Q wave infarction and generally corresponds to infarction confined to the subendocardial layer of ventricular muscle.

The ECG is not infallible. The early stages of transmural ischemia may be expressed by relatively nonspecific features, such as unusually tall T waves. ST elevation and depression may be slight, that is, less than 0.1 mV, and in rare patients the first ECG may even be normal. These problems of sensitivity and specificity are especially common in the diagnosis of subendocardial ischemia. It is of the utmost importance, therefore, to base initial management on a bedside impression of the patient's symptoms and signs, rather than to rely on the ECG to determine whether to admit, discharge, or reassure the patient.

Laboratory Findings

Cardiac cell death causes a characteristic pattern of enzyme release into the bloodstream. The most specific finding is elevation of serum creatine kinase (CK) and its myocardial subfraction, CK-MB. CK-MB usually constitutes 6–15% of myocardial CK and less than 4% of CK from skeletal muscle. Thus, a high CK level with a 12% CK-MB isoenzyme level would ordinarily be considered evidence of myocardial necrosis, but with only a 2% CK-MB level it would be more consistent with skeletal muscle injury. CK-MB fractions of 4% or 5% may be difficult to

A

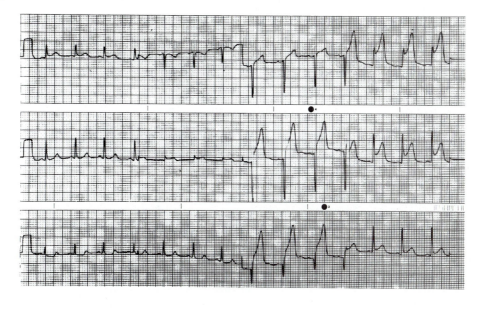

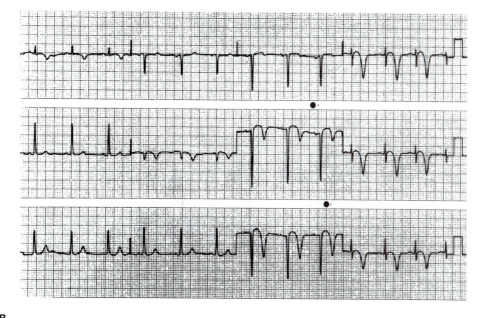

B

Figure 1.3–2. ECGs in anterior myocardial infarction. **A:** On presentation, the patient shows ST elevation in leads aVL and V_1–V_6, with tall (so-called hyperacute) T waves. **B:** The same patient, 2 weeks later, has QS complexes in aVL and V_1–V_3 with extensive anterior T-wave inversion. Persistence of ST elevation in the precordial leads suggests formation of a full-thickness scar and the possibility of aneurysm.

A

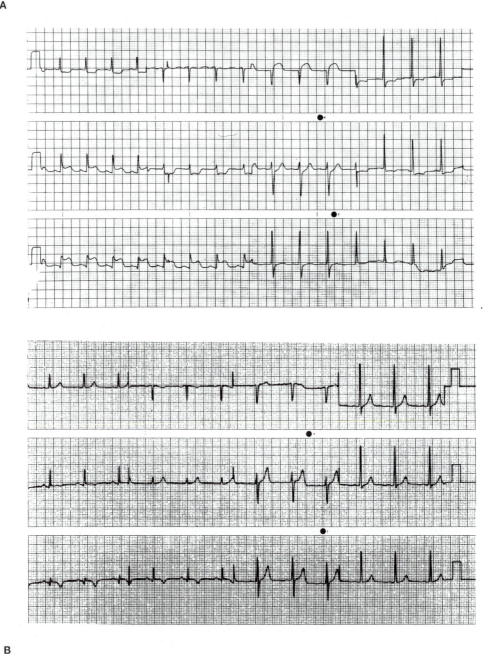

B

Figure 1.3–3. ECGs in inferior myocardial infarction. **A:** Acute changes of ST elevation in the inferior leads—II, aVF, III. **B:** After 10 days, there is T-wave inversion in the inferior leads, with loss of R wave and appearance of a Q wave in lead III.

interpret, particularly when the total CK is only modestly elevated. In these cases, the diagnosis depends on the results of serial ECGs.

Unless the occluded coronary artery is reopened with thrombolytic agents, peak CK levels are observed 20–24 hours after the first symptoms. Reperfusion accelerates

washout of CK and CK-MB. Peak CK and CK-MB levels occur about 6 hours after re␣ usion. Myocytes also contain aspartate transaminase (AST or SGOT) and lactate dehydrogenase (LDH), and elevated levels of these can also be detected, sometimes for a day or two after the CK has returned to normal.

Differential Diagnosis

Not all patients with acute chest pain have MI or unstable angina. The differential diagnosis, like that of exertional angina, encompasses pain originating from all the structures in the thorax, as well as from the chest wall, spine, and upper abdominal viscera (Table 1.3–1).

Aortic Dissection: Aortic dissection is discussed in Chapter 1.4. The tearing pain caused when the aortic media is split is described as extremely intense, usually of very sudden onset, and in dissections involving the descending aorta, often conducted to the back. Most patients with aortic dissection show obvious signs of the severity of their illness: sweating, pronounced pallor, and peripheral cyanosis. Sometimes the symptoms are less severe and the pain is indistinguishable from that of an acute MI. If the dissection extends into the aortic root, it may actually occlude one of the coronary ostia and cause an MI.

Several clinical features of aortic dissection help to differentiate dissection from infarction. Dissection of the aortic root may cause aortic regurgitation, and dissection of the brachiocephalic or left subclavian artery causes differences in blood pressure in the right and left arms. Aortic dissection does not by itself produce ECG changes characteristic of acute MI. Thus, a persistently normal ECG in a patient with protracted severe pain may be helpful in ruling out an MI in patients with aortic dissection alone. On the other hand, among patients with abnormal baseline ECGs or patients with an MI resulting from a dissection, the ECG may be of no value.

The finding of a widened superior mediastinal shadow on a routine chest x-ray suggests dissection. If the diagnosis is suspected, the definitive diagnostic technique is aortography. Transesophageal echocardiography is often performed first because it is quick and very sensitive. Magnetic resonance imaging allows good visualization of many dissections, but it takes too long to be useful in emergencies. Transthoracic echocardiography and CT scanning are of limited reliability for this purpose.

Pulmonary Embolism: Pulmonary embolism should always be kept in mind when evaluating patients with pain in the chest or shortness of breath (Chapter 2.8). The chest pain is usually pleuritic and often accompanied by a pleural friction rub, infiltrates on chest x-ray, and ECG changes that are more commonly nondescript than showing the classic terminal right-axis shift and right ventricular strain pattern. Sometimes this absence of specific ECG findings is of more help than the clinical features; both pulmonary embolism and acute MI cause chest pain, shortness of breath, lung infiltrates, and hypotension, but pulmonary embolism does not by itself cause ST-segment elevations. Even massive pulmonary embolism may cause only minor and nonspecific ST-T wave changes. As a rule, when hypotension and respiratory distress are caused by acute MI, the ST segment shift is widespread and not at all subtle. Thus, chest pain or shortness of breath and hemodynamic instability without striking ECG abnormalities should raise suspicion of a cause other than acute MI.

Table 1.3–1. Differential diagnosis of acute chest pain.

Diagnosis	Pain	ECG	X-Ray	Other
Myocardial infarction	Continuous, crushing	ST elevation or depression	Some acute congestion	CK release
Unstable angina	Intermittent, heavy	ST depression (ST elevation less common)	Normal	No CK release
Aortic dissection	Sudden, intense, terrifying	Usually minor changes, often left ventricular hypertrophy, sometimes inferior infarction	Widened mediastinum	
Pulmonary embolism	Pleuritic; major embolism more likely causes dyspnea, with or without central chest pain	Nonspecific or acute right ventricular strain	Normal, or wedge-shaped infarct	Hemodynamic changes out of proportion to ECG findings
Pericarditis	Pleuritic; affected by position	Characteristic widespread concave ST elevation	Cardiomegaly indicates effusion	Rub (pericarditis may follow an MI)
Pneumothorax	Abrupt, localized	None	Diagnostic	Asthma, asthenic habitus
Pneumomediastinum	Intense, progressive	None	Air in mediastinum	Hamman's sign, crepitus
Esophageal spasm	Can be identical to angina	None, or T inversion	None	Previous indigestion
Herpes zoster	Lateralized; burning and dysesthesia	None	None	Dermatome distribution; rash
Fractured rib	Local tenderness, pleuritic pain	None	Oblique views if in doubt	Sometimes follows only minor trauma, eg, coughing
Costal cartilage pain	Local tenderness, fear of taking a deep breath	None	None	True costochondritis rare; pain common

CK, creatine kinase; MI, myocardial infarction.

Pericarditis: The pain of pericarditis can usually be distinguished from ischemic myocardial pain on the basis of the history alone. Pericardial pain is typically made worse by lying supine and made better by sitting up and leaning forward. Pericardial pain also has a pleuritic component in most cases (ie, it is made worse by deep breathing). A pericardial friction rub helps to establish the diagnosis (Chapter 1.10).

In some patients, serial ECGs and enzyme determinations are required to distinguish pericarditis from MI. Enzyme levels are usually normal in pericarditis, and the ST-segment elevations characteristic of pericarditis have an upward concave contour (Figure 1.10–1). In addition, the ST-segment elevations of pericarditis tend to be widespread, often occurring in the distribution of more than one coronary artery; patients are almost always hemodynamically stable, and the ECG does not evolve over a few hours. This picture contrasts with that of acute ischemia with widespread ST-segment elevations, in which one would expect some evidence of hemodynamic instability, if only sinus tachycardia, and, at least after 1 or 2 hours, loss of R waves and evolution of Q waves.

Pericarditis in a patient who has Q waves that are not known to be old should provoke suspicion of recent infarction and postinfarction pericarditis. Such a patient should be admitted to the hospital.

Other Conditions: Other diseases of the lungs and thoracic cavity may mimic acute MI. These include pneumonia, pneumothorax, and pneumomediastinum. The physical examination and chest x-ray are usually sufficient to establish the diagnosis.

Esophageal spasm and rupture may cause pain that is indistinguishable from that of acute myocardial ischemia, but neither esophageal spasm nor rupture causes ECG changes or CK elevations. Pancreatitis and biliary tract disease may cause low retrosternal and epigastric pain similar to that of an MI and may even cause T-wave inversions or minor ST-segment changes. As with esophageal spasm, however, typical evolutionary ECG changes and enzyme elevations do not occur.

Chest wall abnormalities such as rib fractures or herpes zoster radiculitis may also cause pain similar to that of an MI, but these conditions usually cause chest wall tenderness and should be recognized on physical examination.

MANAGEMENT OF MYOCARDIAL INFARCTION

Initial Measures

Three steps should be taken in the first few minutes of the treatment of patients with acute MI. First, low-flow oxygen should be applied by nasal cannula or face mask. Hypoxemia is common in patients with acute MI and should be corrected, even when not severe. Oxygen therapy also has a useful calming effect and reduces sympathetic tone and myocardial oxygen demand. It is ordinarily continued for 24–48 hours.

Blood pressure permitting, the second step in the treatment of acute MI is to give sublingual nitroglycerin. Sublingual nitroglycerin occasionally interrupts transmural infarctions (because there may be an element of spasm in addition to the thrombosis) and frequently interrupts non-Q wave infarctions. If one or two sublingual nitroglycerin tablets do not abolish the patient's ischemic myocardial pain, thrombolytic therapy (see "Thrombolytic Therapy" below) should be considered.

The third step in initial therapy is to provide adequate analgesia. Patient comfort is of paramount concern, and most patients require opiates—morphine sulfate, or nalbuphine if the blood pressure is low. Although complete relief of pain may not be possible, particularly when opiates cause or aggravate hypotension, most patients can be rendered reasonably comfortable in 20 minutes. Sedation, usually with a benzodiazepine, may also be advisable.

At this point, the patient should be taken to a coronary care unit. This should be a quiet, calm environment where patients can receive close but not intrusive monitoring. The unit should be equipped for emergency resuscitation after cardiac arrest and staffed by nurses who are skilled at recognizing and correcting life-threatening arrhythmias.

Other initial measures that are routinely considered include infusing intravenous nitroglycerin, particularly when there is evidence of continuing ischemia, and giving β-blockers. The value of the latter is supported by evidence from large multicenter clinical trials; but because the reduction in mortality they offer is not large, they are generally reserved for hypertensive patients, who seem to obtain the most benefit. β-Blockers are contraindicated in patients with cardiogenic shock.

With or without concomitant thrombolytic therapy, aspirin reduces the risk of reinfarction and death in patients with acute MI. Full doses of intravenous heparin probably exert a similar favorable effect. Heparin also reduces the incidence of mural thrombus formation and systemic embolization. Thus, most centers advise administering heparin for all patients within the first day or two of infarction, and continue it until a decision is made about long-term anticoagulation. Patients with large anterior MIs are at greatest risk of systemic embolism (usually stroke) after MI and are usually given anticoagulants for at least 3 months.

Thrombolytic Therapy

Patients who come for care within the first few hours after onset of their chest pain, while the ST segments are still elevated, should receive thrombolytic agents to treat their coronary thrombosis. The two drugs usually available are streptokinase and recombinant tissue plasminogen activator (tPA). Either drug can achieve lysis of a coronary thrombus within 1 or 2 hours. It is debatable how often this is in time to save very much myocardium from necrosis. When thrombolytic therapy is started within 1–2 hours of symptom onset, considerable myocardial function is preserved and mortality is strikingly reduced. When treatment is begun after 3 hours, there is still substantial reduction in mortality, even though in about 50% of patients treated at this stage no ischemic myocardium is salvaged. In these patients, the mechanisms of benefit include restoration of flow to the healing area of infarction, thereby allowing it to form a stronger scar (preventing or limiting infarct expansion) and restoring a source of collateral blood supply to other vessel territories adjacent to the region of infarction.

One might imagine that successful thrombolysis would require some secondary procedure directed toward removing the stenosis that formed the site of the original infarct. However, there is no ideal way to achieve this, and routine follow-up revascularization, whether by angioplasty or by surgical bypass, confers no additional benefit after thrombolysis. These procedures are performed when there are additional clinical indications that they are required, based on the patient's course after the acute phase of the infarction.

Thrombolytic treatment is not without risks, the most feared of which is intracerebral hemorrhage. This occurs in 0.5% of patients treated, more in elderly patients and those with hypertension or a history of stroke. These conditions, or any other obvious reason that a patient is at special risk from thrombolytic treatment, are contraindications to taking these drugs. The potential benefit of thrombolysis lessens somewhat with time from the onset of symptoms, and if the coronary thrombosis occurred more than 6 hours previously, the drugs are given only if the infarct is large or there is clinical evidence of persisting ischemia.

Complications

The complications of MI can be grouped under four categories: arrhythmias, left ventricular failure, recurrent ischemia, and miscellaneous complications (Table 1.3–2).

Arrhythmias:

Ventricular tachyarrhythmias: One patient in 20 admitted with acute MI develops cardiac arrest from ventricular fibrillation. Prompt electrical defibrillation is almost always life-saving, and thus represents the fundamental

Table 1.3–2. Complications of myocardial infarction.

Arrhythmias
  Ventricular tachycardia
  Ventricular fibrillation
  Atrial arrhythmias
  Atrioventricular block
Left ventricular failure
Structural catastrophes
  Mitral regurgitation
  Rupture of the septum (ventricular septal defect)
  Rupture of the free wall
Right ventricular infarction
Recurrent ischemia
Postinfarction angina
Reinfarction
Late complications
  Pericarditis
  Dressler's syndrome
  Left ventricular aneurysm

raison d'être for modern coronary care units. The risk of ventricular fibrillation is related directly to the size of the ischemic region, so that those most at risk are patients with ischemic myocardial pain and widespread ST-T abnormalities.

Patients who have ventricular tachycardia or who have already suffered ventricular fibrillation are treated with intravenous lidocaine or sometimes another antiarrhythmic drug such as procainamide. Lidocaine is usually continued for 18–24 hours because ventricular fibrillation is most likely within the first few hours of infarction. It is not necessary to give prophylactic lidocaine to all patients who have suffered MI, since the drug causes some cardiac and mental depression, but prophylactic use is advisable in some patients with frequent or paired ventricular ectopic beats, those with runs of ventricular tachycardia, and those in whom the premature beats occur during the terminal half of the T wave. The dispersion of ventricular refractoriness is greatest during this time, and during acute ischemia premature ventricular beats introduced during the terminal portion of the T wave (the "R on T phenomenon") may induce ventricular fibrillation.

Atrial arrhythmias: Sinus bradycardia is seen in many patients with inferior infarctions. It may be the result of ischemia of the sinoatrial node or of negative chronotropic and vasodepressor reflexes activated by ischemia of the basilar portion of the inferior wall. Atropine is usually effective treatment and should be given if sinus bradycardia causes hypotension or impaired organ perfusion.

Sinus tachycardia, premature atrial contractions, and atrial fibrillation are also common after MI because of atrial distention from elevated left ventricular diastolic pressure. These rhythms may be the first clinical manifestations of heart failure and demand serious attention. Alternatively, premature atrial beats and atrial fibrillation may result from postinfarction pericarditis that extends to the atrial surface. True atrial infarctions are uncommon and lack specific clinical features.

Heart block: Of the several conduction disturbances common after acute MI, high-grade AV nodal block is potentially the most serious. It is more common as a complication of inferior infarction than anterior, since in 90% of persons the AV node is perfused by the right coronary artery. Ischemia of the AV node after inferior infarction often causes first-degree and Mobitz I heart block before complete heart block (Chapter 1.9). If complete heart block develops, subsidiary pacemaker tissue low in the AV node or the bundle of His often emerges to maintain an adequate ventricular escape rhythm. AV nodal dysfunction usually resolves within 1 week, and few patients need artificial pacemakers. The inferior MI itself need not be particularly large to be accompanied by AV block, and the prognosis for patients with heart block after inferior MIs is generally good.

When complete heart block complicates anterior infarctions, the prognosis is much worse. Such block implies extensive necrosis of the septum and anterior wall, affecting conduction through the distal portion of the bundle of

His and the proximal portions of the right and left bundles. In addition, subsidiary pacemakers may not emerge, and the AV block of an anterior MI may lead to cardiac arrest. After anterior infarction, therefore, any suspicious sign that complete heart block is imminent, such as alternating bundle branch block or bifascicular block, warrants prophylactic pacing. In inferior infarction, by contrast, pacing may not be required even if the patient does develop complete heart block.

Other arrhythmias: Accelerated AV nodal rhythm and accelerated idioventricular rhythm are common in the first 1 or 2 days after acute MI. Usually they are best left untreated and simply observed. Treatment is indicated when the loss of synchronized AV conduction lowers the cardiac output. Atropine is usually given first to increase the sinus rate. Lidocaine may suppress idioventricular rhythms. However, when the stability of the sinus node is in doubt, lidocaine should not be given until after a temporary pacemaker has been inserted, in case the drug suppresses the only remaining locus of impulse generation.

Left Ventricular Failure:

Pulmonary edema, hypotension, and cardiogenic shock: The most common mechanical complication of MI is left ventricular dysfunction, the signs of which may range from symptomless basilar lung congestion to cardiogenic shock. In the early hours after MI, pulmonary congestion is common, and although it signifies that there has been substantial myocardial necrosis, most patients who have pulmonary edema early after MI can be treated successfully. In a few, however, persistent severe pump failure leads to the syndrome of cardiogenic shock. This implies persistent low cardiac output, together with hypotension, and is the result of extensive and potentially fatal infarction. It carries a very poor prognosis, unless it proves to have a repairable mechanical cause such as acute mitral valve regurgitation.

Hypotension alone does not always indicate extensive myocardial damage. In addition to left ventricular pump failure, the differential diagnosis of hypotension includes inappropriate vasodilatation caused by reflex mechanisms; hypovolemia; right ventricular infarction; and circulatory depression caused by medication, particularly morphine or nitrates. In a patient who is hypotensive but who otherwise seems well, the first step is to infuse several hundred milliliters of saline. This should be sufficient to correct the relative intravascular fluid depletion underlying these causes of hypotension. If it is not sufficient, the next step should be to perform simple hemodynamic studies using a Swan-Ganz catheter placed in the pulmonary artery. This permits estimating the cardiac output and left atrial pressure (from the wedged pulmonary artery pressure) to determine whether hypotension reflects inadequate left ventricular filling, reduced cardiac output, or low arterial resistance.

After an MI, pulmonary edema may occur after MI in association with normal cardiac output and adequate blood pressure, because of an abrupt rise in left ventricular end-diastolic pressure. Under such circumstances, pulmonary edema is treated with diuretics and vasodilators, usually nitroglycerin. Nitroglycerin has relatively greater venodilator properties than many other arterial vasodilators; besides lowering blood pressure, and with it cardiac work, it also exerts a specific beneficial effect on the central venous pressures. If pulmonary edema persists despite these measures, then one should measure the left atrial pressure with a Swan-Ganz catheter and try to adjust it to about 15–20 mm Hg.

Cardiogenic shock occurs when cardiac pump function is reduced to the point that even with the highest tolerable filling pressures, left ventricular stroke output is insufficient to meet the body's metabolic need. It is the most feared complication of MI. The early stages may not always be obvious, because the signs are so similar to the hyperadrenergic state seen in most patients with acute infarction during pain. However, cool, clammy skin, sinus tachycardia, sweating, and restlessness are ominous signs in a patient who is pain-free, even without obvious respiratory insufficiency or hypotension. In more extreme cases, severe lung congestion, livedo reticularis, metabolic acidosis, oliguria, and hypotension supervene.

Management of cardiogenic shock complicating MI is a matter of optimizing the patient's oxygenation and fluid balance and manipulating the circulation to achieve the best cardiac output with the least additional demand on the remaining viable myocardium. Generally, this entails using vasodilators, often with additional inotropic therapy in the form of dopamine or similar agents. Digitalis is not effective in this setting. Left atrial pressure is monitored with a Swan-Ganz catheter and usually has to be brought up to 20–25 mm Hg. Some patients benefit from mechanical assistance in the form of an intra-aortic balloon pump. Other forms of temporary mechanical assistance are being developed, but their application is always limited by the fact that so little viable myocardium can be recovered at this stage, even with emergency revascularization by coronary bypass surgery or angioplasty.

Mitral regurgitation: This occasionally complicates MI and is most often caused by ischemia of the posterior papillary muscle or surrounding areas of the inferior wall. Rupture of the head of a papillary muscle occurs infrequently but is a catastrophic event, producing immediate and overwhelming pulmonary edema in association with hypotension and cardiogenic shock.

The murmur of acute papillary muscle dysfunction is usually most prominent at the apex, with radiation to the axilla, but may be loudest along the left parasternal area, with radiation to the base. More important, the murmur often has a decrescendo quality, because the left atrium has not had time to dilate and a relatively small regurgitant volume may suffice to bring left ventricular and left atrial pressures into equilibrium. Severe acute ischemic mitral regurgitation may thus be associated with a murmur that is only grade I or II in intensity and not truly pansystolic. In such cases, the diagnosis is confirmed by tall V waves in a wedged pulmonary artery catheter pressure tracing.

Surgical replacement of the mitral valve is required for severe acute mitral regurgitation and is often extremely rewarding. Many of the patients who sustain this complication have had only moderate-sized infarcts, and valve replacement may then allow a good recovery.

Ventricular septal defect: Rupture of the interventricular septum can complicate anterior or inferior infarction, typically 2–5 days after the infarction, later than acute mitral regurgitation. In most instances, the rupture is devastating, causing severe lung congestion and, in many patients, cardiogenic shock.

Diagnosis depends on finding a new systolic murmur, usually loudest along the left sternal border and often indistinguishable from that of mitral regurgitation. The ventricular septal defect is confirmed by finding an increase in oxygen saturation in the right ventricle. This can be achieved by drawing blood gas samples from a pulmonary artery catheter as it is passed from right atrium to right ventricle to pulmonary artery.

The treatment of ventricular septal defect is urgent surgical repair. The results are not as good as for mitral replacement, but without repair the lesion is almost always fatal.

Ventricular rupture: Rupture of the free wall of the left ventricle is an unusual and, in most cases, immediately lethal complication of transmural infarction. Like rupture of the interventricular septum, it tends to occur 2–5 days after infarction. In rare cases, pericardial adhesions adjacent to the infarct confine the hemopericardium to a small area. This condition, known as *left ventricular pseudoaneurysm*, requires urgent surgical correction.

Left ventricular aneurysm: Many transmural infarctions heal with only mild distortion of the cardiac ventricular shape. In a few cases, usually of anterior MI, the infarcted segment bulges out under the systolic ventricular pressure, and as it heals, forms a large segment that can stretch during systole. Such aneurysms, in contrast to false aneurysms or aortic aneurysms, seldom rupture; if a myocardial infarct ruptures, it does so before forming an aneurysmal scar. However, aneurysms can cause a volume loading effect on left ventricular function, and anterior aneurysms may need surgical resection. Posterior aneurysms are rare and should usually be left alone. Sometimes, even when an aneurysm is not causing mechanical problems, it may need surgical resection if it becomes the origin of dangerous ventricular tachyarrhythmias.

Right ventricular infarction: The right ventricle is perfused by branches of the right coronary artery. In about one-third of inferior infarcts, the right coronary artery is occluded proximal to these branches and causes right ventricular necrosis. The primary clinical manifestation of right ventricular infarction is a low-output state (ie, tachycardia and hypotension) that is out of proportion to left ventricular failure. Some lung congestion may be present, because of infarction of the inferior wall of the left ventricle, but this is ordinarily not severe.

ST-segment elevation in lead V_4R (an electrode placed in the right fifth intercostal space at the midclavicular line) has been used to identify patients with right ventricular infarction. However, the diagnosis is usually based on clinical grounds. It may be confirmed by the demonstra-

tion of a high central venous pressure and low wedge pressure on pulmonary artery catheterization.

The hypotension of right ventricular infarction usually responds to intravenous fluids. Large quantities (1–5 L) of normal saline are typically required.

Recurrent Ischemia: Unstable angina and postinfarction angina have similar pathophysiology, and their management is also similar. Each of these syndromes implies that there is an unstable coronary plaque, still subject to transient occlusions and that there is healthy myocardium whose blood supply is in jeopardy. Unstable angina carries the threat of MI; postinfarction angina carries the threat of reinfarction or extension of infarction.

At least 15% of patients develop angina at rest or with slight exertion in the first few days after MI. Usually the cause is threatened reocclusion of the infarct-related artery, and the risk to the patient is greatest when reocclusion threatens a large mass of myocardium that has been salvaged by timely thrombolytic therapy or when the ischemia occurs in a vascular territory other than that of the infarct. Either of these situations carries the risk that reocclusion of the artery will considerably increase the size of a patient's infarct.

Treatment of unstable angina: Medical therapy for unstable and postinfarction angina is directed at inhibiting the interaction of platelets and thrombin with disrupted endothelium, with the expectation that a new layer of endothelium will cover the surface of an unstable plaque. Aspirin reduces the incidence of nonfatal infarction or cardiac death by about 50% in patients with unstable angina. This benefit lasts for at least 18 months and is presumed to persist indefinitely. Heparin is at least as effective as aspirin, provided that it is administered by continuous intravenous infusion in a dose sufficient to prolong the activated partial thromboplastin time 1.5- to 2-fold. In hospital practice, heparin has a practical advantage over aspirin: If the patient needs to undergo bypass surgery, the effect of heparin ceases soon after the infusion is stopped, whereas aspirin may leave the patient with a clotting defect that lasts for several days. Nitrates and beta-blockers are also given to patients with unstable angina to reduce myocardial oxygen demand and coronary spasm. Nifedipine is beneficial as long as it does not cause a reflex tachycardia, an untoward effect that can be prevented by simultaneous administration of a β-blocker.

Thrombolytic therapy has not been shown to be of benefit for more than a few hours in unstable angina. This may be due to the primacy of platelets, as opposed to protein-mediated hemostasis, in the pathophysiology of unstable angina. Alternatively, to whatever extent fibrin deposition occurs without platelet activation, thrombolytic therapy may merely dissolve an existing thrombus and reexpose the underlying thrombogenic plaque surface.

The choice of medications given to patients with unstable angina depends in part on the presentation. Patients with pain at rest or after MI are usually given heparin, nitrates, and a β-blocker, with a calcium antagonist added and urgent catheterization performed in the event of recurrent ischemia. Aspirin is usually substituted for heparin after a few days. At the other extreme, patients with new-onset or progressive exertional angina, who also fit the definition of unstable angina but have less threat of MI, may simply be placed on aspirin and a β-blocker if their exercise capacity is well preserved. Attacks of Prinzmetal's angina usually respond to sublingual nitroglycerin and may be prevented with long-acting nitrates or calcium antagonists.

Patients with postinfarction angina have a high risk of a second infarction; in one study, patients with ECG changes accompanying their postinfarction angina had a 30% risk of reinfarction or death in the next 2 weeks. Thus, this syndrome demands urgent cardiac catheterization, with a view to performing bypass surgery or angioplasty. Patients with unstable angina who have not sustained an MI face a moderate risk of nonfatal infarction or cardiac death in the ensuing weeks and months. Cardiac catheterization is probably not necessary for all patients with unstable angina, but may be reserved for those whose presentation suggests life-threatening coronary disease. This would include patients who become hemodynamically compromised (hypotension or pulmonary edema) during episodes of ischemia, those with serious arrhythmias (ventricular tachycardia or ventricular fibrillation) during ischemia, and those with widespread ST-segment changes or T-wave inversions during ischemia. The ECG can be a very useful diagnostic aid in this case because widespread and extreme deviations of the ST segment from the isoelectric point reflect widespread and severe myocardial ischemia. Catheterization is also required in patients who have recurrent episodes of ischemia despite a reasonable, comprehensive antianginal medical regimen. Stated more bluntly, these are patients who either look bad or whose ECGs look bad during ischemic episodes or who have exhausted their options for continued medical therapy. The remaining patients can be followed on medical therapy and should undergo cardiac catheterization if they cease responding to their oral medications.

Miscellaneous Complications: Pericarditis occurs in many patients 1–4 days after transmural MI. The clinical features are similar to those of pericarditis from other causes: pleuropericardial pain, a pericardial rub, fever, and ST-segment elevations. Pericarditis may be treated with indomethacin. Corticosteroids should not be used because they promote left ventricular aneurysm formation.

Fever and leukocytosis are expected in the first few days after infarction, particularly in patients with large infarcts.

Postmyocardial infarction syndrome, also called Dressler's syndrome, is the development of pericarditis, fever, and pulmonary infiltrates a few weeks after MI. It is analogous to the postcardiotomy syndrome discussed in Chapter 1.10, in that it seems to be caused by an autoimmune reaction triggered by the original myocardial injury. It is treated with nonsteroidal anti-inflammatory drugs and usually resolves after a few days or weeks. Rare cases run a more protracted, relapsing course.

LONG-TERM CARE

General Considerations

Fifteen years ago, death rates among infarct survivors were about 10% during the first year and 3–5% for each of the next several years. Thrombolytic therapy and the introduction of angiotensin converting enzyme inhibitors for patients with moderate or severe heart failure have reduced these figures by 30–50%. The single most important predictor of survival is residual left ventricular function. Whereas patients with ejection fractions of 60% or greater have 1-year mortality rates of about 2% and those with ejection fractions of 40–59% have only a small additional risk, nearly 50% of the patients with ejection fractions of less than 20% die in the first year after their infarctions (Figure 1.3–4).

The number and severity of coronary artery stenoses also predict the risk of dying in the years after an MI; hence the widespread adoption of stress testing to screen for myocardial ischemia before discharge. Frequent premature ventricular contractions (PVCs) also indicate a poor prognosis, but suppressing them with antiarrhythmic drugs does not reduce the late mortality. The implication is that PVCs are not an independent risk factor, but rather a sign of extensive myocardial scarring.

Low-Level Stress Testing

Patients in whom myocardial ischemia is provoked by a low-level stress test (eg, target heart rate that is 70% of the age-predicted maximum) performed 1–3 weeks after an acute MI have a 20% risk of recurrent infarction or death over the next year, whereas those without ischemia have a mortality risk of 2–5%. It is therefore common practice to perform coronary arteriography in patients with ischemic responses, with a view to performing coronary angioplasty or bypass surgery. It is not known whether such

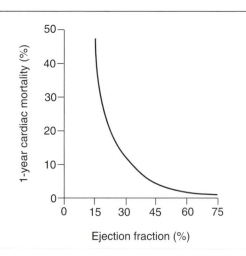

Figure 1.3–4. Effect of left ventricular ejection fraction on prognosis after myocardial infarction.

patients can be treated as effectively with antianginal therapy followed by angioplasty or surgery in the event of failure of medical therapy.

β-Blockers

Long-term treatment with β-blockers, initiated 1–4 weeks after infarction, has been shown repeatedly to reduce mortality rates among selected survivors of infarction (ie, those with no contraindication to β-blockade) by about one-third. This improvement in mortality persists for at least 3 years and is primarily due to reduction in sudden cardiac death among patients with arrhythmias or mild left ventricular failure during the in-hospital phase of their infarction, that is, patients with moderate impairment of left ventricular function.

Aspirin

Several large studies have tested the hypothesis that antiplatelet therapy with aspirin can reduce the incidence of recurrent infarction and death. Although these studies had provided conflicting results, a recent analysis of pooled data from these trials concluded that aspirin reduces the risk of death, stroke, or nonfatal reinfarction by 20%.

Rehabilitation

Treatment of the patient with acute MI does not stop when the patient leaves the hospital. General rehabilitative measures should be aimed at restoring physical and social function and, where possible, eliminating risk factors for atherosclerosis.

Most patients can begin walking on the third or fourth hospital day and can be discharged 1 week after the infarction. Low-level predischarge exercise testing is useful, because apart from long-term prognostic information, it provides specific guidelines about safe or unsafe physical activity.

Because 6 or more weeks is needed for a transmural infarct to be completely replaced by scar tissue, patients are usually advised to avoid strenuous exercise and, in particular, isometric effort during this period. They may walk and do stretching exercises and light household chores. Sexual activity is permitted, generally after some delay to build confidence. The cardiovascular demands of sexual intercourse are ordinarily equivalent to walking at a brisk pace or climbing two flights of stairs.

Depending on the size of the infarct and the nature of the patient's work, most patients can return to work 1–3 months after an MI. Patients with large infarcts and poor left ventricular function should not resume strenuous physical labor. Some patients may benefit from supervised exercise in formal rehabilitation programs. The major advantage of these programs is that they can restore confidence. Controlling hypertension, stopping smoking, and lowering cholesterol levels reduce mortality rates after acute MI by at least as much as therapy with aspirin or β-blockers.

In addition to anxiety about the safety of daily activities, depression and denial are common problems after MI. Most patients respond to a sympathetic and frank appraisal of their physical limitations and prognosis. Those who do not respond usually react favorably to professional counseling. Every effort should be made to return the patient to a normal social and economic life.

SUMMARY

▶ Myocardial infarction follows extended interruption of coronary blood supply by vascular spasm and coronary thrombosis. Unstable angina is caused by brief interruptions with the same underlying mechanisms.

▶ Patients presenting with cardiac pain and ECG evidence of ischemia are treated with nitrates, analgesics, and oxygen, followed by thrombolytic drugs. They are cared for in a cardiac care unit.

▶ Hospital mortality after myocardial infarction is caused by cardiogenic shock, ventricular rupture, and reinfarction. Arrhythmias, mitral regurgitation, ventricular septal defect, and postinfarction angina are usually treatable complications.

▶ Unstable angina and postinfarction angina are treated with nitrates and other agents to prevent coronary spasm, together with anticoagulants and β-blocking agents. Many patients require revascularization and should therefore be studied by coronary angiography.

▶ Follow-up care after myocardial infarction includes stress testing to detect residual ischemia, treatment with aspirin and β-blockers, reducing risk factors for atherosclerosis, and rehabilitation.

SUGGESTED READING

Braunwald E: Unstable angina: A classification. Circulation 1989;80:410.

Comparison of invasive and conservative strategies after treatment with intravenous tissue plasminogen activator in acute myocardial infarction: Results of the thrombolysis in myocardial infarction (TIMI) phase II trial: The TIMI Study Group. N Engl J Med 1989;320:618.

DeBusk RF et al: Identification and treatment of low-risk patients after acute myocardial infarction and coronary-artery bypass graft surgery. N Engl J Med 1986;314:161.

Randomized trial of intravenous streptokinase, oral aspirin, both, or neither among 17,187 cases of suspected acute myocardial infarction: ISIS-2 (Second International Study of Infarct Survival) Collaborative Group. Lancet 1988;2:349.

1.4

Aortic Dissection

Stephen C. Achuff, MD

Aortic dissection is a catastrophic condition that requires urgent medical and, often, surgical treatment. Before current methods of management were developed, the outlook for patients with acute dissection was dismal. Natural history studies documented mortality rates of about 25% in the first 24 hours after onset of symptoms, 50% within 2 days, and 80% in the first week. Many more lives can now be saved because of modern imaging techniques, which provide rapid, accurate definition of the disrupted aorta and give the physician a rational basis for choosing therapy. The unchanging element in this process, however, is the clinician's high index of suspicion when evaluating a patient who presents with symptoms and signs compatible with aortic dissection. This chapter addresses the key factors for prompt clinical recognition of aortic dissection, choice of tests, indications for surgery, or continued medical therapy, and the short- and long-term results of both forms of treatment.

PATHOPHYSIOLOGY

Aortic dissection begins as a transverse intimal tear that permits pulsatile blood to enter the media. The resulting hematoma propagates itself (dissects) in a longitudinal fashion distally, as well as proximally in some patients, and may involve virtually the entire length of the aorta including multiple side branches. Many patients have a distal reentry tear, so that the false lumen of the now double-barreled aorta is decompressed into the true lumen. The most common site of origin of dissections is several centimeters above the aortic valve; the second most common is the region of the ligamentum arteriosum just distal to the left subclavian artery. In vitro and animal studies have shown an important relation between aortic pulse-wave characteristics, particularly dp/dt, and the extent of dissection. This relation has direct clinical application: It should influence physicians' choice of drug treatment (see "Management" below). Aortic dissections are not true aneurysms, and although they may distort the aorta to aneurysmal proportions, the old term "dissecting

aneurysm of the aorta" is a misnomer. An acceptable alternative term, which graphically reflects the pathophysiology of the condition, is *dissecting hematoma of the aorta*.

Aortic dissections occur primarily in the fifth through seventh decades and at least twice as often in men as in women. Most patients have a history of hypertension, but atherosclerosis does not appear to be an independent risk factor. Most younger people with dissection have readily apparent congenital abnormalities or inherited defects of connective tissue. These include coarctation of the aorta (with or without underlying Turner's syndrome), bicuspid aortic valve, Ehlers-Danlos syndrome, and Marfan's syndrome. Patients with Marfan's syndrome may have pre-existing true aneurysms, which, after having reached a certain size (6 cm in the ascending aorta), are highly likely to dissect or rupture. For totally unknown reasons, pregnancy is a risk factor for aortic as well as coronary artery dissection. Finally, iatrogenic conditions can cause dissection; the most common is aortic cannulation for cardiopulmonary bypass.

CLASSIFICATION

The traditional DeBakey system classifies three types of aortic dissection, defined according to the site of the intimal tear and extent of dissection (Figure 1.4–1). Type I dissections originate in the ascending aorta and extend into the descending aorta, type II dissections are limited to the ascending aorta and arch, and type III dissections begin at or just beyond the left subclavian artery and extend distally. The simplified and currently preferred Stanford classification divides dissections into two types: those involving the ascending aorta to any degree (type A) and those limited to the descending aorta (type B). The importance of this distinction cannot be overemphasized: It reflects the great differences among the clinical manifestations, prognosis, and management principles of ascending and descending aortic dissections.

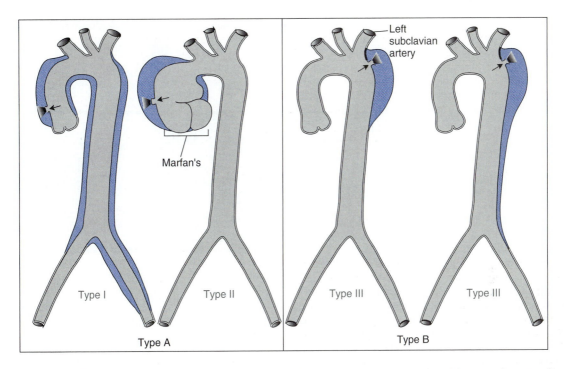

Figure 1.4–1. Classification of aortic dissection. Stanford type A (DeBakey types I and II) is a dissection of the ascending aorta. Stanford type B (DeBakey type III) is a dissection beginning distal to the left subclavian artery in the descending thoracic aorta.

EVALUATION

History

By far, the most common presenting symptom of aortic dissection is chest pain. This is generally so severe that patients use terms such as "the worst-ever pain," "excruciating," or "unbearable." The quality of the pain may be described as "tearing," "ripping," or "stabbing," but it seldom has the intense pressure or constricting sensation experienced by patients with myocardial infarction. The location of the pain tends to track the origin of the dissection: anterior chest pain in patients with ascending dissections, interscapular back pain in those with descending dissections. The pain may radiate or migrate as the process extends distally. The pain begins suddenly and reaches its greatest magnitude within seconds or minutes, but, remarkably, may resolve considerably even before the patient reaches medical attention. Occasional truly painless dissections are said to occur, but probably patients do not report pain because of some complication of the process, such as shock, cerebrovascular accident, or pulmonary edema that renders them unable to provide a lucid history.

Physical Examination

Hypertension is an initial finding in 70–80% of patients with aortic dissection, especially type B dissection. The absence of hypertension in a patient with an otherwise compatible clinical presentation should stimulate the ex-

aminer to look for complications of the dissection, such as cardiac tamponade, acute myocardial infarction, or occlusion of a brachiocephalic artery causing hypotension in the affected limb only. Other abnormalities that may be detected at the bedside (depending on the type and extent of dissection) are elevated jugular venous pressure, pulsus paradoxus, pericardial friction rub, the murmur of aortic regurgitation, neurologic deficits relating to aortic arch vessel or spinal cord involvement, and signs of a left pleural effusion. Rare patients manifest such oddities as superior vena cava obstruction, Horner's syndrome, hoarseness caused by left recurrent laryngeal nerve compression, and hemoptysis from the dissection leaking into a bronchus.

Complications

Most of the important complications of aortic dissection have already been mentioned. The clinician must be aware of these manifold potential problems for two reasons. First, the secondary effects of the dissection (eg, acute myocardial infarction, pericarditis, stroke) may dominate the clinical picture and mislead the physician from recognizing the primary process. Second, by making serial observations, the vigilant physician will be alert to new symptoms and signs that signal extension of the dissection and thus the need for a change of therapy. Type A dissections tend to propagate retrograde and produce aortic regurgitation, occlude a coronary artery (usually the right coronary) at its origin, or rupture into the pericardial space and cause tamponade. In the natural history studies mentioned above, pericardial tamponade was the most common cause of death. The second most frequent mortal complication was, and probably continues to be, rupture into the left pleural space from a descending aortic dissection. All branches of the aorta are susceptible to occlusion by the dissecting hematoma, and the physician must frequently reassess perfusion to the limbs, viscera, and central nervous system.

Laboratory Tests

Patients presenting with acute, severe chest pain should have an ECG performed immediately after the physician has obtained the history and performed the relevant physical exam. In most patients with aortic dissection, the ECG shows nothing diagnostic, although this in itself is helpful in excluding other causes of chest pain. One important source of potential confusion should be noted: About 2% of type A dissections involve one or both coronary artery ostia, more often the right. Thus, a patient with other historical and physical findings of aortic dissection whose ECG shows an acute myocardial infarction should be evaluated and treated for *both* conditions, at least until the situation is fully clarified. Thrombolytic therapy would, of course, be contraindicated in this setting.

The only other relevant laboratory test performed as part of the initial evaluation is a chest x-ray. This is most helpful when a previous film is available for comparison and shows interval widening of the mediastinal shadow, cardiomegaly, or a new left pleural effusion. A normal plain chest x-ray does not exclude aortic dissection.

Because aortic dissections are highly lethal, a definitive diagnosis needs to be made with all due haste. A patient with this condition represents a true medical emergency, and a coordinated multidisciplinary effort must be mounted to maximize the chances of survival. Because many patients are hemodynamically unstable and need constant monitoring, the optimal diagnostic study should be accurate, specific, and atraumatic, and the results available within minutes. No current imaging technique fulfills all these criteria, and each hospital must develop its own strategy for dealing with aortic dissections. For many years, retrograde aortography was considered the gold standard for diagnosis, but this is an invasive procedure, performed in a radiology laboratory, and it requires contrast dye—all factors that may further compromise an unstable patient. Computed tomography (CT) and magnetic resonance imaging (MRI) share the advantage of being noninvasive; MRI does not require contrast dye, but gives excellent image quality in multiple planes of the aorta (Figure 1.4–2). The principal drawbacks to MRI are that it is relatively time-consuming and the imaging facilities are usually distant from intensive care units and operating rooms. In general, the logistic difficulties involved in obtaining MRI scans safely make it less than the ideal technique for critically ill patients. However, both MRI and CT are acceptable for serial follow-up of stable patients.

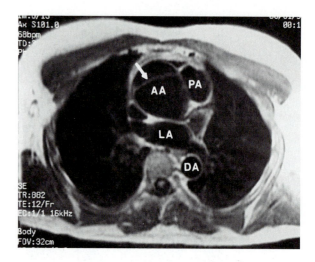

Figure 1.4–2. MRI scan showing type A (ascending) aortic dissection in a patient with Marfan's syndrome. Intimal flap (arrow) separates the true lumen below from the false lumen above. AA, ascending aorta; PA, pulmonary artery; LA, left atrium; DA, descending aorta. (Courtesy of Elias A. Zerhouni, MD.)

Probably the most attractive test for accurate, safe, and prompt definitive diagnosis of aortic dissection is echocardiography, in particular, transesophageal echo (TEE) combined with color-flow Doppler imaging (Figure 1.4–3). In addition to excellent anatomic detail of the entire thoracic aorta, TEE provides real-time information about left ventricular function, presence of pericardial effusion, and aortic valve structure and integrity. Often the echo shows the proximal coronary arteries and the origins of the arch vessels. Furthermore, echocardiography is a bedside technique, which does not require transporting the patient or interrupting intensive monitoring.

Whichever technique is used for imaging the aorta, the following are critical questions in planning management: Does the patient have aortic dissection? If so, is it type A or type B? Where is the intimal flap or site of entry of the dissection? What are the distal and proximal extents of the dissection? Is any branch vessel involved along the course of the dissection? With these questions answered, the clinician can develop an appropriate therapeutic plan.

MANAGEMENT

Any patient suspected of having an acute aortic dissection should be admitted to an intensive care unit. The initial goals of therapy include lowering blood pressure (assuming the patient is hypertensive or normotensive) to a level commensurate with adequate organ perfusion, and lowering heart rate and left ventricular dp/dt. Ordinarily, a short-acting β-blocker is given first, either by intravenous injection (eg, propranolol) or continuous infusion (es-

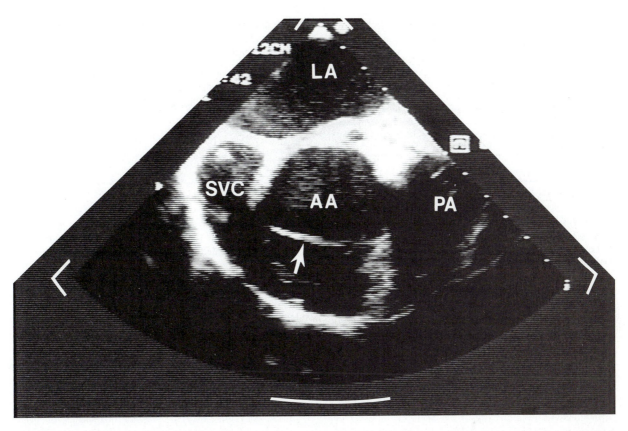

Figure 1.4–3. Preoperative transesophageal echocardiogram showing type A (ascending) aortic dissection in a hypertensive patient. The intimal flap (arrow) separating the true lumen from the false lumen is pathognomonic for aortic dissection. The photograph does not make clear which lumen is the true one. The true lumen expands during systole, a feature that can be seen only during real-time motion pictures. LA, left atrium; SVC, superior vena cava with Swan-Ganz catheter in place; AA, ascending aorta; PA, pulmonary artery. (Courtesy of Joao A. C. Lima, MD.)

molol), and then a vasodilator (eg, nitroprusside) by infusion. This sequence prevents the reflex tachycardia that might result from the vasodilator alone. After taking these measures and stabilizing the patient as much as possible given the emergency, the physician can begin a definitive evaluation (see "Laboratory Tests" above). If a type A dissection is found, the patient should have immediate cardiothoracic surgical consultation. Assuming that no contraindications to major surgery exist, the patient should be operated on within hours. The objective of surgery is to excise and replace the segment of aorta where the dissection originated, not to replace the entire dissected aorta. A woven Dacron graft (and sometimes a composite graft containing an aortic valve prosthesis if the patient has severe aortic regurgitation) is inserted and the coronary arteries reimplanted or bypassed. Hospital mortality for this type of procedure should be no higher than 10–15%. Mortality for medically treated type A dissections, by contrast, is 60% or more.

Patients with type B dissections generally do well with continued medical therapy. About 85–90% survive to be discharged from the hospital. Before discharge, their regimen is converted to oral antihypertensive medications, which should include a β-blocker. Failure of medical therapy is defined as continuing evidence of dissection, such as new pleural effusion or new branch-vessel occlusion, enlarging aortic silhouette on x-ray or other imaging techniques, or unremitting pain or intractable hypertension despite appropriate medications. Surgical mortality for these patients with type B dissection may be as high as 45–50%.

Regardless of the type of dissection or the form of treatment, patients with an acute aortic dissection remain at risk for future problems. Roughly 30% of discharged patients suffer a complication of their original dissection or a new dissection within 5 years. Many of these complications are fatal, and at least theoretically preventable by meticulous medical follow-up. All reasonable efforts should be made to keep blood pressure within normal limits, and MRI or CT scans should be performed every 6–12 months for at least the first few years.

SUMMARY

▶ Aortic dissection is a life-threatening emergency that demands a high index of clinical suspicion and prompt evaluation.

▶ The choice of appropriate therapy depends on imaging techniques that delineate the aortic anatomy unambiguously. Patients with ascending aorta involvement require surgical intervention, while those with dissections limited to the descending aorta do well with medical therapy.

▶ The high incidence of late complications of aortic dissections necessitates regular and meticulous follow-up, with particular emphasis on control of hypertension.

SUGGESTED READING

Cigarroa JE et al: Diagnostic imaging in the evaluation of suspected aortic dissection: Old standards and new directions. N Engl J Med 1993;328:35.

DeSanctis RW et al: Aortic dissection. N Engl J Med 1987; 317:1060.

Doroghazi RM et al: Long-term survival of patients with treated aortic dissection. J Am Coll Cardiol 1984;3:1026.

Spittell PC et al: Clinical features and differential diagnosis of aortic dissection: Experience with 236 cases (1980 through 1990). Mayo Clin Proc 1993;68:642.

Treasure T, Raphael MJ: Investigation of suspected dissection of the thoracic aorta. Lancet 1991;338:490.

1.5

Left Ventricular Dysfunction: Mechanisms and Symptoms

Thomas A. Traill, FRCP

Abnormal heart function can be caused by a wide range of myocardial abnormalities, valve diseases, congenital lesions, and pericardial diseases, yet has a rather restricted repertoire of effects on the patient. These effects stem from the fact that all causes of left heart dysfunction adversely affect the relation between cardiac output and left atrial pressure. Low output causes fatigue, high left atrial pressure causes breathlessness, and together they cause impaired exercise capacity and fluid retention. Thus, confronted with a patient who has dyspnea, edema, and fatigue, the physician may easily recognize heart disease, and then faces the harder task of identifying its nature and cause. The next pages deal with mechanisms of myocardial dysfunction and the symptoms that are common to all of them. The succeeding three chapters deal with specific groupings of myocardial and pericardial disease, and their distinguishing pathophysiologic and clinical characteristics.

Breathlessness in patients with left heart dysfunction is caused by increased pressure in the left atrium and pulmonary veins. Its severity ranges from a sensation of dyspnea during moderate physical exercise to the desperate sensation of near-drowning during episodes of acute pulmonary edema. Because cardiac dyspnea reflects increased filling pressure of the left heart, it is aggravated by any increase in venous return. Therefore, most patients with symptoms of left ventricular dysfunction complain of orthopnea, the sensation of breathlessness on recumbency, relieved by sitting up. Often the patient reports needing to use extra pillows at night and may even reach the point of preferring to sleep in a chair or slumped forward over a bed-table. Careful inquiry into a patient's night time symptoms is the best way to distinguish breathlessness caused by heart disease from airways obstruction or restrictive lung disease.

Everyone experiences fatigue from time to time, and fatigue as a symptom lacks specificity. However, the severity and debilitating effect of the fatigue experienced by patients with severe heart disease should not be underestimated. The sense of being unable to complete simple household tasks or of no longer enjoying outdoor leisure activities may lead to profound changes in lifestyle and can mislead the physician by masking more obvious breathlessness. Particularly when chronic valvular heart disease is the cause of left heart dysfunction, breathlessness may seem mild because activity level is reduced; in this case, increasing fatigue may become the reason to recommend valve replacement.

Patients with cardiac dysfunction retain salt and water. The mechanisms include simple hydrostatic effects of increased pressure in the systemic venous system; changes in the endocrine control of water balance, involving aldosterone, antidiuretic hormone, and atrial natriuretic peptide; and changes in the intrarenal circulation that increase tubular reabsorption of salt and water. These changes cause peripheral edema and contribute to elevation of left and right atrial pressures. When fluid retention is severe, patients develop anasarca, generalized tissue edema, with serous effusions causing ascites, and pleural and pericardial effusions. When William Withering first experimented with digitalis as treatment for dropsy, he was not in a position to distinguish between the several causes of edema and anasarca. Besides treating patients with heart disease, he also used the drug, apparently successfully, in patients with acute glomerulonephritis, and less successfully in patients with ascites caused by cancer. The differential diagnosis of fluid retention includes heart disease, hypoalbuminemia (from nephrotic syndrome, liver disease, or malnutrition), and acute and chronic renal failure. Other causes of edema are venous or lymphatic obstruction, and cellulitis.

There are other symptoms, besides the triad of breathlessness, fatigue, and edema, that may point to left heart dysfunction. These include cough, nocturia, and nocturnal angina. Particularly in patients whose increase in pulmonary venous pressure comes on quite rapidly, dyspnea may be accompanied by a troublesome cough, which, like the breathlessness, may be aggravated by recumbency. Similarly, angina that is aggravated by lying down (angina decubitus) indicates that in addition to having coronary artery disease, a patient has increased left ventricular filling pressure. Nocturia is caused by an increase in cardiac output and renal perfusion at night in response to the increase in venous return that occurs on lying down.

The symptoms described in the preceding paragraphs constitute a syndrome. In clinical practice they are referred to collectively as heart failure or left heart failure. Although these expressions are imprecise and difficult to define, they are useful, and therefore are found in numerous places throughout this book. It is important to recognize that heart failure describes a clinical presentation, not one specific physiologic disturbance. The physician must keep separate the concepts of left ventricular dysfunction, defined in terms of a measured variable, and left ventricular failure, defined more loosely by a patient's symptoms and signs.

CAUSES OF HEART FAILURE

The physician confronted by a patient with symptoms of left heart dysfunction has two tasks: first, to assign the patient's left heart disorder to a pathophysiologic group, whether it is valvular disease, pericardial disease, or one of three pathophysiologic groups of heart muscle dysfunction (cardiomyopathy), and, second, to identify the nature and cause of the underlying disease. For example, left heart failure may develop in a patient whose several myocardial infarctions have produced such extensive scarring in the left ventricle as to cause symptoms. Such a patient may present with fatigue, dyspnea, orthopnea, edema, and episodes of paroxysmal nocturnal dyspnea, and it should be easy to draw the clinical conclusion that they suffer from chronic left ventricular failure. Clinical insight, perhaps combined with noninvasive tests of heart function, allows the physician to determine that the patient suffers from myocardial disease rather than, for example, mitral regurgitation caused by papillary muscle damage. This kind of heart muscle disease, in which the myocardium is extensively weakened by scarring or some other diffuse injury, is termed *dilated cardiomyopathy*. Last, by taking this patient's history, the physician should have little difficulty in identifying the disease underlying the cardiomyopathy as ischemic damage caused by coronary artery disease. The patient's illness can be summed up as a syndrome of chronic left ventricular failure caused by ischemic dilated cardiomyopathy.

Cardiomyopathy

There are three pathophysiologic types of heart muscle disorder, referred to collectively as cardiomyopathy: dilated, hypertrophic, and restrictive cardiomyopathy. The differences between them are defined by their pathophysiologic nature (Table 1.5–1), not by the particular diseases that underlie them. The most common—dilated cardiomyopathy—encompasses the diseases that weaken heart muscle. Along with reduced contractile strength, they cause left ventricular dilatation; left ventricular diastolic volume and pressure are increased. This increase in diastolic cavity size and filling pressure can be seen as a compensatory mechanism, in the sense that increased end-diastolic length and tension increase stroke work, but it is the increase in end-diastolic left ventricular pressure that causes symptoms of pulmonary venous hypertension. The most common cause of dilated cardiomyopathy is ischemic heart disease, with diffuse or patchy scarring caused by coronary occlusions. Other causes are specific toxins, such as alcohol, and infections of the heart muscle, for the most part viral. Many patients have "idiopathic" cardiomyopathy, for which no cause is established. In dilated cardiomyopathy the heart is enlarged, sometimes greatly, and because the left ventricle has impaired contractile strength, the end-systolic volume is a large proportion of the end-diastolic volume. The ejection fraction is low.

Hypertrophic cardiomyopathy is a group of diseases characterized by left ventricular hypertrophy and normal or reduced diastolic cavity size. Such hypertrophy can be the result of hypertension, aortic stenosis, or congenital heart muscle disease, and leads to clinical disease primarily by its effects on diastolic function of the ventricle. The pathognomonic diastolic abnormality is impaired left ventricular relaxation, such that the normal rapid filling period of early diastole is replaced by delayed, slow, and protracted filling. At the end of diastole, when the ventricle behaves as a passive structure, atrial systole causes a rapid and excessive rise in pressure because of reduced distensibility of the ventricular myocardium. In hypertrophic cardiomyopathy, by definition, the heart has thick-

Table 1.5–1. Classification of cardiomyopathy.

Defect	Dilated Contractility	Hypertrophic Relaxation	Restrictive Passive Elasticity
Diastolic cavity size	↑↑	↓	↑
End-systolic cavity size	↑↑	↓↓	↑
Ejection fraction	↓↓	↑	↓
Wall thickness	↓	↑↑	↑
Rate of pressure fall	Normal	↓	Normal
LV end-diastolic pressure	↑	↑	↑↑
Jugular venous pressure	↑	±	↑↑
Third heart sound	Common	Never	Common

LV, left ventricular.

ened left ventricular walls, sometimes in a patchy distribution, and characteristically has a very small end-systolic cavity size and hence a high ejection fraction. Abnormal relaxation of the left ventricular myocardium may be detected by moment-to-moment imaging of the heart cavities, either by echocardiography or by gated blood-pool scanning.

Restrictive cardiomyopathy is best exemplified by a number of diseases, notably amyloidosis, which cause infiltration of heart muscle and thereby interfere both with its systolic function, and, even more strikingly, with its diastolic properties. The diastolic pressure-volume relationship of the left ventricle is abnormally steep, so that there is a large increase in diastolic pressure for any small increase in volume. This is the result of abnormal passive elasticity, not slow relaxation as in hypertrophic diseases. The typical heart with restrictive cardiomyopathy is only slightly larger than normal, but it has thick walls, mild reduction in ejection fraction, and extraordinarily high filling pressures, comparable even to those found in constrictive pericardial disease.

Valvular Heart Disease

The simplest example of valvular heart disease causing pulmonary venous hypertension, breathlessness, and fatigue is mitral stenosis. The effects of this lesion are increased left atrial pressure, generally caused by a pressure gradient between the left atrium and ventricle, and restricted cardiac output. Because patients with mitral stenosis have slow left ventricular filling, like patients with hypertrophic cardiomyopathy, they are particularly intolerant of tachycardia. They may experience their worst symptoms during rapid atrial fibrillation. Some patients with mitral stenosis have abnormal myocardial function, but their symptoms are caused by the valve lesion. They would have the same symptoms whether or not their heart muscle function was abnormal.

In mitral regurgitation, left atrial pressure rises as a result of the regurgitant stream from the left ventricle. The valve fails to maintain the usual systolic pressure difference between the two chambers. This causes breathlessness through a large increase in height of the left atrial V wave, transmitted to the pulmonary veins. In chronic mitral regurgitation, the direct effect of mitral regurgitation on pulmonary venous pressure is aggravated by two additional problems: pulmonary hypertension, caused by reactive changes in the pulmonary vasculature, and left ventricular myocardial dysfunction, the consequence of chronic volume overload. In mitral regurgitation, the ejection fraction is a particularly unreliable guide to the strength of left ventricular contraction, since a leak into the low-pressure left atrium allows the ventricle to contract to a lower end-systolic volume than it would under normal loading conditions.

Aortic regurgitation, like mitral regurgitation, has direct hemodynamic effects that lead to symptoms of heart failure: a rise in left ventricular end-diastolic pressure and resulting elevation of left atrial and pulmonary venous

pressure. In most patients with chronic aortic regurgitation, these effects are mitigated by a fall in arterial resistance and arterial diastolic pressure and by an increase in left ventricular cavity size. Eventually, however, in patients with severe chronic aortic regurgitation, left ventricular function deteriorates because of the chronic volume overload, left atrial pressure rises, and the patient finally becomes symptomatic. The heart in chronic aortic regurgitation is dilated and hypertrophied, with a normal ejection fraction.

Aortic stenosis causes a hypertrophic cardiomyopathy. Except in babies, the mere presence of the valve lesion is seldom enough to cause symptoms directly. Over the years, however, chronic elevation of the left ventricular systolic pressure to levels of 200 mm Hg or so leads to marked left ventricular hypertrophy, just as might be encountered in severe hypertension. This hypertrophy is accompanied by the same symptoms as in idiopathic or familial hypertrophic cardiomyopathy, namely, dyspnea, angina, and syncope.

Pericardial Disease

Pericardial compression of the heart causes two syndromes, cardiac tamponade and chronic constrictive pericardial disease. Each type of cardiac compression reduces the cardiac output and increases the diastolic pressure in all four cardiac chambers. Tamponade is almost always the result of rapid accumulation of a pericardial effusion. As the pericardial pressure exceeds about 20 mm Hg, right heart filling is slowed and eventually halted. Breathlessness is a lesser feature than low cardiac output, which ultimately progresses to cardiogenic shock. The heart is small but the cardiac silhouette on x-ray is usually very large, since the previously normal pericardium can accommodate a prodigious volume of fluid before the pressure increases enough to obstruct the circulation.

In constrictive pericarditis, the process is much more chronic. The cardiac filling pressures increase gradually, often over a period of years, to levels considerably higher than would be tolerable acutely. As a result, the predominant clinical effects are those of systemic venous congestion: massive fluid retention, anasarca, edema, and hepatomegaly. In this disease, there is no pericardial fluid, just an unyielding envelope around the heart. The ventricles are small, the cardiac silhouette normal or only slightly enlarged, and the atria generally large. The physician may have difficulty distinguishing chronic constrictive pericarditis from restrictive cardiomyopathy; the fundamental difference is that in constrictive disease, heart muscle function is normal.

High-Output States

Certain conditions chronically increase left ventricular stroke volume. Two of them are aortic and mitral regurgitation (discussed above in "Valvular Heart Disease"). Others are diseases in which cardiac output is chronically increased in response to increased demand, for example, chronic anemia (most notably sickle cell disease) and hyperthyroidism. Arteriovenous fistulas, such as those used for renal dialysis, have the same effect. A rarer cause is Paget's disease, in which multiple arteriovenous fistulas open in affected bone. All of these causes of chronic high cardiac output eventually lead to increased left ventricular size and increased left ventricular end-diastolic volume. Stroke volume is increased, but ejection fraction may be reduced. In many cases this remodeling takes place without symptoms or physiologic changes of heart failure, but a few patients develop fluid retention and dyspnea. In these few, high-output heart *disease* has then led to symptoms of high-output *failure*. The expansion of extracellular fluid volume in pregnancy has a similar mechanism; for the cardiologist, the physiology of pregnancy is best thought of as the opening of a substantial arteriovenous fistula, in the form of the placenta. Fortunately, most pregnant women tolerate the change without difficulty, but the increased cardiac output and blood volume can cause problems for women with cardiomyopathy or valvular obstruction.

CLINICAL MANIFESTATIONS OF HEART FAILURE

Cardiac Dyspnea

Breathlessness in heart disease is caused by increased left atrial pressure. Any increase above normal in the pulmonary venous pressure disturbs the normal Starling relation between arterial pressure, venous pressure, and extracellular fluid distribution, and thereby increases total lung water. This in turn causes a change in lung turgor and an increase in the work and therefore the perceived effort of breathing. Breathlessness may be aggravated by a reduction in bronchial caliber, and sometimes by acute bronchial spasm. When pulmonary venous pressure exceeds some critical threshold, typically about 25 mm Hg, the increase in tissue fluid leads to transudation into the alveolar air spaces. This alveolar edema corresponds to the clinical syndrome of acute pulmonary edema, with crackles, acute breathlessness, and frothy sputum, but it is important to recognize that interstitial edema can also cause severe symptoms, although without obvious physical findings.

When breathlessness is a chief complaint, the most important aspect that allows it to be identified as cardiac is the effect of recumbency. Orthopnea and episodic nocturnal pulmonary edema (paroxysmal nocturnal dyspnea) are usually easy to find out about, but it is important also to ask about nocturnal cough, nocturnal angina, and just night time restlessness. Someone who sleeps in the same room can help by describing the patient's night time breathing pattern, or may report that the patient becomes restless after slipping off the pillows. Restless sleep and nocturnal dyspnea have causes besides heart disease; the differential diagnosis includes sleep apnea, orthopnea in bronchial asthma, and esophageal reflux with aspiration.

Examination of the patient with chronic left ventricular dysfunction is devoted to confirming the impression that breathlessness has a cardiac cause and identifying the nature of left ventricular disease. Pulmonary crackles are the best-known sign of pulmonary edema, but especially in the patient with chronic or fairly stable disease, they are an unreliable guide to its severity. They are not present when edema is interstitial, and a patient with desperately severe exercise intolerance may not have them at rest. Elevation of the right atrial pressure is easy to identify, simply by looking at the jugular pulse. Examining the heart yields signs of cardiomegaly in patients with dilated cardiomyopathy, left ventricular aneurysm, and mitral or aortic regurgitation, but not in patients with pure concentric hypertrophy, whose overall heart size may be normal. Auscultation is performed to find characteristic murmurs, or to identify gallops. The fourth heart sound reflects a high atrial contribution to the left ventricular end-diastolic pressure. It is never present in atrial fibrillation, of course, and it is not a normal finding. The most common causes of the increased atrial kick that generates fourth sounds are hypertensive hypertrophy and ischemic heart damage. A fourth sound is not a sign of heart failure, but rather a sign of left ventricular dysfunction. The third sound occurs at the end of the rapid filling period, generated by an oscillation of the myocardium after its early diastolic elastic recoil. The third sound is less commonly heard than the fourth sound and is a feature of dilated, weak, or hyperdynamic ventricles.

Acute Pulmonary Edema

Sudden transudation of fluid into the alveolar air spaces happens unpredictably in patients with heart disease. It may be the culmination of gradually worsening heart failure, typically because of progressive fluid retention, or it may be the immediate response to an abrupt change in left atrial pressure. Such abrupt hemodynamic changes can be caused by acute myocardial infarction, or mitral valve rupture, but may also occur in patients who have unstable angina, and in a few patients who have acute papillary muscle ischemia. Immediate treatment is similar, whatever the cause and progression, but the long-term management for a patient with chronic left ventricular dysfunction who slipped gradually into heart failure and developed acute pulmonary edema differs considerably from treatment for someone in whom pulmonary edema was the first manifestation of disease.

Patients with acute pulmonary edema are in unmistakable respiratory distress. They are tachypneic and display labored breathing, often with a surprising and potentially misleading degree of bronchospasm—hence the old expression "cardiac asthma." Patients with acute pulmonary edema may complain of cough; if the cough is productive, it is likely to yield frothy, watery sputum, unlike the sputum of asthma or acute bronchitis. Sometimes the sputum is pink because of some alveolar bleeding, but obvious hemoptysis is unusual. Hemoptysis with blood clots in a patient with acute dyspnea should suggest pulmonary embolism or pneumonia.

The chest x-ray is usually characteristic (Figure 1.5–1). Pulmonary edema causes a diffuse "ground-glass" infiltrate. When severe, it extends outward from the hila in a pattern that has been likened to a bat's wing and can be accompanied by an air bronchogram. Particularly when there has been chronic pulmonary venous hypertension, the infiltrate may be superimposed on other evidence of left heart dysfunction, including prominence of the upper lobe vessels from redistribution of pulmonary blood flow and engorgement of the septal lymphatics. This lymphatic congestion appears as linear shadows perpendicular to the pleural surface, mostly at the bases, called *Kerley lines*. Besides confirming the clinical suspicion of pulmonary edema by examining the lung fields, the physician should look at the cardiac shadow for evidence of left atrial enlargement and at overall heart size. Cardiac enlargement favors a diagnosis of chronic left heart dysfunction as the cause of pulmonary edema. A smaller cardiac silhouette should raise the suspicion of an acute process such as myocardial infarction or valve rupture.

The differential diagnosis of acute pulmonary edema includes all causes of acute breathlessness. Of particular concern are pulmonary embolism, asthma, pneumonia, and adult respiratory distress syndrome. If the clinical circumstances and findings are unclear, the x-ray usually gives the answer, except when atypical pneumonia or adult respiratory distress syndrome causes diffuse infiltrates. Atypical pneumonia can usually be distinguished from pulmonary edema because of its gradual onset, accompanied by fever; only in patients with subacute mitral chordal rupture does heart disease present in this fashion. In patients with sepsis causing acute respiratory distress syndrome, further tests of cardiac function may be needed, in the form of echocardiography or right heart catheterization.

Management of a patient with acute pulmonary edema begins with urgent lowering of the left atrial pressure. This can generally be achieved with a combination of nitroglycerin, which increases venous capacitance and thereby reduces venous return pressure, and diuretics. The price of lowering left atrial pressure may be that cardiac output is reduced to the point of dropping arterial pressure to an unacceptable level, especially if nitroglycerin is given. It may then prove necessary to increase contractil-

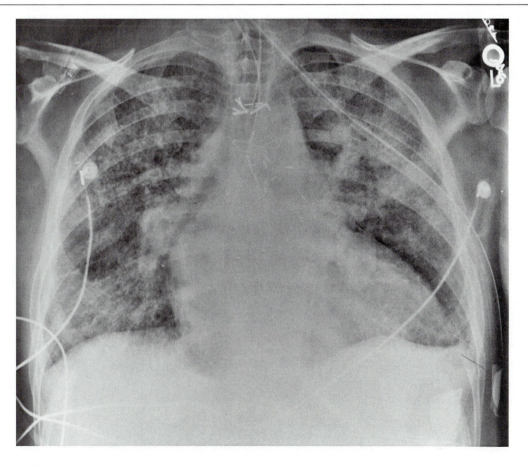

Figure 1.5–1. Chest x-ray of a patient with acute pulmonary edema, showing diffuse bilateral infiltrates spreading from the hila.

ity with intravenous pressors in the form of sympath-omimetic amines—dopamine and dobutamine are most often used. Whether or not the patient has had a myocardial infarction, the physician should look for a reversible mechanical cause such as acute mitral regurgitation.

Low-Output State

Particularly when heart dysfunction begins suddenly because of myocardial infarction or acute valvular rupture, the effect may be low cardiac output more than acutely elevated filling pressures. In this state, signs and symptoms of low flow predominate over signs of pulmonary or systemic venous congestion. Patients have small-volume pulses, are cool and sweaty, and may have evidence of inadequate organ perfusion, including oliguria, liver cell dysfunction, and confusion. If patients are dyspneic, the cause is both increased pulmonary venous pressure and "air hunger" caused by profound restriction in oxygen carrying capacity. Treating acute low-output state, also called "cardiogenic shock," consists of giving positive inotropic agents and vasodilators, and avoiding too much lowering of filling pressures (Chapter 15.4).

Other patients may have a chronic low-output state that is less severe than cardiogenic shock. This chronic reduction of cardiac output is typical of dilated cardiomyopathy and mitral stenosis. Patients may be breathless, but their chief chronic complaints are fatigue, low stamina, and lack of energy. Patients with this syndrome often lose weight, especially if low output is combined with a degree of passive congestion of the liver and splanchnic veins, sometimes to the point of so-called cardiac cachexia. This important indicator of the severity of chronic left heart dysfunction may be masked when loss of dry weight is offset by fluid retention. If patients have not lost weight on the scales, it is helpful to ask whether they look thin, to themselves or to their family.

Fluid Retention in Heart Disease

Patients with left ventricular failure retain salt and water and may develop peripheral edema, ascites, or pleural effusions (Figure 1.5–2). When the right atrial pressure is increased, increased hydrostatic pressure in venules acts against the oncotic pressure gradient and reduces reabsorption of tissue fluid according to the Starling equation. Before long, beginning usually in the ankles (or the sacral area in a bed-bound patient), there develops observable pitting edema. In heart failure, this transudation of edema into the peripheral tissue spaces does not occur at the expense of the intravascular compartment—if it did, the ventricular filling pressures would be reduced rather than increased—because it is accompanied by considerable overall expansion of the extracellular fluid volume. Specifically, for patients to have demonstrable edema they must have retained at least 3 L of fluid and are thus 3 kg or more above their dry weight.

Expansion of the extracellular fluid compartment permits the atrial pressures to rise and thus tends to maintain cardiac output. Sodium and water retention are mediated by the renin-angiotensin-aldosterone axis, by intrarenal mechanisms, and by release of antidiuretic hormone (ADH). In response to reduced arterial perfusion and increased adrenergic stimulation, the juxtaglomerular apparatus increases renin secretion, and this in turn causes local and systemic effects as a result of increased angiotensin levels. Locally, by constricting the efferent glomerular arteriole, angiotensin increases the volume of ultrafiltrate in the proximal tubule and lowers the tonicity

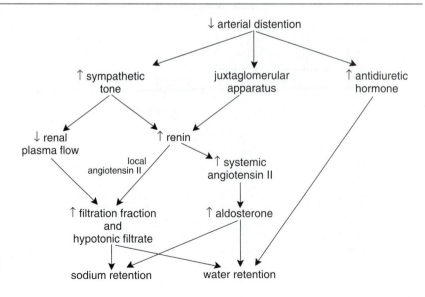

Figure 1.5–2. Fluid retention in patients with heart disease.

and hydrostatic pressure in the peritubular capillaries. The result is an increase in the forces favoring tubular reabsorption of sodium. Systemically, increased angiotensin II levels stimulate aldosterone production and increase peripheral resistance. In patients with symptomatic fluid retention, reduced sodium intake and administration of diuretics further stimulate renin production. Antidiuretic hormone production is increased in patients with left heart dysfunction, and reduces free water clearance by the kidney, thereby contributing to the hyponatremia found in patients with severe cardiac dysfunction. This reduction in serum sodium levels is particularly marked ($\leq$120 mEq/L) in patients who have severely impaired cardiac output and who are also receiving large doses of diuretic to prevent pulmonary edema. Severe hyponatremia is thus a poor prognostic sign and often represents an indication to begin treatment with intravenous inotropic agents.

Atrial natriuretic peptide, normally responsible for excretion of excessive isotonic intravascular fluid loads, is increased in patients with heart failure, as would be expected with increased atrial pressure. However, it is ineffective in reversing the effects of the salt-retaining humoral mechanisms.

Increased circulating levels of angiotensin and increased adrenergic tone contribute to a pronounced increase in peripheral resistance in patients with left heart dysfunction. This occurs even before symptoms develop and may aggravate cardiac disease by imposing additional load on the weakened left ventricle. Evidence is accumulating that increased levels of angiotensin II are linked to a worse prognosis in patients with left heart dysfunction, and that the natural history of dilated cardiomyopathy in particular can be improved by giving angiotensin converting enzyme inhibitors.

MEASURING HEART FUNCTION

Hemodynamics is the measurement and study of pressure and flow in the circulation. Much like the clinical assessment of patients with cardiac dysfunction, hemodynamic studies may be performed either to define the nature of a patient's overall circulatory disturbance or to investigate the nature of the heart disease causing it. In a patient with the clinical findings of heart failure, assessing left atrial pressure and cardiac output gives a measure of the severity of the problem and allows the physician to gauge the effects of treatment. Estimating peripheral resistance, by combining the cardiac output measurement with arterial pressure, provides further information about the intensity of sympathetic nervous system compensation and may help by suggesting noncardiac causes for a patient's shock (Chapter 15.4). Typically, such measurements are required for patients who are acutely ill, in settings where the nature of their heart disease is already clear, such as in a coronary care unit after myocardial infarction.

In outpatients being evaluated for symptoms of chronic or progressive cardiac dysfunction, identifying the nature

of the underlying disorder may require measurements of individual aspects of left heart function. Here, echocardiography or other imaging methods are used to estimate left ventricular chamber size and ejection fraction, to measure myocardial wall thickness, or to assess diastolic left ventricular function. It is important not to make unwarranted extrapolations from aspects of cardiac performance to the performance of the heart as a whole. Having a low ejection fraction tells us that the patient probably has a dilated cardiomyopathy, and allows an assessment of its severity and likely prognosis but does not tell us what the cardiac output or left atrial pressure is.

Cardiac Output

Reliable measurement of cardiac output requires cardiac catheterization. The usual methods use either the Fick principle or indicator dilution. The Fick principle relates the arteriovenous difference in oxygen content to the cardiac output and the rate of oxygen uptake and delivery. For any given stable value of oxygen consumption, the higher the cardiac output, the lower is the arteriovenous oxygen difference; conversely, when mixed venous oxygen saturation falls below a typical normal value of 65–70%, cardiac output is low relative to oxygen consumption. Indicator dilution techniques used to be performed with dyes and colorimetry, but today the technique finds its most convenient application using heat as the "indicator" with a so-called thermodilution catheter. Such catheters are available with balloons (the Swan-Ganz catheter) to assist in positioning in the right heart and pulmonary artery. Swan-Ganz catheters are used to obtain one or multiple measurements of cardiac output, either to guide treatment or as the basis for estimates of stroke volume, vascular resistance, or valve orifice size.

Cardiac output by itself is not a very useful index of heart function. For most patients who are up and about, cardiac output, at least at rest, is normal or only mildly reduced, set as it is by the circulation as a whole. Only in patients with cardiogenic shock is the cardiac output at rest truly limited by heart function; in other patients with heart disease, it is the increased left atrial pressure that is the chief source of symptoms.

Left Atrial Pressure

Measuring left atrial pressure is fundamental to assessing left ventricular function. Clinical clues to a high left atrial pressure are a patient's complaints of dyspnea, orthopnea, and paroxysmal nocturnal dyspnea; rales (crackles) in an acutely breathless patient; and supporting evidence provided by the x-ray. Measuring left atrial pressure directly is difficult; to get a catheter into the left atrium entails puncturing the atrial septum with a special catheter-directed needle—the "transseptal" technique. The alternative, which is very widely used in intensive care units, is to wedge a Swan-Ganz catheter in the pulmonary artery by inflating the balloon, so as to record the downstream pressure in the pulmonary veins. Pulmonary venous pressure is usually an excellent approximation to left atrial pressure.

End-Diastolic Volume, End-Systolic Volume, and Ejection Fraction

Measuring chamber size and ejection fraction is fundamental to identifying the reason for dysfunction of the left ventricular myocardium and for gauging its severity. Measurements can be obtained by contrast angiography, and most reference values have been derived from such estimates, using various formulas to convert data from two-dimensional images to volumes. However, the same information can be obtained more easily for the patient by noninvasive methods, particularly echocardiography and blood pool scanning. Of these two, scanning is probably more reproducible and accurate, but echocardiography is usually preferred because it provides so much additional information about valve function, wall thickness, and cavity shape. Indeed, it is rare for any clinical decision to rest upon an exact value for left ventricular chamber size or ejection fraction. The concepts are important in describing heart diseases, but accurate measurements of individual values are seldom critical. Low ejection fraction and increased end-diastolic volume are the defining abnormalities in dilated cardiomyopathy. However, ejection fraction is too heavily dependent on arterial pressure to be reliable as an index of heart function, whether for comparing different patients or for serial observations in an individual.

Diastolic Function

Certain diseases cause heart dysfunction not by interfering with systolic function, as in dilated cardiomyopathy, but by interfering with filling. In a way, trying to separate systolic from diastolic function is artificial, since even in disorders considered "purely systolic" it is the elevated diastolic pressure in the ventricle that leads to symptoms. Nevertheless, in patients with myocardial diseases who have high left atrial pressures and ostensibly normal systolic function, it becomes important to dissect out the nature of their filling disorder. In hypertrophic cardiomyopathy, a reduced rate of fall in left ventricular pressure in early diastole can be measured with special high-fidelity catheters, but this has not proved clinically applicable. Such catheters are also used to make plots of left ventricular pressure against volume. Families of these pressure-volume loops, obtained under variable loading conditions, are a theoretically attractive approach to clinical studies of abnormal diastolic function. Again, however, the relative complexity of the methods, and some difficulties of interpretation, have stood in the way of their being applied clinically. Usually, mechanisms of abnormal diastolic function are assessed by using echocardiography and Doppler ultrasound. These can be used to examine filling pattern and rates of early-diastolic wall dynamics.

Other Aspects of Left Ventricular Function

Individual measures of heart function correlate poorly with one another. It is impossible to predict from the ejection fraction, or even from some elaborately derived functional index, what is likely to be the value of the end-diastolic pressure, how breathless patients are, or their probable functional capacity. The difficulty in extrapolating from simple measures of chamber function to the whole patient stems partly from the variability in neural and endocrine responses that govern the state of fluid retention and the peripheral vasculature. There is also variability in aspects of left ventricular function that are not described by the conventional indices of function.

Some patients whose ejection fraction is less than 15% remain fully functional, with normal resting cardiac output and only minimal increase in left ventricular end-diastolic pressure. Other patients may be in cardiogenic shock despite ejection fraction values of 20–30% or more. A major source of this discrepancy has to do with coordination of ventricular function. Two examples of clinical effects of incoordination are the fall in blood pressure that accompanies electrical pacing via the right ventricle and the effect of ventricular aneurysms. In each case, reduced stroke volume is the result of incoordinate ventricular activation and contraction. The same mechanism is at work in patients with acute myocardial infarction. Although it is difficult to quantify this aspect of ventricular dysfunction, incoordination is easy to identify when examining echocardiographic or angiographic displays of ventricular wall movement. This, and other disturbances in the complex integration of ventricular pumping such as changes in overall cavity shape, account for the fact that there is no single scale of heart function along which diseases can be quantified and no one test that predicts a patient's functional state and prognosis.

SUMMARY

▶ Left heart failure is the syndrome of dyspnea, fatigue, and fluid retention caused by a disturbed relationship between cardiac output and left atrial pressure. Careful inquiry into a patient's night time symptoms is the best way to distinguish breathlessness caused by heart disease from airways obstruction or restrictive lung disease.

▶ Confronted by symptoms of left heart failure, the physician must first assign the patient's left heart disorder to a pathophysiologic group: valvular disease, pericardial disease, or one of three types of cardiomyopathy. The second task is to identify the nature and cause of the underlying disease.

▶ There is no single index of left ventricular function. Cardiac output and left atrial pressure measurements describe how heart disease affects the whole patient, but say little about specific abnormalities of ventricular function. They do not correlate with ejection fraction.

▶ Echocardiography is used to diagnose the nature of cardiac muscle disorders by estimating chamber size, ejection fraction, and abnormalities of filling. Displaying the ventricular pressure-volume relation yields a more comprehensive view of the interactions between systolic and diastolic function, but requires cardiac catheterization.

SUGGESTED READING

Anand IS et al: Edema of cardiac origin: Studies of body water and sodium, renal function, hemodynamic indexes, and plasma hormones in untreated congestive cardiac failure. Circulation 1989;80:299.

Braunwald E, Ross J Jr: The ventricular end-diastolic pressure: Appraisal of its value in the recognition of ventricular failure in man. Am J Med 1963;34:147.

Goodwin JF: Overview and classification of the cardiomyopathies. Cardiovasc Clin 1988;19:3.

Keren A, Popp RL: Assignment of patients into the classification of cardiomyopathies. Circulation 1992;86:1622.

Packer M: The neurohormonal hypothesis: A theory to explain the mechanism of disease progression in heart failure. J Am Coll Cardiol 1992;20:248.

Pak PH, Kass DA: Assessment of ventricular function in dilated cardiomyopathies. Curr Opin Cardiol 1995;10:339.

1.6

Systolic Dysfunction: The Dilated Left Ventricle

Kenneth L. Baughman, MD

Cardiomyopathy, disease of the heart muscle, can be divided into three pathophysiologic types, distinguished by their effects on left ventricular chamber size, wall thickness, and function. Dilated cardiomyopathy, the most common of the three, encompasses all the diseases that, by reducing the strength of contraction of heart muscle, lead to dilatation of the left ventricle. In dilated cardiomyopathy, the left ventricular ejection fraction is reduced, and typically the left ventricular myocardium is thinner than normal. About 95% of all cardiomyopathies are of the dilated type, whereas 4% are hypertrophic and 1% restrictive. Left ventricular dysfunction and dilatation need not cause symptoms at first, but if the underlying disease progresses, eventually patients complain of symptoms of left heart failure.

The rate at which symptoms develop and the nature of the symptoms depend on how quickly left ventricular function deteriorates. In patients whose left ventricular damage occurs rapidly, left heart failure presents most typically with pulmonary edema. Occasionally, for example, in acute infectious myocarditis, a sudden generalized loss of contractile function can present as cardiogenic shock, mimicking massive infarction. In patients whose left ventricular insult is more gradual, perhaps from accumulation of drug toxicity or alcoholism, the presentation is more likely to be with fatigue, exertional breathlessness, and edema. Sometimes, in patients who develop pulmonary hypertension without ever experiencing the acute effects of left atrial hypertension, right-sided signs and symptoms predominate, and the patient may complain principally of fluid retention and right upper quadrant pain from hepatic congestion. Other symptoms innclude dizziness or syncope, reflecting the fact that arrhythmias are common in these diseases, and chest pain. Pain does not always imply that the cause is coronary disease, because patients with very high left ventricular end-diastolic pressure may have reduced subendocardial perfusion from this

alone. Dilated cardiomyopathy is seldom detected in a presymptomatic phase. Only among patients with ischemic heart disease do we follow some with reduced ejection fraction after myocardial infarction who eventually develop symptoms of left ventricular failure and worsening left ventricular dilatation.

Symptoms of heart failure tell little about its cause, so that identifying the type of cardiomyopathy depends on the physical findings and tests of left ventricular size and function. In many patients with dilated cardiomyopathy, ventricular enlargement and dysfunction are obvious from a displaced point of maximal impulse, decreased forcefulness of contraction, and gallop rhythms, usually an S_3 and often an S_4. The most important differential diagnostic considerations are valvular heart disease, particularly chronic aortic and mitral regurgitation, and left ventricular aneurysm.

Usually, valvular disease is signaled by an obvious murmur, but occasionally the signs are subtle, and it may be easy to underestimate the importance of one or another of the regurgitant lesions. Many patients with dilated cardiomyopathy have functional mitral regurgitation, caused by dilatation of the valve ring and elongation of the cavity; in recognizing this functional mitral regurgitation, it is important not to miss the occasional patient in whom the lesion is severe and correctable. Left ventricular aneurysm may be accompanied by findings identical with those of dilated cardiomyopathy, so that in a patient who has left ventricular failure and whose history and electrocardiogram (ECG) imply a previous large anterior myocardial infarction, it is important to rule out the possibility of a resectable aneurysm by echocardiography or angiography. Some patients can have severe left ventricular dysfunction and dilatation but show virtually nothing on the exam. In these, x-ray and echocardiogram may be needed to diagnose the cause of heart failure.

Once myocardial disease has been identified as the

Table 1.6–1. Common causes of dilated cardiomyopathy.

Idiopathic
Ischemic
Inflammatory
  Viral myocarditis
  Autoimmune disease
  Peripartum cardiomyopathy
  Lyme disease
Toxic
  Alcohol
  Cocaine
Drugs
  Doxorubicin
  Drug hypersensitivity
Iron storage disease
Nutritional
  Beriberi heart disease
Collagen vascular disease
  Systemic lupus erythematosus
Sarcoidosis
Pheochromocytoma
Thyroid disease

cause of left heart failure, the physician must identify the cause of cardiomyopathy (Table 1.6–1) and institute treatment. Treatment entails correcting or optimizing the hemodynamic picture, using therapies that apply to any cause of dilatation, and sometimes giving disease-specific treatment, aimed at reversing or halting the underlying pathologic condition.

CAUSES OF CARDIOMYOPATHY

Idiopathic

In about 50% of patients presenting with a dilated cardiomyopathy, no cause is identified, even after a detailed history, physical examination, and laboratory evaluation, including heart biopsy. This represents a deficiency in our ability to understand the nature of heart muscle dysfunction at the cellular and subcellular level. About 5% of these patients prove to have a familial disorder; genetic loci have been identified in a few families, but the genetic mechanisms remain elusive. Others are believed to have their chronic disease as a result of a discrete previous myocardial insult, perhaps viral infection (see "Myocarditis" below).

Ischemic

Left ventricular dysfunction may be caused by epicardial coronary artery obstruction leading to myocardial cell loss and replacement by fibrous scarring. Sometimes the severity of epicardial coronary disease, seen at coronary angiography in the catheterization laboratory, seems insufficient to account for the severity of left ventricular dysfunction. This may be because of diffuse disease in vessels that are too small to be obvious angiographically or because there is another process that remains undetected, for example, in the patient who has had one small infarction and happens also to have alcoholism.

There are many mechanisms by which epicardial coronary disease can cause ventricular compromise. This may include one major symptomatic event, recurrent symptomatic events, or recurrent asymptomatic ischemic events. Obstruction of the left anterior descending coronary artery proximal to the septal and diagonal branches may produce a massive area of ventricular compromise, often with aneurysmal dilatation. Patients with multiple areas of epicardial obstruction may experience serial myocardial infarctions whose cumulative effects result in left ventricular dysfunction. Similarly, patients with multiple coronary artery obstructions may have episodes of severe ventricular ischemia but display no symptoms until they develop those of heart failure. The end result of any of these mechanisms of ventricular compromise is a decrease in contractility, and dilatation of the left ventricle.

Patients with cardiomyopathy should be queried concerning previous symptoms of coronary artery disease. Note that patients presenting with ventricular compromise may be confused with regard to their history. Patients hospitalized for left ventricular failure frequently believe that they have suffered a myocardial infarction or "heart attack." Therefore, before adopting this diagnosis, the physician must investigate this history by obtaining the past laboratory data to determine whether the creatine phosphokinase became elevated or the ECG changed. Patients with risk factors for coronary atherosclerosis should be investigated with coronary arteriography, assuming that no other cause is apparent. Risk factors include age greater than 35 years, tobacco abuse, hypercholesterolemia, adult-onset diabetes, history of hypertension, or family history of premature atherosclerosis (before age 55).

Inflammatory

Myocarditis: Myocarditis is associated with several potential causes of cardiomyopathy including collagen vascular diseases, human immunodeficiency virus (HIV), sarcoidosis, and Lyme disease. "Primary" myocarditis is often presumed to have a viral origin that led to postviral immunologically induced cardiac dysfunction. Both RNA and DNA viruses may be responsible. The most common is Coxsackie group B. Cardiac dysfunction may occur secondary to myocyte infection or myocardial inflammation, but more likely occurs because of an immune response directed against the sarcolemma, β-receptor, the calcium channel or mitochondrial components.

Like hepatitis, there are several clinicopathologic forms of myocarditis: fulminant myocarditis, acute myocarditis, chronic active myocarditis, and chronic persistent myocarditis—each with distinguishing features (Table 1.6–2).

Fulminant myocarditis is nearly always heralded by a flu-like illness occurring within the few weeks before the patient's presentation. Patients present with profound left ventricular dysfunction, often in cardiogenic shock, requiring pressor and mechanical support. The left ventricle is usually not markedly dilated but has a dramatic loss of function and may appear thickened because of myocardial

Table 1.6–2. Clinicopathologic classification of myocarditis.

	Fulminant	Acute	Chronic Active	Chronic Persistent
Onset of symptoms	Abrupt	Recent	Indistinct	Often no symptoms
Presentation	Cardiogenic shock	LV failure	LV failure	Normal LV function
Biopsy	Multiple foci of myocardial inflammation	Active or borderline myocarditis	Active or borderline myocarditis	Active or borderline myocarditis
Natural history	Complete recovery or death	Incomplete recovery, dilated cardiomyopathy	Dilated cardiomyopathy	Normal heart function
Follow-up biopsy	Complete resolution	Complete resolution	Ongoing or resolving myocarditis; fibrosis, giant cells	Ongoing or resolving myocarditis

LV, left ventricular.

edema. Patients may also have other acute viral symptoms including headache, hepatic inflammation, or rash. Patients either die or recover within 1 month.

The other forms of myocarditis (acute, chronic active, and chronic persistent) have a less obvious onset. Acute myocarditis may or may not progress to dilated cardiomyopathy, whereas chronic active myocarditis patients have recurrent symptomatic or asymptomatic episodes of myocardial inflammation that lead to patchy scarring and compensatory left ventricular hypertrophy within 1–3 years. The result is a minimally dilated severe cardiomyopathy with profound hypofunction and markedly elevated filling pressures. Chronic persistent myocarditis patients have normal left ventricular function; their myocarditis is detected by endomyocardial biopsy performed to investigate palpitations, atypical chest pain, or release of creatine phosphokinase.

Although a history of a flu-like illness should be sought in anyone who presents for the first time with cardiomyopathy, its presence is not specific; only endomyocardial biopsy can establish or refute the diagnosis of myocarditis. The physician must be cautioned that a "flu-like" illness is often misinterpreted. Young patients presenting with a cough and treated with antibiotics for a presumed pneumonitis may prove to have pulmonary edema as opposed to a viral pneumonia. Patients presenting with a cough should also be questioned about fever, myalgia, and arthralgia before they are assigned the diagnosis of a premonitory infectious process.

Peripartum Cardiomyopathy: Dilated cardiomyopathy that develops in the last month of pregnancy or within 5 months postpartum is termed a peripartum cardiomyopathy. It is important to ask female patients with dilated cardiomyopathy about recent pregnancy. The illness can occur during any pregnancy. There may or may not have been associated preeclampsia, twin births, or nutritional deficiencies.

In 75% of patients with peripartum cardiomyopathy, there is myocarditis, demonstrable by biopsy. The inciting pathogen is unknown. Possibly, these patients are predisposed to viral infection by immune suppression during pregnancy. It is also possible that a placental or other antigen induces an autoimmune myocarditis. Women who

present less than 1 month after delivery have a 75% chance of spontaneous recovery of ventricular function. Those who present between 1 and 4 months may recover spontaneously; if they do not recover spontaneously, those with myocarditis usually respond to immunosuppressive treatment. Those who present more than 4 months postpartum with left ventricular failure do not recover spontaneously and are unlikely to respond to immunosuppressive agents. The presence or absence of myocarditis on biopsy is not in itself a prognostic indicator.

If the left ventricle recovers to normal function, further pregnancies may be attempted under close supervision. Those who do not recover normal left ventricular function (recovery may occur with or without myocarditis) have a poor prognosis, and repeat pregnancy carries a significant risk of deterioration or death.

When a woman is found to have cardiomyopathy, it sometimes emerges that symptoms began during or after a past pregnancy. This does not always imply peripartum cardiomyopathy, since the hemodynamic stress of pregnancy may have simply brought to light preexisting left ventricular dysfunction. This usually occurs at the time of maximum volume loading of the ventricle, near the beginning of the third trimester. Not all dilated cardiomyopathies in pregnancy are peripartum cardiomyopathies.

Lyme Cardiomyopathy: Lyme disease, like sarcoidosis, may present with heart block or, very rarely, with dilated cardiomyopathy. A prior history of erythema chronicum migrans or systemic flu-like symptoms days after a tick bite or exposure in an endemic area is recalled by 60–70% of patients with secondary Lyme manifestations. Cardiac involvement is a secondary manifestation of this pathogen and presents weeks after the initial event with histologic evidence of myocardial inflammation. Clinical cardiac involvement is usually characterized by atrioventricular block with normal ventricular function that resolves spontaneously. Very rarely, Lyme disease may be associated with dilated cardiomyopathy, presumably secondary to the primary infection or an immunologic response to it. Other secondary manifestations of Lyme disease involvement may accompany the cardiac presentation, including central nervous system dysfunction, arthritis, or both.

A positive Lyme disease titer does not ensure that the

agent is responsible for the dilated cardiomyopathy. Unfortunately, there are no definitive methods to verify that the exposure to Lyme disease and cardiomyopathy are correlated, since it is often impossible to identify the organism even in direct myocardial samples.

Treatment of patients with Lyme disease carditis with antibiotics may result in improvement in ventricular performance. Patients with atrioventricular block may recover antegrade conduction more rapidly with corticosteroids.

Toxins

Alcohol: Many patients who have dilated cardiomyopathy prove to have a history of excessive alcohol consumption, and it has long been suspected that alcohol, whether in the form of hard liquor or more dilute beverages, is a cause of cardiomyopathy. Proving this causal relationship has been difficult, because alcoholics so frequently have other medical problems that could lead to cardiac dysfunction, particularly malnutrition, hypertension, and cigarette smoking. However, it is clear that acute alcohol intoxication causes left ventricular dysfunction and that there is a dose-dependent relation between chronic alcohol use and left ventricular dysfunction that is not accounted for by other causes of heart muscle disease. This dose dependency—and the frequent observation that left ventricular function can improve if affected patients stop drinking—is the best evidence for a causal relation between alcohol abuse and cardiomyopathy. Alcohol has several demonstrated deleterious effects on the metabolic machinery of the myocardial cell.

A careful history should be taken from the patient and family to document the degree of alcohol consumption. More than 8 ounces of alcohol per day, history of withdrawal symptoms, or treatment of delirium tremens all suggest that alcohol may be responsible. Other causes must be ruled out, even in the person who meets the foregoing criteria for alcoholic cardiomyopathy. Alcoholic cardiomyopathy is not particularly associated with alcoholic liver disease; these conditions may coexist, but they more frequently occur singly, with different drinkers being more susceptible to one or the other consequence of their habit. When cardiomyopathy is accompanied by alcoholic liver disease, the reduced systemic vascular resistance seen in liver disease patients may mask the severity of left ventricular dysfunction.

The treatment is abstention from alcohol. When affected patients manage to quit drinking, particularly early in the course of heart failure and dilated cardiomyopathy, left ventricular function may improve over six to 12 months.

In the past, alcoholic drinks contained additional myocardial poisons, causing cardiomyopathy in particular groups of drinkers. These epidemics have included poisoning with cobalt (added to induce foam) in beer drinkers, lead intoxication in those distilling their own hard alcohol in lead pots, and arsenic poisoning in wine drinkers.

Cocaine: Taking cocaine can have three effects on the heart. The best-recognized is acute myocardial infarction, the result of coronary spasm, often occurring after taking a larger dose than usual. Some patients who take large doses may develop arrhythmias, and these can include lethal ventricular tachycardia or fibrillation. Chronic cocaine use also seems to be associated with a cardiomyopathy, often characterized histologically by patchy fibrosis, a picture that raises the suspicion of multiple subclinical episodes of ischemia in its pathogenesis.

Medications

Several medications, particularly sulfa drugs, can cause an eosinophilic myocarditis that may progress to left ventricular dysfunction. It is important to take a careful drug history when evaluating a new patient with cardiomyopathy. Many drugs, particularly antiarrhythmic agents, β-blockers, and calcium channel blockers, exert negative inotropic effects on the myocardium; however, this is a reversible pharmacologic side effect, not a cardiomyopathy. A few drugs, notably lithium, can cause irreversible or partially reversible left ventricular dysfunction by damaging the contractile machinery of the cell.

Doxorubicin (Adriamycin): Several drugs can irreversibly depress myocardial function (Table 1.6–3). Doxorubicin is an antibiotic with potent antitumor effects used in several chemotherapeutic regimens for cancer. The drug is toxic to the myocardium and leads to a dose-dependent cardiomyopathy in any patient who receives a large enough cumulative dose. Left ventricular dysfunction usually starts to be demonstrable after a total dose of 350 mg/m^2, but some patients have an idiosyncratic reaction to the drug and develop cardiomyopathy at lower doses. Patients are predisposed to left ventricular dysfunction from Adriamycin by age, previous radiation therapy, cyclophosphamide use, or preexisting ventricular dysfunction. The toxicity may be associated with myocardial inflammation, but doxorubicin-induced cardiomyopathy rarely resolves.

Radiation Therapy

Only rarely does radiation treatment have any direct clinically apparent effect on the myocardium. About 10% of patients whose radiation treatment involves the heart

Table 1.6–3. Drugs causing cardiomyopathy.

Drug toxicity
Doxorubicin
Emetine
Cyclophosphamide
Chloroquine
Phenothiazines

Drug hypersensitivity
Methyldopa
Penicillin
Sulfonamides
Tetracycline
Phenylbutazone
Antituberculous medications

may have subclinical reduction in ejection fraction. Therapeutic radiation doses may, by causing endothelial injury, set the stage for premature coronary artery disease in subsequent years and may also cause pericarditis that can progress slowly to a chronic constrictive-effusive picture (Chapter 1.10).

Beriberi Heart Disease: Thiamine deficiency may cause a high-output state because of vascular dilatation. Altered left ventricular metabolic function can result in a cardiomyopathy and lead to congestive heart failure. Patients in industrialized countries who are likely to be affected include alcoholics, persons on fad diets, and those in intensive care units on glucose replacement and diuretics. Patients may display profound vascular collapse, but remain warm peripherally and have markedly elevated cardiac output by direct measurement. Thiamine replacement corrects both the vascular and myopathic deficiencies. The vascular resistance may normalize before the development of improved left ventricular contractility. This may result in transient worsening of the congestive heart failure, but after a week, cardiac function should have returned to normal.

Pheochromocytoma

Intermittent or persistent release of high levels of norepinephrine causes myocyte hypertrophy and focal necrosis. This may result in a reactive cellular infiltrate and ultimately lead to scar tissue and the development of left ventricular dysfunction. Although a history of repeated episodes of hypertension, diaphoresis, palpitations, and tremor might be anticipated, rare patients may present with a dilated cardiomyopathy without having noted these symptoms. Unfortunately, patients with severe cardiomyopathy from other causes may depend on the sympathetic nervous system (norepinephrine) to maintain blood pressure in the face of a diminished cardiac output. This results in tremor, sweating, and tachycardia. Therefore, pheochromocytoma (Chapter 4.3) should be considered in all patients presenting with dilated cardiomyopathy in whom the cause has not been established.

Thyroid Disease

Both hypothyroidism and hyperthyroidism rarely cause dilated cardiomyopathy; more commonly, they exacerbate intrinsic cardiac diseases. When thyroid disorders are the primary cause of heart disease, profound and prolonged myxedema or thyrotoxicosis is almost invariably clinically obvious. Patients can be screened for thyroid dysfunction by serum thyroid-stimulating hormone (TSH) measurement (see Chapter 4.4 for treatment of these conditions).

The dilated cardiomyopathy associated with hypothyroidism is distinguishable only by accompanying features of myxedema and by its remarkable reversibility with thyroid hormone therapy. More frequently, hypothyroidism exacerbates cardiomyopathy caused by other myocardial diseases; this is particularly common in amiodarone-

treated cardiac patients. Hypothyroidism without significant myocardial dysfunction can also masquerade as left ventricular failure, when a large pericardial effusion causes a widened cardiac silhouette on chest x-ray in a patient who may be complaining of fatigue, dyspnea on exertion, and edema.

Thyrotoxicosis is also rarely a cause of heart failure, particularly when rapid atrial fibrillation reduces left ventricular filling or when left ventricular dilatation leads to functional mitral regurgitation. Although these patients usually have a normal resting ejection fraction, myocardial performance deteriorates with exertion, probably because the thyrotoxic heart is already functioning at the peak of its performance curve.

Acromegaly

Acromegaly causes left ventricular hypertrophy and an increase in left ventricular cavity size, often with some reduction in left ventricular systolic function. This acromegalic cardiomyopathy is seldom severe enough to lead to symptoms.

Sarcoidosis

Patients with systemic sarcoidosis may develop dilated cardiomyopathy. Rarely is sarcoidosis confined to the heart, however, and other systemic features aid in its recognition. These include skin lesions, lower-extremity oligoarticular arthritis, uveitis, fever, or pulmonary involvement with cough, adenopathy, or infiltrate. Cardiac sarcoidosis may result in heart block, mitral or tricuspid regurgitation, or cardiomyopathy, depending on the location and extent of the inflammatory involvement. Patients with active inflammation in the myocardium, as judged by endomyocardial biopsy, angiotensin converting enzyme level, erythrocyte sedimentation rate, or degree of uptake in a gallium scan, may improve with corticosteroid treatment.

Iron Storage Diseases

Hemochromatosis, the result of an inborn error of metabolism (Chapter 7.4), usually affects the heart and may cause a dilated cardiomyopathy or sometimes a restrictive pattern of myocardial disease. Almost always, cardiac involvement in hemochromatosis follows development of liver and pancreatic disease. Therefore, it is very unusual for a patient with this disease to present for the first time with symptoms of left ventricular dysfunction. Transfusion siderosis, the result of obligatory iron overload from multiple transfusions in a patient with a chronic anemia, can and usually does affect the heart before obvious involvement of other organs. Thus, any patient without a source of iron loss (from bleeding), who has received more than 50 units of transfused red cells, is at risk of developing left ventricular dysfunction. Prevention consists of giving iron chelation treatment along with blood transfusions; such treatment has improved the prognosis for patients with hereditary hemolytic anemia such as thalassemia.

Collagen Vascular Disease

A number of rheumatologic disorders may be associated with dilated cardiomyopathy, including systemic lupus erythematosus, polyarteritis nodosa, and progressive systemic sclerosis. Heart disease is virtually never the presenting feature, and other more typical organ afflictions account for the current or previous symptoms. Nonetheless, the degree of cardiac involvement with these disorders is often overlooked or underestimated. Persons with connective tissue disease and unexplained tachycardia, cardiomegaly, or signs and symptoms of congestive heart failure should have noninvasive studies performed to evaluate left ventricular function. Treatment with immunosuppressive agents may result in improvement in ventricular function. This is particularly the case when myocardial inflammation is present on a biopsy.

Other Precursors of Cardiomyopathy

Hypertension precedes the development of congestive heart failure in 75% of patients, according to the Framingham data. Whether hypertension can cause a dilated cardiomyopathy is less clear. Nonetheless, blood pressure elevation greater than 200 mm Hg or poorly controlled hypertension for longer than 5 years can result in a thickened and then dilated left ventricle, and ultimately in dysfunction. The molecular and cellular factors predisposing some patients to this scenario are not clear.

Morbid obesity and a history of asthma are found more often in patients with cardiomyopathy than would be expected by chance alone. How obesity causes cardiomyopathy is uncertain, but the association seems to be stronger than can be accounted for just by the various comorbidities that so frequently accompany obesity. Patients with dilated cardiomyopathy often have a history of bronchial asthma. In some patients, this may merely be misdiagnosis of bronchospasm caused by pulmonary congestion; in others, airways hyperreactivity may be increased by pulmonary congestion. There remains, however, a suspicion on the part of many clinicians that a link exists between left ventricular dysfunction and asthma itself. One possible explanation is that β-adrenergic agonists used to treat bronchial asthma cause cumulative damage to the left ventricular myocardium through a mechanism comparable to that of pheochromocytoma.

DIAGNOSTIC TESTING

The goal of diagnostic and laboratory testing in patients with dilated cardiomyopathy is to confirm the suspicion of a primary heart muscle disorder; to rule out the possibility of a structural lesion that can be repaired, such as aneurysm or mitral regurgitation; and to look for treatable causes of heart failure, particularly treatable forms of infiltrative disorders, steroid-responsive diseases, and pheochromocytoma. By documenting the severity of cir-

culatory dysfunction, laboratory tests, imaging studies, and additional studies may also help by providing prognostic information.

Chest X-Ray

The chest x-ray shows the size of the combined right and left ventricular cavity and helps to indicate the degree of left-sided congestion as evidenced by vascular redistribution, peribronchial cuffing, interstitial infiltrates, or pulmonary edema. Right ventricular failure may be suggested by enlargement of the right ventricle or right atrium, or by engorgement of the superior vena cava. Usually combined right- and left-sided failure is necessary to produce pleural effusions. The chest x-ray may not accurately determine the chamber that accounts for the ventricular enlargement. Clues to the cause of the chamber responsible may be garnered from the x-ray, particularly in those with evidence of coarctation or arteriovenous communications.

Echocardiogram

The echocardiogram is the most sensitive noninvasive test for the determination of the specific cardiac chamber enlargement, ventricular thickness, ventricular function, and presence or absence of intrinsic valvular disease. The echocardiogram can also rule out pericardial effusions or other pathologic conditions that may cause radiographic cardiomegaly and heart failure but are not due to ventricular abnormalities.

Electrocardiogram

The ECG is usually abnormal in patients with cardiomyopathy. These changes may include nonspecific ST-T wave changes. With increasing durations of right or left ventricular dysfunction, right and left ventricular hypertrophy may be evident on the ECG. Similarly, as ventricular diastolic filling pressures are elevated, mean left and right atrial pressure increases and atrial enlargement may occur. Patients with ischemic heart disease may show evidence of a myocardial infarction characterized by Q waves. Other cardiomyopathy patients without coronary disease may appear to have had a myocardial infarction; the evidence is a "pseudoinfarct" pattern that is often seen in infiltrative diseases such as amyloidosis.

Routine Blood Work

Low cardiac output and decreased renal perfusion are often reflected by an increase in the serum urea nitrogen (SUN) and creatinine values. The values of liver function tests are often modestly elevated, including tests for bilirubin, alanine aminotransferase (ALT, or SGOT), and aspartate aminotransferase (AST, or SGPT). These reflect hepatic congestion from increased right atrial pressure. Patients who have elevated venous pressure and then experience transient episodes of very low cardiac output develop ischemic changes within the liver characterized by marked elevations in the transaminase that return to normal rapidly upon correction of perfusion abnormalities.

Specific Tests for the Cause of Cardiomyopathy

The cause of cardiomyopathy should be assessed with specific tests in virtually every patient presenting with a dilated cardiomyopathy. Even in patients whose history implies a straightforward cause, a limited number of laboratory studies should be performed. These include an antinuclear antibody test, a urinary vanillylmandelic acid (VMA) test, and thyroid function tests.

The antinuclear antibody test screens for subtle forms of collagen vascular diseases that may cause systolic dysfunction. Patients with pheochromocytoma may present with dilated cardiomyopathy and are virtually impossible to differentiate from patients with high sympathetic "spillover" due to worsening heart failure. Therefore, urinary analysis for products of norepinephrine secretion should be assessed (by VMA). Similarly, patients with thyroid disease may present with a dilated cardiomyopathy; this disease may be missed if specific studies are not performed. Measurements of serum iron, iron binding, and transferrin may be appropriate to rule out an iron storage disease, but are unnecessary if the patient is to have a biopsy. Other studies depend on specific historical or physical examination features that suggest a specific cause.

Additional Studies

Metabolic exercise stress testing and right heart catheterization may provide additional objective information concerning the functional status of patients with dilated cardiomyopathy and their prognosis.

Metabolic Exercise Stress Test: Regular exercise stress tests in patients with systolic dysfunction may be of some benefit to determine whether patients have ischemic changes with exercise. Patients who have nonspecific ST-T wave changes prior to exercise often have worsening of these changes with exercise, making standard ECG stress testing difficult to interpret without adding more specific scintigraphic testing (thallium) to the exercise. The metabolic exercise stress test, like other exercise stress tests, gathers data on the heart rate, rhythm, and ECG changes with exercise while monitoring blood pressure. In addition, minute-by-minute assessment of oxygen consumption and carbon dioxide production allows the determination of the patient's maximum oxygen consumption and anaerobic threshold. These data provide a reasonably accurate way of objectively determining the functional status of a patient's cardiopulmonary system. Functional exercise tests correlate more closely with the patient's exercise capacity than the determination of the ejection fraction alone. Maximum oxygen consumption (MVO_2) of less than 10 mL/kg/min implies severe cardiopulmonary impairment; 10–15 mL/kg/min implies moderate impairment; and 15–20 mL/kg/min, mild impairment. These objective measures of cardiopulmonary performance correlate well with prognosis and can be used to assess the need for aggressive treatment or cardiac transplantation. The metabolic exercise stress test may also allow an objective assessment of a patient's true exercise capacity.

Endomyocardial Biopsy: The endomyocardial biopsy may establish a histologic diagnosis in certain disorders (Table 1.6–4). This procedure has minimal morbidity and mortality; nonetheless, it requires an expertise not present in every catheterization laboratory. Of equal or greater importance is the experience of the cardiac pathologist who is interpreting the tissue specimens. For patients with a high likelihood of having the disorders listed in Table 1.6–4 and for whom a tissue diagnosis cannot be made or has not been made by any other techniques, endomyocardial biopsy should be considered to establish the diagnosis.

Coronary Arteriography: Coronary arteriography may be performed in patients suspected of having cardiomyopathy due to ischemic heart disease. Patients should be considered as candidates for coronary arteriography if they are older than 35 years of age; have risk factors for coronary atherosclerosis, including hypertension, tobacco abuse, hypercholesterolemia, family history of premature coronary disease, or abnormal cholesterol status; or have evidence in their history that suggests that a myocardial infarction may have occurred with or without ECG confirmation.

The endomyocardial biopsy may suggest ischemic heart disease as the cause of cardiomyopathy by demonstrating large areas of replacement fibrosis as opposed to the usual interstitial fibrosis found in nonspecific heart reaction to dysfunction. Left ventriculography may also be performed with the coronary arteriogram, and provides another measure of ejection fraction and regional left ventricular function. Left heart catheterization and angiography allow further assessment of valvular lesions, which may be particularly hard to quantify by clinical and noninvasive means in patients with very poor left ventricular systolic function.

Table 1.6–4. Diseases detected by endomyocardial biopsy.

Inflammatory
  Myocarditis
  Rheumatic diseases
Vascular
  Ischemic injury
  Thrombotic thrombocytopenic purpura
Infiltrative
  Amyloidosis
  Hemochromatosis
Fibrosis
Sarcoidosis
Endocardial fibrosis
Malignancy
  Primary or secondary tumors
  Carcinoid
  Anthracycline toxicity
  Radiation toxicity

PROGNOSIS

The prognosis for patients with dilated cardiomyopathy is poor and depends in part on the cause of the disease. The 1-year mortality rate is about 30%, and the 5-year mortality rate 80%. About 50% of patients die by sudden death related to arrhythmia, and the remainder by progressive left ventricular dysfunction. Without chronic anticoagulant therapy, 15% have symptomatic embolization.

Prognostic features include (1) severe congestive heart failure by history or examination, (2) older age, (3) the degree of cardiac dilatation by chest x-ray, echocardiogram, or left ventricular angiography, (4) height of the left- and right-sided diastolic filling pressures, (5) the degree of depression of the cardiac output, and most important (6) the ejection fraction. Recently, analysis of neuroendocrine activation in patients with congestive heart failure has added several additional parameters, such as plasma norepinephrine, antidiuretic hormone, and atrial natriuretic factor levels.

MANAGEMENT

Treatment of patients with dilated cardiomyopathy includes correcting the circulatory abnormalities that cause symptoms—reducing the left ventricular filling pressure, "preload," and improving cardiac output—and sometimes additional treatment directed at the primary cause of heart muscle dysfunction.

Preload Reduction

The three ways to lower the left ventricular filling pressure are diuretics, venodilators, and arterial vasodilators. Diuretics are the most effective and direct, and they make up the fundamental treatment for most kinds of heart failure, particularly for dilated cardiomyopathy. Nitrates redistribute blood by venous dilatation, causing pooling of blood in the legs. Narcotics, such as morphine, work in a similar fashion, causing venous pooling. Arterial vasodilators, particularly converting enzyme inhibitors and α-adrenergic blockers (discussed below) also lower the left ventricular filling pressure in dilated cardiomyopathy patients by reducing cardiac stroke work.

Diuretics should be used carefully, especially in patients whose heart disease is severe. When diuresis occurs too rapidly or is excessive, the fall in intravascular volume lowers the filling pressure in the left ventricle too much. This improves symptoms of pulmonary congestion, but may result in an excessive decrease in the cardiac output. Unless fundamental improvement in left ventricular performance accompanies this decrease in left ventricular filling, the diminished cardiac output may result in renal underperfusion as well as symptoms of dizziness, lightheadedness, presyncope, or syncope. Patients with less severe heart failure may undergo diuresis until their edema is absent or their symptoms improve. Patients with life-threatening heart failure and massive edema should undergo diuresis until they begin to develop prerenal azotemia, which defines their "dry" weight, below which further diuresis will only result in progressive renal dysfunction.

Afterload Reduction

Afterload, the resistance presented to left ventricular ejection by the arterial circulation, is usually increased in patients with symptomatic dilated cardiomyopathy, by virtue of increased sympathetic vasomotor tone and increased levels of circulating angiotensin II. Afterload-reducing agents include several categories of drugs, particularly direct-acting agents, calcium channel blockers, and neurohumoral agents. Direct-acting vasodilators include nitroglycerin and hydralazine. These agents act directly on the smooth muscle or specific receptors (such as nitrate receptors) to cause dilatation of the vascular bed. Calcium channel blockers work by prohibiting calcium influx into the vascular cell, resulting in vasodilatation. Neurohumoral agents interfere with some portion of the neuroendocrine axis. This may include α-blockers, which cause α-I or α-II vasodilatation, but more usually angiotensin converting enzyme (ACE) inhibitors. ACE inhibitors have been demonstrated to improve the prognosis for patients with mild and severe systolic dysfunction with or without heart failure. Because of the ability of afterload-reducing agents to improve symptoms of congestion and to improve prognosis, virtually all patients with dilated cardiomyopathy with or without symptoms of left ventricular failure should receive afterload reduction therapy.

Inotropic Agents

Inotropic agents increase contractility by increasing intracellular calcium or intracellular cyclic adenosine monophosphate (AMP) (Figure 1.6–1).

Digoxin: Digoxin interferes with the sodium pump (sodium-potassium ATPase) and makes more sodium available within the cell for passive exchange with extracellular calcium ions. The result is an increase in intracellular calcium concentration and availability. Digoxin does not seem to benefit all patients equally, and even after 200 years of the drug's use, there is still argument about its efficacy and indications. As a general rule, digoxin is of benefit to patients with left heart failure already being treated with vasodilators and diuretics who have persistent cardiomegaly and an S_3 gallop. There is a narrow window between the therapeutic and toxic effects of this drug. Digoxin excess may cause supraventricular and ventricular arrhythmias and may hasten sudden death. Digoxin may also cause gastrointestinal complaints such as nausea and vomiting, alterations in personality, and occasionally complaints by patients that they see yellow halos around bright lights.

Sympathomimetic Agents: Dopamine, dobutamine, norepinephrine, and other sympathomimetic agonists can increase myocardial contractility. These agents stimulate the membrane β_1-receptor and thereby activate the mem-

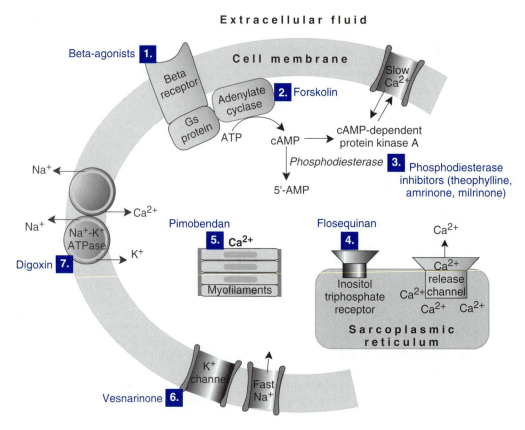

Figure 1.6–1. Sites of action of inotropic drugs in the myocyte.

1. **Beta-agonists:** β_1-agonist receptor stimulation activates the Gs (stimulatory) protein in the myocyte membrane. Gs activates membrane-bound adenylate cyclase, which increases cyclic AMP (cAMP). Agents that increase intracellular cAMP activate protein kinase A and thereby increase the force of contraction.
2. **Forskolin** increases contractility by stimulating adenylate cyclase.
3. **Phosphodiesterase inhibitors:** Phosphodiesterase degrades cAMP. If phosphodiesterase is inhibited, cAMP increases and contractility increases. Clinically available phosphodiesterase inhibitors include theophylline, amrinone, and milrinone. Amrinone and milrinone are used only for brief intravenous treatment; in studies of long-term treatment, oral milrinone increased mortality in patients with heart failure.
4. **Flosequinan:** Like cAMP, inositol triphosphate is a messenger system that may increase contractility. Flosequinan appears to act in part by stimulating inositol triphosphate. Although studies of short-term flosequinan use were encouraging, long-term use increased mortality.
5. **Pimobendan** appears to increase contractility by increasing myofilament sensitivity to calcium.
6. **Vesnarinone** increases contractility by inhibiting phosphodiesterase and prolonging the action potential duration (by increasing inward Ca^{2+} currents and inhibiting repolarizing K^+ currents).
7. **Digoxin** "poisons" the sodium-potassium ATPase pump, thereby increasing intracellular sodium. Increased intracellular sodium increases the passive exchange between intracellular sodium and extracellular calcium. Increased intracellular calcium increases force of contraction.

The slow inward calcium channel and the fast inward sodium channel may also influence contractility. Drugs acting specifically on these channels are not yet available.

brane-bound G protein, which serves to activate membrane-bound adenylate cyclase, thereby producing greater amounts of intracellular cyclic AMP. This increased concentration of cyclic AMP improves contractility. Dopamine not only stimulates the β-receptor, but also activates dopaminergic receptors in the kidneys, brain, and coronary arteries and, at low doses (1–5 μg/kg/min), causes vasodilatation in these vascular beds.

Other Inotropic Agents: Phosphodiesterase inhibitors, including amrinone, milrinone, theophylline, and caffeine, exert their inotropic effect by increasing intracellular levels of cyclic AMP and thus also cause vasodilatation. Trials of these drugs given orally to outpatients have demonstrated that they increase mortality. Intravenous amrinone is available for short-term use (48 hours) and is an effective vasodilator and inotropic agent, but prolonged intravenous treatment with this agent may cause hepatic and platelet dysfunction and, as with all inotropes, tachyphylaxis or down-regulation may occur. Another drug, vesnarinone, shows more promise as an inotropic stimulant, but experience with it is still limited and experimental.

Anticoagulation

Patients with systolic dysfunction from any cause are predisposed to venous stasis. This is particularly so in patients with lower-extremity edema or right heart dilation. These patients may be at high risk for pulmonary emboli.

Patients with diminished ejection fraction and left ventricular dilatation are also predisposed to systemic embolization. There is a 10–15% chance of systemic symptomatic embolization in patients with dilated cardiomyopathy not treated with anticoagulant therapy. The risk of embolization can be reduced dramatically with oral anticoagulant agents. We therefore place on anticoagulant therapy those patients with diminished systolic function who have an ejection fraction below 30%, particularly those with dilated hearts and congestive heart failure. The benefit of anticoagulant therapy must be balanced against the potential risk. Patients on chronic anticoagulant therapy are at increased risk for bleeding episodes, and those who are noncompliant or who cannot follow a medical regimen are considered to be at too high a risk for this form of therapy. Aspirin may be of some benefit for patients in the latter category, although the protective anticoagulant effect is considered to be incomplete.

Antiarrhythmics

Patients with diminished systolic function and dilated cardiomyopathy have supraventricular and ventricular arrhythmias. Their prognoses are inversely related to the presence and severity of their arrhythmias, from atrial premature contraction to paroxysmal atrial tachycardia, atrial fibrillation, atrial flutter, ventricular premature contractions, ventricular couplets, and bursts of nonsustained ventricular tachycardia. About 50% of patients with diminished systolic function and dilated cardiomyopathy experience sudden death. These sudden deaths are thought to be caused by ventricular tachycardia, ventricular fibrillation, or sudden bradyarrhythmia.

The patients' risk for sudden death has not been demonstrated to be altered by treatment of supraventricular or ventricular arrhythmias, but rather is inexorably associated with the severity of ventricular dysfunction. Amiodarone and β-blockade are the only forms of medical treatment that appear to have any influence on the risk of sudden death in patients with diminished systolic function. Some studies of amiodarone have shown a decreased risk of sudden death with its use. Amiodarone has significant cumulative toxicity, including ophthalmologic corneal deposition, hepatitis, pulmonary dysfunction affecting the interstitium or causing acute pneumonitis, and skin infiltration causing discoloration. Some patients become hypothyroid on amiodarone treatment, while a few develop hyperthyroidism. Because of the potential toxicity of this medication, its use is avoided except where significant arrhythmias and ventricular compromise coexist without benefit of other drugs. Preliminary studies with β-blocking drugs have suggested that they may improve the prognosis of patients with dilated cardiomyopathy. Because these drugs stabilize the myocyte membrane and relieve ischemia, and as most patients with dilated cardiomyopathy have some degree of subendocardial ischemia as a result of high wall stress and heart rate, it is reasonable to expect that β-receptor antagonists may be somewhat effective. Because of the negative inotropic effect of β-receptor antagonist on systolic function, patients may not be able to tolerate institution of even low doses of therapy. Over the next several years, specific trials of amiodarone and β-receptor antagonists are anticipated to answer the question as to the appropriate use of these agents.

Other forms of antiarrhythmic therapy, and amiodarone itself, may cause a prorhythmic effect in up to 10–15% of patients. The prorhythmic effect results in a worsening of the ventricular arrhythmia that the antiarrhythmic medicines were intended to treat. Therefore, institution of any antiarrhythmic agent must be done under controlled circumstances, with the patient hospitalized and monitored. Prolongation of QT intervals with antiarrhythmic therapy heralds prorhythmic effects.

Transplantation

Few patients with dilated cardiomyopathy can expect useful improvement in their left ventricular function. The ones who can are those with viral and postpartum myocarditis, alcoholic cardiomyopathy, and some with cardiac sarcoid or other treatable diseases. Among the majority of patients in whom left ventricular failure gradually progresses, a few cases progress to the point at which transplantation offers the only chance for extending survival. Although the surgery to replace a heart is not especially complicated, the medical aspects of transplantation have been worked out satisfactorily over about only the last 10 or 12 years.

The main advances that have allowed proper medical understanding and application of heart transplantation have been the development of effective immunosuppressive drugs and the simple technology that allows monitoring of cardiac histology by biopsies performed transvenously every few weeks or months. Immunosuppressive regimens typically include substantial doses of corticosteroids, combined with one or both of azathioprine and cyclosporine. Such treatment carries considerable side effects, including susceptibility to infection, being cushingoid, osteoporosis, avascular necrosis of the femoral heads, hypertension, and chronic renal insufficiency. Less common problems include increased incidence of lymphoma, skin cancer, and other malignant growths of the kinds associated with immunosuppression. Patients for transplantation must be under age 60, free of complicating medical conditions, and prepared to withstand the rigor of the post-transplantation regimen. This requires being psychologically robust and having adequate family or other social support. In well-selected patients who undergo transplantation, the long-term results are good, with 5-year survival rate in the region of 70%.

SUMMARY

▶ Dilated cardiomyopathy is the most common of the three types of heart muscle disease; it is characterized by left ventricular enlargement and reduced left ventricular ejection fraction.

▶ Causes of dilated cardiomyopathy include ischemic left ventricular damage, myocarditis, alcohol, and cocaine. In most patients with dilated cardiomyopathy, none of these is found and the disease is labeled idiopathic.

▶ Treatable causes of dilated cardiomyopathy are thyroid disease, lupus, pheochromocytoma, and sarcoidosis.

▶ The hemodynamic abnormalities associated with dilated cardiomyopathy are managed with diuretics, vasodilators, and inotropic agents. In good candidates, transplantation offers a better chance of survival.

SUGGESTED READING

Effect of enalapril on mortality and the development of heart failure in asymptomatic patients with reduced left ventricular ejection fractions. The SOLVD Investigators. N Engl J Med 1992;327:685.

Effects of enalapril on mortality in severe congestive heart failure: Results of the Cooperative North Scandinavian Enalapril Survival Study (CONSENSUS). N Engl J Med 1987;316:1429.

Manolio TA et al: Prevalence and etiology of idiopathic dilated cardiomyopathy (summary of a National Heart, Lung, and Blood Institute workshop). Am J Cardiol 1992;69:1458.

McKee PA et al: The natural history of congestive heart failure: The Framingham study. N Engl J Med 1971;285:1441.

O'Connell JB et al: Cardiac transplantation: Recipient selection, donor procurement, and medical follow-up. Circulation 1992;86:1061.

1.7

Hypertrophic and Restrictive Cardiomyopathy

Thomas A. Traill, FRCP

Hypertrophic and restrictive cardiomyopathy are diseases in which abnormal diastolic function of the left ventricle is much more conspicuous than defects of systolic function. In each of these conditions, the left ventricular diastolic pressure is increased, as the primary consequence of the myocardial disorder, while measures of systolic function are relatively unaffected. This is in contrast to dilated cardiomyopathy (Chapter 1.6), the more common kind of heart muscle disorder, in which increased left atrial pressure reflects the increased end-diastolic cavity size of the left ventricle and can be considered as a compensatory mechanism. Thus, hypertrophic and restrictive disease cause symptoms of heart failure—breathlessness, pulmonary congestion, and fluid retention—without left ventricular dilatation. Patients with hypertrophic cardiomyopathy may also present with angina or syncope, or even experience sudden death.

Hypertrophic cardiomyopathy and restrictive cardiomyopathy differ in that restrictive disease causes increased left ventricular filling pressure exclusively by virtue of impaired elasticity, a purely physical property of the heart muscle. In hypertrophic cardiomyopathy, the physiologic process of myocardial relaxation is impaired, such that with each heartbeat the myocardium takes an abnormally long time to make the transition from its systolic, contracting state to its diastolic state. This impaired relaxation is compounded by the fact that hypertrophied muscle, like the muscle of restrictive disorders, is also inelastic. In many cases, architectural distortion of the left ventricular cavity, the result of regional hypertrophy, adds further complexity.

Hypertrophic cardiomyopathy is not a single disease; it is a pathophysiologic grouping, just as dilated cardiomyopathy is. Any of several stimuli to left ventricular hypertrophy can be the cause, particularly hypertension and aortic stenosis. The disease also occurs as a familial disorder caused by mutations affecting the contractile proteins.

Indeed, it was the familial form of hypertrophic cardiomyopathy that was first identified as a distinct kind of heart muscle disorder and in which the pathophysiology was first worked out. Only later was it recognized that the same pathophysiology applied in secondary forms of hypertrophy as well. Patients with hypertrophic cardiomyopathy have pulmonary congestion, angina, and syncope as their chief symptoms. Treatment is directed toward slowing the heart rate, to allow time for their slow ventricular relaxation to be completed, and toward making the left ventricular cavity larger, using negative inotropic drugs. Treating the syndrome of "heart failure" with drugs that depress myocardial contractility may seem paradoxical, but makes complete sense when it is appreciated that relaxation rather than systolic contractility is the problem. Negative inotropic drugs are clearly not the treatment for either dilated or restrictive disease.

Restrictive cardiomyopathy is uncommon. Most cases are caused when infiltration of the myocardium causes changes in the elasticity of its connective tissue matrix, for example, in amyloidosis and hemochromatosis. Other causes are characterized by interstitial fibrosis, for example, the cardiomyopathy seen in Friedreich's ataxia and many idiopathic cases. Rarely, restrictive cardiomyopathy runs in families, but no genetic loci have yet been identified. Patients with restrictive cardiomyopathy have striking elevation of filling pressures in both sides of the heart, without necessarily showing cavity dilatation. They present with breathlessness, a striking increase in jugular venous pressure, and severe fluid retention. Usually, affected patients prove to have abnormally thick ventricular myocardium, but it is essential to distinguish them from patients with hypertrophic disorders because their treatment is utterly different.

Although patients with restrictive myocardial disease have impaired elasticity, relaxation is not prolonged, so they do not benefit from slowing the heart rate. Like patients with dilated cardiomyopathy, they require diuretics and may benefit from vasodilators and positive inotropic drugs. In practice, it is seldom difficult to distinguish restrictive disorders from the other kinds of cardiomyopathy; the resemblance between restrictive disease and chronic constrictive pericarditis is a more common source of difficulty.

HYPERTROPHIC CARDIOMYOPATHY

Familial Hypertrophic Cardiomyopathy

Familial hypertrophic cardiomyopathy is a disease that affects young adults and may cause angina, syncope, left ventricular failure, or sudden death. The disease is inherited as an autosomal dominant. A number of patients have heart muscle abnormalities identical with those of the familial disorders but no family history of the disease; some of these patients must have new mutations. In these patients with no family history, the disease is considered idiopathic. The appearance of the heart muscle is usually characteristic, with massive hypertrophy that affects the septum more than other parts of the heart (Figure 1.7–1). The result is that the left ventricular cavity is small and distorted. At end-systole, the walls in the middle of the chamber may be in contact, leaving only the base of the ventricle around the mitral valve, and in some patients a small portion of the apex still containing blood. This phenomenon is often described as "cavity obliteration." From this very low end-systolic volume, the ventricle relaxes slowly, so that the duration of isovolumic relaxation is prolonged, mitral valve opening is delayed, and filling is slow and protracted (Table 1.7–1). The passive distensibility of the heart muscle is also abnormal in this disease, so that in addition to slow filling, there is an abnormally abrupt rise in diastolic pressure at the moment of atrial systole.

Clinical Findings: Hypertrophic cardiomyopathy may be detected when a heart murmur is discovered, or it may manifest with angina or syncope. In the differential diagnosis of syncope in a young adult or teenager, hypertrophic cardiomyopathy should be considered along with fainting, arrhythmias, and aortic stenosis (Chapter 1.9). Hypertrophic cardiomyopathy and aortic stenosis are almost the only causes of angina in young patients. In older patients with angina, coronary artery disease may be the first diagnosis suspected. Left ventricular failure is not usually a presenting feature of the familial disease, but it may develop, often after some years.

The clinical features of familial hypertrophic cardiomyopathy are predictable from the pathophysiologic abnormalities. The arterial pulses are forceful, with sharp upstrokes consistent with rapid ejection of blood from a small, hypercontractile ventricle. Left ventricular ejection often stops abruptly in midsystole, as the midportion of the cavity obliterates; this may lend a bisferiens character to the carotid pulses. The jugular pulse often has a promi-

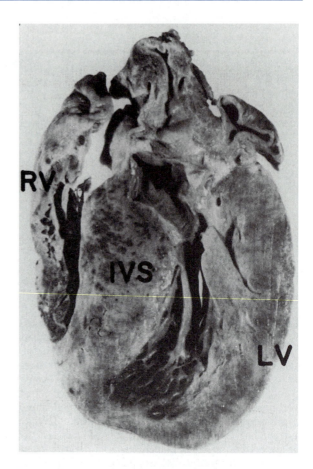

Figure 1.7–1. Familial hypertrophic cardiomyopathy. Pathologic specimen shows disproportionate hypertrophy in the interventricular septum. (Reproduced, with permission, from Hutchins GM, Bulkley BH: Catenoid shape of the interventricular septum: Possible cause of idiopathic hypertrophic subaortic stenosis. Circulation 1978;58:392.)

nent a wave, which reflects the increased pressure generated by left atrial systole as it is transmitted across the atrial septum. The cardiac impulse is sustained and forceful, but not necessarily displaced and may also have a palpable a wave. On auscultation, there is often a fourth heart sound, again reflecting the height of the atrial contribution to the left ventricular end-diastolic pressure. Characteristically a long systolic murmur is heard all over the precordium. This can be generated by turbulence from rapid ejection through the narrow left ventricular outflow tract, but may also be caused by mitral regurgitation.

Mitral regurgitation in hypertrophic cardiomyopathy is another effect of the left ventricle's tendency to midcavity obliteration during systole. The much-reduced end-systolic volume leaves some of the mitral subvalve apparatus redundant. At the same time, the anterior mitral leaflet is pulled into the outflow part of the ventricle by a Venturi

Table 1.7–1. Distinguishing causes of abnormal diastolic function.

	Hypertrophic Cardiomyopathy	Restrictive Cardiomyopathy	Dilated Cardiomyopathy	Mitral Stenosis
Jugular venous pressure	a wave	Steep, short y descent	a wave	Depends on pulmonary artery pressure
Cardiac impulse	Sustained, not displaced	Quiet	Displaced, prominent early diastolic retraction	Tapping S1; quiet LV impulse
Third sound	Rare	Usual	Usual	Rare
Fourth sound	Common	Sometimes	Common	Presystolic murmur
Isovolumic relaxation	Prolonged	Short	Short	Short
Filling	Slow	Abbreviated	Normal	Slow
Cardiac catheterization	LV outflow gradient; small LV	High pressures in both atria	Dilated, hypodynamic LV	Mitral valve gradient

LV, left ventricle, left ventricular.

suction effect caused by rapid ejection through a narrow left ventricular outflow tract. Diastolic murmurs are not heard; there is no reason for aortic regurgitation in this disease. If there is an aortic diastolic murmur, the physician should suspect intrinsic aortic valve disease or discrete subaortic stenosis in the form of a subaortic membrane (Chapter 1.11).

The electrocardiogram (ECG) in familial hypertrophic cardiomyopathy shows left ventricular hypertrophy, often with rather unusual septal forces that give deep Q waves in the inferior leads, or tall, narrow initial R waves in the right precordial leads V1 and V2.

Echocardiography: Echocardiography is the diagnostic test for hypertrophic cardiomyopathy; it displays the abnormal anatomy and characterizes almost all of the physiologic disturbances in this condition (Figure 1.7–2). The

most obvious findings are the anatomic ones. The hallmark of the disease is regional hypertrophy, characteristically in the mid- and proximal septum, but in some patients affecting other parts of the ventricle, such as the apex. Usually, the remainder of the ventricle displays a mild degree of hypertrophy, and sometimes the abnormality is diffuse. The left ventricular diastolic and systolic cavity size is strikingly reduced.

The physiologic abnormalities are a little more subtle. Abnormally slow relaxation can be recognized from delay in mitral valve opening and the subsequent reduced rate of increase in cavity size; the pattern of filling can look like that of mitral stenosis. During systole, as the ventricular cavity becomes small and distorted, the mitral chordae become redundant and the anterior mitral leaflet may flip forward into the outflow tract. This phenomenon, called *systolic anterior movement* (SAM) of the mitral valve, may be seen in any condition associated with either distortion of the end-systolic outline of the left ventricle or over-rapid ejection.

Doppler echocardiography can be used to display the filling abnormalities, showing reduced rate of filling in early diastole (the E wave) and more filling at the time of atrial systole (A)—often referred to as reversal of the E/A ratio. Again, although this is usual in hypertrophic cardiomyopathy, it has several other causes and should not be regarded as a specific finding. The Doppler study also shows the rapidity of ejection, and, by showing a high velocity in the left ventricular outflow tract, implies a pressure gradient within the cavity of the left ventricle during systole.

This pressure gradient is real; it can be demonstrated by cardiac catheterization, with catheters placed at the left ventricular apex and in either the outflow tract or the aorta. The usual mechanism is that after obliteration of the midcavity in midsystole, the apex continues to contract and thus compresses a small apical chamber to pressures that exceed the blood pressure. In some cases, there seems to be transient obstruction to ejection, caused by the bulging septum or the protruding anterior mitral valve leaflet. It is important to recognize, however, that this ob-

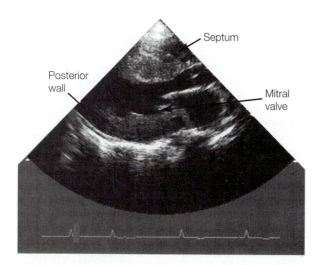

Figure 1.7–2. Echocardiogram in a patient with hypertrophic cardiomyopathy.

struction is a consequence of the primary hypertrophic disorder, not its cause; in no sense is this disease a form of aortic stenosis.

Treatment: Symptoms of familial hypertrophic cardiomyopathy are mediated by the combination of a tiny cavity, hypercontractile state, and slow filling. Treatment therefore consists of enlarging the cavity, using negative inotropic agents that increase the end-diastolic and end-systolic volume, and slowing the heart rate to extend the period of diastole available for filling. Medications that combine these properties to good effect are verapamil, a calcium channel blocker with pronounced negative inotropic activity, and the β-blockers such as propranolol and atenolol. Certain antiarrhythmic agents, such as disopyramide and amiodarone, have negative inotropic properties that can also be put to use in this setting.

The alternative to medication, usually reserved for only the most refractory symptoms, is enlarging the cavity surgically. A piece of the bulging proximal septum is removed through the aortic valve, a technique known as *myectomy.* A somewhat similar effect can be achieved by inserting a transvenous pacemaker, thereby moving the point of activation of the ventricles to the right ventricular apex. This effectively causes left bundle branch block, and by delaying septal activation may enlarge the end-systolic left ventricular cavity.

The hearts of patients with hypertrophic cardiomyopathy have slow filling and a steep diastolic pressure-volume relation, which make them sensitive to reductions in ventricular filling pressure. Therefore, patients should not be allowed to become hypovolemic. Diuretics are rarely indicated, and nitrates can cause irreversible hypotension. Patients should also not be exposed to the increase in inotropic state brought on by overvigorous exercise, and they are ordinarily advised against competitive sports. They are also especially sensitive to the effects of tachycardia on filling, and they tolerate atrial fibrillation and other tachyarrhythmias poorly. Although patients with familial hypertrophic cardiomyopathy should not ordinarily receive drugs that increase myocardial contractility, they can be given digitalis, if needed, to control atrial fibrillation; the disadvantage of its slight positive inotropic effect is insignificant compared with the importance of slowing the ventricular rate.

Patients with hypertrophic cardiomyopathy have a risk of sudden death, sometimes but not necessarily in the context of exertion. In recently diagnosed teenagers, this risk is about 3% per year. In older patients, who have stood the test of time, the risk is lower. Syncope and ventricular arrhythmias are both adverse prognostic signs; none of the hemodynamic abnormalities or ventriculographic findings in this disease predict poor prognosis nearly as accurately as ventricular tachycardia recorded on a 24-hour Holter monitor. It is always tempting to assume that when sudden death is a possibility and arrhythmias are known to occur, the two are causally related; but it turns out that, with the possible exception of amiodarone, treatment with

antiarrhythmic drugs is not particularly effective in reducing patients' risk of death. In the few patients who have died suddenly while under electrocardiographic surveillance, primary arrhythmias have often not been the terminal event. The ECG gives little clue to what happened, and we are left speculating about ischemia, neurogenic cardiac depression, or complete failure of filling as mechanisms leading to hypotension and cardiac arrest. Since there is no medication that in controlled studies prolongs survival in this disease, the mechanisms of death are still uncertain.

Genetics: Familial hypertrophic cardiomyopathy is inherited as a mendelian dominant with complete penetrance; anyone who has the mutation has an abnormal myocardium. The disease has proved to be genetically heterogeneous. Loci have been identified on chromosomes 14, 11, 15, and 1. The locus on chromosome 14, which is the most common, is the gene that codes for the cardiac β-myosin heavy chain; genes at two of the other loci code for components of the troponin-tropomyosin complex. It should come as no surprise that this disease can be the result of a congenital abnormality of the contractile proteins. The abnormalities encountered in different families vary in severity; different mutations, even within the same β-myosin gene, are associated with strikingly diverse natural histories.

In families with identified mutations, it is possible to study natural history more fully than in sporadic cases or in families in which detection depends only on the clinical findings. Very few mutations cause clinically detectable disease in childhood; most affected patients begin to develop hypertrophy only around the time of puberty. An abnormal ECG is often the first outward sign of the disease, followed by a wide-ranging spectrum of echocardiographic abnormalities ranging from "classic" bulging of the proximal septum to milder forms of regional hypertrophy affecting other parts of the left ventricle. In patients who survive to middle life, the hemodynamic picture may gradually evolve from the most typical kind of hypercontractile state to a more normal end-systolic cavity size, but still with very pronounced filling abnormalities. Thus, this disease is both genetically and phenotypically heterogeneous.

Secondary Hypertrophic Cardiomyopathy

Left ventricular hypertrophy caused by hypertension or aortic stenosis can be accompanied by the same physiologic disturbances as familial or idiopathic hypertrophic cardiomyopathy. Such secondary hypertrophic cardiomyopathy is more common than the primary form. A typical presentation is the elderly patient with a long history of moderate hypertension who is seen for angina or breathlessness. First on the differential diagnosis might well be coronary artery disease, perhaps with ischemic left ventricular dysfunction from previous infarctions. However, the echocardiogram shows a normal or supernormal left ventricular ejection fraction, and, instead of being dilated, the left ventricular cavity is small, with the same abnormalities of diastole as found in patients with familial hypertrophic disease. Treatment for such a patient is different from the usual treatment for ischemic heart disease. Patients with pulmonary congestion caused by secondary hypertrophic cardiomyopathy may not tolerate vasodilators and diuretics, since these may aggravate diastolic dysfunction and cause dangerous hypotension. Similarly, angina caused by hypertrophic cardiomyopathy responds better to β-blockers or verapamil than to nitroglycerin and nitrates.

RESTRICTIVE CARDIOMYOPATHY

The defining characteristic of restrictive cardiomyopathy is a very steep diastolic pressure-volume relationship, such that for any increase in diastolic volume there is a disproportionate rise in diastolic pressure. Relaxation is not prolonged, and systolic function is usually somewhat depressed. The result is that patients have very high filling pressures on both sides of the heart. They present with dyspnea, pulmonary congestion, and, after the early stages, severe fluid retention. Restrictive cardiomyopathy is not likely to be mistaken for dilated or hypertrophic cardiomyopathy, once the patient has been studied by echocardiography. The left ventricular walls are thickened but not hypercontractile like a hypertrophied heart, and the cavity is seldom dilated. The chief diagnostic problem in restrictive disease is distinguishing it from chronic pericardial constriction, in which the clinical, echocardiographic, and even hemodynamic findings may be similar (Table 1.7–2; Chapter 1.10).

Some cases of restrictive cardiomyopathy are idiopathic, and a few familial cases have been described. However, more than in either of the other two cardiomyopathy groups, restrictive cardiomyopathy is often part of a systemic disease. The most common systemic disease causing—and often presenting with—restrictive myocardial disease is amyloidosis, either primary or in associa-

tion with plasma cell dyscrasia. Particularly in elderly patients, cardiac amyloidosis may present as a virtually isolated disorder, without clinical involvement of other organs. Hemochromatosis and transfusion siderosis cause restrictive cardiomyopathy, and a few patients with cardiac sarcoidosis develop restrictive pathophysiology. Diseases of the endocardium can cause restriction from within, as in endomyocardial fibrosis, a disease of tropical countries; in Loeffler's eosinophilic endocarditis, a very rare condition; and in endocardial fibroelastosis, which is a disease of infancy. Friedreich's ataxia causes restrictive cardiomyopathy, as does scleroderma. In many patients, therefore, restrictive cardiomyopathy is diagnosed by detecting the underlying disease, as in amyloidosis, by Congo red staining of a fat pad aspirate or rectal biopsy or by the results of serum protein electrophoresis.

Hemochromatosis patients do not present with cardiomyopathy; involvement of the heart follows liver disease and diabetes mellitus. Secondary iron storage disease, however, caused by multiple transfusions in patients with chronic anemia, typically first appears as heart disease. Restrictive cardiomyopathy remains the usual cause of death, therefore, in some of the heritable hemolytic disorders and is also seen in older patients with acquired anemia. Anyone who has received more than 50 units of transfused blood, over whatever time period, and who has no identifiable source of iron loss is at risk from transfusion siderosis.

Clinical and Hemodynamic Findings

When the underlying disease is not identified, diagnosis of restrictive cardiomyopathy depends on careful analysis of the hemodynamics as revealed by the jugular pulse, the echocardiogram, and, if needed, a cardiac catheterization. The characteristic abnormality of the atrial pressure pulse is a steep fall and rise during early diastole. This "square root sign" resembles the atrial pressure wave in constrictive pericarditis, whether recorded on a strip chart from an intravascular catheter or observed in the neck veins (Friedreich's sign). The first deflection of the square root sign is the steep, abbreviated y descent of the jugular pulse. In constrictive disease, the two atrial pressures are identical; in diastole, when the atrioventricular valves are open, all the pressures in the heart become equal.

The echocardiogram is not good at looking at the pericardium directly—for that we use computed tomography (CT) or magnetic resonance imaging (MRI)—but may help by showing whether myocardial function is abnormal. In amyloidosis, the echocardiogram is often diagnostic, since the myocardium in these patients has a characteristic gray, glittery appearance on the video image. In constrictive pericarditis, the ejection fraction should be normal or high; in most restrictive diseases, the ejection fraction is low. Isovolumic contraction may be prolonged in restrictive myocardial disorders, and isovolumic relaxation, prolonged in hypertrophic disease, is always short in restrictive myopathy. Restrictive cardiomyopathy and pericarditis both cause a third heart

Table 1.7–2. Distinguishing restrictive cardiomyopathy from constrictive pericarditis.

	Restrictive Cardiomyopathy	Constrictive Pericarditis
X-ray	Big heart	Normal or small heart; calcification in 25% of patients
Atrial size on echo	Big	May be small
Ejection fraction	Often reduced	Normal or high
CT or MRI	Normal pericardium; thick heart	Thick pericardium
Heart biopsy	Specific disease	Normal
Equal atrial pressures	Sometimes	Usual

sound, called a *pericardial knock* in the case of pericarditis; this is never heard in hypertrophic cardiomyopathy.

In some patients, it is impossible to distinguish restrictive cardiomyopathy from constrictive pericarditis by any indirect means. Then the only possibilities are to biopsy the heart, which is a simple outpatient procedure when performed via the jugular vein, or to inspect the pericardium directly by a limited thoracotomy, usually performed by resecting the fourth left costal cartilage. It is essential to make the distinction accurately because constrictive pericarditis is an eminently treatable condition, whereas the prognosis and opportunities to improve the patient with restrictive cardiomyopathy are very limited.

Treatment

Treatment of restrictive cardiomyopathy includes treating the underlying disease, which may halt progression of the myocardial dysfunction but seldom reverses it, and treating the patient's fluid retention and pulmonary congestion. Diastolic dysfunction in this disease does not respond to negative inotropic agents, so that treatment of pulmonary congestion is similar to that of dilated cardiomyopathy. Generally, patients tolerate only moderate control of their fluid overload. If the jugular pressure is restored to normal, patients are likely to develop low cardiac output and hypotension; therefore, management consists in finding what level of jugular pressure suits the patient best.

The prognosis for patients with restrictive cardiomyopathy is generally not very good. When transplantation is not contraindicated by an underlying systemic disease, it may be the only option.

SUMMARY

▶ Hypertrophic and restrictive cardiomyopathy are pathophysiologic groups of heart muscle disease in which the primary abnormalities lie with diastolic function of the myocardium.

▶ Hypertrophic cardiomyopathy is characterized by impaired ventricular relaxation; patients are sensitive to tachycardia and lowered filling pressure. Familial hypertrophic cardiomyopathy is the paradigm, but secondary hypertrophy from hypertension and aortic stenosis is more common.

▶ Treatment of familial, idiopathic, or secondary hypertrophic cardiomyopathy consists in slowing the heart rate and decreasing the inotropic state of the myocardium with verapamil or a β-blocker.

▶ Restrictive cardiomyopathy is characterized by impaired elasticity of the myocardium. It is usually caused by systemic diseases, particularly amyloidosis. Diuretics are the mainstay of treatment, and the prognosis is generally poor.

SUGGESTED READING

Katritsis D et al: Primary restrictive cardiomyopathy: Clinical and pathologic characteristics. J Am Coll Cardiol 1991;18: 1230.

Kelly DP, Strauss AW: Inherited cardiomyopathies. N Engl J Med 1994;330:913.

Sanderson JE et al: Left ventricular relaxation and filling in hypertrophic cardiomyopathy: An echocardiographic study. Br Heart J 1978;40:596.

Teare D: Asymmetrical hypertrophy of the heart in young adults. Br Heart J 1958;20:1.

Topol EJ, Traill TA, Fortuin NJ: Hypertensive hypertrophic cardiomyopathy of the elderly. N Engl J Med 1985;312:277.

Watkins H et al: Mutations in the genes for cardiac troponin T and α-tropomyosin in hypertrophic cardiomyopathy. N Engl J Med 1995;332:1058.

Valvular Heart Disease

Nicholas J. Fortuin, MD

Cardiac valve lesions cause heart murmurs. Patients with valvular lesions may come to medical attention because of a murmur found at a routine examination or because heart function has been affected and symptoms have appeared. In either case, the physician's responsibility is to determine the nature of the valvular lesion, its severity, and its effect on overall cardiovascular function. The keys are the history, physical examination, and simple laboratory procedures such as the electrocardiogram (ECG), chest x-ray, and echocardiogram. These tests should allow the clinician to arrive at precise conclusions about the patient's condition without having to resort to more elaborate technology such as catheterization. Indeed, when cardiologists evaluate hemodynamics in the absence of clinical information, they can be misled.

EVALUATION

Faced with the patient who has valvular disease, the clinician needs to answer eight questions.

1. What is the lesion? The major valvular lesions—aortic stenosis, aortic regurgitation, mitral stenosis, and mitral regurgitation—can almost always be identified by auscultation.
2. What is the cause of the valvular lesion? Fifty years ago, most valvular disease followed rheumatic fever, so other causes of valvular lesions were not recognized until the prevalence of rheumatic heart disease had declined. Understanding the origin helps to predict the natural history and to plan management.
3. How severe is the lesion? The answer determines when to recommend surgery. Assessing the severity of mitral regurgitation is important in deciding whether the lesion represents a primary valve disorder or is secondary to left ventricular muscle disease in the patient with cardiomyopathy.
4. How has the lesion affected other parts of the circulation, particularly the left ventricle and pulmonary circulation? The prognosis is determined primarily by how well the left ventricle functions. Successful management of the valvular problem may not be effective if the left ventricle has been severely damaged. On the other hand, even a moderate valvular lesion may be poorly tolerated by a dysfunctional ventricle and thus prompt earlier surgery. Changes in the pulmonary vasculature caused by longstanding pulmonary venous hypertension may not be reversible even with successful valve surgery.
5. Does the patient have other valve lesions, and, if so, are they severe enough to contribute to cardiac malfunction? Some valvular lesions may be missed in the presence of another lesion that produces a loud murmur. For example, mitral stenosis may be difficult to recognize when aortic stenosis dominates the presentation.
6. Does the patient have other heart disease? Many patients with valvular heart disease present in middle life, and they may have coronary artery disease. Symptoms and physical findings alone may not enable the physician to determine whether coronary vascular lesions are playing a role in the patient's presentation.
7. Where does this patient stand in the natural history of the lesion? Specific valvular lesions have distinctive natural histories. For example, the natural history of mitral stenosis is predictably long, with many periods of improvement and deterioration. This means that for most patients there is little urgency about deciding when to perform valve surgery. In contrast, in a patient with valvular aortic stenosis, rapid progression and death may follow soon after the first symptoms.
8. What is the patient's overall medical condition? In patients debilitated by other medical problems, correction of even severe valvular lesions may have to be postponed or canceled if the other medical problems cannot be treated.

History

Assessing the degree of disability that patients suffer as a result of a valvular problem is critical to planning their management, and depends entirely on the history. Objective tests of effort tolerance are ineffective in this setting.

The predominant symptoms are those of left heart dysfunction—fatigue, breathlessness, and fluid retention. It is important to keep questions specific, asking what activities patients tolerate and for how long, and how this compares with previous years. In some patients with valvular heart disease, particularly those with mitral stenosis, incapacity evolves so gradually that the patient is unaware of the change. Such patients may think that they have "just gotten old." Others may not complain of symptoms because they have gradually learned to accommodate to inadequate cardiac reserve by withdrawing from activities. These patients deny that they are breathless, because they have learned to avoid activities that produce shortness of breath. Subtle changes in exercise capacity, even in patients who still enjoy a full spectrum of activities, are sometimes a tipoff to changing heart function, even before changes in objective laboratory measurements of ventricular size or function are noted.

Other symptoms of valvular disease are as follows:

1. Angina, which may occur in the absence of coronary disease because of increased demands on a normal coronary circulation in patients with aortic stenosis.
2. Syncope, typically exertional, also in patients with aortic stenosis.
3. Palpitation from premature beats, or "fluttering" due to rapid flutter or fibrillation may herald worsening mitral valve disease.
4. Systemic emboli to any organ, particularly the cerebral circulation, may produce the first symptoms in occult mitral disease.

The family history may reveal that other family members have valvular disease or heart murmurs, as in patients with mitral prolapse or Marfan's syndrome. The past medical history should include questions about rheumatic fever; although this disease is rare in developed countries today, older patients may recall it, particularly when cardinal manifestations are described to them. On the other hand, many patients with heart murmurs have been told incorrectly that they had rheumatic fever, just because of the old belief that all valvular disease was likely to have a rheumatic origin. It is important to establish when the patient first became aware of a murmur. School and military physicals, insurance exams, exams during pregnancy, or routine health evaluations may have detected the murmur years before the patient comes for evaluation.

Physical Examination

Although the obvious manifestations of valvular lesions are the murmurs they produce, the answers to the eight questions posed earlier are usually found through the other aspects of the physical examination. First, the physician should observe the patient's overall condition, looking for signs of a systemic disease or heritable syndrome, evidence of infection, cyanosis, pulmonary congestion, or fluid retention. Then, proceed by inspection and palpation from the periphery to the central arterial and venous pulses of the neck, and then to the precordium, where careful inspection and palpation provide information about size and function of right and left ventricles.

Only then, armed with a clear expectation of what is to be found and where to put special attention, can the examiner proceed to auscultation. For example, having palpated a displaced and sustained apex impulse, indicating left ventricular dilatation, not much time would be spent searching for auscultatory signs of mitral stenosis, because in this condition the left ventricle is small. Again, having identified a systolic jugular pulse wave of tricuspid regurgitation, the examiner knows that the patient has pulmonary hypertension or right ventricular dysfunction. Specific physical findings relevant to each of the valvular lesions are discussed in the following sections.

Laboratory Tests

Laboratory findings augment those of the examination. The ECG is important in describing the cardiac rhythm and providing evidence of right or left ventricular hypertrophy. Because ECG sensitivity for hypertrophy is only fair, ventricular hypertrophy shown by ECG is clear-cut evidence that the problem is severe. The chest x-ray may be useful to assess the degree of pulmonary venous congestion or the effects of pulmonary arterial hypertension on central and peripheral vasculature. It shows overall heart size, but is unreliable for detecting specific chamber enlargement. For that purpose the echocardiogram is superior.

The intracardiac imaging provided by echocardiography shows cardiac structures in motion and in two dimensions and permits accurate measurements of distance. Thus, the examiner can visualize valvular pathologic conditions and determine individual cardiac chamber sizes and thickness of walls. The Doppler technique is used to display abnormal flow patterns in the heart in regurgitant lesions and to measure the abnormal flow velocities across stenotic valves. It is possible to predict pressures remarkably accurately with this technique, but as with catheterization, hemodynamic information must be integrated with other clinical findings to be of value in clinical decision making.

The elegant imaging of structure, function, and flow patterns by the echocardiogram can beguile the clinician by suggesting that the other clinical information is less important and that the technology can answer the questions posed by the patient with a valvular lesion. It does not deny the importance of technology to state that this is most certainly not the case. The technology achieves its purpose only when it is part of the patient's overall clinical evaluation.

For most patients with valvular heart disease, the evaluation previously described is sufficient to answer the eight questions posed earlier in the chapter. Occasionally, cardiac catheterization is needed to provide quantitative information about the nature of a lesion. For most patients, catheterization is performed to check for coronary artery disease and to confirm the clinical impression regarding

Table 1.8–1. Signs of severity in valvular lesions.

	Physical Examination	Echocardiogram	Chest X-Ray	ECG
Aortic stenosis	Late-peaking murmur, absent A2; carotid thrill, low volume retarded carotid upstroke; LV heave	Degree of calcification and immobilization of valve; LVH, LV dysfunction; high Doppler velocity	Cardiomegaly, aortic valve calcification	LVH
Aortic regurgitation				
Chronic	Wide pulse pressure, low diastolic pressure, collapsing pulse, LV enlargement, Austin Flint murmur, S3 gallop, Duroziez's sign	LV dilatation, valve or root abnormalities	Cardiomegaly	LVH
Acute	Abbreviated diastolic murmur, absent S1, mid-diastolic Austin Flint murmur	Premature mitral closure in mid-diastole, prolapsing aortic leaflets or vegetations	Pulmonary congestion	Not helpful
Mitral stenosis	Short S2-OS interval, loud P2, parasternal heave (RVH)	RVH, LA enlargement, tricuspid regurgitation, reduced valve area and high-velocity inflow by Doppler	Kerley lines, large pulmonary arteries, pulmonary congestion, LA enlargement	RVH, atrial fibrillation
Mitral regurgitation				
Chronic	Enlarged LV, parasternal lift, S3 with mid-diastolic rumble, widely split P2	LV dilatation, LA dilatation, marked leaflet prolapse	Cardiomegaly, LA enlargement	LVH, atrial fibrillation
Acute	Decrescendo murmur, S4 gallop, accentuated P2, parasternal lift	Hyperdynamic LV, LA pulsation, flail leaflet or vegetations	Pulmonary congestion	Not helpful

ECG, electrocardiogram: LA, left atrium; LV, left ventricle; LVH, RVH, left and right ventricular hypertrophy; OS, opening snap; S1, S2, S3, S4, first, second, third, and fourth heart sounds; A2, P2, aortic and pulmonary components of the second heart sound.

the lesion and its effects on the heart. Specific signs indicate the severity of each major valvular lesion as detected by physical exam and laboratory study (Table 1.8–1).

AORTIC STENOSIS

Obstruction to left ventricular outflow is most common at the aortic valve itself, but can also occur above (supravalvular) or below (subvalvular) the aortic valve. Valvular aortic stenosis is usually caused by congenital abnormality of the aortic valve or, in older patients, by calcification of a normal valve. Rheumatic heart disease is a rarer cause, and rheumatic aortic stenosis without mitral stenosis is exceptional. Subvalvular aortic stenosis is a congenital lesion in which a discrete fibrous membrane or tunnel causes obstruction. In patients with familial hypertrophic cardiomyopathy, a pressure gradient may be recorded between the apex of the left ventricle and the area just beneath the aortic valve, but this results from rapid emptying of the ventricle, rather than from any obstruction to ejection (Chapter 1.7). Supravalvular aortic stenosis is also a congenital lesion. It is seen rarely in adult patients, occasionally is familial, and is more usually associated with a characteristic facies (Williams syndrome) that is also seen in the hypercalcemia syndrome of infancy.

Clinical Features

Congenital aortic valve disease in adult patients is usually in the form of a bicuspid valve and produces left ventricular outflow obstruction during two different age periods. Patients with valves that are stenotic from birth usually come to medical attention in childhood or adolescence because of a heart murmur or symptoms of left ventricular outflow obstruction. Such congenitally stenotic valves may show signs of progressive narrowing with age and may need surgical relief of their outflow obstruction in early adult life. A second and larger group of patients with congenitally malformed valves have no outflow tract obstruction in early life. Examination shows a systolic ejection murmur preceded by an ejection sound, or sometimes a diastolic murmur, along with normal carotid pulses. Eventually, often only in the sixth or seventh decade, these patients may develop aortic stenosis from progressive valve calcification. When patients present with aortic stenosis after age 70, the cause is usually calcification of a normal, three-cusped aortic valve. In either case, the important point is that older adults with aortic stenosis get into trouble because of calcification of the valve; absence of valve calcification is evidence against severe aortic obstruction.

Patients tolerate even severe left ventricular outflow obstruction for long periods without symptoms. Left ventricular systolic pressure is increased, and the myocardium becomes hypertrophied as a result. Ultimately, the hypertrophy may alter diastolic function so that pulmonary congestion develops, or the pressure work demanded of the ventricle may outstrip its capacity for hypertrophy. In either case, many patients with aortic stenosis have breathlessness caused by pulmonary congestion as their first symptom. Angina pectoris is also a common symptom, even in the absence of left ventricular dysfunction or coronary atherosclerosis, because left ventricular stroke work and muscle mass are increased, whereas coronary perfusion pressure may diminish with increasing valve obstruction. Since most patients with aortic stenosis are elderly, they may have coexisting coronary artery disease that may contribute to angina or symptoms of left ventricular dysfunction. The third cardinal symptom of aortic stenosis is syncope, usually on exertion. The underlying mechanism may be inability to augment cardiac output because of fixed outflow obstruction or even a reflex-induced fall in cardiac output. In some patients, the cause of syncope is cardiac arrhythmias, either ventricular arrhythmias or heart block. After symptoms develop, progression to more severe symptoms or even sudden death is usually rapid; without surgical treatment, many patients die within 1 year. Sudden death is unlikely to occur before other symptoms, however. Even the mildest symptoms in patients with aortic stenosis demand prompt investigation of its severity.

The severity of aortic stenosis may be accurately assessed at the bedside by proper description and interpretation of the physical findings. The key is the character of the arterial pulse. In severe disease, the carotid pulse is retarded in upstroke and small in volume (pulsus parvus et tardus), and a thrill can be appreciated. In young patients, the systolic pressure and pulse pressure are reduced. In older patients with coexistent sclerosis of large vessels, these arterial signs may not be prominent; the pulse pressure may be wide, the systolic pressure high, and the pulses bounding. Usually, the careful examiner can recognize some degree of retardation of the carotid upstroke. The murmur of aortic stenosis begins after the first heart sound and ends before the second sound. It is an "ejection" or "diamond-shaped" systolic murmur, which means that it rises in crescendo to a peak and then falls off in late systole. This "shape" of the murmur parallels the timing of turbulence produced by blood flow across the stenotic orifice. Typically, the murmur is best heard at the base of the heart and radiates upward into the carotid vessels. However, it is often well appreciated at the cardiac apex, and it is the shape of the murmur, not its location or radiation, that distinguishes it from mitral regurgitation. The character is usually harsh or rasping, but it may be blowing or even musical (Gallavardin murmur), and its quality may be different at the apex than beside the sternum. The intensity of the systolic murmur does not correlate well with severity of the lesion, but the timing of the murmur is helpful in determining its severity. As obstruction becomes more severe, ejection is prolonged and the peak intensity occurs later in systole. The murmur still ends short of the second heart sound and continues to maintain its diamond shape.

Young patients with congenital aortic stenosis have a prominent ejection sound and a loud aortic component of the second heart sound (A_2). An ejection sound occurs immediately after the first heart sound at the moment of doming of the fused aortic leaflets. This is not the case in older adults with calcific aortic disease: Ejection sounds are not heard, and the aortic second sound is absent. A well-maintained A_2 suggests valve mobility and is a strong point against a diagnosis of severe aortic stenosis in older patients. Left ventricular hypertrophy, usually obvious by palpation or indicated by ECG or echocardiogram, suggests severe disease.

The chest x-ray may show cardiomegaly, as well as aortic root enlargement from poststenotic dilatation. Aortic valve calcification is best seen on lateral or oblique projections. The echocardiogram provides the most help in assessing this disorder. The clinician can assess hypertrophy, dilatation, and function of the left ventricle and can see the aortic valve in motion, while looking for mobility, thickness, and calcification of the leaflets. The finding of mobile leaflets without evidence of major thickening is strong evidence against significant aortic stenosis in older patients.

Left ventricular outflow obstruction implies a systolic pressure gradient between the left ventricle and the aorta (Figure 1.8–1). Measuring this gradient, either by catheterization or by Doppler echocardiography, provides an indication of the severity of obstruction. However, the gradient very much depends on the volume of flow through the stenotic orifice. Thus, low stroke volume may be associated with only a small gradient, even in severe aortic stenosis. Only by combining measurements of gradient and stroke volume is it possible to estimate aortic valve orifice area. Catheterization data give the best estimates of aortic valve area, but the abnormal flow velocities recorded by Doppler echocardiography may be extrapolated to give a remarkably accurate estimate of valve area as well. The Doppler technique becomes unreliable only at the extremes of high and low aortic valve flow rates. Rarely is catheterization needed to quantitate severity; usually it is done to check for coronary artery disease in patients who have been referred for surgery.

Treatment

There is little justification for medical therapy for a patient with symptomatic aortic stenosis. Symptoms indicate that left ventricular outflow obstruction is severe and surgery is indicated. In children with mobile, noncalcified valves, a prosthesis is undesirable, and commissurotomy may relieve obstruction sufficiently. In adults, when the valve is calcified, it must be replaced with a prosthesis. Coronary artery disease, left ventricular dysfunction, or other valvular lesions are reasons to proceed quickly to valve surgery because the extra work imposed by aortic stenosis is less well tolerated when these conditions coexist.

Asymptomatic patients without severe left ventricular hypertrophy should be followed carefully, using serial ECGs to monitor for the appearance of left ventricular hypertrophy and periodic echocardiography. Some patients develop evidence of severe outflow obstruction and worsening left ventricular hypertrophy even before they develop symptoms; if these patients are in middle life, otherwise well, and have gradients over about 70 mm Hg, it is prudent to recommend valve replacement surgery. Their operative risk is good, and the prostheses used for valve replacement are effective and extremely durable.

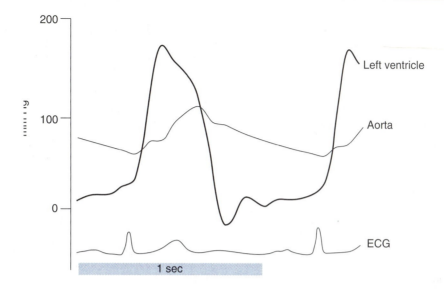

Figure 1.8–1. Pressure tracings recorded at catheterization in a patient with severe aortic valve stenosis. There is a pressure gradient of 80 mm Hg between the left ventricle and aorta during ejection. The tracing also shows the striking retardation of the aortic pressure upstroke that would have been appreciated by feeling the carotid pulse.

The most difficult clinical decisions involve patients with aortic stenosis who are over the age of 80 or 90 years. As the population lives longer, more patients develop aortic disease at later ages, so this problem has become increasingly common. Generally, if the patient's overall medical situation suggests a reasonable likelihood of surviving several years and if the patient accepts the disability and discomfort of surgery, valve replacement should be offered.

AORTIC REGURGITATION

Aortic regurgitation may be caused by diseases affecting the aortic valve leaflets (eg, rheumatic heart disease), supporting structures in the aortic root above the valve (eg, aortic aneurysm), or supporting structures below the valve (high ventricular septal defect; Table 1.8–2).

Chronic Aortic Regurgitation

Understanding the pathophysiology of aortic reflux allows accurate bedside assessment of the severity of the lesion. In chronic aortic regurgitation, left ventricular stroke volume is increased, since cardiac output is maintained despite the volume of flow that refluxes and the left ventricle is correspondingly dilated. The size of the left ventricle, determined by palpation, chest x-ray, or echocardiography, is a guide to the severity of the volume load. Systolic pressure is increased because of the large stroke volume, but patients have reduced peripheral resistance. Aortic diastolic pressure falls in proportion to the severity of the backward diastolic leak, and the pulse pressure is therefore wide. In most cases of severe aortic re-

gurgitation, systolic pressure exceeds 140 mm Hg and diastolic pressure is less than 60 mm Hg. These effects on the circulation are responsible for the hyperkinetic circulatory signs that are so characteristic of this disorder. The peripheral arteries have a collapsing quality because of the rapid upstroke and quick diastolic runoff, whereas the more central carotid pulse is of full volume, with brisk upstroke. The carotid or brachial pulse may have a bifid character, so that the examiner feels a double systolic impulse (pulsus bisferiens). These findings in the peripheral circulation are so characteristic that their absence is evidence against a severe valvular leak.

Aortic regurgitation causes a number of murmurs. Most typical is the high-frequency decrescendo early-diastolic

Table 1.8–2. Causes of aortic regurgitation.

Disease of the aortic valve
  Rheumatic disease
  Congenital deformity
  Infective endocarditis
  Rupture, spontaneous or traumatic
Disease of the aortic root
  Syphilis
  Dissecting aneurysm
  Cystic medial necrosis (Marfan's syndrome)
  Inflammatory disease
    Rheumatoid spondylitis
    Reiter's syndrome
    Relapsing polychondritis
    Giant cell aortitis
    Takayasu's disease
Disease of subvalvular structures
  Aneurysm of the sinus of Valsalva
  High ventricular septal defect
  Discrete, membranous subaortic stenosis

murmur indicative of the aortic reflux itself. This murmur is usually blowing in character, best heard at the base of the heart or along the left sternal edge, and it begins at the time of A_2. The high stroke volume causes turbulence in the outflow area and a systolic ejection murmur even in the absence of aortic obstruction. In severe aortic regurgitation, there may be a low-frequency late- or mid-diastolic rumbling murmur, heard at the apex, with a quality similar to the murmur of mitral stenosis. This murmur, described by Austin Flint in the 19th century, is caused by turbulence from antegrade flow across the mitral leaflets, which are being closed by a rapid rise in left ventricular diastolic pressure caused by the severe aortic reflux.

The echocardiogram is particularly useful in aortic regurgitation. It gives quantitative information about the severity of the volume load by determining the size of the left ventricle. It describes the effects of the volume load on left ventricular pump function. It depicts the pathologic condition of the aortic valve or root that is responsible for the problem. Color-flow imaging with the Doppler technique provides a map of the area of reflux, but has proved to be disappointing as a quantitative tool in this disorder.

Patients tolerate even severe aortic regurgitation for long periods and maintain normal exercise capacity. Symptoms of pulmonary congestion occur when the aortic reflux is overwhelming even to a normal left ventricle or when the left ventricle is impaired and unable to handle the volume load. Left ventricular disease may result from the longstanding volume load or, as occurs more frequently, from previous damage to the ventricle or associated coronary artery disease. As with aortic stenosis, once symptoms appear, the progression to more severe symptoms and death is usually rapid and little affected by medical therapy. Therefore, aortic valve replacement should be recommended for patients at the first sign of symptoms.

The dilemma of when to recommend surgery for the asymptomatic patient with severe aortic regurgitation is one of the more difficult in cardiology, because intervention too early may deny the patient many symptom-free years without a prosthetic valve and anticoagulation, while delaying valve surgery too long may result in irrevocable left ventricular dilatation and dysfunction. Generally, surgery should be considered before symptoms appear once the signs indicate severe regurgitation and the left ventricle is markedly enlarged on x-ray or by echocardiography (> 7.0-cm diastolic dimension) or when there is evidence of left ventricular dysfunction. Surgery is also advisable in asymptomatic patients when aortic root disease is responsible for aortic reflux, as in Marfan's syndrome, when the diameter of the aorta as determined by echocardiography reaches 5.5 cm.

Acute Aortic Regurgitation

Patients with acute aortic valve disruption behave differently from those with chronic aortic regurgitation. Acute aortic regurgitation is most often the consequence of infective endocarditis; the other causes are dissecting aneurysm, chest trauma, or spontaneous rupture of a cusp. In acute aortic regurgitation, the left ventricle has not had time to become dilated. Reflux into a small ventricular chamber causes a very high ventricular diastolic pressure, often as high as 60–70 mm Hg. The aortic diastolic pressure must be at least as high, but the systolic pressure may not be increased and the pulse pressure is likely to be narrow. The characteristic signs of a hyperkinetic circulation are therefore missing. The mitral valve closes early in diastole, because the ventricular filling pressure increases rapidly and comes to exceed left atrial pressure before the onset of ventricular systole. The first heart sound is therefore absent or soft. The aortic diastolic murmur may be low in frequency and soft in intensity, and may end in mid-diastole as aortic and left ventricular pressure equalize.

Because the mitral valve maintains competence, the high diastolic pressure in the left ventricle may not be reflected in the pulmonary circulation, and a few patients appear deceptively well. Others develop severe pulmonary congestion, and some show signs of multiorgan failure as a result of inadequate cardiac output. The echocardiogram reveals premature closure of the mitral valve in mid-diastole and may show disruption of the aortic cusp or a prolapsing vegetation. Surgery is mandatory and should be done promptly, since delay while the patient is given additional medical therapy may allow further deterioration of the hemodynamic state, or systemic embolization.

MITRAL STENOSIS

Pathology and Natural History

In adult patients, the only known cause of mitral stenosis is rheumatic heart disease. Nevertheless, only 50% of patients can recall an attack of acute rheumatic fever in childhood; presumably in the others, rheumatic fever, often a subtle disease, has been subclinical. After the initial acute rheumatic valvulitis and with the passage sometimes of many years, characteristic fusion of the mitral commissures develops. This is followed by fibrosis and ultimately calcification of the leaflets. The subvalvular apparatus is also affected, with fusion and shortening of the chordae tendineae and papillary muscle heads. These changes in the tensor apparatus lead to a second level of obstruction to left ventricular inflow below the orifice of the valve. The reason why valvular obstruction progresses in the years after the initial immunologic insult is either persistent low-grade rheumatic activity or, more commonly, continuous hemodynamic stress to a diseased valve in the form of abnormal turbulence of flow across it. Thus, obstruction may be progressive in spite of adequate prophylaxis against recurrent streptococcal infection. With the virtual elimination of rheumatic fever in many industrialized countries, mitral stenosis has become a rare disorder, but it remains common in the developing world, where poor living conditions and streptococcal infection are widespread. In the latter countries, mitral stenosis is often symptomatic in adolescence or early adulthood, typically when the circulation is subjected to some extra hemodynamic stress, such as pregnancy or extreme exertion. Pulmonary edema and hemoptysis are common early presenting manifestations. In Western society, mitral stenosis has become a disease of the elderly. Many patients first become aware of the problem in their 60's and 70's, and their complaints are less dramatic than those of younger patients. Symptoms related to low cardiac output predominate.

As the mitral orifice narrows, left atrial pressure rises and causes the most common symptom of mitral stenosis—dyspnea on exertion. This may begin acutely, but more frequently the dyspnea develops insidiously and is slowly progressive. When mitral obstruction becomes more severe, cardiac output does not increase in response to demands, giving rise to fatigue. Fatigue may develop so gradually that patients do not realize that their activities have become restricted, and sometimes only in retrospect, after surgical correction, do they recognize how limited they had been. Longstanding left atrial hypertension causes left atrial enlargement and atrial arrhythmias, particularly atrial fibrillation, which further impairs cardiac output. The enlarged fibrillating atrium is a site for mural thrombosis, which may cause systemic embolism. In some patients with severe left atrial hypertension, the pulmonary arteries constrict to produce "reactive" pulmonary hypertension. Such patients may show predominant signs and symptoms of right-sided heart failure early in their course.

Some patients respond to elevated pulmonary venous pressure with bronchospasm, so that asthmatic features may dominate the presentation. Patients with mitral stenosis are particularly susceptible to bronchopulmonary infection and often develop chronic bronchitis and emphysema. Lung disease may obscure the physical signs of mitral stenosis and delay recognition of the valvular lesion as the cause of dyspnea and fluid retention.

Diagnosis

Mitral stenosis is diagnosed by recognizing the characteristic physical findings. The arterial pulses are not abnormal, but the rhythm is often that of atrial fibrillation. The jugular pulse may show signs associated with pulmonary hypertension—a prominent "a" wave caused by increased diastolic pressure in the right ventricle, or a systolic wave reflecting tricuspid regurgitation. The left ventricle is typically quiet to palpation and may be obscured by an enlarged right ventricle that produces a parasternal heave or lift. On auscultation, the first heart sound is accentuated because the mitral leaflets close in systole only after the left ventricular pressure has equaled the high left atrial pressure. The pulmonic component of the second heart sound is increased when there is pulmonary hypertension. The second sound is followed by an opening snap of the fibrotic, mobile mitral valve, a sign that disappears as older patients develop valve calcification. This is fol-

lowed by the characteristic mid-diastolic rumble that leads into a presystolic crescendo rumble in late diastole, usually as a result of atrial systole. The mitral diastolic rumble is difficult to hear because of its low frequency and low intensity. It is best heard with the patient rolled into the left lateral position with the bell of the stethoscope lightly applied to the cardiac apex or beyond, in the axilla.

Assessing the severity of mitral stenosis begins with the understanding that the lesion predominantly affects the lungs and the right side of the heart. Furthermore, dyspnea, generally a good guide to the severity of valvular disease, may be misleading in mitral stenosis. Patients with mild obstruction may develop severe pulmonary congestion during stress or a paroxysm of rapid atrial fibrillation, whereas some patients with severe reactive pulmonary hypertension may be protected from pulmonary congestion and complain only of fatigue, caused by low cardiac output. Signs of pulmonary hypertension on physical examination or chest x-ray or signs of right ventricular hypertrophy by electrocardiography always indicate that the mitral stenosis is severe.

The chest x-ray is invaluable in this setting (Figure 1.8–2). Besides showing overall heart size and left and right atrial enlargement, it shows the severity of pulmonary venous hypertension, ranging from mild degrees characterized by redistribution of pulmonary venous flow patterns to the upper lobes, to more severe forms indicated by Kerley B lines. These thin horizontal lines, seen at the lung bases, suggest that pulmonary venous pressure is

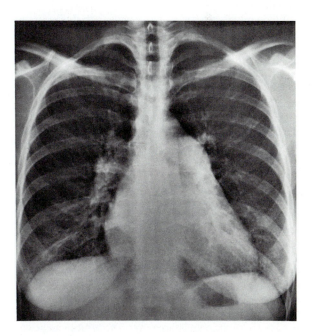

Figure 1.8–2. Chest x-ray of a patient with mitral stenosis, showing enlargement of the left atrium and pulmonary artery and redistribution of blood flow to the upper lobes.

25 mm Hg or higher. The diagnosis of mitral stenosis can always be established by echocardiography. This technique allows characterization of the degree of leaflet thickening, immobilization, and altered motion, all typical of this disorder. Doppler measurement of inflow velocities in the left ventricle may be used to estimate mitral valve gradient and area, but these numbers may not accurately reflect the severity of the whole lesion, especially in patients with extensive subvalvular disease, and they add little to the clinical assessment of disease severity. The echocardiogram shows any other valvular lesions and allows estimation of left atrial size and right ventricular pressure.

Signs of mitral stenosis can be subtle. There are several situations in which mitral stenosis should be looked for carefully:

1. Unexplained pulmonary hypertension
2. Recurrent atrial fibrillation
3. Systemic embolization
4. Asthma with atypical features
5. Chronic obstructive pulmonary disease in which dyspnea is out of proportion to the objective evidence of lung disease
6. Unexplained pulmonary or systemic congestion

It is also important to recognize that the clinical findings of mitral stenosis may be mimicked by other conditions, such as atrial myxoma, atrial septal defect, and even constrictive pericarditis.

Treatment

When mitral stenosis is severe enough to cause loss of exercise capacity or pulmonary hypertension, mechanical enlargement of the mitral orifice is indicated. Atrial fibrillation usually heralds progression of symptoms. Some patients can maintain good functional capacity while the heart is in sinus rhythm, but deteriorate markedly when atrial systole is lost. In such patients, maintaining sinus rhythm with antiarrhythmic drugs may postpone surgical therapy. Patients with atrial fibrillation usually require digoxin to control the ventricular rate, and anticoagulant therapy is mandatory to prevent embolism from the left atrium.

Mitral valve replacement is the surgical procedure of choice for symptomatic older patients with mitral stenosis, since the valves are fibrotic and calcified and cannot be surgically repaired. In younger patients, if the valve leaflets are mobile, the orifice can be enlarged by splitting the fused commissures of the leaflets. The surgeon can do this with the patient on cardiopulmonary bypass under direct vision (open commissurotomy) or, while the heart is beating, using a dilator introduced through the apex of the left ventricle, guided by a finger in the left atrial appendage (closed commissurotomy). The orifice can be enlarged without surgery using inflatable balloons on catheters inserted percutaneously (valvuloplasty). Commissurotomy and valvuloplasty have the advantage of leaving patients with their native valve. Good results may be maintained for 20 or more years after successful surgical commissurotomy. The longevity of balloon valvuloplasty is not yet known.

MITRAL REGURGITATION

Effective closing of the mitral valve requires the interaction of each of the components of the mitral apparatus—the leaflets, chordae tendineae, papillary muscles, anulus, and left ventricular myocardium. Diseases affecting any of these structures may lead to mitral regurgitation. There are several common causes of mitral regurgitation (Table 1.8–3).

Natural History and Diagnosis

Mitral Valve Prolapse: The most common valvular cause of mitral regurgitation is myxomatous change in the leaflets. This lesion, which is also called mitral valve prolapse, or "floppy" mitral valve, can be caused by a generalized connective tissue disorder such as Marfan's syndrome, but occurs most commonly as an isolated abnormality. The mitral regurgitation associated with this lesion is usually mild and nonprogressive. The floppy leaflets produce systolic clicks as they balloon backward into the left atrium, and they allow a small degree of mitral reflux, which results in a characteristic late systolic crescendo murmur. The clicks and murmur vary with position, respiration, and time of day. Sometimes prolapse occurs in mitral valves whose leaflets have minimal if any intrinsic structural abnormality, as a consequence of disproportion between the size of the ventricular cavity and the mitral orifice. This occurs particularly in young patients who are hyper-responsive to endogenous sympathetic stimulation. This hyper-responsiveness leads to palpitations and cardiac awareness, effort intolerance, light-headedness, and sometimes a variety of types of chest pain.

In most patients, mitral valve prolapse pursues a benign course. Some patients are helped by β-blockers. The combination of a mitral valve click or murmur, with quasicardiologic symptoms, is called the mitral valve prolapse syndrome, or sometimes Barlow's syndrome.

Table 1.8–3. Causes of mitral regurgitation.

Mitral valve prolapse (myxomatous degeneration, "floppy" valve)
Rheumatic disease
Ruptured chordae tendineae
Valve perforation or loss of substance (infective endocarditis)
Papillary muscle dysfunction or rupture (ischemic heart disease)
Calcification of the mitral anulus
Dilated or hypertrophic cardiomyopathy
Congenital heart disease
   Endocardial cushion defect
   Corrected transposition of the great vessels
   Anomalous origin of left coronary artery from pulmonary artery
    (Bland-Garland-White syndrome)

Rarely, patients with mitral valve prolapse develop progressive mitral regurgitation. This occurs because of dilatation of the mitral anulus or rupture of chordal structures. Such patients usually show more marked echocardiographic signs of pathologic conditions of the mitral leaflets, in the form of extreme degrees of prolapse and obvious tissue redundancy. Other rare complications in patients with pronounced myxomatous change are systemic emboli, infective endocarditis, and sudden cardiac death. It must be emphasized, however, that mitral prolapse is a common disorder, affecting up to 7% of the population, with a benign natural history in most cases, particularly those with prominent sympathetic manifestations and minor abnormalities on echocardiography.

Chronic Mitral Regurgitation: Of all valvular lesions, chronic mitral regurgitation is the best tolerated. The left ventricle and atrium enlarge gradually to accommodate the regurgitant volume load. Because the left ventricle ejects the extra volume load into a low-resistance chamber, the left atrium, the extra work imposed by the leak is only moderate, much less than the same degree of aortic regurgitation. Because the atrium can expand, pressure in the chamber may remain low even with a large volume of mitral regurgitation, so dyspnea comes late. Mitral regurgitation worsens if floppy leaflets deteriorate, if the anulus dilates, or as the left atrium enlarges and thereby retracts the posterior leaflet.

Patients with chronic mitral regurgitation pursue a slowly progressive course in which symptoms of fatigue and mild breathlessness wax and wane over many years. Signs and symptoms of pulmonary congestion may be lacking because of the compliance and size of the left atrium. Eventually, however, some patients develop low output and pulmonary hypertension, with striking cardiomegaly.

On physical examination, the left ventricular impulse is displaced and hyperkinetic in proportion to the size of the volume load. A parasternal impulse may occur when the enlarged left atrium impinges on the spine and pushes the heart forward as it swells during systole. The murmur of mitral regurgitation is pansystolic, beginning with the first sound and ending with the second, distinct from the ejection murmur of aortic stenosis. It is typically blowing and radiates laterally to the axilla, but may be harsh and radiate to the base of the heart. A third heart sound signifies rapid filling and is not necessarily a sign of ventricular disease. The third sound is usually followed by a rumbling mid-diastolic murmur, which indicates a large volume of flow during the rapid filling phase of diastole. Atrial fibrillation is common. The best clinical guide to severity is the size of the left ventricle, as determined by palpation, echocardiography, or chest x-ray.

Acute Mitral Regurgitation: Acute mitral regurgitation can be caused by infective endocarditis, spontaneous rupture of a chorda tendinea, or infarction of a papillary muscle head. When mitral regurgitation develops acutely, the left atrium cannot expand to accommodate the extra volume load, and left atrial pressure may rise precipitously to high levels even though the regurgitant volume may not be large; left atrial v waves may reach 60–70 mm Hg. Patients with acute mitral regurgitation rapidly develop pulmonary congestion and edema, and severe breathlessness. The heart size may be normal or only slightly enlarged, but the lungs show striking acute congestion on chest x-ray. In chronic mitral regurgitation, the heart is larger, but the lung fields are clearer (Figure 1.8–3).

The physical findings in acute mitral regurgitation also differ from the chronic counterpart. Because the left atrial v wave rises to such high levels of pressure in late systole, regurgitant volume decreases at this time. The murmur

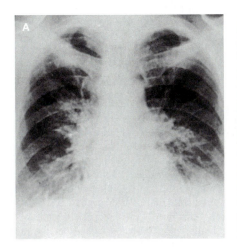 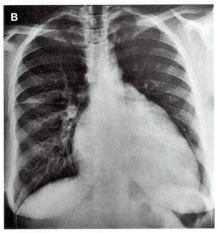

Figure 1.8–3. Chest x-rays in mitral regurgitation. **A:** Acute mitral regurgitation causes pulmonary edema, but the heart is only slightly enlarged. **B:** In the patient with chronic mitral regurgitation, the heart is severely enlarged, but the lung fields do not show acute congestion.

may therefore decrease in late systole, in a decrescendo that can easily be mistaken for the ejection murmur of aortic stenosis. This murmur can radiate toward the upper left sternal edge as a result of impingement of the regurgitant jet on the interatrial septum, and this can further confuse the issue. Because the regurgitant volume is not excessively large, a third sound and rumble may not be present; a fourth sound is often heard. The rhythm is that of sinus tachycardia.

The echocardiogram is useful for determining the pathologic condition of the mitral leaflets, assessing the severity of the volume load by measuring ventricular and left atrial dimensions, and evaluating left ventricular function. Color-flow mapping of the regurgitant velocities by the Doppler technique may be of some value in assessing the severity of the lesion, but is not to be relied on. Right heart catheterization demonstrates the large v waves in the wedge tracing and shows elevation of pulmonary pressure.

Treatment

Severe mitral regurgitation is treated with surgical replacement or repair of the mitral valve. Many patients with mitral regurgitation are candidates for repair of the mitral apparatus; this is particularly true of those with floppy mitral leaflets. The surgeon repairs the valve by resecting the redundant or unsupported parts of the leaflets and then reducing the size of the mitral anulus by suturing in an inelastic ring, to allow proper apposition and closure without leak. This operation has proved to be durable and does not deform the left ventricle by removing subvalvular tissue. If patients can maintain sinus rhythm, they need not receive anticoagulants. The success of valve repair procedures has prompted earlier surgical intervention in patients likely to be candidates, in order to preserve sinus rhythm and left atrial and ventricular architecture.

Replacement is required for severely damaged valves, but carries disadvantages, chiefly the need for anticoagulants. Removing the papillary muscles adversely affects left ventricular function, and mechanical prostheses do not permit as normal a pattern of filling as a well-repaired native valve.

TRICUSPID VALVE DISEASE

Tricuspid regurgitation is a common but infrequently recognized valvular lesion. It is detected at the bedside from the jugular venous pulse, which shows a prominent systolic wave. Severe lesions cause systolic pulsation of the liver. The murmur may be a typical pansystolic regurgitant murmur, but more commonly is truncated in late systole in a decrescendo. The murmur is often said to increase or become more pansystolic with inspiration because of augmented right heart return of blood, but this finding is often lacking, especially when right ventricular pressure is high. Sometimes there is no murmur. The most common cause of tricuspid regurgitation is pulmonary hypertension (Chapter 1.13), in turn the result of left heart disease or pulmonary vascular disease. Thus, tricuspid regurgitation can complicate left ventricular disease with pulmonary venous hypertension, mitral stenosis with pulmonary hypertension, cor pulmonale, or any other form of pulmonary vascular disease leading to pulmonary hypertension. Other causes, in which the right heart pressures are not increased, include congenital tricuspid valve disease, rheumatic heart disease, endocarditis, and carcinoid syndrome.

When right ventricular hypertension is the cause, the lesion is progressive: right ventricular dilatation begets tricuspid regurgitation, tricuspid regurgitation begets right ventricular dilatation, and overall cardiac function deteriorates. This is less the case when tricuspid regurgitation occurs with normal right ventricular pressure, such as when the tricuspid valve is damaged by endocarditis from intravenous drug abuse. In this setting, the lesion is well tolerated and does not lead to progressive cardiac dysfunction. The treatment of refractory endocarditis of the tricuspid valve is to remove it without inserting a prosthesis, and this is generally well tolerated.

Tricuspid stenosis is a rare lesion, most often seen as a consequence of rheumatic fever in association with mitral and aortic involvement. Tricuspid regurgitation or stenosis occurring without other valvular disease or developing later in life should immediately bring to mind a right atrial tumor or the carcinoid syndrome (Chapter 1.12). The features of these lesions are readily apparent on echocardiography. In the carcinoid syndrome, serotonin or possibly some other pharmacologically active tumor product causes fibrosis of the right heart valves. The source of serotonin is liver metastases of a malignant gastrointestinal carcinoid tumor. Patients characteristically show other humoral effects, such as flushing and diarrhea, but sometimes their cancer progresses so slowly that the cardiac effects predominate and they need tricuspid valve surgery as palliation.

ATRIAL TUMORS

Atrial tumors simulate valvular lesions by obstructing inflow to the left or right ventricle. They most commonly arise on the left side of the septum, to which they are attached with a stalk. This allows the tumor to move into the mitral orifice during diastole and obstruct left ventricular inflow. Movement of the tumor may result in fragmentation, leading to systemic emboli. Thus, the presentation is much like that of mitral stenosis, and so are the physical findings, a mid-diastolic rumble and an opening noise or "tumor plop." On the right side, the presentation is also that of inflow obstruction, manifested as neck vein distention and fluid retention. Echocardiography provides excellent images of these intracardiac masses. Surgical removal is curative.

MANAGEMENT

Medical Treatment

Most diseases of the valves produce their effects gradually over many years. First priority must be given to preventing events that accelerate the disease process, such as recurrence of acute rheumatic fever or an attack of infective endocarditis. Recurrences of rheumatic fever are prevented by giving continuous penicillin or sulfa treatment to protect against streptococcal infection, at least until age 40. All patients with valvular lesions should receive prophylaxis against bacterial endocarditis by the use of penicillin or other antibiotics at the time of dental procedures or other potentially contaminating surgery.

Chronic anticoagulant treatment is required for patients with mitral valve disease who are in atrial fibrillation; there is some risk of systemic embolism in patients with mitral stenosis even when their heart rhythm is regular, and many physicians recommend anticoagulant therapy even before atrial fibrillation develops. Other medical treatments include digitalis, used to control the ventricular response in atrial fibrillation and as a positive inotropic agent, and diuretics for fluid retention. In patients with chronic mitral valve disease, progression of symptoms after atrial fibrillation can be postponed by electrical cardioversion and maintaining sinus rhythm with antiarrhythmic drugs.

Surgical Treatment

In general, mechanical problems, such as valvular lesions that cause symptoms or cardiac malfunction, should be treated by mechanical means, that is, valve replacement or repair. In most instances, the patient tells the physician when valve surgery is needed, not directly, but by describing symptoms. It is a mistake to treat symptoms with medications or reassurance for too long. Repair or replacement of cardiac valves has had a major effect in improving the natural history of valvular heart disease. Durable prosthetic devices of excellent hemodynamic design are available for valve replacement, and patients who have surgery have a mortality rate of less than 5%. However, prosthetic valves all have a finite life span and their own complications, and heart surgery continues to carry a certain unavoidable rate of morbidity and mortality. The physician's dilemma about when to recommend valve surgery is compounded by the facts that the minimally diseased native valve may serve the patient better and longer than the best prosthetic device, while the earlier the operation, the lower the operative risk. Intervention too early may deny the patient many years of active life without a valve prosthesis, whereas waiting too long may result in irreversible damage to myocardium or pulmonary vasculature. Left ventricular disease, other valvular lesions, or coronary artery disease is usually reason to proceed earlier to surgery, even though operative risk is higher.

The physician should play an active role with the patient and cardiac surgeon in deciding what type of operative procedure or valve prosthesis is to be used. Repair of a valve is always preferred because the patient's own native valve may function effectively for many years without risk from anticoagulant therapy or other adverse effects associated with prostheses. Valve prostheses made from artificial materials—pyrolytic carbon and metal—have functioned for more than 20 years and thus have proven longevity. Patients with these prostheses in place must take anticoagulant therapy lifelong to avoid thrombosis and embolism. Prostheses made from biologic materials—porcine or human—simulate the normal human valve more closely than those made from artificial materials and do not require instituting anticoagulant measures. However, these valves have a much shorter life expectancy, some failing within 10 years and most by 15 years.

For a middle-aged patient in whom anticoagulant therapy carries only slight risk, artificial mechanical prostheses are often preferred, whereas tissue valves find their main use in patients for whom anticoagulant therapy presents special problems. Such patients include women who plan pregnancy, those whose occupation or recreation puts them at risk of injury, travelers or unreliable patients, and the elderly, for whom the limited life expectancy of a tissue valve is acceptable, given their risk from falls or cerebrovascular accidents while on anticoagulants.

Complications of Prosthetic Valves

Modern prosthetic valves are remarkably free of complications. Most patients live normal lives and are unaware of the prosthesis. However, the following complications may occur.

Thromboembolism: With prostheses used since the 1980's, the incidence of thromboembolism is low, but the complication has not been eliminated. Emboli usually occur because the patient has not maintained an adequate level of anticoagulation (INR [international normalized ratio] of 2.5–3.5). Occasionally, when embolism occurs despite adequate anticoagulation levels, the patient needs an additional platelet-inhibiting agent such as aspirin, ticlopidine, or dipyridamole.

Infection: A foreign body within the circulation is an inevitable target for blood-borne infection. For this reason, patients should be given prophylactic antibiotics during any dental or surgical procedure. Infective endocarditis on a prosthetic valve is a dreaded complication, carrying a mortality rate of more than 25% (Chapter 8.6). Infections acquired soon after surgery are caused by organisms such as *Staphylococcus aureus* and *S epidermidis*, *Candida*, and gram-negative bacteria. They affect the prosthetic valve sewing ring and are difficult to eradicate by antibiotic therapy alone. Because the mortality rate for prosthetic valve endocarditis, which occurs early in the postoperative period, is above 50%, reoperation should be considered early in the course of the infection. Endocarditis occurring more than 3 months postoperatively can sometimes be cured with antibiotic therapy alone, but left ventricular failure, systemic emboli, conduction disturbance, valve dehiscence, or persisting fever or bacteremia during treatment demands surgical removal of the infected prosthesis.

Prosthesis Malfunction: Malfunction of mechanical prosthetic valves is unusual, but may result from thrombus formation (because of inadequate anticoagulation), tissue ingrowth into the prosthetic orifice leading to obstruction, mechanical disruption of the valve struts or disc, or leaks around suture lines (paravalvular leak) or actual dehiscence of the prosthesis. Over their life span of 10–15 years, bioprostheses develop thickening, calcification, and ultimately obstruction or retraction of the leaflets. Malfunction of a prosthetic valve may be sudden, presenting as acute pulmonary edema and low-output state, or it may evolve gradually over months or years. It should be suspected when a patient manifests any of the following:

- Alteration of the timing or quality of opening or closing sounds
- Development of a new regurgitant murmur
- Embolization in the presence of adequate anticoagulant therapy
- Increased severity of intravascular hemolysis
- Development of heart failure or angina after a period of improvement
- Syncope

Recognition of malfunctioning prostheses may by helped by echocardiography and Doppler evaluation of valve function, but some cases escape detection by these techniques. Management is surgical, and patients with acute presentation survive only with immediate surgery. Occasional patients with thrombosed valves who are not good surgical risks may be treated successfully by thrombolytic agents, but with a risk of systemic embolism.

Hemolytic Anemia: The red blood cell survival time is shortened in all patients with prosthetic valves because of battering and destruction of cells by the intravascular foreign body. The hemolysis is usually mild and readily compensated for by increased red cell production. In the unusual patient in whom hemolysis is severe enough to cause anemia, there is generally prosthesis dysfunction or a leak; such patients may need reoperation. Chronic intravascular hemolysis results in urinary iron loss in the form of hemosiderin, and iron deficiency may eventually develop.

SUMMARY

▶ The type and severity of most valvular lesions can be determined by the physical examination, assisted by echocardiography.

▶ The natural history of valvular lesions differs: mitral lesions pursue a slow course after onset of symptoms, whereas aortic lesions progress rapidly, often to death.

▶ Aortic stenosis is the commonest valvular lesion in the elderly; the only successful treatment is surgery, which is well tolerated even by octogenarians.

▶ In aortic regurgitation, it is important to determine the cause, since disease of the aortic root that causes reflux is managed differently from disease of the valve leaflets.

▶ Mitral stenosis is predominantly a disorder of the pulmonary circulation, and its major manifestations will be found there. In industrialized countries, the course is more chronic than in the developing world.

▶ Mitral regurgitation is the best tolerated of all valvular lesions because of the low-impedance circuit (the left atrium) that some of the left ventricular stroke empties into.

▶ When cardiac dysfunction becomes manifest as a result of valvular heart disease, there is little place for medical management. Mechanical problems demand mechanical solutions, namely, valve surgery.

SUGGESTED READING

Baxley WA: Aortic valve disease. Curr Opin Cardiol 1994;9:152.

Oakley CM, Burckhardt D: Optimal timing of surgery for chronic mitral or aortic regurgitation. J Heart Valve Dis 1993;2:223.

Palacios IF: Percutaneous mitral balloon valvotomy for patients with mitral stenosis. Curr Opin Cardiol 1994;9:164.

Pellikka PA et al: The natural history of adults with asymptomatic, hemodynamically significant aortic stenosis. J Am Coll Cardiol 1990;15:1012.

Roberts WC: Morphologic aspects of cardiac valve dysfunction. Am Heart J 1992;123:1610.

Syncope and Cardiac Arrhythmias

Thomas Guarnieri, MD

The three symptoms of cardiac arrhythmia are syncope, palpitations, and light-headedness. Syncope means brief loss of consciousness caused by an abrupt fall in cerebral perfusion pressure. It has several causes besides arrhythmias, particularly fainting, orthostatic hypotension, and sudden severe ventricular dysfunction, as might be seen in aortic stenosis or left main coronary artery disease. Syncope does not include epileptic seizure, the chief other cause of sudden temporary unconsciousness (Chapter 13.3). Although fainting and other benign conditions are more common, arrhythmias are of special concern as a cause of syncope, because of the possibility that they can presage sudden death. Thus, in approaching a patient with syncope as the chief complaint, the physician's concerns are to determine whether the cause is benign, whether there is underlying heart disease, and whether a dangerous arrhythmia has to be considered. When arrhythmias are suspected, further evaluation is essential. This may entail no more than simple electrocardiographic monitoring when a patient has frequent spells. Sometimes, however, attacks are infrequent, and the electrocardiogram (ECG) between episodes contains no clues. Then the patient may need additional studies including electrophysiologic testing in the catheterization laboratory.

Palpitation means awareness of the heart's beating irregularly, rapidly, or unusually forcefully within the chest. It is something that most people experience from time to time, usually in response to exercise, excitement, or too much caffeine. The physician must first determine whether the sensation is caused by an arrhythmia or simply by awareness of forceful contractions, as might occur in anxiety or excitement. Usually, the history is the key, but occasionally help can be supplied by the results of continuous ECG recording, using a Holter monitor.

Light-headedness is an important symptom in a patient with palpitation, since it implies that an arrhythmia is sufficiently serious to cause hypotension. In a patient with episodic loss of consciousness, a history of light-headed spells implies that the attacks have variable severity. This symptom thus points to a circulatory cause in contrast to the all-or-none quality of seizures. Light-headedness is

often a difficult symptom to interpret. The key is to distinguish it from vertigo (both may be called "dizziness") or other symptoms of vestibular or brain-stem dysfunction, such as diplopia (Chapter 13.3).

Many rhythm disturbances do not cause concern on the patient's part, but are discovered on a routine ECG or during monitoring. Some of these need treatment, but it is important to recognize that the threat posed by any rhythm disturbance depends very much on its context. Premature ventricular contractions, for example, occurring in the first hours after myocardial infarction, may presage ventricular fibrillation. Exactly the same rhythm disturbance in a healthy young adult should generally be ignored. Antiarrhythmic drugs have side effects, including the potential for causing further rhythm disturbances, and it is important to resist the temptation to overtreat without regard for clinical context.

This chapter deals with three problems: how to assess a patient who has had syncope, how to assess palpitations, and how to manage arrhythmias identified on an ECG tracing. Wolff-Parkinson-White syndrome and the long QT syndromes, conditions that cause syncope and have specific ECG manifestations, overlap these headings; they are discussed in "Arrhythmias," the ECG-based section.

SYNCOPE

The three main categories of sudden loss of consciousness are syncope, seizures, and transient cerebral ischemic attacks (Table 1.9–1). Metabolic causes, such as hypoglycemia, and rare sleep disorders like narcolepsy seldom cause diagnostic confusion in this setting. Syncope is distinguished from the others by its abruptness, comparable to that of a seizure, but without sustained seizure activity or a postictal state of confusion or paralysis. Many patients with syncope have some brief involuntary clonic movements, but they do not report tongue biting or incontinence. Pallor, sweating, and piloerection—signs of sympathetic discharge—imply hypotension and point to syncope, as does a report of flushing as the patient recov-

Table 1.9–1. Episodic loss of consciousness.

	Syncope	Seizure	Transient Cerebral Ischemic Attack
Onset	Often abrupt, but may have warning	Aura, but unconsciousness abrupt	Abrupt
Prompt waking	Yes	Postictal state	Slow waking
Seizure	No	Yes	No (seizure implies irritation; think of meningitis, abscess)
Pallor	Yes	No	No
Hyperemic flush	Yes	No	No
Associated symptoms	No	Aura	Other cerebral symptoms usual

ers. This flush is caused by reactive hyperemia following skin ischemia and implies a brief severe drop in cardiac output. Transient cerebral ischemic attacks rarely cause loss of consciousness without also causing some other transient and more focal neurologic disturbance.

Causes of recurrent syncope range from orthostatic hypotension and vasomotor depression (the basis of the simple faint) through other reflex mechanisms to arrhythmias, both fast and slow, and certain primary cardiac diseases: aortic stenosis, hypertrophic cardiomyopathy, left main coronary artery disease, and severe pulmonary hypertension (Table 1.9–2). A single syncopal spell may be the first sign of myocardial infarction, pulmonary embolism, or aortic dissection. Distinguishing the cause depends entirely on the history from the patient and any witnesses; additional tests have a low yield, at least until the category of disease has been identified. Questions should be directed to whether the blackouts are abrupt or gradual, whether they have an all-or-none quality, and whether the patient also experiences milder spells in the form of dizzy attacks. Precipitating factors are important, such as exercise, change in posture, or physiologic actions (micturition, coughing, hyperventilation).

Differential Diagnosis of Syncope

Vasodepressor Syncope: The most common cause of transient loss of consciousness is the vasodepressor reflex, which is the basis of the simple faint. The effects of faint-

Table 1.9–2. Causes of recurrent syncope.

Vasodepressor syncope (fainting)
Orthostatic hypotension
Tachyarrhythmia
   Ventricular tachycardia, supraventricular tachycardia
   Ventricular fibrillation
Bradyarrhythmia
   Sick sinus syndrome
   Atrioventricular block
Carotid sinus syncope
Micturition syncope
Tussive syncope
Deglutition syncope
Aortic stenosis
Hypertrophic cardiomyopathy
Left main coronary artery disease
Pulmonary hypertension

ing are better understood than its mechanisms; in response to unpleasant stimulation or reduced venous return, patients develop abrupt circulatory depression, with bradycardia and severe hypotension. They are pale, have vasoconstriction, and often are profusely sweaty. The key to clinical diagnosis is identification of the unpleasant stimulus or the finding of bradycardia, since most other causes of hypotensive collapse cause tachycardia. Hypotension in a patient with cutaneous vasoconstriction results from massive muscle bed dilatation. The efferent pathways for this vasodepressor response are from the vasomotor center of the medulla via the vagus and the autonomic innervation of the vasculature. The afferent mechanisms are complex and not completely understood. The reflex is stimulated by reduced venous return or painful or noxious stimulation. Blood donation combines these in a particularly effective fashion. The threshold varies greatly from person to person and is influenced by cortical factors; by other sources of vagal stimulation, particularly hunger and nausea; and by other sources of general discomfort such as a hot stuffy room. Other common situations involve prolonged immobility while standing upright (eg, on parade on a hot day, or assisting in the operating room), or interrupted venous return in pregnancy.

Fainting can be studied experimentally using lower-body negative pressure chambers that lower venous return, reduce left ventricular end-systolic cavity size, and trigger the reflex in normal people as well as those who are particularly susceptible to fainting. In those who have a tendency to faint, it can be unmasked by testing on a tilt-table. The tilt-table affords a way of moving a patient to an upright position without allowing an increase in venous return via the skeletal muscle pump. There is a growing sense that the afferent arc of the vasodepressor reflex originates in the ventricular myocardium and that the basic peripheral mechanism is excessive left ventricular emptying at end-systole. This may be relevant to the mechanism of syncope in patients with left ventricular hypertrophy.

In some susceptible patients, an unusual sensitivity to fainting is a cause of recurrent syncope. Adult patients with this problem may have a history of fainting frequently during childhood and teen-age years or a history of having a low threshold for feeling faint or queasy during injections. Because sympathetic stimulation probably plays a role in causing the excessive left ventricular emptying that precipitates an attack, β-blockade may afford excellent relief; this is despite the fact that the final event may involve bradycardia.

Orthostatic Hypotension: Orthostatic hypotension is a very common cause of dizzy spells, but in only a few patients is it severe enough to cause syncope. This diagnosis should be considered in anyone with suggestive symptoms and can be checked simply by taking the blood pressure while the patient is supine and then again while standing. Absolute boundaries for changes in blood pressure with posture are difficult to define, but falls of more than 15% are abnormal. Patients who are hypovolemic have orthostatic hypotension from the moment they stand, but patients with autonomic neuropathy may take some time before the blood pressure falls to its nadir; therefore, it is important to take the blood pressure sev-eral times over the course of 5 minutes after the patient stands up.

In older patients, especially those with diabetes, mild autonomic neuropathy is common and may be easily aggravated by diuretic treatment, by medications prescribed for hypertension, or by tricyclic antidepressants. Severe autonomic neuropathy, sometimes with a central basis (Shy-Drager syndrome), is less common, but can occasionally be crippling. Treatment involves maintaining intravascular volume with supplemental synthetic mineralocorticoid, and elastic stockings to shore up venous return during postural shifts.

Other Reflex Mechanisms: Four other—less common—causes of syncope related to circulatory reflex mechanisms are carotid sinus syncope, micturition syncope, tussive (cough) syncope, and deglutition syncope.

Carotid sinus syncope occurs when mechanical stimulation of the carotid sinus baroreceptors, for example, by a stiff collar or rotation of the neck, causes hypotension accompanied by profound sinus bradycardia or arrest. Usually, this hypersensitivity of the baroreflex is at the efferent end. If the history is suggestive, as in syncope while backing up the car or while wearing an especially unyielding collar, the symptoms can often be reproduced with carotid sinus pressure, similar to that used to treat an arrhythmia. Carotid pressure should be done cautiously because susceptible persons may have pauses of several seconds after firm pressure. Treatment with a pacemaker is usually effective, except in patients whose blood pressure falls even when the rhythm is maintained. Carotid sinus hypersensitivity can be seen after radical neck dissection or from a cancer in the neck or at the jugular foramen—settings in which treatment is difficult.

Micturition syncope occurs almost exclusively in men and follows emptying the bladder. The usual circumstances occur at night when awakening with an uncomfortably full bladder (hence, often with a contribution from prostatic hypertrophy). Bladder stretching causes either heightened sympathetic tone or stimulation of vagal afferent nerves, and its sudden release may be accompanied by a sharp fall in blood pressure. For most patients, the problem is infrequent, and they can take steps to avoid it.

Tussive syncope occurs when a paroxysm of coughing causes a sufficiently prolonged Valsalva maneuver to cause hypotension. Susceptible patients are those with chronic bronchitis and left ventricular hypertrophy. Usually, all that is required to prevent extended coughing paroxysms is to avoid irritants, particularly cigarette smoke.

Exertional Syncope: There are five common causes of exertional syncope: aortic stenosis, hypertrophic cardiomyopathy, left main coronary artery disease, severe pulmonary hypertension, and, especially in adolescents, cardiac arrhythmia. The first two causes should present no diagnostic problem because of their characteristic physical findings (Chapters 1.7 and 1.8). Left main coronary artery disease occasionally presents with exertional syncope as its only symptom, but more commonly causes angina or episodes of exertional light-headedness. Once the diagnosis of exertional syncope has been suspected, it can be confirmed with a treadmill test, performed under appropriate supervision. Pulmonary hypertension should be considered in a young patient with fatigue, effort intolerance, and exertional light-headedness and syncope and can be confirmed with the exam, ECG, and echocardiogram. Exercise-induced arrhythmias, sometimes in the setting of cardiomyopathy, Wolff-Parkinson-White syndrome, or congenital long QT syndrome, are an uncommon cause of exertional syncope and should be considered when there is no more obvious explanation, especially in children.

Cardiac Arrhythmia as a Cause of Syncope: When arrhythmias cause syncope, either fast or slow, loss of consciousness is usually sudden. The patient may be apneic and so cyanotic that witnesses may (appropriately) begin cardiopulmonary resuscitation, and it is always worth asking whether, even for a moment, they thought the patient was dead. Injuries, especially to the face, imply that a person was unconscious before falling.

Paroxysmal bradycardia is a common cause of syncope, particularly in elderly patients with conduction disorders. Syncope in a patient with complete heart block is called a *Stokes-Adams attack*. It is usually caused by ventricular standstill (asystole) or less often by ventricular tachycardia. A typical patient might complain of recurrent syncope and dizzy spells and prove on examination to have bradycardia, with a rate of 45 beats per minute. The ECG would confirm the clinical suspicion of complete heart block, and the patient would be admitted urgently for implantation of an artificial pacemaker.

The other main cause of bradycardia sufficient to cause syncope is sick sinus syndrome (see below). This term covers several types of abnormal sinoatrial pathologic conditions and can cause asystole when sinus arrest is compounded by a failure of the atrioventricular (AV) node to function as the backup pacemaker. This carries a much better prognosis than AV block. When symptomatic, it too is treated by pacemaker.

Paroxysmal ventricular tachycardia can cause spells of

unconsciousness identical to the Stokes-Adams attacks caused by complete heart block. Almost always this is in the setting of significant structural heart disease—anything from myocarditis to a left ventricular aneurysm. Patients with normal myocardium and valves may tolerate ventricular tachycardia at heart rates as high as 200 per minute, but the same rhythm at a rate of only 140 per minute may be disastrous to a patient with coronary artery disease and left ventricular dysfunction. Patients with ventricular tachycardia may complain of palpitations, but they often do not. It may be exceedingly difficult to distinguish Stokes-Adams attacks caused by intermittent heart block from syncope caused by ventricular tachycardia without either recording the ECG during a spell or reproducing an attack in the electrophysiology laboratory.

PALPITATIONS

The three causes of palpitations are awareness of sinus rhythm that is accelerated or more forceful because of a change in autonomic tone; an irregular rhythm caused by ectopic beats; and awareness of a tachyarrhythmia, for example, paroxysmal supraventricular tachycardia. Distinguishing these depends primarily on the history—continuous ECG monitoring with a Holter monitor or event recorder is of only limited help. It is usually easy to sort out when a patient's complaint of palpitation refers to the episodic skip or thump caused by ectopic beats. It may be difficult to separate palpitation caused by sinus tachycardia from paroxysmal arrhythmia. The crucial difference is the onset and offset, that is, whether the accelerated heart rate begins and ends suddenly, as in a tachyarrhythmia, or gradually, as in accelerated sinus mechanism. The offset may be more informative than the onset, since awareness is often sudden even when the fast heart rate is not. Thus, the most important question may be, "Did the palpitation settle down gradually, or did it just stop suddenly like turning a switch?" Questions are also directed to whether the rhythm was regular or irregular, and how fast it seemed to be. The patient is invited to tap out the rate and rhythm. Patients sometimes report a sensation of pounding in the neck, and this symptom, caused by atrial contraction against a closed tricuspid valve, is usually evidence of a paroxysmal AV nodal reentry tachycardia.

Paroxysmal supraventricular tachycardia sometimes causes polyuria, presumably through release of atrial natriuretic peptide. When patients report this somewhat unlikely symptom, the diagnosis of paroxysmal tachycardia is almost a certainty.

ARRHYTHMIAS

Identifying the nature of an arrhythmia from an ECG tracing is generally straightforward, based as it is on the simple logic of identifying and relating the P waves and the QRS complexes. The usual source of difficulty is in-

adequate data, and it is important whenever possible to record the onset, the offset, and the full 12-lead ECG during an arrhythmia. There are four steps in the diagnosis of any arrhythmia:

1. Identify the ventricular rate and place the arrhythmia in one of three basic categories: bradycardia, tachycardia, or extrasystoles.
2. Extract all the information possible from the QRS complex. A narrow QRS, less than 120 msec in duration, implies that the ventricles are activated synchronously through the normal conduction system. The rhythm is supraventricular. If the QRS is wide, it may be difficult to determine whether the complex is supraventricular or ventricular in origin (see "Ventricular Tachycardia" below).
3. Seek out all the P waves. This is vital for correctly identifying atrial tachycardia and flutter. Either of these rhythms can be accompanied by a ventricular rate slower than the atrial rate. If all the P waves are not detected, these rhythms may be mistaken for sinus rhythm.
4. Identify which P wave is related to which QRS. This step is critical for identifying the type of heart block.

Ectopic Beats

The simplest abnormal rhythm is the ectopic beat. The expressions "premature atrial contraction" and "premature ventricular contraction" refer to single beats arising from below the sinus node, coming sooner than the next sinus beat would have. Premature atrial contractions often reset the sinus pacemaker, so that the interval between them and the next, normally arising beat is the same as the usual RR interval. Premature ventricular contractions seldom reset the sinus pacemaker, and therefore are often followed by a longer pause, so that two cardiac cycles elapse between the last normal beat and the next. This long interval is referred to as a *compensatory pause*.

Distinguishing premature atrial contractions from premature ventricular contractions is usually straightforward; atrial beats are initiated by a P wave that is usually a little different from the P wave in sinus rhythm, reflecting a different origin in the atria. Atrial beats usually have a narrow (<100 msec) QRS complex, since the activation spreads through the normal pathways to the ventricles, whereas ventricular beats always have a wide QRS complex that looks like bundle branch block. Atrial ectopic beats can have a wide complex if the patient has bundle branch block, or sometimes when an impulse is so premature that it arrives at the bundle of His when either bundle branch is still refractory. This phenomenon is known as *aberrant conduction* (Figure 1.9–1). Sometimes an atrial ectopic beat can be so premature as to find the entire AV junction refractory, in which case it may not be conducted to the ventricles at all. It is described as "blocked."

Not all beats that arise outside the sinus node are premature. An escape beat occurs when for some reason impulse generation or conduction is slowed and a secondary

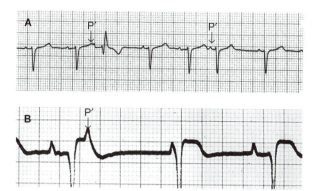

Figure 1.9–1. Atrial ectopic beats (P′) showing aberrant conduction **(A)** and block **(B)** (see text).

pacemaker with intrinsic rhythmicity takes over. Thus, if sinus arrest occurs, there is commonly a nodal escape beat, characterized by having an inverted P wave, or even an escape rhythm.

Bradycardia

Sinus Bradycardia: Sinus bradycardia, defined as a sinus rhythm (inferred from a normal P-wave vector) of less than 60 beats per minute, is not necessarily pathologic. Sinus bradycardia may be present during sleep or in conditioned athletes and is especially common in elderly patients. When it is not part of normal variation, the usual cause is cardioactive medications such as sympathetic blocking agents and antiarrhythmic drugs. Sinus bradycardia may accompany hypothyroidism, hypothermia, or increases in intracranial pressure. The two primary causes are the vasodepressor reflex (see "Vasodepressor Syncope" above), and the sick sinus syndrome.

Sick Sinus Syndrome: The sick sinus syndrome encompasses a variety of disorders of sinus node and atrial function. It may be defined by sinoatrial arrest with resultant asystole, inappropriate sinus bradycardia, variations of sinoatrial block, and asystole following an episode of either atrial fibrillation or atrial tachycardia (tachycardia/bradycardia syndrome). It is generally accompanied by diffuse dysfunction in the conducting system. Without involvement of the AV node, it is difficult for sick sinus syndrome to cause symptoms, because even with sinus arrest or bradycardia, a normal AV node has an intrinsic escape rate fast enough to prevent symptoms. The bradyarrhythmias of sick sinus syndrome carry a generally good prognosis. Sudden death is extremely uncommon; therefore, in patients who are not experiencing symptoms, pauses of a few seconds can be left untreated. When bradyarrhythmias in sick sinus syndrome do cause symptoms, artificial pacing is very effective.

One variant of the sick sinus syndrome is the tachycardia/bradycardia syndrome, seen in some elderly individuals who may have a rapid rate response during atrial fibrillation, yet have long pauses when they convert to sinus rhythm. It is often difficult to treat their tachyarrhythmias without at the same time aggravating their tendency to bradycardia, so pacemaker treatment is usually required in order to make drug treatment possible. The primary morbidity of this variant is the risk of stroke associated with atrial fibrillation (see "Atrial Fibrillation" below).

Junctional Rhythm: Most examples of junctional rhythm are secondary disorders; they occur because the sinus pacemaker has slowed or stopped, or because of AV block. When the junction takes over as a secondary pacemaker, the rhythm is described as an escape rhythm—just as a single escape beat is the first beat to end a protracted pause. The rate and ECG appearance of an escape rhythm depend on its origin: proximal AV junction rhythms have a narrow QRS complex and a rate of 40–60 per minute, and distal rhythms have a wide QRS complex and rates of 20–40 per minute.

The intrinsic junctional rate may accelerate to the point of taking over from the sinus node as the heart's pacemaker in patients with myocardial infarction, in digitalis toxicity, or as a primary phenomenon. Such a junctional pacemaker may or may not conduct retrograde to the atria. If it does, the result is an upside-down P wave often within or following the QRS. If it does not, the atria beat independently, at a slower rate, of course, and the P waves and QRS complexes reveal complete AV dissociation. If the sinus rate accelerates in its turn, it may take over again as the pacemaker for the whole heart, and normal AV conduction is restored. Occasionally, when the sinus rate and junctional rate are about equal, the two may alternate as pacemakers, and the appearance is referred to as *isorhythmic dissociation.*

Atrioventricular Block: AV block can occur at any level in the atrioventricular junction and is classified in three degrees of severity (Figure 1.9–2). First-degree AV block is characterized by slow AV conduction; each atrial beat is followed by a ventricular beat, but with a prolonged PR interval of greater than 0.20 second. The delay is generally in the AV node, above the level of the bundle of His, or in the atrium.

Second-degree AV block is defined by the conduction of only some of the atrial beats to the ventricles. It can occur at the level of the AV node, like first-degree block, or in the distal conducting system. The level of block markedly affects prognosis, and it is helpful to distinguish the two levels by their two ECG types: Mobitz type I and Mobitz type II. Mobitz I, generally corresponding to block at the level of the AV node, is characterized by Wenckebach's phenomenon of progressive lengthening of the AV interval. In Wenckebach block, the QRS complexes are usually normal, but follow the P waves by an interval that progressively increases until after a number of beats one P wave is not conducted to the ventricles. The pattern produced on the ECG is a characteristic group beating pat-

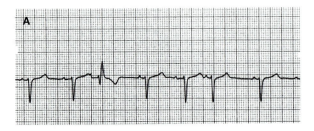

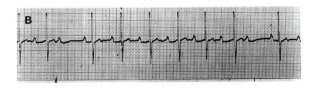

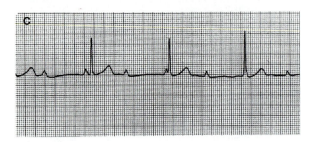

Figure 1.9–2. Atrioventricular block. **A:** First-degree block with prolonged PR interval. **B:** Mobitz type I second-degree block with Wenckebach phenomenon. **C:** Complete heart block.

tern, in which each cycle of beats has one more P wave than QRS. First-degree block and Mobitz I block are common. They may be seen in inferior infarction, acute myocarditis (eg, in viral, rheumatic, or Lyme disease), or as side effects of drugs. The usual offenders are digitalis, β-blockers, calcium channel blockers, and amiodarone.

Mobitz II AV block occurs when there is sudden and abrupt failure of one or more atrial impulses to reach the ventricle without previous prolongation of the PR interval. When more than one successive atrial impulse fails to be conducted, this is called *high-grade AV block.* Mobitz II is often associated with a wide QRS complex, and the site of block is generally distal. When the ratio of P waves to QRS complexes is 4:1 or 3:1, the diagnosis is straightforward, but sometimes every other QRS complex is blocked without changing PR or PP intervals. Such a 2:1 AV block can be either Mobitz type I or type II, and its level may be either in the AV node or in the distal conducting system. Distinguishing them depends on the type of QRS complex present and what other varieties of AV block are seen in the same patient or on the same ECG rhythm strip. A narrow QRS complex suggests AV nodal block, whereas a wide QRS complex suggests block below the bundle of His. When associated with Wenckebach block, the 2:1 conduction pattern is generally at the AV node. When the

2:1 pattern is permanent or associated elsewhere with the drop of two QRS complexes, it is generally in the distal conducting system.

Third-degree AV block is synonymous with complete heart block and implies that there is complete failure of impulse transmission from the atria to the ventricles. It is characterized by complete AV dissociation in which the ventricular rate is regular, uninfluenced by activity in the atria, and thus completely dependent on whatever intrinsic pacemaker tissue is fastest below the site of block. The level of block can be inferred from the width of the QRS complex. Congenital complete heart block occurs at the level of the AV node, and because the site of the block and the source of the escape rhythm are high, the QRS complex is narrow. The same is usually true of transient heart block after inferior myocardial infarction, or heart block in myocarditis. Most other patients with Mobitz II or complete heart block have diffuse conducting tissue disease; the QRS is wide, implying a pacemaker low in the ventricles, and the escape rate correspondingly slow.

Third-degree heart block is only one cause of AV dissociation. To diagnose it requires that the ventricular rate be slow and regular (thus uninfluenced from above), that the atrial rate be faster than the ventricular rate (thus capable of normal conduction), and that the atrial rate be physiologic (thus not a case of atrial tachycardia.)

Patients with chronic complete heart block, with a wide QRS and a slow ventricular escape rate, have a substantial likelihood of progressing to complete ventricular standstill, causing Stokes-Adams attacks or death. Untreated, their 1-year mortality rate is high, especially if they are already having blackouts; this is very different from the outlook in sick sinus syndrome with sinus pauses. Treatment with artificial pacemakers is simple, effective, and therefore very rewarding.

Tachycardia

The slow rhythms discussed in the previous few paragraphs are generally unambiguous on the ECG. Causes of tachycardia are not always so easy to identify (Table 1.9–3), and in some patients whose arrhythmia is so rapid as to cause hypotension and threaten cardiac arrest, it may be necessary to treat first and make a diagnosis second. In others, whose fast rhythm is tolerable for some time, the diagnosis is easy if the QRS is narrow and the P waves are easily identified, but becomes difficult in patients whose QRS complexes are wide, with a bundle branch block pattern, or whose P waves are difficult to find. A wide QRS complex is inevitable if the impulse arises in the ventricles and is thus always present in ventricular tachycardia. The difficulty in making the diagnosis stems from the fact that it sometimes occurs in patients whose arrhythmia arises at the AV node or above, if they have bundle branch block, or if they develop bundle branch block at high heart rates. This phenomenon, in which bundle branch block develops at increased heart rate, or when a single premature beat encounters a partially refractory AV junction, is referred to as *aberrant conduction,* or simply *aberrance.*

Table 1.9–3. Causes of tachycardia.

Diagnosis	Atrial Rate (/min)	Ventricular Rate (/min)	Clinical Setting	ECG Features	Vagal Stimulation
Sinus tachycardia	100–180	Same	Fever, anemia, pain, stress	Normal P waves, gradual onset and offset	Gradual slowing
Ectopic atrial tachycardia	110–200	Same	Isolated, or after myocarditis, stimulants	Regular but abnormal P-wave morphology	No effect
Ectopic atrial tachycardia with AV block	120–220	Fixed fraction of atrial rate	Digitalis	Regular P waves, 2:1 or 3:1 conduction	Further increase in block
Multifocal atrial tachycardia	>100	Same	COPD, theophylline	Multiple P-wave morphologies, variable PP and PR intervals	Slight, if any, slowing
Atrial flutter	220–320	Fixed fraction of atrial rate	LV dysfunction, mitral valve disease, hyperthyroidism, pulmonary embolism, pneumonia; isolated	Sawtooth P-wave pattern; regular QRS; 2:1, 4:1 conduction common	Increase in block; rarely terminates flutter
Atrial fibrillation	Not discernible	40–300		Random low amplitude atrial activity; irregular RR interval	Slows ventricular rate
Paroxysmal supraventricular tachycardia	120–220	Same	Isolated	Regular RR interval, QRS narrow or wide (aberrant); P waves inverted before, during, or after QRS	No effect or terminates (but does not slow)
Nonparoxysmal junctional tachycardia	70–120	Same	Digitalis, inferior myocardial infarction	QRS narrow; sometimes AV dissociation	No effect
Wolff-Parkinson-White syndrome	140–220	Same	Isolated	Regular RR interval, retrograde P waves follow QRS	No effect or terminates
Ventricular tachycardia	60–140	140–280	Acute ischemia, infarction, cardiomyopathy, aneurysm	Wide QRS, P waves often dissociated	No effect
Torsades de pointes	40–140	200–300	Long QT, quinidine	See Figure 1.9–5	No effect
Ventricular fibrillation		>300	Acute ischemia, anoxia, electrocution	Random electrical signal	No effect

AV, atrioventricular; COPD, chronic obstructive pulmonary disease; LV, left ventricular.

Supraventricular Tachycardia: Arrhythmias originating at or above the AV junction with a rate of more than 100 per minute can arise from several different mechanisms. Sinus tachycardia, in which the sinus rate exceeds this arbitrary criterion, under physiologic control, is invariably a sign of some other problem and should never be treated as if it is a primary abnormality to be controlled in its own right. Causes range from increased metabolic demand (eg, exercise, anemia, pregnancy, thyroid disease, fever) to impaired stroke volume (valvular or myocardial disease) to central increase in sympathetic tone (anxiety, excitement). Sinus tachycardia is distinguished from the various arrhythmias that cause supraventricular tachycardia by its gradual onset and offset, by the normal relation of P wave to QRS, and by its physiologic, small, moment-to-moment fluctuations in rate. In pathologic supraventricular tachycardia, other than atrial fibrillation, the ventricular rate is often extremely regular, since it is not subject to moment-to-moment variation in autonomic tone.

The common arrhythmias included in supraventricular tachycardia are ectopic atrial tachycardia, atrial flutter, atrial fibrillation, and paroxysmal supraventricular tachycardia, with or without the preexcitation syndrome.

Ectopic Atrial Tachycardia: Three forms of ectopic atrial tachycardia are encountered in clinical practice: ectopic atrial tachycardia, multifocal atrial tachycardia, and drug-induced atrial tachycardia (sometimes called paroxysmal atrial tachycardia) with or without AV block (Figure 1.9–3).

In ectopic atrial tachycardia, the heart rate is between 110 and 200 beats per minute and may be incessant. The cause is unknown, but this form of tachycardia is frequently seen as a sequela to myocarditis or rheumatic fever, being much more common in children and adolescents. It is characterized by an abnormal P-wave vector preceding each QRS complex. The abnormal P wave is consistent with the site of the tachycardia. There may be various degrees of AV block because of physiologic refractoriness of the AV node.

Multifocal atrial tachycardia is a common form of

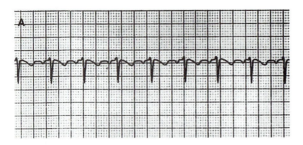

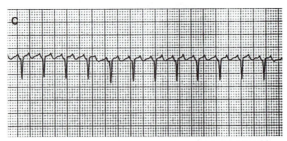

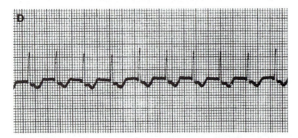

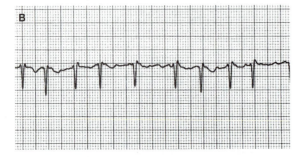

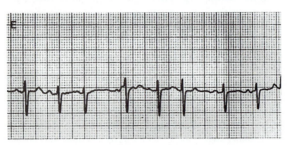

Figure 1.9–3. Supraventricular tachycardia. **A:** Sinus tachycardia. **B:** Atrial fibrillation. **C:** Atrial flutter. **D:** Paroxysmal supraventricular tachycardia (PSVT). **E:** Multifocal atrial tachycardia.

chaotic atrial tachycardia seen in seriously ill patients. It is characterized by a heart rate greater than 100 beats per minute and by at least three forms of P waves with varying PR intervals and RR intervals. Multifocal atrial tachycardia is differentiated from atrial flutter and fibrillation by discrete but chaotic-appearing P waves. It is commonly seen in patients with advanced heart or lung disease.

Drug-induced atrial tachycardia, typically caused by digitalis excess, combines the effects of increased atrial automaticity with block of the atrial impulse in the AV node: hence, the term paroxysmal atrial tachycardia with block. This is a poor term because this tachycardia is not paroxysmal and should not be confused with AV node reentrant tachycardia.

Atrial Flutter: Atrial flutter is a common supraventricular arrhythmia characterized by rapid but organized beating of the atria at a rate between 220 and 360 beats per minute, with the ventricular rate dependent on the refractoriness of the AV node. Atrial flutter produces a characteristic "saw-tooth" or flutter baseline that is best seen in the inferior leads. Carotid sinus massage frequently produces a decrease in the ventricular response rate because of increasing AV node refractoriness, but is very unlikely to terminate the underlying atrial arrhythmia.

Atrial flutter is generally associated with some form of organic heart disease, including myocarditis or coronary disease, but it is occasionally seen in healthy young persons. It is a common rhythm after open heart surgery and after correction of complex congenital heart disease.

Atrial Fibrillation: Atrial fibrillation is the most common of all sustained atrial arrhythmias and is said to be present in 3–4% of the population over the age of 70 years. Chronic atrial fibrillation is generally accompanied by organic heart disease, but can occur in people with no underlying cardiac or other cause. It is then referred to as "lone" atrial fibrillation. It is a common rhythm in patients who have distended atria from valvular heart disease (especially mitral) or ischemic heart disease, or who have had myocardial infarction. In the United States, long-standing, untreated hypertension is probably one of the most common risk factors for the arrhythmia. Atrial fibrillation is common in hyperthyroidism and may also occur in patients with fever or who have overwhelming systemic illness.

New unexplained atrial fibrillation may occur in otherwise normal healthy people, particularly in the context of recent imbibing ("holiday heart"), cocaine use, or even simple fatigue, but it may also be triggered by a pathologic condition within the thorax, particularly pneumonia, pulmonary embolism, or pericarditis. Most people who have an unexplained paroxysmal episode of atrial fibrillation have it only once. A few develop recurrent episodes and may need drug treatment to suppress attacks; some of these patients go on to have other kinds of sinoatrial disease, sometimes including bradycardia/tachycardia syndrome.

Atrial fibrillation is characterized by the absence of P waves and a chaotic, irregularly irregular ventricular rhythm. The irregularity reflects concealed conduction of the disorganized atrial impulses to the AV node. This concealed conduction may result in the ventricular response having a wide QRS complex, called the *Ashman phenomenon.* Ashman beats are frequently confused with premature ventricular beats. Aberrancy is present because the refractoriness of the right bundle is directly proportionate to the duration of the preceding RR interval. Therefore, a long RR cycle may increase the refractoriness of the right bundle, and thus the next conducted beat may be aberrant. Although there are no P waves, the fibrillatory activity of the atria can usually be identified as a low-amplitude vibration of the ECG baseline. Sometimes this can even be organized and resemble the waveform seen in flutter.

Besides the hemodynamic consequences of the rapid ventricular response, the irregular rhythm may pose another risk to the patient: stroke. This is largely related to the common occurrence of mural thrombosis in fibrillating atria, and evidence from long-term epidemiologic studies, including data from the Framingham study, suggests that the risk from stroke in patients with chronic atrial fibrillation is also related to other associated vascular disease. In either case, the evidence strongly points to the advisability of placing patients with chronic atrial fibrillation on anticoagulant therapy.

Paroxysmal Supraventricular Tachycardia: Paroxysmal supraventricular tachycardia (PSVT) is a common atrial arrhythmia. It may also be called paroxysmal junctional tachycardia, circus movement tachycardia, paroxysmal atrial tachycardia (PAT), or AV node reciprocating tachycardia. The mechanism of PSVT is either microreentry about the AV node (about 75% of cases) or macroreentry via a concealed accessory AV connection (about 15–20% of cases [see "Wolff-Parkinson-White Syndrome" below]). Both mechanisms produce a paroxysmal, narrow QRS complex tachycardia, and may be indistinguishable.

The ECG shows a narrow QRS complex tachycardia at a rate of 120–220 beats per minute. In AV node reentrant tachycardia, the P waves are retrograde, buried in the QRS complex, and not visible. In AV reciprocating tachycardia, on the basis of a concealed bypass tract, retrograde P waves are occasionally seen. In some patients with AV reciprocating tachycardia, the QRS axis shifts slightly from beat to beat, giving rise to electrical alternans. Aberrant conduction may occur if the rate is fast, and the arrhythmia may be difficult to distinguish from ventricular tachycardia (see "Ventricular Tachycardia" below). The classic response of PSVT to carotid massage or to a Valsalva maneuver is sudden cessation of the arrhythmia.

PSVT is a common arrhythmia, seen in otherwise healthy persons. It may complicate or be associated with other forms of heart disease, but is generally seen in healthy young people and may be a lifelong nuisance.

Nonparoxysmal Junctional Tachycardia: Nonparoxysmal AV nodal tachycardia is an automatic rhythm originating within the AV junction. The rhythm is recognized as a narrow QRS complex that is considerably slower than PSVT, generally 70–120 beats per minute. There may be retrograde capture of the atrium or, in many cases, AV dissociation. Depending on the site of the automaticity of the arrhythmia, the QRS complex may be either narrow or wide. Unlike PSVT, nonparoxysmal junctional tachycardia is not perturbed by sinus massage. Nonparoxysmal junctional tachycardia is seen most frequently after cardiac surgery but can also be caused by digitalis intoxication or myocardial infarction.

Wolff-Parkinson-White Syndrome: The Wolff-Parkinson-White syndrome is the prototype of the family of preexcitation syndromes, so called because the ventricle is preexcited through an accessory connection. This accessory connection takes the form of normal myocardium (as opposed to the specialized AV nodal fibers) crossing the fibrous separation between the atria and the ventricles. This bypass tract has two important consequences:

- It provides a pathway for AV macroreentrant tachycardia.

- It provides a pathway from the atrium to the ventricle that may bypass the physiologic refractoriness of the AV node, thus allowing for potentially rapid conduction of atrial impulses to the ventricle.

The Wolff-Parkinson-White syndrome produces a characteristic ECG with a short PR interval and a slurred QRS complex (the delta wave; Figure 1.9–4). These two features result from the initial forces of the QRS undergoing preexcitation through the bypass tract. This characteristic ECG is the basis for diagnosis of the Wolff-Parkinson-White syndrome; diagnosis does not depend on any particular type of arrhythmia. In fact, most individuals with this electrocardiographic abnormality are asymptomatic.

Two common arrhythmias are seen in the Wolff-Parkinson-White syndrome. The first is AV reciprocating tachycardia (one of the forms of PSVT). In this tachycardia, there is anterograde conduction over the AV node His-Purkinje system and retrograde reentry over the accessory pathway. In this form of tachycardia, the ECG pattern may be indistinguishable from that of the AV node reentrant tachycardias of PSVT. The second arrhythmia that patients with the Wolff-Parkinson-White syndrome may experience is atrial fibrillation or flutter. In these patients, there may be rapid conduction of the atrial impulses over the accessory pathway, producing a wide and bizarre QRS complex. Atrial fibrillation leading to ventricular fibrillation has been well documented in the Wolff-Parkinson-White syndrome. In some patients with atrial fibrillation, conduction may occur over both the accessory connection and the AV node, producing striking

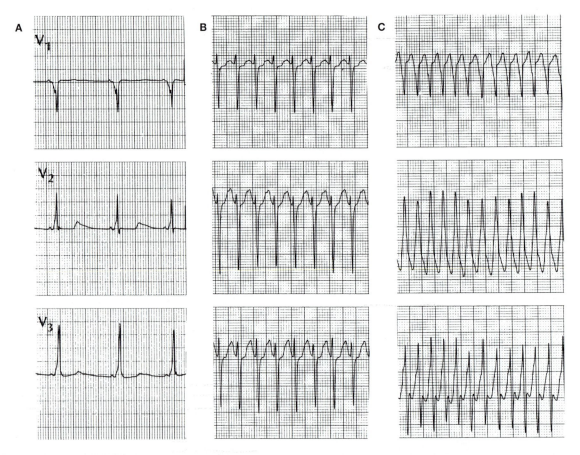

Figure 1.9–4. Wolff-Parkinson-White syndrome. **A:** Sinus rhythm with preexcitation (delta wave). **B:** AV reciprocating tachycardia. The normal QRS duration implies antegrade conduction through the bundle of His. The retrograde part of the reentry circuit is through the accessory pathway. **C:** Atrial fibrillation. The irregular wide QRS complexes result from conduction of atrial activity through the accessory pathway.

variations in the QRS complex. Preexcitation syndromes are generally seen in otherwise healthy persons, and atrial fibrillation in patients with the Wolff-Parkinson-White syndrome may constitute a life-threatening arrhythmia and require immediate treatment.

Treatment of Supraventricular Tachycardia

The approach to the patient with supraventricular tachycardia is predicated on the mechanism and the risk of syncope or stroke. All too often ambulatory recordings are described as displaying "supraventricular tachycardia," which is not a helpful description. For practical purposes, there are three structures generally involved in consideration of diagnosis and management: the atrium, the AV node, and accessory AV connections. It is only by consideration of all three that one can determine the mechanism and adopt appropriate treatment.

In those arrhythmias localized to the atrium (atrial fibrillation or flutter), consideration should be given to inciting factors, such as caffeine, hyperthyroidism, or alcohol

use. In many instances, simple correction of these factors will be sufficient to control the arrhythmia. Although there is little risk of syncope in atrial fibrillation, the clinician must weigh risk for stroke, especially age (>70 years) and underlying heart disease (valvular or hypertensive). In those patients with atrial fibrillation that is not amenable to standard pharmacologic therapy, warfarin should be given.

In general, patients with any of the forms of PSVT (including the Wolff-Parkinson-White syndrome) have unpredictable paroxysms of arrhythmia that appear unrelated to any inciting cause. In these patients, there is little or no risk of stroke, but there may be risk of syncope, especially in the Wolff-Parkinson-White syndrome. Pharmacologic therapy is directed to altering conduction properties of the AV node and the accessory tract. Most clinicians have regarded the AV node as the "weak link" in the reentry circuit and use agents that increase AV node refractoriness, that is, digitalis or β-blockers. In some patients with the Wolff-Parkinson-White syndrome, digitalis and verapamil may paradoxically enhance conduction throughout the bypass tract and thereby render these patients more vulnerable to the risk of rapid conduction of atrial fibrillation. Therefore, in patients with the Wolff-Parkinson-White syndrome, these drugs are used only when a detailed electrophysiologic assessment has been performed.

For young patients with recurrent PSVT, long-term drug treatment is onerous and undesirable. Several of the agents available can cause side effects, and many are contraindicated during pregnancy. The alternative is nonpharmacologic therapy in the form of catheter modification (generally using radiofrequency energy) of the AV node or accessory tract. This procedure has a high success rate, both for treatment of macroreentry through bypass tracts and for treatment of AV nodal reentry, and carries only a low risk of causing conduction block. For younger patients, it has become the treatment of choice.

Ventricular Tachycardia

When three or more ectopic beats arise from below the bundle of His, the abnormality is termed ventricular tachycardia. The rate is greater than 100 beats per minute and generally in the range of 130–200 beats per minute. The QRS complex may be monomorphic (having one form) or polymorphic. In most patients, AV dissociation is present but may not always be recognizable on the ECG. Ventricular tachycardia is usually associated with significant organic heart disease, particularly ischemic heart disease or cardiomyopathy. It may be seen with rheumatic heart disease, digitalis excess, or valvular heart disease. There are occasional patients with ventricular tachycardia who have no underlying organic heart disease. In these patients, the primary question is the risk of cardiac arrest.

All wide QRS tachycardias should be considered ventricular tachycardia until proven otherwise. It cannot be overemphasized that in a patient with a wide-complex tachycardia with a history that suggests organic heart disease, the diagnosis is almost always ventricular tachycardia. The ECG gives several clues to the differential diagnosis of wide-complex tachycardia, depending on whether the rhythm has a right or left bundle branch morphology (Table 1.9–4). Evidence for AV dissociation should be searched for in the physical examination (intermittent "cannon" waves in the jugular pulse, varying first heart sound) and on the ECG. However, absence of AV dissociation does not establish the diagnosis of supraventricular tachycardia, since AV dissociation can be demonstrated on the surface ECG in only about 25% of patients with ventricular tachycardia.

The approach to the patient with ventricular tachycardia is predicated on ventricular function. Most patients with no heart disease and short episodes of nonsustained ventricular tachycardia have little or no risk and require no treatment. Patients need treatment if they have significant heart disease, and present with sustained ventricular tachycardia, particularly with hypotension or syncope. In

Table 1.9–4. Distinguishing the causes of wide-complex tachycardia.

Clues	Ventricular Tachycardia	Supraventricular Tachycardia
History of myocardial infarction	Frequent	Infrequent
Atrioventricular dissociation	Frequent	None
Left bundle branch morphology		
Axis	Left superior	Left
V$_1$	r	R or S
V$_6$	q	R
QRS	≥0.16 sec	<0.16 sec
Right bundle branch morphology		
Axis	Left	Normal
V$_1$	R or RS	RSR
V$_6$	S>R	S<R
QRS	≥0.14 sec	<0.14 sec

V$_1$, V$_6$, precordial leads.

many cases, this may entail revascularization, antiarrhythmic drug treatment, or implantation of an antitachycardia device.

Patients with underlying heart disease who have nonsustained ventricular tachycardia are difficult to manage. In most cases, ventricular tachycardia is an adverse prognostic indicator, whether the underlying disease is ischemia, recent myocardial infarction, dilated cardiomyopathy, or hypertrophic cardiomyopathy. Treatment does not necessarily improve prognosis, however. In the case of myocardial infarction, a multicenter study known as CAST (Cardiac Arrhythmia Survival Study) showed that antiarrhythmic drugs could actually worsen prognosis for patients with myocardial infarction and asymptomatic ventricular arrhythmias.

Torsades de Pointes: Torsades de pointes is a particular form of ventricular tachycardia, defined by the very specific ECG appearance that gives it its name. It is considered distinct from the usual kind of ventricular tachycardia because in addition to its peculiar ECG morphology, the arrhythmia has special clinical associations and causes. The name torsades de pointes, taken from an old French expression for a certain kind of bell-pull, refers to a twisted strip of fabric; the ECG shows a pleomorphic ventricular tachycardia, with an axis that gradually shifts, so that in a recorded lead the QRS repeatedly inverts and then reverts to upright (Figure 1.9–5).

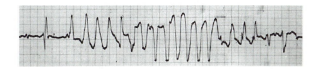

Figure 1.9–5. Torsades de pointes.

Table 1.9–5. Causes of a long QT interval.

Inherited
With hearing loss
Without hearing loss
Acquired
Drugs
Antiarrhythmic type Ia or III (rarely)
Phenothiazine, tricyclic antidepressants
Others: IV erythromycin, gemfibrozil
Electrolytes: hypokalemia, hypocalcemia, hypomagnesemia
Central nervous system: subarachnoid hemorrhage, trauma
Others
Bradycardia (atrioventricular block)
Myocarditis
Mitral valve prolapse

Torsades de pointes may occur as a short burst or may be sustained and induce cardiac arrest.

Torsades de pointes almost always occurs in patients whose resting ECGs show an extended QT interval, typically as long as 0.5–0.6 second. This long QT interval may be congenital or acquired. Congenital long QT interval occurs in the Romano-Ward syndrome, and in other rare mendelian syndromes. Acquired lengthening of the QT interval is much more common and is caused by electrolyte disturbances or drug side effects (Table 1.9–5). The most notorious drug in this regard is quinidine, which causes lengthening of the QT interval in all patients, occasionally to the extent of precipitating torsades de pointes, syncope, or fatal cardiac arrest. Other drugs in the same class of antiarrhythmic agents (type Ia group of drugs) can have the same effect; these include procainamide and disopyramide. Hypocalcemia and hypomagnesemia both cause lengthening of the QT interval and torsades de

pointes; although hypokalemia does not lengthen the QT, it does produce bizarre U waves and lowers the threshold to all cardiac arrhythmias, including torsades de pointes.

Ventricular Fibrillation: Ventricular fibrillation is a chaotic activity of the QRS complex. It is differentiated from ventricular tachycardia by its disorganization. It produces no effective cardiac output, and without immediate cardioversion results in death.

SUMMARY

▶ Syncope can be caused by fainting, other reflex mechanisms, arrhythmias (particularly bradycardia), left main coronary disease, and severe left ventricular hypertrophy.

▶ There are five common causes of exertional syncope: aortic stenosis, hypertrophic cardiomyopathy, left main coronary artery disease, severe pulmonary hypertension, and, especially in adolescents, cardiac arrhythmia.

▶ Chronic complete heart block has a bad prognosis without treatment and is managed with a pacemaker. Sinus pauses need pacing only if they cause symptoms.

▶ To diagnose an arrhythmia, identify (1) the ventricular rate, (2) the QRS duration and morphology, (3) *all* the P waves, and (4) which P wave is related to which QRS.

▶ Tachycardia with a wide QRS complex is usually ventricular tachycardia, rather than supraventricular tachycardia with aberrancy. If there is doubt, the former should always be assumed.

SUGGESTED READING

Almquist A et al: Provocation of bradycardia and hypotension by isoproterenol and upright posture in patients with unexplained syncope. N Engl J Med 1989;320:346.

Curran M et al: Locus heterogeneity of autosomal dominant long QT syndrome. J Clin Invest 1993;92:799.

Echt DS et al: Mortality and morbidity in patients receiving encainide, flecainide, or placebo: The Cardiac Arrhythmia Suppression Trial. N Engl J Med 1991;324:781.

Jackman WM et al: Treatment of supraventricular tachycardia due to atrioventricular nodal reentry, by radiofrequency catheter ablation of slow-pathway conduction. N Engl J Med 1992;327:313.

Jones G et al: A prospective randomized evaluation of implantable cardioverter-defibrillator size on unipolar defibrillation system efficacy. Circulation 1995;92:2540.

Pritchett ELC: Management of atrial fibrillation. N Engl J Med 1992;326:1264.

1.10

Pericardial Disease

James K. Porterfield, MD

Diseases of the pericardium—pericarditis, pericardial effusion, and the pericardial compressive syndromes—can easily be misdiagnosed, with serious consequences. Pericarditis, which is often benign and simple to treat, causes chest pain that can be taken for myocardial infarction or unstable angina. Pericardial tamponade, which can be relieved by pericardiocentesis, may present with cardiogenic shock, and is rapidly fatal if not treated promptly. Chronic pericardial constriction causes severe systemic venous congestion, comparable to the effects of restrictive cardiomyopathy (Chapter 1.7) and can be mistaken for myocardial disease or even for chronic liver disease. Constrictive pericarditis should be treated surgically by pericardiectomy, and the results are gratifying, provided the diagnosis is made promptly, before the pericardium adheres permanently to the epicardium.

In general, the approach to a patient with a pericardial disease parallels the approach to a patient with a disease of the pleura (Chapter 2.10). Pericarditis without an effusion is generally benign, like pleurisy, and can be treated symptomatically. When a patient has an unexplained effusion, the most straightforward diagnostic method is to take a sample for laboratory analysis, provided there is enough fluid. When the cause of a pericardial effusion is known, then the indications for aspirating it, or for some surgical drainage procedure, are mechanical and depend on signs of cardiac compression.

ACUTE PERICARDITIS

Patients with acute pericarditis present with characteristic chest pain, pericardial friction rub, and serial electrocardiographic changes. The most common causes of this syndrome are idiopathic or viral pericarditis, acute myocardial infarction, neoplasm, uremia, and pericardiotomy associated with cardiac surgery (Table 1.10–1). Most forms of acute pericarditis are self-limited, but it is nonetheless important to remember that this syndrome may represent the first or most prominent manifestation of a systemic illness, such as cancer or systemic lupus ery-

thematosus. Sometimes the first sign of pericarditis is a large effusion with tamponade, but usually the mechanical consequences of pericarditis follow the initial presentation.

History

The most common symptom of acute pericarditis is chest pain, typically retrosternal or left precordial, sometimes radiating to the neck, trapezius ridge, or even the back. Pericarditis pain tends to be more sharp or burning than angina and is often exacerbated by deep breathing, coughing, or lying supine. It is typically ameliorated by sitting up and leaning forward. The effect of breathing is like that in pleurisy; hence, the pain is often referred to as "pleuritic" chest pain to distinguish it from "ischemic" chest pain. Nonetheless, the features of pericardial pain can be difficult to distinguish from those of myocardial ischemia or infarction. Table 1.10–2 lists distinguishing features of these two important clinical syndromes, which share some historical and electrocardiographic features. Dyspnea may also be a manifestation of acute pericarditis, most often from restricted inspiratory effort caused by the accompanying chest pain. In a few patients, dyspnea is a direct consequence of cardiac tamponade or pulmonary parenchymal compression from a large pericardial effusion.

Physical Examination

The pathognomonic sign of acute pericarditis is the pericardial friction rub. This is a high-pitched scratching sound that is typically most intense at the lower left sternal border. Although generally attributed to friction between the inflamed pericardial and epicardial surfaces, a pericardial rub may also be heard in a large effusion, even though direct serosal contact is minimal. A pericardial friction rub characteristically has three components, caused by the rapid movements of the ventricles during atrial systole, ventricular systole, and rapid ventricular filling in early diastole. The ventricular systolic component is typically the most prominent part of the friction

Table 1.10–1. Causes of acute pericarditis.

Idiopathic
Infectious causes
   Viral: coxsackievirus, echovirus, HIV
   Purulent: *Staphylococcus aureus, Streptococcus pneumoniae,*
     Neisseria sp, Francisella tularensis
   Fungal: *Histoplasma, Candida, Aspergillus*
   Tuberculous: *Mycobacterium tuberculosis*
Cardiac causes
   Myocardial infarction
     Acute transmural myocardial infarction
     Dressler's syndrome
   After heart surgery (postpericardiotomy)
Neoplastic causes
   Breast cancer
   Lung cancer
   Lymphoma
Rheumatologic causes
   Systemic lupus erythematosus, Still's disease, rheumatoid
     arthritis, scleroderma
   Acute rheumatic fever
Uremia
Hypothyroidism
Drugs
   Procainamide
   Hydralazine
   Phenytoin
   Isoniazid
Radiation

rub; the early diastolic and atrial systolic components may fuse, producing a biphasic "to-and-fro" rub. Friction rubs are often evanescent and therefore heard only intermittently. It is helpful to examine the patient for a pericardial rub first with the breath held and then during quiet respiration, since the rub may be audible only during part of the respiratory cycle. It is important that the stethoscope be in good contact with the chest, to be sure that the noise of the rub is not being simulated by skin moving against the stethoscope.

Table 1.10–2. Distinguishing acute pericarditis from acute myocardial infarction.

	Pericarditis	**Myocardial Infarction**
Location of pain	Retrosternal	Retrosternal
Character of pain	Sharp	Unvarying pressure
Duration of pain	Hours to days	Hours
Thoracic movement	Pain increased by breathing	No effect
Posture	Pain aggravated by recumbency, lessened by leaning forward	No effect
ECG	ST elevation concave upward; T wave inverts late	ST elevation convex; T wave inverts before ST at baseline

Electrocardiogram

The cardiac rhythm in uncomplicated acute pericarditis is most often sinus rhythm, and the development of atrial fibrillation suggests underlying heart disease.

The electrocardiogram (ECG) goes through a characteristic series of stages during acute pericarditis. Recognizing these stages also helps to distinguish this syndrome from acute myocardial infarction. The ECG changes are thought to be the result of superficial myocardial inflammation or epicardial injury resulting in a current of injury. Initially, when chest pain begins, the ST segment is elevated, with a characteristic concave-upward ST segment, often in most or all of the leads that have predominant R waves (Figure 1.10–1). The diffuse nature of the ST segment elevation and the characteristic shape of the ST segment help to distinguish acute pericarditis from the ST-segment elevation associated with acute transmural myocardial infarction. Over the next few days, the ST segment returns to the isoelectric line, and the T waves become flattened. Eventually the T waves invert, but this does not happen until the ST segment has become isoelectric. In contrast, T-wave inversion often develops while the ST segments remain elevated in acute myocardial infarction. Finally, the T waves revert to normal, a change that may occur weeks or months following resolution of the acute illness. Rarely, T-wave inversion persists indefinitely, as in the patient with chronic tuberculous pericarditis. Depression of the PR segment, presumably as a consequence of atrial inflammation, is seen in 80% of patients with acute pericarditis.

ST elevation with a concave-upward contour is a common normal variant in young men, thought to be caused by early repolarization. It can look very like the changes of pericarditis, but it tends to be stable day after day and is most often confined to the precordial leads.

Treatment

Hospitalization is warranted for most patients with acute pericarditis, primarily for bed rest and observation to exclude myocardial infarction and to watch for the development of tamponade. The latter occurs in up to 15% of patients with acute pericarditis.

Treatment with a nonsteroidal anti-inflammatory agent such as aspirin or indomethacin usually alleviates the pain of acute pericarditis. Corticosteroids are generally effective for those patients whose pain is severe or does not respond well to a nonsteroidal anti-inflammatory agent. Anti-inflammatory therapy can be tapered after 5–7 days of treatment in patients whose pain is relieved. The rare patient who develops chronic pain can be given alternate-day corticosteroids. Pericardiectomy has been recommended for patients with refractory or relapsing pericarditis, but has variable success.

For the immunocompetent patient who has uncomplicated acute pericarditis, the diagnostic yield of pericardiocentesis or pericardial biopsy is low. Unless the patient needs relief of tamponade, these tests are recommended only when there is an urgent need to confirm a suspected diagnosis of purulent pericarditis.

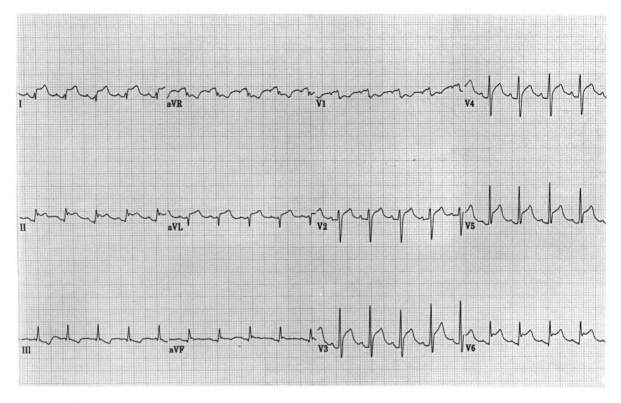

Figure 1.10–1. ECG in acute pericarditis showing ST elevation in almost all leads, with a characteristic concave upward shape. PR depression is seen in the precordial leads.

PERICARDIAL EFFUSION WITHOUT COMPRESSION

Presentation

The pericardial space normally contains 15–50 mL of fluid. Pericardial effusion may develop in response to inflammation or injury of the parietal pericardium. It may be clinically silent, or if intrapericardial pressure rises, it may compress the heart, ultimately causing cardiac tamponade. The rise in intrapericardial pressure depends not only on the size of the effusion, but also on the rate at which it accumulates. In addition, the physical properties of the pericardium, such as fibrosis, also influence the severity of cardiac compression. If fluid accumulates slowly and the pericardium is compliant, the pericardial sac can accommodate up to 2 L, accompanied by an increase in intrapericardial pressure from atmospheric to only the 15–20 mm Hg range. When accumulation is rapid, as for example when aortic dissection ruptures into the pericardial space, tamponade may develop with only 150–200 mL of fluid.

For diagnostic purposes, pericardial effusions may be divided into serous and hemorrhagic effusions. The most common cause of hemorrhagic pericardial effusion in Western countries is direct extension of a local tumor. The other causes of pericardial effusion are all the diseases that can cause pericarditis (see Table 1.10–1).

Patients with pericardial effusion and no elevation in intrapericardial pressure may be asymptomatic. Large effusions cause fatigue and symptoms of limited cardiac output, or symptoms caused by compression of adjacent structures. For example, dysphagia may result from esophageal compression, or epigastric fullness may occur as a result of pressure on abdominal viscera.

Many small pericardial effusions produce no physical signs, but large effusions lead to a number of typical findings. Heart sounds may be soft or distant because of the muffling effect of the pericardial fluid. Rales may be noted over the left lower lung from compression of adjacent lung tissue, and sometimes a focal area of dullness may be appreciated beneath the angle of the left scapula (Ewart's sign).

Laboratory Studies

The chest x-ray may suggest pericardial effusion if there is a rapid increase in the size of the cardiac silhouette without associated pulmonary venous congestion. The cardiac silhouette has an unusually sharp edge (because it is motionless) and may have the characteristic shape described as a "water bottle" configuration, with a broad diaphragmatic surface and narrow upper mediastinum. Magnetic resonance imaging (MRI) not only identifies effusions, but also distinguishes hemorrhagic from serous effusions and can delineate pericardial thickening or masses.

Electrocardiographic changes in pericardial effusion are nonspecific and include reduction in QRS voltage and T-wave flattening. Electrical alternans can accompany a large pericardial effusion and suggests the risk of tamponade.

The echocardiogram is the most useful technique for evaluating pericardial effusion. The distinct acoustic difference between myocardium, pericardial fluid, and the pericardial membrane results in an echo-free space between the myocardium and the pericardium (Figure 1.10–2). Although quantification of pericardial effusion by echocardiography is imprecise, clinically useful indices to estimate size of an effusion have been developed. Very small effusions typically are seen only posteriorly, with separation of epicardium and pericardium only during systole. Moderate-sized effusions can be imaged both anteriorly and posteriorly, with an echo-free space persisting throughout the cardiac cycle. Large effusions are associated with an exaggerated swinging motion of the heart.

Treatment

The management of pericardial effusion depends on the intrapericardial pressure and whether there is evidence of a systemic disease. Pericardiocentesis is indicated when there is evidence of tamponade or when it is important for diagnosis, perhaps to establish the presence of an associated process such as tumor growth.

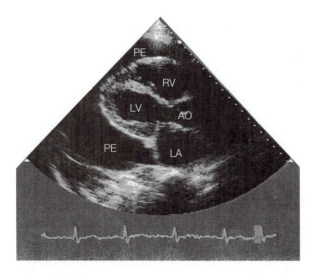

Figure 1.10–2. Echocardiogram showing a large pericardial effusion (PE). RV, right ventricle; LV, left ventricle; LA, left atrium; AO, aorta.

CARDIAC TAMPONADE

Mechanism and Etiology

The mean right atrial pressure is normally about 5 mm Hg, compared with pericardial pressure of about 1 mm Hg, giving a transmural pressure of 4 mm Hg. This transmural pressure may dip to below zero during the y descent; hence, it is possible for the right heart to suck air from an uncapped central venous catheter. When pericardial pressure increases, the right atrial pressure increases along with it; in experimental preparations, the transmural pressure falls, so that as pericardial pressure exceeds about 10 mm Hg, the right atrial and pericardial pressure become almost equal. As right atrial pressure climbs toward 20 mm Hg, it reduces the pressure gradient between the systemic veins and the heart (the mean systemic venous pressure minus the right atrial pressure; Chapter 15.4) and venous return falls. Tamponade refers to a fall in cardiac output to critical levels caused by compression of the heart by a pericardial effusion and typically develops when the pericardial pressure reaches 20–24 mm Hg. The reduction in venous return is initially counterbalanced by a reflex increase in heart rate and contractility. Systemic vascular resistance increases to maintain arterial pressure at the expense of cardiac output. Eventually, as cardiac output falls, the compensatory mechanisms no longer maintain systemic arterial pressure and shock develops. Profound sinus bradycardia often occurs during severe hypotension and precedes the development of electromechanical dissociation and death.

Cardiac tamponade may follow any type of pericardial inflammation or injury. Malignant disease is by far its most common cause, followed by idiopathic pericarditis and bleeding after cardiac surgery, particularly in patients receiving anticoagulants.

Clinical Features

Patients who present with acute cardiac tamponade from perforation or rupture of the heart have a more fulminant presentation than those in whom effusion develops more slowly. The acute type of tamponade is characterized by three findings (Beck's triad): (1) a decline in systemic arterial pressure, (2) elevation of systemic venous pressure, and (3) a small, quiet heart (Table 1.10–3). In this acute type of tamponade, the pericardium is not enlarged or stretched, and quantities of less than 200 mL of blood or fluid can produce severe embarrassment of cardiac function. Profound hypotension is typical, often associated with distant heart sounds, cool, clammy extremities, and anuria.

The patient presenting with the more common clinical scenario of slowly developing tamponade appears acutely ill but not *in extremis*. The major complaint is usually dyspnea. This symptom is usually not accompanied by alveolar edema or hypoxemia and represents "air-hunger" from reduced cardiac output. Vague chest discomfort and profound weakness are also common in patients with this subacute form of cardiac tamponade.

Table 1.10–3. Physical findings in cardiac tamponade and constrictive pericarditis.

	Tamponade	Constrictive Pericarditis
Blood pressure	Low	Normal
Jugular pressure	High	Very high
Dominant jugular venous descent	x descent	y descent
Pulsus paradoxus	Yes	Seldom
Kussmaul's sign	No	Often
Pericardial knock	No	Yes

Physical Examination

Jugular venous distention is the most common physical finding in patients with cardiac tamponade. Not only is the jugular venous pressure elevated, but there is also a characteristic wave form with a prominent systolic x descent and diminutive diastolic y descent. The y descent is attenuated because the high intrapericardial pressure does not fall with opening of the tricuspid valve, so that the usual surge of systemic venous return during early diastole is abolished.

Pulsus Paradoxus

The other vitally important sign found in patients with cardiac tamponade is pulsus paradoxus, an inspiratory fall of aortic systolic pressure by more than 10 mm Hg (Figure 1.10–3). The weakening of the arterial pressure during inspiration was originally described by Kussmaul; the "paradox" was that the pulse disappeared during inspiration but the heart sounds were unchanged. Pulsus paradoxus is really an exaggeration of the normal 3% inspiratory decline of systemic arterial pressure. Inspiration normally increases right ventricular filling, and there is a slight bulging of the interventricular septum to the left, causing a small decrease in left ventricular dimension. When the tight pericardium keeps the total heart volume constant, this ventricular interdependence is exaggerated, and pulsus paradoxus reflects the more pronounced "physiologic" decline in left ventricular dimension. In experimental tamponade in laboratory animals, pulsus paradoxus can be eliminated when right ventricular volume is strictly controlled.

Pulsus paradoxus is measured by inflating a blood pressure cuff 20 mm Hg above systolic pressure and slowly deflating the cuff until Korotkoff's sounds are heard only during expiration. The cuff should then be deflated until Korotkoff's sounds are equally well heard during inspiration and expiration. The difference between these pressures is the estimated magnitude of pulsus paradoxus.

Pulsus paradoxus can also be observed in severe obstructive lung disease, particularly during asthma attacks and in massive pulmonary embolism. It is not usually seen in patients with constrictive pericarditis, because the thick adherent pericardium does not transmit the inspiratory decline in intrathoracic pressure to the heart.

Laboratory Studies

Echocardiography establishes the diagnosis of cardiac tamponade and is generally done before pericardiocentesis, except when the patient is *in extremis*. Not only can the echocardiogram confirm the presence and size of an effusion, it can also give important clues as to whether there is associated tamponade. The most important echocardiographic sign of tamponade is diastolic right ventricular compression or collapse. Taken by itself, this finding is not entirely sensitive or specific, but in a large effusion and high jugular pressure, it confirms the need for pericardial drainage.

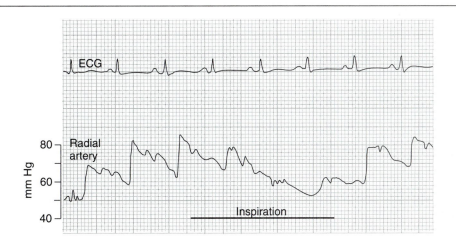

Figure 1.10–3. Pulsus paradoxus in a patient with acute tamponade. During inspiration, there is a fall in systolic pressure and almost complete loss of pulse pressure with no change in heart rhythm.

Treatment

Pending pericardiocentesis, the initial treatment of patients with cardiac tamponade consists of volume expansion with intravenous saline. Vasodilators (with the idea of lowering systemic vascular resistance and increasing cardiac output) should not be given because they simply aggravate systemic hypotension.

Definitive treatment of cardiac tamponade consists of draining the pericardial space. Pericardiocentesis is usually done from a subxiphoid approach with a long needle or a catheter, at the bedside or under fluoroscopic guidance. The infrequent complications are perforation of the right ventricle or epicardial coronary arteries and pneumothorax. To avoid perforating the heart, one can make the needle into an exploring ECG electrode by connecting it to the V lead of an ECG and looking for a current of injury when the needle contacts the epicardium.

Pericardial effusions caused by cancer are likely to recur. This can be managed by repeat pericardiocentesis, sclerosis of the pericardial space, radiation of the pericardium, or pericardiectomy. Limited pericardiectomy, in which a window is created for pericardial fluid to drain into the pleural space, can be done with minimal morbidity, but many patients develop localized fibrosis and recurrent tamponade within a few months. Hence, this operation should be limited to critically ill patients with a poor prognosis. Complete pericardiectomy by a median sternotomy is the more definitive treatment for patients with recurrent tamponade whose anticipated survival is more than 6 months.

CONSTRICTIVE PERICARDITIS

Etiology

When pericardial inflammation continues for months or years, the ensuing process of fibrosis, scarring, and eventual calcification leads to a syndrome of chronic cardiac constriction. As in tamponade, the fundamental hemodynamic problem is increase in right atrial pressure that threatens to prevent venous return, but, because of its chronicity, constrictive pericarditis presents differently (see Table 1.10–3). The pathologic condition typically evolves through stages; the pericardial fluid produced during an acute bout of pericarditis is resorbed and then the visceral and parietal pericardium thicken and fuse. Ultimately, the pericardium becomes calcified and entirely noncompliant. This process is usually symmetric, affecting all four cardiac chambers, but in some patients it is localized to a particular region of the heart such as the right ventricular outflow tract.

The hemodynamic hallmark of chronic constriction is that the diastolic pressures in the two sides of the heart are equal. A characteristic finding is rapid early-diastolic filling of the ventricles, followed by abrupt cessation of diastolic flow as the expanding heart reaches the noncompliant pericardium. This hemodynamic characteristic is the cause of one of the principal physical signs of con-

strictive pericarditis—a prominent diastolic y descent in the jugular pulse (Friedreich's sign).

Until the advent of routine tuberculosis screening and antitubercular chemotherapy, the most common cause of constrictive pericarditis in Western countries was tuberculosis. Tuberculosis remains the most common cause in the Third World and recently has been found with greater frequency in the United States in patients with acquired immune deficiency syndrome (AIDS). At present, the most common cause of constrictive pericarditis in the United States is idiopathic; constriction is presumed to follow a clinically inapparent episode of acute pericarditis. Of roughly equal frequency as causes of constrictive pericarditis are previous cardiac surgery and mediastinal radiation therapy, especially for Hodgkin's disease or breast cancer.

Clinical Features

The presenting symptoms of constrictive pericarditis are a consequence of elevated right heart pressures and simulate features of right ventricular failure or chronic liver disease. Edema, anasarca, and symptoms of hepatic congestion—postprandial fullness, anorexia, and loss of muscle mass—are the usual complaints early in the course of the disease. As constriction progresses, left heart filling pressures rise and patients develop exertional dyspnea, cough, and orthopnea.

The most important physical sign is elevation of jugular venous pressure. Both x and y descents are usually detectable, with the y descent being particularly prominent. Sometimes the jugular pressure may be seen to rise during inspiration (Kussmaul's sign). This probably reflects massive engorgement of the splanchnic veins, such that they are compressed by the inspiratory descent of the diaphragm. Auscultation may reveal an early-diastolic sound called the *pericardial knock*, which corresponds to the sudden cessation of rapid filling. Although its mechanism is similar to that of a normal S_3, the sound has a higher frequency than most third sounds, and because it occurs early, it can be mistaken for the opening snap of mitral stenosis.

Hepatomegaly, typically with prominent hepatic pulsations, is always present in constrictive pericarditis, and liver function tests are usually abnormal. The bilirubin may be very high, and it is not surprising that many patients are evaluated for liver disease before they are recognized to have constrictive pericarditis. Young patients with competent venous valves may have marked abdominal distention from hepatomegaly and ascites in the absence of leg edema. Older patients may have massive leg and scrotal edema in addition to abdominal distention. The torso and upper extremities of patients with constrictive pericarditis often show striking muscle wasting, resulting in a characteristic body habitus of thin arms and chest wall accompanied by massive abdominal and leg swelling.

Diagnosis

The chest x-ray in constrictive pericarditis may demonstrate an egg-shell rim of calcification around the heart (Figure 1.10–4). This is often best seen on the lateral film. Calcification of the heart on chest x-ray is not specific for constrictive pericarditis and may be seen in left ventricular aneurysm with thrombus and in mitral annular or coronary arterial calcification. Fluoroscopy, computed tomography (CT), and MRI scans may be helpful in distinguishing the location of cardiac calcification; imaging scans also show caval and hepatic venous dilatation.

The ECG is not particularly helpful in the diagnosis of constrictive pericarditis. Nearly 50% of patients with constrictive pericarditis have atrial fibrillation, and many have diffuse but nonspecific T-wave abnormalities.

The echocardiogram can be helpful in demonstrating a calcified, thickened pericardium and usually shows normal left ventricular function, which helps to distinguish the disease from restrictive cardiomyopathy (Chapter 1.7). Doppler flow studies can show the rapid but abbreviated early filling pattern, but their specificity in this disease is as yet unproved.

Catheterization

In patients with suspected constrictive pericarditis, right and left heart catheterization should usually be performed to document constrictive hemodynamics and to exclude other causes of elevated systemic venous pressure. Simultaneous pressures in the right and left ventricles should be recorded to look for elevation and near-equalization of diastolic pressures in all four heart chambers and to show the characteristic pressure dip followed by a plateau in both right ventricular and left ventricular diastolic recordings. This is called the "square-root" sign because of its appearance on the tracing. In patients with constriction, the diastolic pressures in the two sides of the heart should be within 5 mm Hg of one another, but in some patients

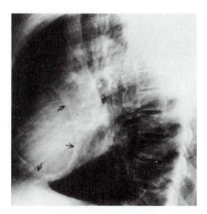

Figure 1.10–4. Lateral chest x-ray in a patient with chronic constrictive pericarditis showing pericardial calcification (arrows). The calcium is usually seen in the region of the atrioventricular groove and on the diaphragmatic surface of the heart.

who have received diuretics and whose constriction is not severe, it may be necessary to give saline to reveal these characteristic hemodynamic findings.

Treatment

The clinical course of untreated constrictive pericarditis is progressive and unaffected by medical therapy. Treatment is complete pericardial resection, by median sternotomy and with cardiopulmonary bypass available. The outcome of surgery depends on the patient's functional status at the time of operation. Because patients in New York Heart Association class IV have a high operative mortality rate and a mediocre long-term result, pericardiectomy should be performed early in the course of constrictive pericarditis.

Effusive-Constrictive Pericarditis

Some patients who have had pericarditis are found after some months, or even a year, to have persistent effusions, markedly thickened pericardium, and early signs of chronic constriction. The jugular pressure is high, edema may be present, and patients may have noticed fatigue and lack of stamina. This is referred to as the syndrome of effusive-constrictive pericarditis and probably represents a stage in the progression to constrictive pericarditis. The most important hemodynamic feature is persistence of right atrial hypertension following pericardiocentesis and can be documented by simultaneous recordings of intrapericardial and right heart pressures. These patients should be treated by pericardiectomy, and they have an excellent long-term outcome.

SPECIFIC TYPES OF PERICARDITIS

Viral Pericarditis

Viral and idiopathic pericarditis are not distinguishable on clinical grounds, and it is conjectured that most cases of idiopathic pericarditis are unrecognized viral infections. Viral pericarditis can be caused by a number of enteroviruses, most frequently coxsackievirus group B and echovirus type B. The incidence is seasonal, with peaks in the spring and fall. In addition to the common viral causes of acute pericarditis, rickettsiae and mycoplasma have been documented as causes. Recently, acute pericarditis has been seen with increasing frequency in patients with AIDS, in whom it may be caused by unusual pathogens such as cytomegalovirus or herpes simplex virus.

Viral pericarditis can be diagnosed by antibody titers in acute and convalescent sera, but in practice this is of limited clinical value in the absence of specific treatment for this generally benign disease.

The course of viral pericarditis is typically self-limited, lasting from 1–3 weeks. Treatment with nonsteroidal antiinflammatory agents is directed at symptoms. Patients should be monitored for the two most serious associated syndromes: acute myocarditis and cardiac tamponade. Occasional patients have periodic recurrences of acute pericarditis over a period of months to years. These patients are often very difficult to manage. Some respond to corticosteroids; others may need pericardiectomy for pain relief.

Bacterial Pericarditis

Purulent pericarditis caused by bacterial infection in the preantibiotic era was most often a consequence of pneumonia, with lymphatic or hematogenous seeding of the pericardial space. Today, bacterial pericarditis is most frequently seen in patients with mediastinitis after cardiac surgery, and the most common pathogen is *Staphylococcus epidermidis*. Other causes are staphylococcal septicemia and intrathoracic malignancy. Treatment requires parenteral antibiotics and early surgical drainage.

Tuberculous Pericarditis

In Western countries, the incidence of tuberculous pericarditis had declined almost to zero in recent decades, until the advent of AIDS. It is now on the rise, seen in patients with AIDS and in immunocompromised patients undergoing chemotherapy for a malignant tumor. In developing countries, particularly in Africa, tuberculosis remains the major cause of pericarditis and is second only to rheumatic heart disease as a cause of heart failure in young adults.

Tuberculous pericarditis typically progresses slowly, causing nonspecific complaints of fever and dyspnea, and the diagnosis is often not established until signs and symptoms of constriction develop. Bacteriologic diagnosis is difficult. Culture of pericardial fluid has a low yield, and caseating granulomas are rare in pericardial biopsy specimens. Often, the diagnosis of tuberculous pericarditis can be confirmed only after pathologic examination of the entire pericardium following pericardiectomy or autopsy. Skin testing is unreliable because anergy is common.

The treatment of tuberculous pericarditis is a prolonged course of triple-drug antitubercular therapy. Corticosteroids given early in the course of antitubercular chemotherapy may reduce pericardial inflammation and enhance pericardial fluid resorption, but it is unclear whether corticosteroids prevent progression to constriction. Pericardiectomy should be performed after 4–6 weeks of antitubercular therapy if the patient develops recurrent effusion or evidence of constriction.

Neoplastic Pericarditis

Neoplastic involvement of the pericardium is the most common cause of hemorrhagic pericardial effusion. Primary neoplasms of the pericardium, such as asbestos-related mesothelioma, are extremely rare. Pericardial metastasis occurs most often by direct extension of a mediastinal tumor, particularly breast or lung carcinoma, but lymphatic or hematogenous seeding of the pericardium can occur, particularly with leukemia, lymphoma, or melanoma.

Malignant pericardial effusions are most often diagnosed only when cardiac compression develops. Treatment—by aspiration, sclerotherapy, or limited surgical drainage—depends on the severity of cardiac compression and the patient's overall prognosis. As in malignant pleural effusions, neoplastic pericarditis does not necessarily indicate imminent death.

Postmyocardial Injury

Pericarditis can develop within days or weeks of cardiac injury, either myocardial infarction or at the time of heart surgery. Pericarditis after myocardial infarction occurs in two clinically distinct forms: acute postinfarction pericarditis, which occurs during the first week after infarction, and Dressler's syndrome, which develops 2 weeks to 6 months after infarction. Early postinfarction pericarditis typically occurs after transmural infarction and is commonly accompanied by pleuritic chest pain, pericardial friction rub, and low-grade fever (Chapter 1.3). Treatment is anti-inflammatory therapy with salicylates, nonsteroidal agents, or a short course of corticosteroids. Salicylates are preferred since either of the other classes of agent may interfere with healing of the infarct. Anticoagulants in patients with early postinfarction pericarditis can cause pericardial hemorrhage and should be discontinued in patients who develop a rub after infarction.

Dressler's syndrome is an uncommon, late complication of myocardial infarction, reported in less than 5% of patients. It is an acute illness that is characterized by fever and pleuropericarditis and is thought to have an autoimmune origin. Antimyocardial antibodies are present in patients with this syndrome, but are also found in patients after infarction or heart surgery who do not have the syndrome. Patients may have recurrent bouts of pleuritic pain, and they can develop constrictive pericarditis.

The postpericardiotomy syndrome is similar to Dressler's syndrome: it occurs after heart surgery and is characterized by fever and pleuropericarditis beginning more than 1 week after the operation. As with the two postmyocardial infarction syndromes, the postpericardiotomy syndrome must be distinguished from the much more common type of pericarditis that occurs within the first several days after cardiac surgery. The cause of the postpericardiotomy syndrome involves an autoimmune mechanism, like Dressler's syndrome, and there is evidence that perioperative viral infections play a role in stimulating this autoimmunity.

Uremic Pericarditis

Pericarditis can complicate chronic renal failure, most often in patients undergoing hemodialysis or about to begin dialysis. The immediate cause has not been established; it is clearly related to azotemia, and typically develops when blood urea nitrogen is greater than 100 mg/dL, but there is no clear correlation between the level of any particular metabolite and the development of pericardial inflammation. Asymptomatic, small pericardial effusions are extremely common in uremic patients, are often transudative (as a result of volume overload), and may require no treatment. Large effusions that persist despite 1–2 weeks of intensive dialysis eventually lead to hemodynamic compromise, particularly during dialysis itself, and hence frequently require intervention. Pericardiocentesis in conjunction with instillation of corticosteroid may reduce the severity and frequency of bouts of uremic pericarditis, but the critical treatment is effective dialysis.

Collagen Vascular Disease

Systemic Lupus Erythematosus: Pericarditis is the most common cardiovascular manifestation of systemic lupus erythematosus (Chapter 3.2). Pericarditis typically develops during flares of the systemic disease and correlates with serologic evidence of increased disease activity. Pericardial effusions are usually serous and have a high protein content, low glucose level, and low complement levels relative to serum values. Occasionally, pericardial effusion, or even tamponade, may be the first sign of the systemic disease.

Rheumatoid Arthritis: As many as 50% of all patients with rheumatoid arthritis (Chapter 3.3) may have some degree of pericardial involvement, but it is usually subclinical. Affected patients usually have severe systemic disease with joint deformity, subcutaneous nodules, and often pneumonitis.

In Still's disease, pericarditis can occur in the absence of active joint involvement. The diagnosis depends on recognizing the triad of high fever, pericarditis, and the characteristic rash.

Acute Rheumatic Fever: Pericardial effusion is common in acute rheumatic carditis (Chapter 8.4), and a few patients develop pain and a rub. Clinically apparent pericarditis is uncommon without a murmur of mitral valvulitis.

Myxedema Pericardial Disease

Serous pericardial effusions, sometimes gelatinous in consistency, may develop in patients with chronic untreated hypothyroidism. Many of these patients have accompanying pleural effusions and ascites, and the pericardial effusion may be massive. Pericardial effusion in patients with myxedema may be overlooked when fatigue and weakness are attributed to the underlying thyroid disorder.

SUMMARY

▶ Pericarditis is distinguished from acute myocardial infarction by the pleuritic nature of the pain, friction rub, and concave ST elevation on the ECG.

▶ The signs of cardiac tamponade are hypotension, high jugular pressure, and pulsus paradoxus; the paradoxical pulse is caused by inspiratory augmentation of right ventricular filling at the expense of the left ventricle.

▶ The most common cause of hemorrhagic pericardial effusion is malignancy. Recurrence of tamponade from malignant effusions is treated with sclerosing agents, or drainage through a pericardial window.

▶ Constrictive pericarditis should be suspected in any patient with anasarca and a high jugular pressure. Distinguishing it from restrictive myocardial disease may require heart biopsy or even thoracotomy.

▶ Because chronic pericardial constriction eventually involves the epicardium, surgical resection should be performed as soon as the diagnosis is established.

SUGGESTED READING

Anguita ZR: Incidence of specific etiology and role of methods for specific etiologic diagnosis of primary acute pericarditis. Am J Cardiol 1995;75:378.

Fowler NO: *The Pericardium in Health and Disease.* Futura, 1984.

Sagrista-Sauleda J, Permanyer-Miralda G, Soler-Soler J: Tuberculous pericarditis: Ten year experience with a prospective protocol for diagnosis and treatment. J Am Coll Cardiol 1988; 11:724.

Singh S et al: Right ventricular and right atrial collapse in patients with cardiac tamponade: A combined echocardiographic and hemodynamic study. Circulation 1984;70:966.

Suwan PK: Predictors of constrictive pericarditis after a tuberculous pericarditis. Br Heart J 1995;73:187.

1.11

Congenital Heart Disease

Thomas A. Traill, FRCP

Today, most congenital heart malformations are identified in children. They often require surgical repair, usually in the early years to avoid interrupting school and to minimize secondary effects of the original lesion. Physicians who take care of adult patients often assume care of people who have had such surgery during childhood. They also encounter some who have congenital heart disease that has not proved appropriate for surgical repair, because the defect is one with a benign natural history or because the lesion is too complex. In some cases, congenital heart disease is first detected during adulthood, usually by discovering a heart murmur in someone with few, if any, symptoms. Atrial septal defect is the most common lesion to be found in this way. Other common diseases that may be detected from symptomless murmurs include bicuspid aortic valve; mitral valve prolapse, arguably a congenital lesion; and idiopathic hypertrophic cardiomyopathy, which is not detected (Chapters 1.7 and 1.8).

ACYANOTIC LESIONS

Left-to-Right Shunts at Atrial Level

Atrial septal defect (ASD) is the most common congenital lesion to be detected in adults. Usually, ASDs are discovered at a routine examination before they have caused symptoms, for example, at entry into military service. In older patients, they eventually cause problems, typically atrial arrhythmias, fluid retention, and breathlessness. Some ASDs are found not because of clinical suspicion, but serendipitously by echocardiography when the test is being performed for some other reason.

The most common kind of ASD is a defect in the fossa ovalis (Figure 1.11–1), usually referred to as an ostium secundum defect. Other sites are the ostium primum defect, which involves the atrioventricular valve rings, and the sinus venosus defect, which lies at the junction of one or other of the venae cavae and is accompanied by an anomalous pulmonary vein. Five percent of adults have a patent foramen ovale; this does not cause a left-to-right shunt and has neither the pathophysiologic nor the clinical effects of ASDs. Rarely, however, a patent foramen ovale provides a pathway for paradoxical embolism from the venous system to the arterial circulation, or is the site of right-to-left shunting in certain patients with cyanotic lesions (see "Cyanotic Lesions" below). Other kinds of ASD all permit left-to-right shunting and thereby cause an increase in right ventricular and pulmonary blood flow. Anomalies of pulmonary venous return, in which one or more of the pulmonary veins drain to the right atrium, typically via the superior vena cava, also increase pulmonary blood flow, and are therefore included with ASDs in the overall category of "left-to-right shunts at atrial level."

The clinical findings reflect right heart enlargement and increased right ventricular stroke volume. The a wave in the jugular pulse is prominent, and there may be a right ventricular lift. The pathognomonic auscultatory finding is wide splitting of the second heart sound with no respiratory variation ("fixed" splitting.) There is usually a systolic ejection murmur caused by increased flow through the right ventricular outflow tract, and there may be an additional diastolic rumble reflecting the increased tricuspid valve flow. In patients with secundum ASD, the electrocardiogram (ECG) typically shows partial or complete right bundle branch block. Left-axis deviation (a superior vector) on the ECG is characteristic of an ostium primum defect, which is the simplest expression of an atrioventricular canal defect (or endocardial cushion defect). This type of defect is associated with abnormalities of the atrioventricular valve ring; the mitral valve is displaced forward and toward the apex, and the leaflets may be cleft or dysplastic. Ostium primum defects are much less common than ostium secundum defects, except in association with Down's syndrome, in which they are the most characteristic heart lesion.

The chest x-ray and the echocardiogram are usually both characteristic (Figures 1.11–2 and 1.11–3). The chest x-ray shows enlargement of the central pulmonary arteries and an increase in vascular markings commensurate with the increase in pulmonary blood flow. The echocardiogram shows increased volume of the right ventricle and usually shows the site and size of the ASD itself. The

Normal

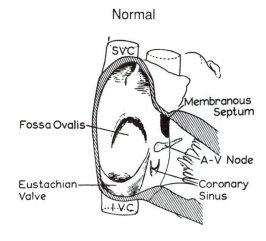

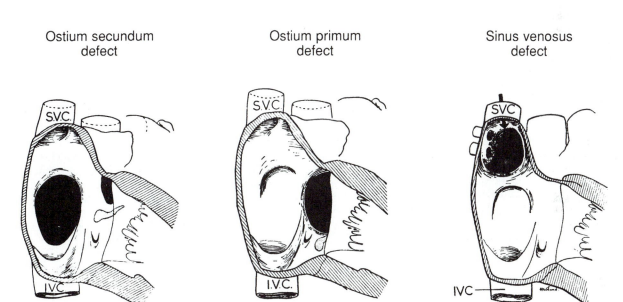

Ostium secundum defect

Ostium primum defect

Sinus venosus defect

SVC, superior vena cava; IVC, inferior vena cava.

Figure 1.11–1. View of the atrial septum from the right side, showing sites of atrial septal defects. (Reproduced, with permission, from Bedford DE et al: Atrial septal defect and its surgical treatment. Lancet 1957;272[1]:1255.)

echocardiogram readily identifies the mitral and tricuspid valve abnormalities associated with an ostium primum lesion and is helpful in assessing the severity of any mitral regurgitation. Sometimes, when the anatomy is in doubt, transesophageal echocardiography may be needed, since this technique provides very clear detailed images of the atrial septum and atrioventricular valves. If necessary, the shunt volume can be measured by cardiac catheterization as the ratio of pulmonary flow to systemic flow, typically between 1.5:1 and 4:1. Such estimates are always approxi-

mate, and it is dangerous to set a particular value of shunt size below which surgical correction is unnecessary. In the young patient whose diagnosis is obvious, there is seldom any need to perform diagnostic catheterization or angiography.

Natural History and Treatment of Atrial Septal Defect: The natural history of ASD dictates that the majority of patients be referred for surgical closure. There have been studies of an umbrella or clam-like closure system

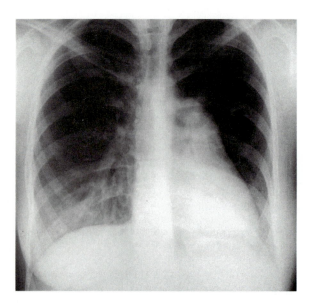

Figure 1.11–2. Chest x-ray of a patient with atrial septal defect, showing enlarged pulmonary arteries and increased pulmonary vascularity.

that can be placed through a cardiac catheter, but this is not yet applicable to adult-sized defects. Although symptoms are rarely present in the young, in patients over the age of 40 the lesion eventually causes fluid retention, atrial arrhythmias, cardiomegaly, and dyspnea. Atrial septal defect in elderly symptomatic patients may mimic the clinical presentation of mitral stenosis, which is easily excluded by echocardiography, or cor pulmonale, a more

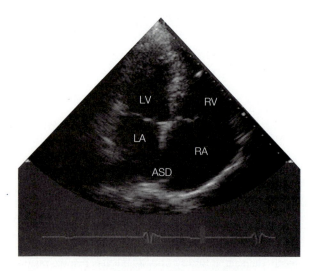

Figure 1.11–3. Echocardiogram (apical view) showing an atrial septal defect (ASD) with enlargement of the right ventricle (RV). RA, right atrium; LA, left atrium; LV, left ventricle.

difficult source of confusion. Although such patients often appear to be unpromising candidates for surgery, operative mortality is low and the benefit of repair, even in the symptomatic stage, is remarkable.

Atrial septal defects can permit paradoxical embolism, that is, passage of an embolus from the systemic venous system into the left heart and thence to a systemic artery. This risk represents another reason to advocate surgical closure. Endocarditis, however, is very rare. Development of pulmonary vascular disease is not as common as in defects at the ventricular or aortic level, nor is it as rapid, and only a few patients are seen, typically in their 20's, with Eisenmenger's syndrome complicating ASD. Surgical repair at this stage is too dangerous to contemplate. Patients who are older, and usually seen because of symptoms, often have moderate pulmonary hypertension, but it seldom approaches the systemic level.

Ventricular Septal Defect

In contrast to ASDs, which generally cause little trouble during childhood and often go undetected, the deciding events in the natural history of ventricular septal defects (VSDs) occur in the first few years of life. By the time VSD patients reach adulthood, their course is generally set, and adult physicians seldom have to apply any judgment to their management. By a patient's teenage years, large VSDs should have been closed surgically, small VSDs are enjoying their benign natural history, and a small number of large defects that went uncorrected or unrecognized in infancy have caused pulmonary vascular disease and a rise in pulmonary vascular resistance that has passed the point of being operable. In these few in whom the opportunity for correction was missed in childhood, pulmonary vascular disease is the eventual cause of death.

Natural History of Ventricular Septal Defect: A VSD comparable in size to the aortic anulus has no pressure difference across it in systole. At birth, as during fetal life, the pulmonary vascular resistance is very high; as a result, despite the high pressure, the volume of pulmonary blood flow is scarcely increased. At this stage there is no murmur and heart disease is not suspected. During the first 2 or 3 days after birth, as the pulmonary vascular resistance falls to perhaps one-tenth the systemic resistance, a large left-to-right shunt develops, to the point where the volume of pulmonary blood flow may be several times the cardiac output. The result is severe pulmonary congestion, and the infant becomes breathless, cannot feed, and fails to gain weight. During the succeeding months one of three things may happen:

1. The defect may be closed surgically (in times past, when infant surgery was more risky, a physiologic means of palliation was to place a constricting band around the main pulmonary artery).
2. The defect may get smaller spontaneously.
3. The pulmonary vascular resistance may rise in reaction to the high flow and pressure.

The initial result of an increase in pulmonary vascular resistance is to reduce the excessive pulmonary blood flow, which initially improves the baby's symptoms. But as the reactive vascular changes progress, they eventually limit pulmonary blood flow to the point at which the left-to-right shunt is replaced by right-to-left shunting and cyanosis develops. This situation is referred to as Eisenmenger's syndrome, which can occur in response to any type of lesion capable of permitting a large left-to-right shunt, such as a persistent ductus arteriosus, aortopulmonary window, single ventricle, or even some ASDs.

In adults, simple VSDs with left-to-right shunts are much less common than in children. Many or most small defects ("pinhole" size up to 3 mm) close in infancy or childhood. A few large defects progress undetected until they reach the stage of Eisenmenger's syndrome. Patients who still have left-to-right shunts in adult life have lesions of intermediate size that are neither very large nor small enough to have closed spontaneously. These patients are asymptomatic and normally developed; the only striking physical finding is a loud pansystolic murmur at the lower left sternal border. The intensity of the murmur is no indication of the size of the defect; indeed, a pinhole defect in the muscular portion of the ventricular septum may cause a palpable thrill. When its intensity rapidly diminishes in late systole, the murmur almost certainly arises from such a small muscular defect that is pinched off by the contracting myocardium.

Thus, most adult patients with VSDs need no special treatment. There are three exceptions to this:

1. Infective endocarditis should be preventable in most patients by good dental hygiene and prophylactic antibiotics, but VSDs should be closed in patients who have endocarditis more than once.
2. Very occasionally, the flow across the defect and the resultant volume load on the left ventricle are sufficient to cause cardiac dilatation and a gradual deterioration in left ventricular function. This situation is analogous to chronic mitral regurgitation of moderate severity and represents a second unusual indication for surgical repair.
3. Aortic regurgitation develops in a few patients with defects immediately beneath the right coronary cusp of the aortic valve.

    These defects allow the aortic leaflet to herniate down into the right ventricle, and if they are not corrected, irreparable damage to the valve is likely and replacement will be required. Operating early usually permits leaving the valve in place. Unless one of these three complications develops, adults with VSDs should be treated conservatively with no restrictions and with antibiotic prophylaxis as their only special precaution.

Persistent Ductus Arteriosus

The ductus arteriosus normally closes within the first day or two of life to become the ligamentum arteriosum. Persistence of the duct represents the most common cause of left-to-right shunting at the level of the great arteries and of a continuous murmur, characteristically the "machinery" murmur heard beneath the left clavicle. Except in a few cases with Eisenmenger's syndrome and in elderly patients, surgical closure of the duct is recommended even in the absence of hemodynamic upset, since the operation is straightforward and the natural history includes a significant risk of bacterial endocarditis.

Left-Sided Obstructive Lesions

Congenital obstructive lesions of the left heart include coarctation of the aorta and various anomalies of the aortic valve, mitral valve, and left atrium.

Coarctation of the Aorta: Coarctation of the aorta should be detected and treated surgically in infancy. It is still occasionally found for the first time in adults, usually when they are being evaluated for hypertension, or much less commonly after they complain of bilateral claudication. The physical findings of coarctation are delay in the femoral pulse compared with the brachial, reduced blood pressure in the legs, a murmur, and evidence of collateral flow through the intercostal arteries to supply the descending aorta. These collateral vessels may cause a continuous murmur over the back, and are sometimes palpable. They are tortuous and cause characteristic "rib-notching" on a chest x-ray. The natural history of coarctation is for hypertension to worsen, and patients should be referred for surgical repair, even though this carries a small risk (<5%) of damage to the anterior spinal artery supply and consequent paraplegia.

Aortic Stenosis: Aortic stenosis may be valvular, typically with a unicuspid or bicuspid valve, or it may occur above the valve (supravalvular aortic stenosis) or below (subaortic stenosis). Fixed subaortic lesions represent a spectrum from a discrete fibrous rim or diaphragm immediately beneath the aortic valve to a tubular fibromuscular constriction extending into the left ventricular cavity. These should not be confused with hypertrophic cardiomyopathy, which may also be accompanied by a systolic pressure gradient between the left ventricle and aorta, but without true obstruction (Chapter 1.7).

Congenital Mitral Stenosis: Congenital mitral stenosis is caused by commissural fusion, very like its acquired counterpart. Other varieties include parachute mitral valve, in which both mitral leaflets are supported by a single papillary muscle, and supravalvular mitral stenosis (cor triatriatum), in which a membrane, often perforated by only a tiny hole, is situated above the mitral valve in the left atrium.

Right-Sided Obstructive Lesions

The physiology of right-sided obstructive lesions differs in some respects from the corresponding abnormalities on the left side, because the structure of the right ventricle is different from that of the left and because the foramen ovale exists as a potential valve allowing right-to-left shunting between the atria when normal flow through the right heart is impeded.

Right Ventricular Outflow Obstruction: The most common kind of pulmonary stenosis is congenital valvular stenosis. The pulmonary valve commissures are fused, so that during ejection the structure forms a dome with a jet of blood leaving through the small central orifice. The valve is mobile and usually creates a characteristic ejection sound as it assumes this shape, preceding a loud ejection systolic murmur. The pulmonary closure sound is typically soft and delayed. Obstruction below the level of the valve can be caused by infundibular stenosis. This type of stenosis, accompanied by a VSD is the most common congenital cause of cyanosis in adults, referred to as *tetralogy of Fallot* (see "Mechanisms of Cyanosis" below).

The natural history of severe isolated right ventricular outflow obstruction is generally predictable from the gradient between the right ventricle and pulmonary artery. When this gradient exceeds about 40 mm Hg, increasing right ventricular hypertrophy, right atrial hypertension, fluid retention, and in some cases syncope may occur, and surgical relief of the obstruction is therefore indicated— either by balloon dilatation in the catheterization lab, or, if this is not feasible, by surgery. When the gradient is smaller, progression is unusual and the natural history is benign. Although definitive assessment often requires catheterization, the ECG is a useful indicator of the severity and progression of right ventricular hypertrophy. A monophasic R wave in V1 is a sure indication that right ventricular pressure is similar to the systemic pressure. A chest x-ray shows normal peripheral pulmonary vessels unless there is an associated shunt. In the case of valvular stenosis, poststenotic dilatation causes widening of the main pulmonary artery shadow.

Right heart obstruction within the body of the right ventricle occurs as a secondary phenomenon when right ventricular hypertrophy causes enlargement of the trabecular system and development of an anomalous right ventricular muscle bundle separating the outlet of the ventricle from the inlet region.

Ebstein's Anomaly: Ebstein's anomaly is the most common congenital lesion of the right ventricle and tricuspid valve. A portion of the valve, usually part of the anteromedial leaflet, is attached in the body of the right ventricle and causes functional obstruction to right ventricular filling, often with tricuspid regurgitation. Ebstein's anomaly causes cyanosis when a patent foramen ovale allows right-to-left shunting across the atrial septum.

The clinical severity of Ebstein's anomaly is extremely variable. Sometimes the lesion causes severe cyanosis and requires surgical treatment in infancy. In this situation, the prognosis is poor. By contrast, many adult patients with Ebstein's anomaly are virtually asymptomatic. They may have considerable cardiomegaly, mainly due to right atrial enlargement, but cyanosis is often mild and may fluctuate in severity over the years. Physical examination reveals a quiet cardiac impulse and the characteristic auscultatory feature of a loud delayed tricuspid closure sound, often referred to as the "sail sound." In addition, there may be a rather nondescript systolic murmur at the base. The ECG is often bizarre, with a very wide right bundle branch block pattern, and arrhythmias are common. The echocardiogram is characteristic, showing a dilated right heart with a large and displaced tricuspid valve.

CYANOTIC CONDITIONS

Mechanisms of Cyanosis

There are three ways that congenital heart abnormalities can allow venous blood to reach the arterial circulation and cause cyanosis. The most common is the right-to-left shunt, in which severe obstruction to pulmonary blood flow is combined with a hole between the two sides of the heart. Tetralogy of Fallot is the most familiar example of this type, in which a VSD is the site of right-to-left shunting caused by severe obstruction to pulmonary flow at the level of the right ventricular infundibulum. A similar mechanism applies in Eisenmenger's syndrome, except that the obstruction to pulmonary flow is the increased resistance in the pulmonary arterial bed.

The second mechanism of cyanosis is that found in transposition of the great arteries, in which the aorta arises from the right ventricle and the pulmonary artery from the left. In this and certain related conditions, the two circulations are effectively in parallel, so that oxygenated blood circulates continuously in the pulmonary circuit, mixing with the systemic circulation only across an ASD and the persistent ductus arteriosus.

The third way for venous blood to reach the systemic circulation is referred to as central mixing, typified by the condition of single ventricle, in which all of the blood from the systemic and pulmonary venous return is mixed together in one chamber before being ejected into the aorta and pulmonary artery. The degree of cyanosis that results depends on the relative contributions of pulmonary venous blood and systemic venous return to the final mixture, in turn determined by the relative flow rates in the two circulations. If there is no resistance to ejection into the pulmonary circuit, pulmonary blood flow is high and the resulting mixture is largely oxygenated blood, so that cyanosis is scarcely detectable. The excessive pulmonary artery pressure and blood flow eventually cause Eisenmenger's syndrome. When there is severe pulmonary stenosis, the physiology is more like that of tetralogy of Fallot. The pulmonary pressure and flow are low, and cyanosis is obvious. These considerations apply regardless of the level of the central mixing and whatever other defects may be present. For example, in tricuspid atresia the pathophysiology is determined not by the absence of the right atrioventricular orifice, but by the presence of a functional single ventricle, with a degree of pulmonary stenosis that varies from patient to patient.

Approach to the Cyanotic Patient

The two fundamental questions to be asked when planning the diagnostic evaluation of a patient with cyanotic congenital heart disease are:

1. Is pulmonary blood flow reduced because of Eisenmenger's syndrome, or because of stenosis at the level of the pulmonary valve?
2. Does the heart contain a complete "set of parts"—two atrioventricular valves, two ventricles, and two great arteries?

The answers to these two questions determine the long-term strategy of treatment. If pulmonary vascular disease is the cause of cyanosis, then the only available treatment is supportive, or eventually transplantation; further diagnostic studies are not required. On the other hand, a patient with low pulmonary arterial resistance and two ventricles, each with an atrioventricular valve, should receive detailed investigation of cardiac anatomy and function, with the possibility in mind of complete surgical correction.

Pulmonary vascular obstructive disease is discussed in Chapter 1.12. The clinical diagnosis of Eisenmenger's syndrome is usually straightforward. In many cases, the history is consistent with the patient having had a left-to-right shunt in childhood, followed by insidious development of cyanosis; the cyanosis is often noticed before any serious impairment of exercise capacity. In addition to cyanosis and finger clubbing, there is right ventricular hypertrophy and a palpable tap at the upper left sternal border, corresponding to a very loud pulmonary valve closure sound. The chest x-ray (Figure 1.11–4) is characteristic, showing enlargement, frequently massive, of the central pulmonary arteries and peripheral "pruning" of the smaller vessels. In contrast, the patient whose obstruction to pulmonary blood flow is at the level of the pulmonary valve

has a soft, delayed, or absent pulmonary closure sound, and the chest x-ray shows a pulmonary artery that is more likely to be reduced in size than enlarged. The history is one of cyanosis since soon after birth and may even include previous palliative surgery in the form of a shunt procedure.

The question of whether the patient has a "complete set of parts" is most easily decided by echocardiography. The ECG may provide a clue—absence of right ventricular hypertrophy in a cyanotic patient often implies a hypoplastic or absent right ventricle. Sometimes a gated magnetic resonance imaging study of the thorax is needed to identify certain parts of the anatomy, in particular, the size and potential for reconnection of the pulmonary arteries in patients with pulmonary atresia.

Tetralogy of Fallot

The most common cyanotic condition in adults, tetralogy of Fallot is characterized by stenosis of the right ventricular infundibulum in association with a VSD straddled by the aorta. The four elements of the tetralogy thus consist of (1) a VSD, (2) pulmonary stenosis, (3) aortic override, and (4) right ventricular hypertrophy. The muscular narrowing of the infundibulum increases as the right ventricle hypertrophies, so that obstruction to pulmonary blood flow tends to worsen with the years. The typical patient is not obviously blue at birth or even in the first months of life, but gradually becomes cyanotic in the first few years. When infundibular stenosis is severe, "cyanotic spells" may ensue, during which spasm of the hypertrophied infundibulum acutely obstructs pulmonary blood flow. Squatting, a maneuver by which the child abruptly increases venous return, temporarily dilating the right ventricle and right ventricular outflow tract, is also a feature of severe right ventricular outflow obstruction. The patient who survives to adult life without corrective or palliative surgery has finger clubbing, polycythemia, often rather pronounced acne, and a degree of exercise impairment by fatigue and dyspnea. Fluid retention and syncope are late manifestations and are rarely seen.

Examination of the heart of a patient with tetralogy of Fallot reveals right ventricular hypertrophy, an easily appreciated aortic closure sound, since it arises closer than normal to the chest wall, and an absent or soft and delayed pulmonary valve closure sound. In the typical case, there is a loud ejection systolic murmur with no ejection click. A quiet heart with a continuous murmur from congenital systemic to pulmonary collateral vessels favors the diagnosis of pulmonary atresia.

The chest x-ray in a patient with tetralogy of Fallot indicates pulmonary oligemia, and the ECG shows right ventricular hypertrophy, confirmed by echocardiography. The latter confirms that there are two ventricles separated by a normally formed septum and that the two great arteries are in approximately their normal spatial relationship. This is in contrast to more complicated diseases with more extreme architectural abnormalities, such as double outlet right ventricle, transposition, single ventricle, and tricuspid atresia.

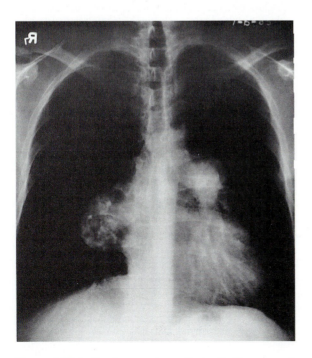

Figure 1.11–4. Chest x-ray of a patient with Eisenmenger's syndrome complicating a ventricular septal defect.

Management

The principles of surgical management of cyanotic lesions follow naturally from the pathophysiology. When cyanosis is the result of inadequate perfusion of the lungs, the first aim of therapy is to increase pulmonary flow. Ideally this can be achieved by total correction. However, when the lesion is too complex, as in single ventricle, or when the pulmonary arteries are absent or hypoplastic, inadequate to allow the right ventricle to pump the entire systemic flow, a systemic-to-pulmonary shunt is created. In the Blalock-Taussig operation, one or other subclavian artery is connected to the ipsilateral pulmonary artery. Other less frequently used shunts include the Waterston-Cooley, in which the ascending aorta is connected to the right pulmonary artery; the Potts procedure, in which the descending aorta is connected to the left pulmonary artery; and the Glenn operation, in which the superior vena cava is joined to the right pulmonary artery. The Glenn operation was a natural predecessor to the Fontan operation for tricuspid atresia, in which the entire systemic venous return is made to bypass the absent right ventricle through a direct connection between the right atrium and the pulmonary artery. Such an approach has proved remarkably successful as treatment for conditions in which the right heart is absent or hypoplastic.

Cyanosis causes polycythemia, and when further management of the cardiac lesion is impossible, an excessive hematocrit is an important source of mortality and morbidity, including complications such as intravascular thrombosis and brain abscess. Routine venesection with clear fluid replacement if necessary, to maintain blood volume, is advocated to keep the hematocrit less than 65–70%.

THE POSTOPERATIVE PATIENT

Many patients who have undergone surgery for congenital heart disease should be regarded as cured; the lesions that can be permanently corrected and that require no long-term follow-up include persistent ductus arteriosus, many ASDs, pulmonary stenosis, and many VSDs. Some other patients may have residual functional abnormalities or minor valvular anomalies that require occasional clinic visits and antibiotic prophylaxis in the case of the valvular lesions but do not interfere with the normal activities of

life, including work, vigorous sports, and pregnancy. These include ostium primum ASD and tetralogy of Fallot. Others have serious residual abnormalities of structure and function. For example, until recently, the most common surgical approach to transposition of the great arteries in babies was to redirect blood flow within the atria so as to divert the pulmonary venous return to the right ventricle, and thus to the aorta, and the systemic venous return to the pulmonary artery via the mitral valve and left ventricle (the Mustard procedure). Not surprisingly, as these patients reach adulthood, they and their doctors face a number of problems related to the long-term effects of requiring the right ventricle to function at systemic pressure. These patients, those who have received Fontan operations, and others who have undergone various types of palliation for very complex defects, require close supervision and may need to have their activities restricted. Ultimately, some need further surgery or even heart transplantation.

SUMMARY

▶ Atrial septal defect is the most common lesion to be detected for the first time in adults. Usually it should be repaired, whether asymptomatic in early adult life, or after causing right heart failure and arrhythmias in an older patient.

▶ The determining events in the natural history of a ventricular septal defect occur in the first 2 years of life. Adult patients with ventricular septal defects either have Eisenmenger's syndrome or small defects with a generally benign course.

▶ Small ventricular septal defects, uncorrected persistent ductus arteriosus, and minor valvular lesions (including bicuspid aortic valve) have benign natural histories, but, in common with all cyanotic conditions, they require antibiotic prophylaxis for potentially contaminating procedures, particularly oral surgery.

▶ The three mechanisms underlying cyanotic congenital heart disease are right-to-left shunting, typified by tetralogy of Fallot; transposition; and central mixing, typified by single ventricle.

SUGGESTED READING

Campbell M, Neill C, Suzman S: The prognosis of atrial septal defect. Br Med J 1957;1:1375.

Konstantinedes S et al: A comparison of surgical and medical therapy for atrial septal defect in adults. New Engl J Med 1995;333:469.

Murphy JG et al: Long-term outcome after surgical repair of isolated atrial septal defect: Follow-up at 27 to 32 years. N Engl J Med 1990;323:1645.

Murphy JG et al: Long-term outcome in patients undergoing surgical repair of tetralogy of Fallot. N Engl J Med 1993;329:593.

Steele PM et al: Isolated atrial septal defect with pulmonary vascular obstructive disease: Long-term follow-up and prediction of outcome after surgical correction. Circulation 1987;76:1037.

Wood P: The Eisenmenger syndrome: Or pulmonary hypertension with reversed central shunt. Br Med J 1958;2:701, 755.

Right Heart Dysfunction

Thomas A. Traill, FRCP

A common presentation of heart disease is with symptoms and signs that reflect a prolonged increase in systemic venous pressure caused by chronic right atrial hypertension. In contrast to the effects of left heart dysfunction, breathlessness is not a prominent symptom, and patients complain of fluid retention, liver enlargement, fatigue, and abdominal discomfort. They have edema (sometimes massive), ascites, and transudative pleural and even pericardial effusions. Pulmonary edema and orthopnea develop only late in their disease, as a consequence of generalized fluid overload. Although their weight may be increased by virtue of retained fluid, patients often lose muscle mass, so that they look thin and wasted in the face and arms, yet develop massive lower body swelling.

Table 1.12–1 lists the differential diagnosis of this predominantly "right-sided" presentation of heart disease. The most common causes are those that lead to pulmonary hypertension, either from intrinsic disease of the pulmonary vessels or because of increased pressure downstream in the pulmonary veins. However, before assuming that patients with right heart dysfunction have pulmonary hypertension, it is important to consider the possibility of atrial septal defect and constrictive pericarditis, since either of these lesions is so eminently treatable. Other diseases that can present in this way are restrictive cardiomyopathy, disease of the tricuspid valve (including carcinoid syndrome), and other sources of right atrial obstruction.

DIFFERENTIAL DIAGNOSIS

The jugular pressure is the starting point in sorting out the hemodynamic cause of anasarca or extensive fluid retention. Examining the jugular pulse allows estimation of right atrial pressure, expressed as centimeters of water measured vertically from the sternal angle (whatever the angle of the patient), and a description of the right atrial pressure waves. Distinguishing jugular pulsations is largely a matter of practice; the experienced observer looks for a characteristic undulating waveform that contrasts with the abrupt outward movement of the arterial

pulse. Often the x or y descent is more obvious to the eye, as an inward motion, than the a or v wave (Figure 1.12–1). It helps to palpate a carotid artery at the same time as inspecting the venous wave to confirm that the timing of the jugular pulse differs from that of the arterial pulse and to identify the predominant wave. The a wave precedes the carotid upstroke, and the v wave follows it. The x descent is synchronous with the arterial upstroke, and the y descent is 180° out of phase.

In chronic pericardial constriction and in restrictive cardiomyopathy, the y descent is the predominant movement in the jugular pulse. In pulmonary hypertension, the a wave is accentuated initially, but as the right ventricle dilates, the v wave enlarges. When tricuspid regurgitation develops, the v wave gives way to a systolic wave with a contour identical with that of the right ventricular pressure. In patients with atrial septal defect, the a wave is often conspicuous during the long asymptomatic phase of the disease, but with the onset of symptoms, usually a v wave or systolic wave becomes more prominent.

PULMONARY HYPERTENSION

Pulmonary hypertension can develop in three ways—because of increased left atrial pressure, increased pulmonary vascular resistance, or a combination of the two. If a patient has a high left atrial pressure, then the pulmonary venous and pulmonary artery pressures must also be high, even if the resistance in the pulmonary circuit is normal; this is by far the most common mechanism of pulmonary hypertension. Most such patients, who have pulmonary hypertension because of left heart dysfunction and a high left atrial pressure, present with symptoms and signs that point to the left heart as the primary problem. A few, however, may have such gradual increases in left atrial pressure that their problem is not detected until they have developed pulmonary hypertension and right-sided signs and symptoms. Mitral stenosis is notorious for presenting in this way, but is nowadays uncommon enough that left ventricular myopathy and even other valvular le-

Table 1.12–1. Causes of chronic right heart failure.

Dilated cardiomyopathy
Pulmonary vascular disease
Mitral stenosis
Atrial septal defect
Restrictive cardiomyopathy
Constrictive pericarditis
Ischemic right ventricular dysfunction
Organic tricuspid valve disease
   Carcinoid syndrome
   Rheumatic disease
Right atrial myxoma
Pulmonary stenosis (or the late effects of surgery for pulmonary
   stenosis)

Table 1.12–2. Causes of pulmonary hypertension.

Left heart dysfunction
   Cardiomyopathy
   Valvular heart disease
Cor pulmonale
Primary pulmonary hypertension
Thromboembolic pulmonary hypertension
Systemic lupus erythematosus
Scleroderma, including CREST syndrome
Eisenmenger's syndrome
Cirrhosis
Schistosomiasis

CREST, calcinosis, Raynaud's phenomenon, esophageal dysfunction, sclerodactyly, telangiectasia.

sions are more common causes of this secondary pulmonary hypertension.

Pulmonary hypertension caused by changes that begin in the pulmonary vessels implies an increase in pulmonary vascular resistance. The pulmonary artery pressure is increased to a level higher than can be explained by the pulmonary venous pressure, because of obstruction within the small vessels of the lung. This may be the result of

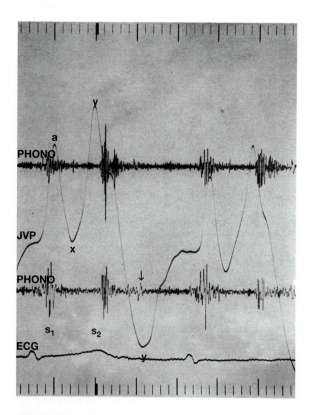

Figure 1.12–1. Jugular pulse tracing from a patient with chronic constrictive pericarditis. The a wave is synchronous with the first heart sound (S$_1$). The y descent marks tricuspid valve opening and the beginning of right ventricular filling. The sound (arrow) in early diastole is a pericardial knock.

spasm and may be potentially reversible, or of pulmonary vascular obstructive diseases, which can be identified histologically. These conditions include pulmonary thromboembolism, chronic respiratory disorders, congenital heart disease, and primary changes in the pulmonary circulation (Table 1.12–2).

Some patients with increased left atrial pressure, such as those with mitral valve disease or a chronic cardiomyopathy, have pulmonary hypertension that is only partly accounted for by their increased pulmonary venous pressure. They have additional obstruction in the pulmonary circulation, which has developed as a secondary reaction to the rise in downstream pressure. This so-called reactive pulmonary hypertension is at first caused by spasm and is reversible, but if left-sided heart disease has been present long enough, some of the reactive changes are permanent. Such reactive pulmonary vascular disease may account for a disappointing result from mitral valve replacement, or it may jeopardize the chance for successful cardiac transplantation in a patient with cardiomyopathy.

Clinical Features of Pulmonary Hypertension

In patients who have mild pulmonary hypertension, features of the primary disease usually determine the clinical picture, and the only clues to pulmonary hypertension may be an accentuated pulmonary closure sound (P2) and subtle evidence of right ventricular hypertrophy. However, as pulmonary vascular disease becomes severe, manifestations of pulmonary hypertension and right heart failure predominate, so that, regardless of the initiating cause, most patients with severe pulmonary vascular disease present in similar fashion.

The earliest symptom is fatigue. Exertional dyspnea begins gradually and is seldom severe until a late stage of the disease. Ankle swelling, abdominal discomfort, and an increase in girth reflect fluid retention and passive hepatic and splanchnic congestion. With further progression of the disease, patients develop anorexia, weight loss, angina from right ventricular ischemia, and syncope. Small hemoptyses are common, particularly in association with respiratory infections. Some patients have massive hemoptysis.

Physical examination reveals a chronically ill patient,

often tired and breathless on crossing the room. Mild cyanosis may be present as a result of right-to-left shunting across the foramen ovale. Severe central cyanosis with finger clubbing usually indicates that the patient has Eisenmenger's syndrome (see "Eisenmenger's Syndrome" below). Peripheral pulses are of small volume. The jugular venous pressure is elevated, often with a systolic wave of tricuspid regurgitation. The precordial impulse includes a prominent right ventricular lift and palpable bulge in the second left intercostal space over the pulmonary outflow tract. On auscultation, the pulmonary closure sound (P2) is accentuated, audible even at the apex, and often preceded by a systolic murmur and an ejection click. In advanced cases, a Graham Steell murmur of acquired pulmonary valve regurgitation may be present.

The heart size on chest x-ray depends on the initiating cause, but is seldom very large. The proximal pulmonary artery segment is prominent, and the distal pulmonary vessels are "pruned" (Figure 1.12–2). The echocardiogram shows a dilated and hypertrophied right ventricle. The short-axis cross section shows flattening of the septum and, in extreme cases, bulging of the septum into the left ventricular cavity (Figure 1.12–3). The most important aspect of the echocardiographic examination is to identify or exclude primary left-sided heart disease, in particular, mitral stenosis or other, rarer causes of left atrial obstruction (left atrial myxoma, congenital membrane within the atrium). It is essential not to overlook

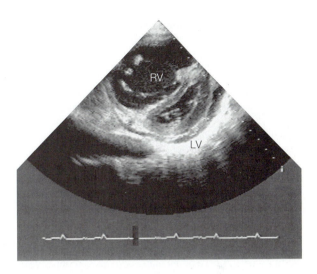

Figure 1.12–3. Echocardiogram of a patient with severe pulmonary hypertension, showing right ventricular enlargement and corresponding distortion of the interventricular septum.

such treatable causes of pulmonary hypertension, and before echocardiography was widely available it was sometimes necessary to perform cardiac catheterization to exclude occult mitral disease. In a few such patients, the only other clue to left-sided disease is left atrial as well as right ventricular hypertrophy on the electrocardiogram.

Primary Pulmonary Hypertension

Several causes of pulmonary vascular disease are associated with identical morphologic changes in the pulmonary arterioles and small pulmonary arteries, best referred to as "plexogenic pulmonary arteriopathy." These changes are seen in Eisenmenger's syndrome, in the pulmonary hypertension that can complicate systemic lupus erythematosus, and in rare patients with hepatic cirrhosis. "Primary pulmonary hypertension" is used to describe the idiopathic form of this kind of vascular disease, in which the disease originates in and is confined to the small pulmonary arteries. In the earlier stages, there is pronounced hypertrophy of the pulmonary arteriolar media, with an "onion-skin" type of intimal fibrosis; in advancing cases, there is fibrinoid necrosis and a lesion characterized by small venous lakes, the so-called plexiform change. These changes may be complicated by intravascular thrombosis and lead to widespread obliteration of small pulmonary vessels.

The pathogenesis of primary pulmonary hypertension is not understood, but it is widely suspected that the initiating event is intense pulmonary arteriolar spasm. Consistent with this view is the association with Raynaud's phenomenon, either in the patient or in the patient's family, and with systemic sclerosis and the CREST syndrome (calcinosis, Raynaud's phenomenon, esophageal involvement, sclerodactyly, telangiectasia; see also Chapter 3.10).

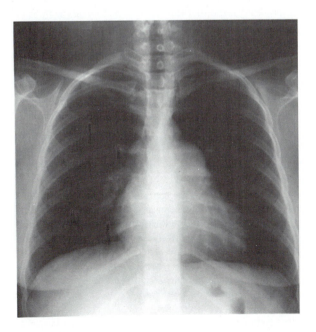

Figure 1.12–2. Chest x-ray of a patient with primary pulmonary hypertension. The central pulmonary artery segments are enlarged, but "pruning" of the peripheral pulmonary vessels is present. The cardiac silhouette is mildly enlarged.

Although it might be supposed that pulmonary hypertension complicating systemic sclerosis is merely secondary to pulmonary fibrosis, plexogenic pulmonary arteriopathy may occur in systemic sclerosis independent of the degree of fibrosis in the parenchyma.

Most patients are young, typically in their early 20's, but the overall age range extends from childhood to late middle life. There is a pronounced female preponderance of 4:1 or 5:1, and familial occurrence is not unusual. The disease is presumed to have a presymptomatic phase during which pulmonary hypertension develops. At the time of presentation, patients often have pulmonary artery resistance and pressure similar to those in the systemic circulation, fixed or reduced cardiac output, right ventricular enlargement, and increased right ventricular filling pressure.

The prognosis for patients with primary pulmonary hypertension is poor. The median survival is about 3 years from the time of diagnosis. Treatment with vasodilators, in particular the calcium channel blocker nifedipine, is helpful in 15–25% of patients. Among those who show a measurable beneficial response to nifedipine, the survival figures are much better. Many physicians advise anticoagulation, both because of the possibility that the patient has chronic thromboembolic disease (see "Chronic Thromboembolic Pulmonary Hypertension" below) and because in situ thrombosis may accelerate the progression of the idiopathic condition. In two uncontrolled studies, patients treated with warfarin survived longer than those not so treated. Currently, the only definitive therapy is transplantation of the lungs, either singly or as a combined heart and lung transplant, but the limited supply of suitable donors has restricted the application of these techniques.

Chronic Thromboembolic Pulmonary Hypertension:

A small number of patients with a clinical presentation identical with that of the idiopathic form of primary pulmonary hypertension prove to have chronic thromboembolic disease (Chapter 2.8). In some patients, this is related to taking oral contraceptives, but only a few have clinical evidence of systemic venous disease or venous thrombosis. The diagnosis is often difficult to make at the bedside, but ventilation-perfusion scans usually reveal multiple perfusion defects. Pulmonary arteriography is hazardous and has its chief value in acute or subacute massive pulmonary embolism when thrombolytic or surgical treatment is under consideration. When patients with chronic thromboembolic pulmonary vascular disease have persistently high pulmonary artery pressure, with systolic pressure greater than 60 mm Hg, the prognosis is poor, comparable to that of primary pulmonary hypertension.

Pulmonary Veno-Occlusive Disease

Obstruction at pulmonary venous level is a very rare cause of pulmonary hypertension. In babies, congenital anomalies of pulmonary venous return may occur with or without an obstructive component. In either case, they require early correction. In a few adults who present with acquired pulmonary hypertension, the diagnosis turns out to be a variant of pulmonary vascular disease known as pulmonary veno-occlusive disease, a fibrosing condition affecting small pulmonary veins and venules. The clinical clue to this condition is a presentation with established pulmonary hypertension and a history of episodic pulmonary edema. Right heart catheterization reveals variable wedge pressures, depending on whether the wedged position communicates with an obstructed or still patent segment of the pulmonary venous system.

Eisenmenger's Syndrome

Eisenmenger's syndrome may be defined as a congenital cardiac defect complicated by irreversible pulmonary vascular disease with a resistance so high that the shunt is bidirectional or reversed. Any of the congenital systemic-to-pulmonary communications that are normally associated with left-to-right shunting may be complicated by Eisenmenger's syndrome, for example, ventricular septal defect, persistent ductus arteriosus, atrial septal defect, or more complex lesions that cannot be surgically corrected in infancy, such as single ventricle. When pulmonary vascular disease complicates congenital heart disease, the pathologic condition resembles plexogenic pulmonary arteriopathy of primary pulmonary hypertension.

One might imagine that modern pediatric and surgical expertise would have made Eisenmenger's syndrome a disease of the past and that children with cardiac defects carrying the potential for pulmonary vascular disease would be detected and treated early in life. However, a number of patients with congenital heart disease continue to present for the first time at ages 5–25 years with established and inoperable pulmonary vascular disease. They come from families at all socioeconomic levels, and it must be assumed that many have been expertly examined as infants or young children. Thus, a proportion of patients develop the Eisenmenger reaction without going through the stage of having a large and clinically apparent left-to-right shunt. One presumes that vasospasm occurs from birth and that the high pulmonary vascular resistance that is normal during intrauterine life does not fall after delivery (Chapter 1.11).

Cor Pulmonale

To the pathologist, the term cor pulmonale means right ventricular enlargement caused by disease of the respiratory system with pulmonary hypertension. In clinical practice, cor pulmonale implies also that there is evidence of right ventricular failure. There are two general mechanisms by which lung disease causes pulmonary hypertension. In a few patients, such as those with fibrosing alveolitis, pulmonary vascular disease is secondary to obliteration of the pulmonary vascular bed as part of the underlying disease of the lung parenchyma. However, simple destruction of the pulmonary vasculature has to be very extensive to cause pulmonary hypertension; for example, pneumonectomy does not of itself cause a rise in pressure in the remaining pulmonary artery. In most patients with cor pulmonale, the primary mechanism is pulmonary artery vasoconstriction from chronic arterial hypoxemia. This, rather than destruction of lung tissue, is the cause of pulmonary hypertension and cor pulmonale in patients with chronic respiratory failure due, for example, to emphysema, chronic bronchitis, sleep apnea, kyphoscoliosis, cystic fibrosis, or muscular dystrophy.

Patients with cor pulmonale usually present with the cardiac complications of their pulmonary disease late in the course of a longstanding respiratory disorder. They develop fluid retention, signs of right ventricular enlargement, and tricuspid regurgitation. The cardiac signs in these patients may be difficult to appreciate clinically because of the chronic changes in the lungs. Echocardiography, which may be difficult, demonstrates right ventricular enlargement and flattening of the septum. On the chest x-ray, enlargement of the main pulmonary artery or the right descending pulmonary artery to 16 mm or more suggests pulmonary hypertension. Patients who develop pulmonary hypertension because of fibrosing alveolitis generally have less than 40% of the predicted vital capacity and diffusing capacity for carbon monoxide. Patients with emphysema and chronic bronchitis who develop pulmonary hypertension usually have PaO_2 values under 60 mm Hg and an FEV_1 value under 1 L.

Chronic respiratory disease is common in the population and can accompany pulmonary hypertension without being its cause. Thus, before diagnosing cor pulmonale it is important to be alert for primary cardiac disease, in particular mitral stenosis or atrial septal defect. Elderly patients with primary cardiac conditions and severe fluid retention frequently appear to be poor candidates for surgical correction, yet may obtain spectacular benefit when an underlying cardiac cause is correctly diagnosed and treated.

Management of cor pulmonale consists of treating the underlying condition and optimizing the patient's oxygenation and fluid balance. Since fluid retention is due both to elevated right heart pressures and to the renal ef-

fects of combined hypoxemia and hypercarbia, treatment directed at reversing the abnormal blood gas values is preferable to over-reliance on diuretics. The patients are sensitive to underfilling of the right heart, and zealous efforts to achieve a normal jugular venous pressure may result in a low cardiac output state and azotemia. Use of digitalis has little to contribute and may be hazardous in chronic hypoxemic states. The only exceptions may be patients with biventricular failure or supraventricular tachycardias. Treatment with oxygen has little effect in patients whose pulmonary hypertension is caused by obliteration of the pulmonary vascular bed, but can be effective in those who have a high pulmonary vascular resistance because of chronic hypoxemia. Patients with chronic lung disease who have a PaO_2 value under 60 mm Hg should be treated with low-flow oxygen. In these patients, continuous use of oxygen selectively vasodilates the pulmonary circulation and lowers pulmonary arterial pressure, thereby improving survival, exercise performance, and quality of life.

SUMMARY

▶ Anasarca and a high jugular pressure are most often caused by pulmonary hypertension, cardiomyopathy, atrial septal defect, or constrictive pericarditis.

▶ The most common cause of pulmonary hypertension is left-sided heart disease. Intrinsic pulmonary vascular disease (plexogenic pulmonary arteriopathy) is seen in cor pulmonale, lupus, chronic thromboembolic disease, and primary pulmonary hypertension.

▶ Oxygen is the only medicine that selectively dilates the pulmonary vascular bed. Calcium channel blockers and anticoagulants benefit some patients with pulmonary vascular disease.

SUGGESTED READING

Case Records of the Massachusetts General Hospital (Case 25–1992): A 33-year-old woman with cirrhosis and right ventricular failure. N Engl J Med 1992;326:1682.

D'Alonzo GE et al: Survival in patients with primary pulmonary hypertension: Results from a national prospective registry. Ann Intern Med 1991;115:343.

Rich S, Kaufmann E, Levy PS: The effect of high doses of cal-

cium-channel blockers on survival in primary pulmonary hypertension. N Engl J Med 1992;327:76.

Rich S et al: Antinuclear antibodies in primary pulmonary hypertension. J Am Coll Cardiol 1986;8:1307.

Rubin LJ: Pathology and pathophysiology of primary pulmonary hypertension. Am J Cardiol 1995;75:51A.

Hypertension

Michael J. Klag, MD, MPH, and Paul K. Whelton, MD, MSc

Hypertension is one of the most common clinical problems encountered by the internist. There are about 50 million patients with hypertension in the United States. Usually, such patients are identified at periodic medical examinations or during care for other medical conditions, but some are detected through community screening programs. The clinical spectrum of hypertension runs the gamut from no symptoms with a minimally elevated blood pressure to markedly elevated levels of blood pressure, acute symptoms, and the need for immediate treatment.

"Essential hypertension" is a misnomer. This term came about because physicians erroneously thought that hypertension was an essential accompaniment of aging, necessary to force blood through atherosclerotic blood vessels. We now know that most hypertension results from physical inactivity, an excessive intake of salt and alcohol, and unhealthy lifestyles that lead to obesity. "Secondary hypertension" refers to cases in which there is an identifiable medical cause for the elevated blood pressure. "Accelerated hypertension" describes markedly elevated blood pressure (diastolic blood pressure >115 mm Hg, usually >130 mm Hg) associated with hemorrhages and exudates in the eyegrounds; the term "malignant hypertension" is used when papilledema is also present. Because the pathophysiology and the treatment implications of the latter two groups are the same, most clinicians lump them together as "accelerated-malignant hypertension." In this chapter, we describe the pathophysiology of hypertension, review the epidemiology of blood pressure, discuss the clinical characteristics and evaluation of patients with hypertension, and provide a framework for selection of antihypertensive drugs.

PATHOPHYSIOLOGY OF ESSENTIAL HYPERTENSION

Development of hypertension is usually a slow and gradual process, and pathophysiologic changes differ in various stages of this disease. Blood pressure is determined by cardiac output and peripheral resistance. A number of factors affect these two variables and may contribute to the pathogenesis of hypertension. Extracellular fluid volume, an essential determinant of cardiac output, is increased in hypertension because of excess intake of sodium, impaired renal sodium excretion, or hormonal changes that lead to conservation of sodium and water by the kidney. The renin-angiotensin-aldosterone system is the major hormone system involved in the control of blood pressure, and increased aldosterone levels are responsible for some of the enhanced renal retention of sodium and water seen in hypertensives.

In recent years, essential hypertension has been linked to insulin resistance. Insulin resistance results from obesity and, possibly, a genetic predisposition. The compensatory hyperinsulinemia associated with insulin resistance stimulates renal sodium reabsorption and sympathetic nervous system activity. Higher Na^+-K^+-ATPase activity in hypertensive patients is also associated with increased renal sodium reabsorption.

Even if hypertension begins because of elevated cardiac output, an increased peripheral resistance is both necessary and sufficient to perpetuate the elevated blood pressure. Peripheral resistance is controlled by neural, local, and humoral factors. All blood vessels are richly supplied by adrenergic nerves that provide for vasoconstriction. Sympathetic nervous activity is increased in patients destined to be hypertensive, even before hypertension is clinically evident. Higher angiotensin II levels and lower kallikrein-kinin system activity also contribute to the increased peripheral resistance in hypertensives. Abnormalities in cation transport in hypertension may increase intracellular concentration of Na^+ and Ca^{2+} and decrease vessel compliance, thereby increasing systemic vascular resistance. Patients with hypertension, as well as their normotensive children, also have impaired endothelium-dependent vasodilatation. This abnormality is thought to be caused by arterial endothelium not producing enough nitric oxide, a vasodilator. This may be another mechanism for hypertensive patients' increased systemic resistance.

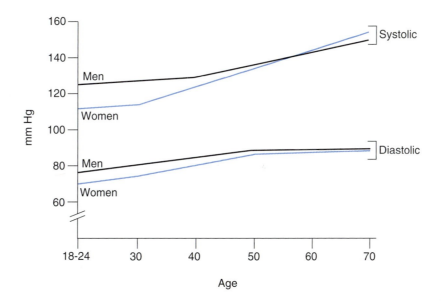

Figure 1.13–1. Mean blood pressure by age and sex in US adults, 1976–80. (Modified from: Blood pressure levels in persons 18–74 years of age in 1976–80, and trends in blood pressure from 1960 to 1980 in the United States. In: *Vital and Health Statistics,* Series 11, No. 234. National Center for Health Statistics, US Department of Health and Human Services Publication No. [PHS] 86-1684, 1986.)

EPIDEMIOLOGY OF BLOOD PRESSURE

Blood Pressure and Aging

Mean blood pressure has been consistently demonstrated to rise with age in westernized societies. The pattern seen in Figure 1.13–1, from a representative sample of the United States population, is typical of the relationship. Both systolic and diastolic blood pressure are higher in men than in women in early adult life, but the reverse is true in later years. In both genders, diastolic blood pressure rises more gradually than systolic pressure with increasing age. As a consequence, pulse pressure widens progressively in the elderly. The typical rise in systolic blood pressure with progressive aging is due, in part, to a decrease in the capacitance of the arterial bed but is not an automatic biologic consequence of aging.

Persons from preindustrial societies who remain physically active and lean, and consume diets with relatively large amounts of potassium and small amounts of sodium, do not show an age-related rise in blood pressure. The strongest argument against regarding the age-related rise in blood pressure as physiologic is the results of the Systolic Hypertension in the Elderly Program. This clinical trial showed that treatment of elevated systolic blood pressure in the setting of normal diastolic blood pressure reduces future risk of coronary heart disease and stroke.

Classification and Prevalence of Hypertension

Hypertension is exceedingly common in all developed countries, and its prevalence, like mean blood pressure, increases with age. Table 1.13–1 gives definitions of the stages and follow-up for hypertension, based on recommendations of the fifth report of the Joint National Committee (JNC V) on Detection, Evaluation, and Treatment of Hypertension. Systolic blood pressure is given equal weight with diastolic blood pressure in this taxonomy.

Table 1.13–1. Blood pressure classification and follow-up recommendations for persons aged ≥18.*

Category	Systolic (mm Hg)	Diastolic (mm Hg)	Recommended Follow-Up
Normal	<130	<85	Recheck in 2 yr
High normal	130–139	85–89	Recheck in 1 yr
Hypertension			
Stage 1 (mild)	140–159	90–99	Confirm within 2 mo
Stage 2 (moderate)	160–179	100–109	Evaluate or refer for care within 1 mo
Stage 3 (severe)	180–209	110–119	Evaluate or refer for care within 1 wk
Stage 4 (very severe)	≥210	≥120	Evaluate or refer for care immediately

*When systolic and diastolic pressures fall into different categories, the higher category should be used.
Modified and reproduced, with permission, from: The fifth report of the Joint National Committee on Detection, Evaluation, and Treatment of High Blood Pressure (JNC V). Arch Intern Med 1993;153:154.

Table 1.13–2. Prevalence of hypertension* by age and race in US adults, 1976–1980.

Age	Whites (%)	Blacks (%)
18–24	1.9	2.9
25–34	6.2	10.0
35–44	10.4	25.5
45–54	23.8	43.4
55–64	33.0	53.8
65–74	43.7	59.9
18–74†	16.8	25.7

*Hypertension is defined as systolic blood pressure ≥160 mm Hg or diastolic blood pressure ≥95 mm Hg at one visit, or the patient is taking antihypertensive medication.
†Age adjusted to the US population.
Modified from: Blood pressure levels in persons 18–74 years of age in 1976–80, and trends in blood pressure from 1960 to 1980 in the United States. In: *Vital and Health Statistics,* Series 11, No. 234. National Center for Health Statistics, US Department of Health and Human Services Publication No. (PHS) 86-1684, 1986.

The term "stage" is used to categorize hypertension because of the chronologic progression of high blood pressure. If persons with any degree of hypertension are not treated, they tend to progress to a higher stage of hypertension. The category of high normal blood pressure is included because persons in this range are at high risk of developing frank hypertension in the near future, and they also have a greater risk of future cardiovascular disease than persons with lower levels of blood pressure.

Estimates of the prevalence of hypertension in the United States based on observations at a single visit are provided in Table 1.13–2. Because of substantial biologic and measurement variability, classification and treatment decisions should normally be based on an average of two to three measurements obtained at each of two or more visits (ie, six to nine blood pressure measurements). At every age, the prevalence of hypertension is higher in blacks than in whites, regardless of differences in body weight and educational level.

Blood Pressure and Cardiovascular Risk

The physician measures blood pressure because of what it implies about risk of future disease as well as the clinical state of the patient. Figure 1.13–2 shows the probability of developing cardiovascular disease by level of systolic blood pressure. Higher blood pressure imparts a higher risk of cardiovascular disease incidence and mortality. The risk is graded, without a threshold, and increases throughout the entire range of blood pressure. When other cardiovascular risk factors are present, the shape of the curve remains the same but the risk of future disease increases further. Thus, the risk of developing cardiovascular disease at a given level of blood pressure can vary 8- to 10-fold, depending on other risk factors.

The risk is similar for systolic and diastolic blood pressure, although we have recently come to realize that systolic blood pressure is somewhat more important. The relative risk of stroke, especially hemorrhagic stroke, associated with hypertension is stronger than the corresponding relative risk of coronary heart disease. Given that coronary heart disease is three to four times more common than stroke, however, the absolute number of blood pressure-related coronary heart disease events is far greater than the corresponding number of blood pressure-related strokes. This is true for both genders and every level of blood pressure and age. Although the risk of cardiovascular disease is greatest at the highest level of blood

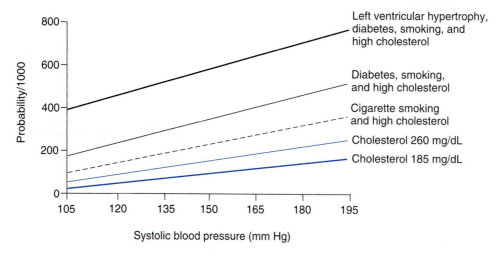

Figure 1.13–2. Cumulative effect of additional risk factors on the probability that a 50-year-old man will develop cardiovascular disease within 8 years, plotted by systolic blood pressure. Almost all the men in this study were white. (Modified from McGee D: The probability of developing certain cardiovascular diseases in eight years at specified values of some characteristics. In: *The Framingham Study: An Epidemiological Investigation of Cardiovascular Disease.* Kannel WB, Gordon T [editors]. US Department of Health, Education and Welfare Publication No. [NIH] 74-618, 1973.)

pressure, few people in the community have such elevated values. Because most of the people in the population are in the high normal range, most cardiovascular disease events attributable to blood pressure occur in this group. To prevent the majority of blood pressure-related cardiovascular disease, therefore, identification and treatment of individual hypertensive patients need to be supplemented with public health interventions designed to lower the blood pressure of the whole population.

Important variables that modify the association of blood pressure with cardiovascular disease are gender and race. Men have a higher risk of disease than women at every level of blood pressure. Blacks also have an increased risk of developing blood pressure-related complications compared with whites. It is unclear whether these racial differences are caused by an increased susceptibility to the harmful effects of high blood pressure or merely reflect longer duration of hypertension and less treatment. The relation of blood pressure to cardiovascular disease is similar for both fatal and nonfatal events. Mortality from all causes is somewhat higher in persons at the lower end of the blood pressure distribution because a number of chronic diseases are associated with lower levels of blood pressure.

EVALUATION OF THE PATIENT WITH HYPERTENSION

Measurement of Blood Pressure

It is important to measure blood pressure carefully or else patients may be inappropriately labeled, or worse still, started on unnecessary lifelong drug therapy. Blood pressure should be measured after the patient has been seated quietly for 5 minutes. The patient's arm should be supported at the level of the heart, and the stethoscope placed over the brachial pulse just distal to the cuff. During inflation, the ipsilateral radial pulse should be palpated and the cuff inflated to a pressure about 20 mm Hg above the point at which the pulse disappears. In some patients, the radial artery can still be palpated even after their pulse disappears (Osler's sign). This reflects the presence of a rigid, calcified radial artery. Resistance of the calcified brachial artery to compression by the arm cuff may, rarely, lead to a falsely elevated blood pressure measurement.

The cuff should be deflated slowly, at a rate of about 2–3 mm Hg/sec. Letting the cuff down more rapidly leads to underestimating systolic and overestimating diastolic blood pressure. Systolic blood pressure should be recorded at the appearance of the first Korotkoff sound, and diastolic pressure at the disappearance of the blood pressure sounds. An appropriately sized cuff should be used in conjunction with a mercury sphygmomanometer. If an aneroid sphygmomanometer is used, it should be calibrated periodically against a mercury sphygmomanometer. Patients should be encouraged to monitor their own blood pressure at home, using a conventional cuff rather than an electronic blood pressure measurement device, since most of these are inaccurate. Ambulatory blood pressure monitors that record repeatedly over a 24-hour period are also available. Although these devices can provide a great deal of information, it is not known whether ambulatory blood pressure measurements will prove better than office readings for predicting future cardiovascular disease and for routinely managing hypertensive patients. Their use in clinical practice should probably be limited to management of patients with a marked discrepancy between their office and home blood pressure measurements.

History, Physical Examination, and Laboratory Studies

The physician should have three goals in mind when assessing a new patient with hypertension. The first is to determine whether the patient has suffered *target organ damage* from hypertension. If so, this provides a strong indication for pharmacologic antihypertensive therapy. The second goal is to determine whether there are any indications of *secondary hypertension*. Because the prevalence of secondary hypertension is low, further evaluation should be based on the signs, symptoms, or laboratory findings indicating an increased likelihood of secondary hypertension. Lastly, other *cardiovascular disease risk factors* should be assessed because the probability of developing future cardiovascular disease depends not only on the patient's level of blood pressure but also other risk indicators as well. The eyes should be examined for signs of hypertensive retinal vascular changes (see Color Plates). A urinalysis should be performed, serum potassium and creatinine levels should be measured, and an ECG should be obtained. A complete blood count should also be obtained if any antihypertensive drug therapy is contemplated. Echocardiography is indicated to look for left ventricular hypertrophy, if left ventricular enlargement would influence whether to treat, for example, in an asymptomatic patient whose blood pressure is mildly elevated.

Secondary Hypertension

Less than 5% of patients with established hypertension have a secondary form of hypertension, that is, an underlying structural or hormonal abnormality that causes the high blood pressure. Correction of the abnormality often leads to normalization of the patient's blood pressure. Common causes of secondary hypertension are listed in Table 1.13–3. Because the prevalence of secondary hypertension is low, evaluating all patients with an elevated blood pressure would yield many false-positive results and generate excessive costs and anxiety. Therefore, secondary causes of hypertension should be sought selectively, in patients in whom there is a reasonable chance of their being found.

Drinking more than two alcoholic beverages a day, although not usually listed as a cause of secondary hypertension, is a behavior that accounts for 6–11% of

Table 1.13–3. Causes of secondary hypertension.

Renovascular disease
Renal parenchymal disease
Pheochromocytoma
Medications and drugs
    Oral contraceptives
    Sympathomimetic drugs (decongestants, cocaine,
       amphetamines)
    Alcohol
Pregnancy
Coarctation of the aorta
Aortic insufficiency
Endocrine disorders
    Acromegaly
    Hyperthyroidism, hypothyroidism
    Mineralocorticoid excess
    Glucocorticoid excess
    Hyperparathyroidism

hypertension in men. Renal artery stenosis is the cause of about 1% of hypertension. All the other causes of secondary hypertension are much less common.

Several factors in the medical history suggest the possibility of secondary hypertension: severe hypertension in a young person, especially with a negative family history of hypertension; a poor response to therapy, as indicated by stage 3 or stage 4 levels of hypertension on three or more antihypertensive drugs; accelerated or malignant hypertension; and, in an older person, sudden onset of severe hypertension or a worsening of blood pressure control in the setting of previously well-controlled hypertension. The diagnosis of renal artery stenosis secondary to fibromuscular dysplasia should be considered in women less than age 40 with diastolic blood pressure of 110 mm Hg or higher. Recent onset or worsening of hypertension in the elderly suggests a diagnosis of renal artery stenosis secondary to atherosclerotic disease, especially if there is evidence of large vessel atherosclerotic disease elsewhere.

A history of orthostatic symptoms, palpitations, "spells," and labile hypertension raises the suspicion of pheochromocytoma. Increasing ring and shoe size, headaches, and a history of diabetes suggest acromegaly. Temperature intolerance, changes in hair and skin, changes in bowel habits, and other symptoms of thyroid disease should be ascertained. Hyperthyroidism is usually associated with systolic hypertension because of increased cardiac output. Hypothyroidism causes diastolic hypertension secondary to increased peripheral vascular resistance. Truncal obesity, purple striae, and other signs of glucocorticoid excess point to a diagnosis of Cushing's syndrome. Patients with primary hyperaldosteronism and other causes of mineralocorticoid excess may note muscle weakness caused by hypokalemia. Patients with hyperparathyroidism have numerous symptoms attributable to an excess of parathyroid hormone.

At the first evaluation, blood pressure should be measured in both arms to make certain that it is equal. Blood pressure should also be measured in the popliteal artery to rule out coarctation of the aorta. Signs of end-organ dis-

ease and causes of secondary hypertension, listed in Table 1.13–3, should be specifically sought, and careful auscultation for a renal artery bruit performed. If the initial evaluation suggests that an underlying cause of hypertension is present, the diagnosis should be thoroughly pursued.

TREATMENT OF HYPERTENSION

Lifestyle Changes

Weight loss, increased physical activity, reduced salt intake (≤100 mmol sodium or 6 g salt per day), and moderation of alcohol consumption (no more than two drinks per day) are recommended for persons with high normal blood pressure as well as for those with established hypertension (Figure 1.13–3). Nonpharmacologic interventions lower blood pressure, regardless of its severity. With lifestyle modification, antihypertensive drug therapy can be reduced or even stopped in well-controlled hyperten-

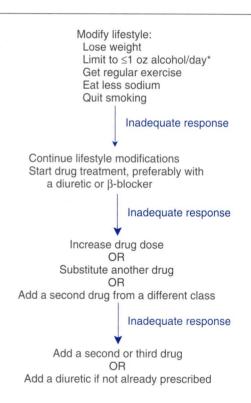

*1 oz alcohol = beer 24 oz, wine 8 oz, or 100 proof whiskey 2 oz.

Figure 1.13–3. Treatment algorithm for hypertension. An adequate response is defined as reaching or making considerable progress toward reaching target blood pressure. (Modified and reproduced, with permission, from: The Fifth Report of the Joint National Committee on Detection, Evaluation, and Treatment of High Blood Pressure [JNC V]. Arch Intern Med 1993;153:154.)

sive patients. The prospect of stopping their drug therapy may help motivate patients to achieve and maintain the desired change in lifestyle.

Several principles are helpful in achieving success with nonpharmacologic intervention. Reasonable, attainable short-term goals should be established in collaboration with the patient. Over time, short-term success can build incrementally toward the patient's overall goal. Patients should be seen frequently for short visits to provide feedback pertinent to the intervention (eg, weight, urine sodium concentration) as well as positive reinforcement and problem solving. The family, especially the food preparer, should be involved, and other health professionals, particularly nutritionists and nurses, or community resources such as weight loss centers, can play a part. Successful lifestyle interventions take time.

Other nonpharmacologic interventions such as potassium supplementation, omega-3 fatty acids, and calcium and magnesium supplementation require further study before they can be recommended for widespread use.

Rationale and Benefits of Drug Treatment

The availability of effective, well-tolerated pharmacologic treatment for hypertension is one of the success stories of modern medicine. Mortality from hypertension and blood pressure-associated diseases, such as coronary heart disease and stroke, have fallen markedly in the United States over the last 20 years. Improved detection and treatment of hypertension have undoubtedly played a major role in these beneficial trends. Antihypertensive drug treatment of malignant or accelerated hypertension has obvious effects on mortality from stroke, renal disease, and congestive heart failure. Treatment of mild-to-moderate hypertension has also been shown to prevent blood pressure-related complications such as congestive heart failure and stroke. Treatment also reduces the risk of atherosclerotic complications of mild-to-moderate hypertension, although the benefit is less pronounced.

Table 1.13–4 represents an overview of the results of 14 randomized clinical trials of antihypertensive drug therapy in patients with mild and mild-to-moderate hypertension. Most of these trials used a stepped-care approach in which diuretics were the initial form of drug treatment. Overall, drug therapy resulted in a 42% reduction in the risk of stroke, similar to the 35–40% expected from the average reduction in blood pressure. Coronary heart disease risk was reduced by 14%, which, although significant, is somewhat less than the 20–25% expected based on observational studies. This lower-than-expected effect of treatment on coronary heart disease has variously been attributed to an inadequate length of follow-up, chance, and the harmful metabolic side effects of diuretics. Recent clinical trials, however, have demonstrated that low doses of thiazide diuretics (eg, chlorthalidone 12.5 mg a day) result in much more substantial reductions in coronary heart disease incidence. β-Blockers, surprisingly, do not appear to be consistently better than diuretics in the primary prevention of coronary heart disease. Clinical trials compar-

Table 1.13–4. Summary of 14 randomized trials of antihypertensive drug therapy.*

	Total Events (Fatal Events)		
	Treatment Groups	Control Groups	Reduction in Risk
Stroke	289 (87)	484 (160)	42% (45%)
Coronary heart disease	671 (316)	771 (356)	14% (11%)
Other vascular deaths	86	97	—
All vascular deaths	489	613	(21%)
All other deaths	396	401	(1%)

*The 36,908 patients were evenly randomized to treatment and control groups. The mean diastolic blood pressure of the treatment groups was 5–6 mm Hg lower than that of the control groups. Average follow-up was 5 years.
Modified and reproduced with permission, from Collins R et al: Blood pressure, stroke, and coronary heart disease (Part 2). Lancet 1990;335:827. Copyright by The Lancet Ltd.

ing the effects of newer classes of drugs, such as calcium channel blockers and angiotensin converting enzyme (ACE) inhibitors, on clinical cardiovascular disease end points such as stroke, coronary heart disease, and kidney disease are now underway. Such trials are necessary to determine whether these new, usually more expensive, classes of drugs provide an improved level of disease prevention.

When to Start

Patients with an average systolic blood pressure of 140 mm Hg or higher or an average diastolic blood pressure of 90 mm Hg or higher on three or more visits should be started on drug therapy. Physicians may decide to delay drug therapy and closely observe patients with an average blood pressure in the 90–94 mm Hg diastolic or 140–149 mm Hg systolic range. Such patients should be started on medication if they have other cardiovascular disease risk factors or end-organ damage. The goal of antihypertensive treatment is to prevent future cardiovascular disease with a minimum of side effects. Many physicians have expressed concern that excessive lowering of diastolic blood pressure may increase the risk of myocardial infarction, but the basis for this conclusion is questionable. A diastolic blood pressure between 80 and 90 mm Hg on treatment appears to be an appropriate goal in most patients.

Choice of Drug for Initial Therapy

Most antihypertensive drugs lower blood pressure effectively when given as monotherapy. Ideally, selection of a particular drug should be based on demonstrated ability of the agent to prevent future sequelae of hypertension. Evidence for a reduction in cardiovascular disease with the use of antihypertensive drugs suitable for monotherapy is, however, available only for thiazide diuretics and β-blockers. Thus, the recent JNC V report recommends these classes as the drugs of choice for initial treatment in patients with uncomplicated hypertension (see Figure

1.13–3). Clinicians often choose other antihypertensive drugs based on a presumed special benefit in a given clinical situation or to minimize side effects. Once-a-day dosage, a favorable side-effect profile, and cheaper cost are characteristics that enhance compliance and should influence choice of antihypertensive agent. Although the large number of drugs precludes a detailed discussion of each agent, broad recommendations can be made regarding the classes of drugs available for monotherapy of hypertension (Table 1.13–5).

Thiazide Diuretics: Thiazide diuretics were the first available effective form of pharmacologic therapy for hypertension. A major advantage of diuretics is the large amount of information available on their efficacy and side effects. Diuretics can be used in almost any patient with hypertension, and they are often considered the treatment of choice for patients with isolated systolic hypertension, for elderly hypertensives, and for hypertensive patients who have trouble paying for their medications. A month's supply of thiazide diuretics costs only a few dollars. Thiazide diuretics are particularly effective in lowering blood pressure among elderly and black patients. A disadvantage of these drugs is the potential for metabolic side effects during chronic therapy. Because they can cause hypokalemia and hypomagnesemia, thiazide diuretics should be given in low doses, preferably in combination with a potassium-sparing agent. Other metabolic side effects include hyperglycemia, hyperuricemia, and elevations of total and very low density lipoprotein (VLDL) cholesterol.

Diuretics can worsen glucose intolerance in persons with diabetes and increase the risk of developing diabetes mellitus in patients free of the disease. Thiazide diuretics should not be prescribed for patients with a history of gout, in whom they may precipitate an acute attack, and in patients with hyperlipidemia. The effect of these drugs on the lipid profile can be blunted by instructing patients how to adopt a step I American Heart Association diet.

β-Blockers: β-Blockers lower blood pressure in most patients but are somewhat less effective than diuretics in the elderly and in blacks. β-Blockers are effective in secondary prevention of myocardial infarction and should be used in hypertensive patients with a previous myocardial infarction unless there is a contraindication to their administration. β-Blockers are effective in the treatment of angina pectoris and prevention of migraine headaches and are often a good choice for the treatment of hypertensive patients with these conditions. Generic β-blockers are available at fairly low cost.

Because of their negative inotropic properties, β-blockers should be avoided when there is evidence of left ventricular pump failure. They can also worsen cardiac conduction delays. Because they can cause bronchoconstriction, β-blockers should be avoided in persons with a history of childhood or adult asthma and in those who have signs or symptoms of chronic obstructive pulmonary disease. Selective β_1-blockers, although safer than nonselective β-blockers in these settings, may also cause pulmonary symptoms and should not be prescribed. Despite their effectiveness in the secondary prevention of myocardial infarction, these drugs tend to lower high-density lipoprotein (HDL) cholesterol. Agents with intrinsic sympathomimetic activity (pindolol, acebutolol) are an exception to this rule. β-Blockers decrease cardiac output, increase systemic vascular resistance, and may worsen symptoms of peripheral vascular disease. Like thiazide diuretics, β-blockers increase the risk of developing diabetes. They may also mask symptoms of hypoglycemia in poorly controlled diabetics. Other drugs are more appropriate choices for first-line therapy in diabetics.

Angiotensin Converting Enzyme (ACE) Inhibitors: In persons with high renin hypertension, secondary to either large- or small-vessel renal disease, ACE inhibitors are the treatment of choice. ACE inhibitors decrease mortality in patients with dilated cardiomyopathy more than treatment with nitrates or other vasodilators. Thus, in patients

Table 1.13–5. Overview of factors influencing choice of monotherapy for hypertension.

Drug Class	Pro	Con
Thiazide diuretics	Elderly and black patients, low cost	Coronary artery disease, diabetes mellitus, gout, hyperlipidemia
β-blockers	Coronary artery disease (especially post-MI), congestive heart failure (diastolic dysfunction), migraine, low cost	Congestive heart failure (systolic dysfunction), asthma, COPD, cardiac conduction defects, peripheral vascular disease, diabetes
ACE inhibitors	Congestive heart failure (systolic dysfunction), high renin hypertension, diabetes, renal disease	Bilateral renal artery stenosis, high cost, pregnancy
Calcium channel blockers	Elderly and black patients, congestive heart failure (diastolic dysfunction), angina, vasospastic disease (especially Prinzmetal's angina), peripheral vascular disease, migraine, cardiovascular disease	Congestive heart failure (systolic dysfunction), cardiac conduction defects, high cost
α_1-blockers	Hyperlipidemia, benign prostatic hypertrophy, diabetes	Elderly patients, high cost
Central sympatholytics (α_2-agonists)	Poor control with 2-drug regimen, low cost	Elderly patients, depression, poor tolerance by most persons

ACE, angiotensin converting enzyme; COPD, chronic obstructive pulmonary disease; MI, myocardial infarction.

who have both hypertension and left ventricular systolic dysfunction, ACE inhibitors are the drugs of choice. ACE inhibitors are also the best drugs to use in patients with type I diabetes because they decrease the transglomerular pressure gradient and thus reduce proteinuria in patients with diabetic renal disease. ACE inhibitors also retard progression of renal disease in type I diabetics with proteinuria. These drugs have also been shown, in insulin clamp studies, to improve insulin resistance. If insulin resistance is one of the underlying mechanisms of essential hypertension, as has been suggested, use of these drugs would represent an approach to ameliorating the underlying metabolic disturbance in essential hypertension.

ACE inhibitors may cause dangerous hypotension when maintenance of blood pressure is highly dependent on the renin-angiotensin axis, as in patients on high doses of diuretics and in those with congestive heart failure. To avoid this problem, diuretics should be discontinued 2–3 days prior to starting patients on ACE inhibitors. If discontinuation is not possible, the dose of diuretics should be cut in half. In the setting of bilateral renal artery stenosis, hypotension and acute renal failure may occur promptly after starting ACE inhibitors. If this condition is suspected, other drugs should be used pending a more complete evaluation. ACE inhibitors may worsen renal failure in a patient with preexisting renal disease, but especially nephrosclerosis and polycystic kidney disease. One of the most common adverse effects of these drugs is chronic cough. It is unclear whether persons with preexisting pulmonary disease are at increased risk of the development of this problem, but it is probably wise to avoid using ACE inhibitors in such patients. ACE inhibitors are absolutely contraindicated during pregnancy, because they cause fetal and neonatal morbidity and death.

Calcium Channel Blockers: Calcium channel blockers comprise dihydropiridines (nifedipine, nicardipine, isradipine, and others), diltiazem, and verapamil. Like thiazide diuretics, calcium channel blockers are especially effective in lowering blood pressure in elderly persons and in blacks. Verapamil causes significantly better regression of left ventricular hypertrophy than β-blockers and other calcium channel blockers in patients with hypertensive cardiac hypertrophy. Like β-blockers, these drugs are effective in the treatment of angina and migraine headaches. Because they decrease systemic vascular resistance, they do not worsen peripheral vascular disease. Animal studies have suggested that dihydropiridines reduce ischemic stroke infarct size, but studies in humans have been disappointing.

In the past, dihydropiridines have been used as vasodilators to decrease systemic vascular resistance and to "unload" the left ventricle in persons with congestive heart failure. However, these drugs do have some negative inotropic activity, and studies have suggested that nifedipine may increase mortality in patients with left ventricular pump failure. This finding, in addition to the demonstrated benefit of ACE inhibitors in this setting, argues for

avoiding the prescribing of dihydropiridines in patients with hypertension and systolic dysfunction. A relatively new dihydropyridine, amlodipine, is probably the safest calcium channel blocker in this setting. In terms of cost, calcium channel blockers are the most expensive group of drugs. However, a long-acting generic preparation of verapamil is available.

α-1-Blockers: Although α_1-blockers are less commonly used by physicians than other classes of antihypertensive drug therapy, they are an effective form of therapy for many patients. In a number of studies α_1-blockers have been shown to have a beneficial effect on the lipid profile by raising HDL and lowering total cholesterol. Thus, they are the therapeutic agents of choice in treatment of hypertension when hyperlipidemia is present. In theory, these beneficial lipid effects should result in a much larger reduction of coronary heart disease than can be achieved with other forms of antihypertensive therapy, but this notion is only now being tested in clinical trials. α_1-Blockers improve symptoms of bladder outlet obstruction in men with benign prostatic hypertrophy. Finally, preliminary studies have suggested that α_1-blockers, like ACE inhibitors, may improve insulin resistance. This finding requires confirmation.

A major problem with α_1-blockers is the occurrence of orthostatic symptoms, especially following administration of the first dose. Hypotension is less common when the initial dose is minimized, when the patient is supine, and probably when longer-acting preparations (terazosin, doxazosin) are used.

Central Sympatholytics: Central sympatholytics are very effective hypotensive agents and were the mainstay of antihypertensive therapy for many years. They block some symptoms of opiate and nicotine withdrawal and are very effective in causing regression of left ventricular hypertrophy. However, their side-effect profile is less favorable than other classes of drug therapy, such as ACE inhibitors, calcium channel blockers, and α_1-blockers. For this reason, use of central sympatholytics should probably be limited to persons whose blood pressure is inadequately controlled with a two-drug regimen and to those who have a contraindication to administration of other drugs. Because these drugs impair cognition, the clinician should not prescribe them for elderly patients. Because of secondary hyperaldosteronism, they also tend to lose their effectiveness when used alone. These drugs are available in generic form and are inexpensive.

Compliance with Medical Therapy

The most common reason for poor control of hypertension is noncompliance with therapy, not secondary hypertension. Persons who miss follow-up appointments or who drop out of care are most likely to be noncompliant. Compliance can be assessed by asking patients in a nonjudgmental fashion whether they ever miss taking their medications and, if so, how often. Although not very sensitive (it detects only about 50% of noncompliers), this approach is very specific (close to 100% of those who answer "no" are, indeed, compliant). Drug compliance can also be evaluated by pill counting and by testing for drug metabolites in the blood or urine. Urine toxicology screens are also useful when surreptitious use of stimulants is suspected.

Hypertensive Urgencies and Emergencies

Moderate or severe elevations of blood pressure sometimes place patients at imminent risk of a hypertensive complication unless their blood pressure is promptly lowered. The rapidity with which blood pressure should be lowered depends not only on the patient's blood pressure level but also on other findings that may influence the likelihood of an acute hypertensive complication. Situations in which blood pressure must be lowered within 2 hours are often termed *hypertensive emergencies.*

Most patients with a hypertensive emergency have symptoms and signs of central nervous system or cardiovascular disease, including alteration in mental status, papilledema, focal neurologic deficits, angina pectoris, dyspnea, rales, and acute changes on the ECG. Examples of a hypertensive emergency include (1) hypertensive encephalopathy, (2) hypertension-induced angina pectoris, intracranial hemorrhage, acute left ventricular failure with pulmonary edema, or type B aortic dissection, and (3) severe hypertension associated with acute myocardial infarction, toxemia of pregnancy, or extensive burns or head trauma.

Situations that are less dramatic but nevertheless mandate control of blood pressure within a 24-hour period are commonly referred to as *hypertensive urgencies.* These include accelerated or malignant hypertension in a patient without evidence of an impending complication and moderate or severe hypertension in the perioperative period or in patients requiring surgery. It is not always possible to make a clear distinction between a hypertensive urgency and a hypertensive emergency.

Most patients with the above conditions and all patients with hypertensive encephalopathy have impaired cerebral autoregulation. In the face of a fall in systemic blood pressure, cerebral blood flow may fall, causing cerebral ischemia and stroke. For safety reasons, patients with hypertensive emergencies should be admitted to the hospital and treated with a parenteral agent to initially lower dias-

tolic blood pressure to about 110 mm Hg. After several days, diastolic blood pressure can gradually be lowered to a more normal level. Intravenous nitroprusside is probably the therapy of choice for the initial lowering of blood pressure because it allows minute-to-minute control of blood pressure. A variety of other parenteral drugs including other direct vasodilators, α-blockers, β-blockers, and $\alpha\beta$-blockers (labetalol) can also be used. When pheochromocytoma is suspected, phentolamine is the drug of choice.

Most patients with hypertensive urgencies can be treated with oral medications. Because ACE inhibitors preserve cerebral autoregulation, they are probably the oral drugs of choice. Sublingual nifedipine and oral clonidine can also be used to lower blood pressure rapidly in such patients. However, use of these drugs is not without problems. There have been several case reports of myocardial ischemia or infarction with the use of oral nifedipine in this setting. Rapid titration of blood pressure with clonidine causes sedation, and many patients are continued on this medication chronically. Because rebound hypertension may occur with discontinuation of clonidine and noncompliance is common in patients who develop accelerated hypertension, use of clonidine in this setting may not be a wise choice.

SUMMARY

▶ Treatment of hypertension, both systolic and diastolic, reduces a person's risk of developing cardiovascular disease.

▶ The initial assessment of a patient with hypertension should focus on assessing other cardiovascular disease risk factors, detecting end-organ disease from elevated blood pressure, and screening for secondary forms of hypertension.

▶ Thiazide diuretics and β-blockers should receive first consideration when selecting antihypertensive medications because their efficacy and safety have been shown in long-term trials. Newer classes of drugs should be used in clinical situations in which they may have special benefit.

SUGGESTED READING

The fifth report of the Joint National Committee on Detection, Evaluation, and Treatment of High Blood Pressure (JNC V). Arch Intern Med 1993;153:154.

Hebert PR et al: Recent evidence on drug therapy of mild to moderate hypertension and decreased risk of coronary heart disease. Arch Intern Med 1993;153:578.

Kaplan NM: *Clinical Hypertension*, 6th ed. Williams & Wilkins, 1994.

Materson BJ, Reda DJ, Cushman W: Department of Veterans Affairs: Single drug therapy of hypertension study revised figures and new data. Am J Hypertens 1995;8:183.

National High Blood Pressure Education Program Working Group report on primary prevention of hypertension. Arch Intern Med 1993;153:186.

1.14

Cardiac Arrest

Nisha Chibber Chandra, MD

One of the most critical situations that any physician can encounter is having to respond to a patient who suddenly collapses, unresponsive. This patient may have fainted, had a seizure, become hypotensive from several possible causes (including blood loss, allergic reaction, response to medications, an arrhythmia, or a myocardial infarction), had a pulmonary catastrophe (pulmonary embolism, pneumothorax), or be in respiratory or cardiac arrest. This chapter gives an approach to the patient in cardiac arrest. First-responder actions and diagnosis, major mechanisms of cardiac arrest, and the treatment and subsequent clinical course of survivors will be discussed. In addition, mechanisms of blood flow during cardiopulmonary resuscitation (CPR) will be reviewed to clarify therapeutic interventions during resuscitation. (For more detailed information, the interested reader may wish to refer to the Guidelines for Cardiopulmonary Resuscitation and Emergency Cardiac Care listed in the "Suggested Reading" section at the end of this chapter.)

ESTABLISHING THE DIAGNOSIS OF CARDIAC ARREST

Cardiac arrest should be considered in the differential diagnosis of sudden collapse or unresponsiveness. The diagnosis is confirmed by pulseless major vessels (carotid or femoral arteries) and absent heart sounds. Agonal respiration may continue for several minutes, but the cardiac arrest victim rapidly becomes cyanotic and loses consciousness. If respirations are feeble but a pulse is present, the patient probably has respiratory arrest. This is most often caused by acute airway blockage. It requires specific, but simple, management designed to maintain airway patency and assist breathing.

ACUTE RESPIRATORY ARREST

Respiratory arrest is the cessation of effective respiratory effort, and it is a common result of airway obstruction by a foreign body or other causes such as drowning, drug overdose, head trauma, smoke inhalation, cerebrovascular accidents, or suffocation. In an inpatient, causes to consider are acute respiratory failure in obstructive airways disease, neuromuscular disorders, and pharmacologic sedation.

The Heimlich maneuver is recommended for relieving foreign body airway obstruction. The maneuver is performed by standing behind the victim and delivering a series of sharp thrusts to the upper abdomen with a closed fist. Abdominal thrusts can also be used directly in the unconscious supine victim to help dislodge a suspected foreign body. (The maneuver can be self-administered by placing the fist between the xiphoid process and the navel and delivering a series of quick upward thrusts.) If incorrectly administered, this maneuver can lead to visceral damage. When properly used, it is both safe and effective. Manual removal of a foreign body should be used only in the unconscious victim. In adults, back blows are not as effective as the Heimlich maneuver.

MECHANISM OF BLOOD FLOW DURING CARDIOPULMONARY RESUSCITATION

CPR as we practice it today was developed in the early 1960s. Studies in the last 20 years have defined and elaborated the mechanism of blood flow during CPR. Understanding the physiology of blood flow during resuscitation has led to a more focused strategy of therapeutic and mechanical interventions. There are two mechanisms of blood flow during CPR: movement of blood by manipulation of intrathoracic pressure and direct cardiac or vascular compression. There are no conclusive data regarding the dominant mechanism or the interrelationship of these mechanisms in humans. However, the fact that patients can maintain consciousness by coughing alone when in ventricular fibrillation is convincing evidence that movement of blood by manipulation of intrathoracic pressure is a viable mechanism in humans, since the vital aspect of a cough is a rise in intrathoracic pressure rather than direct cardiac compression.

These studies have also shown that vital organ perfusion

is dependent on pressure gradients. Blood flow to the heart during resuscitation depends on the gradient between the aorta and the right atrium during the release phase of chest compression, and blood flow to the brain depends on the gradient between the carotid and the intracranial pressure during chest compression. Epinephrine has been shown to increase coronary and brain blood flow in animal models of cardiac arrest. In limited human studies, epinephrine has also been shown to increase coronary perfusion pressure.

Understanding the physiology of blood flow during resuscitation has led to the recommendation for faster chest compression rates (which facilitates a prolonged compression phase), emphasis on the early use of epinephrine, and the recommendation to avoid vasodilators such as isoproterenol, which would lower the coronary perfusion pressure gradient. These studies have also helped to clarify the role of acid-base buffers such as sodium bicarbonate and have discouraged their early use because they often cause metabolic alkalosis, hypernatremia, and hyperosmolality. The metabolic acidosis associated with cardiac arrest is best treated with CO_2 removal by effective hyperventilation. In addition, these studies have led to several investigational CPR techniques that have been shown in limited studies to improve hemodynamics during resuscitation. The results, however, are preliminary, and clinical application of these techniques must await more detailed human survival studies.

BASIC CARDIOPULMONARY SUPPORT

One person should assume responsibility for directing resuscitation, using an organized, calm approach. The key to successful resuscitation lies in rapid implementation of the "chain of survival"—early identification of cardiopulmonary arrest and collapse, early basic life support, early defibrillation, and early advanced life support. A physician encountering a victim of cardiac arrest in a nonhospital setting must rapidly establish a diagnosis and then, if alone, *first* activate the emergency medical system by calling 911 (or your emergency number) and then initiate CPR. If the physician is with someone, that person has to call the emergency medical system immediately while the physician initiates rescue support. Basic life support comprises opening the airway, supporting ventilation by breathing into the patient, and supporting circulation by rhythmic chest compression.

Clearing the Airway

It is of utmost importance to clear the airway and remove foreign bodies, loose dentures, or any other oral obstruction. Then the airway should be opened by lifting the chin forward with the fingers of one hand supporting the victim's jaw while tilting the head back by placing the other hand on the forehead. Alternatively, the airway may be opened by tilting the victim's head backward with one hand on the forehead while placing the other hand behind the neck, lifting it upward.

Restoring Breathing

If no spontaneous respirations are present, mouth-to-mouth or mouth-to-nose ventilation should be immediately initiated by delivering two slow ($1^1/_2$- to 2-second) breaths. Slow breaths minimize gastric distention. The adequacy of ventilation should be judged by the rise and fall of the patient's chest with each breath.

When possible, rescuers and those in hospitals should use a barrier device or a bag-mask technique of ventilation, together with a plastic oral airway, which keeps the tongue forward. Adequate ventilation is difficult with the bag-mask technique because a single operator often has difficulty maintaining an airtight seal on the face. Several invasive airway adjuncts are available that facilitate opening the airway, for use primarily in the prehospital setting. Endotracheal intubation is the optimal technique for ensuring adequate ventilation during resuscitation, and it can be rapidly implemented both in the prehospital scenario and in the hospital by trained persons. However, much valuable time is often wasted by repeated unskilled attempts at intubation.

Bag-valve-mask ventilation, if correctly administered, is often sufficient to maintain oxygenation until intubation can be achieved. During attempts at intubation, CPR should be discontinued for no more than 20 seconds. If more than 20 seconds elapse without successful intubation, the laryngoscope should be withdrawn and CPR reinstituted promptly. When resuscitative efforts are prolonged, or probably will have to be restarted, a nasal gastric tube should be inserted to drain the stomach and reduce the chance of aspiration. Patients should be ventilated with 10–12 slow ventilatory breaths per minute.

Chest Compressions During Cardiopulmonary Resuscitation

Chest compression during CPR requires compressing the lower end of the sternum 80–100 times per minute, with each compression and relaxation phase being of equal duration. Every five chest compressions should be followed by one slow ventilation ($1^1/_2$–2 seconds) if two trained rescuers are performing CPR, but if one rescuer is doing CPR, every 15 chest compressions should be followed by two slow ventilations.

DEFINITIVE THERAPY FOR CARDIAC ARREST

A "practical" new classification for the various drugs and procedures used during the definitive therapy of cardiac arrest came into use in 1992. This classification allows a relative value to be assigned to a therapeutic endeavor. For purposes of this chapter, only the most imperative therapies will be highlighted.

During cardiac arrest, the electrocardiogram (ECG) commonly shows rapid ventricular tachycardia or fibrillation, asystole, or heart block, or it may be near normal. The rhythm can be rapidly ascertained by using "quick-look" paddles that are now commonly found on most *de-*

fibrillators. Quick-look paddles serve a dual purpose: as defibrillation electrodes and as electrodes to monitor the ECG without placing additional electrodes. Hospitals occasionally have an earlier version of a defibrillator that allows defibrillation but not immediate ECG visualization. In this situation, the patient should undergo defibrillation and be treated as if in ventricular fibrillation, since this is the most likely rhythm. Despite the availability of quick-look paddles, some physicians are not used to using them, leading to a common mistake: They often delay life-saving therapeutic procedures to obtain an ECG that can take several minutes. Physicians should familiarize themselves with the equipment available at their hospital.

Ventricular Tachycardia or Fibrillation

In cases of ventricular fibrillation or ventricular tachycardia associated with lack of a pulse, the treatment of choice is immediate electrical defibrillation. Successful defibrillation is facilitated if transthoracic impedance is reduced. Transthoracic impedance can be reduced by using saline-soaked gauze pads or a gel or cream between the electrode and the skin and applying firm pressure on the hand-held electrodes. Proper electrode paddle placement is also important to maximally reduce transthoracic impedance; an anterolateral paddle position is commonly used. Alternatively, by placing preadhesive electrodes, the physician can also use the anteroposterior electrode approach: one electrode is placed over the left precordium and the other behind the heart in the right infrascapular location. Defibrillation requires giving the patient up to three successive rapid defibrillatory shocks: 200 joules initially, followed by a second 200–300-joule shock if the first shock is unsuccessful, followed, if necessary, by a 300–360-joule shock. Eighty-five to ninety percent of successful defibrillation is usually achieved using only 200 joules in patients weighing up to 90 kg (200 lb). High-energy defibrillation may cause more cardiac injury, and there is no clear evidence that it increases the frequency of successful resuscitation. An important evolving concept that incorporates the role of transthoracic impedance is that of current-based defibrillation. Here, the physician selects an electrical current (amperes) rather than energy (joules). Such an approach avoids the problem of using unnecessarily low energy selections in patients with high thoracic impedance (with a consequent failure to defibrillate secondary to low current flow) or unnecessarily high energy selection in patients with low impedance, which could result in excessive current flow, failure to defibrillate, and myocardial injury.

When the initial ECG shows fine fibrillation waves (low-amplitude ventricular fibrillation) or when initial defibrillation efforts are unsuccessful, administration of epinephrine intravenously may result in a more vigorous and coarse fibrillation (high-amplitude fibrillation) that is more responsive to defibrillation (Figure 1.14–1). This effect is probably a consequence of the improved coronary flow following epinephrine administration (as previously described). If defibrillation is unsuccessful, it is likely that

marked acidosis or hypoxemia is present. Treatment should then include hyperventilation with supplemental oxygen to correct both hypoxemia and metabolic acidosis. Sodium bicarbonate might then be administered to aid in the management of acidosis. Defibrillation should be repeated with 300–360 joules.

For recurrent ventricular fibrillation, intravenous administration of lidocaine followed by repeat defibrillation may improve the likelihood of returning to a stable rhythm (see Figure 1.14–1). Lidocaine is the antiarrhythmic agent of choice for recurrent ventricular fibrillation. Bretylium tosylate and procainamide are second-line drugs. For recurrent ventricular fibrillation, especially in patients with primary ventricular fibrillation complicating acute myocardial infarction, propranolol given intravenously may be a particularly helpful agent. Magnesium sulfate can also be administered, especially if the patient has torsades de pointes or if hypomagnesemia is suspected (such as in patients on diuretics). After successful cardioversion, an intravenous infusion of either lidocaine, bretylium, or procainamide should be maintained for at least 24 hours. Factors that perpetuate ectopy, such as ischemia, hypokalemia, hypomagnesemia, or hypoxemia, should be sought and treated.

Hyperkalemia as a cause of ventricular fibrillation is not uncommon, especially in an inpatient setting and in patients with severe renal disease. An ECG diagnosis can be made on the basis of tall peaked T waves with a normal QT interval or a sine wave ventricular tachycardia on prearrest tracings. Hyperkalemia can result in atrioventricular block, intra-atrial or intraventricular conduction delays, ventricular fibrillation, and, infrequently, asystole. Life-threatening hyperkalemia is best treated by an intravenous infusion of calcium gluconate with ECG monitoring. Calcium counteracts the adverse effects of potassium at the neuromuscular membrane by competitive inhibition, but does not alter plasma potassium levels. Hyperkalemia should be subsequently treated using sodium bicarbonate, glucose-insulin infusions, or ion-exchange resins.

Until it came under dispute in the 1992 resuscitation guidelines, a sharp blow to the precordium (precordial thump) was recommended for the initial treatment of ventricular tachycardia or ventricular fibrillation while the patient was being prepared for defibrillation. A forceful rhythmic cough has also been shown in rare instances to convert ventricular tachycardia to a supraventricular rhythm, and repeated coughing can maintain consciousness as a result of the rise in intrathoracic pressure if cardiac arrest is recognized before loss of consciousness occurs. This technique is usually not an option in most clinical situations, except in controlled environments such as the exercise stress laboratory or the catheterization laboratory.

Asystole or Heart Block

In patients with prehospital cardiac arrest, asystole has been shown to be an ominous rhythm, associated with a very low likelihood of successful resuscitation. In the hospital, however, asystole due to vagal stimulation is the

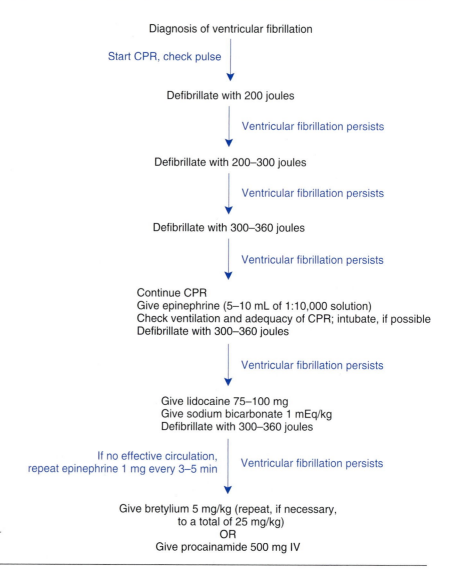

Diagnosis of ventricular fibrillation

Start CPR, check pulse

Defibrillate with 200 joules

Ventricular fibrillation persists

Defibrillate with 200–300 joules

Ventricular fibrillation persists

Defibrillate with 300–360 joules

Ventricular fibrillation persists

Continue CPR
Give epinephrine (5–10 mL of 1:10,000 solution)
Check ventilation and adequacy of CPR; intubate, if possible
Defibrillate with 300–360 joules

Ventricular fibrillation persists

Give lidocaine 75–100 mg
Give sodium bicarbonate 1 mEq/kg
Defibrillate with 300–360 joules

If no effective circulation,
repeat epinephrine 1 mg every 3–5 min   Ventricular fibrillation persists

Give bretylium 5 mg/kg (repeat, if necessary,
to a total of 25 mg/kg)
OR
Give procainamide 500 mg IV

Figure 1.14–1. Flow chart for management of ventricular fibrillation.

most common cause of cardiac arrest associated with anesthesia induction and surgical procedures. Asystole can also occur as a result of heart block or sinus node disease. Atropine given intravenously and repeated in 5 minutes can successfully prevent and reverse brad-yarrhythmias in such situations. Dopamine may also be useful in such patients. Again, if the patient is conscious, rhythmic forceful coughing can maintain adequate vital organ perfusion until definitive treatment can be initiated. In rare instances, rhythmic precordial percussion "fist pacing" may also be useful. If chest blows fail and there is no palpable pulse, CPR should be immediately initiated and intravenous epinephrine administered.

Other possible treatable causes of asystole should be considered (eg, acidosis, hypoxemia, hypo- or hyper-kalemia, hypothermia) and appropriately treated. If cal-cium channel blocker overdose is suspected, calcium chloride may be extremely effective. Resuscitation measures may result in the return of a slow ventricular rhythm, which can subsequently be supported with at-ropine until a temporary pacemaker is placed. Routine use of calcium for asystole is discouraged. In a patient who is pulseless, there is no role for isoproterenol since, as a va-sodilator, it will further worsen coronary flow.

Temporary pacing is the optimal treatment of true asystole or profound bradycardia. Considerable skill and training are needed for temporary transvenous pacer placement. However, transcutaneous pacing offers a simpler, noninvasive approach that can be rapidly implemented in such situations. The technique uses external surface electrodes with a high-voltage pacing source. As a consequence, the technique is painful and should therefore be used only in unconscious patients. The energy delivered by this technique is variable, as is its efficacy. Clinical evidence does not support routine use of pacing in all patients with asystole. A recently reported prehospital study demonstrates no benefit of early transcutaneous pacing in patients with out-of-hospital cardiac arrest who were in pulseless electrical activity or asystole.

In rare instances, fine ventricular fibrillation may masquerade as asystole. In such cases in which the diagnosis of asystole is in question, a perpendicular ECG lead should be viewed. If using quick-look paddles, this is easily accomplished by rotating them 90 degrees. If ventricular fibrillation is present, the perpendicular ECG lead will demonstrate a typical fibrillation pattern, whereas in true asystole, a straight line will be seen. If ventricular fibrillation is diagnosed, the initial treatment should be similar to that described above, that is, three successive countershocks. There is little value or harm in defibrillating true asystole.

Pulseless Electrical Activity

Pulseless electrical activity (PEA) encompasses all organized electrical activity on the ECG at a reasonable rate without effective perfusion (no pulse or blood pressure). Hypovolemia, tension pneumothorax, pulmonary embolism, and pericardial tamponade are among the most treatable and common causes of this condition. After the diagnosis of PEA is made during a resuscitation effort, respective clinical features of these treatable conditions should be sought by looking for sudden severe blood loss (eg, sudden gastrointestinal bleeding or vascular injuries following catheter placement); by assessing for adequacy of breath sounds bilaterally; by checking arterial blood gases to rule out severe hypoxemia; or by emergency chest x-ray or emergency two-dimensional echocardiographic evaluation. If appropriate, definitive therapy should be accordingly directed with intravenous fluids or blood replacement, chest tube placement, or pericardiocentesis. If PEA is due to primary myocardial failure, the prognosis is grim; epinephrine should be administered, and ventilation optimized. There is no role for the routine administration of calcium in this setting. Occasionally, in patients with acute myocardial infarction, sudden PEA may represent myocardial rupture. Emergency pericardiocentesis followed by surgical repair may sometimes be successful in such patients.

ESTABLISHING AN INTRAVENOUS ROUTE

Once CPR has been initiated, an intravenous line is necessary for definitive drug therapy. However, venous access may be difficult. Several emergency drugs can be effectively administered via the endotracheal tube pending successful venous cannulation. Epinephrine, lidocaine, and atropine can be administered through the endotracheal tube into the bronchial tree. Sodium bicarbonate should never be given via the endotracheal tube. Drugs given

through the endotracheal tube should be injected through a long catheter, passed beyond the tip of the tube. If this technique is used, chest compression should be temporarily withheld, and several insufflations of a ventilator bag should immediately follow drug administration to facilitate drug delivery and absorption through aerosolization.

If a peripheral vein is cannulated, every effort should be made to find a source above the diaphragm, since there is little cephalad blood flow from veins situated below the diaphragm. If a peripheral route is used, drugs should be given by bolus injection and followed by a 20-mL bolus of intravenous fluid and elevation of the extremity. If a peripheral vein cannot be cannulated, a central venous line should be placed by the percutaneous route. If CPR is properly performed, central line placement has little advantage over a peripheral line in terms of rapidity of drug circulation. Drugs administered via peripheral line will reach the arterial circulation within 15–30 seconds. Central lines should be placed only by skilled personnel because serious complications such as pneumothorax, arterial laceration, or nerve injury can occur.

Intracardiac injections should be avoided if possible since they can result in coronary laceration. Intraosseous infusion of drugs is often practiced in pediatric patients. Its role in adults is limited. Most intravenous lines are started with 5% dextrose in water or with normal saline. Patients in whom hypovolemia is suspected may benefit from volume expansion with appropriate fluids, such as blood or lactated Ringer's solution.

TERMINATING CARDIOPULMONARY RESUSCITATION

Despite aggressive efforts at resuscitation, patients in cardiac arrest may not regain spontaneous circulation. The decision to terminate resuscitative efforts is difficult and should be based on the physician's assessment of the cause of the arrest and the cerebral, cardiovascular, and general status of the patient. If organized ECG activity does not return after 15–20 minutes of adequate CPR and appropriate definitive therapy, severe brain injury or death is likely. Persistent, deep unconsciousness accompanied by absence of respirations and reflexes suggests profound cerebral ischemia, and prolonged resuscitative efforts are usually unsuccessful. These broad guidelines, however, must be altered in patients with hypothermia, barbiturate overdose, and electrocution since recovery with return of good cerebral function has been documented in such cases hours after beginning resuscitation.

POSTARREST CARE AND OUTCOME OF RESUSCITATION

Recent data suggest that over 35% of all patients experiencing out-of-hospital cardiac arrests can be successfully resuscitated and can survive to hospital admission. Of

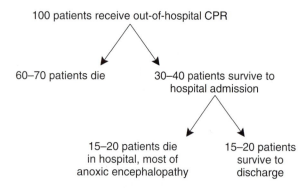

Figure 1.14–2. Outcomes of cardiopulmonary resuscitation (CPR) for 100 hypothetical out-of-hospital cardiac arrest victims in a city with an emergency medical system that is capable of a fast response.

these initial survivors, many die in the hospital, primarily from anoxic encephalopathy. A small percentage of the survivors are discharged home (Figure 1.14–2). Several therapeutic strategies, including using barbiturates, lidoflazine, and hypothermia, have been studied in an attempt to reduce cerebral anoxic injury, a common sequela of prolonged resuscitation. None of these strategies has been shown to be beneficial.

Following successful resuscitation, the patient should be monitored in an intensive care unit. Most patients will be comatose and require respiratory support and frequent arterial blood gas determinations to better treat the hypoxemia and acidosis that cardiac arrest often causes. To manage fluid status correctly and optimize cardiopulmonary function, pulmonary artery catheterization may be required. Renal failure, pneumonia, bowel ischemia, limb ischemia, and sepsis are other common postresuscitation complications that require early and aggressive management.

If recovery does occur, postarrest amnesia, behavioral disturbances, or neurologic deficits may be manifest. Failure to recover neurologic function within 24 hours of resuscitation is an ominous sign. Recent data suggest that oculo-evoked potentials may be highly predictive of outcomes as early as 48 hours after admission.

Prompt CPR and early defibrillation remain the most powerful predictors of successful recovery following arrest. Family and friends of high-risk patients should be trained in basic life support, and first-responder emergency medical systems should be equipped for defibrillation, since such strategies have clearly been shown to save lives and improve neurologic outcome.

An often-neglected issue in resuscitative efforts is the psychological impact on the rescuers. Many members of the health care team may suffer from guilt, especially if the resuscitative effort is unsuccessful. It is highly recommended that physician leaders implement an "arrest debriefing" after CPR efforts, to deal with such issues.

SUMMARY

▶ Blood flow during CPR depends more on generating high intrathoracic pressures than on direct cardiac compression and is augmented by maintaining arterial tone with epinephrine.

▶ The key to successful resuscitation lies in rapid implementation of the "chain of survival"—early identification of cardiopulmonary arrest or collapse, early basic life support, early defibrillation, and early advanced life support.

▶ If a peripheral vein is cannulated, every effort should be made to find a source above the diaphragm, since there is little cephalad blood flow from veins situated below the diaphragm.

▶ Long-term survival after out-of-hospital cardiac arrest should be 15–20% and is confined virtually to patients with ventricular tachycardia or ventricular fibrillation on presentation.

SUGGESTED READING

Cobb LA, Werner JA, Trobaugh GB: Sudden cardiac death. Mod Concepts Cardiovasc Dis 1980;49:31, 37.

Eisenberg MS, Hallstrom A, Bergner L: Long-term survival after out-of-hospital cardiac arrest. N Engl J Med 1982;306:1340.

Guidelines for cardiopulmonary resuscitation and emergency cardiac care: Emergency Cardiac Care Committee and Subcommittees, American Heart Association. JAMA 1992;268:2171.

Heimlich HJ: A life-saving maneuver to prevent food-choking. JAMA 1975;234:398.

Madl C et al: Early prediction of individual outcome after cardiopulmonary resuscitation. Lancet 1993;341:855.

Section 2

Pulmonary Disease

Thomas A. Traill, FRCP, Section Editor

2.1

Approach to the Patient with Pulmonary Disease

Wilmot C. Ball, Jr, MD

The most common symptoms of lung disease are cough, shortness of breath, and chest pain. Many patients presenting with these complaints have one of the following common conditions: asthma, chronic obstructive pulmonary disease (COPD), acute viral and bacterial upper and lower respiratory tract infections, or lung cancer. Chest radiographs taken for other reasons in a patient with no symptoms sometimes show a pulmonary abnormality. This then becomes the presenting manifestation requiring diagnostic study.

The internist evaluates and manages the care of many patients with pulmonary disease. Requests for pulmonary consultation are appropriate (1) when the history and physical findings, basic laboratory assessment, posteroanterior and lateral chest films, and, in some instances, basic pulmonary function testing have been carried out but do not establish a working diagnosis; (2) when treatment expected to cure or improve the patient has proved to be ineffective; (3) when a case is unusually complex because of multiple medical problems (eg, coexisting heart and lung disease); or (4) when a diagnostic procedure such as bronchoscopy or pleural biopsy is indicated. When the diagnosis must account for significant abnormalities in the chest film, the radiologist can often suggest one or more likely diagnoses or recommend additional imaging studies (such as computed tomography [CT]) to clarify the anatomic abnormality.

SIGNS AND SYMPTOMS

A careful history sometimes leads directly to a diagnosis that requires little verification. For example, the diagnosis of asthma can be confidently made from a history of episodic wheezing and dyspnea associated with cough and nasal obstruction in a patient with multiple allergies. In other instances, the history simply suggests the direction that investigation must take to establish a diagnosis.

In the clinical evaluation of a patient with suspected lung disease, it is also important to ask about past illnesses such as pneumonia, pleurisy, and tuberculosis, and to explore important risk factors such as cigarette smoking and occupational exposure to dust, fumes, and asbestos. Information about past x-ray examinations may be useful in evaluating current radiographic abnormalities.

Dyspnea

Shortness of breath is a subjective sensation more often related to abnormalities of pulmonary mechanics than to abnormal arterial blood gas tensions. The most frequently seen pattern is dyspnea during exercise. The most common causes are obstructive pulmonary disease (eg, emphysema, chronic bronchitis, asthma), restrictive lung disease, upper airway obstruction, heart failure, and pulmonary vascular disease such as multiple pulmonary emboli. There may be many contributing causes, and physical deconditioning may compound the problem. In the patient presenting with a single acute episode of shortness of breath, the main possibilities are spontaneous pneumothorax, pulmonary embolism, asthma attack, pulmonary edema, and aspiration.

If recurrent acute attacks of dyspnea occur, asthma, left ventricular dysfunction with bouts of pulmonary congestion, intermittent upper airway obstruction, recurrent pulmonary embolism, and anxiety-hyperventilation syndrome should be considered.

The cause of dyspnea is often clear from the history and physical examination. In difficult cases or when quantification of impairment is needed, pulmonary function testing, cardiac function evaluation, and, in some cases, formal exercise testing are necessary.

Cough

With rare exceptions, cough is caused by stimulation of receptors in the airway mucosa or in the interstitium of the lung. If the cough is productive of sputum, the problem is to determine the cause of excess mucus production or, in the case of hemoptysis, the source of the bleeding. Characteristics of the sputum may be important in diagnosis. An abnormality seen on chest x-ray may completely reorient the differential diagnosis. When a patient with chronic productive cough has an entirely normal chest film, the most likely causes are asthma, bronchitis, and bronchiectasis. The most common cause of acute or short-term productive cough is bronchitis due to viral or bacterial respiratory infection.

Dry or nonproductive cough may also result from a variety of parenchymal disorders. Examples are nonbacterial pneumonia, interstitial fibrosis, and infiltrating tumor. Long-term dry cough in a patient with a normal chest film may be caused by an occult endobronchial lesion such as primary lung cancer, treatment with angiotensin converting enzyme (ACE) inhibitors, or an inhaled foreign body. In most cases, the cause will prove to be a variant of asthma, postnasal drip, or reflux of gastric contents into the esophagus, with or without aspiration. In these cases, the diagnosis is sometimes made by methacholine challenge, by ENT evaluation, or by tests to identify reflux and disorders of swallowing, respectively. Alternatively, a therapeutic trial of aerosol bronchodilators, antihistamine-decongestants, or antireflux measures may be chosen.

Hemoptysis

Blood-streaked purulent sputum lasting only a few days and associated with symptoms of upper respiratory tract infection is usually caused by bronchial infection. If there are no clinical signs of more serious lung disease and the chest x-ray is normal, patients at low risk for lung cancer need no further studies. Persistent or recurrent blood streaking may be a manifestation of lung cancer, tuberculosis, or one of many other focal pulmonary infections. Findings on chest x-ray often narrow the range of possibilities, but full investigation including bronchoscopy is needed in most instances. Coughing up a large amount of blood suggests bronchiectasis, lung cancer, pulmonary infarction, tuberculosis, aspergilloma within a lung cavity, or diffuse alveolar bleeding, as seen in mitral stenosis, pulmonary edema, vasculitis, idiopathic pulmonary hemosiderosis, and Goodpasture's syndrome.

Bronchoscopy during an episode of profuse bleeding is usually not diagnostically helpful. It is important to distinguish true hemoptysis from a source of bleeding in the upper airway with secondary aspiration of blood.

Chest Pain

There are so many causes of pain in the chest that differential diagnosis is a common problem. A detailed characterization of the location, intensity, character, and timing of the pain usually allows the pain to be categorized correctly. *Pleurisy* is chest pain caused by stimulation of pain fibers in the parietal pleura. This pain is usually described as sharp or stabbing, is typically made much worse by deep breathing, coughing, or sneezing, and is most often located over the lower portion of the chest. Pleurisy is usually caused by pleural inflammation from viral, bacterial, or tuberculous infection, connective tissue disease such as acute lupus erythematosus, or pulmonary infarction. Pain simulating pleurisy but arising in other chest wall structures may be caused by pneumothorax, rib fracture, costochondritis and other chest wall syndromes, and nerve root pain from herpes zoster infection or vertebral body collapse.

Pain of cardiovascular origin is usually central and diffuse, often described as pressing or squeezing rather than sharp. It may radiate to the neck, jaw, or arms and may worsen with exertion. Examples are angina, acute myocardial infarction, dissecting aortic aneurysm, and pulmonary hypertension. Pericardial pain is like pleurisy, but is generally felt in the anterior chest and the back, and is often aggravated by lying supine. Chronic chest pain is rarely caused by parenchymal lung disease, since there are no pain fibers in the lung or visceral pleura. Causes include respiratory muscle fatigue in chronic respiratory insufficiency, esophageal or gastric disease, empyema, malignant tumor invading the chest wall from the lung or a rib, and other chest wall syndromes. Diagnosis can usually be made from a careful history, associated clinical findings, and radiographic examination.

PHYSICAL EXAMINATION

While the history is being obtained, the examiner will note the presence or absence of respiratory distress, cyanosis, and cough. Abnormal mucus production can be accurately assessed by the sound of the cough. The position of the trachea in the neck is noted, and the configuration and symmetry of the chest are observed during full inspiration. Percussion (direct or indirect) over the lung fields allows evaluation of the position of the diaphragms and detection of pleural effusion, consolidated or atelectatic lung, or a large mass near the chest wall. While the patient breathes more deeply than normal and with the mouth open, breath sounds are evaluated by listening over multiple areas of the chest, including the axillae, and by comparing one side with the other. If the breath sounds are thought to be abnormal, additional information may be obtained by listening during deep breathing and after cough, by testing for vocal fremitus, and by listening to spoken or whispered voice sounds. Finally, to test for airways obstruction and assess its severity, it is important to watch the chest move and listen over the lung bases during forced expiration.

Abnormal findings on physical examination may provide the information necessary to establish a diagnosis or at least suggest a list of possibilities. Displacement of the trachea may be caused by direct pressure on the trachea by a mass in the superior mediastinum. More frequently, it results from shift of the mediastinum brought about by unequal pleural pressure on the two sides. Pneumothorax and large pleural effusion shift the mediastinum and trachea away from the affected side, whereas atelectasis causes a shift toward the lesion.

Unequal expansion of the chest with inspiration may be caused by decreased compliance of the lung or chest wall on one side, as seen in pneumonia, bronchial obstruction, atelectasis, pleural effusion, or pleural thickening. Hemiparesis after a stroke also produces asymmetric chest movement. A dull percussion note is caused by dense lung, fluid, or a mass against the chest wall, where it prevents sustained vibration after the chest is struck. Examples are pleural effusion, pneumonia, large tumor, and elevated diaphragm. In contrast, a hyperresonant percussion note is caused by loss of the damping effect produced by normal lung. It is seen in pneumothorax, emphysema, and the hyperinflation of severe asthma.

Listening to breath sounds at the mouth may help to distinguish asthma and bronchitis from emphysema. In asthma and bronchitis, an abnormally loud breath sound at the mouth is caused by high flow velocity through narrowed large and medium-sized airways. In emphysema, the large airways have normal caliber. Diminished breath sounds on auscultation of the lungs can be caused by reduced production of sound (diminished air movement), by reduced transmission of sound through the airways (obstruction of a large airway by tumor or mucus plug), or by interruption of the sound between medium airways and the chest wall (large mass, pleural effusion, thickened pleura, pneumothorax). A four-fold asymmetry of breath sound intensity is occasionally seen in normal subjects, so an isolated reduction should not be overinterpreted.

Bronchial breath sounds are similar to the breath sounds heard by listening over the trachea in the neck. The inspiratory component is louder than normal and contains more high-pitched components, and the expiratory sound is very prominent. The change results from transmission of sound generated by turbulent flow in the central airways through lung that is consolidated or otherwise abnormally stiff or dense. Bronchial breathing is heard in patients with pneumonia, atelectasis (provided that the airway is open), and advanced pulmonary fibrosis.

Bronchophony refers to an altered quality of spoken voice sounds as they are transmitted through consolidated lung. The voice is less muffled than normal and may take on a nasal quality. Another variation may be heard when the patient is asked to whisper. These sounds, normally almost inaudible, come through the consolidated lung with clarity. *Egophony* is an exaggerated form of bronchophony, in which the spoken letter E sounds like A. This is heard over compressed lung above a large pleural effusion and in some patients with pneumonia.

Wheezes are discrete, high-pitched musical sounds, heard predominantly in expiration and caused by vibration of airway walls during flow-limitation. They denote airways obstruction, as in asthma and bronchitis. *Rhonchi* are low-pitched vibratory sounds, often heard in both inspiration and expiration. They are usually caused by mucus in the airways and may be abolished or altered by coughing. A *squeak* is a very brief high-pitched musical sound heard in mid- to late inspiration. The mechanism is not fully understood, but it is probably related to vibration of the walls of small airways. The squeak is typically heard over only a small area on the chest wall and is often transient. It may be heard in patients with bronchiolitis, bronchiolitis obliterans, bronchiolitis obliterans organizing pneumonia, interstitial diseases, especially idiopathic pulmonary fibrosis and hypersensitivity pneumonitis, and sometimes bronchiectasis. *Fine crackles* are momentary clicking sounds caused by popping open of closed small airways; they are heard in conditions that favor abnormal airway closure. Fine crackles are usually end-inspiratory or pan-inspiratory. They are common in patients with early pneumonia, congestive heart failure, and any form of interstitial lung disease. *Coarse crackles* sound more muffled, and the individual clicking sounds are louder and fewer in number. Early inspiratory coarse crackles are common in patients with severe COPD and should not be interpreted as evidence of bronchitis, pneumonia, or heart failure. Pan-inspiratory or inspiratory-and-expiratory coarse crackles are heard in patients with pulmonary edema, but are usually caused by mucus in the airways. They are often present in bronchitis, pneumonia, especially during the clearing phase, and bronchiectasis. These crackles are often associated with rhonchi and may clear with cough.

X-RAY AND OTHER IMAGING STUDIES

Because of the air they contain, the lungs are unique in the detail with which they can be imaged by x-ray techniques. Plain films of the chest may be normal in some patients with obstructive lung diseases, pulmonary embolism, and the earliest stages of various conditions. For most lung diseases, however, radiographs of good quality are an essential component of the pulmonary examination, because they provide information about the gross anatomy of the lesion. An important rule for the clinician to observe is that when the anatomic features of a radiographic abnormality are not clearly defined on available films, additional imaging is required. Poor-quality radiographs should be repeated, and sometimes extra views (eg, apical lordotic, oblique, and decubitus films) need to be taken.

CT is perhaps the most helpful supplemental imaging technique because it effectively separates lung and mediastinal, pleural, and chest wall structures, and may reveal important information about the fine structure of the lung. Magnetic resonance imaging (MRI) is sometimes useful for visualizing lesions in the apex of the lung, when coronal sections are required to show structural relations, when vascular shadows must be separated from lymph nodes in the mediastinum, and when a malignant tumor may be directly invading the heart or pericardium. Ultrasound examinations are of limited usefulness, but may be appropriate for localizing small collections of pleural fluid for aspiration.

Ventilation-perfusion (V/Q) radionuclide scans are used in conjunction with clinical evidence to evaluate the likelihood of pulmonary embolism (Chapter 2.8). The V/Q scan is very sensitive but not very specific, and when there is still substantial uncertainty about the diagnosis after V/Q scanning, a pulmonary arteriogram may be necessary. Gallium radionuclide scans are sometimes useful in determining the activity of an inflammatory process such as sarcoidosis or idiopathic pulmonary fibrosis, or of a localized infectious process in the lung.

PULMONARY FUNCTION TESTING

Quantitative assessment of the mechanical and gas exchange properties of the lung by means of pulmonary function studies is often useful in the evaluation of patients with lung disease. The most commonly used studies are spirometry, lung volumes, diffusing capacity, and arterial blood gases. *Spirograms* allow measurement of the vital capacity and the forced expiratory volume in 1 second (FEV_1), which detect and quantify airways obstruction. Spirograms may be repeated after aerosol bronchodilator to assess reversibility of the obstruction. A low vital capacity alone suggests a restrictive ventilatory defect, which can be confirmed by measuring lung volumes with a gas dilution method. *Diffusing capacity,* usually measured using the single-breath carbon monoxide method, is a test of the integrity of the gas exchange function of the lung and is usually abnormal in diffuse lung disease even when lung volumes are normal. Arterial blood gas measurement can enable diagnosis of alveolar hyper- and hypoventilation (low or high PCO_2) and detection of hypoxemia resulting from lung disease. Many additional tests—some complex or specialized—may have application in specific clinical problems.

Evaluation of Dyspnea

When the cause of dyspnea is not clear from clinical examination, spirograms, lung volumes, diffusing capacity, and arterial blood gases may be ordered. If all these are normal, it is most unlikely that the dyspnea is caused by lung disease. Flow-volume loops may be obtained to exclude upper airway obstruction. An exercise test is necessary to determine whether exercise limitation is caused by disease of the lungs, heart, or other abnormality.

Evaluation of Obstructive Pulmonary Disease

Spirograms are used to quantify the obstruction. FEV_1 is the best measure of severity because its absolute value in liters correlates well with exercise tolerance. This value is used to follow the progress of the disease over time or to evaluate therapy. For asthma or other labile airways disease, the peak flow meter may be used instead of a spirometer to measure serial changes in function. The advantage is that much less effort by the patient is required,

and the patient can be taught to perform the test several times each day and chart the results for review by the physician. Lung volumes and diffusing capacity measurements can be used to distinguish emphysema and chronic bronchitis. If the FEV_1 is less than 1.2 L or if respiratory failure is suspected on clinical grounds, arterial blood gases are obtained to detect carbon dioxide retention and to evaluate the need for supplemental oxygen.

Evaluation of Diffuse Restrictive Lung Disease

To follow the progress of diffuse interstitial disease or monitor the effect of treatment, serial spirograms and diffusing capacity tests are basic. Arterial blood gases or even exercise tests are sometimes more sensitive indicators.

Evaluation of Operative Risk

The most common problem is evaluation of the older patient or the patient with known lung disease when surgery under general anesthesia, especially abdominal surgery, is planned (Chapter 15.2). Spirograms alone in conjunction with a clinical assessment are often adequate for such an evaluation. The risk of postoperative complications increases progressively in patients with increasing degrees of airways obstruction, especially if there is labile airways disease or sputum production. Patients with CO_2 retention pose a high anesthetic risk. When lung resection is contemplated, more elaborate studies including a quantitative V/Q scan help to estimate the permanent effect of surgery on lung function.

SUMMARY

▶ Patients with pulmonary diseases present with dyspnea, cough, and chest pain. Most of these patients prove to have asthma, chronic obstructive pulmonary disease (COPD), acute viral and bacterial upper and lower respiratory tract infections, or lung cancer.

▶ Dyspnea usually reflects a change in the mechanics of breathing rather than abnormal blood gas tensions. The most common causes of exertional breathlessness are obstructive pulmonary disease, restrictive lung disease, upper airway obstruction, heart failure, and pulmonary vascular disease such as multiple pulmonary emboli.

▶ Productive cough with a normal chest radiograph is usually caused by asthma, bronchitis, or bronchiectasis. The most common cause of acute productive cough is bronchitis due to viral or bacterial infection. In contrast, there are many causes of chronic, nonproductive cough.

▶ The clinician should order additional imaging when in doubt about the cause of an abnormal chest radiograph. CT is perhaps the most helpful of these techniques because it effectively separates lung and mediastinal, pleural, and chest wall structures, and may reveal important information about the fine structure of the lung.

SUGGESTED READING

Bates DV: *Respiratory Function in Disease,* 3rd ed. WB Saunders, 1989.

Baum GL, Wolinsky E: *Textbook of Pulmonary Diseases,* 5th ed. Little, Brown & Co, 1994.

Murray, JF, Nadel JA: *Textbook of Respiratory Medicine.* WB Saunders, 1988.

Pneumonia and Pneumonitis

Peter B. Terry, MD, and Augustine M. K. Choi, MD

Pneumonia denotes inflammation in the alveoli or interstitium (or both) of the lung caused by microorganisms. This definition has evolved from the original Greek usage in which the word simply meant disease of the lungs. Although we tend to think of pneumonia in terms of infectious agents, a number of noninfectious diseases can cause inflammation in the lung and may have a radiographic picture indistinguishable from pneumonia caused by infectious agents (Table 2.2–1). The term *pneumonitis,* often used synonymously with pneumonia, should be reserved for noninfectious inflammatory reactions.

Types of pneumonia have been given a variety of names in the past, some of which serve only to confuse. Specific radiographic patterns suggest causes or categories of disease, such as lobar (bacterial [Figure 2.2–1]), bronchopneumonia (bacterial), interstitial (viral [Figure 2.2–2]), and migratory (mycoplasmal). The common term "atypical pneumonia" implies a clinical presentation not characteristic of lobar pneumococcal pneumonia. Organisms usually associated with this atypical presentation are *Mycoplasma pneumoniae,* viruses, and *Rickettsia.*

Pneumonia currently ranks as the primary cause of mortality from infectious diseases in the United States in spite of newer antibiotics and more aggressive prophylactic and therapeutic approaches. It will remain a serious health problem because of the expanding geriatric population; the growing number of immunosuppressed patients with AIDS, cancer, and transplanted organs; and increased world travel.

The aims of this chapter are (1) to introduce the clinical approach to diagnosis and treatment of patients with infectious pneumonia and (2) to draw attention to the diseases that can masquerade as infectious pneumonias. It is important to be able to distinguish infectious pneumonia from pneumonitis and other lung diseases, because an early decision must be made about appropriate treatment to prevent unnecessary morbidity or even death. Distinguishing factors in the history, physical examination, radiologic pattern, microbiologic studies, and diagnostic testing are stressed.

ACUTE PNEUMONIA

Presentation

A patient with a typical presentation of acute pneumonia has a 1–10-day history of increasing cough, yellow sputum, shortness of breath, a temperature as high as 104°F (40°C), tachycardia, increased respiratory rate, and an appearance of being sick. The affected person may be a susceptible host, for example, with a history of alcoholism, HIV infection, or seizures. Physical examination may reveal dullness to percussion and bronchial breaths sounds over an area of consolidation, and the chest x-ray may show a dense lobar infiltrate (see Figure 2.2–1).

Clinical Considerations

Pneumonia is the result of an interaction between a host and an organism. Therefore, knowing the characteristics of both can be helpful in predicting the infecting organism. A reasonable generalization is that bacterial pneumonias are more common in persons with previous viral infections, chronic obstructive lung disease, mechanical airways obstruction, a propensity to aspirate, or impaired host defenses. Alcoholics, who are especially susceptible to lobar pneumonia, have both impaired host defenses and a tendency to aspirate.

It is important to differentiate community-acquired pneumonia from hospital-acquired pneumonia because each is likely to have different causative agents (see also Chapter 8.5). A *community-acquired pneumonia* in a normal host implies an inhaled organism with relatively high virulence (Table 2.2–2). Included in this group are the respiratory viruses, in particular the influenza, rubeola, and rubella viruses; *Mycoplasma pneumoniae; Streptococcus pneumoniae; Legionella* sp; *Mycobacterium tuberculosis;* some respiratory mycoses; *Chlamydia psittaci* and *Coxiella burnetti.* Young healthy adults tend to have pneumonias that reflect casual first contact with community organisms. These are usually viruses, mycoplasma, postviral bacterial pneumonia, or *Chlamydia* infections. Middle-aged and older healthy persons are less likely to

Table 2.2–1. Diseases radiographically mimicking pneumonia.

Alveolar filling diseases
  Cells
    Bronchoalveolar cell carcinoma
    Desquamative interstitial pneumonitis
    Eosinophilic pneumonias
  Protein
    Alveolar proteinosis
  Water
    Pulmonary edema
  Blood
    Systemic lupus erythematosus
    Goodpasture's syndrome
    Idiopathic pulmonary hemosiderosis

Interstitial diseases
  Granulomatous diseases
    Sarcoidosis
    Wegener's granulomatosis
    Eosinophilic granuloma
    Hypersensitivity pneumonitis
  Occupational lung diseases
  Drug ingestions
  Radiation
  Collagen vascular diseases

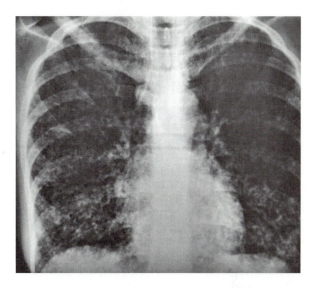

Figure 2.2–2. Chest x-ray of a patient with interstitial (atypical) pneumonia, showing bilateral diffuse pulmonary infiltrates.

have *Mycoplasma* infections and more likely to have viral or bacterial pneumonia.

Pneumonia in patients with altered immune status often reflects the underlying immune deficit. Thus, persons with reduced B-cell function (as with multiple myeloma) are likely to have bacterial pneumonia, whereas those with

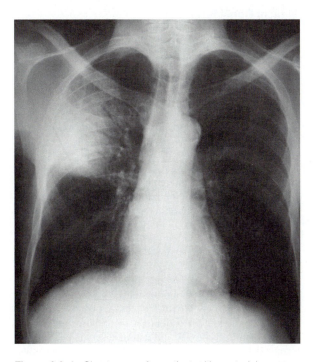

Figure 2.2–1. Chest x-ray of a patient with acute lobar pneumonia, showing a dense infiltrate in the right upper lobe.

markedly reduced T-cell function (as with late-stage AIDS) have more viral, fungal, and other opportunistic infections. Other circumstances such as corticosteroid therapy or environmental exposure may alter host defenses or present the patient with unique infectious agent exposures.

Patients with underlying obstructive lung diseases tend to have recurrent episodes of acute viral or bacterial bronchitis superimposed on a background of chronic bronchitis or bronchiectasis. If untreated, these episodes may progress to pneumonia. If suspicion of bacterial bronchitis or pneumonia is great, antibiotics should be instituted after sputum is obtained for analysis. Common organisms seen in acute exacerbations of bronchitis are respiratory viruses, *Haemophilus* sp, *S pneumoniae, Branhamella catarrhalis,* and *Legionella* sp. An occupational and travel history or an animal or avian exposure history may be invaluable in raising the suspicion of less common offending organisms (see Table 2.2–2).

Hospital-acquired pneumonia is caused by organisms that colonize ill patients, staff, and equipment. After colonization of the oropharynx, the organisms are aspirated. *Staphylococcus aureus* and gram-negative bacilli including *Pseudomonas* sp are of particular concern.

Bacterial, viral, rickettsial, and protozoal pneumonias are associated with characteristic symptoms and signs, some of which reflect the virulence of the organism and some of which reflect the host's response. Frequently, these symptoms and signs overlap, and their specificity is therefore limited.

Bacterial pneumonias are usually associated with an abrupt onset of symptoms, which may include chills, cough, headache, pleuritic pain and, especially in older persons, confusion. Gradual onset of symptoms should suggest anaerobic, mycobacterial, or actinomycotic pneu-

Table 2.2–2. Diagnosis of infectious pneumonia.

	Symptoms and Signs
Common causes	
Typical pneumonia	Productive cough, fever (often
Streptococcus	abrupt in onset), chills, pleuritic
pneumoniae	chest pain, pulmonary
Haemophilus influenzae	consolidation
Staphylococcus aureus	
Legionella	
Gram-negative bacilli	
Atypical pneumonia	Nonproductive cough, fever; chills
Mycoplasma	uncommon; pleuritic chest pain
Viruses	uncommon; myalgia, headache,
	fatigue common; minimal or
	absent pulmonary consolidation;
	scattered rhonchi, rales, or
	wheezes
Uncommon causes	
Bacterial infection	
Anthrax: wool,	Insidious fever, nonproductive
animal hides,	cough, diffuse edema of neck
fertilizer	and chest
Brucella sp: meat	Subacute fever, headache, malaise
processing, farming,	
veterinarians	
Francisella tularensis:	Fever, chills, ulceroglandular
animal, bird contact	infection
Yersinia pestis: rodent,	Hemoptysis, adenopathy,
flea contact	productive cough
Fungal infection	Common in immunocompromised
	patients
Candida	Nonspecific symptoms: fever and
	cough
Blastomycosis	Abrupt onset of fever, chills;
	arthralgia
Cryptococcosis	Symptomatic pulmonary disease
	uncommon in normal host
Mucormycosis	Black eschar; rhinocerebral
	mucormycosis in diabetic
	ketoacidosis
Histoplasmosis	
Rickettsiae	
Q fever	Chills, fever, myalgia, headache,
	stiff neck; rash uncommon
Rocky Mountain	Fever, chills, headache, rash
spotted fever	
Scrub typhus	Fever, rash, lymphadenopathy
Epidemic typhus	Abrupt onset of headache, fever,
	chills

monias. Certain bacteria are associated with the presence or absence of specific symptoms. Thus, pneumonia caused by *S pneumoniae* commonly leads to a single shaking chill (rigor), whereas pneumonia caused by anaerobic organisms is rarely associated with rigors. Headaches, confusion, and gastrointestinal symptoms are commonly seen in those with *Legionella* pneumonia. The most reliable signs of bacterial pneumonias are fever, sputum, and the physical findings on chest examination of inspiratory crackles or consolidation.

Viral pneumonias are frequently associated with extrathoracic symptoms such as coryza, sore throat, headache, myalgia, and arthralgias. Signs may include a relative bradycardia, scanty or no sputum, and an irritating nonproductive cough.

Occasionally, symptoms including chills and fever together with infiltrates seen on chest x-ray suggest an infectious pneumonia when in fact the patient has suffered an acute inhalational injury from a chemical or toxin or has had a drug reaction. Examples are hypersensitivity pneumonitis in pigeon breeders, heavy metal inhalation, and nitrofurantoin ingestion. In these cases, antibiotics should be withheld. Only careful questioning of the patient will uncover the inciting agent.

CHRONIC PNEUMONIA AND PNEUMONITIS

Presentation

In patients with a noninfectious pneumonitis or those who have a chronic infectious pneumonia, the clinical presentation is usually subacute; typically, symptoms may have developed over a period of weeks to several months. Vital signs may be normal, except for an increase in respiratory rate and possibly a low-grade fever. Rather than signs of lobar consolidation, the lung examination may reveal fine inspiratory crackles, typically over the lower parts of both lung fields at the back. The chest x-ray shows infiltrates that are patchy or diffuse. When the presentation suggests a chronic, progressive process, absence of fever or sputum should raise the possibility that the process is not infectious.

Clinical Considerations

Infectious agents that result in an indolent course of pneumonia are usually not bacteria—anaerobes and mycobacteria being exceptions—but are more likely to be fungi, parasites, or *Nocardia* sp. Noninfectious causes of chronic pneumonitis include eosinophilic pneumonitis, pulmonary infarction, primary and secondary neoplasms, noninfectious granulomatous diseases, lipoid pneumonia, collagen vascular diseases, drug-induced pneumonia, occupational lung diseases, or those of unknown etiology (eg, alveolar proteinosis).

A chronic productive cough is more suggestive of an infectious cause than an environmental or work-related disorder or one of unknown etiology. Alveolar proteinosis and alveolar cell carcinoma are exceptions, being occasionally associated with a productive cough. Pleuritic pain is more common with infectious agents. Exceptions to this rule are pleuritic pain caused by pulmonary infarction, lupus pneumonitis, mesothelioma, and a benign asbestos-related effusion. Continuous thoracic pain lasting for 1 month or more, without trauma or signs of infection, is nearly always caused by cancer. Dyspnea is a more common complaint in patients with noninfectious pneumonitis than in those with infectious diseases because the former disease generally causes greater physiologic dysfunction.

PHYSICAL EXAMINATION: PNEUMONIA AND PNEUMONITIS

The most reliable physical findings in patients with bacterial pneumonia are fever of 100–104°F (38–40°C), tachypnea, cough, and crackles (rales), and evidence of consolidation. However, these findings are not specific to infectious pneumonias; hypersensitivity pneumonitis, lupus pneumonitis, and metal fume fever may cause similar signs and symptoms. Patients with more severe cases of bacterial pneumonia may be hypotensive, cyanotic, and jaundiced, with a "toxic" appearance. These findings are not characteristic of noninfectious pneumonitis. Relative bradycardia is commonly seen in viral pneumonias and *Legionella* pneumonia; the latter is more commonly associated with signs of consolidation. An inspiratory squeak, heard on auscultation, may differentiate bronchiolitis obliterans organizing pneumonia from bacterial pneumonias.

Extrapulmonary physical findings may suggest specific causes of pneumonia or help differentiate infectious processes from other pulmonary diseases. Clubbing, commonly seen in patients with idiopathic pulmonary fibrosis, an uncommon scarring disease of the lungs (Chapter 2.5), is not seen in patients with acute pneumonia; other pulmonary causes of clubbing are cancer, bronchiectasis, lung abscess, and empyema. Skin rashes may be seen in patients with rickettsial, fungal, viral, and some bacterial infections. The character of the rash usually distinguishes an infectious disease from other noninfectious causes of pulmocutaneous syndromes. Neurologic deficits are generally nonspecific, being found in both infectious causes of pneumonias and in some noninfectious causes of pneumonitis. Splenomegaly is not uncommon in rickettsial infections, psittacosis, or sarcoidosis.

Radiographic Patterns

Bacterial pneumonias usually are seen on x-ray as localized patchy alveolar infiltrates (Chapter 8.5). Noninfectious processes with a similar radiographic pattern include pulmonary infarction, neoplasms, eosinophilic pneumonia, and lipoid pneumonia. Occasionally, patients with bacterial pneumonias may present with lobar consolidation, which should suggest infection with *S pneumoniae, S aureus, Klebsiella,* or *Legionella* sp. Noninfectious causes of lobar consolidation include alveolar cell carcinoma and the "drown lobe" syndrome secondary to an obstructing carcinoma. Bacterial pneumonias tend to be radiographically more dense and more asymmetric then their viral counterparts, which tend to appear as diffuse symmetric interstitial infiltrates. *Pneumocystis carinii* pneumonia characteristically presents with a symmetric interstitial process.

Aspiration pneumonia usually manifests in parts of the lung that are dependent at the time of aspiration. Thus, in the somnolent alcoholic infiltrates are often found in the posterior segment of the right upper lobe, the superior segment of the right lower lobe, or the basal segments of both lobes. Aspiration of lipids (eg, nose drops, cathartics) may lead to a discrete circumscribed lesion, which is radiographically similar to a neoplasm.

Pleural effusions are more common with bacterial and mycoplasmal infections than with viral pneumonias. Noninfectious causes of pneumonitis with pleural effusion include immunologic diseases (eg, systemic lupus erythematosus), neoplastic diseases (eg, lung cancer), pulmonary embolism, and trauma.

Cavitation indicates a necrotizing process and occurs most commonly with bacterial pneumonias, especially *S aureus, Pseudomonas, Klebsiella* infections, and *M tuberculosis.* Most cavitating bacterial pneumonias have an air-fluid level seen on the radiograph, but only one-third of tuberculous lesions show air-fluid levels. The most common noninfectious cause of a cavitating lesion is primary lung cancer.

Diagnostic Workup

Sputum Specimen: Examination of expectorated sputum is the most important and least invasive method to recover the pathogen from the lower respiratory tract in suspected pneumonia; 50% of routinely collected samples are ultimately helpful in the diagnosis of acute bacterial pneumonia. It is critical to obtain a good specimen—sputum that is clearly derived from the lung and not contaminated by oropharyngeal flora or saliva. Fewer than 10 squamous epithelial cells and more than 25 leukocytes per high-power field indicates that the specimen represents lower respiratory tract secretions.

After an adequate sputum specimen is obtained, its color, quality, and odor may be helpful in determining the causal agent. For instance, yellow mucopurulent sputum suggests a bacterial pneumonia, whereas a scant and watery sputum suggests a viral or atypical pneumonia with an organism such as *Mycoplasma* or *Legionella* pneumonia. Classically, a rust-colored sputum suggests pneumococcus, whereas dark mucoid "currant jelly" sputum favors *Klebsiella* pneumonia. Foul-smelling sputum is found in about 50% of anaerobic pulmonary infections. Absence of any secretions is characteristic of pneumonitis; striking exceptions are pulmonary alveolar proteinosis and alveolar cell carcinoma, both of which often may cause copious secretions.

Gram's stain of the sputum is paramount in the initial microbiologic analysis. For example, the pneumococcus is an unmistakable gram-positive, lancet-shaped diplococcal organism. In addition to noting the morphology and gram-staining characteristics of the predominant organism, polymorphonuclear leukocytes with intracellular organisms should also be sought. Other stains should be performed as well if the differential diagnosis includes infection such as *M tuberculosis* (stain for acid-fast bacilli), fungi (KOH prep), or *P carinii* (methenamine-silver nitrate stain). Although cultures of sputum are less reliable than microscopic examination, all adequate specimens should be sent for culture and sensitivity to provide conclusive identification of the pathogen. A Gram's stain and culture should be done on sputum obtained before antibiotic therapy is begun. If the suspicion of malignancy is high, cytologic analysis of sputum should be performed. Sputum analysis revealing a high eosinophil count can sometimes help in diagnosing noninfectious disorders such as drug-induced pneumonitis. Atypical histiocytes with X bodies by electron microscopy are characteristic of eosinophilic granuloma. If sputum is too scanty or is contaminated by oropharyngeal secretions, several more invasive procedures are available if clinical circumstances warrant.

Bronchoscopy: Although fiberoptic bronchoscopy is well tolerated by most patients, it has significant limitations when used to recover lower respiratory bacterial pathogens. The bronchoscope is often contaminated during passage though the upper airway, making the results of routine culture unreliable and difficult to interpret. Quantitative cultures of specimen obtained by bronchoscopy and introduction of a protected catheter brush have been reported to reduce both false-positive and negative results. Generally, bronchoscopy should be reserved for evaluation of immunocompromised patients who are at high risk for becoming infected by nonbacterial pathogens including viruses, *M tuberculosis, P carinii,* and fungi.

Bronchoalveolar Lavage: A procedure to obtain alveolar fluid after instillation of normal saline (usually 100–200 mL), bronchoalveolar lavage is often performed during the course of fiberoptic bronchoscopy. It is very effective in diagnosing *P carinii* pneumonia. Lavage specimens are especially helpful during the workup of patients with noninfectious pneumonitis such as pulmonary hemorrhage syndromes, eosinophilic granuloma, sarcoidosis, drug-induced lung injury, and hypersensitivity pneumonitis.

Open Biopsy: Open lung biopsy should be reserved for severely ill immunocompromised patients who are not responding to appropriate antimicrobial therapy. The role of open lung biopsy in the diagnosis of pneumonia even in this patient population is highly controversial, because the risk of the invasive procedure often outweighs the benefit of the test. Usually, the data obtained from open lung biopsy does not alter the eventual outcome of the disease process despite a change of therapy. This type of biopsy should be considered in a patient suspected of having a noninfectious cause of pneumonitis, which has not been diagnosed by less invasive biopsy procedures. If a malignancy is suspected, open lung biopsy should be restricted to patients with surgically resectable lesions (Chapter 2.9). Transthoracic needle aspiration, although more commonly used for diagnosis of malignancy, can be used for infectious pathogens, especially if the lesion is peripheral.

Thoracentesis: Thoracentesis should be performed in all patients with pneumonia associated with pleural effusion. Parapneumonic effusions are common and represent the most common causes of exudative effusions. Patients with anaerobic, pneumococcal, and gram-negative pneumonias are at high risk for developing parapneumonic effusions. If the parapneumonic pleural fluid is infected (empyema), with rare exceptions, a chest tube must be placed. Undrained empyema is seldom cured with antibiotics alone and eventually leads to bacteremia and sepsis.

Transtracheal Aspiration: An alternative method for obtaining material from the lower respiratory tract is through puncture of the trachea. Although the technique is considered a "gold standard" for identifying the causal pathogen, it is not without risk and should not be performed in patients with significant coagulopathy or thrombocytopenia. Complications of transtracheal aspiration include paratracheal infection, pneumothorax, mediastinal emphysema, and death. This technique, uncommonly used, may be helpful in patients who are unable to produce sputum but who have obvious clinical and radiographic findings of pneumonia, poor response to antibiotics, or a question of superinfection.

Laboratory Data

Complete laboratory testing including blood cell count, serum electrolytes, liver function test, and urinalysis should be performed in every patient suspected of having pneumonia. The white blood cell count and its differential are helpful in distinguishing bacterial pneumonia from atypical pneumonia or noninfectious pneumonitis. A marked leukocytosis with leftward shift is often observed in pneumococcal, *Haemophilus,* and other gram-negative bacillus infections; viral and mycoplasmal infections are often associated with leukopenia, a normal, or only a slight elevation of the white blood cell count. In a patient with bacterial pneumonia, leukopenia usually denotes an overwhelming bacterial infection and suggests a poor outcome. It is often seen in alcoholic patients bacteremic with *S pneumoniae* or gram-negative bacilli. Eosinophilia is uncommon in infectious pneumonia and, when present, should alert the physician to noninfectious processes such as a drug reaction, Löffler's syndrome, or chronic eosinophilic pneumonitis. Serum electrolyte abnormalities (especially hyponatremia), abnormal liver function tests, and abnormal urinalysis are often seen as systemic manifestations of bacterial pneumonias such as *Legionella* pneumonia.

Arterial blood gases or oximetry should be performed if the patient shows signs of respiratory compromise in the form of tachypnea, dyspnea, or cyanosis. Hypoxemia can arise from shunting of venous blood through areas of pneumonia or pneumonitis. It may be associated with a fairly normal-appearing chest x-ray and is often seen in noninfectious disorders such as pulmonary embolus and

Table 2.2–3. Causes and treatment of pneumonia.

Syndrome	Usual Pathogens	Therapy
Community-acquired The "common four"	*Streptococcus pneumoniae* *Legionella* *Mycoplasma* Virus	Erythromycin, penicillin Erythromycin Erythromycin No current treatment
Postviral influenza	*Staphylococcus* *Haemophilus influenzae*	Nafcillin Cephalosporin
Aspiration or lung abscess	Anaerobes	Penicillin, clindamycin
Chronic bronchitis	*S pneumoniae, H influenzae*	Cephalosporin, erythromycin, trimethoprim-sulfamethoxazole
Alcoholic or drug addict	*S pneumoniae, Staphylococcus, Klebsiella*	Aminoglycoside, cephalosporin
Immunocompromised host	*Staphylococcus* Gram-negative bacilli Fungus Virus *Pneumocystis carinii*	Vancomycin Cephalosporin Amphotericin B Acyclovir Trimethoprim-sulfamethoxazole
Hospital-acquired Usual nosocomial	*Staphylococcus* Gram-negative bacilli	Vancomycin Aminoglycoside
Immunocompromised host	Fungus	Amphotericin B

pulmonary alveolar proteinosis, or with *P carinii* pneumonia. Conversely, relatively "good" oxygenation in the setting of a markedly abnormal chest x-ray is suggestive of sarcoidosis or pulmonary hemorrhage syndromes. Hypocarbia is common in patients with acute pneumonia or noninfectious diseases leading to extensive interstitial fibrosis. Hypercarbia is an ominous sign implying respiratory failure.

Pulmonary function tests are not routinely used in the diagnostic workup of patients with pneumonia. An exception to this rule may be the HIV-positive patient at high risk for developing *P carinii* pneumonia, since a decreased diffusing capacity is often seen in patients with early *P carinii* pneumonia. Amiodarone-induced pneumonitis is also associated with a reduction in the diffusing capacity. Pulmonary function tests are useful in patients who have underlying lung disease and are recovering from recent bouts of pneumonia, because these tests allow the physician to determine whether the patient has returned to baseline lung function.

TREATMENT

Specific therapy for pneumonia can be guided by the clinical and laboratory data. Common causes of pneumonia and their treatment are found in Table 2.2–3. When selecting an antibiotic, the physician should make sure that it is appropriate for the suspected pathogen and that it is not one to which the patient may be allergic.

PREVENTION

Basic good hygiene must be practiced by patients, family members, and health care providers to minimize spread of infectious pathogens, especially in trying to reduce the incidence of nosocomial pneumonia. Adhering to effective hand-washing techniques and proper handling of equipment such as ventilator tubing are simple but effective modes of prevention. Prophylactic influenza vaccinations should be available yearly both to high-risk patients (eg, those with COPD, cardiovascular disease, or renal failure) and to the elderly population. Although its efficacy is controversial, pneumococcal vaccine is generally recommended for patients at risk for pneumococcal infection (COPD, splenectomy, or immunosuppressed patients).

SUMMARY

▶ Acute infectious pneumonia is marked by increasing cough, purulent sputum, dyspnea, fever, and signs of consolidation. The likely organism is predicted by the host, the patient's immune status, and source of the infection.

▶ Community-acquired pneumonia is caused by an inhaled organism of high virulence, such as viruses, *Pneumococcus, Legionella,* and mycoplasma. Hospital-acquired pneumonia is more likely to be caused by *Staphylococcus aureus* or gram-negative organisms.

▶ Infectious causes of chronic pneumonitis are often not bacteria; fungi, *Nocardia,* and parasites should be considered along with anaerobic organisms and mycobacteria.

▶ Noninfectious causes of chronic pneumonitis include pulmonary infarction, cancer and secondary tumors, granulomatous disorders, eosinophilic pneumonitis,

drug-induced disease, and occupation diseases. Productive cough is common in chronic infections and in alveolar proteinosis and some forms of lung cancer.

▶ Thorough examination of a good-quality sputum specimen is the most valuable aspect of workup for pneumonia. All pleural effusions associated with pneumonia should be aspirated. Bronchoscopy and biopsy techniques are required only infrequently.

SUGGESTED READING

Cook DJ et al: Evaluation of new diagnostic technologies: Bronchoalveolar lavage and the diagnosis of ventilator-associated pneumonia. Crit Care Med 1994;22:1314.

Fang GD et al: New and emerging etiologies for community-acquired pneumonia with implications for therapy. Medicine 1990;69:307.

MacFarlane JT et al: Prospective study of etiology and outcome of adult lower-respiratory-tract infections in the community. Lancet 1993;341:511.

Swartz MN: Approach to the patient with pulmonary infections. In: *Pulmonary Diseases and Disorders.* Fishman A (editor). McGraw-Hill, 1988:1375.

Wilson WR et al: Pulmonary disease in the immunocompromised host. Mayo Clin Proc 1985;60:473,610.

Yungbluth M: The laboratory diagnosis of pneumonia: The role of the community hospital pathologist. Clin Lab Med 1995;15:209.

Chronic Obstructive Pulmonary Disease

Robert A. Wise, MD, and Gail G. Weinmann, MD

Patients with chronic obstructive pulmonary disease (COPD) can present to the physician with slowly progressive exertional dyspnea or as an emergency with rapidly developing respiratory failure. COPD is a clinical and pathophysiologic syndrome comprising three diseases: emphysema, chronic bronchitis, and asthma. These three disorders have overlapping features, and because patients often have characteristics of more than one disorder, all three are classified together as COPD. In common use, the term COPD is applied to patients who demonstrate chronic, incompletely reversible airflow obstruction on forced expiration. This working definition excludes many patients with asthma (Chapter 2.4). This chapter covers COPD caused by pulmonary emphysema and chronic bronchitis.

DEFINITION

Emphysema of the lung is a condition in which the air spaces are enlarged as a consequence of destruction of alveolar septa. Mild emphysema is evident only under the microscope as enlarged alveoli, whereas advanced emphysema causes large, thin-walled air spaces called *bullae*. Bullae may range in diameter from a few millimeters to the span of the entire hemithorax. Chronic bronchitis is a disease characterized by a chronic cough productive of phlegm. The standard definition of chronic bronchitis is a productive cough occurring on most days for 3 months of the year for 2 or more consecutive years, without an otherwise defined acute cause. Most patients with chronic bronchitis have had daily cough and phlegm throughout the year for many years. Both emphysema and chronic bronchitis, however, lead to a common pathophysiologic abnormality—chronic airflow obstruction. Both conditions are produced by cigarette smoking, and both often coexist in the same patient. A component of reversible airway obstruction may also be present, giving rise to the term *asthmatic bronchitis*.

RISK FACTORS

Cigarette smoking is the overwhelming risk factor for COPD; 90% of COPD can be attributed to smoking. Although most persons with COPD have smoked cigarettes, only one in seven smokers develops COPD. Why only some smokers develop COPD depends on other risk factors, particularly male gender, a history of childhood respiratory illness, low socioeconomic status, and a family history of COPD. Most patients with COPD show increased reactivity of the airways when challenged with inhaled constricting agents such as methacholine or histamine. Whether airway hyperreactivity predisposes these persons to COPD or whether it is the consequence of COPD is not known.

About 1 in 2500 whites is homozygous for a single gene mutation that prevents hepatic secretion of the antiprotease enzyme, α_1-antitrypsin. Persons with less than 10% of the normal levels of this enzyme are at particular risk for developing premature emphysema, particularly if they smoke.

PATHOGENESIS

The mechanism by which cigarette smoking leads to emphysema is not known. Because emphysema is associated with a decrease in lung elastin content, because elastase induces emphysema in animals, and because deficiency of the elastase inhibitor α_1-antitrypsin leads to premature emphysema, many believe that elastase or other protease enzymes such as cathepsin B play a central role in the development of emphysema.

Cigarette smoking causes inflammation of the peripheral airways with infiltration by cells that release proteolytic enzymes into the air spaces. Cigarette smoke inactivates antiprotease enzymes and increases the permeability of the epithelial barrier to elastolytic enzymes. The imbalance between protease activity and antiprotease activity is thought to lead to degradation of elastin in the alveolar walls, hence to destruction of alveolar septa. Inflammation of the peripheral airways eventually causes distortion, edema, and fibrosis of the distal airways, which increases their resistance to airflow and increases their tendency to collapse.

The anatomy of emphysema from smoking is different from the anatomy of emphysema caused by α_1-antitrypsin deficiency. With cigarette smoking, the distribution of emphysema follows the distribution of ventilation, that is, centrilobular with the apex of the lung affected more than the base. In contrast, in α_1-antitrypsin deficiency, the distribution of emphysema follows the distribution of blood flow; the emphysema is panacinar and involves the base of the lung more than the apex.

Alveolar destruction and airway inflammation and fibrosis lead to reduction in airflow during forced expiration, hyperinflation of the lung, air trapping, and hypoxemia as a consequence of ventilation-perfusion mismatch. With prolonged hypoxemia, pulmonary hypertension develops and leads to right ventricular dysfunction and fluid retention, referred to as cor pulmonale (Chapter 1.12). In some persons (typically the "blue bloaters"; see "Physical Examination" below), alveolar hypoventilation causing hypercapnia is present. In others ("pink puffers"), alveolar hyperventilation and hypocapnia are present until the disease is far advanced.

CLINICAL EVALUATION

In patients with symptomatic COPD, the history, physical examination, and selected laboratory studies should be directed to assess the severity of disease, exclude other causes of breathlessness, and evaluate the response to treatment.

History

Patients with COPD are usually over the age of 50 years when they present to the physician. A person who starts smoking in adolescence or young adulthood develops a chronic productive cough, most frequently in the morning, which is dismissed as an innocent "smoker's cough." Over several decades, there is accelerated decline in pulmonary function. The volume of air expired in 1 second during a forced expiration, FEV_1, is used to track the course of this disease. Whereas the normal age-related decline in FEV_1 is about 30 mL per year, patients who develop COPD have declines of 50–80 mL per year (Figure 2.3–1). When the FEV_1 falls to about 50% of the predicted level, the person notices exertional breathlessness, but often attributes it to deconditioning. Exertion levels are gradually reduced to accommodate this dyspnea. Chest infections or episodes of acute bronchitis become more frequent and prolonged. It is not until the FEV_1 reaches about 30% of predicted that shortness of breath interferes with the usual activities of daily living. Many patients spontaneously stop smoking at this point, and at this advanced symptomatic stage the patient often seeks medical attention. In other cases, the diagnosis is made when the person develops a severe respiratory infection or exacerbation that leads to hospitalization.

In advanced stages, exacerbations are more frequent, with progressive incapacity from dyspnea. Cor pulmonale supervenes, and death is the eventual result of worsening cardiac and respiratory failure. Fifty percent of patients with COPD die within 10 years after the initial diagnosis. Patients with worse lung function or low arterial oxygen tensions have shorter survival.

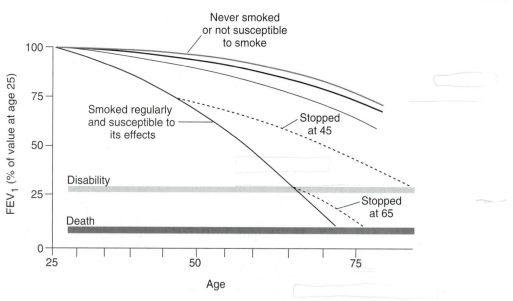

Figure 2.3–1. The natural history of several typical persons. In nonsmokers and in smokers who are not prone to develop COPD, the FEV_1 declines about 30 mL/yr from normal aging. Thus, at the age of 75, nonsmokers and smokers not susceptible to COPD have lost about 25% of their early adult lung function. In susceptible smokers, the decline in lung function is accelerated two- to three-fold. This leads to serious impairment in lung function by middle age. A smoker who stops smoking at any point reduces the decline in lung function to the normal aging rate. (Reproduced, with permission, from Fletcher C, Peto R: The natural history of chronic airflow obstruction. Br Med J 1977;1:1645.)

Physical Examination

The physical examination of a patient with advanced COPD shows an asthenic person with well-developed neck and abdominal muscles, dyspneic, with pursed lip breathing or grunting expirations. Speech is punctuated by frequent inspirations, so-called "telegraphic" speech. The patient leans forward on the elbows in a "tripod" position to stabilize the shoulder girdle, allowing the accessory muscles of respiration in the neck to elevate the rib cage with inspiration. The sternomastoid muscles contract with each inspiration. This is the typical appearance of the so-called "pink puffer," whose oxygenation is maintained by virtue of continued respiratory effort. In contrast, the "blue bloater" with COPD tends to be obese, with less dyspnea, but showing peripheral cyanosis and edema. Blue bloaters are usually in chronic respiratory failure, with hypercarbia, reduced central respiratory drive, and arterial desaturation. Clubbing of the nails is rare with uncomplicated COPD and should alert the physician to the possibility of carcinoma of the lung or bronchiectasis.

Chest examination shows signs of hyperinflation, with increase in the anteroposterior dimension and elevation of the clavicles. Percussion of the thorax shows increased resonance. The diaphragm is low and moves poorly with full inspiration. Auscultation of the lungs reveals decreased breath sounds over areas with emphysematous bullae. Early inspiratory crackles are common. Wheezes may not be present at rest, but can usually be evoked by forced expiration. The duration of expiration is prolonged, typically more than three times the duration of inspiration. The duration of a forced vital capacity expiration is prolonged. Listening with a stethoscope over the trachea, expiratory airflow can be heard for more than 6 seconds. In patients with chronic bronchitis, rhonchi reflect secretions in the airways. The breathing of a patient with chronic bronchitis is typically raspy and loud when the stethoscope is placed a few inches in front of the mouth.

The cardiac examination shows soft, muffled heart sounds, with the maximum cardiac impulse palpated best in the subxiphoid region. When cor pulmonale has developed, present are elevated venous pressure, peripheral edema, a loud pulmonic second heart sound, and a murmur of tricuspid regurgitation.

Chest X-Ray

Although the chest x-ray may suggest COPD, it is neither sensitive enough to serve as a screening test nor specific enough to serve as a diagnostic test for this condition. Typically, the chest x-ray of a person with COPD shows hyperinflation of the lungs with flat diaphragms; the anterior and retrocardiac air spaces are enlarged, and the costophrenic and sternophrenic angles are widened (Figure 2.3–2). The lung fields show a paucity of vessels. The cardiac silhouette is long and narrow. Patients with chronic bronchitis may show an increase in reticular and nodular markings in the lower lung zones, and sometimes thickened bronchial walls can be seen. In some patients with emphysema, thin-walled bullae can be seen on the chest x-ray. Computed tomography (CT) of the lung,

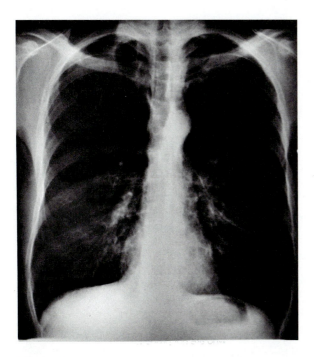
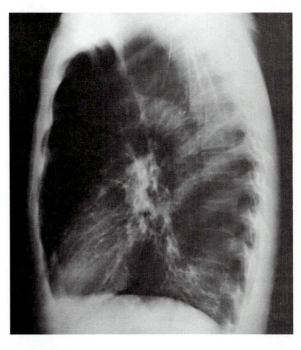

Figure 2.3–2. Chest x-rays of a patient with COPD, showing hyperlucent lungs with a paucity of blood vessels. The diaphragms are flat, making a wide angle with the rib cage. The anterior and posterior air spaces are enlarged. The heart is narrow and elongated. The central pulmonary vessels are prominent. Large bullae in the right and left upper lobes cause crowding of lung markings in both lower lung fields.

particularly with high-resolution techniques, is an accurate method of determining the presence and extent of anatomic emphysema.

Pulmonary Function Testing

The diagnosis of COPD rests on demonstrating airflow obstruction on forced expiratory spirometry. This is defined by a reduction in the FEV_1 compared with the forced vital capacity (FVC). Thus, the FEV_1/FVC ratio is decreased. The severity of the functional impairment and the prognosis for survival are best determined from the FEV_1. Displaying the forced expiratory maneuver as a flow-volume loop is helpful in excluding upper airway obstruction as a cause of reduced airflow (Figure 2.3–3). A reduced FVC is common because of the increase in air trapped in the lung at residual volume (RV). To distinguish this reduction in FVC by air trapping from restrictive lung disease requires lung volume measurements by helium dilution or body plethysmography. The carbon monoxide diffusing capacity (Dco) is reduced with emphysema and correlates with the anatomic extent of disease. When the Dco is greater than 50% of that predicted, the arterial oxygen saturation is not likely to fall significantly with exercise; when it is below this level, about 50% of patients desaturate with exercise.

Arterial blood gas measurements are helpful when the FEV_1 is less than 40% of that predicted, in order to assess the presence of hypoxemia or hypercapnia. Exercise testing with room air and oxygen is useful to determine the extent of disability and whether oxygen supplementation improves exercise tolerance.

A complete physiologic assessment including spirometry, lung volumes, and diffusing capacity is helpful during the initial assessment of patients with COPD to establish the diagnosis, evaluate severity, and exclude other causes of dyspnea. Once the disease severity and diagnosis are established, however, forced expiratory spirometry is usually sufficient to follow the course of disease and the response to treatment. In patients with borderline or established hypoxemia, arterial blood gas studies are useful to assess the requirement for oxygen and to titrate the dose.

Other Laboratory Tests

A complete blood count may show polycythemia caused by chronic hypoxemia, but this is often absent even with prolonged hypoxemia. Eosinophilia suggests an

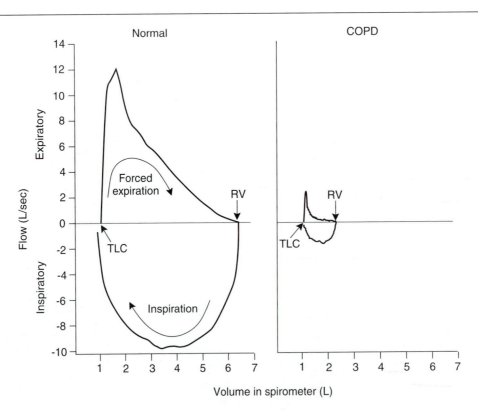

Figure 2.3–3. Flow-volume tracings of a normal person and a person with COPD. Both tracings are shown on the same scale. COPD causes severe reduction in both airflow (ordinate) and vital capacity (abscissa). The patient with COPD has both a higher total lung capacity (TLC) and a higher residual volume (RV).

allergic component to the disease. α_1-antitrypsin levels should be measured in smokers who show advanced COPD before the age of 50 or in nonsmokers who develop COPD at any age. The electrocardiogram typically shows low voltage with a vertical or rightward axis and clockwise rotation. Cor pulmonale is suggested by tall peaked P waves (P pulmonale) indicating right atrial enlargement, right axis deviation, and right ventricular hypertrophy (Chapter 1.12).

DIFFERENTIAL DIAGNOSIS

Disorders that can be confused with COPD include asthma, left ventricular failure, upper airway obstruction, vocal cord paralysis, diaphragm paralysis, obesity-hypoventilation syndrome, bronchiolitis obliterans, unilateral hyperlucent

lung syndrome, sarcoidosis, bronchiectasis, cystic fibrosis, hypogammaglobulinemia, and lymphangioleiomyomatosis (Table 2.3–1). These disorders can usually be distinguished from COPD on the basis of the history, physical examination, chest x-ray, and pulmonary function testing, but it is important to consider other less common diagnoses before assuming that a patient with chronic dyspnea has simple COPD.

TREATMENT

Asymptomatic Disease

COPD has a known reversible major risk factor—smoking—and a long asymptomatic period during which the disease is detectable by a simple and inexpensive test,

Table 2.3–1. Differential diagnosis of COPD.

Disorder	History	Physical Examination	Laboratory Findings
Asthma	Episodic dyspnea;trigger factors such as cold air, allergic exposures; nocturnal symptoms frequent	Usually normal examination between attacks	Positive allergy skin testing; sputum eosinophilia; normal or elevated diffusing capacity
Left ventricular failure	Orthopnea, paroxysmal nocturnal dyspnea	Paninspiratory crackles, normal or increased breath sounds, abnormal cardiac impulse	Cardiomegaly and pulmonary vascular congestion on chest x-ray; restriction on lung function tests
Upper airway obstruction		Inspiratory wheeze or stridor; normal lung sounds	Peak flows decreased on flow-volume loop
Vocal cord paralysis	Exertional dyspnea only; hoarseness or impaired singing	Inability to sustain "Z" sound as long as "S" sound; failure to oppose cords on laryngoscopy	Inspiratory flows decreased on flow-volume loop
Diaphragm paralysis	Orthopnea	Paradoxical inward movement of abdomen on inspiration	Reduced maximum inspiratory mouth pressures; elevated diaphragms on chest x-ray
Obesity-hypoventilation syndrome	Hypersomnolence	Massive obesity, peripheral edema	Hypercapnia; mild-moderate restrictive ventilatory defect
Bronchiolitis obliterans	Preceding acute viral illness, toxic inhalation exposure, or rheumatic disease	Diffuse paninspiratory crackles	Reticular or ground-glass diffuse infiltrates on chest x-ray
Unilateral hyper-lucent lung syndrome	Childhood respiratory illness	Asymmetric breath sounds	Unilateral bullae; severely reduced perfusion to affected lung on radionuclide perfusion scanning
Sarcoidosis	Erythema nodosum	Skin, mucous membrane, joint involvement	Hilar lymphadenopathy, noncaseating granulomas on biopsy of lung or other organ
Bronchiectasis	Chronic, purulent sputum	Localized chest crackles, clubbing	Dilated, tortuous airways on chest CT scan
Cystic fibrosis	Childhood onset; family history		Elevated sweat chloride, *Pseudomonas* colonization of sputum
Hypogamma-globulinemia (common variable immuno-deficiency)	Childhood onset of recurrent chest infections		Reduced serum gamma globulin, or deficient IgG subtypes
Lymphangioleio-myomatosis	Occurs in premenopausal women only		Characteristic "Swiss-cheese" appearance on CT

forced expiratory spirometry. Early detection of COPD with spirometry in persons at risk allows vigorous efforts at smoking cessation to be directed to those who show early lung damage. A sympathetic but strong personalized antismoking message delivered by the physician, supported by individual or group counseling and, in some patients, nicotine replacement therapy, can enable about 40% of smokers to quit and thus diminish the rate of decline of lung function.

Chronic Symptomatic Disease

When the patient develops symptomatic COPD, the main goals of treatment are to improve functional state and relieve symptoms. Smoking cessation is important, although many persons will have stopped spontaneously by the time the disease has progressed this far. Regular prudent exercise should be encouraged. Reassuring the patient and family that exertional dyspnea is not dangerous helps to encourage exercise. Proper nutrition with adequate caloric intake can improve functional state. Prophylactic influenza vaccine in the autumn is recommended. Pneumococcal vaccine may also be of value.

Bronchodilators can reverse some airflow obstruction and can also improve symptoms even when there is little objective evidence of bronchodilation. Bronchodilators of choice are inhaled anticholinergic agents, inhaled selective β-sympathomimetics, and long-acting oral theophylline, in that order. Metered-dose inhalers (MDI) are effective delivery systems for inhaled bronchodilators, but patients should be trained to use them properly. A reservoir or spacer attached to the metered-dose inhaler improves aerosol delivery and should be used by patients who have difficulty coordinating the use of an inhaler. Home nebulizers are reserved for patients who are unable to use a metered-dose inhaler despite repeated training sessions. Some patients benefit from corticosteroids, which should be instituted when other medications have not proved to be helpful and after an individualized trial with monitoring of lung function and symptoms.

Acute chest infections, heralded by a change in the color, consistency, or quantity of phlegm, should be treated promptly with a 10–14-day course of oral antibiotics such as tetracycline, amoxicillin, trimethoprim-sulfamethoxazole, or erythromycin. More expensive and broad-spectrum antibiotics such as cephalosporins and ciprofloxacin should be reserved for resistant organisms. About 50% of acute bronchial infections are caused by the common bacterial pathogens *Haemophilus influenzae, Streptococcus pneumoniae,* and *Branhamella catarrhalis.* The remainder are caused by *Mycoplasma* and viruses. It is not usually necessary to culture the sputum unless there is evidence of pneumonia or resistant infection.

Continuous low-flow oxygen by nasal cannula is indicated when the arterial PaO_2 is below 55 mm Hg despite 1 month of treatment or when the arterial PaO_2 is less than 60 mm Hg with signs of pulmonary hypertension, right heart failure, or neuropsychological dysfunction. Continu-

ous use of low-flow oxygen in hypoxemic patients is the only intervention to date that has proved to improve survival in advanced COPD. Patients should be encouraged to use their oxygen for 18 hours or more per day and should understand that it is used to treat and prevent pulmonary hypertension rather than to treat symptoms of dyspnea.

In patients with cor pulmonale, diuretics are used to control peripheral edema, but care should be taken to avoid excessive diuresis because patients with right ventricular failure tolerate hypovolemia poorly. Digitalis has little role other than for rapid atrial fibrillation. Pulmonary vasodilators, other than oxygen, have not been shown to have long-term efficacy (Chapter 1.12).

Other treatments that may benefit some patients, but are not widely used, are respiratory muscle training, intermittent respiratory muscle rest with an external cuirass ventilator, specialized low carbohydrate diets, mucolytic agents, and low-dose narcotics to relieve dyspnea. In patients with α_1-antitrypsin deficiency, intravenous enzyme replacement therapy should be considered.

Acute Exacerbations

Worsening of COPD may be caused by respiratory infections, exposure to respiratory irritants leading to bronchospasm, or pulmonary vascular congestion (Table 2.3–2). In most cases, the decline in respiratory status is subacute, occurring over days or weeks with no apparent cause. If worsening of dyspnea is sudden, myocardial infarction, pulmonary embolism, pneumonia, atelectasis, and pneumothorax should be considered possible causes. Treatment of acute exacerbations should be guided by the severity of the exacerbation and the patient's response to therapy. Spirometry and arterial blood gas monitoring provide useful guides to the success of treatment.

Bronchodilators should be administered by nebulizer when the patient is too dyspneic to use a metered-dose inhaler. Theophylline by intravenous infusion is commonly prescribed, but the beneficial effects are probably small in relation to the potential toxicity. Corticosteroids are fre-

Table 2.3–2. Causes of sudden worsening of COPD.

Cause	Characteristic Features
Acute bronchitis	Change in sputum volume, color, or consistency
Bronchospasm	Wheezing during tidal breathing; reduced FEV_1
Pulmonary vascular congestion	Weight gain, ankle edema, increased vascularity on chest x-ray
Myocardial infarction	Sudden onset; chest pain or pressure, ECG changes, enzyme changes
Pulmonary embolism	Suggestive ventilation-perfusion scan; diagnostic pulmonary angiogram
Pneumonia	Fever, leukocytosis, pulmonary infiltrates
Atelectasis	Atelectasis on chest x-ray
Pneumothorax	Sudden onset; asymmetric breath sounds; diagnostic chest x-ray

quently given during an acute exacerbation and may speed recovery. Antibiotics should usually be started, the choice being guided by the sputum Gram's stain and culture. Oxygen should be administered to overcome hypoxemia. During institution of oxygen, a face mask with a Venturi inflow nozzle allows precise adjustment of oxygen concentration, since too much oxygen may depress respiratory drive and aggravate respiratory failure (Chapter 2.7). Later, the more comfortable nasal cannula allows the patient to speak and eat. Respiratory acidosis with arterial pH greater than 7.20 is acceptable if the oxygen saturation can be maintained above 90%.

When hypoxemia cannot be corrected without severe respiratory acidosis, ventilatory support with a mechanical ventilator is necessary. In some instances, support by means of a tight-fitting nasal mask may be adequate, but endotracheal intubation is usually required if ventilatory support is required for more than 24 hours (Chapter 2.7).

SUMMARY

▶ COPD is a common chronic progressive disease caused mainly by smoking, characterized histologically by emphysema and symptomatically by chronic bronchitis.

▶ Risk factors for developing COPD include cigarette smoking, advanced age, male sex, low socioeconomic status, childhood respiratory infections, bronchial hyperreactivity, and deficiency of α_1-antitrypsin.

▶ COPD causes functional deterioration with progressive cough and dyspnea, punctuated by exacerbations, culminating in cor pulmonale and death.

▶ Smoking cessation in the early phases of COPD can halt progression of the disease. In the advanced stages, therapy is directed toward alleviation of symptoms and prevention and treatment of complications.

SUGGESTED READING

American Thoracic Society: Standards for the diagnosis and care of patients with chronic obstructive pulmonary disease. Am J Respir Crit Care Med 1995;152:S78.

Burrows B et al: The course and prognosis of different forms of chronic airways obstruction in a sample from the general population. N Engl J Med 1987;317:1309.

Ferguson GT, Cherniack RM: Management of chronic obstructive pulmonary disease. N Engl J Med 1993;328:1017.

Fletcher C, Peto R: The natural history of chronic airflow obstruction. Br Med J 1977;1:1645.

Asthma

David B. Jacoby, MD, and Mark C. Liu, MD

Asthma is a chronic obstructive disease of the airways. It is the most common disease of the lower respiratory tract, affecting 3–5% of the population in the United States or about 10 million people. It was once regarded as a nonlethal disease. William Osler said, "The asthmatic pants into old age." Nonetheless people do die of asthma and despite advances in treatment, the incidence of asthma as well as hospitalizations and death from the disease have been increasing since about 1980, especially among young blacks, the elderly, and the poor. The causes of these increases are unknown, but the trends in the United States reflect worldwide trends in asthma prevalence and severity.

Asthma is characterized by three components. (1) Obstruction to airflow is due to widespread narrowing of the airways, which is reversible either spontaneously or with treatment. Obstruction may be due to airway smooth muscle contraction, airway edema, or mucus. (2) Bronchial hyperreactivity describes an exaggerated tendency of the airways of asthmatic patients to constrict to a variety of physical or chemical stimuli such as exercise, hyperventilation, cold air, cigarette smoke, or chemical mediators (eg, methacholine, histamine). (3) Inflammation of the airways has long been recognized in fatal asthma where there is marked infiltration of the airways with inflammatory cells, particularly eosinophils. Other prominent pathologic changes include infiltration of the airways with lymphocytes, epithelial damage with subepithelial fibrosis, smooth muscle and mucous gland hyperplasia, and airway plugging with tenacious material consisting of exudated plasma proteins, mucus, and cellular debris. Active airway inflammation accounts for the sputum findings described historically in asthmatic patients, including "Creola bodies," composed of desquamated aggregates of epithelial cells, "Curschmann's spirals," representing mucous casts of small airways, and Charcot-Leyden crystals, composed of the crystallized enzyme, lysophospholipase, derived from the eosinophil granule. Recent techniques using bronchoscopy to examine airway tissues obtained from living patients with asthma have provided direct evidence of airway inflammation in virtually all patients with asthma, even in those with mild asymptomatic disease.

An important therapeutic implication of the chronic inflammatory basis for asthma is the recognition that bronchodilators, such as adrenergic agents and theophylline, may improve symptoms by reversing bronchospasm but do not alter the inflammatory process that underlies the disease. Hence, the trend in asthma management today is toward early treatment with anti-inflammatory agents such as glucocorticoids and cromolyn sodium.

Asthma is characterized by intermittent occurrence of cough, chest tightness, breathlessness, and wheezing with periods of being relatively symptom-free between attacks. This pattern helps to distinguish asthma from other chronic obstructive pulmonary diseases such as emphysema and chronic bronchitis, but because these diseases are also subject to exacerbations and remissions, clear distinctions may sometimes be difficult. Chronic bronchitis (sputum production complicated by progressive airways obstruction) and emphysema (destruction of pulmonary parenchyma with associated airflow obstruction) are discussed in Chapter 2.3. The demonstration of improved lung function following bronchodilator administration and of bronchial hyperreactivity on provocative testing supports the diagnosis of asthma.

Depending on the severity and duration of disease, between attacks the person with asthma may feel completely normal with normal pulmonary function, may feel normal despite decreased pulmonary function, or may experience persistent breathlessness and decreased pulmonary function. The frequent lack of correlation of clinical symptoms with the severity of airways obstruction in asthma underscores the need for objective measures of pulmonary function not only to establish the diagnosis, but also to follow the disease and assess management.

ASTHMA SYNDROMES

Asthma may be classified into several categories based on clinical associations or precipitating factors. Although assignment to a single category may be possible in about 50% of patients with asthma, there are large degrees of overlap.

Extrinsic Allergic Asthma

Symptomatic asthma clearly precipitated by exposure to specific allergens constitutes only 10% of the asthmatic population. Precipitating exposures include seasonal allergens such as tree and grass pollen in the spring, ragweed pollen in the fall, and perennial allergens such as animal danders or insect detritus (dust mite, cockroach). Asthma symptoms begin during childhood and are often associated with other allergic diseases such as allergic rhinitis, eczema, and urticaria. There is usually a family history of allergic disease. Immediate-type skin testing by intradermal injection of specific allergens causes a wheal-and-flare reaction through mediator release from mast cells sensitized with specific IgE antibody. Patients have elevated total IgE levels and eosinophilia consistent with an underlying allergic state.

Allergic Bronchopulmonary Aspergillosis

In a small proportion of patients with asthma, chronic colonization of the airways with *Aspergillus* plays a prominent role in the disease process. There is usually a long history of asthma that is often steroid-dependent and associated with radiographic findings of central bronchiectasis and recurrent pulmonary infiltrates. Brown mucous plugs composed of aggregated *Aspergillus* may be expectorated. Positive, immediate-type skin tests to *Aspergillus* and very high levels of total serum IgE are characteristic. Precipitins to *Aspergillus* may also be found.

Intrinsic Asthma

The most common type of asthma is characterized by persistent airway hyperreactivity to nonallergic stimuli. Although specific antigen exposure may trigger an occasional asthma attack, the clinical course does not correlate with allergic hypersensitivities. Instead, asthma is dominated by poorly defined "intrinsic" factors that mediate exacerbations related to infection, irritants, exercise, or psychological factors. Symptoms may begin at any age, but most often in adulthood. A viral upper respiratory tract infection may precede the initial episode. Immediate-type skin test reactivity is absent or minimal; however, elevated total IgE and eosinophilia are often present. Symptomatic periods tend to be prolonged in this group with many patients going on from their initial episode to develop chronic symptomatic disease.

Extrinsic Nonallergic Asthma

Asthma occurring in occupational settings may not have an immunologic basis, although in some cases, sensitization and an immunologic response have been demonstrated (eg, toluene-diisocyanate [TDI] and phthalic anhydride used in the manufacture of plastics and polyurethane foams). Examples of occupational exposures causing bronchospasm include metal fumes (chromium, nickel), wood (oak and western red cedar), grain, coffee dusts, and soybeans (baker's asthma), industrial chemicals (epoxy resins, soldering fluxes), detergent enzymes derived from bacteria *(Bacillus subtilis)*, and pharmaceutical agents (penicillin and pancreatic enzymes).

Aspirin Sensitivity

Aspirin and related compounds such as other non-steroidal anti-inflammatory drugs (NSAIDs) can precipitate asthma in 5% of asthmatics. This sensitivity is often associated with sinusitis and nasal polyps. This triad of asthma, aspirin sensitivity, and nasal polyps (Samter's triad) occurs more often in women. Although the basis of aspirin sensitivity is unknown, it is thought not to be immunologic and may be related to excessive production of leukotrienes induced by inhibition of the cyclooxygenase pathway of arachidonic acid metabolism. Asthma begins within 2 hours of aspirin ingestion and may result in respiratory failure, vascular collapse, and, rarely, death. Patients with asthma should be cautioned about using these agents.

Exercise-Induced Asthma

Most patients with asthma may precipitate an attack with exercise, and in some, this is the major manifestation of their disease. Asthma induced by exercise is directly related to heat and water loss from the airways. The mechanisms may involve changes in the osmolarity of airway secretions that induce release of inflammatory mediators or neuropeptides. Activities that promote heat loss from the airways such as running in a cold environment are more likely to precipitate asthma than is swimming where the environment is usually warm and humid.

Asthma Associated with Chronic Obstructive Pulmonary Disease

The course of chronic obstructive pulmonary disease (COPD) is often characterized by attacks of asthma, with greater or lesser degrees of reversible airways obstruction. Although the prognosis of COPD is dominated by the progressive decline of pulmonary function, airway hyperreactivity may be a risk factor in the development and progression of COPD. This reversible component of chronic airway obstruction should be managed in the same way as typical asthma.

DIFFERENTIAL DIAGNOSIS

Chronic Obstructive Pulmonary Disease

Asthma must be distinguished from chronic bronchitis and emphysema (Table 2.4–1). This distinction is frequently blurred because patients with COPD often have bronchial hyperreactivity and may have substantial improvements in pulmonary function after bronchodilator treatments.

The history is often important in making this distinction, since most patients with COPD are current or former cigarette smokers, whereas patients with significant asthma rarely tolerate smoking and are frequently bothered by the

Table 2.4–1. Differential diagnosis of wheezing.

Asthma
Acute infectious diseases
    Bronchiolitis
    Bronchitis
Chronic obstructive pulmonary disease
    Chronic bronchitis
    Emphysema
    Bronchiectasis
    α_1-antitrypsin deficiency
    Cystic fibrosis
    Immunoglobulin deficiency
Left heart failure
Pulmonary embolism
Anatomic upper airway obstruction
    Tumor
    Abscess
    Extrinsic compression
    Laryngeal edema
    Epiglottitis
    Bilateral vocal cord paralysis
Functional upper airway obstruction
    Paradoxical vocal cord dysfunction
Large airway obstruction
    Tumor
    Foreign body
Drug side effects

cigarette smoke of others. Cystic fibrosis, α_1-antitrypsin deficiency, and immunoglobulin deficiency are underlying causes of progressive lung disease, which should be sought in patients under 40 years old who present with COPD. Pulmonary function testing may demonstrate a low diffusing capacity in patients with emphysema, whereas in asthmatics, the diffusing capacity is normal or elevated.

Left Heart Failure

Patients with left-sided heart failure frequently wheeze—hence the term "cardiac asthma"—and asthmatic patients are often orthopneic. In patients with pulmonary venous congestion, lung function tests may demonstrate airway obstruction, decreased vital capacity and bronchial hyperresponsiveness. Nevertheless differentiating heart failure from asthma is usually obvious from the other signs or symptoms of heart disease or from the chest x-ray, but occasionally depends on objective tests of heart function, such as echocardiography. Sometimes a therapeutic trial of diuretics is needed to make the distinction.

Pulmonary Embolism

A clot lodging in the pulmonary circulation frequently causes wheezing and cough as well as acute shortness of breath and may therefore be confused with asthma. When such symptoms arise in a patient not previously known to have pulmonary problems, the diagnosis of pulmonary embolism is frequently considered. However, in a patient who has asthma or COPD, the occurrence of these symptoms will generally be ascribed to their underlying lung disease. Thus, pulmonary emboli may be overlooked, a serious mistake in view of the high mortality of recurrent emboli.

The finding of a low diffusing capacity may prompt the physician to consider the diagnosis of pulmonary embolism, as should associated findings suggesting deep venous thrombosis. Acute asthma may cause abnormalities in the ventilation-perfusion scan making interpretation difficult. If pulmonary embolism is being considered seriously and if the ventilation-perfusion scan is nondiagnostic, pulmonary arteriography may be required to establish the diagnosis.

Anatomic Upper Airway Obstruction

A cursory auscultation of the chest may fail to distinguish between wheezing coming from the chest and transmitted wheezing coming from the upper airway. Obstruction in the trachea or larynx causes stridor, a wheezing sound usually heard during both inspiration and expiration and heard most loudly over the anterior neck. The stridor associated with extrathoracic large airway obstruction is often louder during inspiration, whereas that associated with intrathoracic airway obstruction is often louder during expiration.

If large airway obstruction is suspected on clinical grounds, flow-volume loops can be examined to confirm this diagnosis. Extrathoracic large airway obstruction causes a plateau in inspiratory flows, whereas intrathoracic large airway obstruction causes a plateau in expiratory flows.

The differential diagnosis of large airway obstruction includes tracheal and laryngeal tumors, compression of the airways by extrinsic masses, airway edema, epiglottitis, tracheomalacia, tracheal stenosis, vocal cord paralysis, and foreign bodies. The difference in management between asthma and upper airway obstruction emphasizes the importance of routinely auscultating the anterior neck in wheezing patients.

Functional Upper Airway Obstruction

In some patients presenting with wheezing and shortness of breath, the cause of airway obstruction is vocal cord closure during respiration, particularly "paradoxical" vocal cord closure, or adduction during inspiration. This mimic of asthma is most common in young or middle-aged women who are often refractory to usual asthma management regimens. Flow-volume loops or direct laryngoscopy or both are needed to confirm the diagnosis, but these tests are often normal in the absence of symptoms. Thought to be psychogenic, paradoxical vocal cord movement usually responds to counseling and speech therapy.

Drug Side Effects

Medications used in the management of glaucoma, heart disease, and hypertension may cause cough and symptoms of asthma. β-blockers may induce attacks in some patients with asthma. Angiotensin converting enzyme (ACE) inhibitors may cause cough.

MANAGEMENT OF SEVERE ACUTE ASTHMA

Signs of Asthma Severity

More than 4000 deaths per year are caused by acute asthma in the United States. Many of these deaths occur at home before the patient reaches the hospital, but some occur during treatment. The relative contributions of severe airway obstruction and the complications of therapy to asthma death are matters of debate, and either or both may be responsible for the recent rise in asthma mortality.

The fact that asthma can be fatal emphasizes the importance of recognizing patients with severe attacks and treating them intensively, while at the same time attempting to minimize the complications of treatment. In evaluating patients during acute attacks, neither the patient's perception of the severity of the attack nor the intensity of wheezing heard by auscultation of the chest are reliable indicators of the degree of airway obstruction. A severe attack is suggested by sweating, fatigue or lethargy, and difficulty speaking in complete sentences.

Objective physical findings indicating a severe asthma attack are shown in Table 2.4–2. Severity can be assessed quickly by focused observation of the patient and vital signs. The normal fall in systolic blood pressure during inspiration is exaggerated during severe asthma attacks (pulsus paradoxus) because of the more negative intrathoracic pressures needed to breathe at high lung volumes. The chest x-ray may reveal findings that cause or complicate severe asthma and that may not be detected by physical examination, particularly pneumonia or pneumothorax.

A measure of pulmonary function is often helpful, both in assessing the severity of the attack and in following the response to treatment. Spirometry with 1-second forced expiratory volume (FEV_1) and forced vital capacity (FVC) and peak expiratory flow rate (PEFR) are the most easily measured and used in the acute setting. Pulmonary functions less than 25% of predicted (based on age, height and weight) indicate a severe attack, and FEV_1 values of less than 1.0 L, FVC of less than 1.5 L, or PEFR of less than 150 L per minute should prompt urgent attention.

Arterial blood gas measurements are useful as indicators of acute asthma severity and should be obtained in all but the mildest of attacks. A decreased PO_2 and low PCO_2 (respiratory alkalosis) is typical in mild-moderate acute asthma. Hypoxemia is usually due to ventilation-perfusion mismatching and readily responds to supplemental O_2. Not uncommonly, hypoxemia worsens transiently as the acute asthma attack resolves. Although a normal or elevated PCO_2 may indicate fatigue or progressive respiratory failure, the need for intubation and mechanical ventilation in hypercapnic patients must be evaluated in association with other signs of impending respiratory failure, such as obvious fatigue, lethargy, change in mental status, and worsening CO_2 retention.

In patients who are intubated, a common mistake is rapidly to normalize the patient's PCO_2 or to allow the patient to hyperventilate on assisted ventilation. Mechanical ventilation may result in higher tidal volumes or respiratory rates than can be maintained in a patient with severe airway obstruction. Thus, each mechanical breath is delivered before the previous one has been completely exhaled. The result of this "stacking" of breaths is a gradual increase in intrathoracic pressure, which impairs venous return and cardiac output, sometimes with catastrophic hemodynamic effects. Hence, ventilatory parameters must be carefully adjusted to avoid breath stacking leading to increased risks of hypotension and barotrauma, with normalization of the PCO_2 being of secondary importance. Achieving these goals may require paralysis and sedation of the patient until airway obstruction responds to therapy.

TREATMENT OF ACUTE ASTHMA

The primary goals of acute asthma management are to relieve airway obstruction and to maintain adequate oxygenation and ventilation. An outline of treatment is presented in Table 2.4–3.

Supplemental oxygen should be given to maintain PO_2 higher than 60 mm Hg or saturations over 90%. Usually, low flow rates of 2–4 L per minute by nasal cannula are sufficient. Dehydration caused by poor fluid intake or respiratory losses should be corrected; however, there is no evidence that excessive hydration improves mucous clearance. Mucolytic agents may cause airway irritation and should not be used. Antibiotics appropriate for bronchitis, sinusitis, or pneumonia may be administered as indicated.

Bronchodilators

β₂-Adrenergic Agonists: β₂-agonists that directly relax airway smooth muscle are the most effective bronchodilators for management of the acute asthma attack. Although

---

Table 2.4–2. Indications of severe asthma.

Physical examination
    Wheezes heard by auscultation: unreliable
    Sweating
    Pulse >120/min
    Respiratory rate >30/min
    Pulsus paradoxus >18 mm Hg
    Use of accessory muscles of respiration (ie, sternocleido-
        mastoid or abdominal)

Laboratory
    Pulmonary function
        FEV_1 <1.0 L or 25% predicted
        PEFR <150 L/min or 25% predicted
    Arterial blood gas
        PO_2 <60 mm Hg
        PCO_2 >40 mm Hg, particularly if rising
    Chest x-ray
        Pneumonia
        Atelectasis
        Pneumothorax
        Pneumomediastinum

FEV_1, 1-second forced expiratory volume; PEFR, peak expiratory flow rate.

Table 2.4–3. Treatment of acute asthma.

Selective β_2-agonist by inhalation
   Dose 3 ×/hr as needed
   Subcutaneous injection is alternative but less effective with
     more side effects
   Maintain every 2–4 hr as needed
Anticholinergics by inhalation
Theophylline
   Loading dose: 5–6 mg/kg IV; maintenance: 0.5–0.6 mg/kg/hr
Systemic glucocorticoids
   Methylprednisolone 60–80 mg or equivalent IV every 6–8 hr
     initially, with rapid taper
Oxygen
Antibiotics
Hydration

these medications are available for aerosolized, parenteral, or oral use, the preferred route of administration is an inhaled form that minimizes the risk of systemic side effects, including tachyarrhythmias, tremor, and nervousness. Subcutaneous administration of medications is usually unnecessary if aerosol therapy is promptly delivered. Oral therapy has no role in acute management.

Administration of aerosol by metered dose inhaler (MDI) is the preferred route of delivery, and use of the MDI with a spacer device or reservoir may improve drug distribution and effectiveness. Selective β_2-agonists with durations of action from 4–6 hours are available in MDI form, including albuterol, metaproterenol sulfate, and terbutaline. Less selective β-adrenergic agonists with shorter durations of action such as isoproterenol and epinephrine are also available but carry greater risks of side effects. In the acute setting, with adequate supervision, β_2 selective agonists may be started with 2–4 puffs, followed by 1–2 puffs every 10–20 minutes until side effects such as tremor, arrhythmia, or tachycardia are encountered. Therapy can be maintained with administration every 2–4 hours as necessary.

β_2-agonists are commonly delivered by nebulizer in emergency or hospital settings where patients may be unable to achieve adequate response with MDI use because of their respiratory distress. Continuously nebulized medication is inhaled during tidal breathing over 5–15 minutes. Albuterol, metaproterenol, or isoetharine are diluted for nebulizer use. Initial treatment can be repeated every 15–20 minutes for three doses before maintenance every 2–4 hours as necessary.

Injection of adrenergic agents subcutaneously is not usually indicated when aerosol therapy is available. However, epinephrine (0.3 mL 1:1000 subcutaneously) or terbutaline repeated every 15–20 minutes for three doses can be used.

Anticholinergics: Although atropine is sometimes administered as an aerosol bronchodilator, its use for this indication is not officially approved by the Food and Drug Administration. Side effects include dry mouth, blurred vision, urinary retention, and cardiac and central nervous

system stimulation. Ipratropium bromide, an anticholinergic quaternary ammonium compound is administered by MDI. Although useful in COPD, ipratropium is less effective in asthma and is less potent than β_2-agonists in the acute setting. A nebulized form is available.

Theophylline: A weak bronchodilator, theophylline is a phosphodiesterase inhibitor and adenosine receptor antagonist. In the acute setting, theophylline is generally administered intravenously in the water-soluble form of aminophylline. However, continuing oral therapy in patients already on theophylline is an acceptable alternative. Infusion rates should be reduced for patients with heart failure or liver disease or those who take medications that decrease metabolism (eg, cimetidine, propranolol, erythromycin, allopurinol); rates are increased in young patients, smokers, and patients on medications that increase metabolism (eg, phenobarbital, phenytoin, rifampin). Theophylline levels should be monitored and levels maintained at 10–20 mg/L. Side effects are dose-related and include nausea, vomiting, diarrhea, insomnia, headache, nervousness, and atrial arrhythmias, which may occur at therapeutic doses. More serious toxicity, causing seizures and ventricular arrhythmias, can develop at levels above 30 mg/L.

Anti-Inflammatory Agents

Corticosteroids: Systemic corticosteroids improve airway obstruction by reducing airway inflammation. Pure glucocorticoids are preferred for their reduced effects on salt and water metabolism. They have no direct effect on airway smooth muscle, and effects take 4–6 hours to become apparent. Any patient who fails to respond promptly to bronchodilator therapy or who is hospitalized for asthma should receive systemic corticosteroids. Optimal doses and frequency of administration are unknown, but an initial dose of 60–80 mg methylprednisolone (or equivalent) intravenously every 6–8 hours is recommended. Larger or more frequent doses have not clearly demonstrated improved outcomes. Initial high doses can be rapidly tapered to 40–80 mg/day, depending on response, in anticipation of continuing oral therapy. If the duration of systemic corticosteroid therapy is less than 2 weeks, gradual reduction in dosages is probably unnecessary. However, if response to therapy is slow or incomplete, prolonged administration of corticosteroids may be indicated requiring gradual decreases in dosage while adjusting concurrent therapy.

MANAGEMENT OF CHRONIC ASTHMA

The long-term goal of asthma therapy is to maintain a stable condition free of symptoms with the best possible pulmonary function using a minimum of medication. In some cases, environmental control measures and avoiding known precipitating factors, irritants, or allergens provide adequate relief from asthma; however, medications are usually necessary.

Since the treatment of asthma relies heavily on the use of MDI, proper inhaler technique can be as important as the choice of medication. A suggested technique is as follows: After shaking the inhaler, the opening is positioned 2 fingerbreadths (3–4 cm) in front of the open mouth with tongue down. One dose of the MDI is discharged at the beginning of a normal inspiration (ie, at functional residual capacity). Slow inspiration, taking 5 seconds to reach total lung capacity, optimizes particle distribution to the lower airways. Holding the breath 5–10 seconds allows particles that have reached the lower airways to settle. In patients unable to coordinate inhalation with the brief MDI discharge, spacers (tubes that serve as chambers into which medications can be sprayed) allow the patient to inhale suspended medications at will.

The first-line therapy for rapid, symptomatic improvement of asthma is an inhaled β_2-adrenergic agonist. If symptoms are mild or infrequent, this may be all that is necessary. In the circumstances of asthma limited to specific stimuli such as exercise or allergen, use of a β-agonist before such exposures may prevent acute attacks.

If symptoms are prolonged or require β_2-agonist use more than several times per week, anti-inflammatory therapy should be started with inhaled cromolyn sodium or inhaled glucocorticoids.

Cromolyn Sodium: Cromolyn sodium and the related compound, nedocromil, are classified as mast cell stabilizers and anti-allergic medications that improve lung function and may reduce airway hyperreactivity. These agents are most effective in patients with mild asthma or disease related to allergen exposure. Although not as effective as inhaled corticosteroids for chronic management of asthma, cromolyn sodium and nedocromil are virtually free of side effects. They have the added advantage of blocking acute asthma precipitants such as exercise and allergen exposure, if used prophylactically. A 4–6-week trial of therapy is needed to assess beneficial effects in patients with regular symptoms.

Inhaled Glucocorticoids: Inhaled glucocorticoids are the most beneficial anti-inflammatory agents for chronic asthma management. Their use reduces the frequency of asthma attacks, the degree of bronchial hyperreactivity, and the need for concurrent medications such as bronchodilators, and especially systemic corticosteroids. Available preparations are beclomethasone dipropionate, triamcinolone acetonide, and flunisolide. All appear to be similarly effective. Beneficial effects on asthma usually occur within 2 weeks and reach a maximum sometimes after months of treatment.

The effects of inhaled corticosteroids are dose-dependent, and dosages more than twice the recommended maximum may be needed to control unstable asthma. Oral candidiasis, dysphonia, cough, and sore throat are the major untoward side effects. These effects are largely due to upper airway deposition of medication and can be prevented by gargling after use or by using a spacer device.

Local antifungal therapy is usually effective in managing thrush. Absorption of inhaled corticosteroids does occur, but at recommended doses this is not enough to suppress adrenal function, to interfere with bone metabolism and growth in children, or to cause skin changes or cataracts. In patients who may require chronic corticosteroid administration, topical application, even at high doses, causes fewer side effects than continuous systemic use of corticosteroids for equivalent control of asthma.

Systemic Therapy: In patients with sufficient severity of asthma symptoms or decreased lung function, systemic corticosteroids at doses of prednisone, 40–80 mg/day, may achieve rapid relief while allowing concurrent medications to take effect. These measures should include inhaled anti-inflammatory therapy and may use theophylline or oral β_2-agonists, particularly before bedtime for management of nocturnal symptoms. Oral theophylline may be used continually or as an adjunct therapy to treat mild exacerbations. Many preparations are available with short-acting, generic aminophylline for acute use, and long-acting 12-hour preparations available for long-term or nocturnal use. When converting from intravenous to oral therapy, 80% of the daily intravenous requirement in divided oral doses is usually adequate. A long-acting inhaled β_2-agonist, salmeterol xinafoate, with a 12-hour duration of action, is also available for long-term therapy.

A combination of therapies is usually necessary to achieve optimal asthma control, and regular measures of lung function with a peak flow meter or spirometry are necessary to guide therapy. A symptom diary documenting medication use and daily peak flow rates is most helpful in assessing the objective response to treatment or in detecting early deterioration in a stable patient who is experiencing an exacerbation or is being weaned from a medication such as systemic corticosteroid. After stable control of asthma has been achieved, medications should be reduced or discontinued as tolerated, beginning with medications with the greatest potential for toxicity. Inhaled anti-inflammatory medications should be the last treatments withdrawn. The patient can use peak flow measures to notify the physician and to institute a course of treatment such as systemic corticosteroids if peak flows fall below a certain level. Patients who have required hospitalization or mechanical ventilation are especially at risk of developing recurrent life-threatening asthma. These patients should be carefully followed up, and exacerbations should be managed early with systemic corticosteroids. Patient education is particularly important in this group.

SUMMARY

▶ Asthma is a chronic inflammatory disease of the airways characterized by bronchial hyperreactivity and variable airflow obstruction.

▶ Inhaled corticosteroids are the most effective anti-inflammatory medications for asthma management and avoid most of the side effects associated with systemic corticosteroid use.

▶ Optimal asthma management should include daily measurements of pulmonary function with a peak flow meter or spirometry, and appropriate adjustments of medications based on these measurements.

SUGGESTED READING

Barnes PJ: Inhaled glucocorticoids for asthma. N Engl J Med 1995;332:868.

Corbridge TC, Hall JB: The assessment and management of adults with status asthmaticus. Am J Respir Crit Care Med 1995;151:1296.

Guidelines for the diagnosis and management of asthma: National Asthma Education Program expert panel report. National Heart, Lung, and Blood Institute, National Institutes of Health, Bethesda, MD 20892 (August 1991, NIH publication No. 91-3042).

McFadden ER, Gilbert IA: Asthma. N Engl J Med 1992;327: 1928.

Schlosberg M, Liu MC, Bochner BS: Pathophysiology of asthma. Immunol Allergy Clin North Am 1993;13:721.

2.5

Interstitial Lung Disease

David R. Moller, MD, and Carol Johnson Johns, MD

A common clinical pulmonary problem is that of persistent, often progressive, cough and shortness of breath. This can relate to a large and heterogeneous group of chronic diseases characterized by diffuse infiltration of the lung parenchyma involving the alveolar walls and air spaces. Sarcoidosis is a common and prototypic example (Table 2.5–1). These diffuse interstitial lung diseases are grouped together because they share many common clinical and pathologic features. Diffuse radiographic infiltrates are seen in most cases. Systemic manifestations of illness such as fever, fatigue, anorexia, and weight loss predominate in some disorders. Occasionally, a patient may be asymptomatic, referred because of an abnormal chest x-ray. In other instances, diffuse lung disease may exist without radiographic changes. Characteristically, the abnormalities of the interstitium and alveolar air space lead to stiff lungs and hypoxemia.

The natural course of interstitial lung disorders may be one of spontaneous remission, as is common in sarcoidosis, or persistent inflammation and progressive fibrosis leading to chronic respiratory failure, cor pulmonale, and death. The physician must therefore make an accurate diagnosis whenever possible to identify treatable disorders. Successful treatment may allow the patient to live a normal lifestyle for many years and prevent the progression to respiratory failure.

INITIAL ASSESSMENT

The chest x-ray is frequently the first indication that symptoms of dyspnea, cough, or hemoptysis are the result of a diffuse infiltrative disease of the lung rather than obstructive airway disease, congestive heart failure, or a localized pulmonary process such as infection, embolus, or tumor. Whenever possible, serial x-rays should be reviewed to assess the rapidity of the disease process and associated abnormalities. Rapid changes in symptoms and radiologic progression are unusual except for pulmonary edema, pneumonia, or hemorrhage. When the clinical setting suggests chronic diffuse lung disease, a systematic approach is needed to distinguish the various possibilities.

History

The first points to be gathered from the history are (1) the duration and severity of dyspnea and cough to provide an indication of the progression or remission of the underlying disease and (2) the presence or absence of systemic symptoms. These can give clues to the underlying disorder (Table 2.5–2). For example, fever associated with dyspnea or cough suggests an infectious process, sarcoidosis, rheumatologic disorder, malignancy, hypersensitivity pneumonitis, or drug reaction. Dyspnea associated with arthritis should lead to a consideration of collagen vascular disease or pulmonary vasculitis. Hemoptysis may be a dominant feature in advanced fibrocystic sarcoid, bronchiectasis, or pulmonary vasculitis such as in Wegener's granulomatosis and Goodpasture's syndrome.

A comprehensive occupational, environmental, and drug history must be obtained. The importance of this line of questioning cannot be overemphasized, since the information can provide critical evidence for a treatable disorder. A detailed occupational history involves asking questions of all current and past jobs; specific tasks performed; exposures to dusts, chemicals, and fumes; and symptoms related to the work, home, or hobby environment. Occupational exposure to asbestos, silica dust, or coal dust raises the possibility of asbestosis, silicosis, or coal workers' pneumoconiosis. Farmers who are exposed to moldy hay or people who keep pigeons or other birds may have hypersensitivity pneumonitis. A person with eosinophilic granuloma of the lung almost always has a history of smoking.

A positive family history may suggest familial pulmonary fibrosis or another rare cause of interstitial lung disease. Sarcoidosis and collagen vascular disorders may also cluster in some families. The possibility of a shared infection such as tuberculosis should also be considered.

Finally, after a detailed inquiry for known causes of dif-

Table 2.5–1. Major causes of diffuse interstitial lung disease.

Familial or congenital pulmonary fibrosis

Infections

Environmental lung disease
Inorganic dust diseases (pneumoconioses)
Asbestosis
Silicosis
Coal workers' pneumoconiosis (progressive massive fibrosis)
Siderosis
Talcosis
Hard metal disease
Hypersensitivity pneumonitis
Moldy compost (farmer's lung, bagassosis, mushroom workers' lung)
Contaminated ventilation system (ventilation pneumonitis)
Avian dust (bird breeder's disease)
Chemicals (eg, isocyanates)
Chronic beryllium disease
Chemical fumes (eg, nitrogen dioxide, polyvinyl chloride)

Drugs
Illicit drugs (eg, heroin, cocaine)
Chemotherapeutic agents (eg, bleomycin, nitrosoureas, methotrexate)
Antiarrhythmic drugs (eg, amiodarone, procainamide)
Antibiotics (eg, nitrofurantoin, penicillins, sulfa drugs)
Anti-inflammatory agents (eg, gold, D-penicillamine)

Physical agents
Radiation pneumonitis
Oxygen toxicity

Primary eosinophilic pneumonias
Löffler's syndrome
Chronic eosinophilic pneumonia
Allergic bronchopulmonary aspergillosis
Tropical pulmonary eosinophilia
Churg-Strauss syndrome (vasculitis)
Hypereosinophilic syndrome

Miscellaneous disorders of unknown etiology
Sarcoidosis
Idiopathic pulmonary fibrosis
Collagen vascular lung disease
Bronchiolitis obliterans organizing pneumonia (BOOP)
Eosinophilic granuloma of the lung (histiocytosis X)
Pulmonary vasculitis
Wegener's granulomatosis
Goodpasture's syndrome
Systemic necrotizing vasculitis
Hypersensitivity vasculitis
Lymphomatoid granulomatosis
Lymphocytic infiltrative disorders
Idiopathic pulmonary hemosiderosis
Lymphangioleiomyomatosis
Amyloidosis
Pulmonary alveolar proteinosis

Table 2.5–2. Diagnostic features of diffuse interstitial lung disease.

Often asymptomatic
Sarcoidosis
Siderosis (arc welders)
Eosinophilic granuloma (histiocytosis X)
Löffler's syndrome
Alveolar proteinosis (minimal infiltrates)

Fever
Infections, especially tuberculosis
Hypersensitivity pneumonitis
Sarcoidosis
Collagen vascular lung disease
Drug reactions

Hemoptysis
Fibrocystic sarcoidosis or tuberculosis
Bronchiectasis
Idiopathic pulmonary hemosiderosis
Vasculitis (Wegener's granulomatosis, Goodpasture's syndrome)

Airway obstruction
Fibrocystic sarcoidosis or tuberculosis
Eosinophilic granuloma (histiocytosis X)
Wegener's granulomatosis
Lymphangioleiomyomatosis
Tropical eosinophilia
Hypersensitivity pneumonitis (uncommon)

Pneumothorax
Eosinophilic granuloma (histiocytosis X)
Fibrocystic sarcoidosis or tuberculosis

fuse lung disorders, the physician must complete a thorough review of systems to search for additional clues to the disease process.

Physical Examination

The physical examination may provide useful information in the evaluation of persons with diffuse lung disease. Pulmonary fibrosis associated with idiopathic pulmonary fibrosis, collagen vascular diseases, or asbestosis is frequently associated with end-inspiratory "Velcro" crackles. Short, musical mid-inspiratory squeaks are a clue to bronchiolitis obliterans (often associated with organizing pneumonia) or, uncommonly, hypersensitivity pneumonitis, bronchiectasis, or pulmonary fibrosis. Findings may be limited to restriction of lung expansion. Finger clubbing is seen in 10–15% of patients with advanced pulmonary fibrosis but is more common in those with chronic bronchiectasis, cystic fibrosis, or as a congenital abnormality. With advanced pulmonary fibrosis, cardiac involvement is common with evidence of pulmonary hypertension and right heart failure.

Chest X-Ray

Although the radiographic picture is often nonspecific, characteristic patterns in the lung fields can provide important clues to a diagnosis of interstitial lung disease (Table 2.5–3). Disorders with predominantly interstitial involvement are associated with reticular, reticulonodular, or nodular patterns or a "ground-glass" appearance of the lung fields. Alveolar filling processes are associated with ill-defined nodular or acinar infiltrates, which may become confluent to form large areas of consolidation with air bronchograms and loss of the border outlines of normal structures. The distribution of infiltrates can provide helpful information. For example, upper lobe reticulonodular infiltrates are characteristic of tuberculosis, sarcoidosis, silicosis, and coal workers' pneumoconiosis. Lower lobe involvement is typically seen in cases of asbestosis and scleroderma and in most cases of idiopathic

Table 2.5–3. Radiographic features of diffuse lung disease.

Predominantly interstitial pattern
Sarcoidosis
Idiopathic pulmonary fibrosis
Collagen vascular lung disease
Pneumoconiosis (eg, asbestosis, silicosis)
Eosinophilic granuloma (histiocytosis X)
Hypersensitivity pneumonitis
Radiation pneumonitis
Bronchiolitis obliterans organizing pneumonia (mixed pattern)
Lymphangitic spread of tumor

Predominantly alveolar pattern
Pulmonary edema (cardiogenic, noncardiogenic)
Diffuse pulmonary hemorrhage (eg, Goodpasture's syndrome,
   idiopathic pulmonary hemosiderosis, vasculitis)
Infectious pneumonias
Pulmonary alveolar proteinosis
Sarcoidosis (occasionally)
Idiopathic pulmonary fibrosis (desquamative phase)
Neoplastic disease (bronchoalveolar cell carcinoma, metastatic
   disease)

Cystic spaces
Sarcoidosis
Silicosis (complicated form)
Eosinophilic granuloma
Lymphangioleiomyomatosis

Mediastinal adenopathy
Sarcoidosis
Granulomatous infections (tuberculosis, fungal disease)
Lymphoma
Silicosis
Wegener's granulomatosis (uncommon)

Pleural disease (effusions and thickening)
Tuberculosis
Collagen vascular lung disease
Asbestos-related disease
Malignancy
Pulmonary edema
Fibrocystic sarcoidosis with *Aspergillus* infection (thickening)

pulmonary fibrosis. Peripheral patchy alveolar infiltrates are characteristics of eosinophilic pneumonia. Although diffuse infiltrates can be seen in patients with Wegener's granulomatosis, cavitating infiltrates are more typical in this disorder.

Many of the chronic interstitial diseases may eventually progress to diffuse cystic dilatation of distal air spaces, and a nonspecific radiographic pattern known as "honeycomb" lung is seen. Large cystic spaces are common in sarcoidosis patients and may become the sites of mycetomas.

Clues to a specific diagnosis should be searched for outside the radiographic lung fields. Mediastinal adenopathy is common in sarcoidosis, lymphoma, granulomatous infections, lymphangitic carcinomatosis, silicosis, chronic beryllium disease, and amyloidosis; adenopathy is uncommon in Wegener's granulomatosis. Pleural effusions associated with an interstitial radiographic pattern are frequently seen in those with tuberculosis and other infections, rheumatologic diseases, asbestos-related disease, lymphangitic carcinomatosis, and, uncommonly, lymphangioleiomyomatosis (chylous effusion) and nitrofurantoin drug reaction. Calcified hilar and mediastinal nodes

are seen in silicosis (egg-shell pattern), tuberculosis, fungal diseases, and occasionally in sarcoidosis. Bilateral calcification of diaphragmatic pleural plaques is essentially pathognomonic of asbestos-related diseases, and lung parenchymal calcification can occur in longstanding sarcoidosis.

Pulmonary Function Tests

Diffuse interstitial and alveolar air space disorders characteristically cause restrictive lung impairment by virtue of the deposition of cells, matrix, or fluid in the lung parenchyma. The forced vital capacity (FVC) and 1-second forced expiratory volume (FEV_1) are reduced proportionally. If the FEV_1 is reduced more than the FVC, there is associated obstructive airway disease. Lung volumes (total lung capacity, vital capacity, and residual volumes) and lung compliance are reduced. Typically, reduction of the diffusing capacity (D_{CO}) and increase in the difference between alveolar and arterial oxygen tension ($P_AO_2 - PaO_2$) are noted. Hypoxemia is the result of mismatching of ventilation and perfusion and, in alveolar filing processes, of effective venous shunt. Alveolar hyperventilation with respiratory alkalosis is typical. Respiratory acidosis may occur with advanced disease or with significant airway obstruction.

Obstructive lung impairment is common in patients with eosinophilic granuloma of the lung, with lymphangioleiomyomatosis, and in the late stages of chronic interstitial fibrosis when fibrocystic or fibrobullous changes are prominent. Such a course is seen in advanced fibrocystic sarcoidosis. Intermittent reversible airways obstruction caused by bronchial hyperresponsiveness is not uncommon in interstitial lung disease and is superimposed on the underlying stiff lungs.

APPROACH TO DIAGNOSIS

The initial history, physical examination, previous and current chest x-rays, and pulmonary function tests should be reviewed before proceeding with further diagnostic tests. With this information, the differential diagnosis can often be sharply narrowed.

Acute interstitial and alveolar lung diseases are characterized by rapid changes in symptoms and radiographic patterns within hours or days. Common causes are pulmonary edema, hemorrhage, and pneumonia. Acute drug reactions or hypersensitivity pneumonitis can also behave this way in patients with relevant exposures. When acute dyspnea and diffuse pulmonary infiltration are seen in an immunocompromised patient, the clinician should be alert to the likelihood of an opportunistic infection, pulmonary edema or hemorrhage, or drug reaction.

In some instances, the presentation of a person with chronic interstitial lung disease is so characteristic that it is diagnostic. For example, a young black woman who presents with fever, erythema nodosum, uveitis, and a chest x-ray demonstrating bilateral hilar and right paratracheal adenopathy with reticulonodular infiltrates and

Table 2.5–4. Therapy of some treatable diffuse interstitial lung diseases.

Disorder	Primary Treatment	Secondary Treatment
Infections	Specific antimicrobials	
Pneumoconiosis	Removal from exposure	
Hypersensitivity pneumonitis	Removal from exposure	Corticosteroids
Drug reactions	Discontinuation of drugs	Corticosteroids
Chronic eosinophilic pneumonia	Corticosteroids	
Tropical pulmonary eosinophilia	Diethylcarbamazine	
Sarcoidosis	Corticosteroids	Chloroquine for mucocutaneous sarcoid
Idiopathic pulmonary fibrosis	Corticosteroids	Cytotoxic agents, eg, cyclophosphamide
Bronchiolitis obliterans organizing pneumonia	Corticosteroids	
Eosinophilic granuloma (histiocytosis X)	Cessation of smoking	Corticosteroids
Wegener's granulomatosis	Corticosteroids plus cytotoxic agents	Trimethoprim-sulfamethoxazole?
Goodpasture's syndrome	Plasmapheresis, corticosteroids	Cytotoxic agents
Pulmonary alveolar proteinosis	Whole lung lavage	
Neoplastic disease	Chemotherapeutic agents, hormonal agents (eg, for breast carcinoma)	

mild restrictive lung impairment almost certainly has sarcoidosis. A compatible occupational history, characteristic chest x-ray, and lung function tests may be sufficient for a clinical diagnosis of coal workers' pneumoconiosis, silicosis, or asbestosis; unexpected clinical or radiographic progression would make it necessary to exclude superimposed left heart failure, infection, or malignancy.

Fever, eosinophilia, and migratory alveolar infiltrates on chest x-ray in a person with minimal pulmonary symptoms suggest Löffler's syndrome, perhaps caused by a prescription drug. Persistent or progressive symptoms mandate further diagnostic evaluation. Rheumatologic disorders associated with lung disease may be clinically apparent with arthritis or may be suggested by serology. However, in most cases of diffuse lung disease, further evaluation is needed to establish a specific diagnosis or to exclude treatable causes of progressive lung disease. Specific attention should be directed to establishing a diagnosis of potentially treatable disorders (Table 2.5–4).

DIAGNOSTIC PROCEDURES

A specific diagnosis can sometimes be confirmed by first-line tests. For example, appropriate sputum smears and cultures can establish a diagnosis of tuberculosis, fungal pneumonia, or *Pneumocystis carinii* pneumonia. Sputum cytology may reveal tumor cells. Biopsy of a superficial lymph node or skin lesion can provide a specific diagnosis of sarcoidosis, lymphoma, tuberculosis, or fungal disease. Note that bacterial and mycobacterial cultures are mandatory for any biopsy material to exclude infection. Serologic testing can confirm the diagnosis of a rheumatologic disease such as rheumatoid arthritis or lupus erythematosus. If a diagnosis is not forthcoming from these tests, further studies are indicated.

Computed Tomography

The use of computed tomography (CT) of the chest has been an important advance in the diagnostic evaluation of diffuse lung disorders. The evaluation of patients with in-terstitial and alveolar lung disease is best performed using high-resolution, thin-section (1–2 mm thick slices) CT techniques because of the improved ability to distinguish specific patterns of diffuse lung disorders. For example, patients with idiopathic pulmonary fibrosis demonstrate a characteristic patchy, peripheral predominance of interstitial opacities intermingled with small cystic spaces. Asbestosis may cause a similar pattern, often associated with pleural thickening or calcified pleural plaques. Sarcoidosis, silicosis, hypersensitivity pneumonitis, and lymphangitic carcinomatosis demonstrate nodular opacities, often with reticular infiltrates.

Compared with standard chest x-rays, CT also provides superior diagnostic information about mediastinal structures. For example, mediastinal, hilar, or subcarinal adenopathy are better shown by CT scans and can suggest the possibility of granulomatous lung disease or lymphoma (see Table 2.5–3). A chest CT scan can also be helpful when planning a biopsy of these tissues by demonstrating the feasibility of a bronchoscopic approach to a lymph node biopsy, thereby avoiding mediastinoscopy. Occasionally, a lymph node biopsy by mediastinoscopy may be required to exclude definitively lymphoma or malignancy. This is rarely necessary in sarcoidosis patients.

Fiberoptic Bronchoscopy and Lung Biopsy

Many patients with diffuse pulmonary infiltration need fiberoptic bronchoscopy and bronchoscopic lung biopsy before a specific diagnosis can be reached. Four or five transbronchial biopsies are obtained from different sites and sent for histologic examination and microbiologic culture. Characteristic noncaseating granulomas are seen in 80% of patients with sarcoidosis (See Color Plates). Needle aspiration biopsy of enlarged paratracheal, subcarinal, or hilar nodes may provide useful cytologic material that allows diagnosis of a granulomatous or neoplastic process. Bronchoscopic biopsy procedures have proved to be very effective in diagnosing infectious diseases such as tuberculosis, fungal infections, and *Pneumocystis* infections. These procedures also are highly likely to provide a specific diagnosis in those with lymphangitic carcinomatosis, pulmonary alveolar proteinosis, eosinophilic pneumonia, and, less certainly, Wegener's granulomatosis, Goodpasture's syndrome, eosinophilic granuloma, and bronchiolitis obliterans organizing pneumonia. The risk associated with fiberoptic bronchoscopy, bronchoscopic biopsies, and bronchoalveolar lavage is small when performed by experienced bronchoscopists. Serious bleeding is unusual, provided that a bleeding diathesis is excluded before the biopsy procedure.

Bronchoalveolar Lavage

Bronchoalveolar lavage (BAL) can provide important diagnostic information with appropriate microbiologic and cytologic analyses of the fluid and is an important research tool in understanding the pathogenesis of diseases such as sarcoidosis. The differential cell count of BAL specimens frequently shows characteristic profiles in many of the noninfectious, nonmalignant, interstitial lung diseases. For example, sarcoidosis and chronic beryllium disease typically have increased proportions of total and CD4+ T cells in BAL fluid; hypersensitivity pneumonitis usually is characterized by increased proportions of total and CD8+ T cells in BAL fluid. Although results compatible with a specific disease can support a specific diagnosis, such findings alone are not diagnostic of interstitial lung disease.

Open Biopsy

An open lung biopsy is occasionally necessary to establish a definitive histologic diagnosis when simpler diagnostic procedures are inadequate. This procedure is most frequently performed to establish a diagnosis of idiopathic pulmonary fibrosis before beginning high-dose corticosteroid or cytotoxic therapy. In this instance, the information may be not only diagnostic but helpful in predicting the patient's response to therapy. Occasionally, an open lung biopsy is performed to confirm a diagnosis of eosinophilic granuloma of the lung, hypersensitivity pneumonitis, or bronchiolitis obliterans organizing pneumonia. More recently, thoracoscopic lung biopsy has been used to obtain adequate tissue for a definitive diagnosis of diffuse lung disease when bronchoscopic biopsy is inadequate. In all cases, a lung biopsy is not justified if the findings will not alter the approach to treatment.

SPECIFIC LUNG DISEASE

Sarcoidosis

Sarcoidosis is a multiorgan disease of unknown etiology characterized by noncaseating granulomatous inflammation in affected organs such as the lungs, lymph nodes, eyes, skin, liver, spleen, salivary glands, heart, and nervous system. Young adults are more frequently affected, often presenting with bilateral hilar adenopathy and erythema nodosum or uveitis. Spontaneous remissions are common with mild asymptomatic disease. In the United States, sarcoidosis is more common and severe in black patients of African-Caribbean origin. Although the in-

citing stimulus is unknown, activated macrophages and CD4+ lymphocytes accumulate in discrete granulomas at sites of disease, distort normal tissue architecture, and release inflammatory mediators that can result in fibrosis.

Presentation: Common respiratory symptoms of sarcoidosis include cough, dyspnea, and chest discomfort. Symptoms and pulmonary function abnormalities may be minimal, even with significant radiographic changes in white patients. Chest x-rays often demonstrate symmetric bilateral hilar and right paratracheal adenopathy, interstitial infiltrates, or both, although adenopathy may disappear (Figure 2.5–1). Involvement of other organs may be obvious from hepatosplenomegaly or in cardiac sarcoidosis from arrhythmias or cardiomyopathy. These conditions may occur in the absence of lung disease. Cutaneous anergy to recall antigens such as tuberculin, *Candida,* and mumps is characteristic.

The diagnosis of sarcoidosis depends on a compatible clinical and radiographic picture and a tissue biopsy showing noncaseating granulomas with no evidence of other causes of granulomatous reactions such as tuberculous, fungal, or malignant disease. Biopsy of the skin, palpable lymph node, or conjunctivae should be attempted when visible abnormalities are present. Transbronchial biopsy of the lung parenchyma or bronchoscopic needle

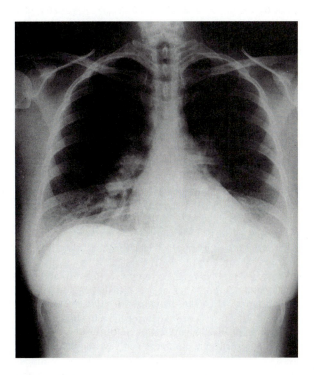

Figure 2.5–1. Chest x-ray of a 32-year-old black woman with sarcoidosis, showing bilateral hilar adenopathy, right paratracheal adenopathy, and increased interstitial opacities in the lower lung zones. Characteristically, the hilar nodes stand away from the cardiac borders.

biopsy of mediastinal nodes can confirm the diagnosis in a high percentage of cases. Mediastinoscopy is occasionally indicated if lymphoma or tuberculosis remain possibilities.

Treatment: Ninety percent of patients with sarcoidosis are very responsive to corticosteroids, and the disease is easily controlled on modest maintenance doses of prednisone, 10–15 mg daily, which allow serious side effects to be minimized. Any patient with established or strongly suspected pulmonary sarcoidosis, who has significant interference with their normal life, should receive a trial of corticosteroids for at least 2–4 months, unless there is strong evidence that the disease is old and inactive with only residual changes. A negative gallium scan may confirm disease inactivity, but gallium scans should not be used routinely because of their radioactivity, nonspecificity, and expense. Because of the frequency of spontaneous remissions, especially in white patients, patients who have minimal symptoms and little or no disability, can be observed for a period of 6 months to 2 years, rather than undergoing immediate treatment. Patients who have spontaneous remission without treatment rarely relapse. Review of symptoms, serial radiographs, and serial measurement of ventilatory function and carbon monoxide diffusing capacity usually clearly indicate the course of the disease.

Corticosteroid treatment should not be given in too-large doses for too long. An example of a regimen is the following:

Treat for 2 weeks at each dose level of 40, 30, 25, and 20 mg prednisone daily.
Continue 15 mg daily (10 mg may be sufficient) for 6 months. Taper by 2.5 mg monthly after total of 8 months of treatment.
Observe for potential relapse and reinstitute treatment, if necessary.

Relapse may occur as corticosteroids are reduced below the daily equivalent of 15 mg. This may occur even after 10–20 years of long-term maintenance dosage of prednisone at 10 mg daily. Following relapse, treatment should be reinstituted at a dosage known previously to control the disease, usually 10–15 mg daily. Severe progressive fibrocystic disease may result if such patients are left untreated, but irreversible lung damage is not helped by excessively aggressive use of corticosteroids. In addition, other immunosuppressive agents usually provide little or no further benefit. Clinical worsening on a maintenance dose of 15 mg or more of prednisone is most likely caused by noncompliance, complicating infection, or left heart failure, rather than exacerbation of disease. It is clearly demonstrated that the benefits of corticosteroid treatment exceed the risks (Chapter 4.3), provided that dosages are modest and patients receive careful long-term follow-up.

Chloroquine (or hydroxychloroquine) may be helpful in patients with chronic indolent mucocutaneous sarcoidosis, but it is disappointing in those with pulmonary disease.

Ocular toxicity is a concern but rarely a problem and is obviated by giving intermittent treatment for alternating 6-month periods with ophthalmologic observation before each course.

Chronic fibrocystic sarcoidosis leads to a clinical picture that resembles bronchiectasis, with chronic productive cough. A mycetoma can form in the cystic spaces, often from colonization with *Aspergillus fumigatus.* The organisms are readily identified in sputum or with bronchoscopy, or diagnosed by serum precipitins. Invasive aspergillosis is exceptional, and amphotericin is generally not used because it does not reach the central portion of the mycetoma to eradicate the organism.

Hemoptysis can occur in sarcoidosis patients, as in those with bronchiectasis, and is sometimes life-threatening. Hemorrhage can usually be managed conservatively with broad-spectrum antibiotics to control the bacterial infections of the cystic space, which typically precipitate bleeding. Therapeutic embolization of dilated bronchial arteries supplying the inflamed areas of the lung can be helpful, at least temporarily. However, recurrence of bleeding is common and is best prevented by reducing infection with continuous rotating antibiotics.

Surgery is to be avoided except in the most extreme circumstances because the severe underlying diffuse, bilateral restrictive fibrosis prevents the lung from expanding to fill the space created by partial resection. Persistent air leaks, chronic pneumothorax, bronchopleurocutaneous fistula, and empyema are life-threatening complications. If surgery is performed, thoracoplasty may be necessary to collapse the unfilled space.

Idiopathic Pulmonary Fibrosis

Idiopathic pulmonary fibrosis (IPF) is a chronic immunologic and inflammatory reaction of the lung interstitium with progressive fibrosis and distortion of the pulmonary architecture. The typical clinical presentation is one of gradual, progressive dyspnea and cough in a person 40–70 years of age, with reticulonodular infiltrates most prominent in the lower lung field, and restrictive lung impairment. Bronchoalveolar lavage characteristically shows an increased proportion of polymorphonuclear neutrophils and eosinophils. Diagnosis of IPF depends on the lung biopsy and exclusion of other diseases that may cause a similar clinical picture. Most persons with IPF progress to severe respiratory impairment and death within 2–10 years of diagnosis. A minority have a favorable response to corticosteroid, cytotoxic agents, or both.

Treatment of IPF patients is usually begun with high doses of corticosteroids, with immunosuppressive agents such as cyclophosphamide or azathioprine, or with corticosteroids and immunosuppressive agents. A similar chronic fibrosing interstitial disease process is sometimes seen in association with rheumatoid arthritis and scleroderma. The course of "rheumatoid" and "scleroderma" lung disease varies greatly but generally is not as aggressive as that of IPF and is not as responsive to treatment.

Environmental Lung Disorders

Interstitial fibrosis caused by cumulative exposure to asbestos over many years results in *asbestosis,* most commonly found in workers involved in asbestos mining and manufacturing, construction, shipbuilding, and automobile and railroad engine maintenance. A 10–20-year latency period is necessary for the parenchymal fibrosis to manifest radiographically. Asbestos exposure is also associated with lung cancer and pleural mesotheliomas, benign calcified pleural plaques, and effusions.

Silicosis is a nodular, fibrotic disease of the lungs, which results from exposure to high concentrations of airborne crystalline silicon dioxide. Sandblasters, miners, and workers involved with manufacturing of glass, pottery, and abrasives may be at risk. The incidence of the disease is declining with improved industrial hygiene. As with asbestosis, a latent period of 10–20 years is characteristic before the disease is clinically or radiographically apparent. *Chronic beryllium disease* is the result of exposure to beryllium dust used primarily in high technology metallurgy, particularly in the aerospace industry. Beryllium causes a granulomatous pulmonary disease very similar to pulmonary sarcoidosis in about 10% of exposed persons.

Hypersensitivity pneumonitis is a lymphocytic-monocytic immunologic reaction to repeated inhalation of one of a variety of organic dusts or inorganic chemicals. This diagnosis must be vigorously pursued, since removal of the patient from exposure to the implicated agent prevents progressive, irreversible pulmonary fibrosis and respiratory failure. The occupational origins of many of the agents have led to descriptive names such as farmer's lung (caused by thermophilic actinomycetes spores from moldy hay), bird breeder's disease (caused by avian proteins from avian dust and droppings), and plastics worker's lung (caused by exposure to isocyanates used as plastic curing agents or paint hardeners). The acute form is characterized by fever, chills, dyspnea, and cough 4–12 hours after exposure. A chronic form causes insidious progression of dyspnea, cough, and progressive interstitial fibrosis. Corticosteroids may hasten recovery.

Drug-Induced Interstitial Lung Disorders

Drugs can cause several distinct pathophysiologic reactions such as a chronic interstitial pneumonitis with fibrosis, hypersensitivity reactions, pulmonary infiltrates with eosinophilia, drug-induced lupus syndromes, and diffuse alveolar hemorrhage. The key to making a diagnosis is a careful history of medication use and knowledge of the potential reactions caused by the drug.

Chronic interstitial pneumonitis and fibrosis caused by drugs is manifested by insidious respiratory symptoms and bilateral radiographic reticulonodular infiltrates, often most prominent in the lower lobes. The most common offending drugs are bleomycin, busulfan, nitrosourea compounds, amiodarone, and nitrofurantoin.

Hypersensitivity drug reactions may be characterized by fever, arthralgias, occasionally pleuritis and peripheral eosinophilia with radiographic alveolar and interstitial infiltrates. Nitrofurantoin, sulfonamides, amiodarone, methotrexate, gold salts, and salicylates are most commonly implicated. Corticosteroids may be helpful in alleviating symptoms in hypersensitivity drug reactions; exacerbations may occur when corticosteroid dose is reduced.

Primary Eosinophilic Pneumonias

Primary eosinophilic pneumonias are characterized by pulmonary infiltration by eosinophils with or without peripheral blood eosinophilia. *Löffler's syndrome* is associated with transient pulmonary infiltrates and mild or no symptoms. Many causes are likely due to unrecognized drug reactions, parasitic infestations, or allergic bronchopulmonary aspergillosis.

Chronic eosinophilic pneumonia is most commonly seen in middle-aged women, who present with dyspnea, cough, fever, night sweats, and often wheezing. A characteristic radiographic pattern of peripheral alveolar infiltrates termed the "photographic negative of pulmonary edema" is highly suggestive of the disorder. Patients with this disorder are exquisitely responsive to corticosteroid therapy.

Allergic bronchopulmonary aspergillosis should be considered in any asthmatic with pulmonary infiltrates; eosinophilia, high serum IgE levels, positive immediate skin test, and serum precipitins to *Aspergillus* sp are typical. Treatment consists of corticosteroids in addition to bronchodilator therapy.

Tropical pulmonary eosinophilia is caused by a local hypersensitivity response in the lung due to migration of microfilaria through the lungs. Persons from India, Sri Lanka, Southeast Asia, and Indonesia are at risk. Asthma, severe cough, chest pain, and hemoptysis are characteristically worse at night; marked peripheral eosinophilia, elevated IgE levels, and high titers of antifilarial antibodies are present. The antifilarial drug diethylcarbamazine is used to treat tropical pulmonary eosinophilia. *Churg-Strauss syndrome* is a rare, systemic vasculitis discussed in Chapter 3.5.

Miscellaneous Disorders of Unknown Cause

Patients with *bronchiolitis obliterans organizing pneumonia* (BOOP) usually present with a poorly resolving pneumonia with persistent, patchy, bilateral ground-glass opacities in the lower lung fields and midinspiratory squeaks on auscultation of the lungs. CT scans often show a distinctive pattern of infiltrates juxtaposed to normal or hyperlucent areas. Transbronchial biopsies may show organizing pneumonia but often miss the obliterative bronchiolitis. Treatment with corticosteroids is usually effective, but exacerbations are common as the dose is tapered.

Eosinophilic granuloma of the lung (adult form of histiocytosis X) is characterized by an abnormal accumulation in the lung of atypical histiocytes in stellate granulomatous lesions and is associated with fibrocystic changes.

Most patients are 20–40 years old and present with cough, dyspnea, fever, and weight loss. A history of pneumothorax or diabetes insipidus may be present. Over 90% of affected persons smoke, leading to the hypothesis that the disease is caused by a reaction to a component in cigarette smoke. Corticosteroids are of questionable effectiveness but should be tried in progressive disease.

Pulmonary alveolar proteinosis is a disease in which lipoproteinaceous surfactant material accumulates in alveoli. Affected persons typically present with cough, dyspnea, and diffuse fluffy, alveolar infiltrates, often in a perihilar or lower zone distribution. Repeated whole-lung lavage with saline is often helpful in ameliorating symptoms; occasionally, the patient undergoes remission.

GENERAL MANAGEMENT PRINCIPLES

Review of all clinical and laboratory information can lead to a specific diagnosis that is amenable to specific treatment, such as appropriate antibiotic agents for infections, or corticosteroids (see Table 2.5–4). The importance of avoiding agents responsible for hypersensitivity pneumonitis, pneumoconiosis, or drug-induced lung disorders must be emphasized in order to minimize progressive lung dysfunction.

The patient is best monitored by means of assessment of symptoms, pulmonary function tests, and chest radiographs. Exercise studis may be sensitive for finding small changes in pulmonary function but are not routinely required. Such studies may be particularly valuable in evaluating the response to therapy in patients with IPF in whom even small objective signs of improvement are an indication to continue potentially toxic therapy.

In many cases of interstitial lung disease there is no specific treatment, or irreversible damage has occurred,

and the physician is left with providing compassionate, supportive therapy. General supportive measures include supplemental oxygen for hypoxemia and good nutrition. Adjusting life patterns and circumstances to accommodate the degree of incapacity is an essential feature in enabling patients to live productively. Patients benefit if they can avoid chronic invalidism and remain active within their own limitations.

SUMMARY

▶ Interstitial lung disease is characterized by diffuse infiltration of the alveolar walls and alveolar air spaces, resulting in stiff lungs and hypoxemia. Presentation is with persistent cough and dyspnea, usually without evidence of airflow obstruction.

▶ The patient's history and review of serial chest radiographs are central to establishing the cause and course of interstitial lung disease. Environmental, occupational, and drug histories may indicate a specific cause.

▶ If a diagnosis is not reached after first-line clinical tests, a transbronchial lung biopsy should be performed. Surgical lung biopsy is sometimes required but should not be pursued unless it will change the approach to therapy.

▶ The natural course of many interstitial lung diseases is one of persistent inflammation and fibrosis leading to chronic respiratory failure, unless a treatable cause can be identified. In certain diseases, especially sarcoidosis, corticosteroids significantly suppress the damaging inflammation. Long-term treatment may be required.

SUGGESTED READING

Crystal RG et al: Interstitial lung disease of unknown cause: Disorders characterized by chronic inflammation of the lower respiratory tract. Parts 1 and 2. N Engl J Med 1984;310:154,235.

Johns CJ, Scott PP, Schonfeld SA: Sarcoidosis. Annu Rev Med 1989;40:353.

Schwartz MI, King TE Jr: *Interstitial Lung Disease.* Mosby-Year Book, 1993.

Turner-Warwick M: Widespread pulmonary fibrosis. In: *Pulmonary Diseases and Disorders,* 2nd ed, vol I. Fishman AP (editor). McGraw-Hill, 1988.

Sleep Apnea and Other Disorders of Ventilatory Control

Philip L. Smith, MD, and Alan R. Schwartz, MD

Diseases that affect the control of ventilation can cause either an elevation in carbon dioxide level (PCO_2) during wakefulness or a change in breathing pattern during sleep. During wakefulness, chronic obstructive lung disease is the most common cause of acute or chronic hypercarbia (Chapter 2.3); this chapter discusses other types of disorders that interfere with the overall integration of breathing.

By definition, a rise in PCO_2 indicates hypoventilation in its physiologic sense of reduced effective (alveolar) ventilation (Chapter 2.7). In general, it is useful to consider patients' inability to maintain a normal resting PCO_2 as a result of either "can't breathe"—a defect in the respiratory muscles or apparatus—or "won't breathe"—a defect in the chemical control of breathing. For example, patients "can't" eliminate carbon dioxide, because of either abnormal muscles that easily fatigue (eg, in myasthenia gravis) or normal muscles that cannot cope with increases in the work of breathing (eg, in severe obstructive airways disease). In contrast, patients "won't breathe" because of either a defect in the chemical drive to breathe (eg, in primary alveolar hypoventilation) or depression of the central nervous system (eg, in drug overdoses). In some patients, this distinction can become blurred; for example, patients with morbid obesity (pickwickian syndrome) probably have both alterations in the mechanics of breathing, because their excess weight increases the work of breathing, and a resetting of the chemical control of respiration.

CONTROL OF BREATHING

Regulation of arterial carbon dioxide is a function of the amount produced by the tissues and eliminated by the lungs:

$$PaCO_2 = K \cdot \frac{\dot{V}CO_2}{V_A}$$

where $\dot{V}CO_2$ = CO_2 production, V_A = alveolar ventilation, and K = constant.

Two aspects of this equation are worth emphasizing. First, at constant levels of CO_2 production, any reduction in alveolar ventilation leads to a rise in PCO_2. Since the equation takes the form of a hyperbolic relationship, reducing the alveolar ventilation 50% doubles the normal arterial PCO_2 from 40 to 80 mm Hg. In practical terms, patients who can't breathe have severe and rather obvious clinical illness when their alveolar ventilation is reduced by 50%. On the other hand, many persons who won't breathe have remarkably elevated levels of carbon dioxide but appear normal on initial evaluation. Second, since overall ventilation can be partitioned into effective (alveolar) and ineffective (dead space), measuring total minute ventilation is not useful in determining the primary causes of elevations in carbon dioxide. In fact, minute ventilation can be normal or even elevated in patients with increased dead space, for example, those with severe obstructive airways disease. Thus, it is more practical to determine the defect in ventilatory control by systematically reviewing the components of the respiratory system.

Control of ventilation depends on complex interaction among the various proprioceptive and chemical stimuli to the central nervous system and the neural output to the muscles of respiration. A simplified scheme of the components of the respiratory system is outlined in Figure 2.6–1. The respiratory system appears to have a hierarchical response to different types of mechanical and chemical stimuli. In normal persons, CO_2 levels in the blood and medulla are closely coupled, and the brain-stem chemoreceptors are exquisitely sensitive to changes in PCO_2 (Figure 2.6–2A). The feedback gain is high; an increase in

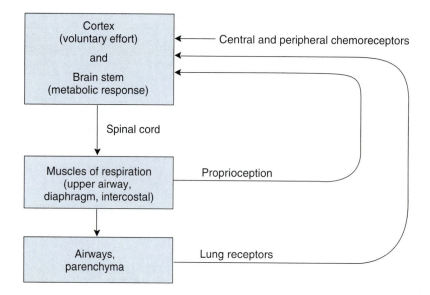

Figure 2.6–1. Components of the system for respiratory control. The respiratory center in the brain stem integrates the input from central and peripheral chemoreceptors, voluntary control of respiratory effort, and afferent impulses from the lung and chest wall.

arterial PCO_2 of about 5 mm Hg approximately doubles minute ventilation. Therefore, arterial blood PCO_2 is tightly controlled, and a change of as little as 2–4 mm Hg in blood CO_2 should be taken as evidence of significant disruption.

Hypoxemia increases ventilation and the sensitivity of

the ventilatory versus CO_2 response, but the effects of hypoxemia do not become very significant until arterial oxygen falls to about 60 mm Hg (see Figure 2.6–2B). However, as can be seen in Figure 2.6–2A, under conditions of low levels of arterial oxygen tension, marked interaction with CO_2 is shown by the leftward shift and

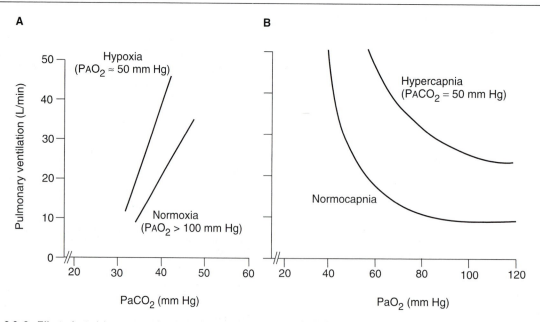

Figure 2.6–2. Effect of arterial oxygen and carbon dioxide levels on minute ventilation. **A:** Arterial carbon dioxide level is tightly controlled by virtue of the steep relationship between $PaCO_2$ and minute ventilation. Sensitivity to $PaCO_2$ level is increased by hypoxia. **B:** Effect of hypoxia on minute ventilation. Under normal conditions of arterial $PaCO_2$, there is little effect of hypoxia above PaO_2 levels of 60 mm Hg. When the $PaCO_2$ level is increased, the sensitivity and threshold of hypoxic drive are increased.

increased slope of the CO_2-ventilatory response. The hypoxic-hypercarbic interaction has major clinical implications. For example, in a patient who is maintaining a given level of PCO_2 under hypoxic conditions, removal of the hypoxic stimulus by supplemental oxygen can cause marked hypercarbia.

Clinical Features

In general, for a given level of hypercarbia, patients who "can't breathe" complain of dyspnea either at rest or on exertion. In contrast, patients who "won't breathe" experience minimal if any respiratory discomfort. For example, in patients with chronic obstructive pulmonary disease, dyspnea on exertion is the major presenting symptom. Early in the course of neuromuscular disorders such as poliomyelitis and myasthenia gravis, significant muscle weakness as well as dyspnea is apparent, even though resting levels of CO_2 may be only slightly increased. In progressive neuromuscular diseases such as Guillain-Barré syndrome or acute poliomyelitis, profound peripheral muscle weakness may be the dominant presenting symptom. Under these circumstances, because exertion is not possible, the patient may not be dyspneic.

Patients with hypoventilation who "won't breathe" typically present with the mental status changes associated with CO_2 retention, and with cardiovascular effects of chronic reduction in arterial oxygen. Because hypercarbia and hypoxia occur in combination, it is often difficult to distinguish which is the primary cause of the clinical manifestations. In general, the degree of central nervous system and hemodynamic alterations is proportional to the chemical abnormalities; thus, patients with mildly elevated CO_2 (≤ 50 mm Hg) have no clinical illness. With increased rises in CO_2, patients develop fatigue, lethargy, confusion, morning headache, and poor sleep (Table 2.6–1). As hypoventilation worsens, leading to hypoxemia of <55 mm Hg, patients develop additional signs of cardiovascular decompensation, including pulmonary hypertension and right-sided heart failure.

Evaluation

Evaluation of patients with alveolar hypoventilation begins with the history and physical examination, which may initially suggest which component of the respiratory system has failed. With simple pulmonary function testing, it should be possible to determine whether the

primary defect resides in the chemical control system (won't), the neuromuscular (can't), or the mechanical apparatus (can't) (Table 2.6–2).

Chemical Control: Primary defects involving the central or peripheral chemoreceptors (eg, primary alveolar hypoventilation) are rare. Patients appear normal on physical examination, and their pulmonary function studies show normal mechanics and a normal A-a gradient (Table 2.6–3; Chapter 2.7). Only if ventilation is so reduced that portions of lung develop atelectasis do patients have an increased A-a gradient, from $\dot{V}/Q$ mismatch. During sleep, the effects of these areas of low $\dot{V}/Q$ can be magnified and accelerate faster development of right-sided heart failure and peripheral edema. Because the brain-stem involuntary

Table 2.6–1. Symptoms and signs of respiratory failure.

Hypercarbia
  Headache
  Confusion
  Poor sleep

Hypoxemia
  Cyanosis
  Polycythemia
  Pulmonary hypertension
  Cor pulmonale

Table 2.6–2. Conditions affecting specific components of the respiratory system.

Component	Condition
Sensors	
Chemosensors	Metabolic alkalosis
Nervous system	
Brain stem	Alveolar hypoventilation (primary)
	Bulbar poliomyelitis
	Demyelinating syndromes
	Vascular (stroke)
	Respiratory depression caused by sedatives or hypnotics
Spinal cord	Amyotrophic lateral sclerosis
	Trauma (cervical)
	Poliomyelitis
Nerves	Guillain-Barré syndrome
Muscles	
Neuromuscular	Myasthenia gravis
Muscular	Muscular dystrophy
Mechanics	
Chest wall	Kyphoscoliosis
	Ankylosing spondylitis
	Thoracoplasty
	Osteogenesis imperfecta
Obesity	Obesity hypoventilation
Lung and airways	Obstructive airways disease
	Restrictive lung disease

Table 2.6–3. Pulmonary function in alveolar hypoventilation.

	Gas Exchange	Mechanics		
	A-a Gradient	FEV$_1$/FVC	FVC	MIP
Can't breathe				
Neuromuscular	Normal	Normal	↓	↓
Chest wall	Normal	Normal	↓	Normal
Lungs	↑	Normal/↓	↓	Normal
Won't breathe				
Chemical control	Normal	Normal	Normal	Normal

A-a, alveolar-arterial; FEV$_1$, forced expired volume in 1 second; FVC, forced vital capacity; MIP, maximal inspiratory pressure.

components of the system are disturbed, patients who won't breathe can bypass the chemical control system and voluntarily reduce their PCO_2 on command.

Neuromuscular Defects: Patients with neuromuscular disorders presenting with hypoventilation, such as those with Guillain-Barré syndrome and amyotrophic lateral sclerosis, are picked up by a careful history and physical examination. The hallmark is acute or chronic muscle weakness. Although nonspecific, dyspnea and tachypnea clearly indicate an inability of the respiratory muscles to respond to increased work of breathing during exertion. In addition, careful examination of accessory muscles of respiration often reveals retractions of either the intercostal or sternocleidomastoid muscles. A particularly useful maneuver is to palpate the scalenus muscle deep in the neck; this muscle is often activated at rest, to compensate for weak diaphragmatic contraction. Normally, the thorax and abdomen move in synchrony during respiration; however, paradoxical motion of the thorax and abdomen can be seen in patients with advanced respiratory fatigue involving the diaphragm.

Additional simple measurements of lung mechanics reveal clear evidence of diaphragmatic weakness manifested by reduced maximal inspiratory force. In general, maximal inspiratory pressures are obviously reduced even with minimal increases in PCO_2. In spite of elevations in CO_2, patients maintain a normal A-a gradient unless they have significant atelectasis and changes in compliance. In this situation, the FVC is mildly reduced.

Mechanical Changes: Patients with an elevated CO_2 caused primarily by defects in the chest wall or by intrinsic airways disease complain of dyspnea and have obvious changes on physical examination. The physician can easily see significant kyphoscoliosis or distortions of the chest wall, for example, from thoracoplasty. Auscultation reveals markedly diminished breath sounds in patients with emphysema, or wheezing in patients with bronchospastic airways disease. Spirometry shows marked reductions in forced expiratory volume in 1 second (FEV_1) and forced vital capacity (FVC), as well as an elevated A-a gradient on blood gas test.

Management

Treatment of alveolar hypoventilation is directed at correcting the hypercarbia and its associated hypoxemia. Note that chronic elevations of CO_2 by itself, even to levels of 70–80 mm Hg, impose little immediate clinical consequence. However, the concomitant decreases in oxygenation below 55 mm Hg that accompany marked elevations of CO_2 must be corrected by either increasing alveolar ventilation or giving supplemental oxygen.

When the patient "won't" breathe, drugs can often stimulate the central nervous system. In both acute and chronic medical settings, respiratory stimulants can reduce the CO_2 by 10–20 mm Hg. However, drugs are not effective against acute CO_2 retention in patients who "can't" breathe, for example, because of end-stage

chronic obstructive lung disease; their central nervous system is already maximally stimulated and their ventilatory apparatus can no longer respond. Mechanical ventilation should be considered for these patients if their CO_2 retention is acute and life-threatening. It may be possible to ventilate patients intermittently at home during wakefulness or sleep to rest the respiratory muscles and thus lower CO_2.

Whether or not the elevated PCO_2 is corrected, hypoxemia must be treated immediately. When oxygen is administered to patients with hypercapnic respiratory failure, further rises in CO_2 should be expected as the hypoxic stimulus to breathe is removed. Nevertheless, it is a fundamental principle of therapy that hypoxemia must always be corrected regardless of the effect on overall ventilation. If the carbon dioxide rises significantly, ventilatory support should be provided. It is inadvisable to permit low levels of oxygen (<50 mm Hg) to serve as the stimulus to breathe. This situation generally occurs when high concentrations of oxygen have been given and the patient becomes hypercarbic, thus prompting sudden removal of the supplemental oxygen. When oxygen is withdrawn precipitously, the patient can become acutely worse, since the high partial pressure of carbon dioxide in the alveoli results in dangerously low levels of oxygen, which can lead to acute cardiac or respiratory arrest.

SLEEP APNEA

During wakefulness, normal respiratory control involves sensory input that is integrated with the neural and mechanical apparatus of breathing. During sleep, however, important cortical activity is removed and waking stimulatory influences decrease. The chemical control system (brain stem) assumes a more prominent role in regulating respiration, and breathing patterns are altered. Sleep apnea represents the major clinical syndrome of altered control of ventilation, and the sleep state also alters ventilation and gas exchange in patients with underlying lung disease.

The two types of abnormal breathing patterns during sleep are cessation of respiration (apnea) and periods of hypoventilation alternating with hyperventilation (Cheyne-Stokes respiration). Conventionally, sleep apnea has been classified by descriptive features. A *central apnea* is defined as complete cessation of airflow and respiratory effort for at least 10 seconds; an *obstructive apnea* is cessation of airflow despite continued respiratory effort (Figure 2.6–3). *Mixed apneas* are combinations of central and obstructive apnea. Cheyne-Stokes respiration is seen most often in association with central apnea. However, all variations in respiratory pattern involve a central component, since all aspects of respiration are modulated by the central nervous system through the brain stem. As with hypercapnic respiratory failure, it is useful to think of the alterations in control as "can't breathe" and "won't breathe." Despite a normal drive to breathe, patients with obstructive apneas can't breathe because of upper airway

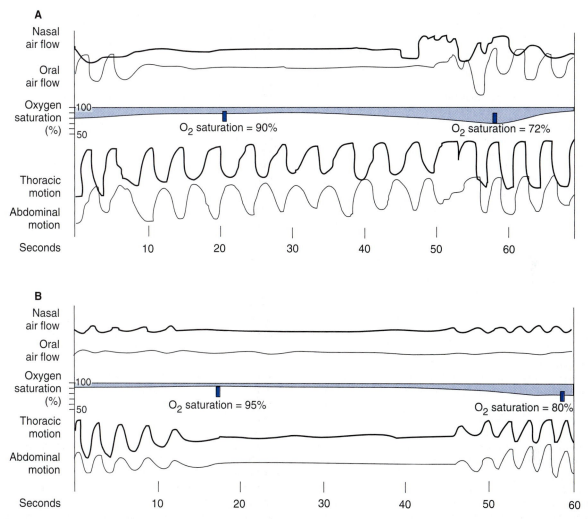

Figure 2.6–3. Multichannel recordings from sleep studies showing apneic spells. **A:** Obstructive sleep apnea. While airflow ceases, respiratory efforts (thoracic and abdominal motion) persist. Eventually, after almost 50 seconds, when oxygen saturation falls, the obstruction is cleared and respiration resumes. **B:** Central apnea. Respiratory effort ceases for 30 seconds and resumes gradually as arterial oxygen saturation falls. (Reproduced, with permission, from Smith PL: Sleep apnea syndromes. The Johns Hopkins Medical Grand Rounds [slide-tape series] 1982;9[3]:21.)

occlusion; patients with central apnea won't breathe because of alterations in the integration of central nervous output.

Clinical Features

The clinical manifestations of sleep apnea are caused primarily by the hypoxemia and microarousal that terminates the apneas. Thus, the symptoms fall into three broad categories.

First, patients complain of daytime sleepiness caused by the recurrent arousals that fragment and reduce their total sleep. When apnea occurs relatively infrequently, patients have daytime sleepiness only during sedentary activities such as watching television or reading. But as apnea becomes more frequent and severe, daytime sleepi-

ness worsens in proportion to the fragmentation of sleep at night. Patients with very severe apnea have pathologic hypersomnolence and may fall asleep while driving a car or even while talking.

Second, patients whose sleep apnea is predominantly obstructive may have loud snoring punctuated by witnessed apneas. Some patients recall awakening for 5–10 seconds, sometimes with no distinct precipitation, but occasionally with choking or gasping. A spouse may report loud snoring and accurately describe periods of apnea that are terminated by loud snorting and gasping. The spouse often reports body movements and arousal that the patient does not remember.

Third, patients may present with cardiovascular effects of their nocturnal hypoxemia. These can take the form of arrhythmias during periods of marked desaturation, most commonly sinus arrest and other bradyarrhythmias, sometimes atrial fibrillation. Arrhythmias generally imply severe chronic sleep apnea. Pulmonary hypertension and cor pulmonale may be seen, probably only in patients whose sleep apnea accompanies daytime hypoxemia, and many patients have systemic hypertension.

The chief difference between central sleep apnea with Cheyne-Stokes breathing and the more common kinds of sleep apnea in which obstruction predominates is that central apnea and Cheyne-Stokes respiration most commonly result from known neurologic or circulatory dysfunction. The periodicity of apneas is proportional to the severity of the underlying heart disease or brain lesion. Therefore, unlike patients with obstructive sleep apnea, patients with Cheyne-Stokes respiration often present with evidence of either right or left ventricular failure. Similarly, patients with brain-stem dysfunction from cerebrovascular events such as cerebral thrombosis present with obvious evidence of a recent neurologic event preceding the onset of irregular breathing during sleep.

Evaluation

Patients with predominantly obstructive apnea are typically overweight middle-aged men or overweight postmenopausal women, who complain of breathing problems during their sleep or excessive daytime sleepiness. Since patients are often unaware of many of the signs and may not complain of daytime hypersomnolence, obtaining a history from the family or other observers is crucial if the diagnosis is not be missed. The physical examination is most often normal in patients with obstructive sleep apnea, although examination of the upper airway occasionally reveals marked narrowing of the oropharynx from tonsillar hypertrophy or other mechanical conditions such as lymphomas or hemangiomas of the tongue. In contrast, most patients with central sleep apnea and Cheyne-Stokes breathing present with a history of recent neurologic event (stroke) or evidence of an underlying cardiopulmonary or neurologic disorder such as congestive heart failure.

The specific diagnosis and characterization of the respiratory pattern during sleep can be made only by a polygraphic recording made during sleep. Waking measurements of lung mechanics, diffusion, or gas exchange do not correlate with patterns during sleep, and thus serve no useful screening purpose. A sleep study simultaneously monitors the electroencephalogram to stage sleep, an electrocardiogram to monitor cardiac rhythm, ear oximetry to determine oxygenation, and respiratory gauges to determine airflow and respiratory effort.

Management

Treatment of sleep-related breathing problems depends on the clinical severity as well as the specific type of breathing abnormality found on the sleep study. At one extreme are patients with obstructive sleep apnea who have minimal symptoms and relatively infrequent apneas that cause only infrequent arousals and minimal desaturation; most of these patients are managed conservatively, perhaps only with observation or weight loss. At the other extreme, symptomatic persons with severe apnea and hypoxemia may need aggressive medical and surgical measures.

For patients with obstructive sleep apnea, the major goal is reversing the upper airway obstruction. This can be done several ways. All patients should lose weight and avoid sedative hypnotics. Patients with severe apnea and symptoms may need constant positive airway pressure (CPAP) applied to the upper airway to prevent upper airway collapse and eliminate apneas. This is achieved by sleeping with a tight-fitting mask on, and the treatment works only if the patient is willing to persist with this inconvenience. If CPAP is unsuccessful, reconstruction of the upper airway (uvulopalatopharyngoplasty) may be possible or tracheostomy can be attempted to bypass the area of pharyngeal collapse. Although respiratory stimulants and supplemental oxygen can improve oxygenation somewhat, in most patients they do not significantly reduce upper airway collapse.

Management of central sleep apnea and Cheyne-Stokes breathing requires treatment of the underlying condition. For patients who have recently had a cerebrovascular event, the sleep problems may resolve with recovery from the event. Many other patients with Cheyne-Stokes respiration have irreversible cardiac and neurologic disease for which there is no specific therapy. For these patients, the physician may simply try to treat the apnea or hypoxemia directly. Supplemental oxygen can be very effective not only in reducing the severity of the oxyhemoglobin desaturation, but also in decreasing the frequency of the apneas and arousals. Respiratory stimulants have not been useful; however, newer techniques of nocturnal assisted ventilation may prove effective. Whatever the treatment, if the periodicity of the arousals that terminate central apnea can be substantially reduced, sleepiness can often be alleviated.

SUMMARY

▶ During wakefulness, chronic respiratory failure that presents with CO_2 retention indicates alveolar hypoventilation and thus a disorder of control of respiration.

▶ Control of breathing can be altered in two major ways: patients either "can't breathe" in response to a normal or increased stimulus from the central nervous system or "won't breathe" because the central nervous system stimulus is reduced or absent.

▶ Treatment for hypoventilation depends on identifying the specific defect in the respiratory system.

▶ The major disorder of control of ventilation during sleep is sleep apnea, characterized by snoring, disruption of sleep, and daytime sleepiness.

▶ Obstructive sleep apnea is treated by relieving upper airway obstruction, using CPAP, uvulopalatopharyngoplasty, or tracheostomy. Central sleep apnea is treated by reversing the cardiac or neurologic cause or by giving supportive therapy for the apnea's cardiopulmonary consequences.

SUGGESTED READING

Lyons HA, Huang CT: Therapeutic use of progesterone in alveolar hypoventilation associated with obesity. Am J Med 1968; 44:881.

Remmers JE et al: Pathogenesis of upper airway occlusion during sleep. J Appl Physiol 1978;44:931.

Rochester DF, Enson Y: Current concepts in the pathogenesis of the obesity-hypoventilation syndrome. Am J Med 1974;57:402.

Smith PL et al: Upper airway pressure-flow relationships in obstructive sleep apnea. J Appl Physiol 1988;64:789.

Sullivan CE et al: Reversal of obstructive sleep apnea by continuous positive airway pressure applied through the nares. Lancet 1981;1:862.

Young T et al: The occurrence of sleep-disordered breathing among middle-aged adults. N Engl J Med 1993;328:1230.

2.7

Acute Respiratory Failure

David B. Pearse, MD, and J. T. Sylvester, MD

Maintaining normal arterial oxygen and carbon dioxide tensions requires adequate minute ventilation, appropriate distribution of gas within the lung, and normal perfusion through alveolar capillaries. A defect in any of these steps can cause respiratory failure, which is defined as inability to maintain normal arterial gas tensions.

Acute respiratory failure can develop so quickly that within hours patients suffer irreversible hypoxic injury or die; identifying and treating respiratory failure is an emergency. Care of these patients can be very rewarding, since many are critically ill, requiring all the resources of the intensive care unit, yet have a pulmonary condition that is completely reversible. There is always the potential to restore patients to their former state of health. For this to happen, the physician must make an accurate diagnosis of the type of functional abnormality, identify its cause, and provide whatever respiratory assistance the patient needs.

ETIOLOGY

Causes of respiratory failure fall into two fundamental categories: failure of oxygenation and impaired ventilation. These are distinguished by the pattern of arterial blood gas abnormality. *Hypoxemic respiratory failure* is caused by parenchymal lung diseases and is characterized by reduction in the arterial PO_2. As long as ventilation is maintained, carbon dioxide clearance is unimpaired and the blood carbon dioxide level is either normal or, in the breathless patient, low. Hypoxemic respiratory failure occurs in acute pulmonary edema caused by heart disease (Chapter 1.5), adult respiratory distress syndrome (ARDS, discussed below), and other diffuse lung injuries such as an extensive pneumonia.

An increased PCO_2 implies failure of alveolar ventilation, and is called *hypercapnic respiratory failure*. Alveolar ventilation can fail because of either reduced minute ventilation or increased dead space ventilation. In other words, hypercapnic failure can develop either because a patient is not breathing or because inspired gas does not reach the functioning alveoli. Causes range from central

depression of breathing (eg, by narcotic overdose) to neuromuscular and skeletal abnormalities to acute asthma. In patients with chronic obstructive pulmonary disease (COPD), acute hypercapnic respiratory failure is generally superimposed on chronic respiratory failure.

Distinguishing hypoxemic from hypercapnic respiratory failure is the first step toward making a diagnosis of its cause. It is also critically important in designing respiratory support. Hypoxemic respiratory failure must be treated with increasing concentrations of inspired oxygen. Ventilator treatment is not the initial choice, but may be required to achieve the highest inspired oxygen concentrations or to increase airway pressure and improve aeration of lung units. Hypercapnic failure is caused by reduced alveolar ventilation and cannot be corrected by changing the inspired gas concentrations. Correct treatment is to increase minute ventilation, which may require early mechanical assistance.

ACUTE HYPOXEMIC RESPIRATORY FAILURE

Five mechanisms can cause hypoxemia (Table 2.7–1). Most patients with acute hypoxemic failure have a right-to-left intrapulmonary shunt and some degree of ventilation-perfusion mismatch. Intrapulmonary shunting is defined as blood flow past unventilated alveoli. Ventilation-perfusion mismatch occurs when areas of lung receive decreased ventilation relative to perfusion. This distinction, between shunt and mismatch, is of physiologic importance, since hypoxia caused by intrapulmonary shunting, like that of intracardiac shunting, is refractory to increasing alveolar oxygen tension. The effect of ventilation-perfusion mismatch can be decreased by increasing FiO_2. Alveolar hypoventilation causes hypoxemia as part of hypercapnic respiratory failure (see below). Decreased diffusion, even when severe, rarely causes hypoxemia at rest, but it can cause hypoxemia during the increased demand imposed by exercise. Hypoxemia from breathing low concentrations of inspired oxygen is unusual but can occur at high altitude or during toxic gas asphyxiation.

Table 2.7–1. Causes of hypoxemia.

Right-to-left shunt
Ventilation-perfusion mismatch
Alveolar hypoventilation
Decreased diffusion
Decreased inspired oxygen concentration

The findings on chest x-ray provide a framework for the differential diagnosis of acute hypoxemic respiratory failure (Table 2.7–2). Acute hypoxemia in radiographically clear lung fields suggests microatelectasis, pulmonary emboli, or an intracardiac right-to-left shunt such as through a patent foramen ovale. More often, acute hypoxemic respiratory failure is accompanied by diffuse alveolar infiltrates on the x-ray, indicating an alveolar filling process. Although alveoli can be filled with blood, as in diffuse alveolar hemorrhage, or with pus, as in a diffuse pneumonia, the most common cause of acute respiratory failure with alveolar infiltrates is edema-filled alveoli from left heart failure (cardiogenic edema) or the adult respiratory distress syndrome (permeability edema).

Adult Respiratory Distress Syndrome

The adult respiratory distress syndrome (ARDS) is defined by severe dyspnea, diffuse alveolar infiltration on chest x-ray, and marked hypoxemia that is refractory to increases in inspired oxygen concentration, all in the absence of left heart failure. The underlying abnormality is increased permeability of alveolar capillary membranes and development of protein-rich pulmonary edema in response to several types of lung injury.

Causes: ARDS is caused by diverse disorders, which can be categorized by route of injury (Table 2.7–3). Disorders such as sepsis and nonthoracic trauma injure the lung by blood-borne mechanisms. Other disorders injure the lung through the airways. Finally, the lung can be injured directly by lung contusion or radiation.

Three clinical settings account for 75% of cases of ARDS. The most important single cause is the *sepsis syndrome,* defined as a serious infection associated with hypotension or metabolic acidosis. About 40% of patients with the sepsis syndrome develop ARDS. The other two common settings are severe multiple trauma and aspiration of gastric contents. With multiple predisposing conditions, the risk of ARDS increases geometrically. Most

Table 2.7–2. Causes of acute hypoxemic respiratory failure.

Clear lungs on x-ray
  Microatelectasis
  Pulmonary emboli
  Intracardiac right-to-left shunt

Diffuse alveolar infiltrates
  Cardiogenic pulmonary edema
  Adult respiratory distress syndrome (ARDS)
  Diffuse pneumonia
  Alveolar hemorrhage

Table 2.7–3. Disorders leading to adult respiratory distress syndrome (ARDS).

Source of Lung Injury	Conditions
Blood	Sepsis* Trauma* Multiple transfusions Disseminated intravascular coagulation Pancreatitis Cardiopulmonary bypass Fat embolism Venous air embolism Drug overdose
Airway	Aspiration of gastric contents* Diffuse pneumonia* Near drowning Irritant gas inhalation (NO_2, Cl_2, SO_2, NH_3) Smoke inhalation O_2 toxicity
Direct injury	Lung contusion Radiation High altitude

*Common cause of ARDS.

patients who develop ARDS are already in the hospital for the disorder that ARDS complicates, but in some the cause is not found. About 90% of patients who develop ARDS require mechanical ventilation within 3 days of the initiating insult.

Pathophysiology: In a normal lung, the interstitium remains free of excess fluid because vascular endothelial permeability to water and protein is low, a significant colloid osmotic pressure gradient between the blood and interstitial fluid tends to return fluid to the vasculature, and lymphatic drainage clears the remaining excess. In ARDS, endothelial permeability is increased. The intravascular hydrostatic pressure may also be increased because of pulmonary venoconstriction. As a result, protein-rich fluid enters the interstitium at an increased rate. When the capacity of the lymphatics to remove fluid is exceeded, fluid collects in the interstitial space around vessels and airways and may then overflow into the alveoli.

Alveolar flooding and collapse lead to profound gas exchange abnormalities. Right-to-left shunts caused by perfused but unventilated alveoli produce severe hypoxemia that is refractory to increases in inspired oxygen concentration. Interstitial edema, intraluminal fluid, and bronchospasm narrow small airways, decreasing regional ventilation. Despite loss of surface area for gas exchange, impaired diffusion does not contribute to hypoxemia in the resting patient at sea level. Neither does hypoventilation, as is indicated by the usually low arterial PCO_2.

As edema fluid collects in the interstitium and alveoli, the lungs become smaller and stiffer. Surface tension at air-liquid interfaces increases because of dilution and alteration of surfactant. Inspissated fluid, peribronchial edema, and bronchospasm increase airways resistance. With pulmonary compliance and lung volume reduced and airways resistance increased, the patient must work harder to maintain an adequate lung volume and ventilation. The increased work of breathing can lead to respiratory muscle fatigue, further decreases in lung volume, and worsening hypoxemia.

The processes causing endothelial injury are not completely understood. Some conditions that cause ARDS, such as lung contusion and aspiration from the stomach, directly injure the lung parenchyma, whereas others, such as sepsis, shock, and nonthoracic trauma, activate indirect mechanisms that may involve cellular and humoral mediators. There is much clinical and experimental evidence to suggest that activated polymorphonuclear leukocytes and macrophages partially mediate the damage, but the occurrence of ARDS in patients rendered neutropenic by treatment for hematologic malignancy, implies pathways of injury other than the neutrophil.

Clinical Features: Early in the evolution of ARDS, there is often a latent period when patients are stable, with no respiratory signs or symptoms. Tachypnea develops gradually, with hypocapnia and mild hypoxemia. Physical examination may at first be normal, and the chest x-ray may be normal or show only minimal infiltration. As ARDS progresses, the patient develops acute respiratory distress, frothy pink or red sputum, diffuse rales, and widespread infiltrates on chest x-ray (Figure 2.7–1). Many patients are cyanotic, and increasingly severe hypoxemia is refractory to administered oxygen.

Distinguishing ARDS from pulmonary edema caused by left heart failure depends on the clinical findings, elec-

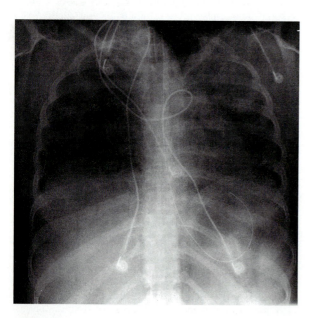

Figure 2.7–1. Chest x-ray of a 30-year-old woman with adult respiratory distress syndrome caused by *Staphylococcus aureus* sepsis.

trocardiogram, echocardiogram, and chest x-ray. In left heart failure, the x-ray shows cardiomegaly, preferential blood flow to the upper lung regions, perihilar distribution of alveolar infiltrates, and pleural effusions. In ARDS patients, heart size and blood flow distribution are usually normal, and few patients have significant pleural effusions. Infiltrates tend to be peripheral and are likely to include radiolucent outlines of the air-filled bronchi (air bronchograms). In many patients, however, ARDS and left heart failure can be distinguished only by pulmonary artery catheterization. The pulmonary capillary wedge pressure, reflecting left atrial pressure, is normal in ARDS but high in left heart failure.

Mortality rate from ARDS is 60–70%. The high death rate reflects the severity of the predisposing conditions. One-third of the deaths occur within 3 days as a direct result of the underlying illness. Most of the remaining deaths occur within 2 weeks and are caused by infection and multiple organ failure (Chapter 15.4). With advances in respiratory care, few patients now die as a direct consequence of respiratory failure. The prognosis for survivors is good. Few are symptomatic, and any residual pulmonary function abnormalities are usually mild.

HYPERCAPNIC RESPIRATORY FAILURE

Pathophysiology

Arterial CO_2 tension is determined by the balance between CO_2 production by the tissues and CO_2 excretion in the alveolar gas. Even in shunting, diffusion impairment, and ventilation-perfusion mismatch, there is a linear inverse proportion between alveolar ventilation and arterial CO_2 tension. Thus, a rise in arterial CO_2 tension above its normal level of 45 mm Hg always indicates decreased alveolar ventilation. Faced with a hypercapnic patient, the physician asks three questions as an initial assessment:

1. Is the hypercapnia caused by reduced minute ventilation or by increased dead space?
2. Is the hypoxemia attributable only to reduced alveolar ventilation, or is gas exchange abnormal as well?
3. Is the reduced alveolar ventilation acute or chronic?

Alveolar ventilation can be decreased in two ways. First, total minute ventilation can be decreased by nonpulmonary disorders affecting the central nervous system, respiratory nerves and muscles, chest wall, or upper airway. Second, dead space ventilation (ventilation not distributed to perfused alveoli) can be increased as a result of lung disease. Measuring total minute ventilation and dead space ventilation may therefore distinguish pulmonary from nonpulmonary causes of hypercapnic respiratory failure. For example, many patients with acute respiratory failure secondary to COPD have dead space-to-tidal volume ratios that exceed 0.60 (normal = 0.25). In asthma, dead space ventilation as well as airway resistance is increased; at first, patients are able to perform the excess work of breathing, but when they become fatigued, their minute ventilation may fall causing retention of CO_2. This grave sign may signal the need for mechanical ventilation.

If a patient is breathing room air, hypoventilation always causes hypoxemia. This is because the sum of the partial pressures of gases in the alveoli must equal atmospheric pressure; when alveolar CO_2 rises, alveolar O_2 tension (and therefore arterial O_2 tension) falls. It is important to note that the hypoxemia associated with hypercapnic respiratory failure is often secondary to a combination of hypoventilation and an additional pulmonary parenchymal abnormality. To decide whether this is the case, the alveolar-arterial PO_2 difference should be calculated, often called the "A-a gradient." The measured arterial PO_2 is subtracted from the alveolar PO_2 (PAO_2), calculated as:

$$PAO_2 = FiO_2 \ (P_B - P_W) - \frac{PACO_2}{R}$$

where FiO_2 is the fractional inspired O_2 concentration, P_B is the barometric pressure (760 mm Hg at sea level), P_W is the water vapor pressure at the patient's temperature (47 mm Hg at 37°C [98.6°F]), $PACO_2$ is the arterial CO_2, and R is the ratio of CO_2 production to O_2 consumption (usually 0.8). The alveolar-arterial PO_2 difference expresses the efficiency with which a lung exchanges oxygen. In a perfect lung, this difference would be 0; however, slight shunting and imperfect ventilation-perfusion matching cause the alveolar-arterial PO_2 difference to be as large as 10 mm Hg in healthy young adults breathing room air. Because it increases with FiO_2, the alveolar-arterial PO_2 difference should ideally be measured with the patient breathing room air. A normal alveolar-arterial PO_2 difference in a hypoxemic, hypercapnic patient indicates that hypoventilation is the sole cause of hypoxemia. If the alveolar-arterial difference is elevated, shunt or ventilation-perfusion mismatch is also contributing.

An acute increase in arterial CO_2 caused by hypoventilation leads to respiratory acidosis. Acute hypoventilation in a previously normal patient decreases the pH by 0.008 for every 1 mm Hg increase in $PACO_2$. A pH change lower than this suggests that the patient has been hypoventilating long enough (3–5 days) for there to be a compensatory increase in plasma bicarbonate concentration, the result of increased acid excretion by the kidneys. Knowing the patient's plasma bicarbonate and history usually allows the physician to determine whether hypercapnic respiratory failure is acute or chronic or is an acute exacerbation of a chronic process.

Causes and Clinical Features

The clinical features of acute hypercapnic respiratory failure depend in part on the underlying disorder. Acute hypercapnia quickly causes pronounced central nervous system narcosis. Confusion, obtundation, and even coma

may develop during severe respiratory acidosis. Thus, acute hypercapnic respiratory failure should be considered in any patient with impaired consciousness. The clinical suspicion of acute hypercapnia is heightened by evidence of respiratory distress or by a concurrent disorder (eg, drug overdose) that is known to cause alveolar hypoventilation. Acidosis causes vasodilatation, and many patients with acute CO_2 narcosis have warm vasodilated peripheries.

Patients with hypercapnic respiratory failure caused by central nervous system disorders or neuromuscular disease may not complain of dyspnea or develop respiratory distress. A decrease in respiratory rate or in the inspiratory excursion of the chest and abdomen may be the only clue to their alveolar hypoventilation. In patients with acute neuromuscular diseases such as Guillain-Barré syndrome and myasthenic crisis, life-threatening hypercapnia and respiratory arrest can develop rapidly and without warning. Such patients require careful monitoring of respiratory function and arterial blood gases. They should be treated in an intensive care unit, even early in their illness.

Patients with intrinsic lung, airway, or chest wall disorders generally complain of dyspnea and are noticeably breathless. The effort required to maintain a normal level of alveolar ventilation may be seen in the accessory inspiratory muscles, particularly the sternocleidomastoids. Muscles of the abdominal wall may be recruited to aid expiration. When inspiratory effort becomes excessive or the respiratory muscles become fatigued, the patient may develop paradoxical abdominal motion. Normally, as the diaphragm descends during inspiration, the abdomen moves outward. Paradoxical abdominal motion is inward movement of the anterior abdominal wall during inspiration, caused by the fatigued, noncontracting diaphragm being pulled into the thorax. This physical finding, also seen in patients with isolated diaphragm dysfunction, is usually a sign that the patient needs mechanical ventilatory support.

Differential Diagnosis

The differential diagnosis of hypercapnic respiratory failure is categorized according to the component of the respiratory system affected (Table 2.7–4).

Lung Diseases: Lung diseases cause hypercapnic respiratory failure primarily by increasing pulmonary dead space. Obstructive lung diseases are the most common causes of hypercapnic failure. In patients with COPD, acute respiratory failure usually develops as an exacerbation of chronic respiratory failure and may be precipitated by systemic or respiratory tract infections, left heart failure, pulmonary embolism, or pneumothorax. Indirect causes of acute failure must also be considered. For example, overuse of sedatives can depress respiratory drive and decrease minute ventilation.

Patients with COPD typically present with a recent history of worsening dyspnea, confusion, and agitation. Physical examination reveals that respiratory rate is usually increased, and the patient is using accessory respira-

Table 2.7–4. Common causes of hypercapnic respiratory failure.

Lung diseases
  Chronic bronchitis and emphysema
  Cystic fibrosis
  Asthma
  Pulmonary edema

Upper airway obstruction
  Foreign body
  Epiglottitis
  Tumor
  Goiter
  Bilateral vocal cord paralysis
  Inhalation injury (thermal, chemical)
  Laryngospasm and hereditary angioedema

Chest wall abnormalities
  Kyphoscoliosis
  Flail chest

Disorders of respiratory muscles and nerves
  Myasthenia gravis
  Muscular dystrophy
  Guillain-Barré syndrome (acute polyneuritis)
  Phrenic nerve abnormalities
  Polymyositis

Central nervous system disorders
  Sedative drug overdose
  Head injury
  Stroke
  Spinal cord injury at or above C3–5
  Demyelinating diseases and amyotrophic lateral sclerosis

tory muscles. There may be signs of right ventricular failure caused by cor pulmonale. Severe hypercapnia and hypoxemia can lead to coma. Adults with end-stage cystic fibrosis can present in similar fashion. In severe asthma, an increase in arterial CO_2 tension is a grave sign, indicating that respiratory muscle fatigue is preventing the patient from maintaining adequate minute ventilation to overcome the increased dead space and that respiratory collapse may be imminent.

In patients with acute pulmonary edema, the major gas exchange abnormality is severe hypoxemia from intrapulmonary right-to-left shunt, but it is often complicated by additional hypercapnic failure. About 50% of patients have a respiratory acidosis from both increased dead space and increased CO_2 production secondary to increased work of breathing. Similarly, the increase in dead space and work of breathing associated with chronic interstitial lung diseases, such as idiopathic pulmonary fibrosis, may be complicated by acute hypercapnic failure when increased ventilatory demands exceed the capabilities of the respiratory muscles.

Upper Airway Obstruction: Any narrowing of the upper airway, from the oropharynx to the carina, can lead to hypercapnic respiratory failure. As the airway lumen is narrowed, resistance to airflow and the work of breathing increase until the patient is unable to maintain an adequate minute ventilation. In addition, fractional dead space ventilation increases as tidal volume decreases relative to the fixed volume of anatomic dead space in the conducting

airways. Patients with acute upper airway obstruction present with severe dyspnea, tachypnea, and anxiety. If the airway obstruction is extrathoracic (above the vocal cords), loud, high-pitched, stridorous breath sounds that are more pronounced during inspiration may be audible over the throat. A critical obstruction between the carina and larynx, however, may produce inspiratory and expiratory wheezes over the chest that are indistinguishable from acute asthma. Clues to upper airway obstruction in such a case are normal lung volumes on chest x-ray and the characteristic reduction in inspiratory flow rate on pulmonary function tests.

Upper airway obstruction has a broad differential diagnosis (see Table 2.7–4). Obstruction from a foreign body is most common in children, but adults occasionally occlude their upper airway with aspirated food, producing the so-called "café coronary." Bacterial epiglottitis, although uncommon in adults, can occur, usually after symptoms of an upper respiratory infection. The most common presenting symptom is a sore throat, variably accompanied by dyspnea, fever, difficulty swallowing, and drooling. In patients without respiratory distress, a prompt diagnosis by lateral neck x-ray or pharyngoscopy is crucial because of the potential for rapid airway occlusion.

Another cause of edema and obstruction is thermal or chemical injury of the upper airway after inhalation of steam, smoke, or noxious chemicals. Patients with accompanying skin burns who receive rapid fluid replacement are at risk for laryngeal edema. Thus, burn patients with evidence of inhalation injury, such as hoarseness or soot in the nose or mouth, should have prophylactic tracheal intubation to protect the airway.

Chest Wall Abnormalities: Kyphoscoliosis reduces lung volumes and increases the stiffness (reduces the compliance) of the chest wall; lung compliance is also decreased because of progressive atelectasis. Patients with severe kyphoscoliosis therefore have increased work of breathing, a fall in minute ventilation, and eventually chronic hypercapnic respiratory failure. Acute respiratory failure precipitated by infection, bronchospasm, or heart failure often complicates this chronic deterioration in lung function.

A sudden increase in chest wall compliance can also disrupt normal ventilation. For example, multiple rib fractures may make part of the chest wall unstable ("flail chest"). The paradoxical respiratory motion of the unstable section of chest wall and the severe pain of breathing can cause hypoventilation and atelectasis. An adjacent lung contusion can further aggravate abnormal gas exchange if focal pulmonary edema develops. Many patients need ventilatory assistance and pain control until the chest wall is stabilized.

Disorders of Respiratory Muscles and Nerves: Many disorders interfere with the function of respiratory muscles and nerves. Diaphragmatic contraction may be impaired by myasthenia gravis, muscular dystrophy, or polymyositis. Phrenic nerve palsy may be caused by Guillain-Barré syndrome, peripheral neuropathy, trauma, or malignancy, but seldom leads to hypercapnic respiratory failure unless both phrenic nerves are affected. Patients with respiratory muscle weakness complain of dyspnea and difficulty in coughing, not always in proportion to the severity of their illness. Worrisome signs are ineffective cough, difficulty in handling secretions and swallowing, and increasing respiratory rate. Arterial blood gases reveal hypoxemia caused by atelectasis. The $PaCO_2$ may be unexpectedly low at first, indicating alveolar hyperventilation. As the respiratory muscles weaken, the $PaCO_2$ slowly rises into the normal range. Serial measurements of vital capacity and inspiratory force are the most sensitive indices of respiratory muscle strength and impending respiratory failure. Measurements of $PaCO_2$ are less useful because hypercapnia may not develop until vital capacity and respiratory muscle strength are well below 50% of their predicted values and respiratory arrest is imminent.

Central Nervous System Disorders: Hypercapnic respiratory failure often complicates disorders that interfere with function of the brain stem respiratory center or transmission of efferent impulses in the cervical spinal cord. Overdose of central nervous system depressants, such as sedatives, narcotics, or barbiturates, is the most common cause of respiratory center suppression. Patients are typically comatose, with a decreased respiratory rate, but no focal neurologic signs. Patients can develop hypercapnic failure because of head trauma, intracerebral hemorrhage, or a stroke that involves the respiratory center or compresses the brain stem. These patients are also comatose, but examination usually reveals focal neurologic signs. Trauma to the cervical cord is the spinal disorder that most often causes respiratory failure. The diaphragm is innervated from the third through fifth cervical nerve roots. Cord injuries at or above this level cause paralysis of the diaphragm. Patients with diaphragmatic paralysis present with dyspnea that is characteristically worsened by the supine position. These patients use accessory respiratory muscles, and many have paradoxical abdominal motion. Other causes of spinal cord disease that can impair function of the diaphragm include amyotrophic lateral sclerosis and demyelinating syndromes such as multiple sclerosis.

MANAGEMENT

To manage acute respiratory failure successfully, the physician must accomplish four goals: (1) establish an airway; (2) administer the appropriate amount of oxygen; (3) maintain adequate alveolar ventilation; and (4) identify and treat the underlying cause of respiratory failure.

Airway Management

The physician should consider the possibility of upper airway obstruction in every patient with acute respiratory failure. Stridorous breath sounds or a history compatible with upper airway pathology such as a sore throat with fever should prompt an upper airway examination by the most experienced person available. If epiglottitis is suspected, the examination is often performed in the operating room, because of the possibility that an instrument introduced into the upper airway may make it close completely. For the same reason, patients with signs and symptoms of inhalation injury from smoke or noxious chemicals undergo prophylactic tracheal intubation. In these situations, the primary goal of therapy is to establish an open airway. If an endotracheal tube cannot be placed, patients should undergo emergency cricothyroid intubation or tracheostomy.

In an unconscious patient without upper airway obstruction, an oropharyngeal airway may improve the effectiveness of spontaneous ventilation or ventilation assisted by a bag-and-mask system. The oropharyngeal tube is a temporary measure; if the patient does not improve, an endotracheal tube is needed.

Oxygen Therapy

The aims of giving supplemental oxygen are to increase arterial oxygenation without thereby depressing hypoxemic respiratory drive, and, in patients with pulmonary hypertension, to reduce pulmonary vascular resistance. Too much oxygen can be harmful. The most common ill effect is respiratory depression, seen in hypercapnic patients whose medullary chemoreceptors no longer respond to hypercapnia and acidosis, and whose ventilation therefore depends on hypoxemic drive. Besides this, oxygen in high concentrations is directly toxic to the lungs, through such products such as the superoxide anion, hydrogen peroxide, and the hydroxyl radical. Damaged lungs seem to be particularly susceptible to oxygen toxicity. High concentrations of oxygen can also aggravate mismatch and lead to intrapulmonary shunting by the mechanism of absorption atelectasis. This occurs in perfused, but poorly ventilated lung units, containing only CO_2, oxygen, and water vapor, which collapse after oxygen is absorbed. Therefore, the physician should use the lowest oxygen concentration that produces an arterial oxygen saturation of 90%. When pH, $PaCO_2$, and temperature are normal, this corresponds to a PaO_2 of 60 mm Hg. With lower pH or higher temperature, the PaO_2 at 90% saturation is increased because of a shift in the oxyhemoglobin dissociation curve to higher partial pressures. Under these circumstances, the therapeutic goal should be a PaO_2 of 70–80 mm Hg.

Patients who are breathing spontaneously can receive oxygen by nasal cannula or face mask. Nasal cannulae, with oxygen flow rates of up to 4 L/min, are comfortable and convenient, but rather unreliable. The inspired oxygen concentration may be too low or too high. Cannulae are therefore reserved for patients whose oxygen needs are not critical and who are not at risk for respiratory depression.

Face masks can give more carefully metered oxygen therapy. "Venturi" masks allow selection of FiO_2 concentrations between 24% and 40% and are unaffected by the patient's minute ventilation. These masks allow titration of FiO_2 in patients at risk for respiratory depression and are thus of particular value in those with COPD. Hypoxemia from ventilation-perfusion mismatch—the predominant cause of hypoxemia in these patients—usually responds to very small increments in inspired oxygen concentration. Treatment begins at an inspired oxygen concentration of 24%, which is increased stepwise with repeated checks of the arterial blood gases for worsening hypercapnia. Oxygen concentrations higher than 40% are given through a different, tight-fitting mask with a reservoir bag and valves that theoretically keep out room air. Even with this mask, it can be difficult to exceed a concentration of 70%, particularly in patients with high minute ventilation. In general, patients who require an inspired oxygen concentration over 50% should be considered for tracheal intubation.

Mechanical Ventilation

Ventilator Setup: Mechanical ventilation offers the means to optimize minute volume, precisely control inspired gas concentrations, and adjust airway pressure, usually by adding positive end-expiratory pressure. Ventilation is indicated when patients are manifestly not breathing or are breathing ineffectually, or when blood gas measurements show worsening respiratory failure. Typical conditions are drug overdose, flail chest, ARDS with progressive hypoxemia, and asthma with a rising $PaCO_2$.

Most ventilators used in medical intensive care units are volume-cycled and pressure-limited. They deliver a preset tidal volume unless an adjustable upper limit for airway pressure is reached. Most patients are started in the ventilator's "assist-control" mode. The patient's respiratory effort triggers each breath from the ventilator. The threshold of the trigger is adjustable. If the patient does not make inspiratory efforts, the ventilator delivers breaths at a specified tidal volume and frequency. The assist-control mode allows the inspiratory muscles to rest, because the only work they have to do is activate the trigger.

Positive End-Expiratory Pressure (PEEP): Most patients with hypoxic respiratory failure have widespread alveolar edema. Simply controlling minute volume and inspired oxygen concentration may not be enough to improve their oxygenation unless it is also possible to improve alveolar aeration. In this setting, PEEP can inflate atelectatic alveoli and thus rapidly improve shunting and oxygenation. This is true whether the alveolar edema is caused by left heart failure or by the excessive capillary permeability of ARDS.

PEEP is usually begun at 3–5 cm H_2O and increased by increments until oxygenation improves. PEEP should not exceed 20 cm H_2O. During these adjustments, inspired oxygen concentration should be held constant. When oxygenation improves, it is sometimes possible to reduce PEEP by about 5 cm H_2O, because the transpulmonary pressure necessary to open collapsed alveoli is usually greater than that required to keep them open. As with oxygen, it is important to use the lowest level of PEEP needed for adequate oxygenation.

The potential adverse effects of PEEP are decreased venous return, caused by compression of the right atrium and great veins, pneumothorax, pneumomediastinum, and increased dead space ventilation because of decreased blood flow to ventilated alveoli from capillary compression. Correcting hypoxemia may be of no benefit if the cost is a lowered cardiac output, since the transport of oxygen from the lung to the tissues must be maintained. Cardiac output is seldom affected by PEEP of less than 15 cm H_2O, as long as adequate vascular volume is maintained. A fall in cardiac output can be reversed by giving intravenous fluid. PEEP is contraindicated in patients with hyperinflated lungs and is not helpful when the pulmonary process is focal.

In some patients, incorrect ventilator settings can create PEEP inadvertently, sometimes to the extent of severely compromising cardiac output. This phenomenon, known as "auto-PEEP," occurs when too-rapid ventilation does not allow time for passive expiration between breaths. The lungs are progressively hyperinflated, expiratory pressure increases, and venous return falls. Auto-PEEP is particularly likely in patients with obstructive airways disease and can be relieved by increasing the time available for expiration. This entails decreasing respiratory frequency or increasing the inspiratory flow rate to reduce the inspiration:expiration ratio. Normally, this ratio is about 1:2. With obstructive airways disease, a value of 1:4 or greater is more reasonable.

Weaning: After a period of mechanical ventilation, often in the setting of a catastrophic illness, a number of factors may prevent a patient from breathing again unaided. The most common factors are malnutrition, fluid and electrolyte imbalance, heart failure, depressed mental status, fever, and pain. These conditions must be corrected before the patient can be weaned from the ventilator. Predictors from measurements of respiratory mechanics that a patient may be successfully weaned include vital capacity greater than 10 mL/kg, a maximum inspiratory pressure more negative than –20 cm H_2O, FiO_2 less than 0.5, ratio of dead space to total ventilation less than 0.6, and ratio of respiratory rate to tidal volume less than 105 breaths/min/L. In patients who chronically hypoventilate, the arterial CO_2 tension should be near the baseline level, with the pH normal and the oxygen tension 60–70 mm Hg before weaning is attempted.

There are two ways to wean from the ventilator. One is to have the patient breathe unaided for increasingly long spells, with rest periods in between; the other is to gradually reduce the number of breaths supplied by the machine. In the first method, mechanical ventilation is stopped for 15–30 minutes while the physician monitors vital signs and arterial oxygen saturation with a pulse or ear oximeter. If the patient becomes desaturated or hypotensive or develops respiratory muscle fatigue, mechanical ventilation should be resumed. If possible, an arterial blood sample should be drawn before mechanical ventilation is restarted to quantify hypoxemia and hypoventilation. If this initial trial is successful, the ventilator should be periodically withdrawn for longer periods, interposed by periods of full ventilatory support to allow adequate rest. The other approach to weaning is gradually to decrease the frequency of breaths delivered by the ventilator, thereby increasing the work done by the patient. In both approaches, patients should receive full mechanical ventilation at night so that they can sleep.

Hemodynamic Management

Careful hemodynamic management is essential for treating acute respiratory failure. During acute respiratory distress, as much as 20% of the cardiac output may be diverted to the respiratory muscles, and inadequate cardiac function can significantly impede the respiratory system from maintaining adequate alveolar ventilation. Moreover, cardiac output can greatly influence arterial oxygen content through its effect on systemic mixed venous oxygen saturation. In a patient with significant ventilation-perfusion mismatch or intrapulmonary right-to-left shunting, the mixed venous oxygen saturation, which varies directly with cardiac output, becomes an important determinant of systemic arterial oxygen saturation. Left ventricular dysfunction can also worsen respiratory failure by increasing pulmonary vascular blood volume and edema, both of which decrease lung compliance and increase ventilation-perfusion mismatch. This is particularly important in patients with ARDS, whose increased pulmonary vascular permeability makes the rate of edema formation exquisitely sensitive to changes in pulmonary venous pressure.

Hemodynamic management of patients with acute respiratory failure frequently requires catheterization of the pulmonary artery with a Swan-Ganz thermistor-tipped balloon catheter capable of measuring pulmonary artery and wedge pressures, mixed venous oxygen content, and cardiac output. In patients with ARDS, pulmonary wedge pressure should be kept as low as possible by careful fluid management and judicious use of diuretics to limit edema formation. This strategy is balanced against the need to maintain adequate oxygen transport to the tissues. Thus, hemodynamic management includes repeated clinical evaluation of systemic organ function. Measuring mixed venous oxygen content may be helpful in this regard. For example, if oxygen consumption is constant or increasing, an increase in mixed venous oxygen content indicates improved tissue perfusion.

Bronchodilators

Bronchodilators are the mainstay of pharmacologic therapy for acute respiratory failure from asthma and COPD. In both disorders, a β-adrenergic agent such as metaproterenol or albuterol is administered by inhalation, along with intravenous theophylline, which provides additional bronchodilation and may enhance diaphragmatic function. Patients with severe asthma, who are generally younger than patients with COPD, are often treated initially by subcutaneous injections of β-adrenergic epinephrine or terbutaline. Inhaled anticholinergic drugs are not used routinely in asthma; their value in acute respiratory failure from COPD remains to be determined, despite their proven effectiveness as bronchodilators in patients with stable COPD. Bronchodilators may not play much of a role early in ARDS, but they are often used later to treat wheezing and to maximize pulmonary function during weaning from mechanical ventilation.

Corticosteroids

Corticosteroids are of unquestioned value in hastening recovery of pulmonary function in patients with acute respiratory failure from asthma. They also decrease the airflow obstruction that many patients suffer during acute exacerbations of COPD. Corticosteroids are not useful in patients with ARDS; in controlled studies, they neither decreased the incidence of ARDS in patients at risk nor reduced mortality from established ARDS.

Antibiotics

Secondary bacterial infections such as gram-negative pneumonia are a major cause of death in patients with ARDS—thus, the importance of careful bacteriologic surveillance, early diagnosis of infection, and appropriate antibiotic treatment. Antibiotics should be given routinely during acute exacerbations of COPD. In other patients with acute respiratory failure, antibiotics should be given only when there is proof of bacterial infection.

Management of Tracheal Secretions

Tracheal secretions can be a serious problem in patients with chronic bronchitis or bronchiectasis and in patients with respiratory muscle weakness and ineffective cough. Mucolytic agents are of no proven benefit. Chest physiotherapy (postural drainage and chest percussion) is useful only in patients who are producing at least 30 mL of sputum per day. Intubated patients with obstructive lung disease may initially need frequent tracheal suction, but the need typically diminishes with antibiotic and bronchodilator therapy. Too-frequent suction can irritate the trachea and stimulate further secretion, creating a vicious cycle.

Prophylactic Measures

Gastrointestinal Bleeding: Upper gastrointestinal bleeding from stress ulcers in the gastroduodenal mucosa is a common complication in mechanically ventilated patients.

Stress ulcers can be reduced by keeping gastric pH above 4 with antacids or H_2 antagonists. Unfortunately, raising gastric pH has been shown to increase both gram-negative colonization of the upper gastrointestinal tract and the incidence of nosocomial pneumonia. A reasonable alternative drug for stress ulcer prophylaxis may be sucralfate.

Pulmonary Embolism: Prolonged bed rest is a risk factor for deep vein thrombosis and pulmonary thromboembolic disease. The risk is increased by right heart failure, sedation, and paralysis, as well as by femoral vein catheters. To reduce the risk, patients with acute respiratory failure should receive prophylactic subcutaneous heparin. The platelet count should be monitored to prevent heparin-induced thrombocytopenia.

Feeding: Patients who require mechanical ventilation for more than a short time need a means to receive adequate nutrition (Chapter 4.10). Enteral feeding by a tube in the stomach or jejunum is advantageous because it decreases gastrointestinal mucosal atrophy and stress ulcers without the complications of parenteral nutrition. Patients who cannot tolerate enteral feeding are given parenteral hyperalimentation through a central venous catheter. In either case, note that food stimulates CO_2 production and may aggravate hypercapnic respiratory failure or interfere with weaning from the ventilator. Although nutritional formulas with large carbohydrate components have been thought to aggravate this phenomenon, not overfeeding the patient is probably more important than the type of calories given.

SUMMARY

▶ Acute respiratory failure is classified as hypoxemic, caused by abnormal gas exchange within the lung, or hypercapnic, caused by reduced alveolar ventilation.

▶ Acute hypoxemic respiratory failure is best exemplified by the adult respiratory distress syndrome (ARDS), which is characterized by acute respiratory distress, diffuse alveolar infiltrates, refractory hypoxemia, and the absence of left heart failure. The most common causes of ARDS are sepsis, aspiration of gastric contents, and trauma.

▶ Acute hypercapnic respiratory failure can be caused by disorders that decrease total minute ventilation (eg, abnormalities of the central nervous system, respiratory nerves and muscles, chest wall, upper airway) and by disorders that increase dead space ventilation (eg, chronic obstructive pulmonary disease, asthma).

▶ Acute hypoxemic failure is treated with supplemental oxygen and often requires mechanical ventilation. Positive end-expiratory pressure (PEEP) is added to recruit collapsed lung units. The goal is an arterial O_2 saturation of 90% (PaO_2 ~60 mm Hg). Acute hypercapnic failure is treated by reversing alveolar hypoventilation with either mechanical ventilatory support or drugs that restore minute ventilation or reduce dead space ventilation.

SUGGESTED READING

Curtis JR, Hudson LD: Emergent assessment and management of acute respiratory failure in COPD. Clin Chest Med 1994; 15:481.

Hollingsworth HM, Irwin RS: Extrapulmonary causes of respiratory failure. In: *Intensive Care Medicine,* 2nd ed. Rippe JM et al (editors). Little, Brown, 1991.

Marinelli WA, Ingbar DH: Diagnosis and management of acute lung injury. Clin Chest Med 1994;15:517.

Pepe PE et al: Clinical predictors of the adult respiratory distress syndrome. Am J Surg 1982;144:124.

Weinberger SE, Schwartzstein RM, Weiss JW: Hypercapnia. N Engl J Med 1989;321:1223.

Venous Thrombosis and Pulmonary Embolism

William R. Bell, MD

Despite enormous technologic advances since its recognition at the end of the 11th century, venous thromboembolism remains one of the common yet most difficult diagnostic problems in all clinical medicine. Patients with embolism of venous thrombus to the lungs can present with any of three related clinical syndromes. The most common and most important is acute pulmonary embolism, typically causing sudden breathlessness with some degree of hemodynamic disturbance from the obstruction to pulmonary blood flow. The expression "massive pulmonary embolism" refers to emboli large enough to occlude the pulmonary arteries centrally near their origin and which thus cause hypotension or cardiogenic shock. Infarction of lung is less common with such central emboli than with smaller more peripheral emboli in which there is less opportunity for collateral supply to the affected segment of lung from the bronchial circulation. Patients with smaller pulmonary emboli that may cause pulmonary infarction, may present with a clinical picture of pneumonitis affecting a pleural-based segment of lung. The presenting complaint may be pleuritic pain and breathlessness, with a chest x-ray that demonstrates a wedge-shaped shadow in the periphery of the lung.

A few patients present with chronic or subacute thromboembolic disease, in which individual episodes of pulmonary embolism are unnoticed or barely noticeable, until their cumulative effect causes pulmonary hypertension and right heart failure. This type of presentation most closely resembles that of primary pulmonary hypertension (Chapter 1.12).

Reasonable estimates of the frequency of venous thromboembolism in the United States indicate that annually 5 million people experience an episode of venous thrombosis and approximately 500,000 (10%) suffer pulmonary embolic events, of which 50,000 patients (10%) die. The mortality is five- to six-fold greater in patients when the diagnosis is not established and appropriate treatment is not instituted. Less than 10% of patients with pulmonary emboli have associated incurable disease; the remainder can be completely salvaged when there is early accurate diagnosis followed by prompt treatment.

PATHOPHYSIOLOGY

With rare exceptions, pulmonary emboli originate from sites distant and distal to the right side of the heart, most commonly from the venous network of the pelvis and legs. Almost all pulmonary emboli consist of intravascular thrombotic material (fibrin, red cells, white cells, and platelets), but on rare occasions, nonthrombotic materials such as fat, bone marrow, air, amniotic fluid, tumor, and even exogenous foreign bodies may embolize into the lungs. Most venous thrombi originate as a platelet nidus on the undersurface of the venous valves (valvular pockets) in the legs. The precise reason for thrombus to begin forming varies from patient to patient.

Turbulence on the undersurface of the valves may damage the endothelium, expose subendothelial collagen, and initiate platelet nidus formation. Venous hypertension stretches the venous walls, increases turbulence, disrupts the endothelium, and may thus stimulate thrombus formation. Thrombus grows by accretion of platelets, fibrinogen-fibrin, and adhesive proteins (von Willebrand protein, fibronectin, vitronectin). As it encompasses the valve, it moves to the superior valve surface and extends proximally up the venous lumen. As growth progresses, the vessel may be completely occluded and all or a portion of the thrombus may detach and embolize to the terminal vasculature of the lungs. If the venous thrombus remains uninhibited or unaltered it becomes organized, retracts, is incorporated into the venous wall, irreversibly damages the valve structure and function, and induces local stasis.

Along with intimal damage and local stasis, alterations

in coagulation proteins may contribute to initiation of venous thrombus formation. Alteration in coagulation proteins is described by the term hypercoagulability; although hypercoagulability at some point in time clearly exists, the nature of the hypercoagulable state remains ill defined. Several individual but uncommon aberrations in procoagulant proteins have been identified that are associated with a tendency to thrombus formation. These changes include deficiency in antithrombin III and proteins C and S, dysplasminogenemia, dysfibrinogenemia and abnormal increases in plasminogen activator inhibitor 1 (PAI-1), resistance to activated protein C, and a lupus-like inhibitor. However, these abnormalities are identified in only 20–40% of patients who develop venous thrombosis; most patients have no presently identifiable coagulation protein defect.

Impaction of embolic material in the pulmonary vasculature and consequent complete or partial obstruction to right heart blood flow have serious consequences for respiratory and cardiac function. The major acute respiratory effects are induction of an alveolar dead space, pneumoconstriction, hypoxemia, and hyperventilation, regional loss of surfactant and, infrequently, pulmonary macroinfarction.

The hemodynamic consequences of the reduction in cross-sectional area of the pulmonary vascular bed are an increase in pulmonary vascular resistance, an increase in pulmonary artery pressure, and vascular distention. These may lead to right ventricular failure. Many factors conditionally determine the severity of the hemodynamic compromise. The reserve capacity of the arterial pulmonary vascular bed in normals is extensive and can accommodate substantial degrees of obstruction, frequently with only minimal rise in right ventricular pressure. One entire lung can be obstructed or removed, and this can be tolerated with a minimal rise in pulmonary artery pressure in the resting state.

Several additional factors contribute to a greater rise in resistance than is explained simply by the anatomic degree of obstruction. Neural reflexes or vasobronchoconstriction by humoral mediators such as fibrinopeptides A and B from fibrinogen, vasoactive amines, serotonin, bradykinin, and prostaglandin derivatives are responsible for resistance to blood flow. An additional contributing factor is the cardiopulmonary status before the arrival of embolic material. In patients with preexisting cardiopulmonary disease, even a small amount of embolic material in the absence of cardiopulmonary reserve induces severe incapacitating or even fatal consequences. The oxygen requirements of the right ventricle increase, and oxygen dependence on coronary artery perfusion becomes critical. In this situation, when systemic arterial pressure declines, thus reducing cardiac output, right ventricular performance may deteriorate to complete failure. Under certain circumstances, pulmonary artery pressure therefore may not reflect the full degree of cardiopulmonary insult. As the right ventricle fails, cardiac output declines and the pulmonary artery pressure falls despite enormously elevated pulmonary vascular resistance. Thus, in patients with acutely compromised cardiopulmonary function, the rise in pulmonary artery pressure may be modest and is thus a poor guide to the severity of pulmonary embolic obstruction.

Coexisting Risk Factors

Most patients with venous thromboembolism have an underlying disease. The most common coexisting condition is immobilization caused by a disabling illness. The next most common problem is peripheral venous disease including thrombophlebitis, venous varicosities with accompanying insufficiency and stasis, chronic cardiopulmonary disease, procoagulant protein disorders, use of oral contraceptives, recent surgery (especially orthopedic or pelvic procedures), and possibly obesity. Less common coexisting illnesses include endocrine and metabolic diseases, pelvic disease with obliterative congestion, arterial hypertension, the postpartum period, and malignant neoplasia. Only 20–30% of patients with venous thromboembolic disease have no recognizable concurrent or recent illness.

CLINICAL FEATURES

Signs and symptoms of thrombus in the superficial or deep veins of the arms or legs may be obvious, subtle, or absent. The affected limb may be the site of aches, pains, muscle tenderness, swelling, hyperthermia, pitting edema, or tenderness within vascular compartments. Homans' sign, (sensation of tightening and pain during dorsiflexion of the foot), Moses' sign (tenderness upon anteroposterior and not on lateral calf compression), Lowenberg's sign (extreme tenderness on 180 mm Hg circumferential compression of calf or thigh), Peabody's sign (spasm of calf muscles with leg elevation and extension of foot), and Pratt's sign (distention of pretibial veins when patient is supine) may be elicited.

However, none of the signs of venous thrombosis are specific; all these features of a hot, painful, swollen calf may be caused by other conditions affecting the calf muscles, particularly cellulitis, gastrocnemius bleed, and rupture of a Baker's cyst. The only physical finding that is truly specific is a venous cord that can be grasped by the fingers of the examiner. With this exception, all described clinical features of venous thrombosis in the extremities border on useless for determination of venous thrombosis or thrombophlebitis. For diagnosis, reliance must be placed on objective laboratory techniques.

Regardless of the clinical setting or associated symptoms or signs in the legs, pulmonary thromboembolism usually presents abruptly. Most patients experience chest pain—more commonly pleuritic than nonpleuritic—tachypnea, and dyspnea. These symptoms are so common that the absence of dyspnea, chest pain, or tachypnea makes the diagnosis of pulmonary emboli unlikely. Other common symptoms are diaphoresis, cough and hemoptysis, and apprehension. In some patients, leg cramps, palpitations, syncope, nausea, vomiting, chills, and angina occur. Occasionally, these symptoms are noted intermittently for several days before the diagnosis is established.

Physical examination commonly reveals tachypnea, fever, and tachycardia. Hypotension is common; shock is usually a sign of massive embolism (greater than two lobar arteries occluded). Most patients have the combination of rales, rhonchi, wheezes (most likely secondary to bronchospasm), and a pleural friction rub. Cardiac signs, which may call attention to right heart involvement, include increased jugular venous pressure, accentuated pulmonic component of S_2, right ventricular lift, S_4 gallop, ejection murmur at left sternal edge, and signs of systemic venous congestion. Clinically evident thrombophlebitis of the lower extremities is not usually found at the time of diagnosis. Unilateral leg swelling, determined visually or by circumferential measurements at defined positions above and below the knee, suggests deep vein thrombosis. More commonly observed are signs of chronic venous disease such as tortuous varicosities, mild edema, and skin changes of stasis.

None of the above-mentioned signs or symptoms are specific for pulmonary emboli. They are present in many other diseases, including congestive heart failure, pneumonia, chronic lung disease, and myocardial infarction. It is difficult to establish the diagnosis of pulmonary emboli from clinical findings alone.

DIAGNOSTIC STUDIES

Electrocardiogram

In more than one-third of patients with pulmonary emboli, the electrocardiogram (ECG) is normal, whereas in others there are nonspecific abnormalities that are not helpful in making the diagnosis. The changes observed in the ECG do not correlate with the size or location of the emboli or the hemodynamic alterations. The most common ECG abnormalities are changes in the ST segment and T wave in right precordial leads. P pulmonale, peaking of P wave, right axis deviation, $S_1Q_3T_3$ pattern, atrial fibrillation, and changes of right ventricular hypertrophy have often been described but are observed only occasionally. Almost all the ECG abnormalities are transient, lasting only a few hours or days. Although the ECG may not provide specific diagnostic information, abnormalities noted here may provide a clue that an acute cardiopulmonary event has occurred. The ECG is especially useful in excluding myocardial infarction.

Chest X-Ray

Intravascular thrombi have the same radiodensity as the blood and surrounding tissues and cannot be visualized on plain radiographs. The most frequently observed abnormalities are the secondary pulmonary parenchymal changes of consolidation and atelectasis often with unilateral diaphragmatic elevation. Pleural effusion occurs in

about one-third of the patients and may be bilateral. In 60% of patients, the effusion contains red blood cells. Increase in major vessel and cardiac chamber size may occur, but is rare. Infrequently, changes compatible with pulmonary parenchymal infarction (pleural based, triangular, wedge-shaped density), abrupt vessel cutoff, and large areas of radiolucency secondary to oligemia are seen. Changes of parenchymal infarction, when present, usually occur 18–36 hours after the embolic event. The chest radiograph is normal in about 50% of patients with documented pulmonary thromboembolic disease.

A normal chest radiograph in a patient suspected of having emboli provides most helpful information because it excludes parenchymal disease and pneumothorax. The combination of a normal chest radiograph and an abnormal lung isotope perfusion scan should heighten the suspicion of pulmonary embolism.

Hematology and Coagulation Studies

The erythrocyte sedimentation rate and white blood cell count may be minimally elevated. Infrequently, the white blood cell count (with a normal differential distribution) may increase to 15,000–20,000/mm^3. The platelet count and the plasma fibrinogen concentration are either normal or moderately elevated. Fibrinogen-fibrin degradation products may be elevated at some time in the course of the illness, but are not elevated at the time of the acute event and therefore are not helpful in making the diagnosis or in making the decision to institute therapy.

Blood Chemistry Studies

Measurement of serum enzymes or isoenzymes offers little diagnostic help in patients with pulmonary emboli. Although minimal elevations in bilirubin, alkaline phosphatase, LDH (lactate dehydrogenase), SGOT (serum glutamate oxaloacetate transaminase), and SGPT (serum glutamate pyruvate transaminase) can be detected, they are transient and do not occur with any predictability. No biochemical test is available that is specific for making or supporting the diagnosis of pulmonary thromboembolism.

Arterial Blood Gas Measurements

Although about 80% of patients with pulmonary emboli have a reduced PaO$_2$ on room air, this test has several limitations for diagnosis. At least 15% of patients with even massive emboli have PaO$_2$ levels of 90 mm Hg or greater. In diseases such as acute and chronic lung disease and cardiac disease in which pulmonary embolism is common, the PaO$_2$ level may already be reduced before the suspicious event. If a recent normal set of arterial blood gas determinations is available for comparison, repeat study at the time of symptoms suggestive of emboli may provide evidence favoring the diagnosis.

Isotope Lung Scanning

Pulmonary isotopic perfusion lung scanning is a valuable technique in the investigation of a patient with suspected pulmonary emboli. This technique is sensitive and provides accurate information about blood flow in pulmonary vessels as small as 4–7 μm in diameter. It is performed by injecting isotopically labeled denatured protein particles (microspheres) into a peripheral vein. When the microspheres reach the lung, they are held up transiently in capillaries, allowing external gamma detectors to image the distribution pattern of radioactivity in the lung.

The detectors image six different views of the lungs: anterior, posterior, right and left lateral, and right and left oblique (Figure 2.8–1). This technique can be performed easily and quickly, without discomfort or morbidity to the most seriously ill patient. The diagnostic usefulness of this technique is severely limited because of its lack of specificity. Anything that alters blood flow, such as infectious processes, congestive heart failure, infiltrative neoplasms, or asthma as well as intraluminal vascular obstruction, can yield an abnormal distribution pattern of radioactivity in the lungs. If a properly performed lung scan (six views) reveals bilateral segmental defects, at best this can strongly suggest but not confirm the diagnosis of pulmonary emboli.

The greater usefulness of the lung perfusion scan is in excluding the diagnosis of pulmonary emboli. Because of its sensitivity, a normal perfusion scan effectively excludes the diagnosis of pulmonary emboli. An inconclusive, abnormal scan is helpful at the time of angiography to direct the angiographer to look closely at abnormal areas suspected to be caused by emboli.

The inhalation of radioactive gas (xenon) can be used to examine the function of the ventilatory compartments of the lung and is often performed after the perfusion scan to determine whether ventilatory abnormalities are responsible for perfusion defects. Theoretically, if there is intraluminal obstruction due to thrombi, the perfusion scan is abnormal, but the ventilation scan is normal. In a patient with pulmonary emboli, the defects seen on perfusion scan are not matched by defects on the ventilation scan. Unfortunately, this ideal situation is not always present. If the blood vessels are damaged by extensive embolic obstruction, the adjacent ventilatory compartments may be deranged. The defect seen on perfusion scan may be matched by a similar defect on ventilation scan; such a combination may be interpreted erroneously as pulmonary parenchymal disease and not thromboembolism. The combination of ventilation plus perfusion lung scanning has modestly improved the diagnostic accuracy over perfusion scanning alone.

NONINVASIVE TECHNIQUES

Popularized during the past two decades have been a number of noninvasive techniques used to identify venous thrombosis. ^{125}I-fibrinogen uptake scanning, phleborrheography, Doppler ultrasonography, impedance plethysmography, photoplethysmography, radionuclide venography, duplex β-mode, and real-time ultrasonography have been evaluated in appreciable numbers of patients. Some investigators have suggested that these techniques are precise with excellent accuracy. However, recognize that all these techniques are flow-dependent and do not differentiate thrombotic intraluminal from nonthrombotic extravascular obstruction. Certain of these techniques are sensitive for thrombotic detection in selective anatomic sites and completely insensitive in other anatomic regions. All these techniques—some more than others—are operator-dependent and require considerable skill.

Noninvasive techniques for the detection of pulmonary emboli have not demonstrated great success. Digital substraction angiography, CT, and MRI are frequently inac-

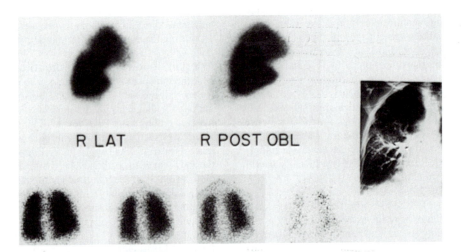

Figure 2.8–1. Ventilation and perfusion scans shown in conjunction with selective right lower lobe pulmonary arteriogram in patient with pulmonary emboli. Segmental perfusion defect in the right midlung field is seen in right lateral and right posterior oblique views of perfusion scan (top). Ventilation scan (bottom) is normal. Arteriogram (right) demonstrates emboli in artery to right midlung field.

curate when direct comparison has been made with angiography yielding similar numbers of false-positive and false-negative results. Spiral rapid sequence CT scanning may provide greater accuracy for detection of thrombi and emboli than the above-mentioned techniques.

Angiography

In both the upper and lower extremities, ascending venography remains the reference standard for establishing the diagnosis of venous thrombosis. It is a relatively noninvasive technique and is routinely performed on an outpatient basis. Properly performed, ascending venography depicts the intraluminal space in the entire deep venous system in the lower and upper extremities, including the external and common iliac veins as well as the renal veins and inferior vena cava. Complications with this procedure including phlebitis, hypersensitivity reactions, and local skin necrosis from dye extravasation are very rare (<1%).

Pulmonary angiography is the best available reference standard to establish the presence of pulmonary emboli. Although the technique is not infallible, studies have demonstrated that the occurrence of false-negatives and false-positives is rare. Discomfort to the patient is minimal. The number of personnel, expense of equipment, and time required limit the availability and routine use of this technique. Associated morbidity and mortality rates are less than 1%.

DIAGNOSTIC APPROACH

When the patient presents with symptoms (aches, pains, tenderness, increase in size, discoloration) or signs (eg, erythema, edema, hyperthermia, venous cords, positive Homans' test) of deep venous thrombosis, it is reasonable to use a noninvasive technique (impedance plethysmography, Doppler ultrasonography, duplex β-mode ultrasonography), provided that the laboratory performing the technique has validated its accuracy with various prospective, randomized, blinded, appropriately controlled comparative studies performed against ascending venography. If the test is unequivocally positive, it is reasonable to accept the result and institute therapy. If there is any question about the result or the interpretation or correlation with the clinical findings, ascending venography should be performed.

If the history and physical examination suggest emboli, the patient should receive a lung perfusion scan directly. An arterial blood gas determination may be helpful. If the lung perfusion scan is normal, the investigation can cease; pulmonary emboli are excluded. If the lung perfusion scan is abnormal, a ventilation scan should be performed. If the ventilation scan is normal and clinical features are appropriate, it is reasonable to accept the diagnosis of emboli and institute therapy. If the interpretation of the perfusion and ventilation scans is abnormal and compatible with

emboli, but there are additional problems such as congestive heart failure, chronic lung disease, and asthma, angiography should be performed to settle the issue.

There are other clinical situations in which confirmation of the diagnosis by angiography is important. These include a past history of bleeding or untoward reaction to anticoagulants; before any surgical procedure, including umbrella insertion; a past history of recurrent pulmonary emboli without angiographic documentation; or deterioration in a patient who has been placed on optimal medical management without substantiating the diagnosis.

Angiography is not available at all hospitals. Even when angiography is available, it is not possible to perform this study in every patient suspected of having venous thromboembolic disease. The combination of ventilation perfusion lung scanning along with Doppler ultrasonography and impedance plethysmography performed on the lower extremities provides evidence of an accurate diagnosis in 80–89% of patients. An arterial PO2 greater than 85 mm Hg plus a low probability lung ventilation perfusion scan have a negative predictive value of 98%.

MANAGEMENT

When the diagnosis of venous thrombosis is made in the deep venous system of the legs or arms, treatment (with extreme exceptions) should be instituted promptly. If thrombus is small (millimeters), limited to one vessel below the knee, and asymptomatic, elevation and external heat may suffice. If the diagnosis is superficial venous thrombosis/thrombophlebitis and the patient is asymptomatic, elevation, anti-inflammatory agents, and external heat are adequate. However, if either of the aforementioned conditions are associated with systemic findings (fever, diaphoresis, inability to bear weight without pain and tenderness of the involved limb), systemic treatment is needed.

If the amount of thrombus formation is moderate and mainly confined below the knee with minimal extension into the vessels of the thigh or from the forearm into the arm, intravenous heparin followed by oral warfarin therapy for a total of 3–4 weeks is the treatment of choice. If thrombus formation is extensive, that is, extending through the thigh vessels to or above the inguinal ligament or through the arm into the axillary vessels and more proximally, thrombolytic therapy (streptokinase or urokinase) followed by heparin and then warfarin for 2–3 weeks is the treatment regimen of choice.

When the diagnosis of pulmonary emboli is made, the most important initial step in treatment is administration of adequate fluid volume in order to increase the venous pressure in order to promote maximal blood return to the right heart. Anticoagulant or thrombolytic therapy should be instituted as soon as the diagnosis is made. In addition, supportive measures such as oxygen, minimal effective doses of analgesics if indicated, aminophylline for bronchospasm, and vasopressors for hypotension should be administered. For patients with uncomplicated pulmonary emboli, the initial agent of choice is intravenous heparin, which should be administered for 10–14 days.

Before discontinuation of heparin, oral anticoagulants should be instituted and continued for 3 to 6 months or longer. The duration of oral anticoagulation must be guided by the status of the patient. In patients with risk factors such as obesity, congestive heart failure, venous disease of the lower extremities, or a history of recurrent thrombotic disease, oral anticoagulation may be continued indefinitely. In patients who are temporarily immobilized, oral anticoagulant therapy should continue until the patient is fully ambulatory.

In patients with massive or submassive emboli who experience cardiopulmonary compromise, prompt restoration of blood flow is needed to return the cardiac index to normal. Thrombolytic agents, streptokinase, urokinase, recombinant tissue plasminogen activator, infused for 12–24 hours, can induce thrombus dissolution and return cardiopulmonary hemodynamics to normal within hours, which does not occur with heparin therapy. In these situations, available data indicate thrombolytic agents to be the initial treatment of choice.

Surgical embolectomy should be considered in the patient who is receiving optimal medical therapy but shows clinical deterioration or persisting hypotension. If, as rarely happens, anticoagulation is ineffective in preventing recurrent embolic episodes, as documented by pulmonary angiography, or the patient is experiencing active hemorrhage and cannot receive thrombolytic or anticoagulant agents, vena caval interruption (usually by insertion of a filter device that can be placed by means of a catheter) may be recommended. These sieve-like devices may prevent the migration of thrombo emboli from the legs into the lungs. In time, when the devices become obstructed, blood flow ceases, collateral veins develop, and the protective effect is lost. Placement of a filter does not obviate the need for anticoagulants. The results of vena caval interruption have generally been disappointing. Recurrent emboli may occur because of the development of collateral vessels within 6–8 days. Occasionally, however, these procedures have been lifesaving.

In the overall management of thromboembolic disease, prophylaxis in patients at risk is critical. Early ambulation after surgical procedures or parturition help to eliminate venous stasis. In patients who must remain immobilized for long periods, such as those recovering from orthopedic procedures or those who require prolonged bed rest for treatment of heart failure or myocardial infarction, low-dose heparin, cyclic alternating compression boots, or oral anticoagulation may be effective in preventing venous thrombosis. Elastic support stockings may promote venous flow in the legs in the same way as leg muscle contraction against resistance will increase venous flow.

SUMMARY

▶ The presentation of pulmonary embolism is occasionally dramatic, but more often subtle. Eighty to ninety percent of patients experience chest pain, shortness of breath, and tachypnea.

▶ No routine study of the blood or urine makes the diagnosis of pulmonary embolism. More than 85% of patients have a reduced arterial PaO_2. The combination of ventilation/perfusion pulmonary scanning may yield findings that strongly support the diagnosis but only pulmonary arteriography can establish the diagnosis.

▶ Treatment of acute pulmonary embolism is with thrombolytic therapy followed by anticoagulation with heparin and then warfarin. The duration of therapy may be a few months if the cause is known and can be removed, longer if the cause cannot be removed.

SUGGESTED READING

Bell WR, Bartholomew JR: Pulmonary thromboembolic disease. In: *Current Problems in Cardiology,* vol 10. Year Book Medical Publishers, 1985.

Bell WR, Simon TL: A comparative analysis of pulmonary perfusion scans with pulmonary angiograms. Am Heart J 1976; 92:700.

Bell WR, Simon TL: Current status of pulmonary thromboembolic disease: Pathophysiology, diagnosis, prevention and treatment. Am Heart J 1982;103:239.

Kelley MA et al: Diagnosing pulmonary embolism: New facts and strategies. Ann Intern Med 1991;114:300.

PIOPED Investigators: Value of the ventilation/perfusion scan in acute pulmonary embolism: Results of the prospective investigation of pulmonary embolism diagnosis (PIOPED). JAMA 1990;263:2753.

Wagenvoort CA: Pathology of pulmonary embolism. Chest 1995;107(Suppl 1):10.

Nodules and Masses in the Lung and Mediastinum

Peter B. Terry, MD

A patient newly discovered on chest x-ray to have a lung nodule or mass may prove to have cancer, with surgical resection as the only hope for cure. On the other hand, many lesions are benign and should not be resected. Therefore, it is important to make an accurate diagnosis before resorting to thoracotomy.

The chest x-ray is the starting point, often taken as part of routine screening before surgery or during evaluation of a new patient. Seldom is the x-ray taken because of complaints related to the chest. Lung masses can become surprisingly large before they cause symptoms because there are few pain fibers in the lung and mediastinum to signal their development. Furthermore, the large thoracic air space and lung reserves allow masses to grow dramatically without the patient noticing any dysfunction. When masses do cause symptoms, they do so in one of three ways: through the airways by causing cough, sputum, or hemoptysis; from adjacent structures by causing pain; or by producing systemic manifestations such as weight loss or other paraneoplastic syndromes.

A pulmonary nodule or mass appears on x-ray as a "coin lesion"; in contrast to an infiltrate, it is a discrete spherical or ovoid lesion with a definable border. Nodules (less than 4 cm in diameter) are distinguished from masses (4 cm or greater) because the differential diagnosis of lung masses is more extensive. Nodules and masses in the mediastinum have different causes from those in the lung and will be discussed separately.

LUNG NODULES AND MASSES

Solitary Lesions

The differential diagnosis of pulmonary nodules and masses is broad (Table 2.9–1). Neoplastic lesions include (1) primary and secondary malignant tumors and (2) hamartomas, which are benign. The most common non-neoplastic lesions are granulomas, usually caused by tuberculosis or histoplasmosis. Less commonly, a solitary nodule proves to be a bronchogenic cyst, pulmonary infarct, rheumatoid nodule, or pulmonary arteriovenous malformation. The differential diagnosis of pulmonary masses includes most of the entities that cause pulmonary nodules, as well as fibroma, sarcoma, silicosis (which can cause discrete nodules or masses) (Chapter 2.5), mucoid impaction syndrome (in patients with asthma) (Chapter 2.4), and pulmonary sequestration. The last is an uncommon congenital anomaly in which a portion of lung develops independently from the midgut so that its air spaces may not communicate with the bronchial tree.

The goals of the initial evaluation of a lung nodule are to determine whether the patient has a malignant or a benign lesion and to use the least invasive diagnostic methods. Relevant aspects of the history are the patient's age, smoking history, family history, and possible exposures to infectious diseases or occupational hazards.

Lung cancer is uncommon in patients who have never smoked, especially when they are younger than 35 years old. In such patients, a positive skin test for tuberculosis, exposure to persons infected with tuberculosis, exposure to avian sources of *Histoplasma capsulatum,* or a history of rheumatoid arthritis suggests that the pulmonary nodule has a benign cause. Features that suggest a primary lung cancer are a history of smoking, age over 40 years, male sex, a family history of lung cancer, exposure to asbestos, or the mining or refining of certain metals. In a smoker, it is prudent to suspect the worst and ignore circumstantial evidence favoring histoplasmosis or tuberculosis unless the x-rays suggest that the lesion is benign (see "Laboratory Studies" below).

Only 10% of solitary lung nodules are metastases from extrathoracic cancer; metastases to the lung are usually multiple. Therefore, patients with a solitary lung lesion should not be worked up for a primary extrathoracic can-

Table 2.9–1. Short differential diagnosis of solitary lung nodules.

Type of Nodule	Clues to Diagnosis
Common causes	
Granulomas (50% of all nodules)	Calcification common; layered or bull's-eye pattern pathognomonic
Histoplasmosis	
Tuberculosis	
Neoplasms	
Malignant	Calcification rare (see Figure 2.9–2)
Bronchogenic (25%)	
Metastatic (10%)	Metastases most often multiple
Benign	
Hamartoma (5%)	Sharp outline, often perfectly round
Uncommon causes (10%)	
Bronchogenic cyst	Paratracheal position
Pulmonary sequestration	Usually in basal segments of left lower lobe
Round pneumonia	
Pulmonary infarction	Pleural-based
Round atelectasis	Pleural-based, in setting of asbestos-related disease; on CT, characteristic swirling pattern toward hilum
Rheumatoid nodule	High titers of rheumatoid factor, prominent subcutaneous nodules
Arteriovenous malformation	Sometimes multiple; on x-ray or CT, large vein draining toward hilum
Wegener's granulomatosis	Usually multiple, often with different-sized lesions, sometimes cavitating
Septic emboli	Usually multiple, sometimes cavitating
Progressive massive fibrosis	Large lesion in setting of diffuse disease

cer unless they have localizing symptoms or signs, or abnormal urinalysis, positive stool test for occult blood, or abnormal routine blood studies.

Multiple Lesions

Multiple pulmonary nodules are most commonly metastatic lesions from extrathoracic sites. Less often, they represent infectious diseases (eg, histoplasmosis, septic emboli), immunologic diseases (eg, Wegener's granulomatosis), or, rarely, congenital lesions (eg, pulmonary arteriovenous fistulas).

An etiology for multiple pulmonary nodules is suggested by a past history of an extrathoracic neoplasm; gastrointestinal, gynecologic, or upper airway complaints; a history of drug abuse leading to right-sided bacterial endocarditis; or a family history of hereditary hemorrhagic telangiectasia.

Physical Examination

The physical examination yields few clues to the presence or nature of a pulmonary nodule, and these are usually in systems other than the lung itself. The physician should look for an enlarged lymph node in the cervical or supraclavicular area, finger clubbing, and pulmonary os-

teoarthropathy—all signs of malignancy. A patient with hereditary hemorrhagic telangiectasia may have cutaneous, mucosal, or conjunctival telangiectasia. Wegener's granulomatosis causes necrotic lesions in the nasal mucosa and sometimes cutaneous vasculitis. A rheumatoid nodule can be diagnosed when the characteristic arthritis is identified.

In patients with multiple pulmonary nodules, the physical examination may suggest the site of a primary malignancy, demonstrate the needle tracks of drug addiction, reveal joint manifestations compatible with rheumatoid arthritis, or show skin lesions compatible with a granulomatous disease (eg, sarcoidosis, Wegener's granulomatosis).

Imaging and Laboratory Studies

The chest x-ray plays the central role in determining the nature of a solitary pulmonary nodule (Figures 2.9–1 and 2.9–2). Evidence of a benign lesion includes no change in radiographic appearance over more than 2 years; an evolving radiographic pattern compatible with an inflammatory lesion; smooth sharp margins; lamellated or diffuse calcification; or a central "bull's-eye" calcification. A doubling of the lesion's volume in less than 30 days or more than 460 days also suggests a benign lesion. The only malignant lesions that can double in less than 30 days are choriocarcinomas, some sarcomas, and an occasional small cell carcinoma.

Chest computerized tomographic (CT) scans are particularly helpful in defining the nature of a solitary pulmonary nodule. A lesion that the CT scan measures as high density is nearly always benign. Areas of extremely low density suggest fat and are characteristic of a hamartoma. The CT scan may unexpectedly show additional nodules not visible on plain x-ray, or mediastinal adenopathy that may alter the diagnostic and therapeutic approach.

Cytologic examination of sputum can seldom diagnose lung cancer in solitary peripheral nodules. The yield is so low that repeatedly positive sputum cytology studies should not suggest a malignant lung nodule so much as prompt a search for an occult proximal airway, laryngeal, or pharyngeal cancer shedding malignant cells. Likewise, sputum examination rarely helps to diagnose multiple pulmonary nodules, unless Gram's stain or a culture demonstrates organisms that can cause septic emboli. A positive serum antineutrophil cytoplasmic antibody study suggests Wegener's granulomatosis, whereas hyperglobulinemia suggests multiple myeloma with a plasmacytoma. CT, magnetic resonance imaging (MRI), and radionuclide thyroid scans may aid in discovering a primary extrathoracic neoplasm.

Blood studies sometimes show that a solitary pulmonary nodule has caused a paraneoplastic process, particularly hypercalcemia caused by ectopic parathormone production, hyponatremia caused by the syndrome of inappropriate antidiuretic hormone (ADH) production, or hypokalemia and Cushing's syndrome caused by ectopic adrenocorticotropic hormone (ACTH) production. On oc-

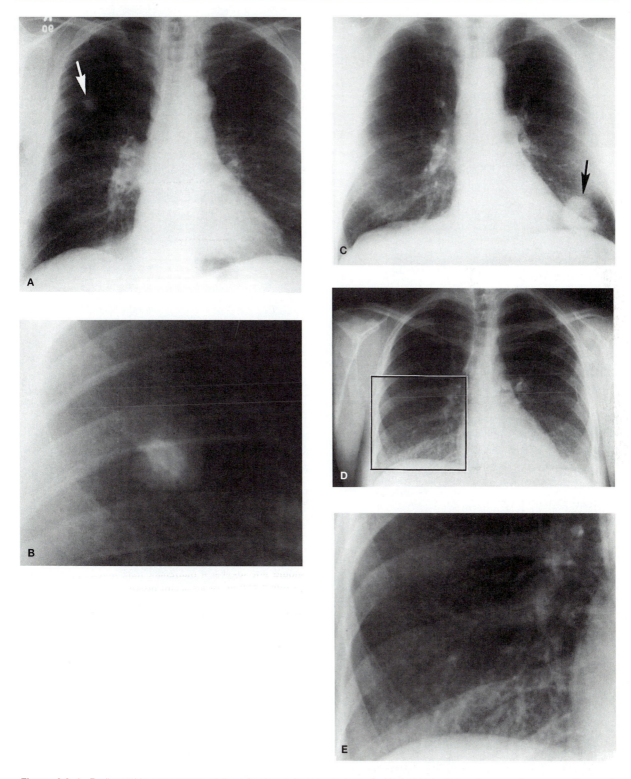

Figure 2.9–1. Radiographic appearance of three benign pulmonary lesions. **A:** Healed histoplasmosis presenting as a solitary pulmonary nodule, with central bull's eye calcification in the right upper lobe. **B:** Detail of Panel A: histoplasmoma. **C:** 4.5-cm hamartoma in the left lower lobe. **D:** Miliary tuberculosis presenting with multiple 1–2-mm nodules throughout the lower lung fields. **E:** Detail of Panel D: miliary tuberculosis in the right lower lobe.

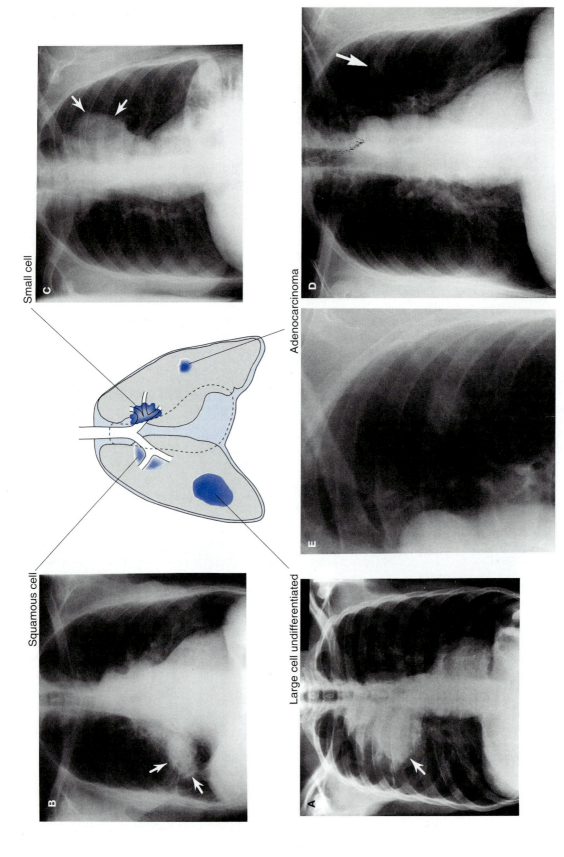

Figure 2.9–2. Typical radiographic presentations of lung cancers. **A:** Large cell undifferentiated carcinoma in the right upper lobe, abutting the right peritracheal area. (Courtesy of Anne McB. Curtis, MD, Professor of Diagnostic Radiology, Yale University School of Medicine.) **B:** Squamous cell carcinoma involving the right lower lobe. **C:** Small cell carcinoma in the left hilar and peritracheal area, with left hemidiaphragm paralysis indicating phrenic nerve involvement. **D:** Adenocarcinoma in the left upper lobe. **E:** Detail of Panel D: adenocarcinoma.

Small cell

Adenocarcinoma

Squamous cell

Large cell undifferentiated

casion, thrombocytosis or abnormal liver function tests suggest a neoplastic origin.

Some congenital sequestrations derive their arterial supply from the aorta. Arteriography reveals these anomalies, as it does pulmonary arteriovenous malformations.

Biopsy Procedures

Every effort should be made to confirm the diagnosis of a solitary pulmonary nodule without recourse to thoracotomy. A lesion that proves to be benign does not require resection, except in the rare case of an enlarging hamartoma or bronchogenic cyst compressing an airway. Even a malignant lesion requires that the patient undergo further evaluation before the decision is made to resect. In particular, diagnosis of a peripheral and therefore potentially resectable small cell cancer requires a thorough search for silent metastasis before surgery can be advised. The advent of transthoracic and transbronchial biopsy techniques has prevented many unnecessary and potentially dangerous thoracotomies.

Each biopsy technique offers advantages under specific circumstances. Transthoracic needle biopsy is appropriate when the lesion is small (6–20 mm in diameter) and in the lung periphery of a patient who does not have significant emphysema. Bronchoscopic biopsy is most effective when the lesion is in the midlung field or adjacent to an airway. Bronchoscopy may also be preferable when paratracheal or mediastinal nodes are enlarged, since these can be aspirated through the bronchoscope using a transbronchial needle.

The major risks of biopsy procedures are pneumothorax and bleeding. Pneumothorax occurs in about 15% of patients undergoing transthoracic needle biopsy of a nodule, but in less than 5% of patients undergoing a bronchoscopic biopsy. Emphysema, in which the likelihood and potential harm of pneumothorax are both increased, may therefore be a reason to favor the transbronchial approach. Many patients have slight bleeding from either procedure, but few lose enough blood to require transfusion.

The diagnostic yield from transthoracic needle biopsy of a peripheral lesion should be as high as 80% when the lesion is malignant, lower for benign diseases. When a peripheral nodule is too small to biopsy or sometimes when the tissue obtained is thought not to represent the whole lesion, thoracotomy may be indicated without proof of malignancy if the clinical presentation suggests a cancer. The morbidity and mortality rates of traditional thoracotomy have to be taken into account: Mortality is about 1% in otherwise healthy young persons, 4% in healthy older persons, and higher in patients with emphysema, angina, previous myocardial infarction, or other causes of myocardial dysfunction. Even after successful resection, patients do not recover their former level of function for 3–6 months.

Multiple pulmonary nodules are usually metastatic disease and should always be diagnosed by biopsy. Thoracotomy is seldom if ever indicated, since resection is not curative.

Mass lesions are usually approached by transthoracic needle biopsy or, occasionally, bronchoscopy. Paradoxically, the larger the lesion, the less likely that bronchoscopic biopsy will be successful in obtaining diagnostic tissue, because the airways through which the biopsy forceps travel often go around large lesions.

Treatment

To understand the treatment of a patient with a primary lung neoplasm presenting as a solitary pulmonary nodule, one must understand histologic and TNM (tumor-node-metastasis) classification, as well as the prognosis associated with each type of neoplasm.

Clinicians divide lung cancers into four cell types: squamous cell carcinoma, adenocarcinoma, large cell undifferentiated carcinoma, and small cell (sometimes still called "oat cell") carcinoma. Occasional tumors contain mixed cell types. Small cell carcinoma is the most aggressive of the four, with a tendency for rapid growth and early metastasis. The others, often collectively described as *non-small cell carcinoma,* vary in their locations and growth characteristics. Characteristic radiographic presentations of the four cell types are shown in Figure 2.9–2.

The interval between the development of the first lung cancer cell and clinical presentation of the disease has been estimated at 5–10 years. This delay in recognition usually allows ample time for metastasis and explains why 75% of all lung cancers are already not resectable when they are diagnosed. Small cell carcinoma, the most aggressive cell type, can least often be resected, primarily because it usually presents with mediastinal node metastasis.

Primary lung cancers are rarely cured by radiation therapy or chemotherapy. At present, the only hope for long-term survival lies with surgical resection, which requires evidence of limited or no spread beyond the primary lesion. Correlation of tumor spread with survival is reflected in the TNM classification of lung cancer. In this system, long-term survival of non-small cell lung cancers is predicted by tumor size and evidence of invasion of adjacent structures (T), by lymph node involvement (N), and by metastasis (M) to the mediastinum or more distant sites (Table 2.9–2; Figure 2.9–3). Most primary lung cancers are diagnosed at a stage beyond being resectable, but about 75% of small malignant pulmonary nodules (less

Table 2.9–2. Staging of non-small cell lung cancer, based on the TNM (tumor-node-metastasis) system.

Stage I	Tumor of any size in the lung or involving visceral pleura, at least 2 cm from the carina, with no involvement of lymph nodes
Stage II	Metastasis confined to peribronchial and hilar lymph nodes on the side of the tumor
Stage III	Invasion of the diaphragm, chest wall (including malignant effusion), pericardium, or within 2 cm of the carina, or: Involvement of nodes outside the peribronchial and ipsilateral hilar nodes
Stage IV	Distant metastasis

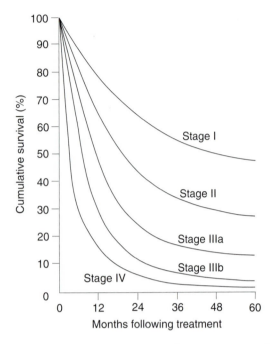

Figure 2.9–3. Survival after diagnosis of lung cancer, according to clinical stage. (Modified and reproduced, with permission, from Mountain CF: A new international staging system for lung cancer. Chest 1986;89:225S.)

than 3 cm in diameter) can be resected, with 5-year survival rates of 40–50%. Detection of tumors at this small size reduces the likelihood of occult nodal or extrathoracic metastasis.

Solitary pulmonary nodules that are primary non-small cell lung cancers without evidence of metastasis should be resected unless the risk of thoracotomy is unacceptable to the patient or the loss of lung function is judged unacceptable by the physician. If thoracotomy is ruled out, the physician may recommend radiation therapy to the lesion, recognizing that treatment may not be curative and that it will cause some local lung damage and dysfunction.

Small cell carcinoma of the lung tends to metastasize early; it seldom presents as a solitary pulmonary nodule. Indeed, when biopsy of a nodule that seems to be solitary reveals small cell carcinoma, the likelihood of there being distant spread is very high. The patient should be evaluated extensively for metastasis before being considered for resection.

Patients with tuberculosis or histoplasmosis presenting with a solitary pulmonary nodule may or may not require treatment at time of diagnosis, depending on the likelihood of active infection and on whether the benefits of therapy exceed the risks. Treatment of the less common causes of pulmonary nodules and masses depends on the nature of the disease. Multiple pulmonary nodules are seldom resected because they are usually metastases from a nonpulmonary primary cancer.

MEDIASTINAL NODULES AND MASSES

The mediastinum is the extrapleural space between the right and left lungs, bordered anteriorly by the sternum and posteriorly by the spine, and extending from the diaphragm to the thoracic inlet. Since the structures in or bounding the mediastinum are the usual sources of mediastinal masses, the location of a mass within the mediastinum is the best clue to its cause (Figure 2.9–4). Anterior mediastinal nodules or masses are most commonly thymoma, germ cell tumor, lymphoma, or substernal thyroid. Posterior mediastinal nodules or masses are usually of neural origin. Middle mediastinal lesions are most often enlarged lymph nodes, caused by metastatic tumor, lymphoma, sarcoidosis, or another granulomatous disease.

Diagnostic Studies

Standard posteroanterior and lateral chest x-rays are usually the first and most helpful study for evaluating a mediastinal nodule or mass. Cysts, calcium, bone erosion, and fatty elements all suggest specific causes. When standard x-rays fail to show these abnormalities, a chest CT scan with contrast material may succeed. MRI scanning is particularly helpful in assessing mediastinal lesions because it differentiates vascular structures from solid tissue. Fluoroscopy may document pulsation or contiguity with the esophagus, aorta, or diaphragm. Barium swallow may show esophageal involvement, and isotope scanning may confirm a thyroid mass.

Many mediastinal lesions have no radiographic characteristics besides location to suggest the diagnosis. Because many of these lesions are treatable, a tissue diagnosis is mandatory unless the patient faces particular risk from an invasive diagnostic procedure or unless other clinical circumstances render the study of no benefit. Anterior mediastinal and right paratracheal lesions can be approached by transthoracic needle biopsy or by mediastinoscopy, a procedure in which a rigid endoscope is inserted through a small incision above the sternum. The limitations are that needle biopsy may not give enough histologic information for diagnosis of lymphomas or germ cell tumors, whereas mediastinoscopy does not allow access to the subcarinal and left paratracheal area below the aortic arch. Middle mediastinal lesions may be approached through a limited parasternal incision (Chamberlain procedure), transbronchial needle biopsy, or, rarely, transthoracic needle biopsy. Posterior mediastinal lesions may be approached by transthoracic needle biopsy. In some patients, particularly those with anterior or posterior mediastinal masses, thoracotomy with open biopsy may prove necessary. Full thoracotomy should be avoided in patients with middle mediastinal masses, since these usually prove to be infectious or neoplastic lymphadenopathy.

Treatment

Mediastinal lesions usually reflect spread of an infectious, malignant, or systemic disease and generally are not

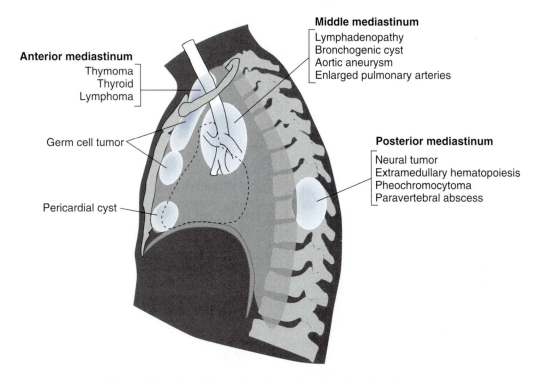

Figure 2.9–4. Lateral chest view of common sites of mediastinal tumors.

amenable to resection. Removal of slow-growing malignant thymomas or thyroid tumors may relieve pain or compression of the trachea.

SUMMARY

▶ Most single pulmonary nodules and masses require biopsy, if possible without thoracotomy, to determine whether they are benign or malignant.

▶ The only hope for long-term survival in patients with

lung cancer is resection at an early stage, but only about 25% of cancers are resectable when first discovered. Small cell cancers are the most aggressive.

▶ Multiple pulmonary nodules are usually malignant and not resectable. Therefore, diagnostic procedures should rarely include a major surgical procedure to determine the cause.

▶ Anatomy is the chief guide to diagnosing a mediastinal mass. Anterior masses are thyroid, thymus, lymphoma, or germ cell tumors. Middle mediastinal masses are most commonly vascular or lymph nodes. Posterior masses often originate from neural tissue.

SUGGESTED READING

Benjamin SP et al: Primary tumors of the mediastinum. Chest 1972;62:297.

Cummings SR, Lillington GA, Richard RJ: Managing solitary pulmonary nodules: The choice of strategy is a "close call." Am Rev Respir Dis 1986;134:453.

Mountain CF: A new international staging system for lung cancer. Chest 1986;89:225S.

Proto AV, Thomas SR: Pulmonary nodules studied by computed tomography. Radiology 1985;156:149.

Swensen SJ et al: An integrated approach to evaluation of the solitary pulmonary nodule. Mayo Clin Proc 1990;65:173.

Wychulis AR et al: Surgical treatment of mediastinal tumors: A 40 year experience. J Thorac Cardiovasc Surg 1971;62:379.

2.10

Pleural Effusions

Wilmot C. Ball, Jr, MD

Pleural effusion may be accompanied by symptoms resulting from inflammation of the parietal pleura or compression of the lung. With a small inflammatory effusion, pleural pain (pleurisy) is often present and a friction rub may be heard. Pleurisy is a sharp, stabbing sensation brought on or intensified by deep breathing. It must be differentiated from other types of pain accentuated by inspiration, such as the pain associated with rib fracture or costochondritis, nerve root compression, herpes zoster, acute bronchitis, and various cardiovascular and esophageal lesions. When there is direct invasion of the parietal pleura by tumor or infection, as in empyema, constant dull aching pain independent of respiration may result.

Large or bilateral pleural effusions may lead to dyspnea, but orthopnea is uncommon in the absence of congestive heart failure. The accumulation of pleural fluid in patients with severe heart disease or chronic obstructive pulmonary disease may result in dyspnea that seems disproportionate to the volume of fluid present. In this group of patients, removal of even small amounts of fluid may produce marked improvement in symptoms. The accumulation of a significant volume of pleural fluid sometimes does not cause symptoms, and the presence of pleural effusion may be first discovered on a routine radiograph of the chest.

PHYSICAL SIGNS

Accumulation of fluid usually occurs first at the bases of the lung, and the earliest physical signs are localized to this area. When the effusion is small, differentiation from elevation of the diaphragm, atelectasis, and consolidation may be difficult. A dull to flat percussion note is usually found over the area of fluid, together with reduced or absent breath sounds in this area. An area of bronchial breathing, accompanied by an alteration of the quality of voice sounds or frank egophony, is sometimes heard over the adjacent compressed lung. When the amount of fluid is large, the volume of the involved hemithorax may appear to be increased, and expansion during inspiration

may be reduced. Unless the mediastinum has become fixed in position by invasion with tumor or unless portions of lung on the affected side have become completely atelectatic, the mediastinum is usually shifted away from the side of a large effusion.

RADIOGRAPHIC APPEARANCE

When there are no adhesions between the visceral and parietal pleura, the earliest signs of fluid in the pleural space that can be appreciated on plain films of the chest are blunting of the costophrenic angle on the posteroanterior view and loss of sharp demarcation of the posterior portion of the diaphragm in the lateral view. With the accumulation of larger volumes of fluid, the outline of the diaphragm in the lateral view is completely lost, and the posteroanterior view shows an area of opacification at the lung base, often tapering up the lateral chest wall in the form of a meniscus. When a major portion of the hemithorax is radiopaque, air-filled bronchi in the compressed and atelectatic lung may be crowded together and displaced into the upper lung field. The heart and other mediastinal structures are typically shifted toward the uninvolved side.

When less than 300 mL of pleural fluid is present, the posteroanterior radiograph may show no abnormality. Furthermore, blunting of the costophrenic angle may be caused by old inflammatory adhesions. Here, lateral decubitus films may be very helpful, since as little as 15 mL of free pleural fluid may be recognized as a layer of density along the inner margin of the dependent chest wall. Examination of the thorax by computed tomography (CT) is also a sensitive method for identifying free pleural fluid. CT may also be useful when plain films do not permit the separation of parenchymal and pleural densities. If previous inflammatory disease has caused adhesions between visceral and parietal pleura, the fluid may be loculated rather than free in the pleural cavity. When it is confined to the area between the lower lobe and the diaphragm (infrapulmonary effusion), the fluid may resemble an elevated diaphragm. The effusion may lie within a fissure (interlobar effusion), most commonly the major fissure on the right. The posteroanterior film in such cases may show a shadow that resembles an intrapulmonary tumor. A loculated pleural effusion may also produce a shadow that lies flat against the pleural surface and bulges into the lung field in one or more locations. The simultaneous presence of fluid and air within the pleural space can be easily identified, because they produce a sharply demarcated horizontal line in an upright film. Placement of a skin marker during fluoroscopy or diagnostic ultrasonography may be used for more accurate localization of loculated fluid to assist in achieving complete removal by thoracentesis.

MECHANISMS OF PLEURAL EFFUSION

The pleural cavity normally contains a small volume of thin serous fluid formed mostly by transudation from the parietal pleural surface. This fluid, including particulate matter and cellular debris, is removed through lymphatic channels that arise from lacunae on the parietal pleural surface.

The visceral pleural surface in man is supplied by the bronchial circulation, but with drainage into the pulmonary veins. The normal balance between formation and removal of fluid may be compromised by a partial or complete obstruction of the lymphatic circulation, by a rise in either the pulmonary venous or the systemic venous pressures, or by a decrease in the colloid oncotic pressure of plasma. In the presence of pulmonary venous hypertension, fluid may also enter the pleural space from the lung surface. Since a significant portion of the lymphatic drainage from the abdomen passes by way of the diaphragm, especially on the right, a variety of inflammatory conditions within the abdomen or the presence of ascites may be accompanied by accumulations of pleural fluid on the right. Small perforations or defects in the diaphragm sometimes allow bulk flow of ascitic fluid from the abdominal cavity into the chest. Accumulation of noninflammatory pleural fluid may therefore occur in any condition that results in ascites, in obstruction to the venous or lymphatic drainage of the lung, or in either isolated left-sided or isolated right-sided congestive failure. The pleural effusion of heart failure occurs most commonly in the presence of combined ventricular failure. A severe reduction in the level of plasma protein concentration may contribute to the accumulation of noninflammatory pleural fluid.

Pleural effusion may result from inflammation of structures adjacent to the pleural space, usually just beneath the visceral pleura within the lung, but occasionally from lesions within the mediastinum, diaphragm, or chest wall. Removal of this fluid by the normal clearing mechanisms may be considerably retarded by the presence of inflammatory obstruction of the lymphatic channels draining the thorax, and secondary inflammation of larger areas of pleural surface may result in the rapid outpouring of fluid.

Unless air has been introduced during thoracentesis or surgery, the simultaneous presence of air and fluid within the pleural cavity almost always implies the presence of a bronchopleural fistula, most commonly from tuberculosis, pyogenic pneumonia, lung abscess, or malignant tumor.

When the thoracic duct is lacerated or interrupted by trauma or obstructed by tumor, lymph may accumulate in the pleural space. This condition is termed *chylothorax* and is identified by the milky appearance of the fluid, by fat droplets on staining with Sudan III, and by a total neutral fat content greater than 0.5 g/dL.

DIAGNOSTIC MEASURES

Unless the cause has been clearly established, the mere presence of fluid within the pleural cavity constitutes an indication for thoracentesis. This simultaneously serves the purpose of providing fluid for examination, permitting better radiographic visualization of the lung following the removal of fluid and relieving symptoms. Thoracentesis is performed by insertion of a short-bevel needle or a catheter threaded through a needle. Although the site of puncture is usually selected with reference to the physical findings and radiographic changes, the incidence of pneumothorax and other complications of the procedure is lower when ultrasound guidance is used. Ultrasonography is especially useful when the amount of fluid is small.

The gross appearance of the fluid should be carefully noted and specimens obtained for various laboratory examinations. A minimum examination would consist of the measurement of total protein and lactic dehydrogenase (LDH) content, the determination of total and differential cell counts, and examination of the spun sediment with Wright's stain. When the cause of the effusion is not firmly established, the fluid should be subjected to appropriate bacteriologic study for pyogenic organisms, fungi, and *Mycobacterium tuberculosis* and to cytologic examination for the presence of malignant cells. Under certain circumstances (see below), it may be useful to analyze the fluid for glucose and amylase and to determine its pH. If the fluid has a milky appearance, which suggests chylothorax, total neutral fat should be measured and the fluid examined for fat droplets by staining with Sudan III.

When an inflammatory effusion is suspected, needle biopsy of the parietal pleura with an Abrams or a Cope instrument may be performed. These biopsies have shown a 60% to 75% positive yield in patients with tuberculosis or malignant pleural effusions and may provide a diagnosis in patients in whom bacteriologic or cytologic examination of the fluid is unrewarding. When biopsy is indicated, it is best performed while free fluid is still present within the pleural cavity, because this protects the lung from being injured by the biopsy instrument. When a diagnosis has not been established despite one or more needle biopsies, thoracoscopy with biopsy of the pleura under direct vision is often successful.

DIFFERENTIAL DIAGNOSIS

In determining the cause of a pleural effusion, it is useful to establish whether the fluid is a transudate or an exudate. Transudative effusions are caused by elevated systemic or pulmonary venous pressure or by decreased plasma oncotic pressure; the pleural surfaces are not directly involved by the primary pathologic process. In contrast, an exudative effusion results from inflammation or other disease of the pleural surface or from lymphatic obstruction.

Table 2.10–1 lists the principal causes of transudative and exudative effusions and also shows a number of less common causes of pleural effusion. Most transudative effusions have protein concentrations of less than 3 g/dL. Exudative effusions usually contain protein concentrations of more than 3 g/dL; those due to tuberculosis or pyogenic infection frequently show a protein concentration of more than 5 g/dL. More reliable separation may be made by measuring the LDH concentration of pleural fluid and serum and by comparing pleural fluid and serum protein concentrations. An LDH concentration greater than two-thirds of the normal serum level, a pleural fluid-to-serum LDH ratio greater than 0.6, or a pleural fluid-to-serum protein ratio greater than 0.5 establishes the presence of an exudative effusion with high reliability. Comparative measurements of cholesterol level may also be useful. The presence of gross blood in the pleural fluid is most common when the effusion is the result of trauma, tumor, or pulmonary infarction. It may also result from bleeding induced at the time of a previous thoracentesis and is occasionally seen in effusions caused by tuberculosis and pneumonia. Blood-tinged fluid with fewer than 10,000 RBCs/μL is commonly found in an inflammatory effusion of any cause and is therefore of little diagnostic aid. Noninflammatory effusions usually contain only small numbers of white blood cells (WBCs), predominantly lymphocytes, whereas total leukocyte counts above 2500/μL are usually seen in inflammatory exudates. Most

Table 2.10–1. Causes of pleural effusion.

Condition	Characteristics
Common causes of transudative effusion	
Congestive heart failure	Usually chronic biventricular failure; usually bilateral; pleuritic pain and friction rub uncommon
Cirrhosis	Ascitic fluid migrates through pores in diaphragm; effusion usually confined to or larger on the right; serum proteins often low
Nephrotic syndrome	Associated with hypoproteinemia and generalized edema and ascites
Common causes of exudative effusion	
Tuberculosis	Effusion usually unilateral, may be asymptomatic; often no parenchymal lesion on x-ray
Bronchogenic carcinoma	Effusion often bloody and large; may recur rapidly after removal
Bacterial pneumonia	Sterile parapneumonic effusion must be differentiated from empyema; fluid frequently loculated
Viral and mycoplasmal pneumonia	Pleurisy and bilateral effusion common
Pulmonary infarction	Pleural pain common; effusion usually small in amount but often bloody
Metastatic tumor	Effusion often bilateral; parenchymal lesions usually apparent
Lymphoma	Most common in Hodgkin's disease; often associated with mediastinal node or parenchymal involvement
Trauma	Associated with intrapleural bleeding
Abdominal surgery	Small effusions common, but usually resolve within 48 hr
Less common disorders in which effusion occurs frequently	
Malignant mesothelioma of the pleura	Fluid protein content high or low; effusion chronic and recurrent, may be bilateral and involve pericardium; irregular thickening of the pleura usually present; history of asbestos exposure
Benign asbestos-related pleural effusion	Recurrent exudative effusion in absence of mesothelioma; may contain many eosinophils
Meigs' syndrome	Benign ovarian or uterine neoplasm with ascites and pleural effusion
Pancreatitis	Effusion more common on left side; fluid amylase higher than in blood, especially in chronic pancreatitis
Dressler's syndrome	Occurs following acute myocardial infarction or cardiac surgery; associated with fever, chest pain, and pericarditis
Systemic lupus erythematosus	Pleuritic pain common; often with areas of plate-like atelectasis on x-ray
Disorders only occasionally accompanied by effusion	
Rheumatoid arthritis	Pleural fluid glucose commonly below 12 mg/dL; LDH usually very high
Other collagen diseases (polyarteritis, scleroderma, Wegener's granulomatosis)	Usually associated with activity of the underlying disease
Fungal infections (actinomycosis, histoplasmosis, coccidioidomycosis)	Effusion or empyema an occasional complication of chronic pulmonary infection
Hypothyroidism	Low-protein effusion possible in absence of congestive failure
Drug reaction	Exudative effusion; may be serosanguineous; with drug-induced lupus, cancer chemotherapy, amiodarone, nitrofurantoin, bromocriptine, minoxidil, others
Sarcoidosis	Rarity of pleural effusion useful in differentiating from tuberculosis

of these cells may be polymorphonuclear leukocytes early in the course of a bacterial or tuberculous infection or following pulmonary infarction, but later in the course of the disease, mononuclear cells predominate. In an occasional patient, the pleural fluid may contain an exceptionally high percentage of eosinophils, even in the absence of blood eosinophilia. This is a relatively nonspecific finding, but is common in benign asbestos-related effusions. It may also be associated with pneumothorax or induced by multiple thoracenteses or intrapleural bleeding. Eosinophilia is unusual in effusions due to tuberculosis and malignancy. Wright's stain of the centrifuged sediment allows identification of mesothelial cells, which are large cells with basophilic cytoplasm, a large nucleus with finely stippled chromatin, and one to three bright blue nucleoli. Tuberculous effusions rarely show more than 1% of mesothelial cells, whereas most nontuberculous effusions contain over 5% of these cells.

Chemical analysis of pleural fluid may provide additional clues to diagnosis. Pleural fluid glucose is only occasionally significantly lower than serum glucose when the effusion is caused by tuberculosis or tumor, but is usually very low (0 to 16 mg/dL) in effusions caused by rheumatoid arthritis and in empyema fluid. The pH of pleural fluid is usually 7.30 or greater; lower values are occasionally seen in tuberculous and malignant effusions. A value below 7.20 in a parapneumonic effusion commonly is associated with the development of an empyema and results from excessive production of carbon dioxide by leukocytes in the fluid. Moderate elevation of pleural fluid amylase is occasionally seen in malignant effusions, but markedly elevated amylase levels indicate either pancreatic disease or rupture of the esophagus with leakage of salivary amylase into the pleural space.

TREATMENT

Effective management requires that the cause of the effusion be established and that specific treatment be applied where possible. In the case of noninflammatory effusions, correction of the underlying abnormality, perhaps accompanied by thoracentesis for removal of the bulk of the fluid, usually results in rapid clearing of the effusion. When pleural inflammation is present, reabsorption of pleural fluid may be slow, and repeated thoracentesis may be required to keep the pleural cavity dry, even after institution of specific therapy. In these cases, reasonable efforts should be made to keep the pleural cavity free of fluid to prevent the development of fibrosis in the pleural space, with subsequent loss of pulmonary function. If this is not done, subsequent surgical decortication may be required.

In tuberculous effusions, once effective antituberculous chemotherapy has been instituted, it may be advisable to administer corticosteroids to hasten resolution of the effusion and prevent pleural fibrosis. When pleural effusion due to malignant disease recurs rapidly, requiring repeated

thoracentesis, reaccumulation may be retarded by insertion of a chest tube and instillation of a sclerosing agent such as doxycycline or talc.

EMPYEMA

Accumulation of pus within the pleural space (empyema) is an occasional complication of bacterial pneumonia or lung abscess and should be distinguished from the more common sterile inflammatory effusion. The fluid is usually thick and has the turbid appearance of frank pus, containing over 30,000 WBCs/µL and often showing the causative bacterial agent on Gram's stain and in culture. Empyema fluid caused by anaerobic organisms, especially *Bacteroides* or streptococci, often has a foul odor. Chronic empyema in a patient already treated with antibiotics may pose a problem in identification, since the fluid may have become thinner and the culture may be sterile. The leukocyte count of the fluid under these circumstances is probably the most reliable distinguishing feature. In addition, pleural fluid with a pH below 7.20 strongly suggests empyema.

The presence of an empyema should be suspected whenever a patient with bacterial pneumonia shows either persistence or recurrence of fever after appropriate antibiotic treatment. Evidence of even a small amount of pleural fluid in this setting requires thoracentesis for diagnosis. Although empyemas usually arise by extension of bacterial infection through the visceral pleura from the lung, they may also result from perforation of the esophagus or from a subphrenic abscess, or as a complication of surgery.

Successful management of the patient with empyema requires both the administration of appropriate antibiotics and the maintenance of effective drainage of the pleural space. Prompt recognition and institution of drainage provide the greatest likelihood that the empyema space will close without becoming chronic. When a small empyema is discovered early in the course of infection, attempts to close the space by repeated thoracentesis may be justified. This is seldom successful, however, and prompt insertion of a chest tube with connection to water-seal drainage is the usual treatment. After several days without adequate drainage, most empyemas become loculated so that a tube is no longer effective, and in this situation prompt thoracotomy with removal of the empyema sac and decortication of the lung results in a more rapid recovery.

SUMMARY

▶ Pleural effusion often produces characteristic symptoms, physical signs, and radiographic changes, but aspiration of pleural fluid for laboratory examination is nearly always necessary to determine the cause of the effusion.

▶ Fluid low in protein and LDH concentration (transudative effusion) is nearly always due to congestive heart failure, hepatic cirrhosis, or the nephrotic syndrome. Protein-rich fluid (exudative effusion) can result from infection, tumor invading the pleura, and a variety of noninfectious inflammatory conditions.

▶ Diagnosis is often facilitated by analysis of pleural fluid for glucose, amylase, and pH by obtaining total and differential leukocyte counts, cytologic examination, and bacteriologic and fungal cultures.

▶ It is important in the patient with pneumonia and pleural fluid to recognize an empyema as early as possible. Early recognition will minimize the likelihood that a chronic drainage procedure or surgical decortication of the affected lung will be required.

SUGGESTED READING

Albertine KH, Wiener-Kronish JP, Staub NC: The structure of the parietal pleura and its relationship to pleural liquid dynamics in sheep. Anat Rec 1984;208:401.

Daniel TM: Diagnostic thoracoscopy for pleural disease (review). Ann Thorac Surg 1993;56:639.

Good JT Jr, Taryle DA, Sahn SA: The pathogenesis of low glucose, low pH malignant effusions. Am Rev Respir Dis 1985; 131:737.

Light RW: *Pleural Diseases.* Lea & Febiger, 1983.

Poe RH et al: Sensitivity, specificity and predictive values of closed pleural biopsy. Arch Intern Med 1984;144:325.

Prakash UBS, Reiman HM: Comparison of needle biopsy with cytologic analysis for the evaluation of pleural effusion. Analysis of 414 cases. Mayo Clin Proc 1985;60:158.

Sahn SA: The pleura (State of the Art). Am Rev Respir Dis 1988;138,184.

Section 3

Rheumatology

David B. Hellmann, MD, Section Editor

3.1

Approach to the Patient with a Rheumatic Disease

David B. Hellmann, MD

Most patients with rheumatic diseases present with either joint pain or inflammation of multiple organs. The multisystem nature of many rheumatic diseases invites physicians to hunt for diagnostic clues from many sources, from the eyelids and nail beds to the peripheral blood smear. Because most patients today do not die from but live with their rheumatic disease, physicians both confront the challenges and enjoy the satisfactions of managing these patients over decades.

This chapter illustrates the general approach to diagnosing and managing patients with rheumatic diseases. Individual diseases are discussed in later chapters.

WHEN TO SUSPECT THAT A PATIENT HAS A RHEUMATIC DISEASE

Many symptoms, signs, and laboratory tests can suggest that a patient has a rheumatic disorder. One cardinal feature of most rheumatic diseases is joint pain, which is called "arthritis" when the joint is swollen or otherwise changed in appearance, and "arthralgia" when the joint looks unchanged. The physician also should suspect a rheumatic disease when a patient has symptoms or findings of a multisystem disorder, particularly with signs of inflammation, such as fever, arthritis, mouth sores, pleuritic chest pain, anemia, and proteinuria. Infections, another cause of multisystem inflammation, often develop abruptly over 1–2 days, whereas systemic rheumatic diseases usually unfold over weeks or months.

In addition to joint pain, symptoms or findings that strongly suggest an underlying rheumatic disease include Raynaud's phenomenon (Chapter 3.10), uveitis (Chapter 3.7), fever of unknown origin (Chapters 3.5 and 8.2), pericarditis (Chapter 1.10), mononeuritis multiplex (Chapters 3.5 and 13.11), and certain rashes, especially photosensitivity or palpable purpura (Chapters 3.5 and 15.5). In a pa-

tient with a strong family history of rheumatic disease, any unexplained symptom should raise suspicion. At times, an occult rheumatic disease is first suggested by a routine laboratory test, such as a biologic false-positive test for syphilis on application for a marriage license or thrombocytopenia on routine preoperative evaluation.

GENERAL APPROACH TO DIFFERENTIAL DIAGNOSIS

Since there are over 100 rheumatic diseases, formulation of a differential diagnosis can at first seem daunting. Yet, by systematically using just clinical information, the physician can often winnow the possibilities to a very few. The two most helpful clinical clues are the joint pattern and extra-articular manifestations (Table 3.1–1).

Joint Pattern

The joint pattern is defined by (1) the presence or absence of inflammation, (2) the number of joints involved, (3) the sites and distribution of affected joints, and (4) the presence or absence of enthesopathy (inflammation at a site in which ligaments, fascia, and tendons insert into bone) (Table 3.1–2).

The hallmarks of inflammatory arthritis are morning stiffness lasting longer than 1 hour and soft tissue swelling accompanied by redness and heat. In contrast, noninflammatory degenerative diseases like osteoarthritis cause morning stiffness for less than 30 minutes and bony joint enlargement with only minimal heat or redness.

Rheumatic diseases can be classified according to the number of joints involved: monoarthritis (one joint), oligoarthritis (two to four joints), and polyarthritis (five or more joints). Some disorders affect characteristic numbers of joints. For example, gout usually presents as a monoarthritis, Reiter's syndrome as an oligoarthritis, and

Table 3.1–1. Clues to the differential diagnosis of rheumatic diseases.

Joint pattern*
Extra-articular manifestations*
Age
Sex
Family history
Onset
Course
Laboratory tests
Response to therapy

*Most common clues.

rheumatoid arthritis as a polyarthritis. However, disorders do not rigidly follow these classifications: Gout can evolve into a polyarthritis, and rheumatoid arthritis can begin as a monoarthritis or oligoarthritis.

The involved joint sites further shape the differential diagnosis. For example, the distal interphalangeal joints are affected almost exclusively by only two disorders: osteoarthritis and psoriatic arthritis. Swelling of the wrists and metacarpophalangeal joints almost always means an inflammatory arthritis such as rheumatoid arthritis or systemic lupus erythematosus.

Table 3.1–2. Differential diagnosis of joint patterns in rheumatic diseases.

Feature	Common Examples
Inflammation (morning stiffness for >1 hr)	
Yes	Rheumatoid arthritis, systemic lupus erythematosus
No	Osteoarthritis
Number of joints involved	
1: Monoarthritis	Infection, crystal disease (gout, pseudogout), trauma
2–4: Oligoarthritis	HLA-B27 diseases: ankylosing spondylitis, Reiter's syndrome, arthritis of inflammatory bowel disease, psoriatic arthritis
≥5: Polyarthritis	Rheumatoid arthritis, systemic lupus erythematosus
Joint sites involved	
Distal interphalangeal joints	Osteoarthritis, psoriatic arthritis
Metacarpophalangeal joints, wrists	Rheumatoid arthritis, systemic lupus erythematosus
First metatarsophalangeal joints	Gout, osteoarthritis
Distribution of involved joints	
Axial	HLA-B27 diseases
Peripheral	Rheumatoid arthritis, systemic lupus erythematosus
Symmetric	Rheumatoid arthritis, systemic lupus erythematosus
Asymmetric	Psoriatic arthritis, Reiter's syndrome
Enthesopathy	
Dactylitis ("sausage digit") Achilles tendon swelling Plantar fasciitis	HLA-B27 diseases

The distribution of joint complaints is also helpful. Axial (spine) involvement is typical of ankylosing spondylitis. The peripheral joints are involved in rheumatoid arthritis and systemic lupus erythematosus. Peripheral arthritis can be either symmetric (as in rheumatoid arthritis, systemic lupus erythematosus) or asymmetric (as in psoriatic arthritis).

Few physical findings are more valuable than enthesopathy. Its presence usually reduces the diagnostic possibilities from over 100, to the four disorders associated with the haplotype HLA-B27–ankylosing spondylitis, Reiter's syndrome, the arthritis of inflammatory bowel disease, and psoriatic arthritis.

Enthesopathy most often appears in one of three ways. The first is dactylitis, a sausage-like swelling of an entire finger or toe. In most forms of arthritis, only the structures immediately around the joint become swollen. But in the HLA-B27 diseases, the surrounding ligaments and tendons also become inflamed, causing the entire digit to swell. A second major form of enthesopathy is plantar fasciitis, heel pain caused by inflammation in which the plantar fascia inserts into the calcaneus; the heel is tender but not swollen. A third major form of enthesopathy is swelling of the Achilles tendon.

Extra-Articular Manifestations

If the first important clue to the diagnosis of rheumatic disease is the joint pattern, the second is the number and types of extra-articular manifestations (Table 3.1–3). One purpose of the history and physical examination is to determine whether the patient has any extra-articular manifestations, and if so, which ones.

The rheumatic diseases cause characteristic extra-articular manifestations that range in severity. At one extreme is osteoarthritis, a disease solely of joints; it does not cause fever, rash, or weight loss. In the middle are disorders that chiefly affect joints but often cause extra-artic-

Table 3.1–3. Extra-articular manifestations of rheumatic diseases: Examples of their diagnostic value.

Extra-Articular Manifestations	Common Disease Associations
Rash	
Malar erythema ("butterfly rash")	Systemic lupus erythematosus
Violaceous eyelids ("heliotrope rash")	Dermatomyositis
Subcutaneous nodules	Rheumatoid arthritis
Palpable purpura	Vasculitis
Ocular findings	
Conjunctivitis	Sjögren's syndrome, Reiter's syndrome
Uveitis	Ankylosing spondylitis, sarcoidosis
Sudden, painless blindness	Temporal arteritis
Raynaud's phenomenon	Scleroderma, systemic lupus erythematosus
Mononeuritis multiplex	Polyarteritis nodosa
Pericarditis	Systemic lupus erythematosus

ular manifestations, such as the subcutaneous nodules in many patients with rheumatoid arthritis. At the other extreme are diseases like systemic lupus erythematosus that affect multiple tissues, only one of which happens to be the joints.

The types of extra-articular manifestations are of diagnostic value (see Table 3.1–3). For example, different rashes are linked to specific diseases. Erythema in a "butterfly" pattern over the cheeks usually means systemic lupus erythematosus. A violaceous discoloration of the eyelids suggests dermatomyositis. Eye manifestations may also signal specific diseases. Conjunctivitis is seen in Sjögren's syndrome; uveitis complicates ankylosing spondylitis. Other extra-articular signs of great value in the differential diagnosis are Raynaud's phenomenon, pericarditis, and mononeuritis multiplex.

Other Clues

Although the joint pattern and extra-articular manifestations are usually the most helpful clues, other features deserve comment (see Table 3.1–1). Rheumatic diseases can affect persons of any age, but certain disorders begin at predictable ages (Figure 3.1–1). The patient's sex may be a clue, because some rheumatic diseases are distributed unequally between men and women. For example, systemic lupus erythematosus affects women nine times more often than men. Many rheumatic diseases, especially autoimmune disorders, have a genetic basis, so a family history of autoimmune diseases like multiple sclerosis, Graves' disease, and pernicious anemia may indicate a familial susceptibility to systemic rheumatic diseases. The onset and course of the arthritis may also be informative. For example, an attack of gout typically begins suddenly and abates after 7–10 days. Laboratory tests help to include some diagnostic possibilities and exclude others. Sometimes the response to therapy, or the lack of therapy, is part of the diagnosis. The patient who does not respond dramatically to prednisone does not have polymyalgia rheumatica.

LABORATORY TESTS

Laboratory tests must be ordered judiciously to allow the physician to confirm or reject the impression created by the history and physical exam. It is worth noting that a patient can have laboratory abnormalities without having disease. For instance, many persons with an elevated serum uric acid do not have gout. Because few laboratory tests are both specific and sensitive, the diagnosis of most rheumatic diseases requires both a compatible clinical picture and supportive laboratory data. The most common tests used in rheumatology are discussed here. Other laboratory tests, including x-rays, are reviewed in the chapters on the specific diseases for which they are used.

Synovial Fluid

Synovial fluid, an ultrafiltrate of blood, normally looks transparent, like raw egg white. A normal joint has too little fluid to be detected on physical exam. Normal synovial fluid has very few cells of any type, with an average of only 65 white blood cells (WBCs)/mm^3. Laboratory analysis of synovial fluid can answer three questions about a joint: Is it inflamed? Is it infected? Does it contain crystals?

A synovial fluid WBC count higher than 3000/mm^3 indicates joint inflammation. Degenerative diseases cause lower counts. Inflammation also decreases the synovial fluid's clarity, increases its volume, and decreases its glucose level, but none of these changes is as specific as a high WBC count.

The most specific tests for joint infection are Gram's stain and culture of the synovial fluid. Although infected synovial fluid has more than 3000 WBCs/mm^3, no particular count is diagnostic of infection. Many pyogenic infections, such as staphylococcus or streptococcus, produce WBC counts greater than 50,000/mm^3. However, noninfectious processes like gout can similarly elevate the synovial fluid WBC count. By contrast, nonpyogenic infections like tuberculosis often produce synovial fluid

1 5 10 15	20 25 30 35 40 45	50 55 60	65 70 75+

Juvenile rheumatoid arthritis
Rheumatic fever
	Autoimmune diseases:
	  Systemic lupus erythematosus
	  Rheumatoid arthritis
	  HLA-B27 diseases (eg, ankylosing
	    spondylitis, Reiter's syndrome)
	  Polymyositis
	  Raynaud's phenomenon
	Scleroderma
	Gonococcal arthritis
	Fibrositis
	Polyarteritis nodosa
	Wegener's granulomatosis
		Gout
		Pseudogout
		Osteoarthritis
		Sjögren's syndrome
			Polymyalgia rheumatica
			Giant cell arteritis

Figure 3.1–1. Typical age of onset for some rheumatic diseases.

occurs in SLE but much less often than is generally believed. Pathologic studies have shown true vasculitis in only 10% of patients with central nervous system SLE. Much more common than vasculitis in SLE is vasculopathy—vascular abnormalities without fibrinoid necrosis.

DIAGNOSIS

SLE is a clinical diagnosis, usually based on a patient's meeting at least 4 of the 11 criteria (Table 3.2–3). These criteria were developed by researchers trying to devise a common classification system. For clinicians, some of the criteria are more important than others. For example, a mouth ulcer or a positive ANA test result is nonspecific, but antibodies to dsDNA are highly specific for SLE. Indeed, the combination of hypocomplementemia (not a criterion) and antibodies to dsDNA is nearly pathognomonic for SLE. The criteria point out that the diagnosis almost always depends on compatible symptoms, signs, and laboratory results.

An important factor in the diagnosis of SLE is time. Some patients have laboratory abnormalities, such as a false-positive test for syphilis, for years or decades before they develop any objective organ damage. Other patients have serologic abnormalities but never develop SLE. This is particularly true for the ANA, which can be positive in about 5% of healthy women. Positive ANAs without SLE

are also found in one-third of first-degree relatives of patients with SLE. Thus, the import of isolated laboratory abnormalities can be determined only over time and should never be the sole basis of a diagnosis, especially one as emotionally charged as SLE.

DIFFERENTIAL DIAGNOSIS

The major entities that can mimic SLE are infections, other rheumatic diseases, and drug reactions (Table 3.2–4). Most infections that cause multisystem disease develop more acutely than SLE, which usually evolves over weeks or months. Patients who can recall the hour or day when they became ill most likely have an infection. Similarly, a fulminant multisystem disease that develops over 2–4 days is most likely an infection, Goodpasture's syndrome, or thrombotic thrombocytopenic purpura. About the only patients with SLE whose first hospital admission is to the intensive care unit are those with acute hypoxia from pulmonary hemorrhage or pneumonitis, and those with tamponade from pericardial effusion. Infections that cause acute multisystem disease include endocarditis, syphilis, Rocky Mountain spotted fever, toxic shock, meningococcemia, salmonellosis, ehrlichiosis, mononucleosis, HIV, malaria, and other forms of sepsis.

Among the rheumatic diseases, early rheumatoid arthritis can be difficult to distinguish from SLE, especially in

Table 3.2–3. Criteria for classification of SLE.*

1. Malar rash
2. Discoid rash
3. Photosensitivity
4. Mouth ulcers
5. Arthritis
6. Serositis
7. Renal disease:
   >0.5 g/day proteinuria, or
   ≥3+ dipstick proteinuria, or
   Cellular casts
8. Neurologic disease:
   Seizures, or
   Psychosis without other cause
9. Hematologic disorder:
   Hemolytic anemia, or
   Leukopenia (<4000/mm^3), or
   Lymphopenia (<1500/mm^3), or
   Thrombocytopenia (<100,000/mm^3)
10. Immunologic abnormality:
    Positive LE cell preparation, or
    Antibody to native DNA, or
    Antibody to Sm, or
    False-positive serologic test for syphilis
11. Positive antinuclear antibody (ANA)

*Patients who have 4 or more of the 11 criteria are considered to have SLE.
Modified and reproduced, with permission, from Tan EM et al: The 1982 revised criteria for the classification of systemic lupus erythematosus. Arthritis Rheum 1982;25:1271.

Table 3.2–4. Differential diagnosis of disorders that can mimic SLE.

Disorder	Distinguishing Features
Infections	
Endocarditis	Sudden onset, positive cultures
Syphilis	Positive VDRL and FTA
Typhoid fever	Positive culture
Mononucleosis	Pharyngitis, positive monospot test
Rheumatic diseases	
Rheumatoid arthritis	Fewer extra-articular findings; bony erosions, deformities not reducible
Dermatomyositis	Rash over knuckles, not between knuckles
Scleroderma	Tight skin
Still's disease	High fever, negative rheumatoid factor
Drugs	
Drug-induced SLE	Older patients, more men, no renal disease, no anti-dsDNA antibody
Allergic reactions	Drug history
Malignancy	
Lymphoma	Histology
Other	
Goodpasture's syndrome	Anti-basement membrane antibodies
Sarcoidosis	Pleural effusions rare
Thrombotic thrombocytopenic purpura	Serologic tests negative

VDRL, Venereal Disease Research Laboratory (test); FTA, fluorescent treponemal antibody.

patients who have few extra-articular manifestations. Both diseases affect the same joints. Swelling tends to be more impressive in rheumatoid arthritis than in SLE, but the difference is not absolute. Nodules, common in rheumatoid arthritis, can also complicate SLE. Later in the course of rheumatoid arthritis, differences in joint involvement emerge: Rheumatoid arthritis is much more likely than SLE to produce bony erosions, and although both diseases can cause deformities, only those in SLE are reducible (the physician can straighten patients' fingers, but patients cannot maintain the position when the physician lets go). The chief clinical difference between SLE and rheumatoid arthritis is SLE's tendency to cause distinctive extra-articular manifestations (see Figure 3.2–1). With some serologic tests, the two conditions can look similar. One-fifth of patients with SLE have rheumatoid factor, and one-third of patients with rheumatoid arthritis are ANA-positive. However, antibodies to ds-DNA or Sm are specific for SLE. Some forms of vasculitis, scleroderma, and polymyositis also share features with SLE.

Several types of drug reactions can mimic SLE. For example, serum sickness from penicillin can cause arthritis, rash, fever, and even proteinuria. In addition, drugs such as isoniazid, hydralazine, and procainamide can cause a syndrome called "drug-induced SLE," which is very similar to idiopathic SLE (Table 3.2–5). One way to distinguish these conditions is by the patient populations affected. The patients who take these drugs and develop lupus are older than patients with idiopathic SLE, and nearly as many are men as women. Other differences are that drug-induced SLE rarely affects the kidneys, rarely triggers production of anti-dsDNA antibodies, and, most important, resolves after the drug is stopped.

Some patients with SLE have such impressive weight loss, fever, and adenopathy that they are first thought to have lymphoma. SLE and sarcoidosis share a number of features, and a patient can have both diseases. But unlike SLE, sarcoidosis rarely produces pleural effusions.

People who present to a doctor with rashes and other features may be suspected of having SLE. For example, acne rosacea causes malar erythema, although, unlike SLE, rosacea often causes pustules, does not spare the nasal labial fold, and does not cause systemic features. Excessive systemic corticosteroids, either from Cushing's syndrome or from prescription, dilate cutaneous blood vessels and cause a malar erythema, but, again unlike SLE, do not spare the nasolabial fold.

COURSE

The course of SLE is most remarkable for repeated spontaneous flares and remissions, their durations unpredictable and highly variable. A few patients have chronic disease, and a few remit for decades. But most patients have an episode once every 1–2 years, particularly during the first 10 years of the disease. After the first decade, flares become less frequent. The severity and duration of attacks depend on treatment (see "Treatment and Monitoring" below).

The first episode of SLE may cause more symptoms than do later flares. A patient may first present with rash, mouth ulcers, pleuritis, arthritis, pericarditis, fever, and glomerulonephritis, but later may experience SLE almost solely as the nephrotic syndrome. Another patient may have multiple admissions for hemolytic anemia or central nervous system involvement. Whatever is the patient's worst problem tends to remain so for the duration of the disease. Treatment probably explains this tendency of SLE to evolve from multiple symptoms at the outset to one or two key problems later in the course, since small doses of prednisone often prevent all but the patient's most resistant problems from manifesting.

TREATMENT AND MONITORING

If one thinks of the inflammation in a patient with SLE as a biologic fire, the physician's role is to play medical fire fighter, determining whether the patient's problem is a conflagration that requires a fire hose or whether it is a small grill fire likely to respond to garden hose therapy. To call the fire department for an ashtray fire has a low benefit-cost ratio. So, too, in SLE the intensity of the treatment must match the severity of the disease.

Minor disease manifestations such as arthralgias and myalgias respond to salicylates or nonsteroidal anti-inflammatory drugs (NSAIDs). Hydroxychloroquine, an antimalarial drug, is effective for the arthritis and rash. Sunscreens, hats, and otherwise avoiding the sun can improve photosensitive rashes.

For major manifestations such as glomerulonephritis, severe thrombocytopenia, hemolytic anemia, and bowel vasculitis, the cornerstone of therapy is a high-dose glucocorticoid. Glucocorticoids in lower dose may also be indicated to treat pleuritis and pericarditis. Although glucocorticoids are effective, they have many side effects (Table 3.2–6). Since the toxicity of prednisone is related to the dose and duration of treatment, the physician must

Table 3.2–5. A sampling of drugs associated with SLE.

Degree of Association	Drugs
Definite	Chlorpromazine, hydralazine, isoniazid, methyldopa, procainamide, quinidine
Possible	Captopril, carbamazepine, cimetidine, hydrazines, levodopa, lithium, nitrofurantoin, penicillamine, phenytoin, propranolol and other β-blockers, propylthiouracil, sulfonamides
Unlikely	Allopurinol, gold salts, oral contraceptives, penicillin

Modified and reproduced, with permission, from Hess EV, Mongey AB: Drug-related lupus. Bull Rhem Dis 1991;40:1.

Table 3.2–6. Side effects of long-term glucocorticoid therapy.

General effects	Increased appetite Weight gain Edema Increased sweating
Skin and appearance	Increased adipose: truncal obesity, moon facies, buffalo hump, enlarged supraclavicular fat pads, increased pericardial fat Skin striae Increased bruisability Rubor Increased facial hair Thinning of scalp hair
Metabolism	Diabetes Hypertension Hypokalemia
Neuromuscular system	Anxiety Mood lability Sleeplessness Psychosis Proximal muscle weakness
Bone	Osteoporosis Avascular necrosis
Immune system	Increased risk of opportunistic infection Lymphopenia
Others	Cataract Peptic ulcer disease

make every effort to give the lowest dose for the shortest time.

Immunosuppressive drugs, especially cyclophosphamide and azathioprine, are being used more and more in the hope that they will prove more effective and less toxic than corticosteroids. Cyclophosphamide, for example, is better than prednisone at preventing renal failure. But cyclophosphamide does not lengthen survival, and it has serious side effects including gonadal failure, hemorrhagic cystitis, and increased risk of opportunistic infection and malignancy.

Laboratory tests help gauge when the patient is improving and therapy may be reduced. The patient with diffuse proliferative glomerulonephritis, for example, may begin with 4 g protein in a 24-hour urine collection, plus red blood cell casts, low complement levels, and high-titer antibody to dsDNA. With adequate treatment, most or all of these abnormalities should improve and may resolve entirely. However, treatment should never be based solely on serologic abnormalities, since, for instance, some patients have high levels of anti-dsDNA antibodies but no objective end-organ inflammation.

As with any chronic disease, a critical part of the physician's job is to provide emotional support for patients and their close friends and family (Chapter 3.1). Most patients start with an excessively negative view of their prognosis and are helped enormously by learning the facts about their disease.

PROGNOSIS

Oliver Wendell Holmes, a physician and Supreme Court justice, noted that the key to longevity is to get a chronic disease and take good care of it. Patients with SLE illustrate his point well. In the 1950's, 50% of patients with SLE died within 4 years; today the 5-year survival rate is 97% and the 10-year survival rate averages 90%.

Only a few factors identifiable at the outset of SLE have prognostic value. One is an elevated serum creatinine; serious renal disease portends a worse outcome. Another is that patients of lower socioeconomic status have a poorer prognosis, as they do with most diseases. Third, some complications carry a poor prognosis; 50% of patients who develop pulmonary hemorrhage die quickly, and abdominal vasculitis can be fatal. Still, an episode of critical end-organ damage does not necessarily portend a poor long-term outcome. Patients with central nervous system SLE, for instance, fare as well as other patients. Many patients now enjoying good control of SLE have recovered from a life-threatening flare.

As treatments for SLE have improved, causes of death have changed. Infection is now the leading cause of death, followed by active disease, chiefly of the kidney or brain. Most fatal infections are opportunistic, striking patients who are taking high-dose glucocorticoids, immunosuppressive drugs, or both. Patients not taking these drugs have no higher rates of important infections than do persons without SLE, with two exceptions: All patients with SLE are at higher-than-normal risk for salmonella and pneumococcal sepsis, perhaps because of hypocomplementemia. But the risk of infection with treatment, particularly prednisone at doses greater than 20 mg/day, underscores the importance of never giving more corticosteroid than the patient needs.

Another change in SLE mortality in the prednisone era has been an increasing rate of coronary artery disease. More 40-year-olds with SLE are now suffering myocardial infarction from atherosclerosis. Beyond the usual risk factors for coronary artery disease, the greatest risk for patients with SLE is longer prednisone treatment.

Thus, most patients treated with prednisone are living longer, but at the cost of higher risk for fatal opportunistic infection and coronary artery disease. The major challenge of treatment today is to preserve the gains of prednisone while minimizing its risks, either by giving less prednisone, especially once the disease has responded, or by identifying drugs that are at least as effective but less toxic.

Having SLE is not now regarded as a contraindication to pregnancy. SLE does tend to flare during or immediately after pregnancy, and the risk of miscarriage and preterm delivery is higher than normal. The best candidate for pregnancy is a woman whose disease is controlled and who has been taking less than 10 mg/day of prednisone for the past 6 months. Passive transplacental passage of anti-Ro antibody can cause the baby to have heart block or a transient rash (neonatal lupus).

SUMMARY

▶ Systemic lupus erythematosus (SLE) is a chronic multisystem autoimmune disease that chiefly affects young women, who most frequently present with rash, joint pain, and fever. The course is marked by repeated flares and remissions.

▶ SLE is diagnosed by a compatible picture of signs and laboratory findings; the diagnosis is never based on serologic abnormalities alone.

▶ The cornerstone of treatment for important SLE flares is glucocorticoids. Glucocorticoids or immunosuppressive drugs should be used in the smallest possible dose for the shortest possible time.

▶ Infection now exceeds active disease as the leading cause of death.

SUGGESTED READING

Balow JE et al: NIH conference: Lupus nephritis. Ann Intern Med 1987;106:79.

Boumpas DT et al: Systemic lupus erythematosus: Emerging concepts. Part 1: Renal, neuropsychiatric, cardiovascular, pulmonary, and hematologic disease, *and* Part 2: Dermatologic and joint disease, the antiphospholipid antibody syndrome, pregnancy and hormonal therapy, morbidity and mortality, and pathogenesis. Ann Intern Med 1995;122:940, and 1995; 123:42.

Hochberg MC et al: Systemic lupus erythematosus: A review of clinico-laboratory features and immunogenetic markers in 150 patients with emphasis on demographic subsets. Medicine 1985;64:285.

Stevens MB: The clinical spectrum of SLE. Md Med J 1991; 40:875.

Rheumatoid Arthritis

Mary Betty Stevens, MD

Rheumatoid arthritis is an inflammatory, immune-mediated, systemic process of unknown cause, primarily targeting the synovial membrane that lines peripheral joints. The chronic inflammatory response—synovial proliferation and hypertrophy, along with release of chemical mediators—can lead to erosion of articular cartilage and bone, disruption of supporting soft tissue structures, and eventual joint deformity and dysfunction. Although systemic features are prominent in some patients, in most the presenting and dominant feature is polyarthritis.

Rheumatoid arthritis is the most common chronic inflammatory arthritis, affecting about 1% of adults. The disease can begin in infancy or as late as the 80's. Peak prevalence is in young and middle-aged adults, with women predominating by 2:1, but when the disease starts at age 60 or later, men and women are equally likely to be affected. All ethnic groups worldwide are at risk. Although the etiology of rheumatoid arthritis is unknown, susceptibility to the disease is genetically determined: Almost all affected patients have a class II human leukocyte antigen (HLA) containing an identical five-amino-acid sequence.

The importance of rheumatoid arthritis is its frequency and potential severity. The diagnosis is primarily clinical, based chiefly on the pattern of joint involvement. Early diagnosis and treatment may help prevent patients from becoming disabled.

CLINICAL MANIFESTATIONS

The early manifestations of rheumatoid arthritis are unpredictable. Some patients have constitutional symptoms—unusual fatigability, lack of energy, and lethargy—for weeks before they develop joint symptoms. In some patients the first manifestation is polymyalgia rheumatica, with its proximal limb and girdle muscle pain. Other patients begin with an acute, refractory monoarthritis. An occasional person has an explosive polyarticular onset. Regardless of the presentation, only when a polyarthritis persists for at least 6 weeks can the diagnosis of rheumatoid arthritis be considered. Premature labeling is hazardous, since so many disorders mimic early rheumatoid arthritis (see "Differential Diagnosis" below).

Articular Features

The hallmark of rheumatoid arthritis is inflammatory arthritis, chiefly involving many of the small joints of the hands (Figure 3.3–1). Specifically, the proximal interphalangeal joints (PIPs), metacarpophalangeal joints (MCPs), and wrists become painful, swollen, warm, and tender; these sites may dominate for months or even years before other peripheral joints become involved. Although rheumatoid arthritis can affect almost any peripheral joint, the distal interphalangeal joints (DIPs) are usually spared. Typically, progression of the synovial inflammation is additive and symmetric, simultaneously affecting the same PIPs and MCPs on both hands. This symmetry is so characteristic of rheumatoid arthritis that it is an important early diagnostic clue. In patients with a monoarticular onset, the knee is a frequent target.

With time and continued inflammation, the synovium hypertrophies and a mass of inflammatory tissue (pannus) develops and extends in from the joint margins to overlie the articular cartilage. Erosions begin at the joint margins and eventually destroy joint structure and alignment. Typical deformities (Figure 3.3–2) result not only from the intra-articular destruction of cartilage and bone, but also from the extra-articular compromise of supporting tendons and ligaments. As deformities worsen, patients lose joint function and range of motion, often to the point of disability. But even in patients who do not respond to treatment, disability develops only after years or decades of smoldering synovial inflammation.

Less often involved than the peripheral joints are the upper cervical segments and the sternoclavicular, cricoarytenoid, and temporomandibular joints. When inflammation at these sites causes clinical problems, they usually emerge late in rheumatoid arthritis. Unlike the spondyloarthropathies, rheumatoid arthritis spares the thoracolumbar spine and sacroiliac joints.

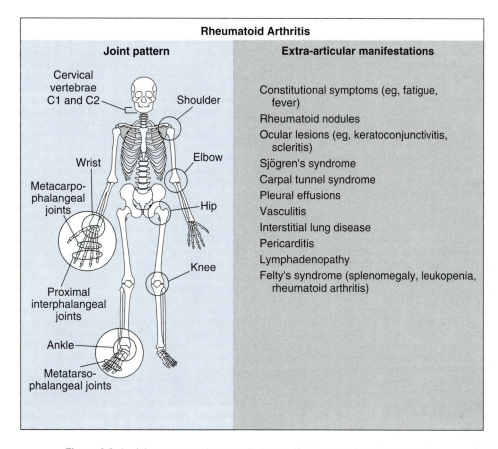

Rheumatoid Arthritis

Joint pattern

- Cervical vertebrae C1 and C2
- Shoulder
- Wrist
- Elbow
- Metacarpo-phalangeal joints
- Hip
- Proximal interphalangeal joints
- Knee
- Ankle
- Metatarso-phalangeal joints

Extra-articular manifestations

Constitutional symptoms (eg, fatigue, fever)
Rheumatoid nodules
Ocular lesions (eg, keratoconjunctivitis, scleritis)
Sjögren's syndrome
Carpal tunnel syndrome
Pleural effusions
Vasculitis
Interstitial lung disease
Pericarditis
Lymphadenopathy
Felty's syndrome (splenomegaly, leukopenia, rheumatoid arthritis)

Figure 3.3–1. Joint pattern and extra-articular manifestations of rheumatoid arthritis.

Periarticular Features

Patients with active disease have the gel phenomenon (stiffness and resistance to movement after a period of immobility). Gelling can be more troublesome than joint pain. Upon arising in the morning, most patients have stiffness lasting longer than 30 minutes; focal (eg, impaired grip, slowed walking) or generalized stiffness may persist for hours. Although morning stiffness is important enough to be a diagnostic criterion for rheumatoid arthritis, gelling develops after immobility as brief as 1–2 hours.

Tenosynovitis (inflammation of a tendon sheath) is especially prominent in the wrists. In addition to palpable hypertrophied synovium—peristyloid and on the dorsum—patients can have tendon sheath effusions and rupture or displacement of the extensor tendons to the fourth and fifth fingers (Figure 3.3–3). The boggy synovium can also encroach upon the median nerve and cause carpal tunnel syndrome (Chapter 3.12). In the early stages of carpal tunnel syndrome, patients often awaken at night with numbness and tingling of the fingers. Later, patients develop weakness of the opponens motion of the thumb, and thenar atrophy.

About 20–30% of patients with rheumatoid arthritis

have periarticular subcutaneous nodules (Figure 3.3–4). Nodules are tissue reactions to a focal arteriolitis. A nodule contains central necrosis and cellular debris surrounded by an encapsulated palisade of inflammatory and epithelioid cells. Nodules typically appear adjacent to inflamed joints and areas of pressure like the Achilles tendons or the periolecranon extensor surface of the forearm. Multiple nodules near the interphalangeal joints can impair digital function. Rheumatoid nodules can develop not only in subcutaneous tissue, but also within the intra-articular synovial mass and in the viscera.

Patients with synovitis of the knees can develop a synovial fluid-filled cyst (Baker's cyst) posteriorly, in or below the popliteal space (Chapter 3.12). In a few patients, the cyst compresses veins or lymphatics, causing lower extremity edema. Far more often, the cyst ruptures or dissects into the calf, causing the pseudothrombophlebitis syndrome. Pseudothrombophlebitis closely mimics true thrombophlebitis, even with a positive Homans' sign, and must be differentiated from deep vein thrombosis because it is treated differently. Although immobilized patients with rheumatoid arthritis are at risk for deep vein thrombosis, very few develop it except after orthopedic surgery; their antirheumatoid drugs may be protective.

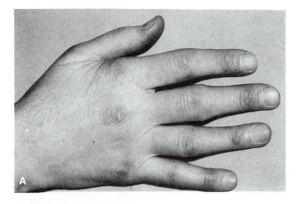

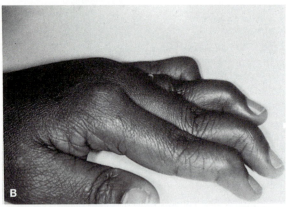

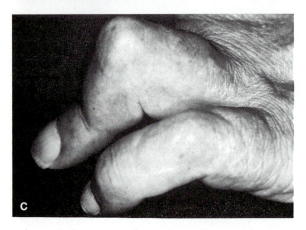

Figure 3.3–2. Joint deformities in rheumatoid arthritis. **A:** Early symmetric proximal interphalangeal joint deformity. **B:** Swan neck deformity. **C:** Boutonnière deformity. (All panels reprinted from the Clinical Slide Collection on the Rheumatic Diseases, copyright 1991. Used by permission of the American College of Rheumatology.)

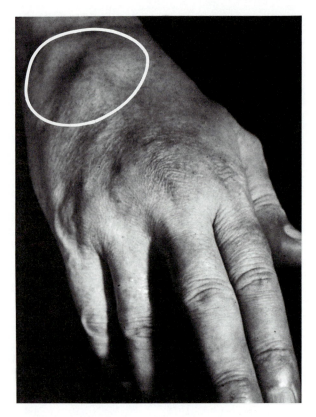

Figure 3.3–3. Extensor tendon rupture of fourth and fifth fingers in rheumatoid arthritis. Within the circle at the wrist are three mounds of inflamed synovium (pannus). (Reprinted from the Clinical Slide Collection on the Rheumatic Diseases, copyright 1991. Used by permission of the American College of Rheumatology.)

Extra-Articular Features

Although a peripheral polyarthritis dominates in most patients, rheumatoid arthritis is a systemic disorder. Constitutional symptoms, especially fatigue and easy tiring, are prominent during active disease and may precede joint inflammation by several weeks. In adults, fever is infrequent and low grade; high fever should alert the physician to an intercurrent problem, especially infection. The only adults likely to present with high fever are those with acute-onset juvenile rheumatoid arthritis (Still's disease), which can begin as late as the fourth decade. In most adults with this unusual variant, joint involvement is overshadowed by a hectic fever (daily fever with severe sweating, chills, and facial flushing) with a double quotidian pattern. Another key sign is a nonpruritic salmon-colored macular rash, chiefly on the trunk; but not every patient has the rash, it may appear only when a patient has a high fever, and it is hard to see in blacks. Adult Still's disease can also cause sore throat, lymphadenopathy, splenomegaly, leukocytosis, and pericarditis.

Muscle wasting and weakness in rheumatoid arthritis are multifactorial and often progressive. The major cause is disuse. Wasting and weakness are worst around involved joints (eg, interossei with digital and wrist inflammation, quadriceps with synovitis of the knees). Tendon contractures can further limit muscle function. Some patients have an inflammatory myopathy.

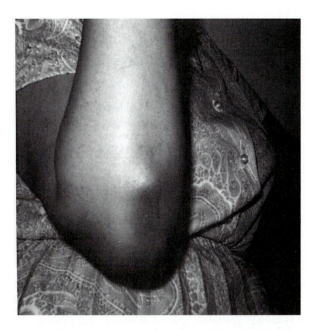

Figure 3.3–4. Subcutaneous nodules in rheumatoid arthritis.

Patients with rheumatoid arthritis may have eye lesions, most commonly keratoconjunctivitis sicca (secondary Sjögren's syndrome; Chapter 3.4). The most characteristic ocular feature, though an infrequent one, is scleral and episcleral inflammation, sometimes with necrotizing scleritis, episcleral granulomatous nodules, or, rarely, scleromalacia perforans. For many children with a monoarticular or oligoarticular onset of rheumatoid arthritis, the most serious part of the disease is a chronic iridocyclitis, often complicated by cataracts and band keratopathy.

The heart and lungs may be involved in rheumatoid arthritis, but not often to the point of causing clinical problems. The most common manifestation, serositis—pericarditis or pleuritis—affects fewer than 10% of patients. Effusions are usually small, but can be large enough to cause cardiac tamponade. The characteristic effusion is mildly exudative, with a moderate leukocytosis, low glucose, elevated protein, and decreased complement level. The low complement supports the theory that immune complexes are injuring the serous membranes. Chronic pleural scarring has been reported, and, rarely, constrictive pericarditis.

Granulomatous nodules, akin to subcutaneous nodules, can develop in the myocardium and on heart valves. Clinical complications are unusual, but patients can develop arrhythmias and rare patients require valve replacement. Most clinical cardiac problems in patients with rheumatoid arthritis are essentially the same as non–arthritis-related heart conditions in the population at large.

Few patients have lesions of the lung parenchyma. The most common lung manifestation, affecting fewer than 5% of patients, is a diffuse interstitial fibrosis that can im-

pair diffusing capacity and alveolar-capillary gas exchange. Rheumatoid granulomatous nodules in the lungs are rare. A rheumatoid arthritis-related pneumoconiosis (Caplan's syndrome), with large silicotic nodules in the lungs, was first described in Welsh miners of soft coal, and is rare in the United States.

About 15–25% of patients with rheumatoid arthritis have lymphadenopathy and 5–10% have splenomegaly. Felty's syndrome is rheumatoid arthritis combined with massive splenomegaly that causes a selective granulocytopenia; patients with this syndrome suffer from refractory leg ulcers and recurrent infections. Especially in early rheumatoid arthritis, a few patients have reticuloendothelial hyperplasia severe enough to suggest lymphoma or sarcoidosis.

Rheumatoid vasculitis (Chapter 3.5) is clinically expressed in several ways, most often the subcutaneous nodule. Other manifestations are periungual infarcts, nailbed splinter hemorrhages, and, in the legs, large indolent ulcers, especially around the distal forelegs and ankles. Inflammation of the nutrient vessels to peripheral nerves leads to peripheral neuropathy. Although rheumatoid vasculitis typically involves the small vessels, an occasional patient has a necrotizing arteritis that perfectly mimics polyarteritis nodosa and may be an "overlap syndrome" of the two disorders.

A few patients with rheumatoid arthritis have Raynaud's phenomenon, but it is usually mild and nonprogressive. It is not related to rheumatoid vasculitis.

DIAGNOSIS

In adults, rheumatoid arthritis is primarily a clinical diagnosis, based on a chronic (at least 6–12 weeks), additive, symmetric peripheral polyarthritis. Serum anti-IgG or rheumatoid factor (see below), especially in high titer, lends diagnostic support but is not specific for rheumatoid arthritis; likewise, seronegativity does not rule out the diagnosis. Subcutaneous nodules rarely develop early, and typical joint erosions appear on x-ray only after months or years. Thus, early diagnosis can be difficult. A process should not be prematurely labeled "rheumatoid arthritis." Some patients carry the designation "unclassified polyarthritis" for months, until the joint pattern of rheumatoid arthritis becomes established or the systemic features of a nonrheumatoid disorder emerge.

Differential Diagnosis

Rheumatoid arthritis must be distinguished from other common conditions that cause chronic polyarthritis (Table 3.3–1). The polyarthritis of systemic lupus erythematosus is usually less severe, rarely causing deformity and almost never producing bony erosions. Instead, lupus is much more likely than rheumatoid arthritis to cause multisystem disease, with photosensitivity, alopecia, central nervous system abnormalities, and kidney disease. Lupus also has distinctive serologic abnormalities (Chapter 3.2).

Osteoarthritis (Chapter 3.9) and rheumatoid arthritis are

Table 3.3–1. Differential diagnosis of common disorders causing chronic polyarthritis.

Condition	How Differs from Rheumatoid Arthritis
Rheumatoid arthritis	
Systemic lupus erythematosus	Arthritis less severe, multisystem disease common
Osteoarthritis	Striking DIP involvement but wrists and MCPs spared, no rheumatoid nodules, no systemic features
Psoriatic arthritis	DIP involvement, rash, nail changes
Gout	History of monoarthritis and synovial urate crystals

DIP, distal interphalangeal joints; MCP, metacarpophalangeal joint.

usually easy to distinguish. Unlike rheumatoid arthritis, osteoarthritis usually affects the distal interphalangeal joints (DIPs), spares the metacarpophalangeal joints (MCPs) and wrists, does not cause subcutaneous nodules, and produces no systemic systems.

Psoriatic arthritis (Chapter 3.7) is notable for its rash and nail changes, predilection for the DIPs, and negative rheumatoid factor test.

Gout (Chapter 3.8) usually begins as an episodic monoarticular disease, but, left untreated, can become a chronic polyarthritis that mimics rheumatoid arthritis. Clues to gout are a long history of episodic monoarthritis and urate crystals in synovial fluid.

Less common conditions that can cause a polyarthritis include sarcoidosis, systemic vasculitis, polymyalgia rheumatica, rheumatic fever, amyloidosis, calcium pyrophosphate dihydrate deposition (CPPD) disease, arthritis associated with malignancy, arthritis of inflammatory bowel disease, and infections, both viral (eg, rubella, parvovirus B19) and bacterial (eg, Lyme disease, secondary syphilis).

Even in patients with clear-cut rheumatoid arthritis, not every clinical event can be attributed to the rheumatoid arthritis. For example, these patients are at high risk for septic arthritis. When they suffer a "flare" in synovitis—especially if monoarticular—the physician must rule out infection before safely assuming an exacerbation of the rheumatoid arthritis. Similarly, although insidious weight loss can be a feature of rheumatoid arthritis, this finding should alert the physician to a possible metabolic disorder or an occult malignancy.

Special Tests

Hematology: Almost 50% of patients with rheumatoid arthritis have anemia, characteristically a mild anemia of chronic disease, with low serum iron and iron-binding capacity. However, with time and treatment, patients may develop a multifactorial anemia; this should be suspected when the hematocrit is less than 30%. Patients with rheumatoid arthritis have a high prevalence of peptic ulcer, made even higher by the ulcerogenic capacity of nonsteroidal anti-inflammatory drugs (NSAIDs); ulcer

bleeding may superimpose iron deficiency on existing anemia. A few patients have chronic folate deficiency or pernicious anemia.

The white blood cell count is usually normal, but may be high or low. The splenomegaly in patients with Felty's syndrome can produce a selective granulocytopenia leading to severe leukopenia. During active rheumatoid arthritis, patients with vasculitis and extra-articular systemic lesions may have eosinophilia and, more likely, thrombocytosis. Other markers of active inflammation are the acute phase reactants C-reactive protein, α_2-globulins, and especially the erythrocyte sedimentation rate, which is valuable in monitoring both rheumatoid arthritis and its response to therapy.

Synovial Fluid: The main reason for testing the synovial fluid is not to diagnose rheumatoid arthritis but to rule out other processes, especially infection and crystal disease. Rheumatoid arthritis produces the same changes as any inflammatory process. The synovial fluid looks grossly turbid. The inflammatory process breaks down the hyaluronate complexes in the synovial fluid, thereby reducing its normal viscosity. The protein level is high and the glucose can be low. A very low glucose may suggest infection, especially when the white blood cell count is high; a polymorphonuclear leukocytosis is the rule, with 5,000–50,000 cells/mm^3.

Serology: The key serologic abnormality in rheumatoid arthritis is rheumatoid factor, an immunoglobulin (usually IgM class) directed against the Fc portion of IgG (Chapter 3.1). About 70–85% of patients with rheumatoid arthritis have rheumatoid factor. It usually appears early in the disease: 75% of those who will ever be seropositive become so within the first year. The prevalence of rheumatoid factor is especially high in patients with subcutaneous nodules, vasculitis, and the variant syndromes (Caplan's, Felty's, Sjögren's), and in patients with x-ray evidence of erosions.

A positive latex agglutination test for rheumatoid factor does not prove rheumatoid arthritis, and must be interpreted in the context of the clinical setting. Part of the problem is that the latex test is positive in many other chronic diseases. For example, 20–50% of patients with systemic lupus erythematosus, subacute bacterial endocarditis, or interstitial pulmonary fibrosis have rheumatoid factor; so do 40% of those with hepatocellular disease. Moreover, rheumatoid factor is found in 5–10% of healthy adults and in even more of the elderly. Patients with rheumatoid arthritis tend to have higher titers than nonrheumatoid individuals.

Antinuclear antibody (ANA) to deoxyribonucleoprotein, detectable by either the lupus erythematosus (LE) cell phenomenon or its immunofluorescent analog (in a homogeneous ANA pattern), can be found in rheumatoid arthritis, usually at a low titer. About 25% of patients have LE cells, and 30–60% have antinuclear antibodies.

Despite the low complement levels in rheumatoid

serous membrane effusions, few patients have hypocomplementemia. Those who do tend to have both advanced disease and rheumatoid vasculitis.

Radiography: Radiographic abnormalities lag months or even years behind the symptoms of synovitis in rheumatoid arthritis and other inflammatory arthropathies (Figure 3.3–5). The earliest x-ray finding in rheumatoid arthritis is periarticular osteopenia, especially PIP and MCP joints. With persistent synovial inflammation and hypertrophy, the articular cartilage is lost and the joint space narrows. Erosions develop and progress in the bone margins. Erosions are worst in the PIPs, MCPs, and wrists, but any peripheral joint can be involved. A late postinflammatory sequela is secondary osteoarthritis.

Biopsy: The histopathology of rheumatoid arthritis, although characteristic, is not diagnostic. Depending on the disease stage, the synovial membrane shows more or less acute and chronic inflammation. Synovial biopsy is of less value in diagnosing rheumatoid arthritis than in ruling out

disorders (eg, gout, sarcoidosis, neoplasia) that mimic it. Even the classic subcutaneous nodule of rheumatoid arthritis is seen in other conditions.

Tissue biopsy can define extra-articular features of rheumatoid arthritis (eg, vasculitis, silicotic pulmonary nodules of Caplan, bone marrow of Felty, salivary gland immunopathology of Sjögren) as well as nonrheumatoid processes (eg, tumor).

COURSE AND PROGNOSIS

On average, patients with rheumatoid arthritis die about 10 years earlier than people who do not have the disease. However, the course of rheumatoid arthritis is highly variable. Patients with high-titer rheumatoid factor, the early appearance of subcutaneous nodules, and articular erosions on x-ray have a poorer prognosis than those who are seronegative and have neither nodules nor erosions. Certain HLA-DRB1 alleles also help to identify patients at risk for severe disease. Patients with a monoarticular onset

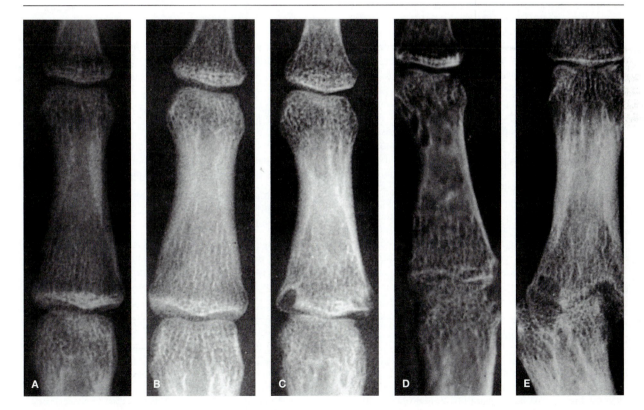

Figure 3.3–5. X-ray progression of rheumatoid arthritis in the proximal interphalangeal (PIP) joint. **A:** Normal phalanx. **B:** Early rheumatoid arthritis. The only abnormality is soft tissue swelling around the joint. **C:** A more advanced lesion. The x-ray shows soft tissue swelling, periarticular osteopenia, and a narrowed joint space. The middle phalanx has a large "punched-out" erosion in the juxta-articular bone; both sides of the joint have irregular small erosions on the articular margins. **D:** Pronounced osteopenia and marked narrowing of the joint space, with ragged surface erosions on both sides of the joint. **E:** Late stage. Both of the articular surfaces and the underlying bone show erosion and destruction. The joint is subluxated.

and an oligoarticular pattern may have a more benign course.

Most patients with rheumatoid arthritis develop deformities in one or more joints, but aggressive early therapy can limit major loss of function to fewer than one-third of patients.

MANAGEMENT

The aims of management are to preserve joint structure and function and to control the systemic features. Fulfilling these aims requires both suppressing the inflammatory process and maintaining the supporting periarticular structures. Comprehensive management includes general health and physical measures, drug therapy, and, for some patients, surgery.

A balanced program of rest and therapeutic exercise should be started early to maintain normal range of motion and preserve muscle strength. Resting involved joints is especially important during active synovitis; splinting can help prevent malalignment and contractures in inflamed joints that are not responding to drug treatment.

Three main classes of drugs are used to suppress the inflammatory process: NSAIDs, remittive (disease-modifying) agents, and corticosteroids. Regimens combining these drugs are designed based on both efficacy and tolerance. Regimens vary from one patient to another, and for the individual patient over time. With early diagnosis and therapy, remissions can be induced for months, even years, especially in seronegative patients who do not have nodules.

NSAIDs offer the primary action of salicylates: inhibition of prostaglandin synthesis. Any advantage that NSAIDs hold over salicylates relates to the NSAIDs' lesser gastrointestinal side-effects; the longer half-life of several NSAIDs, permitting a simpler dosage schedule; and their tolerance by patients who cannot take aspirin and other salicylates. A NSAID is never given together with another NSAID or with aspirin, because this increases toxicity without improving therapeutic benefit. A NSAID alone cannot control rheumatoid arthritis, but must be combined with a remittive agent.

The remittive agents include hydroxychloroquine, gold, D-penicillamine, sulfasalazine, and methotrexate. Despite their chemical diversity, these drugs share a lag time of several weeks to months before they become fully effective. Begun early in the disease, they also share the capacity to induce remissions lasting years. Meager comparative drug trial data, along with the unpredictability and chronicity of rheumatoid arthritis, make it difficult to favor one first-line remittive agent over others. The remittive agents can cause serious side effects, such as cytopenia (gold, penicillamine, sulfasalazine, methotrexate), proteinuria (gold, penicillamine), visual loss (hydroxychloroquine), and liver disease (methotrexate).

Patients may need low-dose corticosteroids to suppress inflammation while a remittive agent is taking effect, or to control systemic disease. Intermittent (pulse) therapy may be less toxic than daily dosing.

Orthopedic surgery is best reserved for the patient with late-stage rheumatoid arthritis who has postinflammatory joint deformity with dysfunction. Total joint replacement of the hip or knee is especially effective at relieving pain and improving the patient's ability to walk.

SUMMARY

▶ Rheumatoid arthritis is diagnosed by its characteristic chronic symmetric inflammatory polyarthritis affecting peripheral joints. Blood tests are nonspecific.

▶ High-titer rheumatoid factor seropositivity (anti-IgG), subcutaneous nodules, and joint erosions seen on x-ray are risk factors for progressive joint disease.

▶ Rheumatoid arthritis can be a systemic disorder, causing fatigue, muscle wasting, eye lesions, heart and lung involvement, and vasculitis.

▶ Management includes physical as well as drug therapy. Early treatment with anti-inflammatory and remittive drugs minimizes the risk of permanent joint deformity.

SUGGESTED READING

Arnett FC et al: The American Rheumatism Association 1987 revised criteria for the classification of rheumatoid arthritis. Arthritis Rheum 1988;31:315.

Felson DT, Anderson JJ, Meenan RF: The comparative efficacy and toxicity of second-line drugs in rheumatoid arthritis: Results of two metaanalyses. Arthritis Rheum 1990;33:1449.

Multiauthored Section IV on Rheumatoid Arthritis. In: *Arthritis and Allied Conditions,* 12th ed. McCarty DJ, Koopman WJ (editors). Lea & Febiger, 1993.

Reginato AJ et al: Adult onset Still's disease: Experience in 23 patients and literature review with emphasis on organ failure. Semin Arthritis Rheum 1987;17:39.

Sjögren's Syndrome

Mary Betty Stevens, MD

Sjögren's syndrome is an autoimmune disease whose cardinal presenting features—dry eyes (xerophthalmia) and dry mouth (xerostomia)—are caused by lymphocytic infiltration and destruction of the lacrimal and salivary glands. Sjögren's syndrome is considered a domain of rheumatologists because many patients have Sjögren's syndrome secondary to another autoimmune disease, usually rheumatoid arthritis or systemic lupus erythematosus. Even without rheumatoid arthritis or lupus, primary Sjögren's syndrome can be complicated by such systemic manifestations as arthralgia, vasculitis, or nervous system involvement (Figure 3.4–1). The physician should be aware of Sjögren's syndrome as a frequent cause of the common symptoms of dry eyes and dry mouth, while recognizing that the systemic manifestations may be serious and that some patients with Sjögren's are at risk of developing lymphoma.

CLINICAL FEATURES

Sjögren's syndrome affects nine times more women than men. It can begin at any time of life, including childhood, but typically starts after age 50. The articular features of primary Sjögren's syndrome are usually minor, often limited to arthralgia; most prominent joint problems are seen in patients who have Sjögren's secondary to rheumatoid arthritis. Sjögren's is dominated by extra-articular manifestations, some caused by sicca (dryness), others by systemic illness.

Sicca Syndrome

The most common presenting complaint of Sjögren's syndrome is xerophthalmia. Patients report a grittiness or a foreign-body sensation in their eyes. They can develop conjunctival and corneal inflammation and even corneal ulcerations (keratoconjunctivitis sicca), which cause photophobia and pain. Few patients lose visual acuity and few are unable to cry. Despite the lymphocytic infiltration, the lacrimal glands are usually not enlarged.

Patients with xerostomia have multiple problems, including difficulty in chewing, inability to swallow dry foods, altered taste, buccal and lip fissures, increased dental cavities, and periodontal inflammation. Normally, saliva inhibits tooth decay by providing both a washing solution and antibacterial salivary IgA. Loss of saliva causes many patients with Sjögren's syndrome to note that after years of having few cavities, they are suddenly developing rampant caries. Patients with severe xerostomia may have impaired phonation. Most patients increase their fluid intake throughout the day and even during the night. Because saliva also plays an important role in clearing acid from the distal esophagus, some patients with Sjögren's have heartburn.

On physical examination, patients have little or no sublingual salivary pool, and the buccal membranes appear dry and lusterless. The tongue is dry and fissured. Fifty percent of patients have enlarged parotid glands, and 20% have enlarged submental salivary glands. The salivary gland enlargement is usually bilateral, symmetric, and nontender. Recurrent enlargement is among the risk factors for lymphoma. When parotid enlargement is unilateral, painful, and tender, the physician should consider an unusual acute suppurative parotitis secondary to inspissated secretions. Similarly, a hard segment of the parotid should arouse suspicion of a tumor.

The dryness of sicca syndrome is not always confined to the conjunctival and buccal membranes, but can involve the entire respiratory tree. Patients may have nasal crusting, nosebleeds, and an altered sense of smell. Hoarseness is unusual. Dryness of the tracheobronchial segments may manifest as a nonproductive cough, bronchitis, or, infrequently, pneumonitis. Many patients have vaginal dryness, resulting in dyspareunia and vaginal candidiasis. Abdominal problems are uncommon, even though achlorhydria can be detected in asymptomatic pa-

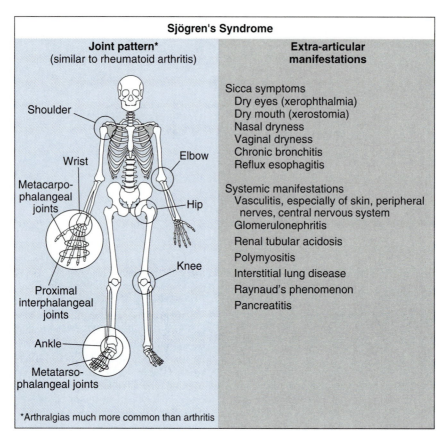

Figure 3.4–1. Joint pattern and extra-articular manifestations of Sjögren's syndrome.

tients. A rare patient develops acute pancreatitis with a lymphocytic infiltration similar to that found in the lacrimal and salivary glands.

Systemic Manifestations

Most patients with primary Sjögren's syndrome, especially older people, have the sicca syndrome alone, with no extraglandular involvement. However, systemic manifestations can be part of the primary syndrome. Many patients have arthralgia; fewer have peripheral polyarthritis. Erosive joint disease and deformities are unusual. About 10% of patients have a myositis that resembles polymyositis. Up to 20% of patients have Raynaud's phenomenon, and some of those have associated esophageal aperistalsis, but without other evidence of scleroderma.

Vasculitis may be seen, especially in patients who have anti-Ro(SSA) antibody (see "Autoantibodies" below). The vasculitis is usually limited to the skin, often appearing as palpable purpura or ulcers. Infrequently, vasculitis in Sjögren's involves the central and peripheral nervous systems, manifested among other ways by cognitive disorders, trigeminal neuralgia, and dysesthesia. Vasculitis is particularly common among patients who will later de-

velop lymphoma. Renal manifestations of Sjögren's syndrome are unusual, but can include renal tubular acidosis and glomerulonephritis. Obstructive or interstitial pulmonary disease can complicate the course of Sjögren's.

In secondary Sjögren's syndrome, the extraglandular features are those of the underlying autoimmune disorder, most often rheumatoid arthritis or systemic lupus erythematosus (Table 3.4–1). Sjögren's is found in over one-third of patients with autoimmune hepatitis and more than half of those with primary biliary cirrhosis. Sjögren's is also seen in patients with autoimmune (Hashimoto's) thyroiditis.

Table 3.4–1. Diseases associated with Sjögren's syndrome.

Rheumatoid arthritis
Systemic lupus erythematosus
Scleroderma
Hashimoto's thyroiditis
Autoimmune hepatitis
Primary biliary cirrhosis
Cryoglobulinemia
Polymyositis

LABORATORY STUDIES

Sicca Complex

Eye dryness is measured objectively by Schirmer's test. The examiner suspends a strip of filter paper from the patient's lower eyelid for 5 minutes and then measures the distance the paper is moistened. A normal person's tears will wet the strip to at least 5 mm, but a patient with xerophthalmia will not reach 5 mm. The examiner can assess the severity of eye dryness by applying a drop of rose bengal solution to the eye. Injured epithelial cells take up the red stain, making corneal defects easily visible.

Salivary function is more difficult to measure and is rarely tested. Lip biopsy of the minor salivary glands is a benign procedure; the degree of lymphocytic infiltration determines whether the biopsy is diagnostic of Sjögren's syndrome. Tissue biopsy of the major salivary glands, especially the parotid, carries significant risk of causing fistulous drainage.

Routine Tests

Hematologic abnormalities are common in primary Sjögren's syndrome. One-third of patients have leukopenia and one-fourth have a mild normochromic, normocytic anemia. Most patients have an elevated erythrocyte sedimentation rate. A few have chemical evidence of renal tubular acidosis and hyperamylasemia, but no clinical signs. Patients who have Sjögren's with autoimmune hepatitis or primary biliary cirrhosis can be expected to have hepatocellular dysfunction.

Serum Proteins

About 50% of patients with primary Sjögren's syndrome have hyperglobulinemia, usually caused by a polyclonal increase in γ-globulins. Less frequent is a monoclonal IgM gammopathy or mixed cryoglobulinemia. Progressive decline in the serum γ-globulin level, development of hypogammaglobulinemia, or loss of rheumatoid factor positivity should alert the physician to the possible emergence of a lymphoma.

Autoantibodies

Patients with Sjögren's syndrome produce autoantibodies. In patients with secondary Sjögren's, the serologic profile reflects both Sjögren's and the associated disorder. Most patients with both primary and secondary Sjögren's, whether or not they also have rheumatoid arthritis, make rheumatoid factor (anti-IgG). Similarly, whether or not patients have systemic lupus erythematosus, a majority make antinuclear antibodies. Anticentromere or anti-Scl-70 antibodies are found only when Sjögren's is superimposed on scleroderma (Chapter 3.10).

Most patients with primary Sjögren's syndrome have antibodies to the nucleoprotein antigens Ro(SSA) and La(SSB). These antibodies are not specific to primary Sjögren's, as was once thought. Anti-Ro(SSA) is also found in 20% of patients who have systemic lupus erythemato-

sus unrelated to the sicca complex and in all mothers of infants with either neonatal lupus or congenital heart block, whether or not the mothers have clinical lupus. These associations have strengthened the evidence for a close immunologic link between primary Sjögren's syndrome and systemic lupus. Furthermore, anti-Ro(SSA) in primary Sjögren's is highly correlated with vasculitis and may signal increased risk for major dysproteinemias and lymphoma.

DIAGNOSIS

Sjögren's syndrome is primarily a clinical diagnosis, first suggested by xerophthalmia, xerostomia, or both. Lacrimal gland failure is usually documented by Schirmer's test of tearing and by rose bengal staining of the cornea (see "Sicca Complex" above). Tissue proof of Sjögren's syndrome comes from a lip biopsy of the minor salivary glands showing the characteristic lymphocytic infiltration. Lip biopsy is needed only when patients present with an unconvincing picture, for example, when their sole symptom is a dry mouth. Buccal membrane dryness is not specific to Sjögren's syndrome. The differential diagnosis of xerostomia includes drugs (especially tricyclic antidepressants and diuretics), chronic mouth breathing, sarcoidosis, head and neck radiation, and type V hyperlipidemia. Likewise, parotid gland enlargement can reflect such processes as suppurative parotitis, sarcoidosis, and neoplasia.

The serologic profile, although nonspecific, can support a diagnosis of Sjögren's, especially when a patient is found to have anti-Ro(SSA). Also supporting the diagnosis are underlying immunologic diseases like systemic lupus erythematosus and rheumatoid arthritis, and associated immunologic conditions like Hashimoto's thyroiditis, autoimmune hepatitis, and primary biliary cirrhosis.

MANAGEMENT

The therapeutic approach to Sjögren's syndrome is twofold, aimed at controlling both the sicca complex and the extraglandular features.

It is easier to wet dry eyes than a dry mouth. Eye drops of artificial tears can relieve symptoms and prevent corneal erosions. Artificial saliva is less well tolerated or effective. Patients can control their xerostomia by increasing their fluid intake and chewing gum and tart sugarless mints. To reduce the risk of cavities, patients should avoid sugary candies, drinks, and desserts. Regular dental visits and fluoride treatments may also help. Secondary oral candidiasis can be treated with antifungal agents.

Although Sjögren's syndrome almost always develops insidiously, the occasional patient with acute parotid enlargement and xerostomia may respond to corticosteroids with improvement in both symptoms and laboratory tests.

For patients with secondary Sjögren's syndrome, treatment of the associated disorder takes priority. This is also true for the few patients with primary Sjögren's who develop dysproteinemia and lymphoma or have associated systemic features, especially vasculitis.

COURSE AND PROGNOSIS

In most patients with primary Sjögren's syndrome, especially older people, the sicca complex usually persists and may slowly worsen. A few patients, especially those with recurrent parotid enlargement, vasculitis, and splenomegaly, develop dysproteinemias and lymphoma. In patients with Sjögren's syndrome secondary to systemic lupus erythematosus, rheumatoid arthritis, or another connective tissue disease, the underlying disorder determines prognosis.

SUMMARY

▶ Sjögren's syndrome (sicca syndrome) is an autoimmune disorder that damages the salivary and lacrimal glands and can cause systemic illness. The cardinal symptoms are dry eyes (xerophthalmia) and dry mouth (xerostomia).

▶ Sjögren's syndrome can occur by itself or accompany other autoimmune diseases, especially rheumatoid arthritis and systemic lupus erythematosus.

▶ Sjögren's syndrome is usually benign. However, a few patients develop serious problems such as vasculitis and lymphoma.

SUGGESTED READING

Alexander EL et al: Sjögren's syndrome: Association of anti-Ro(SSA) antibodies with vasculitis, hematologic abnormalities, and serologic hyperreactivity. Ann Intern Med 1983; 98:155.

Bridges AJ, England DM: Benign lymphoepithelial lesion: Relationship to Sjögren's syndrome and evolving malignant lymphoma. Semin Arthritis Rheum 1989;19:201.

Fox RI (editor): Sjögren's syndrome. Rheum Dis Clin North Am 1992;18:507.

Fox RI et al: Primary Sjögren syndrome: Clinical and immunopathologic features. Semin Arthritis Rheum 1984;14:77.

Marx RE, Hartman KS, Rethman KV: A prospective study comparing incisional labial to incisional parotid biopsies in the detection and confirmation of sarcoidosis, Sjögren's disease, sialosis and lymphoma. J Rheumatol 1988;15:621.

Vasculitis

David B. Hellmann, MD

Vasculitis, an inflammatory destruction of blood vessels, is caused by a heterogeneous group of uncommon disorders. Although the manifestations of the different forms of vasculitis vary greatly, most patients eventually show such signs of multisystem disease as neuropathy, joint pain, pulmonary infiltrates, and skin lesions. Because vasculitis tends to be heralded by nonspecific symptoms like fever, malaise, and weight loss, and because the vascular damage often evolves stealthily over months, vasculitis is one of the great diagnostic puzzles of internal medicine. Solving this puzzle has become rewarding as advances in therapy have transformed the prognosis of vasculitis from certain morbidity and possible death, to near-universal improvement and sometimes cure.

CLASSIFICATION

Since the causes of vasculitis are mostly unknown, the syndromes are classified by a combination of clinical and pathologic features (Table 3.5–1). No single feature is pathognomonic. The size of the affected vessel can provide one level of differentiation. For example, Takayasu's arteritis involves the aorta, polyarteritis nodosa involves small muscular arteries, and hypersensitivity vasculitis involves capillaries and venules. Host factors are also distinctive: Takayasu's arteritis attacks chiefly young women, temporal arteritis afflicts the elderly, and Buerger's disease is limited to heavy smokers. Some syndromes preferentially target certain organs or tissues: Wegener's granulomatosis favors the sinus, lung, and kidney; Cogan's syndrome chiefly affects the cornea, cochlea, and aorta; relapsing polychondritis affects elastic cartilage in the ear and trachea; and Behçet's syndrome almost always produces mouth or genital ulcers or both. Pathologic differences also help in the distinction, since some diseases feature giant cells and granulomas (eg, Takayasu's arteritis, temporal arteritis, Wegener's granu-

lomatosis) and others do not (eg, Behçet's syndrome, Henoch-Schönlein purpura).

Finally, some vasculitic syndromes are associated with other diseases. Churg-Strauss syndrome is usually superimposed on chronic asthma, and some patients develop vasculitis along with malignancies, especially lymphoma and leukemia.

PATHOGENESIS

Although the cause of vasculitis is not well understood, it involves both humoral and cellular immunity. In experimental animals, circulating immune complexes can cause vasculitis by depositing in vascular endothelium, where they activate complement, recruit inflammatory cells, and lead to inflammatory vascular necrosis. In humans, polyarteritis nodosa may be the best example of immune complex-induced vasculitis. Fifty percent of patients have current or past hepatitis B infection, and their vasculitic lesions contain complexes of hepatitis antigen-antibody. Other forms of vasculitis caused by immune complex deposits are hypersensitivity vasculitis and the vasculitis of systemic lupus erythematosus. In contrast, cellular immunity, evidenced by granulomatous inflammation, appears central to the pathogenesis of Wegener's granulomatosis, Takayasu's arteritis, and temporal arteritis. Unfortunately, in none of the granulomatous diseases has an inciting antigen been identified.

PRINCIPLES OF DIAGNOSIS AND TREATMENT

The physician must answer three questions for any patient suspected of having vasculitis. The first is, "How extensive is the vasculitis?" A number of conditions, not discussed in detail here, cause vasculitis only of the skin. Most such conditions have a much better prognosis than systemic vasculitis; few patients need long-term cortico-

Table 3.5–1. Classification and selected clinical features of vasculitis.

Type	Typical Host	Vessels Involved	Target Tissues	Possible Treatment
Polyarteritis nodosa	40-yr-old IV drug abuser	Small muscular arteries	Kidney, nerve, gut, heart	Prednisone + cyclophosphamide
Wegener's granulomatosis	40-yr-old man	Small and medium arteries; veins	Sinus, lung, kidney	Prednisone + cyclophosphamide
Temporal (giant cell) arteritis	>60-yr-old woman or man	Large elastic arteries	Eye	Prednisone
Takayasu's arteritis	20-yr-old woman	Aorta and main branches	Heart, brain, skeletal muscle	Prednisone
Primary angiitis of the CNS	48-yr-old woman	Arterioles, capillaries	Brain	Prednisone + cyclophosphamide
Hypersensitivity vasculitis*	20–50-yr-old woman or man	Capillaries, venules	Skin, kidney, gut, nerve	Prednisone
Vasculitis with connective tissue disease (eg, SLE, rheumatoid arthritis)	35-yr-old woman with SLE	Like polyarteritis nodosa or hypersensitivity vasculitis		Prednisone
Churg-Strauss syndrome	45-yr-old-man with chronic asthma	Like Wegener's granulomatosis	Skin, lung, kidney	Prednisone + cyclophosphamide
Lymphomatoid granulomatosis	50-yr-old man or woman	Like polyarteritis nodosa	Skin, lung, brain	Prednisone + cyclophosphamide
Buerger's disease	35-yr-old male heavy smoker	Arterioles, veins	Skin, digits, muscles	Stop smoking
Cogan's syndrome	50-yr-old man or woman	Aorta, arterioles	Eye, cochlea, heart	Prednisone
Behçet's syndrome	25-yr-old woman	Arterioles, veins	Mouth, genitals, eye, brain	Prednisone or chlorambucil
Vasculitis associated with malignancy	70-yr-old man or woman with lymphoma	Capillaries, veins	Skin	Chemotherapy
Relapsing polychondritis	45-yr-old man or woman	Arterioles	Ear, trachea, eye	Prednisone or dapsone

CNS, central nervous system; SLE, systemic lupus erythematosus.
*Includes serum sickness, Henoch-Schönlein purpura, and cryoglobulinemia.

steroid therapy, and almost none need immunosuppressive treatment. The purpose of the initial history, physical examination, and baseline laboratory tests is to determine whether the patient has an isolated skin condition or systemic vasculitis.

The second question is, "How do I best establish the diagnosis of systemic vasculitis?" Virtually without exception, the diagnosis rests on either biopsies or angiograms. Serologic tests can help, but are not definitive. For example, the antineutrophil cytoplasmic antibody (ANCA) is highly sensitive for Wegener's granulomatosis, but not specific (see "Laboratory Tests" below).

The third question is, "Does the patient need immunosuppressive therapy?" Untreated, systemic vasculitis causes serious illness, and many forms can be fatal. High-dose prednisone improves almost every form of systemic vasculitis. For some forms, such as temporal arteritis and Takayasu's arteritis, patients need only prednisone. For others, such as Wegener's granulomatosis and polyarteritis nodosa, prednisone by itself appears not to produce remission. Patients with these conditions require cyclophosphamide or another immunosuppressive agent.

COMMON FORMS OF SYSTEMIC VASCULITIS

Polyarteritis Nodosa

Polyarteritis nodosa is the prototype of a systemic vasculitis. Polyarteritis nodosa can occur at any age, but usually strikes during the fourth and fifth decades. Men are affected twice as often as women. Fifty percent of patients have an active hepatitis B or hepatitis C infection. The association with hepatitis B and C means that intravenous drug users and patients on chronic renal dialysis are at particular risk for polyarteritis.

Diagnostic Clues: Although the protean manifestations of polyarteritis might at first seem to defy any general guidelines for recognition, several clinical patterns are suggestive (Table 3.5–2). Most patients with polyarteritis have a *multisystem disease* that evolves *subacutely* over weeks or a few months, they show *signs of inflammation,* and they have some kind of *pain,* such as that from neuropathy, arthritis, or an infarcted testicle. Signs of inflammation, along with fever, weight loss, arthritis, and a high erythrocyte sedimentation rate, are common signposts of a

Table 3.5–2. Clues to polyarteritis nodosa.

General
Multisystem disease
Subacute onset
Prominent inflammation
Pain: arthralgia, myalgia, neuralgia

Specific
Peripheral nervous system: mononeuritis multiplex
Skin: palpable purpura, ulcers, livedo reticularis, nodules
Renal: hypertension, proteinuria, hematuria, glomerulonephritis
Gastrointestinal: "abdominal angina," bleeding, gangrene, perforation
Ocular: scleritis
Sudden critical end-organ damage: testicular infarction, myocardial infarction

systemic vasculitis like polyarteritis. The frequency of pain validates the adage that "polyarteritis is a hurting disease." The subacute course helps distinguish polyarteritis and most other systemic forms of vasculitis from acute multisystem diseases such as many bacterial infections, drug reactions, and thrombotic thrombocytopenic purpura (TTP). Systemic vasculitis is rarely fulminant and is seldom first diagnosed in the intensive care unit.

Several signs strongly suggest polyarteritis. One of the most valuable is *mononeuritis multiplex*, which develops in 50% of patients. Mononeuritis multiplex is a distinct peripheral neuropathy in which infarctions of named nerve trunks develop one nerve at a time (Chapter 13.11). In patients who do not have diabetes or trauma, mononeuritis multiplex almost always indicates a systemic vasculitis.

The skin, affected in 20% of patients, often gives early and reliable signs of vasculitis, including *palpable purpura*, ulcers, livedo reticularis, and nodules. Palpable purpura from vasculitis is most often seen on the distal legs and may cause a localized burning sensation. Ulcers and nodules are also common on the legs and are usually painful. Since vasculitis of the skin is so easy to detect, it can be a better clue than some visceral organs that are more commonly but less obviously involved.

Although autopsy studies indicate that all patients have kidney involvement, early kidney disease must usually be inferred from the hypertension that 50% of patients develop. Fifty percent of patients also have gastrointestinal symptoms or signs. Mesenteric vasculitis often produces diffuse abdominal pain that worsens 30–60 minutes after a meal (abdominal angina). Occasionally, vasculitis of the gallbladder mimics cholelithiasis. A few patients have bleeding, gangrene, or perforation of the gut. Even in patients with hepatitis B infection, liver involvement is most often clinically silent. Seventy-five percent of patients have heart involvement, which can cause myocardial infarction or dilated cardiomyopathy. Scleritis is the most common eye manifestation of polyarteritis. Any other sudden ischemic injury to an internal organ, such as testicular infarction, should suggest polyarteritis. The probability of polyarteritis is much higher if a patient has two or more of the signs listed in Table 3.5–2.

Laboratory Tests: On routine laboratory tests, almost all patients with polyarteritis nodosa have an elevated erythrocyte sedimentation rate, three-fourths have a modest leukocytosis, two-thirds have a mild normochromic, normocytic anemia, and half have thrombocytosis. Two-thirds of patients have proteinuria. One-third have an active urine sediment with red blood cell casts. Fifty percent of patients have positive serologies for hepatitis B or hepatitis C infection. A substantial minority have rheumatoid factor and hypocomplementemia. One-third have ANCA. Of the two ANCA patterns, the "P" (perinuclear) pattern is more common in polyarteritis than the "C" (cytoplasmic) pattern (Chapter 3.1).

The diagnosis of polyarteritis nodosa rests on a biopsy showing arteritis or an angiogram showing microaneurysms (Figure 3.5–1). Pathologic changes affect chiefly small- and medium-sized muscular arteries. Depending on the stage of the lesion, changes include endothelial proliferation; infiltration of the vessel wall with first acute, then chronic, inflammatory cells; fibrinoid necrosis; and aneurysms. Angiographically evident aneurysms most often affect the mesenteric, hepatic, or renal arteries. Even in patients who have no abdominal symptoms, mesenteric angiography has a sensitivity of 70%. Biopsy of symptomatic nerve, muscle, or testicle has a similar yield. The biopsy yield at asymptomatic sites is 10–30%.

Course and Treatment: Untreated, polyarteritis nodosa is always fatal. Almost 50% of deaths are from kidney failure; many others are from heart or gastrointestinal complications. With prednisone and immunosuppressive treatment (eg, cyclophosphamide), 5-year survival rate is 80–90%. Hepatitis B-associated polyarteritis nodosa may be treated first with prednisone to reduce vascular inflammation and plasmapheresis to remove immune complexes, and then with interferon to eliminate the hepatitis. Patients also need adjunctive therapy, such as antihypertensive drugs and splints for footdrop.

Temporal Arteritis

Temporal arteritis (also called giant cell arteritis) is a panarteritis of elastin-containing arteries, chiefly affecting the extracranial branches of the carotid artery in the elderly. The importance of temporal arteritis is that without prompt recognition and treatment, it can cause irreversible blindness.

Women are affected twice as often as men. The incidence increases with age: Onset before age 50 is rare, but the annual incidence among octogenarians is 56 of 100,000.

The classic manifestations of temporal arteritis are headache, seen in three-fourths of patients; polymyalgia rheumatica, in almost two-thirds (see "Polymyalgia Rheumatica" below); impaired vision, in one-third; and jaw claudication, in one-fourth. Jaw claudication is pain in the masseter muscles during protracted chewing, as with meats. The pain reflects vasculitis compromising the

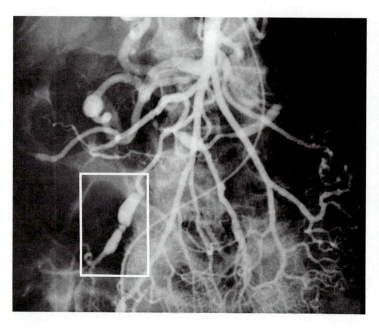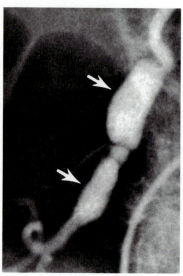

Figure 3.5–1. Polyarteritis nodosa. Mesenteric arteriogram shows multiple diagnostic aneurysmal dilatations, two of which are marked by arrows in the detail panel.

blood supply to the muscles of mastication. One of the major targets of temporal arteritis is the eyes. Patients may report blurred vision, diplopia, or visual loss. The visual loss can be transient, or, typically, permanent. Blindness is the most feared complication of temporal arteritis. Fortunately, visual changes are rarely the disease's first or only manifestation.

Most of the symptoms and signs of temporal arteritis are nonspecific. Many patients present with weight loss and malaise, which may prompt an evaluation for malignancy. One-fifth of patients develop fever, sometimes as their only symptom. In fact, of patients over age 65 who have a fever of unknown origin, one in six has temporal arteritis. The fevers can be as high as 40°C (104°F) and in two-thirds of patients are associated with shaking chills and night sweats, features that make physicians think of infection.

Other symptoms of temporal arteritis are depression, arthralgia (seen more often than arthritis), unexplained cough, throat pain, tongue pain, scalp tenderness, mononeuritis multiplex, and, occasionally, large elastic artery involvement such as aortic regurgitation or aortic aneurysm.

Physical examination in temporal arteritis is usually normal. A few patients have palpable abnormalities of the temporal arteries, caused by thrombosis or nodular swelling. Rare findings are carotid bruits, aortic regurgitation, and synovitis, characteristically affecting the knees, wrists, or sternoclavicular joints.

The laboratory triad of temporal arteritis is (1) a markedly elevated erythrocyte sedimentation rate (typi-

cally >100 mm/hr by the Westergren method) in almost all patients; (2) normochromic, normocytic anemia, in 50% of patients; and (3) a moderately elevated alkaline phosphatase, in one-third of patients. However, these findings are not specific. For example, anemia and a high erythrocyte sedimentation rate are compatible with occult malignancy such as multiple myeloma. The white blood cell count is almost always normal, even in patients whose temporal arteritis has taken the form of fever of unknown origin.

Since the blindness caused by temporal arteritis can be permanent, the patient should be started on high-dose prednisone (40–80 mg/day), as soon as the physician *suspects* the diagnosis, before results of biopsy have been received. The diagnosis is confirmed when a biopsy of the temporal artery shows inflammatory destruction (Figure 3.5–2). It is not known how quickly therapy changes the vessels, but experience has shown that destruction of the elastic lamina is a persistent marker of temporal arteritis, so most biopsies done within 1 week of starting therapy are accurate. Since arteritis often "skips" parts of a vessel, the surgeon should remove a 3–5-cm segment and the pathologist should make multiple sections. Giant cells are not always seen and are not required for the diagnosis. False-negatives occur in 5–15% of patients. Once started on prednisone, most patients feel much better within a few days, and laboratory tests become normal within 1 month. The prednisone can then be tapered slowly over 6–24 months, while the physician monitors the patient's symptoms and erythrocyte sedimentation rate for evidence of reactivation.

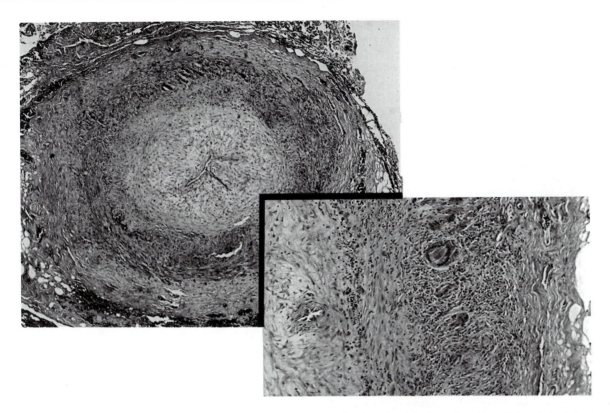

Figure 3.5–2. Temporal arteritis. Biopsy of the temporal artery shows proliferation of endothelium, disruption of internal elastic lamina, and infiltration of media and adventitia by inflammatory and giant cells. Giant cells are especially visible in the detail panel.

Polymyalgia Rheumatica

Polymyalgia rheumatica is a syndrome of pain and stiffness localized around the shoulders and pelvic girdle. It targets the same elderly population as does temporal arteritis. The pain and stiffness of polymyalgia prevent the patient from easily getting out of bed, rising from a chair, combing hair, or putting on a coat. In contrast to polymyositis (Chapter 3.6), polymyalgia rheumatica produces much more pain than weakness.

Fifty percent of patients with temporal arteritis also have polymyalgia rheumatica. The two disorders are closely connected: Some patients who start with polymyalgia alone later develop temporal arteritis. However, two to three times as many patients have polymyalgia by itself, without the characteristic headache, jaw claudication, and visual changes of temporal arteritis.

Temporal arteritis and polymyalgia rheumatica share the same nonspecific symptoms (fatigue, malaise, weight loss, depression), and both produce anemia and a markedly elevated erythrocyte sedimentation rate. These laboratory findings end any possible confusion of polymyalgia with primary depression. Hypothyroidism, a disorder that can cause polymyalgia-like symptoms, is excluded by a normal thyroid-stimulating hormone level.

Patients who have only polymyalgia rheumatica, with

no "above the neck" manifestations of temporal arteritis, are treated with low-dose prednisone (10–20 mg/day). Since almost all such patients respond dramatically within 1–3 days, failure to improve should cast doubt on the diagnosis, which by necessity is a clinical one. The prednisone dose can be reduced over months. When the dose is lowered, some patients' symptoms return, requiring the prednisone to be increased to the lowest dose that controls the symptoms. Follow-up care is also designed to detect and treat the few patients who develop temporal arteritis.

Wegener's Granulomatosis

Wegener's granulomatosis is a granulomatous vasculitis known both for its clinical triad of sinusitis, pulmonary involvement, and glomerulonephritis, and for its dramatically improved prognosis with cyclophosphamide.

Wegener's granulomatosis affects men and women equally often. The age at onset averages 40, but can be at any time of life. Almost all patients present with symptoms in the upper or lower respiratory tracts. Although sinusitis is best known, the upper respiratory tract manifestations can include nasal crusting with congestion; ulceration; epistaxis; otitis media or mastoiditis with hearing loss; subglottic stenosis with stridor; and nasal cartilage inflammation with septal perforation or nasal bridge deformation ("saddle nose" deformity). Lower respiratory tract symptoms are cough, hemoptysis, breathlessness, and pleurisy.

Other common presenting symptoms are nondeforming arthritis or arthralgia, seen in two-thirds of patients; fever, in one-fourth; and in some patients, weight loss, eye involvement (proptosis or scleritis), purpura or skin ulcers, and mononeuritis multiplex. The renal disease usually begins silently. In contrast to polyarteritis nodosa, Wegener's granulomatosis rarely causes hypertension. Although the initial symptoms of Wegener's granulomatosis can be confused with common, self-limited disorders, the symptoms' persistence, severity, and association with other systemic features should lead the physician to suspect vasculitis.

Nonspecific laboratory features of Wegener's granulomatosis include a normochromic, normocytic anemia (mean hematocrit 33); mild leukocytosis (mean white blood cell count 10,500/mm^3); moderate thrombocytosis (mean platelet count 481,000/mm^3); and elevated Westergren erythrocyte sedimentation rate (mean 71 mm/hr). Less than 20% of patients present with an elevated serum creatinine or an active urine sediment with red cells and protein. The chest x-ray is abnormal in 75% of patients, showing nodules, infiltrates, and, occasionally, cavities. Computed tomography (CT) is more sensitive than plain x-ray in showing these abnormalities. Wegener's granulomatosis does not cause hilar adenopathy; large hilar glands should suggest another disease, such as sarcoidosis. On both regular x-ray and CT, the sinusitis looks nonspecific. The ANCA is positive in more than 90% of patients with active disseminated Wegener's granulomatosis, typically in the C (cytoplasmic) pattern rather than the P (perinuclear) pattern. Unfortunately, the ANCA is not specific for Wegener's and can be found in polyarteritis nodosa, a few other rheumatic diseases, and some forms of glomerulonephritis.

Wegener's granulomatosis has three pathologic hallmarks: vasculitis, granulomas, and acute and chronic inflammation associated with necrosis. Only in the lung are all three histologic changes found together. Thus, open or thoracoscopic lung biopsy usually offers the best chance of securing a pathologic diagnosis. Biopsies of the upper respiratory tract rarely show vasculitis, but they can show granulomas and inflammation with necrosis; in a patient with a compatible clinical picture, these changes may be enough to establish the diagnosis. Renal biopsy is less specific, usually showing a focal and segmental glomerulonephritis.

Cyclophosphamide has improved the prognosis of Wegener's granulomatosis from a quickly fatal disease to a manageable chronic condition from which patients can have long-term remissions. Most patients also take prednisone during the first few months. With cyclophosphamide and prednisone, almost all patients improve and 75% achieve initial remission, usually within 1 year. However, as therapy is tapered, 50% of patients have flares. Methotrexate may be less toxic than cyclophosphamide and is effective for Wegener's granulomatosis that is not immediately life-threatening. Twenty-five percent of patients eventually die from the disease or complications of therapy, chiefly infections or malignancy.

Hypersensitivity Vasculitis

Hypersensitivity vasculitis is a family of disorders, among them serum sickness, Henoch-Schönlein purpura, and cryoglobulinemia. All the forms share four features: (1) onset associated with a drug exposure or infection; (2) development of immune complexes that deposit in and cause inflammation of capillaries and venules; (3) prominent skin manifestations, especially palpable purpura; and often (4) visceral involvement that, in contrast to polyarteritis or Wegener's granulomatosis, infrequently threatens life or requires cyclophosphamide therapy.

Upon exposure to a foreign protein, individuals with hypersensitivity vasculitis make antibodies that combine with the protein to form immune complexes. These complexes may deposit in vessels, activate complement, and provoke a transient vasculitic syndrome called serum sickness. The drugs that most commonly provoke hypersensitivity vasculitis are antibiotics, especially the penicillins and sulfonamides; diuretics; and quinidine. Stopping the offending drug is usually the only treatment needed, but severe reactions, with fever, arthralgia, and extensive rash, may necessitate several weeks of prednisone at 20–40 mg/day.

Henoch-Schönlein purpura is distinguished by its predilection for children and young adults (Chapter 5.6); onset after an upper respiratory illness; extensive purpura not only on the legs but classically over the buttocks; abdominal pain that may wax and wane over weeks; and deposition of IgA in skin and glomerular lesions.

Vasculitis caused by cryoglobulinemia is suggested by episodic crops of lower extremity purpura, clinically silent hematuria, and mild sensory neuropathy. The diagnosis is confirmed by a positive serum test for cryoglobulins. A cryoglobulin is an immunoglobulin that precipitates in the cold and solubilizes upon rewarming. Cryoglobulinemia is often associated with hepatitis C or B infection.

Both Henoch-Schönlein purpura and cryoglobulinemia have such a broad range of severity that some patients need no specific treatment, whereas others require prednisone, and a few need immunosuppressive therapy.

SUMMARY

▶ General clues that a patient has systemic vasculitis include evidence of a multisystem disease that evolves subacutely, shows signs of inflammation, and causes pain.

▶ Specific clues to polyarteritis nodosa are neuropathy

(especially mononeuritis multiplex), rash (palpable purpura, ulcers, livedo reticularis, nodules), new hypertension, and "abdominal angina."

▶ The diagnosis of systemic vasculitis requires either positive biopsies or angiograms.

▶ Without prompt recognition and treatment, temporal arteritis (giant cell arteritis) can cause blindness. Since the blindness may be irreversible, patients should be started on high-dose prednisone as soon as temporal arteritis is suspected.

SUGGESTED READING

Cupps TR, Fauci AS: Systemic necrotizing vasculitis of the polyarteritis nodosa group. In: *The Vasculitides.* Cupps TR, Fauci AS (editors). WB Saunders, 1981.

Cupps TR, Fauci AS: Wegener's granulomatosis. In: *The Vasculitides.* Cupps TR, Fauci AS (editors). WB Saunders, 1981.

Guillevin L et al: Prognostic factors in polyarteritis nodosa and Churg-Strauss syndrome: A prospective study of 342 patients. Medicine 1996;75:17.

Hoffman GS et al: Wegener granulomatosis: An analysis of 158 patients. Ann Intern Med 1992;116:488.

Huston KA et al: Temporal arteritis: A 25-year epidemiologic, clinical, and pathologic study. Ann Intern Med 1978; 88:162.

Polymyositis

Mary Betty Stevens, MD

Polymyositis is an unexplained inflammatory process that targets striated muscle. If accompanied by characteristic skin lesions, the disease is called *dermatomyositis.* Both forms of the condition affect skeletal muscle most often, but can also involve myocardium. The inflammation can be so intense that it causes fibrillar necrosis. Not surprisingly, the main presenting feature of polymyositis is muscle weakness. More surprisingly, if patients have any muscle pain at all, it is usually mild, even subtle. Systemic manifestations are protean—from arthritis to interstitial lung disease—and can at first overshadow the muscle inflammation. Because polymyositis and dermatomyositis respond to treatment, especially treatment started early, the physician must recognize the disorder as presented either with subacute generalized weakness or with one of its less common systemic disguises.

CLASSIFICATION

Four subtypes of polymyositis and dermatomyositis have been recognized (Table 3.6–1). In adults, polymyositis or dermatomyositis can appear (1) by itself, (2) with a malignancy, or (3) with another rheumatic disease, most often systemic lupus erythematosus, Sjögren's syndrome, or scleroderma. Each adult subtype has a characteristic age at onset and clinical features. All affected children have dermatomyositis. Children are more likely than adults with dermatomyositis to have contracture, calcinosis, and vasculitis seen on muscle biopsy.

CLINICAL MANIFESTATIONS

Muscles

Symmetric proximal limb girdle muscle weakness is the usual presenting feature of polymyositis and dermatomyositis, as well as the dominant clinical problem. Most often the disease begins insidiously over a few months, with patients noting difficulty ascending stairs or curbs,

changing posture (recumbent to sitting, sitting to standing), or getting out of the bathtub. When the shoulder girdle is involved, it becomes progressively more difficult to lift moderately heavy objects, such as a bag of groceries. Most important, patients become increasingly aware that they cannot perform their usual activities.

In some patients, polymyositis and dermatomyositis present acutely with intense and rapidly progressive muscle weakness, often with muscle pain and tenderness. Patients may have fever and skin lesions. Muscle involvement can include the strap muscles of the neck; the cricopharyngeal muscles, impeding swallowing; and the intercostal muscles and diaphragm, limiting respiratory effort. In patients with cricopharyngeal and respiratory muscle involvement, polymyositis and dermatomyositis can present emergently, with life-threatening risk for aspiration and pneumonia. More often, such a crisis develops later in the disease.

On physical examination, the physician confirms and measures proximal muscle weakness in the legs and arms. The muscles usually look normal, without edema, atrophy (a late complication), or fasciculation. Most patients present with moderate weakness, more evident in the legs than arms. Most cannot do a deep knee bend without help or keep the arms abducted against the examiner's full force. However, the weakness may be subtle, even equivocal, especially in well-muscled, athletic persons whose baseline strength exceeds the norm. Patients may also have distal muscle weakness (eg, handgrip), but it is much less noticeable than their proximal weakness. The muscles of the face, including the eyelids, are spared. Patients with polymyositis or dermatomyositis do not have abnormalities of sensation or of bowel and bladder function. Deep tendon reflexes usually remain normal, being lost only in patients with profound weakness.

The physical findings help distinguish polymyositis from other causes of subacute generalized weakness (Table 3.6–2). Generalized weakness can result from a lesion anywhere in the motor unit (Chapter 13.12), which consists of the motor neuron, peripheral nerve, neuromuscular junction, and muscle. Lesions at different sites give

Table 3.6–1. Subtypes of polymyositis and dermatomyositis.

	Subtype	Age at Onset	Females:Males	Characteristic Features
Adults				
I	Polymyositis or dermatomyositis alone	30–60	3:1	Raynaud's phenomenon in 20% of patients, anti-Jo-1 antibody in 50%
II	Polymyositis or dermatomyositis with malignancy	>45	1:1	Vasculitis in 15% of patients; no Raynaud's phenomenon, no autoantibodies
III	Polymyositis or dermatomyositis with connective tissue disease, most often systemic lupus erythematosus, Sjögren's syndrome, or scleroderma	Depends on connective tissue disease	8:1	Connective tissue disease features dominant
Children				
IV	Dermatomyositis	5–15	1:1	Contracture, calcinosis; vasculitis on biopsy

different findings. For example, amyotrophic lateral sclerosis (ALS), a motor neuron disease, differs from polymyositis and dermatomyositis in producing more distal weakness, fasciculation (often best seen in the tongue), and upper motor neuron signs such as hyperreflexia. Sensory abnormalities are not a feature of muscle diseases, but are characteristic of peripheral neuropathies. Myasthenia gravis, a disorder of neuromuscular transmission, often affects the face and eyes, regions that are never involved in polymyositis and dermatomyositis. Many conditions besides polymyositis and dermatomyositis cause myopathy. Some of these, such as hypothyroidism, can also elevate the creatine kinase (see "Serum Enzymes" below).

Skin

About one-third of adults and all children with polymyositis have the skin lesions of dermatomyositis. Most common is an erythematous maculopapular rash over the face, neck, upper trunk, and proximal extremities; these areas may also be hyperpigmented. Many patients have periungual erythema. Particularly characteristic are erythematous, papular, scaling lesions over the proximal interphalangeal and metacarpophalangeal joints (Gottron's papules; see Color Plates). Periorbital edema with violaceous discoloration of the eyelids (heliotrope lids) is classically described but infrequent. Zonal soft tissue edema and erythema may overlie inflamed muscles in the extremities. About 10% of adults with dermatomyositis

Table 3.6–2. Causes of generalized subacute weakness, with distinguishing clinical features.

Location of Lesion in Motor Unit	Examples	Distribution of Muscle Weakness	Facial Weakness	Fasciculation	Deep Tendon Reflexes	Abnormal Sensation	Creatine Kinase
Motor neuron	Amyotrophic lateral sclerosis	Distal more than proximal	No	Yes	Increased	No	Usually normal[†]
Peripheral nerve	Paraneoplastic syndromes	Distal more than proximal	No	No	Decreased	Yes	Normal
Neuromuscular junction	Myasthenia gravis Lambert-Eaton syndrome	Proximal more than distal	Yes	No	Normal	No	Normal
Muscle	Drugs (eg, alcohol, corticosteroids, *colchicine*)* Endocrine disorders (eg, hyperthyroidism, *hypothyroidism,* Cushing's disease, adrenal insufficiency) Infections (eg, *toxoplasmosis, trichinosis,* HIV) Immune disorders (eg, *polymyositis, dermatomyositis, sarcoidosis, inclusion body myositis*) Heritable disorders (eg, *muscular dystrophy*)	Proximal more than distal	No	No	Normal	No	Usually high

*Conditions set in italic type are associated with an elevated creatine kinase. Conditions in regular type are often associated with a normal creatine kinase.
[†]Fifteen to 30% of patients with amyotrophic lateral sclerosis have an elevated creatine kinase.

have cutaneous vasculitis, manifested by periungual infarcts, digital pad ulcerations, or tender erythematous lesions in the dermis or subcutaneous tissue. Cutaneous vasculitis correlates closely with an occult malignancy.

The skin lesions of dermatomyositis are distinct from skin involvement in subtype III polymyositis (associated with a connective tissue disorder). Subtype III skin lesions are those of the associated disorder, usually systemic lupus erythematosus, Sjögren's syndrome, or scleroderma.

Cardiovascular System

Cardiac muscle is targeted in about one-third of patients with polymyositis or dermatomyositis. The electrocardiographic (ECG) changes are nonspecific and otherwise unexplained. The most common ECG findings are ST-T abnormalities, atrial and ventricular arrhythmias, bundle branch block, and varying degrees of heart block. Few patients develop left heart failure.

About 25% of all patients with polymyositis or dermatomyositis have Raynaud's phenomenon. Raynaud's is seen in more than 50% of patients with subtype III (polymyositis with a connective tissue disorder) but not at all in those with subtype II (polymyositis with malignancy).

Lungs

Polymyositis and dermatomyositis can cause a number of pulmonary problems. Interstitial fibrosis is found on x-ray in up to one-third of patients and is particularly common in patients who have antibodies to Jo-1 (see "Autoantibodies" below). Pulmonary function tests reveal a restrictive ventilatory defect even in asymptomatic patients. In addition, ventilation may be compromised by weakness of the intercostal muscles and diaphragm. This weakness also increases the risk of aspiration in patients with weak cricopharyngeal muscles.

Gastrointestinal Tract

About 40% of patients with each subtype of polymyositis or dermatomyositis have pharyngeal and upper esophageal dysphagia. The main manifestations are difficulty swallowing secretions, and nasal regurgitation of ingested fluids. Lower esophageal (smooth muscle) aperistalsis, most often associated with Raynaud's phenomenon, is particularly prominent in patients with overlapping connective tissue disease. Childhood dermatomyositis can be complicated by perforation of the bowel or gastrointestinal hemorrhage, both secondary to vasculitis; gastrointestinal tract lesions below the esophagus are exceedingly rare in adults.

Joints

About 30–40% of all patients with polymyositis or dermatomyositis first present with polyarthralgia or polyarthritis. Joint involvement is even more common in patients with associated systemic lupus erythematosus. The digits and wrists are involved in all patients, and the knees in some. Joint pain is especially prominent in children when contractures develop and impair joint function. It is interesting that patients with neoplasia can have polymyositis or dermatomyositis, or they can have hypertrophic osteoarthropathy, but not both together.

LABORATORY TESTS

The key laboratory abnormalities of polymyositis and dermatomyositis are predictable for a process characterized by inflammation and necrosis of muscle fibers: leakage of muscle enzymes into the circulation and abnormal electrical activity of damaged muscle fibers. It is curious that the erythrocyte sedimentation rate, usually a sensitive index of tissue inflammation, is normal in many patients and cannot be relied on for monitoring disease activity. When the disease is active, a few patients have mild leukocytosis or thrombocytosis. Anemia is not the rule; when prominent, it should alert the physician to the possibility of tumor or a companion connective tissue disorder, especially systemic lupus erythematosus with hemolysis.

Serum Enzymes

The cardinal laboratory abnormalities in polymyositis and dermatomyositis are serum elevations of one or more muscle enzymes: creatine kinase (CK), the transaminases (AST and ALT, formerly called SGOT and SGPT), aldolase, and lactic dehydrogenase (LDH). The serum AST and ALT rise in both inflammatory muscle disease and hepatitis; some patients with polymyositis or dermatomyositis, especially the elderly, are mistakenly thought to have hepatitis when they present with weakness, weight loss, and overall deterioration and are found to have elevated transaminases. All muscle enzyme levels are usually elevated to some degree with ongoing inflammatory necrosis, and they normalize when the process is suppressed. The CK is the most sensitive marker of disease activity; when disease is active, serum CK levels are very high. However, an elevated CK is not specific for polymyositis and dermatomyositis. Alternative causes must be ruled out, such as rhabdomyolysis, exercise-related muscle injury, hypothyroidism, and hypokalemia. Furthermore, CK fractionation can be key to evaluating whether myocardium is involved in polymyositis and dermatomyositis: An increased MB fraction is characteristic of active myocarditis.

Electromyography

Electromyographic (EMG) abnormalities are characteristic but not specific for polymyositis and dermatomyositis. In up to 90% of patients, polyphasic potentials of low amplitude and short duration are found at symptomatic muscle sites. At rest, most patients have short bursts of rapidly repeating action potentials and spontaneous fibrillation indicating membrane irritability. Most patients have little or no reduction in motor unit potentials on muscle contraction.

Muscle Biopsy

The gold standard for diagnosing polymyositis and dermatomyositis is the finding on muscle biopsy of degeneration and regeneration of muscle fibrils, infiltration with inflammatory cells, muscle fiber necrosis, and marked variation in size and staining of fibers. Postinflammatory interstitial fibrosis can appear late in the course, especially in patients in whom treatment has been delayed. The vasculitis seen on biopsy in childhood dermatomyositis is not a feature of adult disease.

A symptomatic site must be used for biopsy. Shoulder and limb girdle muscle biopsies are preferred because they cause less morbidity than calf biopsies. It is important to avoid sites where EMG testing has been done, because EMG can produce artifactitious myopathic changes. However, because polymyositis and dermatomyositis are usually symmetric, EMG of one limb often indicates a good biopsy site in the other limb. Muscle biopsy is falsely negative in about 30% of patients.

Autoantibodies

Some patients with polymyositis have a broad array of circulating autoantibodies, varying in type and prevalence with the clinical setting. Patients with dermatomyositis are less seroreactive. Least seroreactive are patients with dermatomyositis and malignancy.

Anti-Jo-1 antibody is found in about one-third of patients with polymyositis alone, but it rarely, if ever, occurs in tumor-related dermatomyositis. Interstitial pulmonary fibrosis has been found in more than 50% of patients with anti-Jo-1 antibody-positive polymyositis, but in less than 15% of antibody-negative patients.

Anti-Mi antibody (really two antibodies, Mi-1 and Mi-2) is found in a few patients with myositis; anti-Mi-2 is associated particularly with idiopathic dermatomyositis. Anti-PM-1 and anti-PM-Scl antibodies are found in only about 10% of patients with polymyositis, but in 50% of those with scleroderma-related myositis (Chapter 3.10). Similarly, anti-Sm, anti-nRNP, and anti-DNA antibodies are found in patients who have myositis with systemic lupus erythematosus (Chapter 3.2), and anti-Ro (SSA) and anti-La (SSB) are found in patients who have myositis with systemic lupus eruthematosus and Sjögren's syndrome (Chapter 3.4). The screening antinuclear antibody test (ANA) is occasionally positive in polymyositis alone, but is more likely to be positive in polymyositis with connective tissue disease, especially systemic lupus.

DIAGNOSIS

The diagnosis of polymyositis and dermatomyositis is based primarily on proximal limb girdle muscle weakness. The clinical suspicion is supported by serum muscle en-

zyme elevations, EMG changes, and, ultimately, characteristic inflammatory features on muscle biopsy. The skin features of dermatomyositis are clinically characteristic but histologically nonspecific. Serologic abnormalities are of value not only in defining the subtype and pointing to associated connective tissue disorders, but also in alerting the physician to possible interstitial pulmonary fibrosis in patients with polymyositis alone. Lack of serologic abnormalities points toward malignancy.

Neoplasia

About 15% of patients with polymyositis or dermatomyositis have malignancies. Carcinoma dominates; the most common tumors are those that are most prevalent in general—lung, breast, ovary, prostate, and colon. Raynaud's phenomenon and serologic positivity argue against occult malignancy. Some patients with tumor-related myopathy have cutaneous vasculitis. Patients who have myositis with neoplasms tend to be over 50 years old, they are more likely to have dermatomyositis than polymyositis, and the occult tumor is likely to be clinically expressed within 1 year after the myositis is diagnosed. Childhood dermatomyositis is not tumor-related.

Patients who have polymyositis or dermatomyositis related to neoplasia do not respond to therapy as well as do other patients with myositis, but this does not mean that a neoplasm can be ruled out because patients respond. The physician should consider the patient's risk factors when deciding how aggressively to search for malignancy.

MANAGEMENT, COURSE, AND PROGNOSIS

Polymyositis and dermatomyositis are usually chronic and episodic but suppressible processes. The only patients who may not respond well are those with neoplasia or Sjögren's syndrome. Prognosis worsens with older age at onset, tumor, myocardial involvement, and interstitial pulmonary fibrosis. For all the subtypes, early diagnosis and treatment are key to restoring strength and function.

All patients with polymyositis or dermatomyositis should be given corticosteroids, starting at high doses. Response is measured by a lowering of serum enzyme elevations and by decreased myopathic pain and tenderness. Muscle strength improves more slowly. These improvements may take weeks to months. More than 80% of patients recover on steroids alone; those who do not may respond to cytotoxic therapy, especially methotrexate. Intravenous gamma globulin may also be effective.

In addition to drug treatment, patients with active disease should rest and receive passive physical therapy. As the myositic process is suppressed, intensive active physical therapy maintains or improves muscle strength.

As patients become stronger and their muscle pain and tenderness resolve, their corticosteroids should be tapered slowly and cautiously, with the dose reduced no more than 10% per month. Clinical reevaluations and serum enzyme monitoring are essential guides to the rate and degree of tapering. Patients with malignancy must have their tumor treated. Polymyositis—and more often, dermatomyositis—have been known to resolve with successful treatment of the neoplasm.

A few patients with polymyositis or dermatomyositis present emergently. These are people who have an abrupt onset of disease involving their swallowing and respiratory mechanisms. To prevent aspiration, these patients should not be given anything by mouth. They may also benefit from atropine to minimize their secretions. Patients should be kept sitting up until they can swallow effectively. Rare patients require tracheostomy and assisted ventilation. Some need antibiotics and parenteral nutrition.

About 70–80% of patients are now alive 6–7 years after diagnosis, up from 50% in earlier studies. The improvement may relate to earlier diagnosis and better general medical care. Poor prognosis is signaled by older age at diagnosis and by cardiac involvement. Some patients have remissions and exacerbations, but without treatment the trend is toward increasing impairment.

SUMMARY

▶ Polymyositis and dermatomyositis are the most common inflammatory disorders of muscle.

▶ Proximal limb girdle muscle weakness is the cardinal manifestation, but any striated muscle can be involved, including myocardium, the diaphragm, and cricopharyngeal and intercostal muscles.

▶ Dermatomyositis is more likely than polymyositis to accompany an occult neoplasm, especially in older patients with cutaneous vasculitis.

▶ Elevated muscle enzymes in serum (especially creatine kinase), characteristic electromyographic abnormalities, and muscle biopsy establish the diagnosis of an inflammatory myopathy.

▶ In most patients, the inflammation can be suppressed by corticosteroids.

SUGGESTED READING

Bohan A et al: Computer-assisted analysis of 153 patients with polymyositis and dermatomyositis. Medicine 1977;56:255.

Dalakas MC et al: A controlled trial of high-dose intravenous immune globulin infusions as treatment for dermatomyositis. N Engl J Med 1993;329:1993.

Hochberg MC, Feldman D, Stevens MB: Adult onset polymyositis/dermatomyositis: An analysis of clinical and laboratory features and survival in 76 patients with a review of the literature. Semin Arthritis Rheum 1986;15:168.

Hochberg MC et al: Antibody to Jo-1 in polymyositis/dermatomyositis: Association with interstitial pulmonary disease. J Rheumatol 1984;11:663.

Ramirez G et al: Adult-onset polymyositis-dermatomyositis: Description of 25 patients with emphasis on treatment. Semin Arthritis Rheum 1990;20:114.

Reichlin M, Arnett FC Jr: Multiplicity of antibodies in myositis sera. Arthritis Rheum 1984;27:1150.

Ankylosing Spondylitis and Related Disorders

Carol M. Ziminski, MD

Four rheumatic diseases can cause inflammatory arthritis of the spine: ankylosing spondylitis (the most common), Reiter's syndrome, psoriatic arthritis, and enteropathic arthritis. These spondyloarthropathies are considered together because they share many clinical, radiographic, and genetic features: arthritis of peripheral joints, usually oligoarticular; inflammation at bony insertions of tendons, ligaments, and fascia (enthesopathy); extra-articular inflammation in the eye (anterior uveitis), heart (aortitis), skin, and mucous membranes; predominance in men; onset before age 40 years; and a strong association with the class I human leukocyte antigen HLA-B27.

Most patients with a spondyloarthropathy present with either back pain or peripheral arthritis. Neither symptom alone is specific. Yet, the associated features are so characteristic that often the physician can confidently make the diagnosis at the bedside (Table 3.7–1). After the diagnosis is confirmed, patients are managed with drugs and physical measures.

WHEN TO SUSPECT A SPONDYLOARTHROPATHY

Back pain has many causes (Chapter 3.13). An inflammatory cause—a spondyloarthropathy—is suggested by 4 features: insidious onset over weeks or months, onset before age 40, improvement with exercise, and exacerbation with rest. Since degenerative disorders (mechanical back disease) produce the exact opposite picture, the history alone usually points toward a spondyloarthropathy.

Arthritis of peripheral joints also has many causes (Chapter 3.1). Features suggesting an associated spondyloarthropathy are an inflammatory oligoarthritis of the large joints of the leg (hip, knee, ankle), enthesopathy, and distinctive extra-articular manifestations like anterior uveitis in ankylosing spondylitis and urethritis in Reiter's syndrome (see Table 3.7–1).

Enthesopathy is an especially valuable finding because it is virtually limited to the spondyloarthropathies. Sarcoidosis is the only other process that causes inflammation at the bony insertions of tendons, ligaments, and fascia. Enthesopathy most often manifests as dactylitis, a sausage-like swelling of an entire finger or toe. Swelling of the whole digit reflects the spondyloarthropathies, characteristic inflammation of tendons and ligaments; in contrast, rheumatoid arthritis and systemic lupus erythematosus inflame the synovium, producing swelling just around the joints. Another manifestation of enthesopathy is heel pain, caused by inflammation of the plantar fascia at its insertion into the calcaneus (Chapter 3.1); since degenerative disorders or overuse can also cause heel pain, the physician should suspect a spondyloarthropathy when the patient has other signs of inflammation, like a swollen knee or ankle. A third way that enthesopathy commonly presents is with swelling of the Achilles tendon.

ETIOLOGY

The cause of the spondyloarthropathies is unknown, but both genes and infection seem to play important roles. Almost all patients with a spondyloarthropathy carry the HLA-B27 antigen. This antigen is found in only 4–8% of the normal population, but in over 90% of patients with ankylosing spondylitis (see Table 3.7–1). Since only 10–20% of persons with the gene develop the disorder, the gene is necessary but not sufficient by itself to cause disease. A second factor, most likely infection, also seems to be needed. The importance of infection is most striking in Reiter's syndrome, which often develops after enteritis or nongonococcal urethritis. Although few patients with ankylosing spondylitis report an antecedent infection, transgenic animal models underscore the importance of both genes and infection in the disease. When the human gene for HLA-B27 is introduced in rats, they develop a

Table 3.7–1. Distinguishing features of the spondyloarthropathies.

	Ankylosing Spondylitis	Reiter's Syndrome	Psoriatic Arthritis	Enteropathic Arthritis
Age of onset	Young adult	Young adult	Young adult	Children and young adults
Gender (males:females)	3:1	Endemic disease 9:1 Epidemic disease 1:1	1:1 Patients with spondylitis 2:1	1:1 Patients with spondylitis 2:1
Systemic symptoms	±	++	+	+
Sacroiliitis (% of patients)	100% Bilateral Symmetric	25% Uni- or bilateral Asymmetric	20–40% Uni- or bilateral Asymmetric	10–20% Uni- or bilateral Asymmetric
Peripheral arthritis	Hips, shoulders	Oligoarticular, asymmetric involvement of legs and feet; sausage digits; heel pain	Oligo- or polyarticular asymmetric involvement of distal interphalangeal joints; sausage digits	Symmetric involvement of large joints, especially knees, ankles, wrists
Extra-articular features	Anterior uveitis, aortitis	Anterior uveitis, conjunctivitis, urethritis, cervicitis, keratoderma, balanitis, oral ulcers, nail changes	Psoriasis, nail changes (especially pitting); anterior uveitis and aortitis rare	Anterior uveitis, erythema nodosum, pyoderma gangrenosum
HLA-B27 (% of patients)	90%	75%	Patients with spondylitis 50%	Patients with spondylitis 50%

disease resembling ankylosing spondylitis. However, if the rats are kept in a germ-free environment, they remain free of spondylitis. Few patients with ankylosing spondylitis or Reiter's syndrome appear to have chronic infections. Rather, infection seems to trigger a chronic inflammatory arthritis in genetically susceptible persons.

ANKYLOSING SPONDYLITIS

Ankylosing spondylitis is the prototype spondyloarthropathy characterized by a chronic systemic inflammatory disease dominated by involvement of the axial skeleton (Figure 3.7–1). The disease afflicts about 0.1–0.2% of North American whites, typically begins in early adulthood, and affects men 3 times more often as women.

Clinical Features

Articular Findings: Inflammatory back pain, worse after resting and improved by exercise, may begin in the sacroiliac regions of the buttocks, unilaterally or bilaterally, and may be interpreted as hip pain. Some patients have more generalized stiffness in the lumbar and thoracic areas. Paraspinal muscle spasm may be prominent, as may tenderness over the sacroiliac joints. Many patients report discomfort radiating down the lateral and posterior thigh, sometimes mimicking nerve root compression from intervertebral disk disease.

The physical examination may be relatively normal in early ankylosing spondylitis. However, as the disease progresses, the normal lumbar lordosis becomes flattened. Patients have measurable loss of mobility in lumbar flexion, extension, and lateral bending. In later disease, the thoracic spine assumes an exaggerated kyphotic posture

(hunchback) (Figure 3.7–2). Fusion of the costovertebral joints and the vertebral facet joints restricts chest expansion. Breathing then becomes largely diaphragmatic, although few patients have significantly impaired ventilation. With progressive fusion of the cervical segments, the head assumes a forward flexed position, with vision directed toward the ground. Flexion at hip and knee compensates for spine flexion and can accentuate lower extremity deformities. Although in most patients the disease progresses slowly over many years, rare patients quickly develop severe spinal deformity.

The first manifestation of ankylosing spondylitis may be peripheral joint involvement, usually monoarticular or oligoarticular, and particularly in the lower limbs. Only with time and disease progression may axial symptoms emerge. The most frequently affected peripheral joint is the hip. The problem is not pain so much as limitation of motion, which leads to fixed flexion contractures and progressive disability. The shoulders may lose range of motion, without pain. The small joints of the hands and feet are rarely involved. Sometimes accompanying axial or peripheral arthritis is enthesopathy, in the form of dactylitis, plantar fasciitis, or Achilles tendon swelling.

Extra-Articular Findings: Signs of systemic disease in ankylosing spondylitis are rare, but constitutional manifestations can include fatigue, weight loss, and low-grade fever. Features such as inflammation of the uveal tract (acute anterior uveitis) may develop early or at any time in the disease course. It usually takes years of active disease for patients to develop involvement of the heart (aortic regurgitation, complete heart block), lungs (apical pulmonary fibrosis, extrathoracic restrictive lung disease), or nervous system (cauda equina syndrome, nerve root or cord compression).

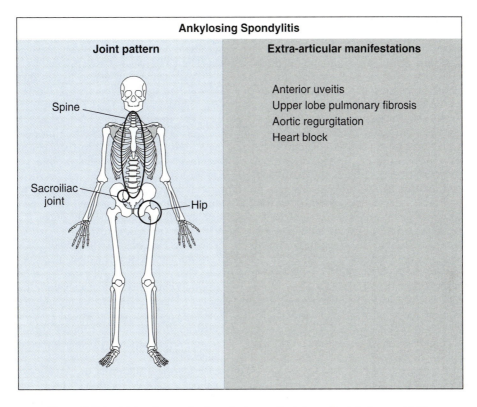

Figure 3.7–1. Joint pattern and extra-articular manifestations of ankylosing spondylitis.

Prognosis

The prognosis in ankylosing spondylitis is generally good. In most patients, the first decade of disease predicts the remainder. Severe disease usually appears early and causes peripheral arthritis, particularly of the hips. For many patients, pain subsides as spinal fusion is completed. Only 6% of patients die from ankylosing spondylitis, primarily from whiplash-induced fracture of the brittle and osteoporotic cervical spine, or from heart disease or secondary amyloidosis.

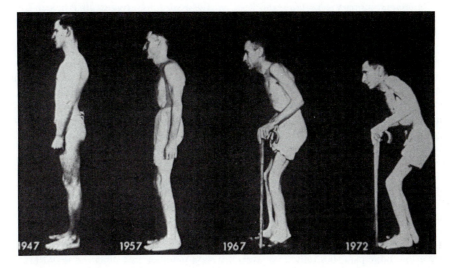

Figure 3.7–2. Progression of ankylosing spondylitis over 25 years. (Reproduced, with permission, from Ogryzlo MA, Rosen PS: Ankylosing [Marie-Strümpell] spondylitis. Postgrad Med 1969;45:182 [panels 1–3] and Syntex Corporation [panel 4]. Figure used courtesy of the Journal of Rheumatology.)

REITER'S SYNDROME

Reiter's syndrome is the most common cause of chronic arthritis in young men. The syndrome was originally described as a triad of arthritis, conjunctivitis, and urethritis or cervicitis, developing after a dysenteric infection. The spectrum of Reiter's syndrome is now known to be broader. Clinical features may also include enthesopathy, uveitis, rash of the glans penis (circinate balanitis), a psoriasis-like rash of the palms or soles (keratoderma blennorrhagicum), and mouth ulcers. The syndrome can be triggered by gastrointestinal and venereal infections. The designations, *incomplete Reiter's* (for patients who do not have the classic triad) and *reactive arthritis,* (for patients with an identified antecedent infection) reflect the struggles of terminology to keep pace with expanding knowledge. Since each term has its faults, the original name, Reiter's syndrome, is used here.

Like those with ankylosing spondylitis, most patients with Reiter's syndrome have the HLA-B27 antigen. They may be susceptible to the syndrome after exposure to certain infections, especially *Chlamydia trachomatis, Shigella, Salmonella, Campylobacter,* and *Yersinia.* It is not known why men are affected 9 times more often than women.

Clinical Features

Classic Symptoms: Typically, symptoms of Reiter's syndrome emerge 2–6 weeks after an initiating infection. By that time, the pathogen can rarely be cultured. Urethritis usually appears first, with mild dysuria, transient mucopurulent discharge, or both. Detecting urethritis may require examining a first-void morning urine for pyuria. This nonspecific urethritis often fails to respond to antibiotic treatment. Men may also have acute or chronic prostatitis, whereas women typically develop cervicitis, vaginitis, or both. Note that these genitourinary symptoms can develop in patients whose antecedent infection was diarrheal and do not necessarily indicate venereal acquisition.

Conjunctivitis, usually bilateral and apparently noninfectious, appears early in the disease and is both mild and transient. Acute anterior uveitis, marked by ocular pain, erythema, and photophobia, may occur at the same time.

Arthritis is usually the last feature of the classic triad to emerge, often lagging several weeks behind the other features. In most patients, the arthritis begins acutely. It is an asymmetric oligo- or polyarthritis that usually affects the lower extremities, especially the knees, ankles, and small joints of the feet. Other peripheral joints are less frequently involved. The arthritis usually persists for several months and then resolves. Recurrent or residual arthritis may lead to joint deformity, although it is seldom as disabling as in rheumatoid arthritis. Many patients with Reiter's syndrome have low back pain, but only 25% ever develop radiographic evidence of sacroiliitis.

Enthesopathy gives rise to more characteristic features.

Many patients have "sausage digits." The most disabling symptom may be the heel pain that 50% the patients suffer because of inflammation at the insertion of the plantar fascia or Achilles tendon ("lover's heel").

Other Features: Keratoderma blennorrhagicum typically appears on the soles or palms and occasionally on the extremities or trunk. Starting as erythematous macules, or as clear vesicles resting on erythematous bases, the lesions later become hyperkeratotic and clinically and histologically indistinguishable from pustular psoriasis. The rash is usually limited and transient, but occasional patients have a generalized psoriasis-like eruption that dominates the clinical picture. Circinate balanitis is painless, superficial, serpiginous ulcers on the glans penis and urethral meatus; dry, scaling plaques similar to keratoderma are characteristic in circumcised men. Some patients develop painless, shallow ulcers of the oral mucosa. Nail changes include yellowish or white discoloration, with thickening and detachment from the nail bed (onycholysis); these abnormalities are clinically indistinguishable from mycotic nail infections. A striking feature of the mucocutaneous features of Reiter's syndrome is that they are not seen in patients with the closely related ankylosing spondylitis.

During the acute onset of Reiter's syndrome, patients may be seriously ill, with high fever, rigors, tachycardia, and exquisitely tender joints. About one-third of patients have significant weight loss. Less common features include cardiac conduction abnormalities and aortitis. With late disease, occasional patients develop aortic regurgitation similar to that seen in ankylosing spondylitis. Rare patients develop amyloidosis, usually only after a prolonged severe course or with acute fulminant illness.

Reiter's syndrome and psoriasis have been reported in patients with AIDS. It is not clear whether Reiter's is more common in patients with HIV infection; however, the association suggests that helper T cells, which HIV infection eliminates, do not play an important role in the pathogenesis of Reiter's syndrome.

Course and Prognosis

The course of Reiter's syndrome is unpredictable. The acute episode usually subsides after several weeks or months. Relapses can occur at varying intervals; patients may have many disease-free years before developing symptoms in previously unaffected joints. Mild chronic symptoms may persist, but a minority of patients suffer an unremitting course.

PSORIATIC ARTHRITIS

Psoriatic arthritis is a syndrome of cutaneous psoriasis and a seronegative inflammatory arthropathy. This definition assumes that other causes of arthritis have been excluded and that the skin and joint manifestations are probably related. Psoriatic arthritis is considered among the seronegative spondyloarthropathies because patients may also have sacroiliitis or arthritis. However, the association with HLA-B27 is weaker than in idiopathic ankylosing spondylitis and Reiter's syndrome; in patients with psoriatic arthritis, B27 correlates with spinal disease, not peripheral arthritis.

Psoriasis vulgaris is a common skin disease that affects about 2% of the world's population. Probably less than 5% of all patients with psoriasis have psoriatic arthritis. Men and women are equally affected. The disease usually begins in early adulthood.

In most patients, the psoriasis begins before or with the arthritis. Less often, but especially in children, arthritis precedes psoriasis, making specific diagnosis difficult or impossible at the outset. In general, the psoriasis does not parallel the activity or severity of the joint disease. Nail changes, particularly nail pitting, occur in 80% of patients with psoriatic arthritis, but in fewer than one-third with psoriasis alone.

Several subtypes of psoriatic arthritis have been described. (1) More than 50% of patients have a peripheral, asymmetric oligoarthritis; characteristically, when fingers or toes are involved, they are sausage-shaped. (2) Almost 25% of patients have a symmetric, rheumatoid-like, but seronegative polyarthritis, which is usually less extensive and deforming than seropositive rheumatoid arthritis. (3) Twenty percent of patients have spinal involvement, especially sacroiliitis. (4) About 5–10% of patients have dominant distal interphalangeal (DIP) joint involvement of fingers or toes, a finding unique to psoriatic arthritis and commonly related to psoriatic nail disease. (5) Rare patients develop arthritis mutilans with severe osteolysis of involved digits.

Systemic manifestations are rare, as are extra-articular features such as uveitis and heart block, which develop only in patients who have spondylitis and the HLA-B27 antigen.

Psoriatic arthritis tends to be indolent and slowly progressive. Severe disease may destroy joints, with or without bony fusion similar to that seen in Reiter's syndrome.

ENTEROPATHIC ARTHRITIS

Enteropathic arthritis is induced by or associated with intestinal disease, usually inflammatory bowel disease (Crohn's disease or ulcerative colitis). Twenty percent of patients with inflammatory bowel disease develop a peripheral oligoarthritis, which typically begins acutely and affects the knees and ankles. The arthritis is transient, often migratory, and not destructive. Episodes of peripheral arthritis often cluster during periods of active bowel disease, although articular symptoms may precede intestinal symptoms, particularly with Crohn's disease. Arthralgias are most common, but some patients develop synovitis with large-joint effusions. Peripheral arthritis may be accompanied by extra-articular manifestations such as fever, painful oral ulcers, uveitis, and skin lesions,

usually erythema nodosum in Crohn's disease and pyoderma gangrenosum in ulcerative colitis.

Less than 20% of patients with inflammatory bowel disease develop sacroiliitis, with or without higher levels of spondylitis. Most of these patients have HLA-B27. Symptoms, signs, and radiographic features are indistinguishable from those of ankylosing spondylitis. The course of enteropathic spondylitis does not parallel fluctuations in bowel disease activity.

The episodes of inflammatory arthritis tend to be worse during the first few years of bowel disease. Attacks often begin abruptly, becoming severe within 1 day. In 50% of patients, episodes last less than 1 month; in 25%, they last 5–9 weeks; and in 20%, they last 2–12 months. The remaining 5% of patients have chronic disease for several years. Most patients recover with no permanent joint damage.

LABORATORY STUDIES

In all types of spondyloarthropathy, the erythrocyte sedimentation rate is often but not always elevated. Occasional patients have a mild normochromic, normocytic anemia. Patients with active psoriasis may have hyperuricemia. Serologic tests for rheumatoid factor and antinuclear antibodies are negative. Synovial fluid is usually highly inflammatory, with a predominance of polymorphonuclear cells. In the United States, the histocompatibility antigen HLA-B27 is found in 90–95% of white patients and 50% of black patients with ankylosing spondylitis, compared with 8% of healthy whites and 4% of healthy blacks. A negative test in a white patient virtually excludes ankylosing spondylitis. HLA-B27 is found somewhat less frequently in the other spondyloarthropathies (see Table 3.7–1).

The earliest radiographic abnormality in ankylosing spondylitis is usually bilateral sacroiliitis, manifested by widening and sclerosis of the joint (Figure 3.7–3). Later, calcification in the anterior spinal ligament and bony bridging (syndesmophytes) of all the vertebral bodies may create the classic though uncommon "bamboo" spine. Reiter's syndrome and psoriatic arthritis are more likely than ankylosing spondylitis to cause unilateral sacroiliitis and spotty involvement of the spine. Psoriatic arthritis also produces distinctive erosions in the small joints of the hands or feet.

MANAGEMENT

Treatment begins with patient education about the natural course of the disease and the rationale for each therapy. The goals of treatment are relief of pain and stiffness by suppression of inflammation, maintenance of as much joint function as possible, and prevention of axial and peripheral joint deformity. Most patients need multifaceted treatment.

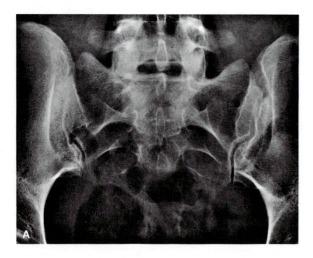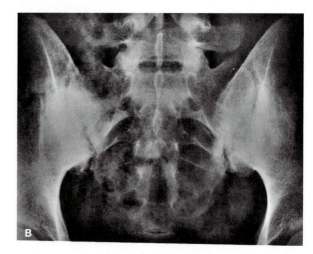

Figure 3.7–3. A: Normal sacroiliac region. **B:** Sacroiliitis in ankylosing spondylitis: Bilateral widening of the sacroiliac joints, with sclerosis and erosions.

Nonsteroidal anti-inflammatory drugs (NSAIDs) are the basic regimen for virtually all patients with these disorders. Since salicylates may relieve pain, they merit trial, but patients may require indomethacin or another NSAID. Patients with peripheral enteropathic arthritis should be given NSAIDs cautiously, since intestinal side-effects may be difficult to distinguish from active bowel disease.

Few patients need systemic corticosteroids for articular disease, but patients may need them to control systemic features. Intra-articular corticosteroids may help reduce joint inflammation that is refractory to other therapy. The antimetabolite methotrexate or azathioprine should be reserved for those few patients with Reiter's syndrome or psoriatic arthritis who have severe and otherwise uncontrollable joint or skin disease. Coexistent HIV infection must be excluded before patients are given any immunosuppressive drugs, including corticosteroids.

As their pain is relieved, patients should begin physical therapy. For ankylosing spondylitis, the major goals are maintenance of normal posture and prevention of spinal deformity. Patients should be told to use a firm mattress, avoid pillows (to reduce cervical deformities), sleep on the back or stomach (not on their side), maintain an erect posture, and sit in chairs with good back support.

SUMMARY

▶ Four rheumatic diseases cause inflammatory arthritis of the spine: ankylosing spondylitis (the most common), Reiter's syndrome, psoriatic arthritis, and enteropathic arthritis.

▶ Back pain caused by inflammation differs from that caused by degenerative diseases in that the pain begins insidiously, usually before age 40 years; it worsens with rest and improves with activity.

▶ The spondyloarthropathies share many other features, including arthritis of peripheral joints; inflammation at bony insertions of tendons, ligaments, and fascia (enthesopathy); extra-articular inflammation (eg, uveitis); predominance in men; onset before age 40; and a strong association with HLA-B27.

▶ Enthesopathy, manifested by a sausage-like digit, plantar fasciitis, or Achilles tendon swelling, almost always signals a spondyloarthropathy.

▶ Reiter's syndrome is the most common chronic arthritis in young men.

SUGGESTED READING

Arnett FC: Seronegative spondyloarthropathies. Bull Rheum Dis 1987;37:1.

Haslock I, Wright V: The musculoskeletal complications of Crohn's disease. Medicine (Baltimore) 1973;52:217.

Keat A: Reiter's syndrome and reactive arthritis in perspective. N Engl J Med 1983;309:1606.

Khan MA, van der Linden SM: A wider spectrum of spondyloarthropathies. Semin Arthritis Rheum 1990;20:107.

Reveille JD, Conant MA, Duvic M: Human immunodeficiency virus-associated psoriasis, psoriatic arthritis, and Reiter's syndrome: A disease continuum? Arthritis Rheum 1990;33:1574.

Gout and Other Crystal Diseases

Ronenn Roubenoff, MD, MHS

Most patients with gout present with intermittent attacks of acute, intense monoarthritis, usually of the great toe. Gout, the most common inflammatory arthritis in men, is caused by uric acid (monosodium urate) crystals deposited in the joint. Other inorganic crystals, such as calcium pyrophosphate dihydrate, can cause a monoarthritis that mimics gout and is known as *pseudogout*.

Gout has fascinated healers since antiquity. The ancients marveled at gout's explosive onset and the bacchanalian habits of some of its victims. Investigators in the 19th century explained gout's proclivity for certain people (see "Clinical Features" below) and made gout one of the few rheumatic diseases whose pathogenesis is now almost fully understood. Current knowledge allows the physician to recognize when a patient with monoarthritis has gout and not some other condition, to identify the few patients with gout who have an important underlying metabolic disorder, and to treat effectively this disabling and very painful arthritis. The physician should also be aware that more than one-third of patients with gout have hypertension and that men with gout have a high prevalence of vascular disease.

CLINICAL FEATURES

Gout is typically an episodic monoarthritis, although about 10% of patients have polyarticular gout, with three or more joints involved (Figure 3.8–1). Men are affected eight times more often than premenopausal women, but after menopause the male:female ratio is narrowed to 3:1. Gout usually begins after age 30 in men and 45 in women. Onset before these ages should raise suspicion of a primary metabolic disturbance (see "Pathogenesis" below).

The pain of acute gout was perhaps best described by Thomas Sydenham in the 17th century:

> The victim goes to bed and sleeps in good health. About two o'clock in the morning he is awakened by a severe pain in the great toe; more rarely in the heel, ankle, or instep. This pain is like that of a dislocation. . . . Then follow chills . . . and a little fever. The pain . . . becomes more intense . . . Now it is a violent stretching and tearing of the ligaments— now it is a gnawing pain, and now a pressure and tightening. So exquisite and lively meanwhile is the feeling of the part affected, that it cannot bear the weight of the bedclothes nor the jar of a person walking in the room. The night is passed in torture. . . .*

Over 50% of patients present with podagra, an acute inflammation of the first metatarsophalangeal (MTP) joint, and 75–90% of patients eventually develop podagra. The first MTP joint is thought to be most susceptible to gout because it is very prone to trauma and to cooling, both of which reduce the solubility of uric acid. After the first MTP, acute gout most commonly involves the ankles, knees, and instep, but it can also affect the wrists, elbows, and small joints of the hands and feet. Large joints such as the hips, shoulders, and vertebral joints are rarely involved. Acute gout can also cause tenosynovitis (inflammation of tendon sheaths) and bursitis. Uric acid crystals can be deposited in the skin, particularly around the foot; these crystals can cause a sterile cellulitis with intense erythema and warmth, even in a person who has no gouty joints.

As Sydenham wrote, gout generally begins explosively, although some patients describe a series of small bouts leading up to a full-scale attack. Untreated gouty arthritis lasts from days to weeks; minor bouts can resolve spontaneously in a few hours. Early in the disease course, the only abnormality that joint x-rays show is soft tissue swelling. If left untreated, acute gout can evolve into a deforming chronic polyarthritis that may be difficult to distinguish from rheumatoid arthritis (Figure 3.8–2) (see "Treatment of Chronic Tophaceous Gout" below).

---

*Sydenham T: *The Works of Thomas Sydenham,* trans RG Latham, vol II. London, Sydenham Society, 1850, page 124.

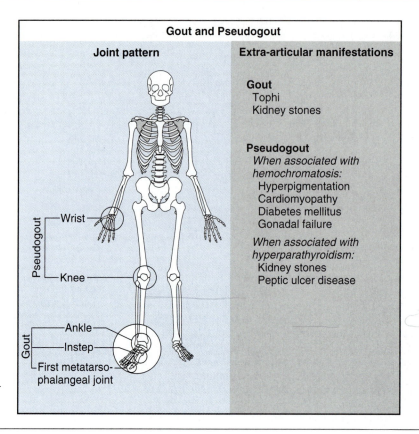

Figure 3.8–1. Joint pattern and extra-articular manifestations of gout and pseudogout.

DIAGNOSIS OF ACUTE GOUT

The three most common causes of monoarthritis are infection, trauma, and gout. The hot red joint looks similar in all three conditions. The way to differentiate them is by analyzing synovial fluid obtained through arthrocentesis. Gout can be documented only when examination of the joint fluid, ideally under a polarizing microscope, shows intracellular or extracellular uric acid crystals. These crystals may be present during the intervals between attacks. They are needle-shaped and 3–20 μm long. They are negatively birefringent: They look yellow when lying parallel with the red compensator on a polarizing microscope and blue when perpendicular (see Color Plates). The calcium pyrophosphate crystals of pseudogout are positively birefringent—yellow when perpendicular to the axis of the red compensator, and blue when parallel. These light properties are the surest way to distinguish gout from pseudogout. A useful mnemonic for the refringent properties of crystals is that "yellow," "parallel," and "allopurinol" all have two L's, and all apply only to gout.

A first attack of monoarthritis is always an indication for arthrocentesis, even if the clinical situation is typical for gout. Synovial fluid obtained by arthrocentesis both confirms gout and allows for cultures to test for infectious arthritis. If there is enough fluid, a cell count is useful, al-though not mandatory. Most patients with gout have elevated synovial leukocyte counts, but the reported range is wide, from 2000 to over 100,000 cells/mm^3. Gout and infection can coexist in a joint, and joint infection can precipitate a gout attack. Thus, even if crystals are found, the physician should test for infection. Possible infection is also the only reason to repeat the arthrocentesis if a patient has further gout attacks. Infection should be suspected in patients who have diabetes, fever, or a high peripheral white blood cell count.

PATHOGENESIS OF GOUT AND HYPERURICEMIA

Gout is caused by uric acid crystals deposited in the joint space. Once phagocytosed by polymorphonuclear leukocytes or macrophages, the crystals initiate an immune response, recruiting white blood cells. The white cells release lysosomal enzymes, as well as tumor necrosis factor and interleukin-1, which recruit more white cells. In addition, ingested uric acid kills the phagocytosing cells, leading to release of the uric acid crystals and more proteolytic enzymes, thus reinforcing the inflammatory condition. The crystals become progressively less inflammatory after several cycles of ingestion and release, and the in-

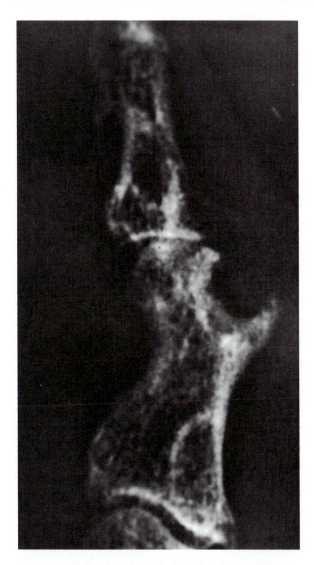

Figure 3.8–2. Tophaceous gout. Finger joint shows characteristic "rat bite" erosion with sclerotic border and overhanging bony edge.

flammation relents over 10–14 days. With repeated gout attacks, however, the lysosomal enzymes destroy cartilage and erode the joint.

Hyperuricemia is a serum uric acid level above the saturation point at 37°C (98.6°F), about 7.0 mg/dL. People who develop gout have had hyperuricemia for years or decades, and most have elevated uric acid levels at the time of the attack. However, only a small percentage of persons with hyperuricemia develop gout. The patients who develop gout may be those whose uric acid solubility in certain joints is reduced by cool temperature (as found in the toe), lead in the synovial fluid, or trauma. The trauma can range from the simple stubbing of a toe to abdominal surgery.

The serum uric acid level is influenced by how much uric acid the body produces, how much uric acid the patient eats, and how much uric acid the kidney excretes (Figure 3.8–3). Uric acid can be overproduced in two ways: (1) Uric acid is a metabolic byproduct of purines, which are essential components of DNA synthesis. Psoriasis, lymphoma, polycythemia, and any other disorder that causes rapid cell turnover can produce hyperuricemia and, eventually, gout. (2) Some patients have intrinsic enzyme defects in purine metabolism, leading to hyperuricemia and gout.

Uric acid, or its precursor purines, are part of a normal diet. Particularly rich in purines are sardines and organ meats like liver, kidney, and sweetbreads. Eating too much of these foods can cause hyperuricemia. Together, overproducing and overeating uric acid account for 15% of cases of gout.

The remaining 85% of cases are caused by too little urinary excretion of uric acid. Most patients with impaired renal clearance of uric acid have no other signs of renal insufficiency. Their serum creatinine and urinalysis are normal. However, patients who have frank renal insufficiency clear uric acid poorly. Renal excretion of uric acid is decreased by drugs, especially thiazide and loop diuretics, and aspirin in doses below 2.5 g/day.

Some factors contribute to gout in more than one way. For example, lead can cause the kidneys to underexcrete uric acid, and can also directly reduce uric acid's solubility in synovial fluid. The gout resulting from lead toxicity is called "saturnine gout." In the past, saturnine gout developed chiefly in people who drank alcohol, especially sherry shipped in lead-lined casks. More recently, saturnine gout has been seen in drinkers of illegal "moonshine" whiskey distilled through lead-lined stills. By itself, excessive alcohol causes hyperuricemia by both increasing uric acid production and inhibiting renal uric acid excretion.

In trying to understand why a patient has developed gout, the physician should review the patient's medical history (eg, renal failure), diet (eg, alcohol and high-purine food intake), medications (eg, aspirin, diuretics, cyclosporine), and exposure history (eg, moonshine). The physical examination may also help identify conditions that overproduce uric acid (eg, polycythemia). The physician should suspect an underlying enzyme defect in purine metabolism (see Figure 3.8–3) if gout begins in someone younger than 30, but most patients with these defects manifest metabolic disorders long before they develop gout. The serum creatinine and complete blood count help identify patients who have occult renal or hematologic disorders.

Renal Manifestations of Hyperuricemia

The most common renal consequence of hyperuricemia is formation of kidney stones (Chapter 5.8). About 5–10% of all renal stones are pure uric acid; uric acid can also serve as a nidus around which calcium stones form. Un-

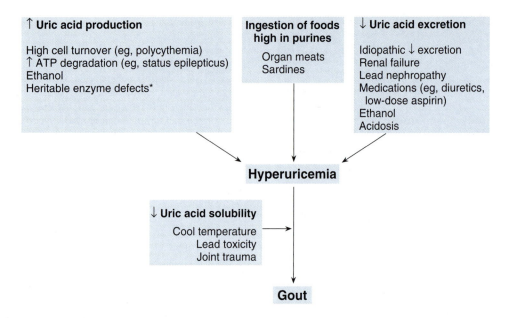

*Hypoxanthine-guanine phosphoribosyltransferase (HGPRT) deficiency, 5-phosphoribosyl-1-pyrophosphate reductase (PRPPr) overactivity, glycogen storage disease type I.

Figure 3.8–3. Conditions leading to the development of gout.

like calcium or mixed calcium-uric acid stones, pure uric acid stones are radiolucent.

Acute uric acid nephropathy is a consequence of cytotoxic chemotherapy in patients who have leukemia or lymphoma with a large tumor burden. If much of the tumor dies all at once, the load of uric acid overwhelms the renal tubules, causing an acute obstructive uropathy and renal failure. Pretreatment with allopurinol, which inhibits the formation of uric acid, has largely eliminated this problem.

Chronic uric acid nephropathy, resulting from years of uric acid deposition into the kidney, rarely causes progressive renal insufficiency. Hypertension, which affects more than one-third of patients with gout, poses a much greater threat to the kidneys and the vascular system. Therefore, long-term management of gout requires at least as much attention to the blood pressure as to the uric acid.

MANAGEMENT

Although gout is one of the most treatable of medical conditions, attacks can be provoked or prolonged by incorrect therapies. The single most common mistake that physicians make is failing to separate the treatment of the acute gouty attack from treatment of the hyperuricemia. Treatment of acute gout should focus on eliminating the inflammation rather than lowering the serum uric acid. Paradoxically, drugs that suddenly lower the serum uric

acid can actually exacerbate an attack. Therefore, the physician should consider treating hyperuricemia only after the attack has resolved.

Management of Acute Gout

For most patients with acute gout, the treatment of choice is a nonsteroidal anti-inflammatory drug (NSAID). Many NSAIDs are effective. The most often used NSAID is indomethacin, which usually greatly relieves the discomfort within 2 days and eliminates it by 5–10 days.

If patients cannot tolerate NSAIDs because of hypersensitivity, fluid overload, or preexisting peptic ulcer disease or renal insufficiency, their two alternatives are colchicine and glucocorticoids. Colchicine is effective, but it has been relegated to secondary status by its toxicity. Many patients taking the high oral doses of colchicine needed to abolish an acute gout attack develop unacceptable side effects, particularly nausea and diarrhea. Whereas patients who cannot take oral medications may respond to intravenous colchicine, intravenous administration should be discouraged because it can have life-threatening side effects, including renal or bone marrow failure. Patients with preexisting kidney or liver disease should never be given intravenous colchicine.

Another problem with colchicine is timing. The drug is most effective when given during the first 24–48 hours of an attack, presumably because it interferes with leukocyte migration and cytokine production. Colchicine no longer works once the inflammation is fully established. In contrast, NSAIDs often work even when started several days into an attack.

The second alternative to NSAIDs is glucocorticoids, which can be given orally, intravenously, or by intra-articular injection. Since gout usually affects one joint, the most effective way to control an attack—often within a few hours—is to inject a long-acting glucocorticoid directly into that joint. A glucocorticoid injection should be given only after the joint fluid has been cultured to exclude septic arthritis masquerading as gout, and patients must be followed up carefully for complications such as joint infection. Persons with multiple inflamed joints should be given a short generous course of oral glucocorticoids. Patients who cannot take oral medicines may be treated intravenously.

Management of Hyperuricemia

After the acute gouty attack has resolved, the physician can consider treating the underlying hyperuricemia. There is no reason to treat hyperuricemia in a person who has no history of gout or uric acid kidney stones. Whether patients with a history of gout should have their hyperuricemia treated depends in large part on their risk of having another attack. Only 50% of patients who have had one attack of gout will have another within 5 years. Therefore, few patients who have had one attack should be started on lifelong therapy, particularly if the uric acid is only minimally elevated or the person has other readily modifiable risk factors such as regular use of low-dose aspirin. However, treatment is indicated for any patient who has had multiple attacks in the past year and anyone who has had a uric acid kidney stone. Treatment should be considered after a single attack in a patient who is at high risk for recurrence because of renal insufficiency, congestive heart failure necessitating long-term diuretics, or a very high serum uric acid (over 12 mg/dL).

Hyperuricemia can be treated by either a uricosuric agent or allopurinol. Uricosuric agents work by enhancing renal excretion of uric acid. The two uricosuric agents available in the United States are probenecid and sulfinpyrazone. (Patients taking these drugs must be urged to drink at least 1 quart of fluid per day to prevent the formation of uric acid kidney stones.) Allopurinol works by inhibiting the enzyme xanthine oxidase; this inhibition reduces production of uric acid and increases production of xanthine, which is many times more soluble than uric acid and is readily excreted.

Which drug to give depends largely on whether patients overproduce or underexcrete uric acid. The physician makes this distinction by measuring how much uric acid patients excrete in the urine over 24 hours while eating their usual diet. If the 24-hour uric acid excretion is less than 700 mg, patients are underexcreters and may first be treated with a uricosuric agent. If the excretion is over 1000 mg, patients are overproducers who require allopurinol. Patients who produce 700–1000 mg of uric acid per day are in a "gray zone" and may be treated with either type of drug.

In certain situations, allopurinol should be given, regardless of how much uric acid the patient excretes. First, allopurinol is indicated for anyone who has had a uric acid kidney stone. Uricosuric agents should not be given, because they move more uric acid into the kidneys. Second, allopurinol is indicated for patients who have renal insufficiency. Since uricosuric agents work through the kidney, they are not effective in these patients. Third, allopurinol is the choice for patients who have developed tophi (see "Treatment of Chronic Tophaceous Gout" below), because these people have a very high total body uric acid load. Lastly, allopurinol is the alternative when uricosuric agents have not worked.

Allopurinol should be used cautiously, especially in the elderly and in people with reduced renal or hepatic function, because the drug's main metabolite, oxypurinol, has a very long half-life. Allopurinol toxicity can cause fever, rash, eosinophilia, and hepatic and renal failure that can, albeit rarely, prove fatal. No one has ever died of gout, but patients have died from complications of allopurinol treatment—most often people with renal insufficiency who are receiving full doses. These complications underscore the importance of not treating asymptomatic hyperuricemia.

When used properly, however, allopurinol is usually safe and effective. As with the uricosuric agents, the allopurinol dose should be built up slowly over several weeks. Patients must be warned that if they develop a rash they should stop taking the drug and call their physician immediately. If for any reason the patient's renal function deteriorates, the dose should be reduced. Allopurinol should be used cautiously in patients taking the purine derivative azathioprine, whose action is greatly potentiated when xanthine oxidase is blocked.

Whether patients take a uricosuric agent or allopurinol, they also need small doses of oral colchicine, because treatment that disturbs body uric acid stores paradoxically increases the frequency of gout attacks. After uric acid levels have fallen to normal, the colchicine can be stopped. Colchicine has no effect on serum uric acid levels, but it reduces the chance that uric acid crystals will trigger an attack. Most people can tolerate long-term small doses of colchicine. Rarely, however, chronic low-dose colchicine causes a myopathy that mimics polymyositis (Chapter 13.12). This complication is limited to patients who are over age 60 and have a serum creatinine above 2.0 mg/dL.

Management of Chronic Tophaceous Gout

Tophaceous gout (a tophus is a subcutaneous deposit of uric acid) develops after an average of 10 years of untreated or inadequately treated gout. Over this time, gout may evolve from an intermittent, intense monoarthritis of the foot to a chronic, deforming polyarthritis, often most strikingly affecting the hands (see Figure 3.8–2). This arthritis can mimic rheumatoid arthritis, although it is usually less symmetric. The radiographic hallmark of tophaceous gout is large, well-demarcated erosions without joint space narrowing (rat bite erosions). Tophi may be found in and around joints, bursae (especially the olecranon), tendons (especially the Achilles and infrapatellar), and the extensor surfaces of the forearms. Less commonly, tophi arise in the cardiac valves, cornea, sclera, nasal cartilage, and pinna of the ear. The diagnosis is confirmed when needle aspiration or spontaneous rupture of a tophus elicits a white, chalky material that microscopy shows to be full of uric acid crystals. All nonallergic patients with tophi should take allopurinol.

CALCIUM PYROPHOSPHATE DIHYDRATE (CPPD) DEPOSITION DISEASE

Deposition of calcium pyrophosphate dihydrate (CPPD) crystals in joints can cause four forms of arthritis, which together are known as CPPD deposition disease. One form so closely resembles gout in its intensity and acuteness of onset that it is called pseudogout (see Figure 3.8–1). Like gout, pseudogout is often precipitated by surgery. However, the two conditions tend to affect different joints: What the great toe and ankle are to gout, the

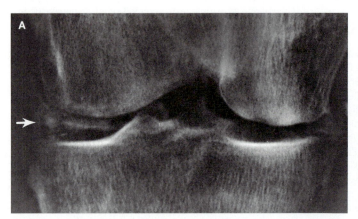

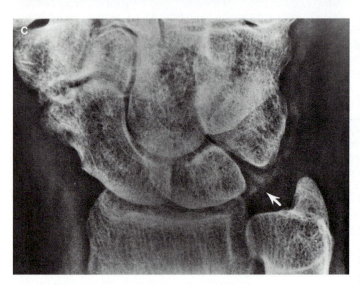

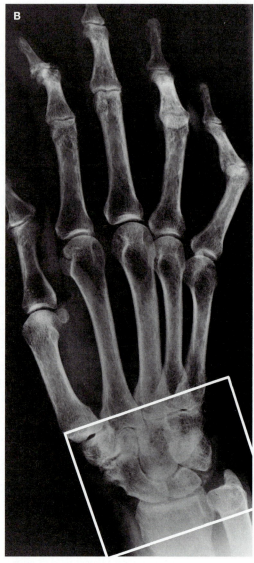

Figure 3.8–4. X-ray signs of chondrocalcinosis in calcium pyrophosphate dihydrate (CPPD) deposition disease. **A:** Articular calcification in knee. **B:** Calcified triangular ligament of wrist. **C:** Detail of panel B. (Courtesy of William W. Scott Jr, MD.)

knee and wrist are to pseudogout. Pseudogout is about half as common as gout, and accounts for up to 20% of CPPD disease. Pseudogout occurs about equally often in men and women, and usually begins after age 65; gout generally begins before 60. Occasionally patients have both gout and pseudogout.

A second, unusual form of CPPD mimics rheumatoid arthritis in that it affects chiefly the wrist and metacarpophalangeal joints, though usually with less striking inflammation than in rheumatoid arthritis. The third and most common form of CPPD mimics osteoarthritis, although unlike osteoarthritis it most often affects the knees and shoulders. The fourth and rarest form produces x-ray changes resembling a Charcot joint, with evidence of bone fragmentation associated with extensive, bizarre hypertrophic bony changes. A true Charcot (neuropathic) joint develops when neuropathy, usually from diabetes, tabes dorsalis, or syringomyelia has disrupted position sense and pain sensation, thereby promoting unrecognized repetitive joint trauma.

All forms of CPPD in symptomatic patients are diagnosed by characteristic x-ray findings or demonstration of CPPD crystals in the synovial fluid of involved joints. X-rays of affected joints typically show linear calcifications in the cartilage, called chondrocalcinosis (Figure 3.8–4). "Chondrocalcinosis" should not be used interchangeably with "CPPD" since many people, especially the elderly, have the x-ray abnormality but no clinical disease. The most common sites of chondrocalcinosis are the knees, triangular ligament of the wrist, and pubic ramus. X-rays of any of these areas offer the best chance of finding chondrocalcinosis to support a diagnosis of CPPD. The definitive diagnosis of CPPD, like that of gout, rests on arthrocentesis. The joint fluid must contain intracellular or extracellular rhomboidal crystals that are positively birefringent, looking blue when parallel with the axis of the red compensator on a polarizing microscope.

CPPD usually occurs spontaneously, but the physician should be aware of its association with certain metabolic conditions, especially hyperparathyroidism and hemochromatosis. CPPD can also be inherited as an autosomal dominant arthropathy.

The inflammation of CPPD is thought to begin when calcium pyrophosphate crystals are shed from joint cartilage into the synovial fluid. Like the uric acid crystals in gout, CPPD crystals are inflammatory. They are phagocytosed by polymorphonuclear leukocytes, which release lysosomal enzymes that damage the joint, whereas chemotactic factors recruit more white cells.

All forms of CPPD are treated with an NSAID or colchicine. Intra-articular corticosteroids are also useful for managing attacks. Colchicine has been shown to prevent pseudogout attacks and improve the more chronic forms of CPPD. However, there is no way to reduce the pyrophosphate concentration in the joint in the same way that allopurinol or uricosuric agents remove uric acid from the body. A patient presenting with CPPD should be evaluated for hyperparathyroidism and hemochromatosis.

SUMMARY

▶ Gout and pseudogout are common causes of acute monoarthritis. Gout most often attacks the great toe; pseudogout, the knee or wrist.

▶ The diagnosis of gout rests on finding uric acid crystals in the synovial fluid, and that of pseudogout on finding calcium pyrophosphate dihydrate crystals.

▶ In a few patients, gout is the first manifestation of a disorder such as polycythemia, and pseudogout is a manifestation of hyperparathyroidism or hemochromatosis.

▶ The treatment of acute gout and the treatment of hyperuricemia are completely separate issues. Treatment of hyperuricemia should be considered only after an acute attack has resolved.

▶ One-third of patients with gout have hypertension, which should be treated whether or not the gout needs treatment.

SUGGESTED READING

Campion EW, Glynn RJ, DeLabry LO: Asymptomatic hyperuricemia: Risks and consequences in the Normative Aging Study. Am J Med 1987;82:421.

Emmerson BT: The management of gout. N Engl J Med 1996;334:445.

Roberge CJ et al: Crystal-induced neutrophil activation: IV. Specific inhibition of tyrosine phosphorylation by colchicine. J Clin Invest 1993;92:1722.

Roubenoff R et al: Incidence and risk factors for gout in white men. JAMA 1991;266:3004.

Singer JZ, Wallace SL: The allopurinol hypersensitivity syndrome: Unnecessary morbidity and mortality. Arthritis Rheum 1986;29:82.

Osteoarthritis

Marc C. Hochberg, MD, MPH

Osteoarthritis is the most common form of arthritis. Osteoarthritis is also called "osteoarthrosis" or "degenerative joint disease," terms reflecting the fact that affected patients are older (most are over 50), develop joint pain insidiously, demonstrate little joint inflammation, and have no systemic symptoms.

For physicians, patients with osteoarthritis present three important challenges. The first is to distinguish osteoarthritis from inflammatory disorders, especially rheumatoid arthritis. The distinction is important because both disorders are so prevalent and their treatments and prognosis are so different. The second challenge is to identify the few patients whose osteoarthritis results from an identifiable and treatable metabolic disorder. The third challenge is to manage patients with the most appropriate medical or surgical options.

PATHOLOGY AND ETIOLOGY

Osteoarthritis is chiefly a disorder of articular cartilage. The pathologic hallmarks (Figure 3.9–1) are focal ulceration and irregularly distributed loss of articular cartilage, plus proliferation of bone at the joint margin (osteophytes, or "bone spurs"). Affected joints have little or no inflammation. Inflammation is not part of the primary disease process, although it can be caused by the body's reaction to joint debris. The lack of inflammation helps distinguish osteoarthritis from the inflammatory disease rheumatoid arthritis.

A number of biochemical changes in articular cartilage precede the development of clinically evident osteoarthritis. Articular cartilage is composed of both collagen, which provides tensile strength, and proteoglycans, which bestow compressibility. The earliest biochemical changes in osteoarthritis are that (1) the cartilage proteoglycan concentration falls; (2) the proteoglycans change in size and aggregation, with a higher concentration of small aggregates and monomers; and (3) water content increases. As the disease progresses, the cartilage surface begins to fragment and ulcerate. Chondrocytes (mature cartilage cells) can repair the cartilage to some degree. When their abilities are exceeded, osteoarthritis develops.

Although the exact cause of osteoarthritis is not known, several lines of evidence indicate that a major factor is structural fatigue (Table 3.9–1). First, the strongest determinant of osteoarthritis is age. Prevalence of disease in all joint groups increases with advancing age. Almost everyone over age 75 has radiographic evidence of osteoarthritis in at least one joint. Second, conditions that alter joint mechanics, such as congenital hip dislocation or previous joint injury, predispose to osteoarthritis. Third, weight loss reduces people's risk of developing symptomatic osteoarthritis in at least one joint, the knee. Fourth, activities like football that unduly stress joints lead to premature osteoarthritis. The fact that jogging does not cause osteoarthritis suggests that oscillating joint movements are less damaging to cartilage than pounding or high impact forces.

Load stresses and joint architecture are not the only factors that can lead to osteoarthritis. Alterations in collagen genes appear to explain some cases of familial osteoarthritis that begin unusually early, before age 45. Systemic metabolic processes such as hemochromatosis, acromegaly, calcium pyrophosphate dihydrate crystal deposition disease, and ochronosis also appear capable of altering cartilage or subchondral bone and causing osteoarthritis. Another risk factor is race. Even after adjustment for other risk factors, osteoarthritis of the knee is more common in black than white American women. Given cartilage's limited range of responses to injury, it is not surprising that the different influences provided by genes, joint architecture, metabolic condition, trauma, and obesity all can lead to the same process of osteoarthritis.

CLINICAL FEATURES

The typical patient with osteoarthritis is a middle-aged or elderly person who presents with gradually worsening pain, stiffness, and loss of function in certain joints. The

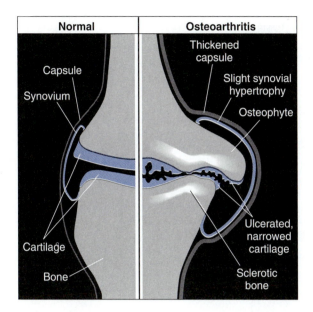

Normal	Osteoarthritis

Figure 3.9–1. Joint structures: normal versus osteoarthritis.

pain begins insidiously. It is usually mild, worsened by use of the involved joints, and improved or relieved with rest. Pain at rest or at night indicates severe disease. The pain of osteoarthritis can be caused by periostitis (inflammation of the connective tissue covering the bone) at sites of bone erosion or proliferation, or by subchondral bone microfractures, joint capsule irritation from osteophytes, periarticular muscle spasm, bone ischemia caused by decreased blood flow and elevated intraosseous pressure, or synovial inflammation accompanied by the release of prostaglandins, leukotrienes, and cytokines.

Osteoarthritis affects a characteristic pattern of joints (Figure 3.9–2). The peripheral joints most commonly involved are the distal interphalangeal joints (DIPs), proximal interphalangeal joints (PIPs), trapezioscaphoid joint, knees, hips, and the first metatarsophalangeal joint. Many patients also develop degenerative disease of the spine, es-

Table 3.9–1. Risk factors for osteoarthritis.

Increasing age
Congenital and developmental bone and joint disorders*
Abnormal joint mechanics*
Prior inflammatory joint disease*
Obesity*
Trauma*
Genetic predisposition
Metabolic disorders (hemochromatosis, ochronosis, acromegaly, calcium pyrophosphate dihydrate crystal deposition disease)
Female sex
Black race
Some occupations, eg, farmers, weavers, dockworkers, football players

*Potentially modifiable or treatable.

pecially the lower cervical and lower lumbar vertebrae. Notably, primary osteoarthritis rarely involves the wrists or metacarpophalangeal joints (MCPs).

The number of affected joints varies. Some patients have disease in only one or two weight-bearing sites, such as one hip and one knee. Other patients have generalized osteoarthritis affecting multiple DIPs, PIPs, and other joints. Generalized disease is more common in women than men.

Many patients report morning stiffness in the affected joints, but this disappears soon, often within 30 minutes—much faster than the stiffness of active rheumatoid arthritis. Many patients also get gel phenomenon (joint stiffness after inactivity), which resolves several minutes after they start moving the joint. As barometric pressure falls, intra-articular pressure rises. Thus, most patients find that their pain and stiffness worsen in damp, cool, rainy weather, and improve when the weather clears. Other complaints depend on the specific joints affected. Osteoarthritis of the knee can cause a sense of instability or buckling. Spinal osteoarthritis can compress neural structures, often causing pain and sometimes weakness or numbness (Chapter 3.13).

Whether a patient loses joint function depends chiefly on whether the osteoarthritis affects weight-bearing joints. Patients with osteoarthritis of the hands rarely lose much function. But degenerative changes in the hips or knees can dramatically reduce a person's ability to walk and lead an active life.

On examination, findings are usually localized to symptomatic joints. Many affected sites show bony enlargement with tenderness at the joint margins and the attachments of the joint capsule and periarticular tendons. Irregular loss of cartilage in the DIPs and PIPs characteristically makes the fingers look like a bent "broken staff" (Figure 3.9–3). The bony spurs at the DIPs are called Heberden's nodes; the same process at the PIPs is called Bouchard's nodes. Mild local inflammation may make a joint feel warm, and joint effusion may swell the surrounding soft tissue. A hot, red, markedly swollen joint is distinctly unusual in osteoarthritis and should suggest gout, pseudogout, or septic arthritis. A joint that locks during range of motion probably has cartilage and bone detritus lodging in the joint space.

The most common finding in osteoarthritis of the knee is crepitation. More than 90% of afflicted patients have the sensation and sound of having crunched potato chips in their knees. Crepitus felt on motion of the joint represents irregularity of the opposing cartilage surfaces, one of the earliest morphologic changes in osteoarthritis. Almost 50% of patients with knee osteoarthritis have malalignment, most typically a varus (bow-legged) deformity caused by loss of articular cartilage in the medial compartment.

One other important clinical feature of osteoarthritis is that it does not cause extra-articular manifestations. Fever, weight loss, and other signs of systemic disease can never be ascribed to osteoarthritis.

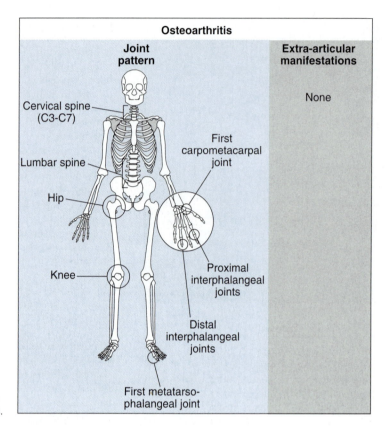

Figure 3.9–2. Joint pattern and extra-articular manifestations of osteoarthritis.

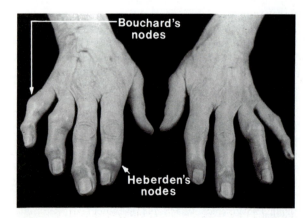

Figure 3.9–3. Characteristic hand deformities in osteoarthritis. Nodules at distal interphalangeal joints are called Heberden's nodes. Nodules at proximal interphalangeal joints are called Bouchard's nodes. (Reprinted from the Clinical Slide Collection on the Rheumatic Diseases, copyright 1991. Used by permission of the American College of Rheumatology.)

DIFFERENTIAL DIAGNOSIS

Osteoarthritis can usually be diagnosed during an office visit, based on the joint pattern and the absence of extra-articular manifestations. The differences between osteoarthritis and rheumatoid arthritis are striking and worth emphasizing (Table 3.9–2). In osteoarthritis, unlike rheumatoid arthritis, the MCPs and wrists are spared, morning stiffness lasts less than 30 minutes, and patients have no subcutaneous nodules or extra-articular manifestations. Psoriatic arthritis is the only disorder besides osteoarthritis that commonly involves the DIPs; psoriatic arthritis can be distinguished by its characteristic rash and nail changes (Chapter 3.7). Both osteoarthritis of the cervical spine and polymyalgia rheumatica can cause neck pain in patients over age 50. Polymyalgia rheumatica is the more likely cause if the patient has stiffness and myalgias involving the shoulder girdle and neck muscles, and an elevated erythrocyte sedimentation rate (Chapter 3.5). Whenever elderly patients develop osteoarthritis at an atypical site such as the shoulder, wrist, or MCPs, the differential diagnosis should include calcium pyrophosphate crystal deposition disease, hemochromatosis, Paget's disease of bone, acromegaly, ochronosis, and malignancy.

Although the risk is low, the physician should suspect that a patient's osteoarthritis is secondary to a metabolic

Table 3.9–2. Differentiating osteoarthritis from rheumatoid arthritis.

Characteristic	Osteoarthritis	Rheumatoid Arthritis
Joints involved		
DIPs	Often	Never
MCPs, wrists	Never	Often
Extra-articular signs	Never	Often
Subcutaneous nodules	Never	Occasionally
Eye inflammation	Never	Occasionally
Morning stiffness	<30 min	>30 min
Rheumatoid factor	<10% of patients	65–80% of patients
X-ray findings	Irregular cartilage loss	Uniform cartilage loss
	Osteophytes	Marginal bone erosions
	Bone sclerosis	Bone demineralization

DIPs, distal interphalangeal joints; MCPs, metacarpophalangeal joints.

disease when the arthritis starts before age 45 or the patient has other features of a metabolic disease (see Table 3.9–1). An important possibility is hemochromatosis, an iron storage disorder usually seen in men (Chapter 7.4). Estimates of gene frequency suggest that many cases go undetected. Hemochromatosis is the only disease that causes degenerative changes at the MCPs, particularly the second and third MCPs. The physician should consider hemochromatosis when a man with knee arthritis also has MCP degeneration, bronzed skin, cardiomyopathy, atrophic testes, late-onset diabetes, or any other feature of excess iron deposition.

LABORATORY FEATURES

X-rays faithfully reflect the pathologic changes of osteoarthritis (Figure 3.9–4). Since cartilage is radiolucent, the irregular cartilage loss must be inferred from irregular joint space narrowing. The second key pathologic feature, bone proliferation at the joint margins, shows up on x-rays as osteophytes (spurs). Proliferation of subchondral bone in areas of deep cartilage ulcers gives the appearance of increased bone density (sclerosis). Bone demineralization and marginal erosions are not radiographic features of osteoarthritis; they strongly suggest rheumatoid arthritis.

Most patients with osteoarthritis have a normal complete blood count, erythrocyte sedimentation rate, blood chemistry tests, and urinalysis. Many patients whose osteoarthritis is secondary to hemochromatosis have elevated liver function tests, and increased serum iron and ferritin levels. The evaluation of patients with arthritis commonly includes a test for rheumatoid factor. Up to 10% of elderly persons with osteoarthritis have a positive

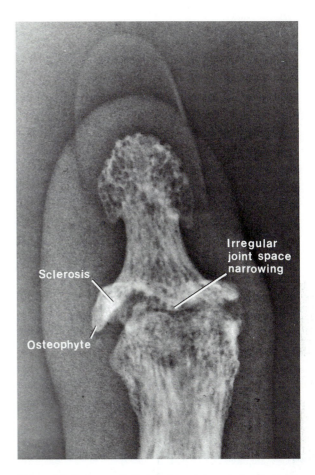

Figure 3.9–4. Osteoarthritis in a finger joint: subchondral bone sclerosis, osteophyte, and irregular joint space narrowing.

test in low titer. Therefore, rheumatoid factor does not exclude osteoarthritis if the patient has a consistent clinical picture and radiographic changes. Because osteoarthritic joints are at most minimally inflamed, the synovial fluid white blood cell count is below 3000/mm^3.

MANAGEMENT

The spectrum of treatment options ranges from "no therapy needed," to medicines and intra-articular injections, to surgical replacement of joints.

Many patients in whom osteoarthritis has caused striking deformities of the fingers, have few if any symptoms. These people seek medical help not for joint pain but because they fear that they have a crippling disease. Most of these patients need only education and reassurance (Chapter 3.1). They should be told that (1) osteoarthritis will not shorten their life span; (2) osteoarthritis in one site, like the fingers, will not necessarily spread to other sites, like the knees; and (3) if therapy is required, effective medical and surgical treatments are available.

Patients with symptomatic osteoarthritis may benefit from occupational and physical therapy. The occupational therapist evaluates how well patients perform such activities of daily living as dressing themselves, brushing their teeth, and handling kitchen utensils. The therapist shows patients how to protect their joints, for example, how to lift a heavy pot by shifting the stress from the affected fingers to the uninvolved shoulder. Patients also learn how to conserve their energy, as by trying to live on one floor and avoid climbing steps. An occupational therapist can also fashion splints to rest finger joints and provide braces, canes, crutches, and walkers to improve mobility. The physical therapist teaches patients the therapeutic use of heat and massage and provides an individualized exercise program that emphasizes range of motion as well as muscle strengthening to stabilize weight-bearing joints.

The main indication for drug therapy in patients with osteoarthritis is pain relief. The most often used classes of drugs are over-the-counter analgesics like acetaminophen, and nonsteroidal anti-inflammatory drugs (NSAIDs) such as aspirin and nonacetylated salicylates. More than a dozen prescription NSAIDs are available in the United States. All are about equally effective. The physician should base the choice of NSAID on dosing frequency, toxicity, and cost.

Intra-articular corticosteroid injections may help when only one or a few joints are warm, tender, and swollen, indicating local inflammation. Injections should be given no more than twice a year, because multiple injections may accelerate damage to cartilage.

Reconstructive joint surgery is an option for patients whose symptoms are not adequately controlled with a medical regimen and for those who have both moderate to severe pain and impaired function, especially with walking. Most patients' joint pain is related to weight bearing.

When patients start having spontaneous joint pain at night, they may be candidates for surgery. Total replacement of knee and hip joints is considered the major advance in the management of osteoarthritis over the past 20 years. In the short term, surgery relieves some or much of patients' pain; in the long term, most patients have significantly improved function. Perioperative mortality rate is generally less than 1%. Fewer than 5% of patients have short-term complications, particularly thromboembolic disease and infection. In some patients, the prosthetic joint loosens after 10–15 years, causing pain and requiring a more difficult and perhaps less successful second operation.

SUMMARY

▶ Osteoarthritis is the most common form of arthritis. The central pathologic features are cartilage ulceration and proliferation of bone at the joint margin (osteophytes). Inflammation, if any, is usually minimal.

▶ In contrast to rheumatoid arthritis, osteoarthritis often involves the distal interphalangeal joints, spares the wrists and metacarpophalangeal joints, causes less than 30 minutes of morning stiffness, and does not produce any extra-articular manifestations.

▶ Hemochromatosis, ochronosis, acromegaly, or calcium pyrophosphate dihydrate crystal deposition disease should be suspected when a person develops osteoarthritis before age 45 or has other manifestations of these metabolic disorders.

▶ The prognosis for those with osteoarthritis is excellent. Survival is not shortened, and any functional impairment can be treated medically and surgically.

SUGGESTED READING

Kuettner KE, Goldberg VM (editors): *Osteoarthritic Disorders.* American Academy of Orthopaedic Surgeons, 1995.

Moskowitz RW (editor): Osteoarthritis. Rheum Dis Clin North Am 1993;19:523.

Pelletier JP (editor): Osteoarthritis: Challenges for the 21st century. J Rheumatol 1995;22(Suppl 43):1.

Pelletier JP (editor): Osteoarthritis: Update on diagnosis and therapy. J Rheumatol 1991;18(Suppl 27):1.

3.10

Raynaud's Phenomenon and Scleroderma

Fredrick M. Wigley, MD

RAYNAUD'S PHENOMENON

Raynaud's phenomenon is an excessive response to cold and emotional stress, manifested by sudden changes in color of the fingers and toes. During cold exposure, the body's normal response is to reduce heat loss by constricting cutaneous arteriovenous shunts; thus, some coolness and discoloration in the fingers and toes are normal. Sympathetic stimuli like emotional stress also provoke this vascular response. Patients with Raynaud's phenomenon, however, have an exaggerated reaction. Even with brief exposure to cool temperatures or stress, some or all of their fingers and toes may be dramatically discolored and cold.

The physician seeing a patient with Raynaud's phenomenon should address one central question: "Does the patient have a systemic disease?" Raynaud's phenomenon is common, occurring in 2–6% of the general population and up to 20% of women of childbearing age. Most affected persons have no systemic disease and are said to have primary (idiopathic) Raynaud's phenomenon. But for some patients, Raynaud's is an early manifestation of a number of systemic diseases (Table 3.10–1), including scleroderma (see below).

Clinical Features and Diagnosis

A classic attack of Raynaud's phenomenon has three phases: (1) The fingers become pale white as vasospasm stops blood flow to the fingers (see Color Plates). (2) The fingers become blue (cyanotic) as blood moving sluggishly through the capillaries of the skin becomes deoxygenated. (3) The fingers turn red as the once-constricted vessels dilate during the hyperemic phase that follows ischemia. During the phases of pallor and cyanosis, many patients complain of a feeling of "pins and needles" over the fingers, a dulled sense of touch, clumsiness of hand function, or pain.

There is no laboratory test that can establish the diagnosis of Raynaud's phenomenon. The diagnosis is made when a patient gives a history of cold hands associated with the typical color changes. However, many patients with Raynaud's do not go through all three phases; in these patients, the defining element is a history of excessive pallor upon exposure to cold. Patients report attacks with what would otherwise be considered mild cold exposure, such as removing a can of juice from the freezer or shopping in the frozen foods section of a grocery store. Anxiety, fear, or anger can also provoke attacks.

Pathophysiology of Primary Raynaud's Phenomenon

Normal control of vascular tone is complex, combining regulation from the central nervous system, hormonal influences, and mediators produced locally by the blood vessel's endothelium. The cause of primary Raynaud's phenomenon is not known; the blood vessels have no morphologic abnormality. Many patients with secondary Raynaud's do have morphologic changes in the vessels, including enlargement or dropout of cutaneous capillary loops, but, again, the cause is unknown.

Differential Diagnosis

Raynaud's phenomenon is classified as either primary (idiopathic Raynaud's disease) or secondary (see Table 3.10–1). Primary Raynaud's phenomenon occurs most commonly in otherwise normal young women; it usually begins after menarche and improves after menopause. Secondary Raynaud's phenomenon can be associated with connective tissue diseases, extrinsic neurovascular compression, intrinsic arterial disease, hematologic disorders, occupational injury, drugs, and toxins. The history and physical examination can distinguish primary from secondary Raynaud's (Table 3.10–2). The physician should suspect secondary Raynaud's if the patient is a man; if the attacks began either during childhood or after age 35 years; if attacks are asymmetrical, unilateral, or intensely painful; or if the patient has symptoms of another disease, eg, malar rash and arthritis suggesting systemic lupus erythematosus. A history of persistent numbness or weakness of the fingers suggests an associated carpal tunnel syndrome, caused by compression of the median nerve at the wrist. β-blockers, sympathomimetic drugs, chemothera-

Table 3.10–1. Causes of Raynaud's phenomenon.

Primary
  Idiopathic (Raynaud's disease)

Secondary
  Systemic sclerosis (scleroderma)
  Systemic lupus erythematosus
  Dermatomyositis
  Extrinsic neurovascular compression
  Carpal tunnel syndrome
  Thoracic outlet syndrome
  Intrinsic arterial disease
  Arteritis
  Occlusive vascular disorders
  Hematologic disorders
  Cryoglobulins
  Polycythemia
  Paraproteins
  Occupational injury (vibration white finger syndrome)
  Drugs and toxins
    Ergotamine
    β-adrenergic blockade
    Polyvinyl chloride exposure
    Sympathomimetic drugs
  Other associations
    Primary pulmonary hypertension
    Migraine headaches
    Coronary artery spasm

peutic agents, and exposure to some toxins can also cause or exacerbate Raynaud's.

Physical findings can help delineate secondary Raynaud's. Ulcerated fingertips and digital gangrene are unusual in primary Raynaud's, and should suggest that the Raynaud's is secondary to a process like scleroderma or vasculitis. Nailfold capillary abnormalities (see Color Plates), chiefly dilatation of some capillaries and disappearance (dropout) of others, are not seen in primary Raynaud's but are common in patients with scleroderma or

dermatomyositis. The best way to assess the nailfold capillaries is to place a drop of immersion oil on the skin at the base of the fingernail and examine the nailfold capillaries with a microscope or ophthalmoscope. Tightness of the skin over the fingers (sclerodactyly; Figure 3.10–1) and telangiectasias (Figure 3.10–2) can be early manifestations of scleroderma.

The physician should look for other stigmata of connective tissue diseases, such as the facial erythema of systemic lupus erythematosus and the lilac-discolored eyelids (heliotrope rash) of dermatomyositis. Discrepant blood pressures between the arms or the legs, loss of pulses, or vascular bruits would argue strongly against primary Raynaud's and suggest diseases of the large arteries, such as Takayasu's aortitis or atherosclerosis. Lymphadenopathy or splenomegaly suggests that Raynaud's phenomenon is caused by hyperviscosity associated with a lymphoproliferative disorder.

Laboratory tests can further help distinguish primary from secondary Raynaud's. The extent of evaluation depends on the patient's presentation and physical findings. A young woman with an unremarkable history and physical examination probably has primary Raynaud's and needs no laboratory studies. A patient with symptoms or signs of secondary Raynaud's should be further evaluated. Most patients with systemic lupus erythematosus, dermatomyositis, or scleroderma have a positive antinuclear antibody test, but so do some patients with primary Raynaud's phenomenon. Certain autoantibodies have greater specificity for certain rheumatic diseases (see Table 3.1–4). Serum immunoelectrophoresis and measurement of serum viscosity identify patients in whom lymphoproliferative disorders are producing monoclonal proteins and hyperviscosity. Cryoglobulins may signal cryoglobulinemia or lymphoma. Low serum complement or an abnormal urinalysis suggests an underlying autoimmune disease.

Table 3.10–2. Clues to secondary Raynaud's phenomenon.

History and host factors
  Male sex
  Sudden onset
  Onset before age 18 or after age 35
  Unilateral Raynaud's
  Symptoms of another disease (eg, photosensitivity of systemic
    lupus erythematosus)

Physical findings
  Nailfold capillary abnormalities
  Digital ulcers or gangrene
  Absent pulses
  Blood pressure discrepancies between arms or between legs
  Arterial bruits
  Findings of another disease (eg, sclerodactyly of scleroderma)

Laboratory tests
  Anticentromere antibody
  Monoclonal gammopathy
  Proteinuria
  Laboratory markers of other diseases (eg, elevated creatine
    kinase from dermatomyositis)

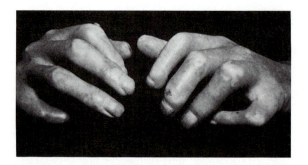

Figure 3.10–1. Sclerodactyly in a patient with scleroderma. Skin tightening has contracted the fingers and erased the creases over the knuckles. (Reprinted from the Clinical Slide Collection on the Rheumatic Diseases, copyright 1991. Used by permission of the American College of Rheumatology.)

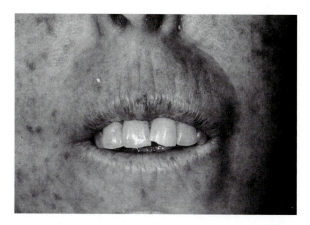

Figure 3.10–2. Telangiectasias on the face of a patient with scleroderma. Note perioral furrowing and small oral aperture.

Management

The mainstay of management for primary Raynaud's phenomenon is avoiding the cold through choices of climate, thermostat settings, and clothes. Patients should also reduce emotional stress and avoid taking β-blockers. Calcium channel blockers, particularly nifedipine, reduce vascular spasm and improve symptoms in the few patients whose lifestyle is significantly hampered by primary Raynaud's. Unfortunately, the calcium channel blockers and other vasodilators are less effective in patients with secondary Raynaud's.

SYSTEMIC SCLEROSIS (SCLERODERMA)

Systemic sclerosis (scleroderma) is an uncommon chronic multisystem disease of unknown etiology, featuring a systemic vasculopathy of small and medium-sized blood vessels, excessive collagen deposition in tissues, and an activated immune system (Figure 3.10–3). Two to three times as many women as men are affected. Most patients with scleroderma present first with Raynaud's phenomenon, followed months to years later by thickening of the skin (scleroderma). However striking the cutaneous findings may be, a patient's prognosis is most influenced by the severity of the visceral manifestations, which can include gastrointestinal, cardiac, renal, and pulmonary complications.

Understanding scleroderma allows the physician to meet at least three important challenges. The first is recognizing when a patient has scleroderma and not simply Raynaud's phenomenon. The second is distinguishing between the two variants of scleroderma—the more benign limited variant (CREST syndrome) and the more severe diffuse scleroderma. This distinction is often made clinically. The third challenge is identifying and managing the visceral complications of scleroderma. Although scleroderma cannot be cured, therapy can greatly improve some of its manifestations.

Clinical Features of Early Disease

The earliest symptoms of scleroderma are usually Raynaud's phenomenon and skin changes, most often on the fingers, forearms, face, and neck. At first the skin is not sclerotic (hard), but it is mildly erythematous, with non-pitting edema caused by excess fluid in the connective tissue. The patient complains of tightness, itching, and restricted motion of the fingers or mouth. Weeks or months later, the skin hardens (scleroderma; see Figure 3.10–1), often with patchy areas of hypo- and hyperpigmentation. The tightening of skin over the face can eliminate facial lines and creases. Taut skin around the mouth thins the vermilion border of the lips, restricts the size of the oral aperture, and produces vertical striations that make the lips look pursed (see Figure 3.10–2). Later, the skin becomes atrophic and loses normal appendages such as hair and sweat glands. Many patients complain about dryness, fissuring, and ulceration of the skin, particularly on the fingertips.

Scleroderma is a clinical diagnosis. It is usually established by finding symmetrical areas of thickened skin on the dorsum of the hand proximal to the metacarpophalangeal joints, or on the forearms, upper arms, face, trunk, or legs. Alternatively, the diagnosis can be made in a patient whose skin changes are limited to the fingers, as long as the patient also has either pitted fingertip ulcers or basilar fibrosis on chest x-ray.

A further important clue is telangiectasias—another early cutaneous manifestation of scleroderma (see Figure 3.10–2). Telangiectasias may appear in patients who have little other skin involvement. Lesions most often develop on the palms, face, mucous membranes of the lips and mouth, and skin of the upper chest. Patients may also have nailfold capillary abnormalities (see Color Plates). Many patients develop subcutaneous calcium deposits, particularly along the fingers and over pressure points.

Patients with scleroderma generally report vague constitutional symptoms such as fatigue, weight loss, and muscular aches, as well as pains that may mimic other rheumatic diseases, especially systemic lupus erythematosus, rheumatoid arthritis, and dermatomyositis. Inflamed, swollen joints are less common in scleroderma than in other rheumatic diseases, but the diffuse swelling of the fingers is often mistaken for arthritis.

Differential Diagnosis

Tight, thickened skin over the fingers (sclerodactyly) is not specific to scleroderma. Sclerodactyly can also be caused by trauma, longstanding insulin-dependent diabetes mellitus, and exposure to toxins like bleomycin and polyvinyl chloride. The hands can also show diffuse swelling with reflex sympathetic dystrophy and with palmar fasciitis, a paraneoplastic condition (most commonly seen in patients with ovarian carcinoma) that produces

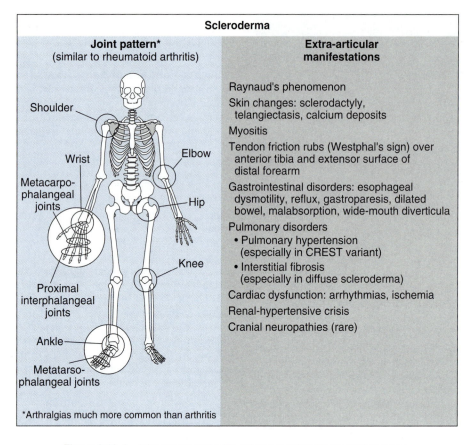

Figure 3.10–3. Joint pattern and extra-articular manifestations of scleroderma.

swelling chiefly of the palms, and finger contraction that resembles scleroderma. However, few patients with these conditions have Raynaud's phenomenon, which nearly always accompanies scleroderma.

Other conditions can cause hardening or swelling of the skin. Morphea is a dermatologic disease with pearly white patches of thickened skin, most often coin-size or larger, but usually no systemic features. Linear scleroderma, as the name indicates, produces a line of hard skin, often the length of a leg or an arm; there are no systemic manifestations, but local tissue damage can be disfiguring and impair function of an extremity.

Eosinophilic fasciitis (Shulman's syndrome) causes skin thickening and swelling that at first glance resemble scleroderma. But in eosinophilic fasciitis the inflammation is deeper, affecting chiefly the fascia and sparing the epidermis. The overlying skin remains soft enough to pinch; the skin in scleroderma is too hard to pinch. The deeper level of inflammation in eosinophilic fasciitis gives it a texture that has aptly been likened to orange peel (peau d'orange). Eosinophilic fasciitis is further distinguished from scleroderma by the absence of Raynaud's phenomenon, the tendency to spare the hands, characteristic inflammatory changes in the fascia, blood eosinophilia, hyperglobulinemia, and a good response to oral cor-

ticosteroids. Other diseases in which thickened skin superficially resembles scleroderma include scleredema, carcinoid syndrome, eosinophilic myalgia syndrome, chronic graft versus host disease, porphyria cutanea tarda, scleromyxedema, and the toxic oil syndrome.

Telangiectasia is not specific for scleroderma. For example, patients with hereditary hemorrhagic telangiectasia (Osler-Weber-Rendu syndrome), an autosomal dominant disorder, have a similar distribution of telangiectasia; but, instead of Raynaud's phenomenon, these patients have gastrointestinal or upper airway bleeding, or arteriovenous malformations. Multiple telangiectasias can also be caused by chronic liver disease, sun exposure, and estrogen use.

Further Evaluation

The treatment and prognosis of scleroderma depend on which visceral organs are involved and whether the scleroderma is limited or diffuse.

Visceral Organ Involvement: The extent of visceral organ involvement in scleroderma is the greatest single determinant of survival (see Figure 3.10–3). Most patients gradually develop dysfunction of the lungs, heart, and gastrointestinal tract. All of the involved organs have similar pathologic changes—vasculopathy and excessive collagen deposition with fibrosis. Rare patients have extensive visceral involvement despite few or no skin changes (systemic sclerosis sine scleroderma).

Types of Scleroderma: Scleroderma has two major forms: limited skin involvement (also known as the CREST syndrome), affecting 60% of patients, and diffuse scleroderma, affecting 40% (Table 3.10–3). CREST is an acronym for the major clinical features of the limited type: Calcinosis, Raynaud's phenomenon, Esophageal dysmotility, Sclerodactyly, and Telangiectasia. These manifestations, with some variation described below, can also be seen in diffuse scleroderma; the chief distinctive feature of limited scleroderma is that the skin changes are generally confined to the hands, feet, and face, and are not seen proximal to the elbows or knees. Patients with limited scleroderma often have Raynaud's phenomenon for years before they develop other manifestations. They generally have less severe visceral involvement than patients with diffuse scleroderma, and they live longer. However, they are more likely to have extensive subcutaneous calcification and ischemic loss of multiple digits, and may develop pulmonary hypertension without lung fibrosis.

Disease with diffuse skin involvement follows a more aggressive course. Skin changes usually begin weeks or months after the onset of Raynaud's phenomenon, and then quickly spread over large areas of the body. Early in the disease, some patients develop life-threatening lung, kidney, gastrointestinal, and heart involvement. Ten-year survival rates average 40–50% in diffuse scleroderma, as against 65–75% in limited (CREST) scleroderma.

Laboratory Findings

Early in scleroderma the blood count, electrolytes, liver function tests, and urinalysis may be normal, but abnormalities develop with late complications. Thyroid function tests may be abnormal because of fibrosis or autoimmune destruction of the gland. Two important laboratory markers of gastrointestinal disease are iron deficiency, caused

by esophagitis and chronic blood loss; and macrocytic anemia, caused by vitamin B_{12} or folate deficiency stemming from malabsorption, bacterial overgrowth, or malnutrition. When hypertensive crisis complicates diffuse scleroderma, the serum creatinine may be elevated.

Skin biopsy shows excess collagen deposition in and thickening of the reticular dermis. A mononuclear cell infiltrate is seen around blood vessels. The papillary dermis and epidermal rete pegs are atrophied. Intimal proliferation and collagen deposition narrow the lumens of arteries and arterioles.

Fifty percent of patients have hypergammaglobulinemia. Most have antinuclear antibody (ANA). The two variants of scleroderma differ in their specific antinuclear antibody associations. Anticentromere antibody is found in 50–90% of patients with CREST but less than 10% of those with diffuse scleroderma. Antibodies to topoisomerase I (Scl-70), which are specific but not sensitive for diffuse disease, are found in 20% of patients. Patients with diffuse disease have also been found to have antibodies to other nucleolar antigens, such as anti-RNA polymerase I, II, and III.

Management

Scleroderma interferes with every aspect of a person's life. Patients may lose their independence. By restricting mobility, the taut skin of the hands and limbs limits patients' ability to dress and care for themselves. They may be unable to fulfill their expected social and sexual roles. Disfiguring changes in the skin and facial features lower their self-image and sense of well-being. The extensive medical care that they need imposes a heavy burden on their time and finances. Coping with this chronic multisystem disease leaves patients depressed, fearful, and frustrated.

The physician caring for a patient with scleroderma must be attuned to patients' range of needs and must provide support. A physical or occupational therapist may help lessen the musculoskeletal pain and weakness, and enable patients to better perform their daily activities. Creating and maintaining an effective support system may require family conferences and counseling for patient and family.

No therapy has been proved to alter the course of scleroderma. D-penicillamine, colchicine, immunosuppressive agents, and antimetabolites have been used, but there is no solid evidence that they can improve outcome. However, a number of the complications are treatable. Raynaud's phenomenon responds partially to calcium channel blockers. Mild esophagitis may respond to H_2-blockers. Severe esophagitis responds dramatically to omeprazole, a drug that almost completely eliminates gastric acid production; omeprazole may also prevent or forestall the development of esophageal stricture. In early disease, symptoms of gastrointestinal dysmotility may be reduced by metoclopramide, erythromycin, somatostatin, or cisapride—all prokinetic agents that enhance gut smooth-muscle contraction. Malabsorption caused by bacterial overgrowth is eliminated by broad-spectrum antibiotics. Many patients with scleroderma have an associated polymyositis, which

Table 3.10–3. Distinguishing features: CREST* variant versus diffuse scleroderma.

Characteristic	CREST Variant	Diffuse Scleroderma
Duration of Raynaud's before other symptoms	Years	Weeks or months
Skin involvement	Fingers and face	Diffuse
Renal involvement	No	Yes
Pulmonary disease	Pulmonary hypertension	Interstitial disease
Prognosis	Good	Variable, poor
Anticentromere antibody	Yes	No
Anti–Scl-70	No	Yes

*CREST, Calcinosis, Raynaud's phenomenon, Esophageal dysmotility, Sclerodactyly, Telangiectasia.

should be detected early and treated aggressively with corticosteroids. Corticosteroids are not effective for other manifestations of scleroderma, and should not be used casually. The angiotensin-converting enzyme inhibitors have been a major advance in treating renal-hypertensive crisis. Anemia, heart failure, kidney failure, pulmonary failure, and the many other complications of scleroderma should be treated as they are in other settings.

SUMMARY

▶ The diagnosis of Raynaud's phenomenon is based on a history of exaggerated sensitivity of the hands to cold exposure.

▶ Raynaud's phenomenon is usually idiopathic and benign, but can develop secondary to systemic diseases, especially scleroderma, systemic lupus erythematosus, and dermatomyositis.

▶ The external manifestations of scleroderma (especially Raynaud's phenomenon and sclerodactyly) first suggest the diagnosis, but the internal complications (renal, cardiac, gastrointestinal, and pulmonary) determine prognosis.

▶ There are two forms of scleroderma. The CREST variant (**C**alcinosis, **R**aynaud's phenomenon, **E**sophageal dysmotility, **S**clerodactyly, **T**elangiectasia) has limited skin changes and less severe visceral involvement. Diffuse scleroderma is more aggressive, with a shorter survival.

SUGGESTED READING

Clements PJ, Furst DE: *Systemic Sclerosis.* Williams & Wilkins, 1996.

Coffman JD: *Raynaud's Phenomenon.* Oxford, 1989.

Klippel JH, Dieppe PA: *Rheumatology.* Mosby, 1994.

LeRoy EC (editor): Scleroderma. Rheum Dis Clin North Am 1990;16:1.

Medsger TA Jr: Treatment of systemic sclerosis. Ann Rheum Dis 1991;50(Suppl 4):877.

Wigley FM, Matsumoto AK: Chapters on "Raynaud's phenomenon" and "Scleroderma." In: *Treatment of the Rheumatic Diseases.* Weisman MH, Weinblatt ME (editors). WB Saunders, 1995.

3.11

Bacterial Arthritis

David B. Hellmann, MD

The terms "bacterial arthritis" and "septic arthritis" describe a joint infected with pyogenic organisms that usually grow rapidly in culture. This definition traditionally excludes some forms of arthritis caused by bacteria: Lyme disease (Chapter 8.16) and syphilis (Chapter 8.9), whose organisms defy routine culturing, and tuberculosis (Chapter 8.14), which is less pyogenic and grows slowly in culture.

Most patients with septic arthritis have at least one feature in common: a hot, swollen joint. How much else they share depends largely on whether they have gonococcal or nongonococcal arthritis (Table 3.11–1). Gonococcal arthritis affects normal people (all sexually active, most younger than 45); patients may present with tenosynovitis or arthritis, respond quickly to treatment, and almost never suffer permanent joint damage. The more serious nongonococcal septic arthritis affects patients with specific risk factors (see "Nongonococcal Septic Arthritis" below) and is caused by pyogenic organisms that must be treated early and intensively to prevent joint destruction and a high risk of death. Given these differences, nongonococcal and gonococcal arthritis are discussed separately.

NONGONOCOCCAL SEPTIC ARTHRITIS

Pathogenesis and Bacteriology

Bacterial arthritis is usually a consequence of hematogenous spread of infection. Normal adults rarely develop bacterial arthritis. People are at risk only when the usual protective mechanisms are breached by abnormal joint anatomy, a prosthesis, or immunosuppression, or they are overwhelmed by persistent bacteremia. This explains why the chief risk factors for nongonococcal bacterial arthritis are rheumatoid arthritis, previous joint trauma or surgery, advanced age, alcoholism, diabetes, cortico-

steroid use, intravenous drug use, and endocarditis. Occasionally, nongonococcal arthritis is caused by organisms directly implanted into joints (eg, through a knife wound, a motorcycle accident, or a joint aspirated through infected skin) or extension of infection from a contiguous site (eg, from a neighboring nidus of osteomyelitis). In whatever way the organisms invade the joint, they first provoke polymorphonuclear cell infiltration of the synovium and vascular congestion, then synovial cell proliferation, granulation tissue, and abscess formation, and ultimately—if the infection is untreated—joint destruction.

Staphylococcus aureus and streptococci account for 80% of cases of nongonococcal bacterial arthritis (Table 3.11–2). *Staphylococcus epidermidis* infection is uncommon except in patients with prosthetic joints. Gram-negative bacilli, which were once rare causes of septic arthritis, have become more common: *Escherichia coli* is seen most often, but *Pseudomonas aeruginosa* is frequently seen in intravenous drug abusers. *Pasteurella multocida* causes 50% of infections from a dog or cat bite. Polymicrobial infections are infrequent (10%) and usually follow penetrating trauma.

Presentation and Diagnosis

Patients with nongonococcal bacterial arthritis typically present with acute monoarthritis. The three most common causes of acute monoarthritis are crystal disease (gout, pseudogout [Chapter 3.8]), trauma, and infection. Until proven otherwise, infection should always be considered the cause of unexplained acute monoarthritis. It is important to remember that infection can be superimposed on other forms of arthritis, especially rheumatoid arthritis. Since active rheumatoid arthritis usually affects more than one joint, an apparent "flare" in a single joint should raise suspicion of septic arthritis. Only about 20% of cases of septic arthritis are polyarticular; multiple joint infection is more common in patients who have rheumatoid arthritis or endocarditis.

The most frequently affected joint is the knee, followed by the hip, shoulder, wrist, ankle, elbow, and small joints

Acknowledgment: John G. Bartlett, MD, provided consultation in the writing of this chapter.

Table 3.11–1. Nongonococcal bacterial arthritis versus disseminated gonococcal infection.

	Nongonococcal Bacterial Arthritis	Disseminated Gonococcal Infection
Host	Person with previous joint damage or abnormal bacteremia (eg, from intravenous drug use)	Healthy young person
Clinical features		
Monoarthritis	80% of patients	33% of patients
Polyarthritis	20%	67%
Skin lesions	Rare	66%
Positive blood cultures	50%	<10%
Positive synovial fluid culture	85–95%	25%
Mortality	10%	None
Complete recovery	66%	>95%

Modified and reproduced, with permission, from Goldenberg DL, Reed JI: Bacterial arthritis. N Engl J Med 1985;312:764.

of the hand or foot. The sternoclavicular joint and sacroiliac joints are rarely involved, except in intravenous drug users. The affected joint is swollen, warm, red, and so painful that patients with knee or hip involvement cannot walk unassisted. In most patients, the pain and swelling reach their peak within 2–7 days. Symptoms and signs are often less dramatic and slower to develop in patients with prosthetic joint infection.

Patients also have decreased function and restricted range of motion—especially helpful findings in diagnosing infection of joints such as the hip, whose swelling cannot be detected by physical examination. Patients with hip disease of any type feel pain chiefly in the groin area and note decreased range of motion. If a patient does not have trouble putting on pants or stockings, important hip disease is very unlikely. When a hip is infected, the groin pain and dysfunction develop over just a few days. When supine, the patient prefers to keep the hip rotated externally and suffers exquisite pain when the physician tries to rotate it internally. If the patient prefers to keep the hip flexed, the physician should suspect psoas abscess, not hip infection.

Like the hip, the sacroiliac joint is too deep to be palpated directly. Infection is suspected when an intravenous

Table 3.11–2. Bacteriology of nongonococcal septic arthritis in adults.

Organism	Frequency (%)
Staphylococcus aureus	40
Streptococcal sp	30
Staphylococcus epidermidis	5
Gram-negative bacilli	20
Streptococcus pneumoniae	5

Modified and reproduced, with permission, from Goldenberg DL, Reed JI: Bacterial arthritis. N Engl J Med 1985;312:764.

drug user, the most common host for this infection, develops fever and sacral or buttock pain that radiates down the posterior thigh to the knee. Although the sternoclavicular joint is easy to palpate, infection there often presents with shoulder pain. Thus, when patients complain of shoulder discomfort, the physician should inspect and palpate the sternoclavicular joint.

Fever almost always complicates septic arthritis, but up to 50% of patients present with a normal temperature—especially patients compromised by age, corticosteroids, liver disease, or alcohol abuse. Therefore, a normal temperature does not exclude infection. Regardless of temperature, any person who develops unexplained acute hip pain that prevents walking must be presumed to have septic arthritis. The rest of the physical exam may give clues to the source of hematogenous infection, such as a murmur or Osler's nodes indicating endocarditis, or track marks from intravenous drug use.

The routine laboratory features of septic arthritis are nonspecific: leukocytosis and an elevated erythrocyte sedimentation rate. Early in the course, plain x-rays of the joint are almost always normal, except that they show effusion. For joints like the hip, effusion shown by computed tomography or magnetic resonance imaging can support a suspicion of infection. A joint without effusion is probably not infected.

Synovial fluid examination is the crucial test for nongonococcal septic arthritis and should be done promptly whenever a patient develops acute monoarthritis of unknown cause. Infected synovial fluid is usually plentiful (over 20 mL) and easily obtained. It looks cloudy and has a white blood cell count of over 3000/mm³. Most patients with staphylococcal or streptococcal infection have synovial fluid white blood cell counts averaging 100,000/mm³, with a majority of polymorphonuclear cells. Gram's stain is positive in 50–75% of patients, and culture is almost always positive. Finding urate or calcium pyrophosphate crystals in the joint does not exclude infection, since infection and crystal disease can coexist. Blood cultures are positive in 50% of patients with septic arthritis; in about 50% of these a primary source of infection is found. Sources include the genitourinary tract, endocarditis, skin abscess or cellulitis, decubitus ulcers, pneumonia, and meningitis.

Management

The mainstays of therapy for nongonococcal septic arthritis are intravenous antibiotics and joint drainage. Choice of initial antibiotics is guided by the bacteriology (see Table 3.11–2), Gram's stain, and host risk factors (Table 3.11–3). All patients with suspected infection should first be given antibiotics (eg, nafcillin) directed against staphylococci and streptococci, since these organisms account for 80% of cases. Coverage for gram-negative bacteria should be added if Gram's stain shows these organisms or if the patient injects illicit drugs. Patients who have recently been hospitalized or had an invasive procedure are at risk for methicillin-resistant *S aureus*; re-

Table 3.11–3. Initial choice of antibiotics for septic arthritis: Role of Gram's stain and risk factors.

	Organisms Suspected	Antibiotics
Synovial fluid Gram's stain		
Negative	Staphylococci, streptococci, aerobic gram-negative bacilli (in injection drug users), *Neisseria gonorrhoeae* (in young, sexually active people)	Penicillinase-resistant penicillin (nafcillin, oxacillin) ± gentamicin or a third-generation cephalosporin OR antibiotics for *N gonorrhoeae* (see below)
Gram-positive organisms	Staphylococci, streptococci	Nafcillin or oxacillin
Gram-negative bacilli	Aerobic gram-negative bacilli	Nafcillin or oxacillin + gentamicin or a third-generation cephalosporin
Gram-negative diplococci	*N gonorrhoeae*	Ceftriaxone, cefotaxime, ceftizoxime, or spectinomycin
Risk factor		
History of prosthetic joint placement, surgery, intravenous line, recent hospitalization	*Staphylococcus epidermidis, Staphylococcus aureus*	Vancomycin OR Vancomycin + rifampin + gentamicin or ceftazidime
Intravenous drug user	Gram-negative bacilli, *S aureus*	Nafcillin or oxacillin + gentamicin or ceftazidime

gardless of the findings on Gram's stain, these patients need vancomycin at least until culture and sensitivity results are available.

For antibiotics to work, the joint must be drained. All antibiotics achieve excellent levels in the synovial fluid, but are effective only if the organism is dividing. In pus under pressure, organisms divide slowly, if at all. Furthermore, polymorphonuclear cells function poorly in pus. Thus, unless the joint is drained, organisms can survive antibiotic treatment. Closed drainage via joint aspiration is effective and is the preferred first step for all joints that are easy to tap. Joint aspirations should be repeated as often as necessary to control swelling; some patients require daily or even twice-daily aspirations. Open surgical drainage is required from the outset for joints (eg, the hip) that are difficult to examine for fluid and difficult to aspirate and for all prosthetic joint infections.

Efficacy of therapy is judged by the patient's clinical picture and repeated joint fluid analysis. Within 2–3 days of starting treatment, the patient should appear more comfortable. Fever may continue but is lower and less constant, and synovial fluid should be less copious, have a lower white blood cell count, and become sterile. A patient who does not improve within 2–3 days despite effective antibiotics and needle drainage needs surgical drainage and débridement. If the infected joint improves but the patient appears toxic, the physician should search for a second site of infection, such as a splenic abscess complicating endocarditis or occult infection of another joint. Debilitated, gravely ill, and poorly responsive patients with rheumatoid arthritis are especially likely to harbor a hidden joint infection.

The acutely infected joint should be rested. Most patients have less pain when the involved joint is slightly flexed, but maintaining that position predisposes to contracture. Therefore, as soon as the joint inflammation begins to improve, passive range-of-motion exercises should

be started to preserve function. Later, patients can do active exercises to improve strength.

Patients with nonprosthetic joint infections receive intravenous antibiotics for an average of 3 weeks; compromised hosts may need treatment longer. Many experts believe that for therapy beyond 3 weeks, patients can be switched to oral antibiotics selected through in vitro sensitivity tests.

Prosthetic Joint Infections

Prosthetic joint infections are caused by *S aureus* (20–30%), *S epidermidis* (20–30%), streptococci (15–25%), gram-negative bacilli (15–25%), and anaerobes (5–10%). Artificial joint infections are classified as (1) acute contiguous infections developing within 6 months of surgery, presumably through contamination at the time of surgery; (2) chronic contiguous infections developing 6–24 months after surgery, presumably also from contamination at surgery; and (3) hematogenous infections that appear more than 2 years after surgery.

Standard therapy is to remove the prosthesis, give intravenous antibiotics for 1 month, continue oral antibiotics for 2–4 months, and then implant a new prosthesis. If patients are poor candidates for surgery and their infections are indolent, they may have no choice but to retain the prosthesis and continue antibiotics for 6 months or longer, depending on whether the infection can be eradicated or simply suppressed. Some centers have had success with a one-stage arthroplasty: removal of the prosthesis and implantation of a new prosthesis with an antibiotic-impregnated cement, followed by a long course of systemic antibiotics.

Prognosis

Nongonococcal septic arthritis causes permanent joint damage in one-third of patients and death in 10% (often from shock lung). Risk factors for morbidity and mortality are age over 65, polyarticular infections, delay in starting treatment, and concurrent conditions, especially rheumatoid arthritis.

GONOCOCCAL ARTHRITIS

Neisseria gonorrhoeae is the most common cause of infectious arthritis and, in contrast to nongonococcal bacterial arthritis, often affects perfectly normal hosts. These people do not have a previously damaged joint or abnormal bacteremia—the usual preconditions for nongonococcal bacterial arthritis. However, patients with gonococcal arthritis have two distinguishing features: They are sexually active and most are young. The condition is rare after age 45.

Gonococcal arthritis can cause considerable damage if not treated properly. Although antibiotics can be effective, the gonococcus's increasing resistance to oral antibiotics requires that treatment begin with parenteral antibiotics and include careful follow-up.

Bacteriology and Pathogenesis

Gonococcal arthritis is caused by dissemination of *N gonorrhoeae,* a gram-negative organism that colonizes or infects chiefly mucous membranes, especially the urethra or cervix, but also the pharynx and rectum. Thus, infection can be spread by oral, vaginal, or anal sexual intercourse that is unprotected by a condom. Young women are twice as likely as men to have disseminated gonococcal infection and are particularly susceptible around their menstrual periods and during pregnancy.

Why some gonococcal infections cause only localized mucosal disease and others disseminate appears linked to differences in gonococcal strains. Compared with strains that cause localized infection, strains that are likely to disseminate have a transparent colony phenotype and are nutritionally deficient; they are also more resistant to the bactericidal effects of serum and complement and more difficult to culture, but more sensitive to antibiotics.

Although all the features of nongonococcal bacterial arthritis are caused by viable organisms, some of the symptoms and signs of gonococcal arthritis result from the patient's immune response to evidently nonviable organisms. To be sure, viable organisms can be identified in many patients with gonococcal arthritis. But in many others, the organism cannot be grown from some inflamed sites. The "sterile" inflammatory features may be explained by a host response to cell wall fragments of dead bacteria or by deposition of immune complexes consisting of antibody and bacterial fragments. The rarity of disseminated gonococcal infection after age 45 presumably reflects either improved host resistance to infection or decreased sexual activity.

Clinical Features

Most patients with disseminated gonococcal infection present with 2–4 days of migratory or additive polyarthralgia, associated with tenosynovitis (pain and swelling along a tendon rather than in a joint). The most commonly affected joints are the wrists, fingers, knees, ankles, and elbows. A few patients have only monoarthralgia. As mentioned, more women than men are affected, and their risk is highest around the menses and during pregnancy. Most patients have constitutional symptoms of mild malaise or fatigue, but, as with nongonococcal arthritis, fewer than 50% present with fever. Less than one-third of patients have any genitourinary symptoms. Thus, the absence of fever or genitourinary discharge does not exclude disseminated gonococcal infection. Similarly, few patients with infection of the throat or rectum report local symptoms.

Within 1–3 days after polyarthralgia starts, one of two patterns usually emerges: (1) the tenosynovitis becomes more prominent and skin lesions appear (in two-thirds of patients) or (2) a monoarthritis develops (in one-third of patients), most often of the knee. Patients who present with monoarthritis are not likely to have tenosynovitis or skin lesions, but presentations vary.

The most common sites of tenosynovitis are around the wrists, fingers, and ankles. The swelling is often visible as a faint "sausage-like" distention of the tendon. Tendon involvement is confirmed if the patient has exquisite pain when trying to flex the involved tendon against resistance.

Skin lesions are extremely helpful in the differential diagnosis, but must be carefully sought since they are often few, small, and asymptomatic. The skin lesions are most often found on the distal extremities, starting as red papules and evolving into pustules on a necrotic base. Most are only a few millimeters in diameter.

The remainder of the physical exam is usually normal. A few patients have a urethral discharge. Few patients have pelvic tenderness or clinically evident pharyngeal or rectal involvement.

Laboratory Features and Diagnosis

Routine tests in patients with disseminated gonococcal infection show only a mild leukocytosis. The synovial white blood cell count is lower than that in nongonococcal bacterial arthritis, averaging 50,000/mm^3. Synovial fluid Gram's stain is positive in less than 25% of patients, and culture is positive in only 50%. Most patients have positive polymerase chain reaction assays for the gonococcus, although this test is not yet widely available. Blood cultures grow *N gonorrhoeae* in fewer than 10% of patients, chiefly those with tenosynovitis and skin lesions; few patients with suppurative arthritis have positive blood cultures. Skin lesions are culture-positive in only 5% of patients. Biopsies of skin lesions may show leukocytoclastic vasculitis; this is evidence that some of the manifestations of disseminated gonococcal infection result from the host's immune response.

Given the low yield from cultures of synovial fluid, skin, and blood, other cultures can help confirm a suspected diagnosis. For example, genitourinary cultures should be done routinely; they are positive in 80% of patients, even though many have no referable symptoms.

Pharyngeal and rectal cultures can also be positive in patients who have no local symptoms or signs. Plain x-rays are normal except for showing effusion.

Congenital complement deficiency of any component of the terminal membrane attack complex is rare, but predisposes affected persons to disseminated gonococcal infections (and *Neisseria* meningitis). The CH50 in such patients is very low.

Differential Diagnosis

Many conditions cause acute arthritis and fever (Table 3.11–4). The disorders that commonly resemble gonococcal arthritis are nongonococcal septic arthritis (especially with endocarditis) and Reiter's syndrome. Endocarditis is favored by a history of injection drug use, a heart murmur, Osler's nodes and Janeway lesions, or illness lasting longer than 2 weeks. Reiter's syndrome can be difficult to distinguish from gonococcal arthritis because both affect young adults and cause fever, arthritis, and urethritis (Chapter 3.7). However, Reiter's syndrome is favored by conjunctivitis, sacroiliitis, heel pain, negative cultures for *N gonorrhoeae*, or failure to improve dramatically after several days of antibiotics.

Management

Gonococcal arthritis is much easier to manage than nongonococcal septic arthritis. Antibiotic treatment lasts only 1 week, and almost no patients require surgical drainage.

Now that the gonococcus is no longer uniformly sensitive to penicillin, patients suspected of having disseminated gonococcal infection should be treated first with intravenous ceftriaxone, cefotaxime, or ceftizoxime. Many patients need to be hospitalized at first, not only for therapy but also to exclude other important differential possibilities such as endocarditis. Patients must undergo needle aspiration for synovial fluid culture, but joint effusions improve so quickly that few patients need either repeat joint aspiration or physical therapy. After the diagnosis of gonococcal arthritis has been established and the improvement from parenteral antibiotics has been sustained for 24–48 hours, patients can be switched to oral cefixime, ciprofloxacin, or ofloxacin to complete a 7-day course. More than 95% of treated patients recover completely.

SUMMARY

▶ Nongonococcal septic arthritis is a life-threatening infection, usually caused by staphylococci or streptococci and presenting as acute monoarthritis, fever, and leukocytosis. Treatment requires intensive drainage and weeks of intravenous antibiotics.

▶ Risk factors for nongonococcal septic arthritis are previous joint injury (eg, rheumatoid arthritis) and per-

Table 3.11–4. Differential diagnosis of acute arthritis and fever: The most common conditions.*

Condition	Joints Involved	Distinguishing Features
Infections		
Bacteria		
Nongonococcal septic arthritis: chiefly staphylococci, streptococci	One	Positive joint culture
Gonococcal arthritis	Few–many	Skin pustules, tenosynovitis
Lyme disease	One	Positive Lyme antibody
Meningococcal arthritis	Few–many	>100 purpuric lesions, positive cultures
Syphilis (secondary stage)	Many	Rash, positive rapid plasma reagin (RPR) test
Postinfectious rheumatic fever	Few–many	Rising antistreptolysin O (ASO) titer, Jones criteria (Chapter 8.4)
Viruses		
Parvovirus B19	Few–many	Rash, positive serology
Hepatitis B	Many	Hives, positive serology
Rubella†	Few–many	Positive serology
Mumps	Few–many	Positive serology
Rheumatic diseases		
Crystal diseases (gout, pseudogout)	One	Crystals in synovial fluid
Reiter's syndrome	Few	Urethritis, conjunctivitis, positive HLA-B27, sacroiliitis
Still's disease	Few–many	Persistent high fever, leukocytosis, negative cultures
Systemic lupus erythematosus	Many	Multisystem disease, positive antinuclear antibody (ANA)
Other		
Sarcoidosis	One–many	Hilar adenopathy
Inflammatory bowel disease	Few	Gastrointestinal symptoms and findings
Familial Mediterranean fever	One	Episodic fever, abdominal pain

*Mycobacterial infections, fungal infections, and vasculitis can cause arthritis and fever, but rarely acutely.
†Arthritis can also follow rubella vaccination.

sistent bacteremia (eg, endocarditis, intravenous drug use).

▶ Gonococcal arthritis begins with polyarthralgia and evolves to either a tenosynovitis with a few small necrotic pustules or to a monoarthritis.

▶ In contrast to nongonococcal septic arthritis, gonococcal arthritis affects chiefly normal persons, responds quickly to brief antibiotic treatment, infrequently requires surgical drainage, and rarely causes joint destruction or death.

SUGGESTED READING

Goldenberg DL: Infectious arthritis complicating rheumatoid arthritis and other chronic rheumatic disorders. Arthritis Rheum 1989;32:496.

Goldenberg DL, Reed JI: Bacterial arthritis. N Engl J Med 1985;312:764.

Mahowald ML: Infectious arthritis: Bacterial agents. In *Primer on the Rheumatic Diseases,* 10th ed. Schumacher HR Jr, Klippel JH, Koopman WJ (editors). Arthritis Foundation, Atlanta, 1993.

Rompalo AM et al: The acute arthritis-dermatitis syndrome: The changing importance of *Neisseria gonorrhoeae* and *Neisseria meningitidis.* Arch Intern Med 1987;147:281.

Soft Tissue Rheumatism

Michelle Petri, MD, MPH

"Soft tissue rheumatism" encompasses common rheumatic disorders such as bursitis, tendinitis, and fibrositis, which affect tissues around joints rather than within them. The cardinal symptom of soft tissue rheumatism is pain. It may be acute and localized, as with olecranon bursitis, or chronic and generalized, as with fibrositis. Often, the physician must distinguish soft tissue rheumatism from inflammatory systemic rheumatic diseases like systemic lupus erythematosus and rheumatoid arthritis, as well as from endocrine, psychiatric, and neoplastic diseases. Making the correct diagnosis allows patients to receive timely, correct therapy, and spares them from seeking unnecessary medical and surgical consultations.

TENDINITIS AND BURSITIS

Tendinitis and bursitis are among the most common forms of soft tissue rheumatism. Tendinitis is tendon inflammation, nodules, or partial tears. Bursitis is inflammation and tenderness in the bursae overlying joints. Symptoms are often triggered by overuse or repetitive trauma. In some patients, bursitis or tendinitis is caused by infection or by a systemic disease like gout or rheumatoid arthritis. If infection has been excluded (see "Painful Elbow" below), treatment has three steps: (1) resting and protecting the area, (2) judicious use of anti-inflammatory agents (NSAIDs), and (3) when pain is severe or has not responded to conservative management, injection with a long-acting glucocorticoid. Deep heat and ultrasound can also be helpful. Many patients with tendinitis or bursitis have recurrences. Thus, the physician's emphasis should be on relieving pain, restoring function, and preventing future episodes. Few patients need surgery.

Painful Shoulder

Except for patients with serious trauma, most individuals presenting with a painful shoulder have rotator cuff tendinitis or subacromial bursitis. These conditions are seen especially often in patients with diabetes mellitus and persons whose jobs, like housepainting, involve repetitive shoulder motion. Typically, the affected shoulder is on the dominant side. Most patients complain of night time pain, but pain may limit use of the shoulder during the day.

Physical examination should determine whether or not the rotator cuff is totally ruptured. The supraspinatus tendon is the major tendon in the rotator cuff and normally assists in abduction (lifting the arm away from the body). Thus, patients with rotator cuff tendinitis experience pain when they abduct the arm (painful arc), either freely or against light resistance applied by the physician. When the rotator cuff is completely ruptured, the physician can abduct the arm to 90°, but the patient cannot sustain the position. When the physician lets go, the patient's arm flops down. A patient with a total rupture of the rotator cuff should be referred to an orthopedic surgeon. Some patients have an impingement syndrome caused by impingement of the acromion on the rotator cuff as the arm is abducted. Patients with the syndrome stop between 90 and 100° when they try to abduct the arm by themselves. Palpating the space between the acromion and humeral head may elicit tenderness in an inflamed subacromial bursa.

The differential diagnosis of painful shoulder includes dislocation and fracture; arthritis, both inflammatory (including rheumatoid arthritis and infectious arthritis) and noninflammatory (osteoarthritis); and referred pain from an internal viscus or tumor. Some patients with polymyalgia rheumatica (Chapter 3.5) complain of shoulder stiffness, but the stiffness is bilateral and worst in the morning; physical exam does not reveal rotator cuff tendinitis, and the erythrocyte sedimentation rate is characteristically high. Many patients with rheumatoid arthritis develop rotator cuff tendinitis as a consequence of the surrounding synovitis.

Several management points deserve emphasis. (1) Treatment is the same for tendinitis, bursitis, or both. (2) Resting the shoulder means using a shoulder sling. However, it is essential to prevent adhesive capsulitis (frozen shoulder). Thus, after patients wear the sling for 48 hours, they should start removing it twice a day for range-of-motion exercises. Patients should slowly move the arm out to the side to the point of pain, then count slowly to 10, and return the arm to the body. This exercise should be done supine, not by the commonly prescribed "walking the fingers up the wall" method. (3) A subacromial bursa injection of the potent glucocorticoid triamcinolone is more effective than an NSAID.

Painful Elbow

Bursitis commonly affects the olecranon, presenting as a swollen sac over the elbow. The differential diagnosis includes trauma, septic bursitis, gout, pseudogout, and inflammatory synovitis such as rheumatoid arthritis or psoriasis. Patients with diabetes mellitus have an usually high occurrence of septic olecranon bursitis. Because the olecranon bursa is so prone to infection, in most patients the bursa should be aspirated to exclude crystal diseases and infection. Fluid obtained is examined under a polarizing microscope for crystals and sent for Gram's stain and bacterial culture. Simple drainage of the accumulated fluid helps relieve the pain of olecranon bursitis, but in most patients the fluid reaccumulates. If the suspicion of infection is high, the patient should be started on antibiotics; these are usually intravenous, emphasizing coverage for *Staphylococcus aureus*. Underlying diseases like gout and rheumatoid arthritis must be controlled to prevent recurrence. If no infection is found, a very effective—if temporary—measure is to inject a long-acting glucocorticoid into the bursa.

Elbow pain can also be caused by epicondylitis, either laterally (tennis elbow) or medially (golfer's elbow). Although epicondylitis is classically related to sports, anyone can develop it from overuse. Physical exam reveals point tenderness over the involved epicondyle. Resisted extension (or flexion) of the wrist causes pain at the lateral (or medial) epicondyle. Velcro support bands can be helpful. Many patients who do not respond to NSAIDs improve after subcutaneous injection of a long-acting glucocorticoid. Such injections should be given carefully to patients with dark skin because superficially injected corticosteroid can cause hypopigmentation. If a sport is to blame for elbow pain, treatment should also include rest and retraining.

Painful Wrist

Carpal Tunnel Syndrome: Carpal tunnel syndrome is a common cause of wrist or hand pain, often with numbness. Patients typically describe the pain as burning or tingling. Many patients awaken at night with the pain and report that it improves after they shake out their hands. The cause is entrapment of the median nerve as it passes the space bounded by the carpal bones and the transverse carpal ligament. Still, few patients can describe numbness limited to the median nerve distribution. Most report that all five fingers are numb.

Carpal tunnel syndrome can develop after repetitive trauma and overuse, but it has a long differential diagnosis that includes diabetes mellitus, hypothyroidism, acromegaly, amyloidosis, pregnancy, oral contraceptives, and inflammatory synovitis (Table 3.12–1). The history is usually more important than physical signs like Tinel's

and Phalen's signs, which lack both sensitivity and specificity. To elicit Tinel's sign, the examiner taps lightly over the carpal tunnel with a reflex hammer and asks whether the patient feels paresthesias (electrical feelings) in the first three fingers, which are innervated by the median nerve. Phalen's maneuver requires patients to press the backs of their hands together at 90° flexion with fingers pointing down (the reverse of holding the hands in prayer) for 60 seconds, to see whether paresthesias appear in the first three fingers.

Patients with carpal tunnel syndrome who do not have a neurologic deficit can be managed initially with a "cock-up" wrist splint that holds the wrist at 10° extension. Most patients are also given an NSAID. Injecting the carpal tunnel with a long-acting glucocorticoid can be helpful, but this is a difficult injection best given by a specialist. A patient with a fixed neurologic deficit should have the diagnosis confirmed with nerve conduction studies and should consult a surgeon about carpal tunnel release.

De Quervain Tenosynovitis: Another cause of wrist pain is inflammation of the tendons near the "snuffbox" (the abductor pollicis longus and extensor pollicis brevis). Overuse is a common precipitant: One patient developed De Quervain tenosynovitis the day after signing all of her Christmas cards. The tendons are usually tender on direct palpation. The physician can elicit tenderness by asking the patient to "hide the thumb" inside a closed fist and then pressing the fist laterally toward the ulna (Finkelstein's test). Treatment requires resting the tendons, but a regular wrist splint is inadequate because it does not immobilize the thumb. An occupational or physical therapist can build up a wrist splint to fix the thumb. Patients whose pain continues after a course of tendon rest and anti-inflammatory drugs may be helped by a subcutaneous injection of long-acting glucocorticoid.

Painful Hip

Inflammation of the trochanteric bursa causes pain over the lateral or posterior aspect of the hip. Patients describe the pain as "aching." It is aggravated by sitting or by lying

Table 3.12–1. Differential diagnosis of carpal tunnel syndrome.

Common causes
Occupational overuse of hands (eg, by typists)
Diabetes
Trauma
Pregnancy
Hypothyroidism
Chronic wrist synovitis (eg, in rheumatoid arthritis, gout, systemic lupus erythematosus, polymyalgia rheumatica)

Less common causes
Amyloidosis
Acromegaly
Sarcoidosis
Granulomatous infection (eg, tuberculosis)
Tumors (eg, leukemia)
Genetic predisposition
Drugs (eg, oral contraceptives, disulfiram)

on the affected side, but not by walking. The area over the trochanter is usually tender to deep palpation; the hip's range of motion is normal and usually painless. In contrast, arthritis of the hip causes inguinal or groin pain that increases with weight bearing; the hip's range of motion is reduced and painful. Most patients with inflammation of the trochanteric bursa are helped by rest, heat, and NSAIDs or bursal injection with glucocorticoid.

Painful Knee

Prepatellar bursitis causes pain, swelling, and redness of a small area right over the patella. The trigger is usually minor trauma, as may result from kneeling on hard floors. However, because the prepatellar bursa gets infected easily, effusions in the area should be aspirated and cultured.

The anserine bursa lies over the anterior medial aspect of the knee, just below the joint space. Anserine bursitis often develops abruptly in middle-aged patients who have a history of degenerative knee arthritis. The pain and swelling do not involve the whole joint, but are restricted to a small area overlying the anserine bursa.

Semimembranous gastrocnemius bursitis (Baker's cyst) develops in patients with chronic knee effusions from either degenerative or rheumatoid arthritis. The cystic swelling behind the knee is best palpated with the patient standing. A Baker's cyst can be asymptomatic, but a large one can produce an uncomfortable sense of fullness behind the knee. If the bursa ruptures, it can cause acute swelling of the lower leg, mimicking thrombophlebitis (pseudothrombophlebitis), or, rarely, so impairs venous return that it causes true thrombophlebitis.

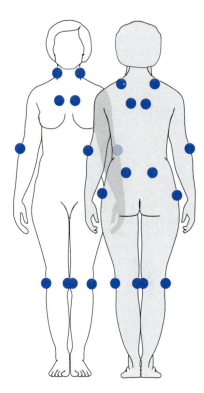

Figure 3.12–1. Common locations of nine paired tender points in fibrositis.

FIBROSITIS

Fibrositis (fibromyalgia) is a common chronic pain syndrome that primarily affects women. Many patients complain of total-body pain; many also have sleep disturbance, vascular headaches, and irritable bowel syndrome. Diagnostic criteria are (1) a history of widespread pain on both the left and right sides, both above and below the waist, specifically including axial skeletal pain, and (2) pain on palpation in at least 11 of 18 tender points. The tender points are discrete areas in muscle or soft tissue that, when palpated with firm pressure, elicit exquisite pain (Figure 3.12–1). The pathophysiology of fibrositis is not understood, but it does not appear to be inflammatory. The syndrome seems to be worsened by two factors: physical deconditioning and nonrefreshing sleep.

The physical exam is remarkable for no objective finding except the tender points. These points are usually symmetric and are concentrated over the muscles of the posterior neck and shoulder girdle. Fibrositis produces no laboratory abnormalities.

The differential diagnosis of chronic, diffuse musculoskeletal pain with no joint findings illustrates some key features of fibrositis (Table 3.12–2). Polymyalgia rheumatica differs from fibrositis in affecting the elderly and in causing anemia and an elevated erythrocyte sedi-

Table 3.12–2. Differential diagnosis of chronic, diffuse musculoskeletal pain with a normal joint examination.

Condition	Some Distinguishing Features
Fibrositis (fibromyalgia)	Young woman with no physical or laboratory findings
Polymyalgia rheumatica	Patient over age 60 with high erythrocyte sedimentation rate
Occult malignancy	Weight loss
Depression	History of depression; demoralization, disturbed sleep, changed eating patterns
Endocrine conditions	
Hypothyroidism	Pale, cool skin; delayed deep tendon reflexes
Panhypopituitarism	Paleness out of proportion to anemia; prostate too small for age
Adrenal insufficiency	Low ACTH-stimulated cortisol
Hyperparathyroidism	High serum calcium and parathyroid hormone
Vitamin D deficiency	Low serum calcium
Polymyositis	Weakness, high creatine kinase
Renal tubular acidosis	Low serum bicarbonate
Postpolio syndrome	History of poliomyelitis
Parkinsonian syndrome	Bradykinesia, resting tremor

mentation rate. Fibrositis almost always begins between ages 18 and 45; the diagnosis should be doubted if symptoms start later. Weight loss, documented fever, lymphadenopathy, or resting tremor would never be expected in fibrositis, but should suggest occult malignancy, endocrine disorders, or parkinsonian syndrome. To verify that the patient has no objective findings takes time. Thus, the diagnosis of fibrositis usually requires more than one evaluation.

An important part of treating fibrositis is reassuring the patient that the disease is not disabling or fatal. Although fibrositis has been reported in patients with hypothyroidism, systemic lupus erythematosus, rheumatoid arthritis, Lyme disease, and HIV infection, most patients do not have any associated condition. Patients must take an active role in controlling the disease by participating in a low-impact aerobic conditioning program like swimming. Low doses of tricyclic antidepressants at bedtime can help the sleep disturbance and reduce pain.

SUMMARY

► Tendinitior bursitis is usually caused by overuse, but it can also be caused by systemic diseases (eg, gout, rheumatoid arthritis) or localized infection.

► The olecranon and prepatellar bursae are the bursae most susceptible to infection. Effusions at these sites should be aspirated, stained for organisms, and cultured.

► The most common causes of carpal tunnel syndrome are repetitive trauma, inflammatory synovitis, diabetes mellitus, pregnancy, and hypothyroidism.

► Fibrositis is a chronic pain syndrome of unknown cause that chiefly affects women, begins between ages 18 and 45, and is not associated with objective physical findings or laboratory abnormalities.

SUGGESTED READING

Petri M et al: Randomized, double-blind, placebo-controlled study of the treatment of the painful shoulder. Arthritis Rheum 1987;30:1040.

Sheon RP, Moskowitz RW, Goldberg VM: *Soft Tissue Rheumatic Pain: Recognition, Management, Prevention,* 2nd ed. Lea & Febiger, 1987.

Wolfe F et al: The American College of Rheumatology 1990 Criteria for the Classification of Fibromyalgia: Report of the Multicenter Criteria Committee. Arthritis Rheum 1990; 33:160.

Low Back Pain

David B. Hellmann, MD

Patients with low back pain are seen in every medical setting—the office, the emergency room, and the hospital ward. This fact reflects both the high prevalence of back pain (80% of the population is affected at some time) and the wide variety of medical conditions, acute and chronic, that cause back pain.

Physicians encountering patients with low back pain have two important goals. The first is to determine whether the patient is likely to have a "serious disorder," one that requires urgent diagnostic assessment and treatment. The second goal is to provide conservative yet effective management for those who do not have emergent conditions. It is a misconception that these goals can be achieved only by a specialist. Indeed, this chapter highlights how the general internist's broad experience is crucially important in the diagnosis and management of patients with low back pain.

DIAGNOSIS

General Approach

The diagnostic approach to the patient with nontraumatic low back pain is dictated by several considerations. First, the differential diagnosis of low back pain is broad and includes systemic diseases (eg, metastatic cancer), primary spine disease (eg, disk herniation, degenerative arthritis), and regional diseases (eg, aortic dissection) that refer pain to the low back (Table 3.13–1). Second, in most patients a precise diagnosis cannot be made. The frequent use of the terms "strain," "sprain," and "lumbago" underscores the common imprecision of diagnosis. Even when patients have anatomic defects, such as a narrowed disk space or a bony spur (osteophyte) on a vertebral body, the physician cannot assume clinical disease, since such "defects" are common in asymptomatic patients. Third, most

patients improve in 1–4 weeks with conservative therapy and need no evaluation beyond the initial history and physical examination. The diagnostic challenge, then, is to use the history and physical exam to identify among the many sufferers of low back pain those few patients who require more extensive or urgent evaluation.

"Serious" disease may be defined as (1) infection, (2) cancer, (3) inflammatory back disease such as ankylosing spondylitis, (4) important regional disease such as dissecting aortic aneurysm, or (5) significant or rapidly progressing neurologic deficits. A patient who does not have evidence of any of these five conditions should be evaluated and treated conservatively.

The most common mistake in evaluating patients with back pain is to focus solely on the back itself. The back symptoms and exam are important, but in themselves do not always distinguish serious from nonserious disorders. Often it is a careful general medical history and physical exam that allow physicians to recognize when a patient has a serious back condition. To be most effective, physicians must seek specific information about the back and general medical knowledge about the patient.

History of Back Symptoms

Anatomy may explain why different back disorders can produce similar symptoms. Many spinal tissues (eg, the facet joint capsules, anulus fibrosus, ligamenta flava, and supraspinous, intraspinous, and longitudinal ligaments) are innervated with nociceptive fibers that can be stimulated by compression, stretching, or inflammation. Stimulation of fibers in any of these tissues reflexively triggers widespread contractions of paraspinal muscles, resulting in diffuse, and nonspecific, low back pain.

Although the way patients describe their pain is not usually distinctive, certain qualities of a patient's pain can indicate a specific diagnosis (Table 3.13–2). Sciatica, low back pain radiating down the buttock along the back of the leg to below the knee, suggests a herniated disk compressing and irritating a lumbar nerve root. Sciatica can also be caused by such conditions as sacroiliitis, degenerative arthritis of facet joints, stenosis of the spinal canal, and

Acknowledgment: This chapter was adapted from Dr. Hellmann's chapter, "Arthritis & Musculoskeletal Disorders," in *Current Medical Diagnosis & Treatment 1995*. Tierney LM Jr, McPhee SJ, Papadakis MA (editors). Appleton & Lange, 1995.

Table 3.13–1. Causes of low back pain.

Indeterminate
  "Lumbago"
  "Back strain"

Degenerative diseases
  Osteoarthritis
  Disk herniation
  Osteoporosis

Systemic diseases
  Infections
    Osteomyelitis
    Epidural abscess
    Endocarditis
  Malignancy
    Metastases
    Multiple myeloma
  Ankylosing spondylitis

Regional conditions causing back pain
  Aortic dissection
  Kidney stones
  Retroperitoneal abscess

even irritation of the sciatic nerve by a bulging wallet. Disk herniation is further suggested by physical exam, and confirmed by imaging techniques (see "Further Examination" below).

Low back pain associated with pseudoclaudication often indicates spinal stenosis, a narrowing of the spinal canal. Since the spinal canal is most commonly narrowed by degenerative changes, which include bony spur formation, disk space narrowing, and ligamentous thickening,

the typical patient is over 60 years old. The patient is bothered less by back pain than by a discomfort in the buttock, thigh, or leg that (like true claudication) is brought on by walking but (unlike claudication) can also be elicited by prolonged standing. The discomfort is often bilateral. The pain has been attributed to arterial ischemia of the lumbar nerve roots, caused by the spinal stenosis. The lumbar spinal canal normally enlarges with flexion and narrows with extension, which is why patients with spinal stenosis often have less difficulty walking uphill than downhill. Some patients complain less about leg discomfort and more about an exercise-dependent weakness or unsteadiness of the legs, often described as "spaghetti legs" or the gait of a "drunken sailor."

Unrelenting low back pain at night, unrelieved by rest or the supine position, should suggest malignancy, either vertebral body metastasis or a cauda equina tumor.

Major quickly evolving neurologic deficits signal that a patient needs urgent evaluation for possible cauda equina tumor, epidural abscess, or, rarely, massive disk herniation (Chapter 13.10). Severe neurologic symptoms with back pain are unusual and should prompt concern. Even with a herniated disk and nerve root impingement, pain is the most prominent symptom; numbness and weakness are less commonly reported and are usually limited to the distribution of a single nerve root. Thus, bilateral leg weakness (from multiple lumbar nerve root compressions), saddle area anesthesia, bowel or bladder incontinence, or impotence (from multiple sacral nerve root compressions) indicates an unusually large neurologic deficit requiring urgent evaluation.

Table 3.13–2. Clinical clues to serious back disorders.

	Infection	Cancer	Inflammatory Back Arthritis	Referred Pain from Regional Disorders	Important Neurologic Deficits
Examples	Vertebral body osteomyelitis	Vertebral body metastasis	Ankylosing spondylitis	Dissecting aortic aneurysm	Cauda equina tumor, epidural hemorrhage
History					
Back symptoms	Back pain unrelated to activity; Nocturnal pain	Back pain unrelated to activity; Nocturnal pain	Back pain improved with activity, aggravated by rest; Insidious onset (>3 months)	Writhing back pain; Sudden onset	Loss of bowel or bladder function; Numbness or weakness in both legs; Progression of neurologic symptoms over hours or days
General history	Rheumatic heart disease; Diabetes; Intravenous drug use; Recent urinary tract infections; Fever (<50% of patients); Corticosteroid use	Age >50; History of cancer or smoking; Weight loss	Age <40; Male sex	History of hypertension or kidney stones	History of cancer
Physical exam	Fever (<50% of patients); Pain localized to 1 vertebral body; Heart murmur	Abnormal lymph nodes; Pallor; Prostate nodule; Ovarian or pelvic mass	Abnormal Schober's test (see text)	Pulsating, enlarged aorta; Loss of pulses; Diaphoresis	Inability to walk because of weakness; Nerve deficits of multiple nerve roots

Low back pain that worsens with rest and improves with activity is characteristic of ankylosing spondylitis or other seronegative spondyloarthropathies, especially when the pain begins before age 40 and the onset is insidious. Most back diseases produce precisely the opposite pattern, with rest alleviating and activity aggravating the pain.

Acute, writhing low back pain, often with sweating, should suggest referred pain from an abdominal catastrophe such as an aortic dissection.

General Medical History

The physician gleans as many clues to possible serious back disease from the general medical history as from the specific history of back symptoms (see Table 3.13–2). For example, the back pain from vertebral body osteomyelitis does not always differ from the pain of strenuous weekend gardening. Yet the likelihood of infection increases if the patient reports a history of risk factors for hematogenous infections, the most common mechanism for the development of vertebral body osteomyelitis. A history of intravenous drug use, endocarditis, rheumatic heart disease, diabetes, immunosuppressive drug treatment, or exposure to tuberculosis increases the risk of vertebral body infection. Since the pelvic veins interconnect with those of the spine through Batson's plexus, a history of urinary tract infections or bladder instrumentation, particularly in a diabetic patient, would further raise suspicions of vertebral body osteomyelitis. Fever should be sought, but is found in only 50% of patients with vertebral body osteomyelitis.

Advanced age or a history of cancer, weight loss, or smoking should raise the possibility that back pain is being caused by primary or metastatic cancer.

Previous problems with kidney stones, or with aortic dissection caused by neglected hypertension, might indicate either disorder as a serious cause of referred back pain. A history of peptic ulcer disease in a patient on chronic prednisone may suggest that the person's refractory back pain is being caused by a perforated gastric ulcer with retroperitoneal abscess.

Physical Examination

Although examination of the back rarely suggests a specific cause for pain, several physical findings should be sought because they help identify those few patients who need more than just conservative management.

Neurologic exam of the lower extremities detects the small deficits produced by disk disease and the large deficits complicating such problems as cauda equina tumors. A positive straight-leg–raising test indicates nerve root irritation. The examiner performs the test by raising the supine patient's extended leg. The test is positive if pain radiates down the leg when it is raised 60 degrees or less. The test is not specific but is 95% sensitive in patients with herniation at the level of L4–L5 or L5–S1 (sites of 95% of disk herniations). The test can be falsely negative, especially in patients with herniation above the L4–L5 level.

The crossed-straight-leg sign is less sensitive but much more specific for disk herniation and is positive when the physician raises the patient's extended unaffected leg and produces sciatica down the affected leg.

Detailed exam of the motor and sensory distributions of the sacral and lumbar nerve roots, especially L5 and S1, is essential for detecting neurologic deficits associated with back pain. Disk herniation produces deficits predictable for the site involved (Table 3.13–3). Deficits of multiple sacral nerve roots, caused by tumors or other processes of the cauda equina, produce the cauda equina syndrome: loss of bowel and bladder function, and anesthesia in the saddle area of both buttocks.

Measuring spinal motion in the patient with acute pain is rarely of diagnostic usefulness and usually just confirms that pain limits motion. An exception to this rule is that decreased range of motion in multiple regions of the spine (cervical, thoracic, and lumbar) indicates a diffuse spinal disease such as ankylosing spondylitis. Unfortunately, by the time the patient has such limits, the diagnosis is usually not a mystery.

If the back pain is not severe and does not itself limit motion, Schober's test of lumbar motion is helpful in early diagnosis of ankylosing spondylitis. In this test, two marks are made on the skin, one 10 cm above S1 and the other 5 cm below. The patient then bends forward as far as possible, and the additional separation between the points is measured. Normally, the points separate at least an additional 5 cm. Anything less indicates reduced lumbar motion, which, in the absence of severe pain, is most commonly caused by ankylosing spondylitis or other seronegative spondyloarthropathies.

Palpation of the spine does not often yield diagnostic information. Point tenderness over a vertebral body is reported to suggest osteomyelitis, but this association appears much tighter in dusty textbooks than in living patients. An abrupt change in vertical alignment between the spinous processes of adjacent vertebral bodies may indicate spondylolisthesis, but the sensitivity of this finding is extremely low. Tenderness of the soft tissue overlying the trochanter is a manifestation of trochanteric bursitis.

Inspection of the spine is not often of value in identifying serious causes of low back pain. The "bamboo-straight" spine of ankylosing spondylitis is a classic but late finding. Mild scoliosis does not increase a patient's risk for clinical back disease. Cutaneous neurofibromas can help the physician identify the very rare patient who has nerve root encasement from paraspinal neurofibromas.

Table 3.13–3. Neurologic testing of lumbosacral nerve roots.

Nerve Root(s) Involved	Motor Deficit	Absent Reflex	Sensory Area
L4	Dorsiflexion of foot	Knee jerk	Medial calf
L5	Dorsiflexion of great toe	None	Medial forefoot
S1	Eversion of foot	Ankle jerk	Lateral foot
S2–S5	Loss of bowel and bladder function	Anal "wink"	"Saddle" area anesthesia

Hip exam should be part of the complete physical. Although hip arthritis usually produces groin pain, some patients have buttock or low back symptoms.

The general physical exam is also of great importance, since fever, elevated blood pressure, pallor, palpable lymph nodes, absent pulses, heart murmur, breast nodules, and pelvic, abdominal, or rectal masses could indicate that a patient's back pain has a serious cause.

Further Examination

If the history and physical exam do not suggest infection, cancer, inflammatory back disease, major neurologic deficits, or pain referred from abdominal or pelvic disease, further evaluation can be eliminated or deferred while conservative therapy is tried. With conservative care, most patients improve spontaneously in 1–4 weeks.

Regular x-rays of the lumbosacral spine give 20 times the radiation dose of a chest film and provide limited, albeit important, information (Figure 3.13–1). Plain spine films have very low sensitivity and specificity for disk disease. Lumbar films are important for detecting vertebral body osteomyelitis, cancer, fractures, and ankylosing spondylitis. Films taken during the first few months of symptoms can be falsely negative. Degenerative changes in the lumbar spine are ubiquitous in patients over 40 and do not prove clinical disease. Thus, plain x-rays are warranted early only for patients suspected of having infection, cancer, fractures, or inflammation, and in selected other patients who fail to improve after 2–4 weeks of conservative therapy.

Magnetic resonance imaging (MRI) and computed tomographic (CT) scanning provide exquisite anatomic detail, but should be reserved for patients in whom the information sought would call for a change in therapy. Sophisticated imaging is needed urgently in any patient suspected of having an epidural mass or cauda equina tumor. On the other hand, sophisticated imaging is not needed early in the course of a patient suspected of having a routine disk herniation. It should be emphasized that disk herniation can be asymptomatic, so that its mere presence on a scan does not always signify clinical disease. Since most patients with disk herniation improve with 4–6 weeks of conservative therapy, imaging should be reserved for patients who have not improved with conservative therapy and who are good surgical candidates. The relative merits of MRI and CT remain controversial.

Radionuclide bone scanning has limited usefulness in the evaluation of low back pain. Radionuclide scans are most useful for early detection of vertebral body osteomyelitis and metastases. The bone scan is often normal in multiple myeloma.

Blood tests (eg, complete blood count, serum calcium, alkaline phosphatase, serum protein electrophoresis, erythrocyte sedimentation rate) and urinalysis should be performed early only in patients suspected of having serious disease. Electrophysiologic testing can be useful in confirming spinal stenosis.

MANAGEMENT

Although any management plan must be individualized, key elements of most conservative treatments for back pain include rest, analgesia, and education. Recent studies suggest that for most patients, continuing daily activities as tolerated is more effective than bed rest. Nonsteroidal anti-inflammatory drugs may be enough to control the pain, but patients with severe pain may require opiates. Rarely does the need for opiates extend beyond 1–2 weeks, and opiates are contraindicated in the management of chronic low back pain.

Limited evidence supports the use of muscle relaxants such as diazepam, cyclobenzaprine, carisoprodol, and methocarbamol. These drugs should also be limited to courses of 1–2 weeks. They should not be given to older patients, who are at risk of falling.

All patients should be taught how to protect the back in daily activities: not to lift heavy objects, to use the legs rather than the back when lifting, to use a chair with arm rests, and to arise from bed by first rolling to one side and then using the arms to push to an upright position. Physical therapists are excellent sources for patient education.

The value of corsets or traction is dubious. Back exercises are contraindicated during acute pain but may have some value in preventing recurrences.

Surgical consultation is needed urgently for any patient with a large or evolving neurologic deficit. Surgery for disk disease is indicated when an imaging procedure documents herniation, the patient has a consistent neurologic deficit on physical exam, and the pain has failed to respond to 4–6 weeks of conservative therapy.

Complaints of a tired, weak back with pain but no ob-

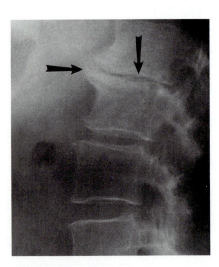

Figure 3.13–1. Lateral x-ray view of lumbar spine, showing changes of osteoarthritis: osteophyte (left arrow) and disk space narrowing (right arrow). (Courtesy of William W. Scott, Jr, MD.)

jective findings may suggest a psychological problem. Hysterical back pain can be severe and dramatically exaggerated. A history of domestic or work-related problems and observation of a flat affect with a bizarre reaction to treatment should reinforce suspicion. Treatment may include reassurance and judicious use of mild analgesics and sedatives.

SUMMARY

► Nontraumatic low back pain is common, rarely serious, and usually self-limited. The initial goal of evaluation is to identify the few patients who have serious conditions.

► Serious low back pain is caused by cancer, infection, ankylosing spondylitis and related diseases, regional diseases that refer pain to the back, and diseases associated with neurologic deficits involving more than one nerve root.

► The general medical history and physical examination are often more important than back symptoms and the back exam in identifying serious disease.

► Plain x-rays have limited diagnostic value, and their use should be limited to patients suspected of having serious disease. MRI and CT scanning are expensive and should usually be restricted to patients who are candidates for surgery.

► Back pain and stiffness that worsen with rest and improve with activity suggest an inflammatory spondyloarthropathy. Back pain that worsens with activity is characteristic of degenerative back disease.

SUGGESTED READING

Deyo RA, Bigos SJ, Maravilla KR: Diagnostic imaging procedures for the lumbar spine. Ann Intern Med 1989;111:865.

Deyo RA, Loeser JD, Bigos SJ: Herniated lumbar intervertebral disk. Ann Intern Med 1990;112:598.

Frymoyer JW: Back pain and sciatica. N Engl J Med 1988; 318:291.

Hall S et al: Lumbar spinal stenosis: Clinical features, diagnostic procedures, and results of surgical treatment in 68 patients. Ann Intern Med 1985;103:271.

Malmivaara A et al: The treatment of acute low back pain: Bed rest, exercises, or ordinary activity? N Engl J Med 1995;332: 351.

Miller GM, Forbes GS, Onofrio BM: Magnetic resonance imaging of the spine. Mayo Clin Proc 1989;64:986.

Endocrinology and Metabolism

Paul W. Ladenson, MD, Section Editor

Approach to the Patient With an Endocrine or Metabolic Disorder

Paul W. Ladenson, MD, and Simeon Margolis, MD, PhD

At least 25% of any physician's patients will have thyroid dysfunction, hyperlipidemia, osteoporosis, or diabetes at some point in their lives. These conditions may be hard to recognize clinically and may require lifelong management. Physicians must also be ready to diagnose rarer but clinically important syndromes of endocrine dysfunction like acromegaly, adrenal insufficiency, and pheochromocytoma. Although these conditions can have striking clinical manifestations, many patients remain undiagnosed for months or years and see several doctors before their illness is recognized.

This chapter covers principles that apply generally to the pathophysiology, diagnosis, and management of the endocrine and metabolic diseases discussed in the rest of the section.

CLINICAL EVALUATION OF ENDOCRINE AND METABOLIC DISORDERS

The clinical diagnosis of endocrine and metabolic disorders can pose several challenges to physicians. First, many of the symptoms and signs caused by hormonal imbalances are common and nonspecific, such as the weakness in patients with adrenal insufficiency or the weight gain in those with hypothyroidism. Such problems may be attributed mistakenly to aging, stress, or other illnesses. Second, the clinical manifestations of many endocrine diseases progress gradually. For example, the slow growth of the face, hands, and feet in acromegaly may go unnoticed by patients, their family, and even their regular physician. Third, metabolic disorders like hypercholesterolemia tend to be entirely silent until they have caused irrevocable harm. Thus, endocrine and metabolic disorders require physicians to maintain a high index of suspicion.

Conscientious physicians suspect and screen for endocrine and metabolic diseases much more often than they ultimately diagnose them. It is important to know which clinical clues should prompt a search for which endocrine and metabolic diseases. For example, most patients with fatigue and weakness do not have adrenal insufficiency, but if they also have weight loss or hyperpigmentation, the physician must consider the diagnosis seriously. Most obese patients with hypertension do not have Cushing's syndrome, but if they also have proximal muscle weakness and wide, purple striae, the diagnosis must be entertained.

Routine laboratory tests often give valuable indications that an endocrine or metabolic disease is the cause of a common clinical complaint or physical finding. For example, a low serum cholesterol concentration may suggest hyperthyroidism in an anxious, sleepless patient. Hypokalemia may mean that hyperaldosteronism is the cause of otherwise routine hypertension. Eosinophilia should raise the possibility of adrenal insufficiency in a patient with vomiting and abdominal pain.

PATHOGENESIS OF ENDOCRINE DISORDERS

Three mechanisms lead to virtually all endocrine gland disorders: deficient hormone action, excessive hormone production and action, and glandular neoplasia (Table 4.1–1). These basic processes can occur in combination, for example, in functioning endocrine tumors that secrete excessive hormone.

Deficient Hormone Action

Hormone action is most often deficient when too little biologically active hormone reaches target tissues. Insufficient hormone production may be explained by primary endocrine gland failure. Such gland hypofunction may be congenital, caused by the gland failing to develop or by a mutant gene for either the hormone or an enzyme respon-

Table 4.1–1. Mechanisms of endocrine pathophysiology.

Deficient hormone action
  Primary gland failure
    Congenital: aplasia and biosynthetic defects
    Acquired: physiologic atrophy, tumor, surgery, inflammation
      (infectious, autoimmune), drug-induced
  Secondary gland failure (lack of tropic hormone)
  Impaired hormone release or activation
  Accelerated hormone metabolism
  Target tissue resistance

Excessive hormone production and action
  Gland autonomy: neoplasia or hyperplasia
  Abnormal stimulation of gland function
  Ectopic hormone production or activation
  Altered hormone metabolism
  Target tissue hypersensitivity

Neoplasia
  Benign and malignant
  Functional and nonfunctional
  Ectopic hormone production
  Sporadic and familial, including the multiple endocrine
    neoplasia syndromes (see Table 4.1–2)

Table 4.1–2. Disorders involving multiple endocrine glands.

Multiple endocrine neoplasia (MEN) syndromes
  MEN I
    Hyperparathyroidism
    Pancreatic adenoma or carcinoma
    Pituitary adenoma
  MEN IIa (also called MEN II)
    Hyperparathyroidism
    Medullary carcinoma of thyroid
    Pheochromocytoma
  MEN IIb (also called MEN III)
    Medullary carcinoma of thyroid
    Pheochromocytoma
    Mucosal neuromas
    Marfanoid habitus

Polyendocrine failure syndromes
  Type I
    Hypoparathyroidism
    Adrenal insufficiency
    Mucocutaneous candidiasis
    Associated conditions: hypogonadism, autoimmune thyroid
      diseases, insulin-dependent diabetes mellitus
  Type II
    Adrenal insufficiency
    Autoimmune thyroid disease
    Associated conditions: insulin-dependent diabetes mellitus,
      primary or secondary gonadal failure

sible for synthesis of the hormone. More often, however, primary gland failure is acquired through physiologic atrophy (eg, menopausal ovarian failure), replacement of normal gland tissue by a tumor, surgical extirpation, effects of pharmacologic or environmental agents, or inflammation. The most common causes of inflammation are autoimmunity and infection. Patients with inflammatory disorders of the thyroid gland may also present with local and constitutional symptoms, such as the neck pain, fever, and malaise that accompany subacute thyroiditis. With some types of injury, the gland transiently releases excess hormone before losing function.

Primary failure can involve more than one endocrine gland (Table 4.1–2). Polyendocrine deficiency syndrome type I, which usually begins in childhood, is characterized by hypoparathyroidism, adrenal insufficiency, and mucocutaneous candidiasis; less common features can include primary gonadal failure, autoimmune thyroid disorders (autoimmune thyroiditis or Graves' disease), and insulin-dependent diabetes mellitus. Polyendocrine deficiency syndrome type II (Schmidt's syndrome) typically presents during the 20's or 30's with adrenal insufficiency and autoimmune thyroid disease; patients may also have insulin-dependent diabetes mellitus and primary or secondary gonadal failure. An autoimmune basis for these syndromes is strongly suggested by circulating antibodies directed against the involved glands, as well as by abnormal suppressor T-cell function and linkage with certain histocompatibility alleles in affected patients and their relatives.

All other kinds of decreased hormone action are much less common. Secondary gland failure is caused by pituitary dysfunction, which can be either congenital or ac-

quired. Another cause of gland hypofunction can be the absence of a factor necessary for hormone secretion; for example, hypomagnesemia can cause a failure of parathyroid hormone release from the parathyroid gland. Defective activation of a hormone precursor or accelerated hormone inactivation can also reduce hormone activity.

Finally, target tissue resistance can cause hormone deficiency states even when concentrations of biologically active hormones are normal or high. Such hormone resistance can be congenital (eg, familial thyroid hormone resistance) or acquired (eg, non–insulin-dependent diabetes mellitus). Target tissues may be unresponsive because of an abnormality in their hormone receptors or in signaling after the hormone-receptor interaction (eg, defects in the guanine nucleotide stimulatory subunit in pseudohypoparathyroidism). Receptor abnormalities may be caused by too few receptors, as in obese patients with non–insulin-dependent diabetes, or by a qualitative defect in receptor function, as in androgen resistance states.

Excessive Hormone Production and Action

Several processes can cause excessive hormone production. A common etiology is autonomous hyperfunction caused by neoplasia arising within an endocrine gland; another etiology is hyperplasia of secretory cells, without a true neoplasm. In some conditions, an abnormal stimulator of gland function causes hyperplasia and hormone overproduction (eg, thyroid-stimulating immunoglobulins in Graves' disease). Ectopic hormone production by nonendocrine tumors can also cause hormonal excess. These tumors may produce either the physiologic hormone itself or, as in the hypercalcemia of malignancy, a product that shares certain biologic properties with parathyroid hormone (Chapter 12.2). Nonglandular tissues may contribute to excessive hormone levels either by increasing hormone activation (eg, activation of vitamin D in sarcoidosis) or by reducing hormone degradation (eg, gynecomastia in cirrhosis caused by decreased estrogen metabolism).

Neoplasia of Endocrine Glands

Endocrine gland tumors are much more commonly benign than malignant. For example, most palpable thyroid nodules are benign, as are most adrenal and virtually all pituitary tumors detected by imaging techniques. Endocrine malignancies display a broad range of clinical behavior, as illustrated by the spectrum of thyroid carcinoma: Well-differentiated thyroid carcinoma grows slowly and is usually curable, whereas anaplastic thyroid cancer progresses quickly and is almost always fatal. Nonfunctional tumors can compromise normal gland function or can spread locally or to distant sites. Because functional tumors typically lack physiologic regulatory mechanisms, their autonomous hormone production causes clinical syndromes of hormonal excess. Syndromes resulting from ectopic hormone production may be the earliest and most distressing manifestations of the tumor, and they must be distinguished from primary endocrine disorders.

Endocrine gland neoplasia may be sporadic or an inherited familial disorder, which can involve one endocrine gland or several (see Table 4.1–2). Three syndromes of multiple endocrine neoplasia are transmitted by autosomal dominant inheritance. Multiple endocrine neoplasia I (MEN I) comprises parathyroid hyperplasia and hyperparathyroidism; pancreatic islet cell tumors that secrete gastrin, insulin, glucagon, or vasoactive intestinal peptide; and pituitary adenomas, which may or may not be secretory. Multiple endocrine neoplasia IIa (also called MEN II) is characterized by hyperparathyroidism, medullary carcinoma of the thyroid, and pheochromocytoma. Patients with the closely related MEN IIb (also called MEN III) have medullary thyroid cancer and pheochromocytoma, along with mucosal neuromas and a marfanoid habitus. Rare patients have crossover syndromes.

PATHOGENESIS OF METABOLIC DISORDERS

Abnormalities of carbohydrate and lipid metabolism can be primary or secondary. Autoimmune destruction of pancreatic islet cells causes insulin-dependent diabetes mellitus, whereas insulin resistance, most often caused by obesity, underlies non–insulin-dependent diabetes mellitus. Diabetes can also be a manifestation of a primary endocrine disease, such as Cushing's syndrome or acromegaly, or a feature of nonimmune destruction of pancreatic islets, as from hemochromatosis or chronic pancreatitis. Fasting hypoglycemia can be the direct consequence of a hormonal abnormality (overproduction of insulin by an insulinoma, or the lack of cortisol in adrenal insufficiency), but more commonly patients develop hy-

poglycemia after receiving too much insulin or drinking alcohol or because they have a malignancy.

Both genetic and environmental factors contribute to hyperlipidemia, which results from either hepatic overproduction of lipoproteins or a defect in their removal from the circulation. The primary hyperlipidemias generally follow an autosomal dominant inheritance pattern, but the abnormality may be expressed only when combined with an unfavorable lifestyle, such as a high-fat diet and alcohol abuse. A defect in the structure of the enzyme lipoprotein lipase, or the absence of its apoprotein activator, always produces severe hypertriglyceridemia. By contrast, familial hypertriglyceridemia may not appear unless overproduction of low-density lipoprotein is triggered by the hyperinsulinemia that accompanies obesity and the early stages of non–insulin-dependent diabetes mellitus. Familial hypercholesterolemia is caused by an abnormality in the receptor for low-density lipoprotein. Secondary hyperlipidemia commonly complicates hypothyroidism, renal failure, and obstructive liver disease, or can be caused by a diet too rich in saturated fat.

ENDOCRINE LABORATORY AND RADIOGRAPHIC TESTS

Laboratory studies of endocrine and metabolic disorders can be categorized as (1) screening tests that reliably exclude the suspected disorders, (2) diagnostic tests that definitively confirm disease, and (3) localizing tests that characterize the specific etiology and site of the disorder.

Direct measurement of circulating hormone concentrations is vital for the accurate diagnosis of most endocrine diseases. Fortunately, highly sensitive and specific tests permit precise measurement of most hormones in blood, despite their low concentrations (10^{-9} to 10^{-12} mol/L). It is important to remember that immunoassays measure immunoreactivity (the ability of a hormone to be recognized by a specific immunoglobulin), not true biologic activity (the hormone's ability to bind to target tissue receptors and initiate actions). Although unusual, dissociation between the immunologic and biological activities of a hormone can confuse the interpretation of immunoassay results. Another potentially confounding issue arises because many circulating hormones are partially bound to protein, with only a fraction of their total blood concentration available to interact with target tissues. The total hormone concentration measured can be particularly misleading if the amount of binding protein changes under physiologic or pathophysiologic influences (eg, an estrogen-induced increase in thyroxine-binding globulin). Because of the potential for misinterpretation, a number of methods have been devised to determine the concentrations of unbound (free) hormones in blood.

By their very nature, endocrine and metabolic parameters respond to both internal rhythms and external stimuli; therefore, circulating levels of hormones and metabolic substrates in healthy persons often fluctuate considerably.

Thus, laboratory tests must be timed correctly, particularly in relation to factors like preceding meals (eg, when measuring serum glucose and insulin), time of day (eg, serum cortisol), and the menstrual cycle (eg, serum estradiol).

In patients with subtle disturbances, hormonal and metabolic measurements taken in the basal state can yield equivocal results. This is particularly true of endocrine systems in which circulating hormone levels show physiologic fluctuations. Provocative endocrine tests are designed to accentuate differences between normal and disease states by manipulating physiologic regulatory mechanisms, for example, the negative feedback that characterizes the hypothalamic-pituitary-adrenal axis (Figure 4.1–1A).

As a general rule, a deficiency in hormone production is revealed by a stimulation test, and excessive or autonomous hormone secretion is revealed by a suppression test. As an example of a stimulation test, patients with possible primary adrenal insufficiency are given adrenocorticotropic hormone (ACTH), and then serial blood measurements are made of their serum cortisol response (see Figure 4.1–1B). An example of a suppression test is evaluation of negative feedback on the hypothalamus and pituitary by giving dexamethasone, a potent synthetic glucocorticoid (see Figure 4.1–1C). Dexamethasone normally suppresses corticotroph and adrenal cortical function, reducing ACTH and cortisol release, respectively. However, hormone release is not suppressed, for example, in patients who have an autonomously functioning adrenal adenoma.

There are several ways to localize the primary abnormality responsible for an endocrine or metabolic disorder. Different etiologies may have characteristic "fingerprints" on provocative endocrine tests, such as those differentiating central from nephrogenic diabetes insipidus (Chapter 4.2), or pituitary from adrenal Cushing's syndrome (Chapter 4.3). Regional blood sampling of local hormone concentrations may lead to a pathogenetic diagnosis as well as the site of involvement. For example, selective venous sampling of parathyroid hormone can differentiate parathyroid hyperplasia from adenoma: Patients with hyperplasia have equal parathyroid hormone levels on both sides of the neck, whereas those with an adenoma have higher levels on the side with the tumor.

Both noninvasive and invasive radiographic studies can help determine the pathogenesis and location of disease. Radionuclide scanning, in particular, provides valuable information about morphology and function, as with the iodine-123 thyroid scan and the iodo-131-cholesterol scan

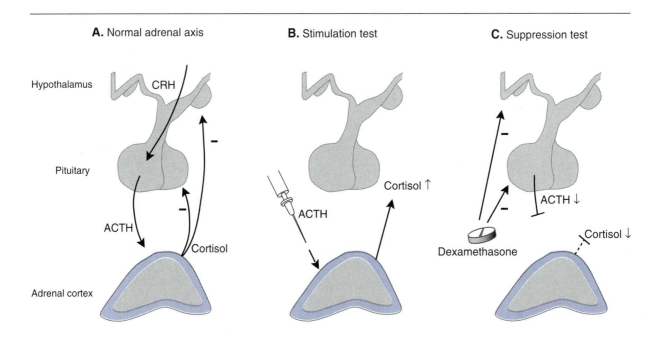

CRH, corticotropin-releasing hormone; ACTH, adrenocorticotropic hormone.

Figure 4.1–1. A: Normal hypothalamic-pituitary-adrenal axis. **B:** ACTH stimulation test for adrenal insufficiency. The serum cortisol concentration is measured before and 30 minutes after the adrenal cortex is stimulated by an injection of synthetic ACTH. A healthy person's serum cortisol should rise. **C:** Dexamethasone suppression test. A healthy person who takes an oral dose of this potent synthetic glucocorticoid should have a drop in serum ACTH and cortisol, reflecting normal glucocorticoid inhibitory feedback on the hypothalamus and pituitary.

of the adrenal cortex. Computed tomography and magnetic resonance imaging have revolutionized the localization of pituitary and adrenal disorders. But because benign nonfunctioning neoplasms of the endocrine glands are relatively common, radiographic findings must be interpreted with great caution in patients with possible or even proven endocrine disease. In general, it is preferable to establish a diagnosis based on hormonal measurements before requesting any localizing radiographic studies.

Pathologic studies also play a role in establishing a specific diagnosis. Routine histopathology can usually distinguish benign from malignant neoplasms, especially when tumor has clearly invaded the gland capsule, blood vessels, or adjacent structures. However, there can be considerable overlap in the histologic features of normal endocrine tissue, hyperplasia, benign neoplasia, and malignancy. These distinctions may ultimately be defined less on histologic appearance than on hormone secretory patterns, gross surgical findings, response to therapy, and the disorder's long-term behavior.

Nonetheless, cytologic analysis of biopsy specimens has proved valuable, for example, with thyroid nodules. Immunochemical techniques, using antisera against hormonal antigens, permit the identification of hormone products in endocrine tissues. This can be extremely valuable in helping the physician pinpoint the diagnosis and plan management. For example, detection of thyroglobulin in a lung metastasis establishes the thyroid gland as the site of the primary tumor and means that the patient may improve if given large doses of radioactive iodine.

PRINCIPLES OF MANAGEMENT FOR ENDOCRINE AND METABOLIC DISORDERS

The paramount goal in treating endocrine and metabolic disorders is to restore normal hormonal and metabolic activity in the tissues. This means establishing normal concentrations of substances in the blood and tissues, and simulating the physiologic responses of these substances to meals, stress, and other life events. For example, insulin treatment must be coordinated with the patient's eating and exercise patterns. Glucocorticoid replacement must be adjusted to mimic the physiologic increase in adrenal glucocorticoid secretion that normally accompanies illness. In metabolic disorders, modifications in diet, physical activity, and body weight are often not only the first line of treatment but may be the only interventions required, as in the management of non–insulin-dependent diabetes mellitus and certain hyperlipidemias. Because therapy almost invariably alters the laboratory parameters needed to confirm the diagnosis, the physician must obtain adequate baseline tests before starting treatment.

SUMMARY

▶ Three fundamental mechanisms underlie endocrine diseases: deficient hormone action in target tissues, excessive hormone production and action, and gland neoplasia.

▶ Because endocrine disorders can cause such nonspecific complaints, physicians must maintain a high index of suspicion for these conditions and know how to use the proper tests to screen possibly affected patients.

▶ Hormone and other biochemical assays are often more accurate than imaging in detecting and localizing an endocrine disorder. Imaging studies may incidentally pick up nonfunctioning, benign endocrine gland tumors that are irrelevant to the diagnosis.

▶ Provocative tests can distinguish between subtle hormonal disorders and physiologic variability by stimulating the release of hormones when baseline levels are too low and by suppressing hormone release when basal levels are too high.

Pituitary Disorders

Gary S. Wand, MD

Patients with disorders of the pituitary gland can present in three ways (Table 4.2–1). First, pituitary adenomas that secrete hormones can cause striking syndromes of hormonal excess, such as Cushing's disease and acromegaly. Second, an expanding mass in the sella turcica can impinge on adjacent structures, causing decreased visual fields and acuity, along with diplopia, headache, and other neurologic syndromes. When chronic, these neurologic syndromes can mimic sinusitis; when caused acutely by hemorrhage, they can be confused with other causes of intracranial bleeding. In the third presentation, compression of normal pituitary tissue by tumors causes hypopituitarism, with a spectrum of problems ranging from nonspecific, slowly progressive constitutional symptoms to acute life-threatening consequences of hormonal deficiencies.

Occasionally, sellar abnormalities are discovered by chance when radiographic tests are done for another reason. In rare patients, pituitary adenoma is part of the familial multiple endocrine neoplasia syndrome, type I (MEN I), which also includes pancreatic islet cell tumors and hyperparathyroidism (Chapter 4.1).

DISORDERS OF THE ANTERIOR PITUITARY

Hypersecretory Syndromes Caused by Pituitary Adenomas

Pituitary adenomas account for 90% of sellar lesions and 10% of intracranial neoplasms. Pituitary adenomas are almost always benign tumors that are classified as microadenomas if their diameter is less than 1 cm, and macroadenomas if they are 1 cm or larger. Prolactin-secreting adenomas are the most common hormone-producing tumors. Less common are growth hormone-secreting adenomas, mixed prolactin- and growth hormone-secreting adenomas, adrenocorticotropin (ACTH)-secreting adenomas, and gonadotropin-secreting adenomas. Rare adenomas secrete thyroid-stimulating hormone (TSH). Although most pituitary tumors synthesize hormones or hormone fragments, many tumors are nonsecretory and produce no clinical syndrome of hormone excess.

Prolactin-Secreting Adenomas and Hyperprolactinemia: Patients with prolactin-secreting pituitary adenomas present with complaints resulting either from the hormonal consequences of hyperprolactinemia or from tumor expansion. The most common symptom is galactorrhea (nonpuerperal lactation). However, this complaint is nonspecific, affecting 20% of all previously pregnant premenopausal women. Most hyperprolactinemic women have irregular menses, with amenorrhea the rule when the serum prolactin exceeds 100 ng/mL. A common scenario is the young woman who takes an oral contraceptive for irregular menses, stops the drug, and does not resume menstruating. Hyperprolactinemia should be ruled out in all nonpregnant women in whom such "post-pill" amenorrhea lasts more than 3 months, by which time virtually all women with a normal prolactin will be menstruating normally.

Although menstrual dysfunction typically leads women to seek medical help and permits early detection of prolactin-secreting adenomas, men are much less likely to complain to their physician about their cardinal symptoms of hyperprolactinemia—impotence with decreased libido. Relatively few men present with galactorrhea and gynecomastia. Thus, men's tumors tend to be larger than women's by the time they are diagnosed. Deficiency of circulating gonadal steroids can cause diminished libido and vasomotor flushing in either sex.

Hyperprolactinemia has other physiologic and pathologic causes (Table 4.2–2). The most common cause in women is pregnancy, which must always be excluded before amenorrheic women undergo radiographic procedures. Other important causes of hyperprolactinemia are (1) any sellar or suprasellar lesion that interferes with the synthesis or secretion of dopamine—lesions such as hypothalamic glioma, craniopharyngioma, and large nonfunctioning pituitary adenoma; (2) several classes of drugs, particularly dopamine antagonists (eg, phenothiazines) and agents that deplete catecholamines (eg, reserpine); (3) kidney failure; (4) liver failure; and (5) hypothyroidism. In rare patients, severe primary hypothyroidism mimics a prolactin-secreting pituitary tumor, with amenorrhea,

Table 4.2–1. Presentations of pituitary tumors.

Increased hormone production
  Hyperprolactinemia
  Acromegaly and gigantism (growth hormone)
  Cushing's disease (adrenocorticotropin [ACTH])
  Hyperthyroidism (thyroid-stimulating hormone [TSH])
Compression of adjacent structures
  Headache
  Visual field defects (classically, superior bitemporal)
  Diplopia
  Diabetes insipidus
Hypopituitarism
Incidental radiographic detection

galactorrhea, and even sellar enlargement caused by hyperplasia of thyrotropin-secreting cells. Thus, all patients with hyperprolactinemia should have their serum TSH tested to exclude primary hypothyroidism. In some patients, hyperprolactinemia is caused by chest wall injury or irritation, which mimics the neurologic input of suckling.

Serum prolactin levels can usually distinguish prolactin-secreting macroadenomas from other causes of hyperprolactinemia. Most macroadenomas produce levels above 250 ng/mL. Levels in microadenomas and other hyperprolactinemic disorders are usually lower.

Prolactinomas should first be treated medically with a dopamine agonist. Bromocriptine and pergolide are dopamine agonists that inhibit prolactin secretion. These drugs normalize the serum prolactin level in more than 90% of patients with microadenomas and in 75% with macroadenomas. In women, symptoms of estrogen deficiency resolve, galactorrhea stops, and ovulatory menstrual cycles return. In men, a normalized serum testosterone restores libido, potency, spermatogenesis, and fertility. In both

Table 4.2–2. Causes of hyperprolactinemia.

Physiologic
  Pregnancy
  Suckling
  Exercise
  Sleep
  Postprandial state

Pathologic
  Prolactin-secreting tumors
  Lesions interfering with hypothalamic dopaminergic tone
    Hypothalamic diseases, eg, sarcoidosis, tumor
    Suprasellar lesions, eg, craniopharyngioma
    Nonfunctioning pituitary adenoma
  Acromegaly (cosecretion of prolactin in 25% of patients)
  Kidney failure
  Liver failure
  Hypothyroidism
  Chest wall stimulation, eg, by herpes zoster, surgery, trauma
  Chronic anovulatory syndrome

Pharmacologic
  Dopamine-blocking agents, eg, phenothiazines, metoclopramide
  Catecholamine-depleting drugs, eg, reserpine
  Certain other intravenous drugs, eg, cimetidine, verapamil

sexes, the drugs reverse the hypogonadotropic hypogonadism that accompanies hyperprolactinemia, unless tumor compression has destroyed gonadotrophs. The drugs can halt or partially reverse hypogonadism's interference with bone mineralization. Lastly, these agents significantly shrink more than two-thirds of prolactin-secreting tumors. Tumors that do not respond to medical therapy should be removed surgically.

Growth Hormone-Secreting Adenomas and Acromegaly: Growth hormone-secreting tumors cause gigantism if long bone epiphyses have not yet fused; after puberty, these tumors cause acromegaly. Acromegaly should be easy to diagnose when the manifestations are severe, but it is rarely recognized early because in most patients it develops insidiously. The changes are so subtle, evolving over years, that not even family members notice how different the patient looks. It is helpful for the physician to see old photographs of the patient. By the time tumors are discovered, many are larger than 1 cm and they may have caused serious local compressive effects. If a pituitary tumor is not found radiographically, the physician must consider hypothalamic overproduction of growth hormone-releasing hormone or ectopic production of this hormone by a tumor.

In patients with acromegaly, soft tissue hypertrophy causes enlargement of hands and feet; thickening of lips, tongue, and skin; and a generalized coarsening of the facial features (Figure 4.2–1). Patients may complain of increasing ring, glove, shoe, or hat size. Malodorous hyperhidrosis (excessive sweating) is an early symptom. Rarely, the intrinsic lactogenic properties of growth hormone produce galactorrhea. Since 40% of growth hormone-secreting tumors also secrete prolactin, patients may present with other manifestations of hyperprolactinemia. Over time, patients develop arthritis, carpal tunnel syndrome, enlargement of the mandible (prognathism), wide spacing of the teeth, hypertrophy of the frontal sinuses (frontal bossing), deepening of the voice (hypertrophy of the vocal cords), and organomegaly. Metabolic abnormalities can include hypertension, glucose intolerance, and hypercalciuria.

Isolated serum growth hormone levels are not very sensitive or specific for acromegaly unless they are markedly elevated, over 10 ng/mL. Glucose challenge testing is more reliable. In normal persons, glucose suppresses growth hormone levels to less than 2 ng/mL, but patients with acromegaly typically have either inadequate suppression or a paradoxical rise. Somatomedin-C (also known as insulin-like growth factor 1, or IGF-1), synthesized in the liver, is a major mediator of growth hormone action. Thus, an elevated plasma somatomedin-C level can also be diagnostic, although elevations are found in some normal young adults.

Growth hormone-secreting tumors are usually first treated surgically, by transsphenoidal resection through the nasal cavity and sphenoid sinus. Patients must be given perioperative glucocorticoids because of the possi-

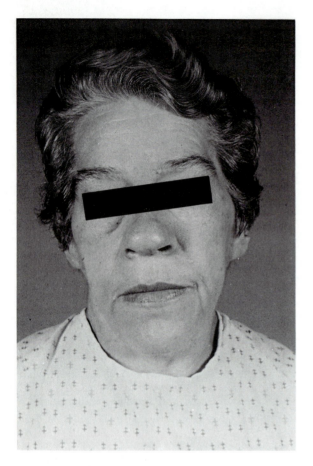

Figure 4.2–1. Coarsening of facial features in a 54-year-old woman with active acromegaly. (Courtesy of David M. Cook, MD, Franklin Square Hospital Department of Medical Communications.)

bility that intraoperative damage to corticotrophs will lead to adrenal insufficiency. Transsphenoidal surgery is the safest approach, with less than 5% of patients suffering neurologic injury, hemorrhage, infection, or a cerebrospinal fluid leak. Trauma to the pituitary stalk causes transient diabetes insipidus in about 25% of patients and permanent diabetes insipidus in less than 1%.

Surgery for growth hormone-secreting tumors cures more than 75% of microadenomas and about 50% of macroadenomas. Patients who still have hypersecretion of growth hormone after surgery can be given a trial of octreotide (the long-acting somatostatin analog) or a dopamine agonist. Bromocriptine lowers the growth hormone level in about one-third of patients, but normalizes it completely in only a few patients. Although bromocriptine can shrink prolactinomas, it rarely shrinks growth hormone-secreting tumors. Octreotide normalizes growth hormone levels in two-thirds of patients and shrinks the tumors in one-third.

When patients are not cured by medical therapy, the re-maining option is radiation therapy. However, radiation may take 2–5 years to work, it does not cure all patients, and it induces hypopituitarism in 30–50% of patients. Radiation therapy of acromegaly is often combined with medical treatment. All patients need periodic follow-up of their pituitary function.

ACTH-Secreting Adenomas and Cushing's Disease: Cushing's *disease* is hypercortisolism caused by excessive pituitary secretion of ACTH, usually by an ACTH-secreting adenoma. Cushing's *syndrome* is hypercortisolism of any source: pituitary ACTH hypersecretion, ectopic production of ACTH by tumors and adrenal overproduction of cortisol, and exogenously administered corticosteroids. Chapter 4.3 covers how to distinguish among the three types of endogenous Cushing's syndrome.

Cushing's disease most often affects women in their child-bearing years. Signs and symptoms include truncal obesity, cervicodorsal fat pad (buffalo hump), moon facies, plethora, purple striae, proximal muscle wasting and weakness, easy bruising, amenorrhea, psychiatric disturbances, and hirsutism. Many ACTH-secreting pituitary adenomas are less than 0.5 cm in diameter and difficult to identify radiographically.

First-line therapy for Cushing's disease is transsphenoidal resection of the tumor; this cures 80% of patients. The remainder can be given a combination of pituitary radiation and "medical adrenalectomy" with one or more drugs that inhibit adrenal glucocorticoid biosynthesis, for example, metyrapone, ketoconazole, aminoglutethimide, trilostane, and o,p'-DDD. However, none of these agents easily normalizes glucocorticoid secretion, and all have side effects. By 5 years, radiation therapy cures only 50% of adults, but more than 50% of children.

If pituitary surgery, radiation therapy, and medical therapy fail to control hypercortisolism, the last option is bilateral adrenalectomy. This commits patients to lifelong glucocorticoid and mineralocorticoid replacement. About 10% of patients who undergo bilateral adrenalectomy develop Nelson's syndrome, which is a progressive enlargement of the pituitary tumor, hyperpigmentation, and very high plasma ACTH levels unleashed by loss of cortisol-negative feedback. Such tumors can be aggressive and difficult to cure. The tumor causing Nelson's syndrome can be detected radiographically as well as by extremely high ACTH levels. All patients who have undergone bilateral adrenalectomy should be monitored closely.

Rare Secretory Tumors: Rare pituitary adenomas (usually macroadenomas) secrete thyroid-stimulating hormone (TSH), which causes hyperthyroidism. Unlike typical patients with primary hyperthyroidism—for example, from Graves' disease, in whom circulating TSH levels are low or undetectable—patients with hyperthyroidism from TSH-secreting adenomas have either elevated or inappropriately normal serum TSH levels at the same time that they have high serum T_4 and T_3 levels. Most TSH-secreting adenomas are managed with surgery and radiation; many patients also need antithyroid drugs and radioactive iodine. Octreotide has been shown to reduce TSH secretion from these tumors.

Many pituitary tumors that secrete luteinizing hormone (LH), follicle-stimulating hormone (FSH), or both are large and cause local compressive symptoms by the time they are discovered. Typical patients present with hypogonadism despite their high serum levels of FSH or LH, because the hormones produced by the tumor are abnormal and hypoactive. These tumors are managed like nonsecretory tumors with surgery followed by radiation therapy.

Other Sellar Lesions: The sellar and suprasellar regions can also harbor primary brain neoplasms such as craniopharyngiomas, which are squamous epithelial tumors that arise from the upper part of the pituitary stalk. Metastases from breast and lung cancers, lymphoma, and melanoma are other uncommon sellar lesions.

Rarely, autoimmune, infiltrative, and infectious diseases involve the pituitary, sometimes mimicking a tumor. Lymphocytic hypophysitis predominantly affects young women in late pregnancy or postpartum and is thought to have an autoimmune pathogenesis. Infiltrative and infectious processes that can damage the pituitary include sarcoidosis, Langerhans' histiocytosis, and tuberculosis. Occasionally, these diseases cause local mass effects and hypopituitarism.

The empty sella syndrome is a symmetric enlargement of the sella turcica caused by cerebrospinal fluid penetrating its diaphragm, putting chronic pressure on adjacent bone, and compressing the pituitary. In spite of this pressure, the pituitary usually functions normally. The empty sella syndrome most often affects obese hypertensive women. It can be distinguished from a pituitary tumor by computed tomography (CT) or magnetic resonance imaging (MRI) of the sella. Pituitary cysts and arterial aneurysms are other conditions that can mimic pituitary tumors and can be differentiated by imaging.

Compression of Surrounding Structures

The signs and symptoms of an impinging sellar mass reflect pituitary anatomy. The pituitary lies within a bony fossa, the sella turcica (Figure 4.2–2). Expanding masses within the sella usually take the path of least resistance, growing superiorly. As a growing lesion stretches the diaphragma sellae, which contains sensory nerves, patients may complain of dull frontal headaches. As the tumor continues to grow superiorly, it compresses the optic nerve and optic chiasm.

Loss of vision is an early—and often the only—symptom of pituitary adenoma. The most subtle visual abnormality is color desaturation in the superior temporal fields, caused by compression of the medial inferior portion of the optic chiasm. However, some patients describe their vision as dim or foggy, or they feel as if they have a veil over their eyes. Many patients have only vague complaints like loss of depth perception. Some are unaware of their visual loss because peripheral vision is typically affected first. However, they may acknowledge problems

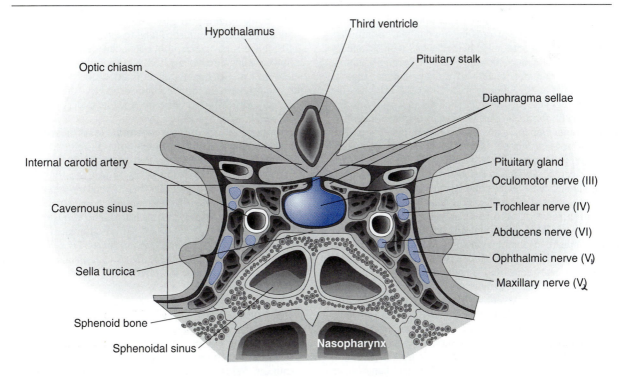

Figure 4.2–2. Anatomy of the sellar region.

with driving, which requires peripheral vision, or they may complain that they are bumping into furniture or other people. If the tumor continues to grow, patients may suffer bitemporal hemianopia, optic atrophy, and loss of visual acuity. Papilledema is rare.

In a few patients, an expanding tumor impinges on the hypothalamus, disturbing consciousness or temperature regulation, or causing hyperphagia. Tumor obstructing the third ventricle and cerebrospinal fluid flow can lead to hydrocephalus.

In a few patients, tumor extends laterally into the cavernous sinuses, where it can compress (1) cranial nerve III, IV, or VI, causing extraocular motor palsies; (2) the parasympathetic fibers in cranial nerve III, causing dilatation of the pupil; and (3) cranial nerve V, causing diplopia and facial numbness. Rarely, tumor erodes down through the floor of the sella and produces cerebrospinal fluid rhinorrhea or epistaxis.

Hypopituitarism

The pituitary is the structure most vulnerable to an enlarging sellar lesion. Compression can damage all types of secretory pituitary cells.

Injury to LH- and FSH-secreting cells causes secondary (central) hypogonadism. In children, this delays puberty. In men, it causes impotence, decreased libido, and infertility. In women, it leads to menstrual irregularities, amenorrhea, infertility, hot flushes, decreased libido, vaginal dryness, and dyspareunia. Deficient prolactin secretion makes women unable to lactate postpartum.

Injury to ACTH-secreting cells causes secondary adrenal insufficiency. Many patients complain of weight loss, anorexia, nausea, weakness, arthralgia, and myalgia. Decreased adrenal androgen production diminishes women's axillary and pubic hair. Patients with secondary adrenal insufficiency do not have hyperpigmentation, which is a common feature of primary adrenal insufficiency (Chapter 4.3). Furthermore, since ACTH is not the primary regulator of the mineralocorticoid axis, few patients with secondary insufficiency have extracellular fluid volume depletion and hyperkalemia, which are often seen in primary adrenal insufficiency. Many patients do have hyponatremia; this is caused by impaired renal free water clearance, which is dependent on glucocorticoid action. Patients are typically sensitive to infection and other stresses, which can quickly precipitate hypoglycemia, hypotension, circulatory collapse, and death.

Injury to TSH-secreting cells causes secondary hypothyroidism. Symptoms include fatigue, cold intolerance, dry skin, constipation, weight gain, impaired mentation, and menstrual irregularities in women. These manifestations resemble those of primary hypothyroidism, but are usually less severe.

Growth hormone deficiency impairs skeletal growth if the epiphyses have not fused. Adults can lose muscle mass and strength and develop hypoglycemia and hyperlipidemia.

From 5% to 20% of pituitary adenomas hemorrhage

spontaneously. About one-third of these hemorrhages are recognizable as pituitary apoplexy, a syndrome of sudden, severe headache, neurologic symptoms and signs, and acute adrenal insufficiency. Neurologic problems characteristically include vision loss, diplopia, ptosis, and pupil abnormalities. Within hours, lack of ACTH and cortisol production causes nausea, vomiting, and hypotension. If necrotic tissue and blood enter the cerebrospinal fluid, the patient may also develop meningismus, hyperpyrexia, and coma. The diagnosis of pituitary apoplexy is often delayed because it can mimic the symptoms of subarachnoid hemorrhage and meningitis; differentiating these disorders requires imaging of the sella. Treatment is emergent surgical decompression of the sella.

Laboratory Tests and Imaging

In addition to a careful history and physical exam, evaluation of patients with a possible sellar lesion usually requires a focused hormone assessment, imaging studies, and visual field analysis.

Hormone Deficiencies: The physician must identify the patient's hormone deficiencies and determine whether they are caused by pituitary failure (secondary, central hormone deficiencies) or target gland dysfunction (primary, peripheral hormone deficiencies). Levels of target gland hormones—T_4, cortisol, and estradiol or testosterone—can be low in both primary and secondary endocrine disorders. Distinguishing between peripheral and central failure depends, therefore, on the level of the pituitary trophic hormone. For example, T_4 levels are low in both primary and secondary hypothyroidism, so one must look to the pituitary trophic hormone, TSH. In primary hypothyroidism, diminished negative feedback causes the TSH to be high, whereas in secondary hypothyroidism, pituitary injury makes the TSH either low or inappropriately normal. Analogous patterns allow the physician to distinguish between primary and secondary adrenal insufficiency and between primary and secondary hypogonadism.

Suspected secondary adrenal insufficiency: A basal morning cortisol is generally not a useful screening test unless the level is high, that is, above 20 μg/dL. In contrast, the rapid ACTH stimulation test usually detects pituitary-adrenal dysfunction when secondary adrenal insufficiency is chronic. Patients are given synthetic ACTH and their serum cortisol is measured 30 or 60 minutes later. Normal people have an ACTH-stimulated serum cortisol level of at least 20 μg/dL. If the ACTH deficiency is less than about 2 weeks old, the adrenal glands may not yet have atrophied and the rapid ACTH stimulation test may be falsely normal.

A more accurate way to diagnose acute secondary adrenal insufficiency is the metyrapone test, which evaluates both the pituitary and the adrenal cortex. Metyrapone reduces serum cortisol by blocking the enzyme 11β-hydroxylase, which catalyzes the last step in cortisol biosynthesis. When cortisol synthesis is inhibited, a normal pituitary responds by secreting more ACTH, thereby raising plasma levels of 11-deoxycortisol, the immediate precursor to cortisol, above 7.5 μg/dL. Patients with secondary adrenal insufficiency have no increase in ACTH and 11-deoxycortisol.

The insulin tolerance test is the gold standard for diagnosing secondary adrenal insufficiency because this test assesses the integrity of the entire hypothalamic-pituitary-adrenal axis. However, this procedure can cause uncomfortable adrenergic symptoms, and a few patients develop hypoglycemia-induced seizures and cardiac complications.

Suspected secondary hypothyroidism: The physician should measure the free T$_4$ (by T$_4$ radioimmunoassay or free T$_4$ index) and serum TSH concentrations. In secondary hypothyroidism, the free thyroxine is low, whereas the serum TSH is low or inappropriately normal. A normal TSH level in a patient with secondary hypothyroidism is explained by the fact that TSH produced in people with pituitary and hypothalamic diseases is less biologically active than normal.

Suspected secondary hypogonadism: The gonadal axis can be evaluated by measuring the LH, FSH, and estradiol or testosterone. Secondary deficiency is marked by LH and FSH levels that are inappropriately low relative to low sex steroid levels. Normal LH and FSH levels in a postmenopausal woman, rather than the expected elevations, also suggest hypopituitarism.

Since few adults are treated for growth hormone deficiency, they do not need their growth hormone measured. Similarly, since the only consequence of low prolactin is impaired lactation, few patients with hypopituitarism need measurement of the serum prolactin.

Imaging and Visual Field Testing: Imaging, preferably by MRI, reveals sellar lesions, defines their size, and occasionally suggests the specific tumor type. For example, a craniopharyngioma can often be predicted by calcification and cystic degeneration as well as by its suprasellar position. Because many people have clinically irrelevant nonsecretory pituitary adenomas, pituitary imaging should be deferred until hormonal or neurologic findings confirm that there is reason to suspect a clinically significant sellar lesion.

If imaging studies show a macroadenoma, the patient should have visual field tests to detect optic nerve abnormalities. Although routine physical exam can reveal gross defects in peripheral vision, formal ophthalmologic evaluation is essential to find subtle abnormalities.

DISORDERS OF THE POSTERIOR PITUITARY

Disorders of the posterior pituitary lead to syndromes caused by excessive or inadequate secretion of antidiuretic hormone (ADH, also called vasopressin).

Diabetes Insipidus

Diabetes insipidus is a polyuric syndrome of excessive excretion of dilute urine, with secondary polydipsia. In general, diabetes insipidus can result from either inadequate central nervous system ADH production or renal disease impairing responsiveness to ADH. Central diabetes insipidus develops when the posterior lobe of the pituitary fails to secrete enough ADH. Most often, the disorder is idiopathic; the major known causes are hypothalamic tumors, head trauma, central nervous system infiltrative disorders (eg, sarcoidosis) or infection (eg, tuberculosis), and transsphenoidal surgery. Primary disease of the pituitary gland is rarely to blame, because the posterior pituitary is merely a storage site for ADH after its synthesis in the hypothalamus. Thus, diabetes insipidus accompanying anterior pituitary dysfunction suggests underlying hypothalamic disease.

In contrast, nephrogenic diabetes insipidus is caused by kidney disorders in which the renal tubules do not respond normally to ADH. The condition can be familial or can be acquired through electrolyte derangements (eg, hypokalemia, hypercalcemia), diseases of the renal interstitium that disrupt medullary concentrating mechanisms, or drugs that impair renal tubular function (eg, demeclocycline, lithium carbonate).

Differential Diagnosis: Polyuria is not pathognomonic for central diabetes insipidus, and the physician must consider other conditions when a patient presents with excessive urination. Polyuria can reflect primary renal diseases, diuretic therapy, and diabetes mellitus. The cause can also be compulsive water drinking, also known as "psychogenic" or primary polydipsia. Such chronic excessive water drinking can lead to temporary loss of renal medullary hypertonicity, which then impairs urine concentration even when the drinking is temporarily interrupted and plasma ADH levels rise. Primary polydipsia is usually diagnosed in young women with known psychiatric disease; in rare patients, the cause is a structural lesion in the hypothalamus.

Diagnosis: The physician evaluating a patient with polyuria must first exclude an osmotic diuresis, such as the glycosuria of diabetes mellitus. The history and routine laboratory findings can generally exclude diabetes mellitus, primary renal diseases, drug effects, and electrolyte disturbances. Special tests are needed for certain systemic diseases that affect renal interstitial function, for example, sickle cell disease, amyloidosis, multiple myeloma, and Sjögren's syndrome.

Most patients need a water deprivation test to confirm diabetes insipidus and to distinguish central from nephrogenic diabetes insipidus. Fluids and food are withheld, starting in the morning to avoid severe nocturnal dehydration. Over the next 4–8 hours, hourly measurements of urine and plasma should show increasing osmolality and a two- to fourfold greater increase in urine osmolality than plasma osmolality. When plasma osmolality exceeds 295 mOsm/L or urine osmolality stops rising, patients are given aqueous ADH or its analog, dDAVP (desmopressin). In normal people, endogenous ADH is already maximally stimulated, so exogenous ADH does not cause further urine concentration. Patients with complete central diabetes insipidus do not concentrate their urine despite a rising plasma osmolality, but do respond to exogenous ADH with a rise in urine concentration. Patients with nephrogenic diabetes insipidus also maintain a dilute urine despite dehydration, and when they receive exogenous ADH, their urine osmolality does not rise above that of plasma.

When central diabetes insipidus is diagnosed, patients should have an MRI scan to check the hypothalamic and pituitary regions for tumor and infiltrative disease.

Patients with primary polydipsia may be difficult to identify with the water deprivation test because chronic dilution of their renal medullary osmolar gradient can prevent them from responding properly to either endogenous or exogenous ADH. However, other features may distinguish primary polydipsia from diabetes insipidus (Table 4.2–3). Polyuria usually begins gradually in primary polydipsia, but suddenly in diabetes insipidus. Patients with primary polydipsia may not have much nocturia, but most patients with diabetes insipidus have a constant urine output. Compulsive water drinkers do not share the high plasma osmolality and inappropriately low urine osmolality seen after overnight fasting in patients with central or nephrogenic diabetes insipidus. Most patients with primary polydipsia have at least one random plasma sample documenting an osmolality below 285 mOsm/L (dilutional hyponatremia). Plasma ADH levels are normal relative to plasma osmolality in patients with primary polydipsia, but are low in patients with central diabetes insipidus.

Management: Patients with mild diabetes insipidus may not need drug treatment as long as they have an intact thirst mechanism and access to water. However, patients with diabetes insipidus who are temporarily deprived of water can quickly develop circulatory collapse and hypertonic encephalopathy. Treatment is usually indicated when urine volumes exceed 5 L per day.

dDAVP, a long-acting synthetic analog of ADH, is the treatment of choice for central diabetes insipidus. The drug is usually given by nasal insufflation or subcutaneous injection. If patients with partial central diabetes insipidus require treatment, many can be successfully managed with chlorpropamide, which augments ADH release and potentiates its action on renal tubular cells. Most patients with normal glucose tolerance can take chlorpropamide in the low dose required without developing symptomatic hypoglycemia. Clofibrate and carbamazepine can also augment ADH release.

Syndrome of Inappropriate Secretion of ADH

Excessive secretion of ADH, termed the syndrome of inappropriate secretion of antidiuretic hormone (SIADH), leads to excessive water retention and hyponatremia. SIADH is the most common cause of noniatrogenic hyponatremia. The major causes of SIADH are ectopic secretion of ADH (eg, by a small cell carcinoma), neurologic disorders, pulmonary diseases, and certain drugs (Table 4.2–4). Cardinal features of the syndrome are hyponatremia and serum hypo-osmolality resulting from an inappropriately concentrated urine.

Patients with mild SIADH may have few symptoms and signs. But when the serum sodium falls below 130 mEq/L, patients can become anorexic, lethargic, and confused, with nausea and muscle cramping. When the serum sodium falls below 115 mEq/L, patients can become obtunded and develop seizures. The severity of symptoms generally corresponds to the degree of hypo-osmolality and the rate at which hyponatremia develops. Premenopausal women seem to be more sensitive to rapid fluxes in serum sodium than are men and postmenopausal women.

Other causes of hyponatremia must be considered in the differential diagnosis of SIADH. The physician should determine clinically whether hyponatremic patients are euvolemic (normal water volume), hypervolemic, or hypovolemic (Chapter 5.2). Although patients with SIADH do have modest volume expansion, they are not edematous; in patients with edema, the physician should consider the major causes of hypervolemic hyponatremia—cirrhosis, heart failure, and kidney failure. Patients with glucocorticoid or thyroid hormone deficiencies can develop hyponatremia because these hormones are essential for normal renal tubular function and free water excretion by the kidney. Thus, the diagnosis of SIADH cannot be established until hypothyroidism has been excluded by measurement of the serum T_4 and TSH concentrations, adrenal insufficiency has been excluded by an ACTH-stimulated serum cortisol level, and kidney disease has been excluded by renal function tests. The physician should also seek a history of medications, neoplasia, pul-

Table 4.2–3. Distinguishing primary polydipsia from diabetes insipidus.

Feature	Primary Polydipsia	Diabetes Insipidus
Onset of polyuria	Gradual	Sudden
Nocturia	Unusual	Common
Random plasma osmolality	Sometimes <285 mOsm/L (normal = 275–295)	Normal or elevated
Morning plasma osmolality	Normal	Elevated
Morning urine osmolality	Normal	Inappropriately low
Plasma ADH concentration	Normal relative to plasma osmolality	Low relative to plasma osmolality (in central diabetes insipidus)

Table 4.2–4. Common causes of the syndrome of inappropriate secretion of antidiuretic hormone (SIADH).

Central nervous system diseases
Meningitis (eg, tuberculous)
Encephalitis
Head injury
Brain abscess
Subarachnoid hemorrhage

Pulmonary disease
Lung abscess
Pneumonia
Positive-pressure ventilation

Tumors
Carcinoma of the lung (especially small cell carcinoma)
Gastrointestinal malignancies (eg, pancreatic cancer)
Prostate cancer
Thymoma
Lymphoma

Drugs
Vincristine
Chlorpropamide
Clofibrate
Carbamazepine
Nicotine
Phenothiazine
Cyclophosphamide

monary disease, and neurologic disorders known to be associated with SIADH.

In SIADH, urine sodium is generally above 20 mEq/L, but it is usually below 20 mEq/L in conditions with intravascular volume contraction or decreased effective plasma volume, for example, congestive heart failure, cirrhosis, and the nephrotic syndrome. The blood urea nitrogen and uric acid are low in SIADH but high in volume-contracted states. Lastly, in SIADH the urine is less than maximally dilute (50–100 mOsm/kg) despite plasma hypo-osmolality.

The aims of treating SIADH are to correct hypo-osmolality and hyponatremia and to diagnose and, when possible, to treat the underlying disorder. For the asymptomatic patient, water restriction to 500–1000 mL/day corrects hyponatremia at a rate of about 5 mEq/L per day. Infusions of normal saline do not correct hyponatremia, because the sodium is promptly excreted in the urine. Symptomatic hyponatremia is treated with hypertonic saline until the serum sodium concentration reaches 125 mEq/L. Then plasma osmolality is restored gradually by water restriction alone or with a loop diuretic. For many patients with chronic SIADH, demeclocycline normalizes serum sodium by inhibiting ADH action in the kidney. Lithium carbonate acts similarly but is rarely used because it can be more toxic.

SUMMARY

▶ Pituitary tumors can present as syndromes of hormone excess, compression of adjacent brain structures, or hypopituitarism.

▶ Patients with clinical features of excessive pituitary hormone production should have relevant hormone levels measured. If an abnormality is confirmed, the sellar region should be imaged.

▶ Hypopituitarism can present as a subtle syndrome of constitutional symptoms or, in pituitary apoplexy, as an acute neurologic and endocrine emergency.

▶ Hallmarks of diabetes insipidus are polyuria, hypertonic serum, and inappropriately dilute urine. Central and nephrogenic diabetes insipidus can be differentiated by the patient's response to exogenous antidiuretic hormone (ADH).

▶ Central nervous system and intrathoracic diseases such as lung tumors and pneumonia can cause the syndrome of inappropriate ADH (SIADH), marked by hypotonic serum with inappropriately concentrated urine in the absence of dehydration, renal disease, adrenal insufficiency, and hypothyroidism.

SUGGESTED READING

Abboud CF, Laws ER Jr: Diagnosis of pituitary tumors. Endocrinol Metab Clin North Am 1988;17:241.
Barkan AL: Acromegaly: Diagnosis and therapy. Endocrinol Metab Clin North Am 1989;18:277.
Dalkin AC, Marshall JC: Medical therapy of hyperprolactinemia. Endocrinol Metab Clin North Am 1989;18:259.

Melmed S (editor): *The Pituitary.* Blackwell Science, 1995.
Vokes TJ, Robertson GL: Disorders of antidiuretic hormone. Endocrinol Metab Clin North Am 1988;17:281.

4.3

Adrenal Disorders

Gary S. Wand, MD, and David S. Cooper, MD

Disorders of the adrenal glands result from overproduction and underproduction of their hormones and from adrenal tumors. Cushing's syndrome, adrenal insufficiency, and other adrenal disorders are rare. However, their symptoms and signs are so common that most of the patients whom a physician sees have one or more complaints that could be attributed to adrenal disease. The physician's first task is to know when to consider an adrenal disorder seriously. Fortunately, there are clues. For example, although many hypertensive patients with diabetes mellitus are overweight or hirsute, the physician should suspect Cushing's syndrome particularly if they have proximal muscle weakness or pigmented striae. Similarly, although many patients feel tired and weak, the physician should consider adrenal insufficiency particularly if they have also lost weight.

Laboratory testing is essential for diagnosing adrenal diseases and determining their underlying causes. Because the adrenal cortex and medulla normally produce different amounts of hormones at different times of day, diagnosis often requires more than measurement of a single random hormone level in blood. Usually, the physician must estimate hormone secretion over time, as by measuring how much hormone patients excrete in their urine, analyzing their response to stimulation or suppression of hormone secretion, or both.

Physicians must be familiar with hormonal and general medical therapy for adrenal disorders, which can require measures ranging from resuscitation to lifelong management. Finally, physicians must understand the actions and side effects of widely used corticosteroid medications.

HYPERCORTISOLISM (CUSHING'S SYNDROME)

Clinical Features

Cushing's syndrome is the clinical manifestation of hypercortisolism. The physician should suspect Cushing's syndrome when a patient presents with obesity, hypertension, and diabetes mellitus. However, this combination of features appears more often from coincidence of independent problems than from hypercortisolism. The most specific physical features of hypercortisolism are proximal muscle weakness and wide pigmented striae.

Evaluation should focus on features that distinguish Cushing's syndrome from simple obesity (Table 4.3–1). In patients with hypercortisolism, body fat is characteristically concentrated in the chest and abdomen (centripetal obesity), supraclavicular and cervicodorsal fat pads (buffalo hump), and face (moon facies) (Figure 4.3–1). With time, muscles in the extremities (especially proximal thigh muscles) become weak and wasted, and the shoulder muscles weaken. The skin becomes thin and easily bruised. Wounds heal poorly. The face may look red (plethoric) because the thin facial skin makes underlying vessels more visible. Most patients develop violaceous striae more than 1 cm wide; these streaks are broader and darker than the "stretch marks" seen in other obese people and pregnant women. Increased adrenal androgen production causes hirsutism and menstrual dysfunction in women and acne and folliculitis in both sexes.

Excess cortisol alters calcium metabolism, causing osteoporosis. Patients may present with pain from vertebral and other fractures. Increased calcium mobilization from bone causes hypercalciuria and kidney stones. Enhanced gluconeogenesis can cause or worsen diabetes mellitus. In ACTH-dependent forms of Cushing's syndrome, hypersecretion of mineralocorticoids can lead to hypertension, peripheral edema, and hypokalemia. Two-thirds of patients have reversible psychiatric manifestations, which can range from emotional lability to frank psychosis. Many patients are depressed.

Causes

Cushing's syndrome is principally the result of chronic glucocorticoid excess (see Table 3.2–6). The most common cause is corticosteroid drugs prescribed to treat other diseases. (Corticosteroids are all 21-carbon adrenal cortical steroids, as opposed to the 19-carbon androgens.) Corticosteroids are subdivided into glucocorticoids and mineralocorticoids based on their relative biological activ-

Table 4.3–1. Characteristic physical findings in hypercortisolism (Cushing's syndrome).

Centripetal obesity
Cervicodorsal fat pad ("buffalo hump")
Moon facies
Plethora
Wide, violaceous striae
Muscle weakness
Easy bruising
Hyperpigmentation
Amenorrhea

ities (Table 4.3–2). Cushing's syndrome is also caused by overproduction of endogenous cortisol through (1) autonomous production by benign and malignant adrenocortical tumors, (2) excessive pituitary secretion of adrenocorticotropic hormone (ACTH) (Cushing's *disease*), and (3) ectopic production of ACTH by nonpituitary tumors, most of which are malignant (Figure 4.3–2).

Adrenocortical tumors account for 25% of cases of endogenous Cushing's syndrome. Benign adenomas, usually appearing singly, cause the normal adrenal cortex to atrophy. The less common adrenocortical carcinomas tend to be aggressive, invading blood vessels and metastasizing to the liver and lungs. Many adrenal cancers produce androgens along with cortisol.

Pituitary Cushing's disease accounts for 60% of cases of endogenous Cushing's syndrome and most often affects premenopausal women. The usual cause is an ACTH-secreting pituitary adenoma, which is less responsive than normal pituitary to negative feedback by corti-sol. Because most such tumors are but a few millimeters in diameter, only one-third can be identified by computed tomography (CT) or magnetic resonance imaging (MRI).

In 15% of patients, endogenous Cushing's syndrome is caused by ectopic production of ACTH by neoplasms arising in organs other than the pituitary. The most commonly implicated tumor is small cell carcinoma of the lung. Pheochromocytoma, pancreatic islet cell tumors, medullary carcinoma of the thyroid, bronchial carcinoid tumors, and thymic carcinoma can also produce ACTH. There have been rare reports of Cushing's syndrome being caused by corticotropin-releasing factor-secreting tumors such as bronchial adenomas.

Occasionally, clinical features suggest the cause of cortisol excess. Adrenal carcinomas can virilize female patients, causing temporal balding, deepening voice, breast atrophy, clitorimegaly, and muscle hypertrophy. Fifty percent of all adrenocortical carcinomas are palpable by the time they are diagnosed. In the ectopic ACTH syndrome, the underlying malignancy and rapid onset of hypercortisolism often produce cachexia rather than centripetal obesity. Some patients with ectopic ACTH present with the metabolic consequences of their hypercortisolism and hyperaldosteronism, primarily hypokalemia, metabolic alkalosis, and hyperglycemia. Many patients have hyperpigmentation.

Laboratory Diagnosis

Laboratory tests (Figure 4.3–3) should address two questions: Does the patient have endogenous hypercortisolism? And if so, what is causing the excess cortisol secretion?

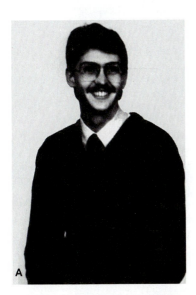 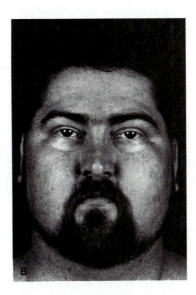 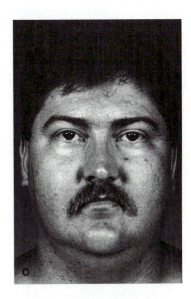

Figure 4.3–1. Young man with pituitary-dependent Cushing's syndrome. **A:** Before (age 19). **B:** During active disease (age 32). **C:** After surgery, improving but not back to baseline (age 33).

Table 4.3–2. Commonly used corticosteroid preparations.

Preparation	Glucocorticoid Potency Relative to Cortisol	Mineralocorticoid Potency Relative to Aldosterone	Biologic Half-life (hours)
Cortisol	1.0	0.005	8–12
Cortisone	0.8	0.004	8–12
Prednisone	4.0	0.004	12–36
Methylprednisolone	5.0	0.0025	12–36
Dexamethasone	25.0	0	36–72
Fludrocortisone	15.0	1.0	8–12

Screening Tests: There are three ways to screen for hypercortisolism. Measuring urine free cortisol excretion over 24 hours is the most sensitive and specific method. Normal adults excrete less than 125 µg/day of unmetabolized free cortisol, but almost all patients with Cushing's syndrome excrete more.

The overnight dexamethasone suppression test is a convenient though less accurate alternative. The potent synthetic glucocorticoid dexamethasone normally suppresses ACTH secretion. A healthy person who takes 1 mg of dexamethasone at bedtime will have a plasma cortisol level below 5 µg/dL at 8:00 the next morning. Patients with Cushing's have a plasma cortisol above 10 µg/dL. False-positives can be caused by obesity, stress, depression, and alcoholism. False-positives can also occur when concurrent diphenylhydantoin therapy accelerates dexamethasone metabolism or when concurrent estrogen therapy or pregnancy elevates the cortisol binding globulin level.

When urine free cortisol levels are elevated or the overnight dexamethasone suppression test is abnormal, a low-dose dexamethasone suppression test should generally be done to confirm hypercortisolism. A baseline 24-hour urine specimen is collected to measure urine free cortisol. At the end of the baseline urine collection, the patient starts taking 0.5 mg dexamethasone every 6 hours. During the second day that the patient takes dexamethasone, another 24-hour urine specimen is obtained. In normal people, urine free cortisol levels fall below 25 µg/day; they remain higher in patients with endogenous Cushing's syndrome.

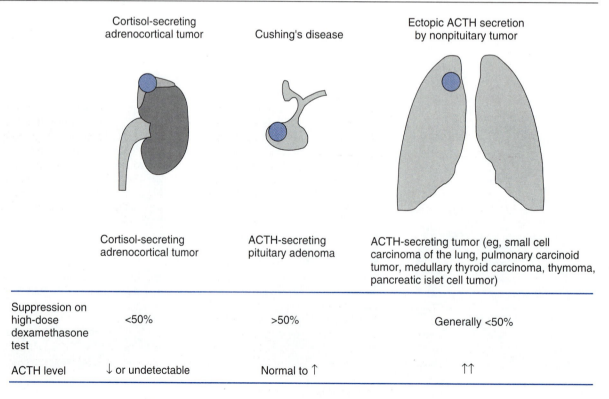

	Cortisol-secreting adrenocortical tumor	Cushing's disease	Ectopic ACTH secretion by nonpituitary tumor
	Cortisol-secreting adrenocortical tumor	ACTH-secreting pituitary adenoma	ACTH-secreting tumor (eg, small cell carcinoma of the lung, pulmonary carcinoid tumor, medullary thyroid carcinoma, thymoma, pancreatic islet cell tumor)
Suppression on high-dose dexamethasone test	<50%	>50%	Generally <50%
ACTH level	↓ or undetectable	Normal to ↑	↑↑

Figure 4.3–2. Primary causes of endogenous Cushing's syndrome.

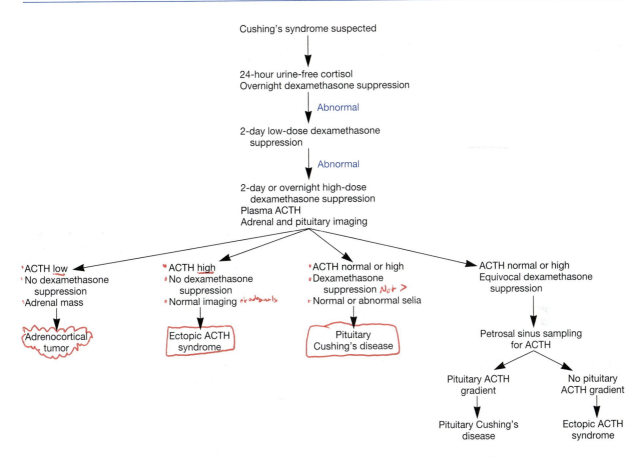

Figure 4.3–3. Evaluation of Cushing's syndrome. (Reproduced, with permission, from Wand GS: Identifying Cushing's syndrome and defining its cause. Med Rounds 1989;2:47.)

Confirming hypercortisolism and finding its cause can be one of the most difficult tasks in clinical endocrinology. Laboratory data can be misleading or conflicting, for two reasons. First, depression, alcohol abuse, and other chronic stresses can increase cortisol production and make it relatively resistant to suppression. After these conditions are controlled, laboratory studies may need to be repeated before a definitive diagnosis can be made. Second, tumors that cause hypercortisolism may secrete only some of the time (periodic hormonogenesis) and thus may cause intermittently false-negative test results.

Etiologic Diagnosis: If the history excludes use of exogenous corticosteroids, the three underlying causes of excessive endogenous glucocorticoid production—adrenocortical tumors, ACTH-secreting pituitary adenomas, and ectopic ACTH production by nonpituitary tumors (see Figure 4.3–2)—can be distinguished by a combination of high-dose dexamethasone suppression testing, plasma ACTH measurement, and imaging.

High-dose glucocorticoids suppress ACTH-secreting pituitary adenomas, but they do not suppress cortisol-secreting adrenocortical tumors and only occasionally suppress ectopic ACTH-secreting tumors, both of which produce hormone autonomously. Thus, the high-dose dexamethasone suppression test can help distinguish pituitary Cushing's disease from the two other types of Cushing's syndrome (see Figure 4.3–2). This test starts with a baseline 24-hour urinary free cortisol collection. Then patients are given 2 mg of dexamethasone every 6 hours for the next 2 days; throughout this period, 24-hour urine specimens continue to be collected. If values of cortisol or its metabolites—the urine free cortisol or 17-hydroxysteroids—fall below 50% of control values during the second day, cortisol secretion is "suppressible" and the patient likely has an ACTH-secreting pituitary tumor. If dexamethasone fails to suppress hypercortisolism, patients probably have an ectopic ACTH-secreting tumor or a cortisol-secreting adrenocortical tumor. These two lesions can be differentiated by plasma ACTH levels: The ACTH is usually low in patients with adrenocortical tumors, but high in patients with the ectopic ACTH syndrome.

A simpler but potentially less accurate way of differentiating pituitary tumors from the other two types is the overnight high-dose dexamethasone suppression test. On the first day of this test, a serum cortisol is obtained between 8:00 and 9:00 AM. Between 11:00 and 12:00 that night, the patient takes 8 mg dexamethasone. The next morning between 8:00 and 9:00 a second serum cortisol is obtained. This test is interpreted like the longer high-dose test described in the previous paragraph.

CT scan of the adrenal glands shows adrenocortical tumors. CT of the chest and abdomen often shows the tumors responsible for ectopic ACTH production. Most ACTH-secreting pituitary tumors are too small to be visualized. Because many people have incidental nonsecreting adrenal and pituitary neoplasms, radiographic procedures should usually be delayed until blood tests are completed.

It can be difficult to differentiate between pituitary and ectopic ACTH production. For example, ACTH-secreting bronchial carcinoid tumors can be small and suppressed by dexamethasone. If clinical and laboratory features are discordant, as sometimes happens, the physician can turn to the "gold standard" for confirming pituitary-dependent Cushing's disease: measuring ACTH levels in the two inferior petrosal sinuses, which carry the venous effluent from each half of the pituitary. A significant difference between the ACTH concentrations in systemic venous blood and either inferior petrosal sinus establishes an ACTH-secreting pituitary adenoma. Furthermore, an ACTH concentration gradient between the two sides localizes the tiny tumor within the pituitary to guide the neurosurgeon. Measuring the plasma ACTH response to exogenous corticotropin-releasing factor can also be helpful in difficult cases. Most patients with pituitary Cushing's disease respond with an exaggerated rise in ACTH, whereas those with the ectopic ACTH syndrome typically have only a slight rise.

Management

Treatment options for pituitary-dependent Cushing's disease are described in Chapter 4.2. Cushing's syndrome caused by adrenocortical adenomas can usually be treated successfully with unilateral adrenalectomy. Inhibitors of adrenal steroid biosynthesis, such as metyrapone, can ameliorate Cushing's syndrome caused by adrenal adenomas preoperatively or when surgery is contraindicated. Adrenocortical carcinomas are also resected when possible. When the lesion is inoperable, hypercortisolism may be partially controlled by inhibitors of adrenal steroid biosynthesis, such as aminoglutethimide and ketoconazole. The cytotoxic agent mitotane can control the progression of some adrenocortical carcinomas.

For patients with the ectopic ACTH syndrome, the treatment of choice is surgical removal of the tumor. When tumors are inoperable, radiation therapy and chemotherapy may be beneficial. Patients who develop serious metabolic complications of the ectopic ACTH syndrome must have their hyperglycemia controlled, potassium replaced, aldosterone blocked, and adrenal corticosteroid production inhibited by aminoglutethimide or ketoconazole.

ADRENAL INSUFFICIENCY

Patients with undiagnosed adrenal insufficiency are in a precarious situation. For most, the disease begins insidiously, with nonspecific complaints like fatigue, weakness, and malaise—common symptoms that are almost always caused by something else. At the same time, because adrenal corticosteroids play such a vital role in coping with stresses like infection, dehydration, injury, and surgery, these hormone deficits can quickly become life-threatening. Physicians must be alert to clinical and laboratory hints that one of their many patients with these common complaints is the rare one with adrenal insufficiency.

Causes

Primary adrenal insufficiency (Addison's disease) is caused by a number of processes that damage the adrenal cortex. The most common form, idiopathic adrenal atrophy, is believed to result from autoimmune inflammation of the adrenal cortex. Affected patients, most often women, may have had either another autoimmune endocrine disease (eg, autoimmune thyroiditis, idiopathic hypoparathyroidism, insulin-dependent diabetes mellitus) or a nonendocrine autoimmune disorder (eg, vitiligo, pernicious anemia). Some patients have circulating anti-adrenal antibodies.

Hemorrhagic destruction of the adrenal may be a complication of anticoagulant therapy or a fulminant infection such as meningococcal or staphylococcal septicemia. Tuberculosis, fungal infections like histoplasmosis, and metastatic tumors can also cause adrenocortical insufficiency. A rare cause in men is adrenoleukodystrophy, an X-linked recessive disorder in which injurious very long-chain fatty acids accumulate in the adrenal cortex and the nervous system.

Secondary adrenocortical insufficiency can be produced when exogenous corticosteroids suppress hypothalamic corticotropin-releasing factor and pituitary ACTH production. The most common cause of adrenal insufficiency is abrupt cessation of glucocorticoid therapy (see "Iatrogenic Cushing's Syndrome" below). For other diseases that damage the hypothalamus or pituitary and secondarily impair adrenal glucocorticoid production, see Chapter 4.2.

Clinical Features

The most common symptoms of adrenal insufficiency are fatigue, weakness, light-headedness, and weight loss, findings that may first suggest chronic infection or malignancy (Table 4.3–3). Weight loss is particularly useful in the differential diagnosis; stable or rising weight makes adrenal insufficiency extremely unlikely. Most patients have myalgias, arthralgias, and muscle weakness. Many report anorexia, nausea, vomiting, and abdominal pain, all of which might suggest an abdominal disorder. Many develop hypersensitive taste, smell, and hearing. Some crave salt. Patients whose adrenal insufficiency is secondary to pituitary or hypothalamic dysfunction may have symptoms and signs of their intracranial disease (Chapter 4.2).

Table 4.3–3. Clinical evaluation of adrenal insufficiency.

Symptoms
  Constitutional
    Fatigue
    Weakness
    Weight loss
    Light-headedness
  Gastrointestinal
    Anorexia
    Nausea and vomiting
    Abdominal pain
  Other
    Myalgias and arthralgias
    Salt craving

History of predisposing factors
  Corticosteroid therapy
  Other autoimmune endocrine diseases, eg, autoimmune
    thyroiditis, idiopathic hypoparathyroidism
  Anticoagulation
  Tuberculosis or AIDS
  Sepsis, especially meningococcal

Signs
  Hypotension, especially postural
  Fever
  Hyperpigmentation*

Routine laboratory findings
  Hyperkalemia*
  Hyponatremia
  Hypoglycemia
  Anemia
  Eosinophilia

*Primary adrenal insufficiency only.

The immediate danger for patients with adrenal insufficiency is that an intercurrent infection or other stress might precipitate acute prostration, hypotension, fever, and hypoglycemia.

Most patients with adrenal insufficiency are hypotensive, particularly when standing. The hypotension is caused primarily by sodium loss and extracellular fluid volume depletion related to a mineralocorticoid deficit. Lack of glucocorticoid-mediated vascular reactivity also contributes to hypotension.

Many patients with primary adrenal insufficiency have hyperpigmented skin because of increased breakdown of proopiomelanocortin (an ACTH precursor) to melanocyte-stimulating hormone. The skin looks dirty, especially over the knees, elbows, and other pressure points. The perineum, areolae, and recent scars show increased pigmentation. Freckles may appear over the forehead, face, and neck. Dark areas may appear on the lips and gums and over the buccal, rectal, and vaginal surfaces.

Patients with secondary adrenal insufficiency may present with muscle weakness, delayed deep-tendon reflexes, and myasthenia-like muscular fatigability, but they do not develop hyperpigmentation.

Laboratory Tests

On routine laboratory tests, glucocorticoid deficiency may be reflected by hypoglycemia, and mineralocorticoid deficiency may be reflected by hyponatremia, hyper-

kalemia, and metabolic acidosis (see Table 4.3–3). Extracellular fluid volume depletion may cause a rise in serum urea nitrogen. Changes in the blood include eosinophilia and anemia, which may become more apparent after the patient is rehydrated.

Other findings point to adrenal insufficiency being secondary. Patients with secondary insufficiency do not develop hyperkalemia; this is because they have relatively unimpaired aldosterone secretion, which is mediated principally by the renin-angiotensin system. However, many patients with secondary insufficiency still have hyponatremia, because cortisol is essential for normal excretion of renal tubular free water. Most patients with secondary insufficiency caused by hypopituitarism have deficiencies of other pituitary hormones. Associated growth hormone deficiency makes hypoglycemia more common in secondary adrenal insufficiency.

The physician who suspects adrenal insufficiency should perform an ACTH stimulation test. The best screen is the short (1-hour) ACTH stimulation test, in which plasma cortisol is measured before and 1 hour after the patient receives intravenous synthetic ACTH. The physician can exclude adrenal insufficiency if the 1-hour cortisol value is above 20 µg/dL and the rise in cortisol exceeds 7 µg/dL. Although this test is excellent for detecting primary adrenal insufficiency, it has a sensitivity of only 90% in detecting adrenocortical failure secondary to hypothalamic or pituitary disease.

If the cortisol does not rise normally, the physician should generally do a long (3-day) ACTH stimulation test to confirm the screening results and distinguish primary from secondary adrenal insufficiency. A basal 24-hour urine is collected to test for free cortisol or 17-hydroxysteroids; then urines are collected for 3 more days while the patient is receiving synthetic ACTH infusions for 8 hours a day. Normal people have a two- to fourfold increase in free cortisol and 17-hydroxysteroids during the first ACTH infusion day. Patients with primary adrenal insufficiency show little or no rise through the 3 days. Patients with secondary adrenal insufficiency have a two- to threefold increase by the third infusion day.

After adrenal insufficiency is confirmed, a clearly high or low plasma ACTH concentration can distinguish primary from secondary adrenal insufficiency. In primary insufficiency, ACTH values typically exceed 100 pg/mL, reflecting lack of negative feedback by cortisol. In contrast, most patients with secondary insufficiency have low or normal ACTH values (0–30 pg/mL), even in the morning.

Management

Primary adrenal insufficiency can be controlled with oral cortisone acetate or hydrocortisone, with two-thirds of the dose taken on awakening and the rest in the late afternoon. The salt-retaining synthetic mineralocorticoid fludrocortisone is usually added when primary adrenal insufficiency causes hypotension or hyperkalemia. Patients with primary adrenal insufficiency should be instructed to increase their glucocorticoid replacement two- to three-fold during periods of stress such as infection or injury. The dose should be increased five- to tenfold for major stresses such as surgery or childbirth. Patients should keep injectable glucocorticoid (eg, methylprednisolone 40 mg) available in case vomiting prevents them from taking their oral dose. They should wear medical identification bracelets stating their need for glucocorticoid therapy in the event of sudden illness or injury.

Acute adrenal insufficiency (addisonian crisis) is a medical emergency characterized by fever, hypotension, and electrolyte disorders (see Table 4.3–3). The patient should be given intravenous glucocorticoid such as hydrocortisone, methylprednisolone, or dexamethasone, along with intravenous saline and glucose. Hypotension caused by adrenal insufficiency typically responds quickly to fluid and steroid replacement; persistent hypotension warrants a search for another cause.

PHARMACOLOGIC USE OF GLUCOCORTICOIDS

Glucocorticoids are often used to control nonendocrine diseases such as asthma, inflammatory bowel disease, collagen vascular disorders, sarcoidosis, nephrotic syndrome, and hypersensitivity reactions. The possible benefits of long-term glucocorticoids must always be weighed against their side effects. To prevent or minimize these complications, the physician should (1) prescribe the lowest effective glucocorticoid dose for the shortest possible time; (2) whenever possible, use preparations and dosing schedules that mimic the normal diurnal rhythm of cortisol secretion; (3) give glucocorticoids every other day when alternate-day regimens have been shown to be effective; and (4) combat the drug's side effects by prescribing exercise, a weight control diet, and oral calcium and vitamin D supplements. Patients who have progressive osteoporosis despite standard treatments might be given bisphosphonate or calcitonin.

Corticosteroid preparations vary in their relative glucocorticoid and mineralocorticoid potencies and their durations of biologic action (see Table 4.3–2). Glucocorticoid preparations with low mineralocorticoid activity (eg, prednisone) do not cause sodium retention, edema, hypertension, or hypokalemia; thus, they are most appropriate for treating inflammatory diseases. Preparations that must be activated in the liver (eg, prednisone, cortisone) may be ineffective for patients with severe liver dysfunction, who are more appropriately treated with methylprednisolone. Preparations with longer durations of action (eg, dexamethasone) provide more sustained therapeutic benefit with less frequent dosing than a short-acting drug like prednisone. However, long-acting steroids are also more likely to produce side effects than is prednisone, which controls some conditions even when given only every 24 or 48 hours.

Iatrogenic Cushing's Syndrome

The clinical features of iatrogenic Cushing's syndrome are identical with those of endogenous hypercortisolism—centripetal obesity, easy bruising, poor wound healing, diabetes mellitus, proximal myopathy, weakness, and osteoporosis. Sustained glucocorticoid therapy can also cause cataracts and aseptic necrosis, an infarction of bones such as the femoral head.

Exogenous glucocorticoids suppress the hypothalamic-pituitary-adrenal axis. If therapy is stopped abruptly or patients develop an intercurrent illness, their suppressed adrenal axis cannot meet the increased glucocorticoid requirement and they can quickly develop manifestations of adrenal insufficiency. The degree of adrenal suppression is related to both the dose and the duration of glucocorticoid therapy.

When patients have received glucocorticoid therapy for longer than 2 weeks, the physician must withdraw the drug gradually, while monitoring both activity of the underlying disease and evidence of adrenal insufficiency. When therapy has continued for months or years, it may be advisable during the final phase of withdrawal to switch patients to a single morning dose of a glucocorticoid that has a shorter half-life to encourage adrenal regulatory mechanisms to awaken.

If symptoms consistent with adrenal insufficiency emerge during withdrawal, the diagnosis should be confirmed with an 8:00 AM plasma cortisol drawn before patients take their glucocorticoid. If the plasma cortisol is less than 10 μg/dL, maintenance hydrocortisone should be given to allow the adrenal axis the weeks or months that it needs to recover. Even after the adrenal axis seems to have recovered completely, patients may need supplemental glucocorticoids if at any point during the next year they have a major illness or surgery. Need can be established by a short ACTH stimulation test.

As glucocorticoids are tapered, some patients develop symptoms like those of adrenal insufficiency, even though they have no biochemical evidence of deficient adrenal secretion. The features of this "steroid withdrawal syndrome" are anorexia, lethargy, malaise, myalgias, weight loss, headache, and fever. If severe symptoms persist for more than a few days, the steroid dose should be increased to its former level. After the symptoms have resolved, the dose can be tapered again, with smaller decrements over a longer time.

DISORDERS OF ALDOSTERONE SECRETION

Primary Hyperaldosteronism (Conn's Syndrome)

Primary hyperaldosteronism is a syndrome of hypertension typically associated with hypokalemia resulting from excessive renal potassium loss. The underlying cause in 60% of patients is a unilateral benign adrenocortical adenoma, and in most others bilateral adrenal cortical hyperplasia (idiopathic hyperaldosteronism). Rare causes are adrenocortical carcinoma and an autosomal dominant glucocorticoid-suppressible hyperaldosteronism.

Primary hyperaldosteronism is responsible for 1–2% of cases of hypertension. The hypertension is usually moderate, seldom severe. It is clinically indistinguishable from other forms of high blood pressure except when it begins at an early age. Potassium depletion, aggravated by diuretics, causes weakness, fatigue, and nocturia in some patients. Occasional patients also have polyuria, intermittent paresthesias, or cardiac arrhythmias. A rare patient presents with flaccid paralysis from severe hypokalemia.

Diagnosis: Primary hyperaldosteronism is established by proof of (1) high aldosterone production that cannot be suppressed and (2) low plasma renin activity that cannot be stimulated. Before these tests are done, potassium depletion must be corrected, because hypokalemia itself lowers plasma aldosterone and raises plasma renin activity, potentially obscuring the diagnosis.

One way to do the tests is to give the patient 80 mg of oral furosemide at 8:00 AM, and at noon measure plasma renin activity and aldosterone with the patient standing. Upright posture normally increases renin production. A suppressed baseline plasma renin (below 1 ng/mL/hr) that remains unstimulated by this volume-depleting maneuver is characteristic of primary hyperaldosteronism. Another method is to show high and autonomous aldosterone production despite extracellular fluid volume expansion. Patients with primary hyperaldosteronism who receive a 2 L infusion of saline over 4 hours still have a plasma aldosterone above 10 ng/dL. Alternatively, patients can be given 12 g of NaCl per day for 4 days. On the fourth day, a 24-hour urinary aldosterone is measured. Patients with hyperaldosteronism have urine aldosterone levels above 14 µg per 24 hours when the urinary sodium is at least 250 mEq/L.

Primary hyperaldosteronism caused by an adrenocortical adenoma is treated differently from that caused by bilateral adrenal hyperplasia, so the two conditions must be differentiated. Many adrenocortical adenomas respond to ACTH, producing a diurnal variation in aldosterone levels that parallels the circadian rhythm of cortisol. Although patients with bilateral adrenal hyperplasia may show the same diurnal changes when supine, they are more sensitive to angiotensin II stimulation, so their plasma aldosterone rises when they stand up. These changes are tested by having patients lie in bed overnight and drawing their blood at 8:00 AM, before they get up. Patients are active for the next 4 hours, and a second sample is drawn at noon. In patients with adrenal hyperplasia, the 8:00 AM plasma aldosterone is less than 20 ng/mL, but the postural change makes it rise sharply in the noon sample. In contrast, patients with adrenal adenomas typically have an 8:00 AM aldosterone above 20 ng/mL and a lower level at noon, reflecting the diurnal fall in ACTH secretion.

CT or MRI is the best initial procedure to localize an adrenal adenoma and further differentiate it from bilateral hyperplasia. Each method is 90% accurate. The most conclusive test is bilateral adrenal venous catheterization. Venous effluent from both adrenal glands and the inferior vena cava is collected and tested for aldosterone to see whether the overproduction is unilateral (adenoma) or bilateral (hyperplasia).

Management: The treatment of choice for aldosterone-secreting adrenocortical adenomas is surgical excision of the adenoma. Resection cures more than 70% of patients and improves the hypertension in 25% more. Preoperatively, patients can be treated with spironolactone to control blood pressure and reverse hypokalemia. This mineralocorticoid antagonist (1) restores the blood pressure to normal and predicts the patient's probable blood pressure and potassium response after surgery, (2) corrects volume expansion and potassium deficits, and (3) reactivates the chronically suppressed renin-angiotensin axis, thereby sparing most patients postoperative hypoaldosteronism and hyperkalemia.

Surgery is of little or no benefit for bilateral adrenal hyperplasia. High-dose spironolactone corrects the hypokalemia but often causes impotence and gynecomastia in men and menstrual dysfunction in women. Many patients need additional antihypertensive medications such as calcium channel blockers and amiloride.

Hyporeninemic Hypoaldosteronism

Hyporeninemic hypoaldosteronism is the most common cause of mineralocorticoid deficiency in adults, causing postural hypotension and hyperkalemia. The main feature is a chronically elevated serum potassium. The hyperkalemia can be worsened by reduced sodium intake and drugs like spironolactone and nonsteroidal anti-inflammatory agents. The hyperkalemia may also be worse in patients with diabetes mellitus, who can have decreased insulin-mediated potassium entry into cells. About 60% of patients have hyponatremia and a hyperchloremic acidosis with a normal anion gap.

The hypoaldosteronism seems to result from inadequate stimulation of the adrenal gland by the renin-angiotensin system. Basal plasma renin activity is low or borderline, and it rises subnormally in response to volume depletion or standing up. Plasma aldosterone is also usually low. It is poorly stimulated by exogenous infusions of ACTH and angiotensin II, probably because of prolonged hyporeninemia.

Most patients with hypoaldosteronism are over 50 years old and have a serum creatinine of 2–4 mg/dL. This mild renal insufficiency is most often caused by diabetes mellitus, but it is also seen with other tubulointerstitial renal conditions such as stones, chronic pyelonephritis, hypertensive nephrosclerosis, and damage by analgesic abuse. Despite patients' mineralocorticoid deficiency, many are hypertensive because of extracellular fluid volume expansion from their renal disease.

Fludrocortisone can correct the hyperkalemia and metabolic acidosis. This synthetic mineralocorticoid can be given with the loop diuretic, furosemide, which also promotes potassium and acid excretion. Mineralocorticoids may not be recommended for patients who have hypertension or diseases that cause extracellular fluid volume expansion; these patients can take furosemide alone.

PHEOCHROMOCYTOMA

Pheochromocytoma, a rare tumor arising from the adrenal medulla, is another of the few potentially curable forms of hypertension. The disorder is also important because unrestrained catecholamine release into the bloodstream can cause cardiomyopathy, myocardial infarction, stroke, and aortic dissection. Finally, a pheochromocytoma can be one manifestation of a genetic multisystem disorder for which patients and their families should be evaluated.

One in 1000 hypertensive persons has a pheochromocytoma. The tumor affects both sexes equally, with a peak incidence during the 20's and 30's. Most pheochromocytomas are sporadic, but about 10% are familial, developing alone or as part of the multiple endocrine neoplasia (MEN) syndromes. In MEN type IIa (also called II), pheochromocytoma is associated with medullary thyroid carcinoma and hyperparathyroidism; in MEN type IIb (also called III), pheochromocytoma is associated with medullary thyroid carcinoma, submucosal neuromas, and a marfanoid body habitus (Chapter 4.1). Familial disease has autosomal dominant inheritance. Pheochromocytoma is also seen with two other autosomal dominant diseases involving neuroectodermal tissues, von Hippel-Lindau disease and neurofibromatosis (von Recklinghausen's disease).

About 90% of pheochromocytomas develop within the adrenal glands, slightly more often on the right side than the left; familial disease is likely to be bilateral. The

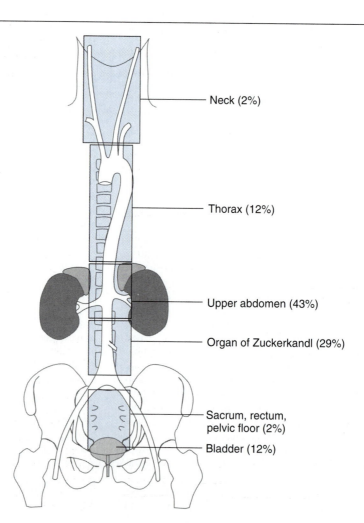

Neck (2%)

Thorax (12%)

Upper abdomen (43%)

Organ of Zuckerkandl (29%)

Sacrum, rectum, pelvic floor (2%)

Bladder (12%)

Figure 4.3–4. Locations of the 10% of pheochromocytomas found outside the adrenal glands. (Modified and reproduced, with permission, from Bergland RM, Gann DS, DeMaria EJ: Pituitary and adrenal. In: *Principles of Surgery,* 5th ed. Schwartz SI [editor]. McGraw-Hill, 1989.)

remaining 10% of patients have extra-adrenal pheochromocytomas, called *paragangliomas* (Figure 4.3–4). Typically, these tumors are found in the abdomen along the sympathetic chains or in the organs of Zuckerkandl (sympathetic tissue around the abdominal aorta, usually disappearing at birth). Pheochromocytomas occasionally develop in the wall of the urinary bladder and, very rarely, along the sympathetic chains in the thorax or elsewhere outside the abdomen.

Only 10% of pheochromocytomas are malignant.

Clinical Features

The symptoms of pheochromocytoma can be among the most dramatic in medicine. The classic paroxysm occurs when the tumor suddenly releases catecholamines, mainly norepinephrine. Attacks cause extremely high blood pressure, severe headache, palpitations, sweating, tremor, and pallor. Patients may have a feeling of dread or "impending doom." Less common paroxysmal symptoms are nausea and vomiting, chest pain, and paresthesias. In an occasional patient, coronary artery spasm causes angina pectoris or myocardial infarction. Atrial or ventricular arrhythmias are also reported. The rare patient with a predominantly epinephrine-secreting pheochromocytoma presents with paroxysmal hypotension from β-adrenergically mediated vasodilatation.

Paroxysms need have no obvious precipitants, although they can be triggered by exercise, straining, bending over, lying in certain positions, and emotional distress. Attacks can also be provoked by the stress of general anesthesia, surgery, or labor, and by drugs (eg, glucocorticoids, opiates, tricyclic antidepressants, radiocontrast dyes). Urination can trigger a paroxysm in a patient with a bladder tumor. A typical paroxysm lasts for 10–30 minutes and leaves the patient very tired. Attacks can occur from several times a day to once every few months. The differential diagnosis of such paroxysmal symptoms includes hypoglycemia, perimenopausal vasomotor instability (hot flushes), hyperthyroidism, and anxiety attacks.

At least 50% of patients with pheochromocytoma never experience a paroxysm. Instead, they have sustained hypertension with periods of further blood pressure elevation. The disease can present with subtle manifestations. For example, in an occasional patient, hypertension and "catecholamine cardiomyopathy" cause congestive heart failure. Paradoxically, many patients complain of orthostatic hypotension, probably because their increased peripheral vascular tone diminishes their circulating plasma volume. Hypermetabolism causes other symptoms such as heat intolerance, excessive sweating, weight loss despite good appetite, and severe constipation caused by diminished gut motility. High circulating catecholamine levels can produce insulin resistance, and 50% of patients have mild glucose intolerance. For unknown reasons, 20% of patients have cholelithiasis. Occasional patients with pheochromocytoma are normotensive and asymptomatic despite their high catecholamine levels; their disease may never be diagnosed.

Physical findings of pheochromocytoma are generally nonspecific. Most patients are hypertensive, and some have hypertensive retinal changes and cardiac findings. An abdominal mass can be palpated in 10% of patients. Café-au-lait spots and neurofibromas may be visible in patients with von Recklinghausen's disease. Thyroid nodules suggesting medullary thyroid carcinoma should be sought in patients suspected of having MEN IIa or IIb.

Diagnosis

Pheochromocytoma should be considered in all patients who get paroxysmal symptoms, especially if they also have sustained hypertension. Diabetes mellitus, hypermetabolic symptoms, and orthostatic hypotension should also raise suspicion. The biochemical diagnosis is made by finding elevated catecholamines or catecholamine metabolites in the urine or blood. Because many people have nonfunctional adrenal masses, imaging studies of the adrenal glands should be delayed until the diagnosis is confirmed biochemically.

The standard laboratory screening test for pheochromocytoma is measurement of the catecholamine metabolites vanillylmandelic acid or metanephrines in an acidified 24-hour urine collection. The tests' sensitivity and specificity exceed 90%, but results may be confounded by concurrent administration of β-adrenergic blocking drugs or radiocontrast dyes. Metanephrine measurement is the more sensitive and specific test, because foods and drugs interfere less with its levels. Catecholamine metabolites are more accurate than total catecholamines.

Plasma catecholamine levels are sometimes a useful adjunct to urinary metabolites. Levels are most helpful if measured during or just after a paroxysm. Because plasma catecholamine levels normally rise in response to pain, anxiety, or postural changes, the test must be done with the patient supine in a restful environment, and the blood samples must be collected through an indwelling catheter inserted at least 30 minutes before sampling. Patients who have only paroxysmal hypertension can get false-negatives.

When urine catecholamine values are equivocal or when drugs interfere with their measurement, a suppression or stimulation test may help. One suppression test uses the central α-adrenergic blocking agent clonidine, which inhibits catecholamine release from normal sympathetic nerve terminals but not from pheochromocytoma cells; in patients with pheochromocytoma, levels either fall only slightly or actually rise. Patients with a highly suggestive clinical syndrome and borderline basal catecholamine levels can be given a stimulation test with glucagon and pentagastrin. However, there is risk of inducing a hypertensive crisis.

When biochemical tests are positive, the next step is imaging studies to localize the tumor. CT and MRI are the procedures of choice. When the tumor cannot be found in the abdomen, scans must be taken of the chest, pelvis, and neck. Another helpful study can be scintigraphy with ^{131}I-labeled metaiodobenzylguanidine (MIBG), a catecholamine precursor that is taken up by chromaffin tissue.

Management

Before patients can have a pheochromocytoma resected, they must be given enough α-adrenergic blockade to prevent (1) catastrophic increases in blood pressure when they are anesthetized and the tumor is manipulated and (2) severe intraoperative hypotension. Most experts give the α-blocker phenoxybenzamine for 1–2 weeks before surgery, to permit adequate vasodilatation and reexpansion of the circulating blood volume. The phenoxybenzamine dose is gradually increased until patients are normotensive. The drug can cause severe orthostatic hypotension; if this happens, patients should also be given intravenous fluids. A β-adrenergic blocker is added to the α-blocker if patients have arrhythmias or the phenoxybenzamine causes reflex tachycardia. Patients with suspected pheochromocytoma should never be given a β-blocker until they have been treated with an α-blocker, because they would risk unopposed α-adrenergic stimulation of peripheral arterioles and worsened hypertension. The α-blocker prazosin and the combined α- and β-blocker labetalol have also been reported useful in preparing patients for surgery, but experience with these drugs is limited.

If oral α-adrenergic blockade has not yet controlled their hypertensive crises, patients should be given intravenous phentolamine. Phentolamine's short half-life makes it unsuitable for chronic use, but it can lower blood pressure quickly. Some patients need a constant infusion of phentolamine or nitroprusside until phenoxybenzamine or other chronic oral therapy has taken effect.

After a pheochromocytoma is localized and the patient is prepared with α-adrenergic blockade, the definitive treatment is surgical resection. In spite of seemingly adequate α-adrenergic blockade, during surgery patients may have marked blood pressure lability and cardiac arrhythmias; they must be monitored by an experienced anesthesiologist. Postoperatively, they may be hypotensive because of blood loss, insensitivity of adrenergic reflexes, and the lingering effects of long-acting α-adrenergic-blocking drugs. Thus, their fluids must be managed carefully. Unfortunately, about 25% of patients remain hypertensive after surgery, presumably because of essential hypertension or acquired renovascular hypertension.

The prognosis for patients with a successfully resected pheochromocytoma is excellent. The 5-year survival rate is greater than 90%. Patients should have their catecholamine metabolites tested every year for several years to detect late recurrences. Patients with familial or genetic syndromes need to be followed up indefinitely because they are at risk for more tumors.

Ten percent of pheochromocytomas are malignant. Metastases typically develop in lymph nodes, lungs, liver, and bone. If at all possible, malignant pheochromocytomas should be resected. Patients with inoperable tumors have been given chemotherapy for palliation. Most patients' symptoms can be controlled with α- and β-blockers. If necessary, blood pressure can usually be further regulated with α-methylparatyrosine, an inhibitor of catecholamine synthesis.

SUMMARY

▶ The most specific clinical features of Cushing's syndrome are muscle weakness, pigmented striae, and centripetal obesity. These signs warrant screening for hypercortisolism with either a 24-hour urine free cortisol or overnight dexamethasone suppression test.

▶ The three endogenous causes of Cushing's syndrome—adrenocortical tumors, ACTH-secreting pituitary adenomas, and ectopic ACTH production by nonpituitary tumors—can be distinguished by a combination of dexamethasone suppressibility, plasma ACTH concentration, and imaging.

▶ Adrenal insufficiency may present as a subtle syndrome of constitutional symptoms or as an acute illness with hypotension, fever, vomiting, and abdominal pain.

▶ Primary hyperaldosteronism, a rare but potentially reversible cause of hypertension, should be suggested by unprovoked hypokalemia. Adrenal adenomas should be distinguished from bilateral adrenal cortical hyperplasia by hormonal and radiographic testing to define the most appropriate treatment.

▶ Pheochromocytoma, a catecholamine-secreting tumor causing hypertension, should be considered in patients with labile high blood pressure and in young people with severe or uncontrolled hypertension.

SUGGESTED READING

Belldegrun A et al: Incidentally discovered mass of the adrenal gland. Surg Gynecol Obstet 1986;163:203.

Carpenter PC: Diagnostic evaluation of Cushing's syndrome. Endocrinol Metab Clin North Am 1988;17:445.

Gifford RW Jr, Manger WM, Bravo EL: Pheochromocytoma. Endocrinol Metab Clin North Am 1994;23:387.

Kailasam MT, O'Connor DT, Parmer RJ: The regulation and role of catecholamines in hypertension and pheochromocytoma. Curr Opin Endocrinol Diabetes 1994;135.

Young WF Jr et al: Primary aldosteronism: Diagnosis and treatment. Mayo Clin Proc 1990;65:96.

4.4

Thyroid Disorders

Paul W. Ladenson, MD

In virtually every clinic session or course of hospital rounds, one or more patients have complaints or physical findings potentially attributable to thyroid disease. Many symptoms and signs of thyroid dysfunction are nonspecific (eg, fatigue and weight change), but laboratory tests can readily distinguish thyroid dysfunction from other conditions. Because thyroid hormones have ubiquitous and tightly regulated tissue actions, any thyroid disorder that alters the gland's function can produce widespread clinical havoc. In addition to the morbidity and even the lethal potential of thyrotoxicosis and hypothyroidism, both can exacerbate other diseases, particularly diseases affecting the cardiovascular system.

Goiter and discrete thyroid masses (nodules) are relatively common, especially in women. Patients with these neoplastic thyroid disorders can present with local obstructive or cosmetic complaints, evidence of associated gland dysfunction, or, in the case of thyroid malignancies, local invasive and distant metastatic complications. Ability to recognize the clinical features and apply the proper biopsy and imaging techniques allows the physician to differentiate benign from malignant lesions.

The most gratifying aspect of diagnosing thyroid disorders is that they are eminently treatable, and the misery they cause patients can almost always be reversed.

THYROTOXICOSIS

Thyrotoxicosis is the metabolic and widespread organ system manifestation of elevated thyroid hormone concentrations. In most patients, thyrotoxicosis is caused by accelerated hormone production by the thyroid gland (hyperthyroidism), as in Graves' disease and toxic nodular goiter; other causes are hormone leakage from an injured thyroid gland and consumption of exogenous thyroid hormone. The term "hyperthyroidism" is most properly reserved for conditions in which hormone synthesis and release by the thyroid gland are abnormally increased, but hyperthyroidism is often used interchangeably with thyrotoxicosis to refer to any condition with thyroid hormone excess.

Clinical Manifestations of Thyrotoxicosis

Thyrotoxic patients can present with pathognomonic symptoms and signs, or they can present with relatively isolated clinical problems affecting a single organ system or with atypical manifestations of thyroid hormone excess. Older patients and those with other diseases are especially likely to develop focused and atypical pictures. Each pattern is discussed below.

Many of the typical symptoms and signs of thyrotoxicosis can be thought of as either being caused by hypermetabolism or mimicking excessive sympathetic nervous system activity (Table 4.4–1). Common clinical features related to increased calorigenesis include heat intolerance, increased sweating, weight loss despite an increased appetite, dyspnea with exertion, insomnia, and hyperactivity despite exhaustion. The patient often feels that "my motor is running too fast." Sympathomimetic clinical features include palpitations (rapid, hard, or irregular heartbeats), tremor, and anxiety. Other common clinical manifestations are chest pain that is precordial, sharp, and ephemeral; hyperdefecation and frequent urination; and muscle weakness, most prominently in the thighs. Many women have oligomenorrhea or amenorrhea, which can cause infertility. Men may develop gynecomastia (from higher circulating estrogen concentrations) and impotence.

In occasional thyrotoxic patients, the clinical picture is dominated by involvement of one organ system. Often this organ's vulnerability to thyrotoxicosis results from some other intrinsic disease. Examples of such focused involvement are atrial arrhythmias, especially atrial fibrillation, sometimes with heart failure; prolonged nausea and recurrent vomiting; psychosis; and several forms of myopathy. In addition to the common proximal skeletal myopathy, muscle involvement may take the form of periodic paralysis, especially in Oriental men; bulbar myopathy in

Table 4.4–1. Important manifestations of thyrotoxicosis.

Organ System	Symptoms	Signs
Constitutional	Fatigue, increased appetite, insomnia, hyperactivity	Weight loss
Cardiovascular	Palpitations, chest pain	Tachycardia, atrial arrhythmias, systolic hypertension
Pulmonary	Dyspnea	
Gastrointestinal	Hyperdefecation, abdominal pain	Borborygmi
Genitourinary	Frequent urination, decreased libido, amenorrhea, or impotence	Gynecomastia
Musculoskeletal	Proximal muscle weakness	Osteopenia
Neuropsychiatric	Tremor, anxiety, depression	Delirium, psychosis
Dermatologic	Increased sweating and oiliness, pruritus	Velvety moist skin, urticaria, acne

older men; or myasthenia gravis, which can be associated with Graves' disease. Because it increases bone resorption, thyroid hormone may cause osteoporosis even when thyroid hormone excess is mild and the patient has no other manifestations of thyrotoxicosis. In most patients with one of these focused presentations, careful evaluation reveals other subtle clinical evidence of thyrotoxicosis.

A minority of thyrotoxic patients have atypical presentations that can lead to misdiagnosis. The best known of these syndromes is apathetic thyrotoxicosis, in which patients lack the characteristic sympathomimetic features of thyroid hormone excess but present with weight loss (often with paradoxical anorexia), myopathy, and an apathetic demeanor. Apathetic thyrotoxicosis is seen most often in elderly persons and patients taking β-adrenergic blocking drugs. Other unusual presentations of thyrotoxicosis include abdominal pain; pruritus, sometimes with urticaria; and lymphadenopathy, splenomegaly, or thymic enlargement, which are seen only in patients with Graves' disease.

Causes of Thyrotoxicosis

Graves' Disease (Diffuse Toxic Goiter): Named for a British physician who was among the first to describe it, Graves' disease causes 90% of cases of thyrotoxicosis. Hyperthyroidism with diffuse gland enlargement is only one aspect of this ailment. Many patients also have a characteristic form of orbital and ocular inflammation (Graves' orbitopathy or ophthalmopathy), and rare patients have a distinctive dermopathy (pretibial myxedema) or acropachy (clubbing).

Graves' disease is an autoimmune disorder in which the body produces immunoglobulins that bind thyroid-stimulating hormone (TSH) receptors and mimic the actions of TSH. Like TSH-mediated gland stimulation, thyroid-stimulating immunoglobulins cause hypertrophy of the gland and increase production of both triiodothyronine (T_3) and thyroxine (T_4).

There is convincing evidence of a genetic predisposition to Graves' disease. First, Graves' disease is particularly common in families with autoimmune thyroid diseases, certain other autoimmune disorders (eg, vitiligo, perni-

cious anemia, myasthenia gravis), and other endocrine diseases in which autoimmunity has been implicated (eg, type I diabetes mellitus, idiopathic adrenal insufficiency). Second, in some populations, Graves' disease has been linked to specific HLA-DR haplotypes. However, it is not known what induces persons with a genetic propensity to produce thyroid autoantibodies. Possibilities include a bacterial infection triggering expression of antibodies that cross-react with the TSH receptor, cigarette smoking, postpartum enhancement of immunosurveillance, and stressful life events, but none of these has been definitively established as the trigger for Graves' disease.

Once started, Graves' disease does not usually resolve on its own; the gradual progression of hyperthyroidism over weeks or months leads to increasingly obvious and severe manifestations of thyrotoxicosis. But the condition does remit spontaneously after several months in 25% of patients, typically persons with a small goiter, mild hyperthyroidism, and no significant orbitopathy.

Other features of Graves' disease: Only 5% of patients with Graves' disease have clinically severe eye involvement. However, sensitive imaging techniques like orbital magnetic resonance reveal subtle extraocular muscle swelling in more than 90% of patients. Graves' orbitopathy generally begins within 1 year after the onset of hyperthyroidism. Rare patients develop orbitopathy with autoimmune thyroiditis (see "Causes of Hypothyroidism" below) or with no apparent thyroid dysfunction, so-called euthyroid Graves' disease.

The proximate cause of Graves' orbitopathy is inflammation of extraocular muscles and orbital fat, a process that is also believed to be autoimmune. It has been postulated that a common antigen is expressed by both extraocular muscle cells and thyrocytes. Lymphocytic infiltration, adipocyte hypertrophy, and edema all conspire to increase the volume of soft tissue in the orbit, a bony cone with only one direction in which pressure can be released. The results are protrusion of the eyes, termed *proptosis* or *exophthalmos* (Figure 4.4–1); increased orbital venous pressure and periorbital edema; and, in the most severe cases, optic nerve compression that can cause visual disturbances ranging from subtly altered color vision to blindness. Eyelid retraction, another aspect of Graves' eye

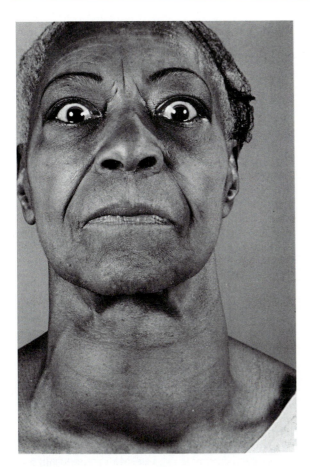

Figure 4.4–1. A 73-year-old woman with hyperthyroid Graves' disease, manifesting signs of goiter, thyrotoxicosis, and ophthalmopathy. (Courtesy of Pablo E. Dibos MD, Franklin Square Hospital Department of Medical Communications.)

disease, is caused by increased muscle tone and fibrosis of the levator palpebrae muscle. An associated sign of thyrotoxic eye involvement is lid lag: The upper lid fails to cover the superior limbal margin continually during vertically descending gaze. The combination of proptosis and lid retraction can lead to exposure keratitis, with symptoms of eye dryness, irritation, redness, and photophobia. A less common complication is corneal ulceration.

Mild to moderate Graves' eye disease is treated by minimizing exposure keratitis with artificial tears and, when necessary, taping the eyelids closed at night. When severe orbitopathy causes diplopia, decreased visual acuity, or cosmetically distressing proptosis, patients can be managed with eyelid or orbital decompression surgery, orbital radiation, or systemic glucocorticoid therapy.

Pretibial myxedema, the characteristic dermopathy of Graves' disease, is an orange peel-like thickening of the skin, usually in the pretibial region. The condition affects less than 1% of patients with Graves' disease. The pathogenesis remains mysterious. Biopsy of early lesions re-

veals a lymphocytic infiltrate; later lesions show mucopolysaccharide deposition. When needed, topical glucocorticoids are moderately effective.

Other Causes of Thyrotoxicosis: Other disorders causing thyrotoxicosis can produce the same symptoms and signs of thyroid hormone excess as Graves' disease, but without its eye and skin manifestations and associated autoimmune disorders. The most common disorders are toxic nodular goiter, the subacute and postpartum forms of thyroiditis, and an excessive dose of thyroid medication.

Toxic nodular goiter: Thyrotoxicosis can develop when either a single thyroid adenoma (toxic adenoma) or several such benign tumors (toxic multinodular goiter) function autonomously, that is, without regard to TSH regulation. When the mass of independently operating thyroid tissue becomes sufficiently large and active, excessive hormone production causes thyrotoxicosis.

Toxic nodular goiter is most common in middle-aged and older persons. Predisposing factors include previous dietary iodine deficiency and neck irradiation in childhood. A high percentage of these tumors have molecular defects in the TSH receptor, leading it to be constitutively activated. Exposure to pharmacologic doses of iodine can provoke thyrotoxicosis in previously euthyroid patients who have autonomously functioning thyroid neoplasms.

Thyroiditis: Acute injury to the thyroid gland can cause uncontrolled leakage of thyroid hormones and a reversible form of thyrotoxicosis that resolves when hormone stores are exhausted. Such thyroiditis can be the result of infection, autoimmunity, or drug toxicity.

Subacute (de Quervain's) thyroiditis is believed to be caused by viral infection, although no pathogen has been established. The clinical syndrome has three components. (1) Many patients have premonitory symptoms suggesting a viral upper respiratory infection, followed by constitutional complaints of fever, chills, malaise, and fatigue. In some patients, these features are severe enough to prompt consideration of serious underlying infection or malignancy. (2) Patients have a characteristic pattern of thyroid dysfunction: transient hyperthyroidism lasting 2–8 weeks, followed by several weeks of hypothyroidism and then a return to normal (Figure 4.4–2). The hypothyroidism develops because the thyroid gland's hormone stores are depleted, TSH has been suppressed by preceding thyrotoxicosis, and the thyroid gland's hormone synthetic capacity has not yet recovered. (3) Most patients have severe thyroid pain, which can radiate to the ears or jaw. The thyroid gland is exquisitely tender, "woody" hard, and moderately enlarged.

Another form of thyroiditis, this one painless, has been called "painless," "silent," or "postpartum" thyroiditis. It mainly afflicts women during the postpartum period and affects 6% of postpartum women. This disorder typically begins 2–8 months after delivery, a time when symptoms of thyroid dysfunction can easily be confused with those common in euthyroid new mothers. In one-third of patients, the pattern of thyroid dysfunction is triphasic—hy-

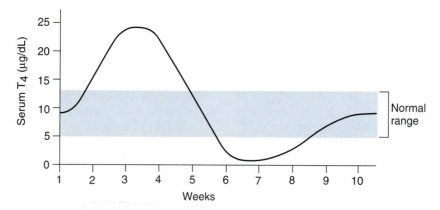

Figure 4.4–2. Characteristic pattern of thyroid dysfunction in subacute thyroiditis and postpartum thyroiditis. Patients with postpartum thyroiditis may have only the hyperthyroid or hypothyroid phase.

perthyroidism followed by hypothyroidism and eventual recovery (see Figure 4.4–2). One-third of patients have only a hyperthyroid phase, and one-third have only a hypothyroid phase. The thyroid gland is nontender and modestly if at all enlarged. Indirect evidence of an autoimmune basis for the disorder includes a lymphocytic glandular infiltrate, associations with preceding Graves' disease and later autoimmune thyroiditis, and the disorder's expression during a postpartum resurgence of immunosurveillance. Subacute thyroiditis can be mimicked by suppurative infections of the thyroid such as *Pneumocystis carinii* infections in immunocompromised patients or by contiguous oropharyngeal spread of streptococcal infections. However, these other disorders cause more severe systemic and local signs of inflammation.

Drug-induced thyrotoxicosis: A common cause of thyrotoxicosis is thyroid hormone preparations taken in excess, whether prescribed by physicians or taken independently by patients—sometimes surreptitiously for weight loss. Hyperthyroidism can also develop when patients receive pharmacologic doses of iodine, amounts 10–1000 times the typical dietary iodine intake, in drugs (eg, amiodarone, certain expectorants) and radiocontrast dyes. Iodine-induced hyperthyroidism is most common in patients with nodular goiters. Amiodarone can also cause a destructive form of thyroiditis with transient thyrotoxicosis.

Rare causes of hyperthyroidism: Excessive TSH production causes hyperthyroidism in two rare disorders, which should be suspected whenever the TSH is not suppressed in a thyrotoxic patient. TSH-secreting pituitary adenomas predictably cause diffuse thyroid gland enlargement and hyperfunction (Chapter 4.2). Isolated pituitary resistance to thyroid hormone is an exceedingly rare familial disorder in which thyrotropic cells are resistant to negative feedback by thyroid hormone, and TSH and thyroid hormone are inappropriately hypersecreted.

Thyrotoxicosis develops in rare women with choriocarcinoma or molar pregnancies, both of which produce human chorionic gonadotropin (hCG), a glycoprotein hor-

mone structurally similar to TSH. The extremely high circulating hCG concentrations in these disorders stimulate TSH receptors and cause hyperthyroidism; variant hCG forms produced by these tumors may also have increased TSH receptor binding activity. Ectopic thyroid tissue can overproduce thyroid hormone itself in women with struma ovarii (a teratoid ovarian tumor) and in rare patients with widespread metastases from follicular thyroid carcinoma.

Laboratory Diagnosis of Thyrotoxicosis

Laboratory tests must always be used to confirm thyrotoxicosis and determine its cause. Most patients with overt thyrotoxicosis have increases in the total and free (unbound) concentrations of both thyroid hormones, T_4 and T_3 (Table 4.4–2). Some thyrotoxic patients have isolated T_3 or T_4 elevations. It is important to remember that high serum total thyroid hormone concentrations can also be caused by factors that increase the thyroxine binding globulin level (eg, pregnancy, estrogen therapy, hepatitis) and by inherited albumin and transthyretin variants that bind circulating thyroxine with unusually high affinity. Therefore, the physician must determine free thyroid hormone concentrations, either by free T_4 immunoassay or indirect T_3 uptake estimates, or by direct equilibrium dialysis measurements.

Since most forms of thyrotoxicosis are accompanied by suppression of pituitary TSH secretion, a low serum TSH concentration is another way of confirming the diagnosis. TSH suppression is the most sensitive laboratory indicator of thyroid hormone excess. The TSH can even be suppressed in patients without overt thyrotoxicosis who have serum T_4 and T_3 concentrations in the high-normal range, a condition termed "subclinical hyperthyroidism." However, a low serum TSH level alone is not pathognomonic for thyrotoxicosis. Other causes are hypothalamic and pituitary diseases, severe nonthyroidal illnesses, and medications such as dopamine, glucocorticoids, and phenytoin.

Other tests and radionuclide studies can define the etiology of thyrotoxicosis when the cause is not clinically

Table 4.4–2. Laboratory features of primary thyroid dysfunction.

Test	Thyrotoxicosis	Hypothyroidism
Thyroid function tests		
Thyrotropin (TSH)	↓	↑
Total thyroxine (T_4)	↑	↓
T_3 uptake	↑	↓
Free T_4	↑	↓
Total and free T_3	↑	↓
Routine tests*		
Hemoglobin	–	↓ (1/3)
Total and LDL cholesterol	↓ (1/3)	↑ (1/3)
Calcium	↑ (1/4)	–
Sodium	–	↓ (1/50)
Prolactin	–	↑ (1/100)

*Approximate incidences of abnormalities are shown in parentheses.

obvious. Circulating thyroid-stimulating and TSH receptor binding immunoglobulins can be detected in most patients with Graves' disease, although the disorder's clinical features usually suffice for diagnosis. The erythrocyte sedimentation rate is markedly elevated in subacute thyroiditis. The pattern and amount of radioactive iodine or technetium pertechnetate isotope uptake by the thyroid gland can also help in the differential diagnosis. The diffuse pattern of tracer uptake in Graves' disease can be diagnostic, as can the focal pattern in toxic nodular goiter; in both disorders, the thyroid takes up large amounts of tracer. In contrast, with thyrotoxicosis caused by thyroiditis or exogenous thyroid hormone, the thyroid gland takes up very little tracer.

Occasionally, thyrotoxicosis is first suspected because of a routine laboratory test abnormality (see Table 4.4–2). A low or declining serum cholesterol concentration is typical. A minority of thyrotoxic patients have hypercalcemia or an elevated serum alkaline phosphatase concentration.

Management of Thyrotoxicosis

Management of thyrotoxic patients entails controlling their symptoms and organ system complications (eg, atrial fibrillation) and reversing hyperthyroidism by decreasing the thyroid gland's overproduction of hormones.

Controlling Symptoms and Complications: β-Adrenergic antagonists are the drugs of choice for managing certain symptoms of thyrotoxicosis and controlling tachyarrhythmias in thyrotoxic patients. Some complaints (eg, tremor, palpitations) improve promptly; others (eg, fatigue, muscle weakness) are relatively unaffected by β-blockers. For patients with spontaneously reversible (eg, postpartum thyroiditis) or drug-induced forms of thyrotoxicosis, β-blockers are the only therapy needed. Patients with thyrotoxic atrial fibrillation may also require digoxin to control ventricular rate and anticoagulation to prevent thromboembolism. Severely ill thyrotoxic patients may

need antipyretics, fluid and electrolyte replacement, and sedatives. It is important for physicians to reassure thyrotoxic patients that their illness is reversible.

Controlling Hyperthyroidism:

Antithyroid drugs: The thionamide compounds methimazole and propylthiouracil (PTU) competitively inhibit two steps essential for thyroid hormone biosynthesis: iodination and coupling of tyrosines in thyroglobulin. Thus, these drugs are useful in controlling conditions with endogenous overproduction of thyroid hormones. Patients should be warned that it may take weeks to start feeling better because these agents do not affect previously synthesized hormone in the gland.

Antithyroid drugs are most often used for temporary control of hyperthyroidism when there is a chance that the underlying condition will remit, as with Graves' disease or iodine-induced hyperthyroidism. Methimazole's longer half-life makes it preferable for most patients. But PTU has some advantages, for example, in pregnant patients, because it does not cross the placenta as well as methimazole, and in those with severe hyperthyroidism, because it also blocks T_4-to-T_3 conversion. Both thionamide compounds occasionally induce hypersensitivity reactions; rarely, both cause reversible agranulocytosis.

Other drugs can be useful to patients with severe hyperthyroidism. Both iodine in milligram amounts and lithium can block release of hormones from the thyroid gland and are indicated as a component of managing patients with severe, complicated hyperthyroidism. Several agents, including β-blockers, glucocorticoids, and sodium ipodate, inhibit extrathyroidal conversion of T_4 to the more metabolically active T_3.

Ablative treatments: Radioactive iodine and surgery: When iodine-131 is concentrated by and irradiates thyroid cells, it permanently reverses hyperthyroidism. Radioactive iodine is an effective, convenient, and relatively inexpensive form of therapy. Its principal side effect is hypothyroidism, which ultimately develops in most patients. No increased risk of malignancy or teratogenicity has been established after radioactive iodine treatment of hyperthyroidism. In thyrotoxic patients who are older or have other cardiopulmonary disease, preliminary antithyroid drug therapy is usually prudent.

Another effective treatment for Graves' disease and toxic nodular goiter is surgical thyroidectomy. However, its inconvenience, discomfort, scar, risk of complications (eg, hypoparathyroidism, recurrent laryngeal nerve injury), and cost all limit its use. Currently, surgery for hyperthyroidism is indicated for only two groups of patients: (1) those who may have thyroid malignancy or a locally obstructive nodular goiter and (2) thyrotoxic pregnant women who have had a severe antithyroid drug side effect, since radioactive iodine can never be given during pregnancy. All thyrotoxic patients must be prepared for thyroidectomy and other surgical procedures with β-blockers and antithyroid drugs.

HYPOTHYROIDISM

Clinical Manifestations of Hypothyroidism

Several factors make clinical diagnosis of patients with hypothyroidism challenging. First, their most common symptoms and signs are nonspecific (eg, fatigue, constipation, depression, weight gain) and are often attributed to other diseases, aging, or life stresses. Second, clinical manifestations of hypothyroidism usually begin and progress gradually. Third, clinical expression of the disorder is highly variable, depending on both the individual patient's organ system vulnerabilities and the severity of thyroid hormone deficiency. The spectrum can range from subclinical thyroid dysfunction, detectable only by laboratory testing, to the striking syndrome of myxedema caused by chronic severe hypothyroidism. Finally, certain neuropsychiatric manifestations of the disorder—impaired mentation and lethargy—can interfere with patients' insight and initiative to seek medical care.

Clinical manifestations of hypothyroidism are caused by hypometabolism and by lack of thyroid hormone actions in particular organ systems. Problems attributable to metabolic slowing include weight gain despite decreased appetite, cold intolerance, and reduced sweating. Important manifestations attributable to specific systemic effects are listed in Table 4.4–3.

Cardiovascular consequences include decreased heart rate and contractility, potentially causing heart failure; peripheral vasoconstriction, leading to diastolic hypertension; and increased interstitial fluid albumin, causing tissue edema and serous effusions in the pericardial, pleural, and abdominal spaces. Ventilatory muscle strength and responsiveness to hypercapnia and hypoxia are reduced; patients may develop sleep apnea. Slowed gastrointestinal motility often causes constipation and in rare patients leads to ileus. Many premenopausal women with hypothyroidism develop menorrhagia; some present with amenorrhea. Some women have hyperprolactinemia and galactorrhea. The neuropsychiatric manifestations of hypothyroidism range from subtle changes like slowed mentation and impaired memory to severe derangements like dementia and coma, which can be confused with primary central nervous system diseases. Emotional changes in affected patients can include depression, irritability, and psychosis, which has been termed myxedema madness.

Causes of Hypothyroidism

In more than 99% of patients, hypothyroidism is primary to the gland and results from one of two insults: (1) autoimmune thyroiditis or previous gland damage from surgery or (2) radiation therapy. Autoimmune thyroiditis (also called chronic lymphocytic thyroiditis or Hashimoto's thyroiditis) is caused by immunologic gland injury, which, although principally cell-mediated, is accompanied by circulating antithyroid antibodies that are diagnostically useful (see "Laboratory Diagnosis of Hypothyroidism" below). This condition is most common in women, increases in frequency with age, runs in families, and is associated with increased risk for other autoimmune disorders such as pernicious anemia, vitiligo, and rheumatoid arthritis. In a minority of patients, autoimmune thyroiditis is associated with other endocrine deficiency states (Chapter 4.1). The specific factors that contribute to a genetic predisposition and those that trigger disease remain unknown. Patients can have a spectrum of thyroid function ranging from euthyroidism to myxedema, and considerable variability in gland size from no palpable thyroid tissue to substantial goiter.

Postablative hypothyroidism is common after surgical treatment of thyroid disease, radioactive iodine therapy of hyperthyroidism, and external-beam irradiation of the thyroid, as is given to treat Hodgkin's disease and neck tumors. Thyroid dysfunction can develop weeks to decades after gland injury.

All other forms of hypothyroidism are rare. Central (secondary) hypothyroidism is thyroid gland failure caused by pituitary or hypothalamic diseases (Chapter 4.2). Certain drugs (eg, interferon-α, aminoglutethimide) and occupational toxins (eg, polybrominated biphenyls) can cause reversible thyroid failure. Congenital defects in organogenesis and biosynthetic enzymes, detected in

Table 4.4–3. Important manifestations of hypothyroidism.

Organ System	Symptoms	Signs
Constitutional	Fatigue, lethargy, decreased appetite	Weight gain
Cardiovascular	Soft tissue swelling	Bradycardia, diastolic hypertension, soft heart sounds, edema
Pulmonary	Snoring	Sleep apnea, hypoventilation
Gastrointestinal	Constipation, abdominal distention	Ileus
Genitourinary	Menorrhagia or amenorrhea	Galactorrhea
Musculoskeletal	Muscle stiffness, cramps	Weakness
Neuropsychiatric	Slowed mentation, memory impairment, anxiety, depression	Hyporeflexia, ataxia, dementia, psychosis, coma
Otolaryngological	Hoarseness, decreased hearing	Middle ear effusion
Dermatologic	Dryness	Swelling, pallor, yellow hue

childhood, require lifelong hormone replacement. Severe dietary iodine deficiency (see "Goiter" below) can cause cretinism, the consequence of untreated fetal and neonatal hypothyroidism. Tissue resistance to thyroid hormone is a rare familial disorder in which people who are clinically either hypothyroid or euthyroid have a variety of mutations in the β_1-isoform of the nuclear T_3 receptor, associated with elevations of circulating thyroid hormones, with an inappropriately high or normal serum TSH level.

Laboratory Diagnosis of Hypothyroidism

Hypothyroidism can be readily confirmed or excluded in the laboratory, and physicians should have a low threshold for pursuing the diagnosis, especially in women. The most sensitive laboratory measure is the serum TSH concentration, which is elevated in patients with primary hypothyroidism. Patients with overt hypothyroidism have low total and free T_4 levels; however, the serum T_3 often remains within the normal range. Persons with the mildest thyroid underactivity, in whom the serum TSH is high despite a low-normal serum free T_4, are said to have subclinical hypothyroidism, even though some may have symptoms that can actually be relieved by thyroid hormone therapy.

Autoimmune thyroiditis can be confirmed by screening the patient's serum for antithyroid peroxidase (formerly called antimicrosomal) and antithyroglobulin antibodies. Most patients with central hypothyroidism have a low or normal serum TSH and a low free T_4. The apparent paradox of a normal TSH level in these patients is explained by the fact that their TSH has decreased biologic activity because of impaired post-translational glycosylation.

Serum thyroid function tests in patients with nonthyroidal systemic illness often mimic the laboratory features of hypothyroidism. The serum total and free T_4 concentrations are low in about 25% of all hospitalized persons, individuals who have no previous history or later proof of thyroid dysfunction. Hypothyroxinemia in this "euthyroid sick syndrome" has been attributed to derangement of T_4 binding to plasma proteins, accelerated thyroid hormone disposal, and cytokine-mediated suppression of pituitary TSH production. A normal serum TSH in patients with systemic illness strongly suggests that their low serum T_4 is not caused by thyroid dysfunction. Patients with other clinical features of central hypothyroidism must have this possibility excluded, usually by pituitary imaging.

Management of Hypothyroidism

Management of hypothyroid patients entails hormone replacement and, occasionally, temporary support for major clinical problems caused by thyroid hormone deficiency. Synthetic thyroxine is the treatment of choice; its convenient 7-day half-life and deiodinative conversion to T_3 in the body restore physiologic thyroid hormone levels in blood and target tissues. Patients need to take a given dosage for 4–6 weeks to reach a steady state and feel the full clinical effects. Since patients' symptoms can be non-

specific, adequacy of treatment is best confirmed by serum TSH measurement.

Potential complications of thyroxine therapy are iatrogenic hyperthyroidism with overtreatment, and certain infrequent problems related to the restoration of euthyroidism. In patients with underlying coronary artery disease, the positive chronotropic and inotropic effects of thyroid hormone can provoke myocardial ischemia. Therefore, the physician should start patients with known or suspected ischemic heart disease on very low thyroxine doses and then increase the dose slightly each month until the patient is euthyroid. In patients with associated adrenal cortical insufficiency, thyroid hormone replacement may accelerate disposal of the residual cortisol still being produced. Hypothyroid patients should be suspected of having adrenal dysfunction in two settings: secondary adrenal insufficiency associated with central hypothyroidism and autoimmune adrenal failure accompanying autoimmune thyroiditis.

The major organ system complications of profound longstanding thyroid hormone deficiency can be life-threatening. The risk is highest in older persons and perioperatively. Myxedematous patients in these categories may require special hemodynamic and ventilatory monitoring and support. Their recovery may be complicated by hypothermia, infection (sometimes occult if it does not cause fever), ileus, drug toxicity caused by slowed clearance, anemia, hyponatremia, and coagulopathy.

THYROID NEOPLASIA

Diffuse or focal enlargement of the thyroid gland is one of the most common endocrine problems in clinical practice. When approaching patients with goiters and thyroid nodules, physicians should ask three questions: (1) Is there malignancy? (2) Does the patient have thyroid dysfunction—thyrotoxicosis or hypothyroidism? (3) Is there significant compression or invasion of adjacent neck structures?

Goiter

Generalized enlargement of the thyroid gland may be the result of inflammation, benign hyperplasia or neoplasia, or malignancy. In autoimmune thyroiditis, a common cause of diffuse goiter, thyromegaly is attributable to infiltration of the gland by lymphocytes and, in the case of a hypofunctioning gland, to TSH stimulation of gland growth. Similarly, in Graves' disease, diffuse goiter is caused by a lymphocytic infiltrate and the TSH-like activity of thyroid-stimulating immunoglobulins. These two conditions illustrate that goiter alone does not define any particular thyroid state.

Goiter may be caused by dietary iodine deficiency. Iodine deficiency is no longer a problem for people in North America or Europe, but it still affects 100 million people around the world, primarily in mountainous or desert regions of underdeveloped countries. Even if pregnant women have only borderline dietary iodine deficiency, their accelerated iodine clearance makes them particularly susceptible to goiter. Inherited defects in the enzymes responsible for thyroid hormone biosynthesis predictably lead to thyroid enlargement that begins in childhood. It has been postulated that goitrogenic substances in food or water, such as resorcinol from Appalachian coal mine tailings, may contribute to thyroid gland enlargement in some populations. Long-term overtreatment with antithyroid drugs can also cause goiter.

In most North American patients, the cause of goiter is unknown. The clinical spectrum of idiopathic thyromegaly ranges from modest, diffuse enlargement (simple goiter) to huge multinodular goiters. Local symptoms may include dysphagia and cough. When goiters extend downward into the thoracic outlet or the substernal space, significant airway obstruction can cause dyspnea; less often, compression of jugular veins or the superior vena cava can cause cervical venous distention and facial edema. A substernal goiter's uptake of radioactive iodine can distinguish it from other anterior mediastinal masses like thymoma, teratoma, and lymphoma. Most patients with nodular goiters are euthyroid, but a small subset have associated hyperthyroidism (see "Toxic Nodular Goiter" above).

Most thyroid malignancies present as discrete nodules, but thyroidal lymphoma and anaplastic, papillary, and medullary cancers can be diffusely infiltrating. Thus, patients with a rapidly enlarging goiter or associated local symptoms suggesting tissue invasion (eg, pain, hoarseness, hemoptysis) should be further evaluated, just like patients with a thyroid nodule (see following section).

Thyroid Nodules

Thyroid nodules are palpable in about 6% of all women and 1% of all men; smaller lesions can be seen by sonography in as many as one-third of women. However, only 5% of palpable thyroid nodules are malignant. Although most thyroid cancers can be effectively treated when diagnosed at an early stage, the morbidity and cost of surgery cannot be justified for all patients. By analyzing clinical evidence, the serum TSH concentration, and fine-needle aspiration cytologic findings, the physician can render surgery unnecessary for most patients and increase the probability of resecting nodules that are thyroid cancers (Figure 4.4–3).

The clinician should first seek symptoms and signs suggesting malignancy: a pattern of growth over weeks or months; pain, hoarseness, hemoptysis, and other local symptoms consistent with tissue invasion; complaints suggesting metastatic disease (eg, cervical lymph node enlargement or bone pain); and a history indicating high thyroid cancer risk (eg, childhood neck irradiation, a family history suggesting features of the multiple endocrine neoplasia II [MEN II] syndrome [Chapter 4.1]). At the same time, some clinical findings can be reassuring, such as a family history of benign goiter or clinical manifestations of thyrotoxicosis (as in toxic nodular goiter) or hypothyroidism (as in autoimmune thyroiditis, which can produce an asymmetric goiter). Serum TSH measurement is the only blood test that is always indicated for thyroid nodules, since it can exclude primary thyroid dysfunction. The physician who suspects autoimmune thyroiditis or medullary thyroid cancer should measure

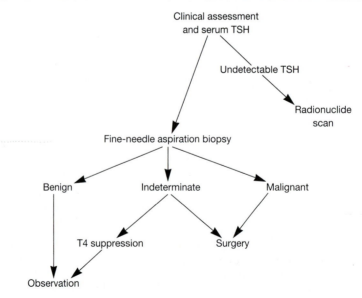

Figure 4.4–3. Diagnostic and therapeutic approach to the patient with a thyroid nodule.

TSH, thyroid-stimulating hormone; T_4, thyroxine.

the patient's antithyroid peroxidase antibody or calcitonin, respectively.

Thyroid fine-needle aspiration biopsy plays a central role in the differential diagnosis of thyroid nodules. The cytopathologic findings can be (1) benign, in which case observation or TSH-suppressive thyroid hormone therapy can be recommended; (2) malignant, in which case surgery is required; or (3) indeterminate. Among the 20% of nodules in this last category, only 20% are thyroid cancers, but surgery is generally required for definitive diagnosis and treatment. Although radionuclide thyroid scanning can define a nodule's function relative to the rest of the gland, only hot nodules—those that concentrate tracer and suppress the rest of the gland—can be assumed to be benign. Thyroid sonography is reassuring only in patients with small, simple cysts; it seldom rules out malignancy in palpable nodules.

Thyroid Cancer

Most cancers arising from thyroid epithelium are well differentiated and slow-growing. In fact, clinically silent microscopic thyroid cancers are often found incidentally at surgery or at autopsy after death from another cause. Papillary thyroid cancer (accounting for 75% of all cases) and minimally invasive follicular thyroid cancer (10% of cases) are both rather indolent tumors that carry an excellent prognosis. At the other extreme, poorly differentiated malignancies, such as the rare anaplastic thyroid cancer, can be among the most aggressive and therapeutically hopeless of all malignancies. Of intermediate severity are invasive follicular and medullary thyroid cancers (10% of cases).

Papillary thyroid cancer affects both young and older people, and, if untreated, spreads by local invasion and lymphatic channels to regional nodes and, less often, to the lungs. Follicular thyroid cancer, which is distinguished histologically from an adenoma by capsular and vascular invasion, is capable not just of local invasion but also of hematogenous spread to lung, bone, and other sites. Three factors predict an increased likelihood of recurrent disease in patients with papillary or follicular thyroid cancer: (1) age over 40; (2) a large primary tumor, especially one greater than 4 cm in diameter; and (3) evidence of local tissue invasion or distant metastases at the time of diagnosis.

Medullary thyroid cancer arises from calcitonin-producing C cells in the gland. This cancer can appear in several ways: sporadically, as an expression of familial medullary thyroid cancer, or as one component of the familial MEN IIa syndrome (medullary thyroid cancer, pheochromocytoma, and hyperparathyroidism). Patients with high calcitonin levels may suffer from diarrhea, flushing, and pruritus. The plasma calcitonin level is a useful tumor marker and can be used to detect subclinical disease in affected family members, as can genetic screening for a specific set of proto-oncogene mutations.

Management of patients with thyroid cancer begins with surgical resection of the tumor along with part or all of the normal thyroid gland. Total or near-total thyroidectomy has the advantages of resecting microscopic tumor foci that may be in the contralateral lobe and of making postoperative monitoring for cancer recurrence (with serum thyroglobulin and radioactive iodine scans) more accurate. However, bilateral neck surgery increases the risk of injury to the recurrent laryngeal nerves and parathyroid glands.

Patients with thyroid cancers of epithelial cell origin (papillary, follicular, and Hürthle cell) require lifelong thyroxine therapy to prevent hypothyroidism and to inhibit pituitary TSH production. TSH-suppressive therapy has been shown to reduce risk of recurrence and disease-related death. Patients with known residual disease or higher risk of recurrence (because of older age, larger tumor size, or locally invasive or metastatic tumor) are also usually scanned with radioactive iodine; iodine-avid tumor and residual normal gland tissue are then ablated with larger doses of iodine-131. Since this radioactive iodine scanning and therapy depend on TSH stimulation of residual thyroid tissue, suppressive thyroxine therapy must be temporarily withdrawn. Administration of human recombinant TSH is being studied as a way of performing such scans without discontinuing thyroxine.

Chemotherapy and external-beam radiation therapy have limited roles in management of thyroid cancers. In patients with anaplastic and other poorly differentiated thyroid malignancies, the only indicated measures may be palliative.

SUMMARY

▶ Hyperthyroidism can present not only with classic symptoms and signs, but with isolated complications affecting a single organ system (eg, atrial fibrillation) and atypical clinical syndromes (eg, apathetic thyrotoxicosis).

▶ Graves' disease is an autoimmune form of hyperthyroidism caused by TSH-receptor antibodies, along with orbital inflammation and, rarely, pretibial myxedema.

▶ Primary hypothyroidism, which is usually caused by autoimmune thyroiditis or previous thyroid radiation, can be clinically subtle but is readily diagnosed by measurement of serum thyroid-stimulating hormone (TSH).

▶ Inflammatory thyroiditis, most often caused by viral infection or postpartum immunologic injury, can produce a triphasic pattern of thyroid dysfunction.

▶ Thyroid nodules are common, but few are cancer. Clinical evaluation, serum TSH measurement, and fine-needle biopsy can be used to select patients for surgery.

SUGGESTED READING

Dulgeroff AJ, Hershman JM: Medical therapy for differentiated thyroid carcinoma. Endocr Rev 1994;15:500.

Franklyn JA: The management of hyperthyroidism. N Engl J Med 1994;330:1731.

Mandel SJ, Brent GA, Larsen PR: Levothyroxine therapy in patients with thyroid disease. Ann Intern Med 1993;119:492.

Mazzaferri EL: Management of a solitary thyroid nodule. N Engl J Med 1993;328:553.

Sherman SI, Ladenson PW: Thyroid gland. In: *Laboratory Medicine: The Selection and Interpretation of Clinical Laboratory Studies.* Noe DA, Rock RC (editors). Williams & Wilkins, 1994.

4.5

Gonadal Disorders

Christine R. Schneyer, MD

Although gonadal disorders are common, their symptoms often go unvoiced by patients and unrecognized by their physicians. Recognition and treatment of gonadal dysfunction are important for two reasons. First, loss of sexual function, infertility, and distressing changes in appearance all can detract from quality of life; once recognized, many of these problems are reversible. Second, clinical features of gonadal dysfunction may provide clues to serious underlying disease. For example, hirsutism in women, in addition to being a disturbing cosmetic concern, can be a sign of otherwise occult disease such as ovarian or adrenal malignancy. Similarly, gynecomastia in men can be a clue to serious liver diseases, hormonal disturbances, drug side effects, or substance abuse. This chapter covers clinical, laboratory, and radiographic means to define the causes of gonadal dysfunction and provides treatment outlines for the responsible diseases.

Two general observations should influence the clinical evaluation of patients with gonadal disorders. First, women are more likely than men to seek medical attention for their symptoms. For example, because amenorrhea and galactorrhea in women are striking changes, affected women usually get medical advice early. In contrast, impotence and loss of libido in men typically begin insidiously; many men are reluctant to mention these complaints and attribute them to psychological factors or aging. Gonadal disorders may also present to physicians when one or both members of a couple complain of infertility—a full discussion of which is beyond the scope of this chapter. Delays in medical attention to the symptoms in either sex can allow underlying diseases, such as pituitary tumors and neuropathic disorders, to progress unchecked.

A second general axiom about gonadal disorders is that symptoms that develop quickly should be taken especially seriously. For example, sudden masculinization in women or gynecomastia in men is likely to reflect serious underlying disease and must be evaluated promptly.

REPRODUCTIVE ENDOCRINE SYNDROMES IN WOMEN

Amenorrhea

Primary amenorrhea is defined as no menarche by age 16; secondary amenorrhea is the absence of menses for 6 months or longer in a woman with previously normal menstrual periods. Loss of menses for less than 6 months is oligomenorrhea. In addition to infertility, amenorrhea can be associated with estrogen deficiency and its potential consequences (see "Menopause" below) or can be a sign of serious diseases affecting the hypothalamic-pituitary-gonadal axis.

Causes: Primary amenorrhea is usually caused by congenital abnormalities of the ovaries or uterovaginal outflow tract (Table 4.5–1). Fifty percent of all cases of primary amenorrhea are caused by Turner's syndrome (ovarian dysgenesis), in which phenotypic females have a single X chromosome (XO karyotype). Turner's syndrome may not be recognized until adulthood, by which time patients may have such complications as osteoporosis or manifestations of coarctation of the aorta. Untreated patients with Turner's syndrome are short and lack features of secondary sexual development: They have prepubertal breasts and sparse pubic and axillary hair. Many patients also have other stigmata such as a webbed neck or shield chest.

Testicular feminization is a rare cause of primary amenorrhea in which XY individuals—genetic males—have complete target tissue resistance to androgen action, leading to development of female external genitalia by default. Cryptorchid testes in these patients may be mistaken for inguinal hernias. Intra-abdominal testes should be resected because they tend to become cancerous.

Secondary amenorrhea is most often the result of pregnancy. Pathologic causes of secondary amenorrhea can be broadly categorized as (1) disorders that directly impair ovarian or uterine function and (2) the more common dis-

Table 4.5–1. Some causes of amenorrhea.

Causes	Clinical Clues
Primary amenorrhea	
Turner's syndrome	Short stature, shield chest, prepubertal breasts, sparse pubic and axillary hair
Testicular feminization	Normal breast development, sparse pubic and axillary hair, inguinal "hernias" (undescended testes)
Congenital anomalies of the uterovaginal outflow tract	Pelvic "mass" (collection of blood)
Secondary amenorrhea	
Primary ovarian failure	
Autoimmune disease	Family history, other autoimmune endocrine disease
Previous oophoritis	History of postpubertal mumps, chemotherapy, radiation
Uterovaginal disturbances	
Intrauterine synechiae	History of endometritis or curettage
Hypothalamic-pituitary disorders	
Functional amenorrhea	Weight loss, systemic illness, sustained strenuous exercise, emotional stress
Hypothalamic sarcoidosis, vasculitis, or tumor	Headache, diabetes insipidus, weight gain, somnolence, multisystem disease
Cranial radiation	
Pituitary disease	Visual field cut, postpartum hemorrhage
Obesity	
Hyperprolactinemic states (see Table 4.5–2)	Galactorrhea, visual field cut, phenothiazine therapy, primary hypothyroidism, chest wall disease
Hyperandrogenemic states	
Chronic anovulatory syndrome	Obesity, hirsutism, family history
Ovarian tumor	Explosive onset, virilization
Nonclassic 21-hydroxylase deficiency	Family history, Ashkenazic Jews
Cushing's syndrome	Hypertension, muscle weakness, easy bruisability

orders that alter hypothalamic or pituitary regulation of ovarian function. Diseases causing hypothalamic-pituitary disturbances can be divided into (a) processes that directly affect these essential regulatory centers and (b) disorders that arise from primary hormonal disturbances elsewhere, for example, hyperprolactinemia, hyperandrogenism, and hypercortisolism, which secondarily disrupt hypothalamic-pituitary regulatory function.

Premature ovarian failure (menopause in a woman younger than age 40) and primary uterine infections and injuries are relatively uncommon causes of secondary amenorrhea. The ovaries may fail prematurely because of oophoritis, caused either by an idiopathic condition (often associated with other autoimmune gland inflammation such as Hashimoto's thyroiditis) or by infection (particularly mumps). Ovarian function may also be lost permanently after irradiation of the ovaries or exposure to toxic chemicals, especially alkylating agents used in chemotherapy. Damage to the endometrium can interfere with its normal responsiveness to cyclical hormonal changes and lead to amenorrhea; this happens in Asherman's syndrome, in which intrauterine synechiae develop after curettage or endometritis.

Reversible hypothalamic dysfunction, also called functional amenorrhea, is caused by changes in the normal pulsatile pattern of gonadotropin-releasing hormone (GnRH) secretion with or without frankly low serum gonadotropin levels. These changes can be caused by systemic illnesses, emotional stress, weight loss from dieting (eg, in patients with anorexia nervosa), and sustained strenuous physical training (eg, in ballerinas, competitive runners, gymnasts). GnRH and gonadotropins can become deficient when hypothalamic or pituitary tissues are compressed by tumor, granulomatous disease, previous surgery or radiation therapy, or postpartum necrosis of the pituitary (Sheehan's syndrome).

Hyperprolactinemia is another relatively common cause of secondary amenorrhea, accounting for 20% of cases (Table 4.5–2). The probable mechanism is disruption of the normal pattern of pulsatile GnRH secretion. Besides pregnancy, the prolactin can be elevated by prolactin-producing pituitary tumors and by drugs like phenothiazines and metoclopramide that deplete or interfere with the action of dopamine, the physiologic inhibitor of prolactin release. Other causes of hyperprolactinemia are hypothalamic disorders that damage dopamine-producing neurons; suprasellar masses (eg, craniopharyngiomas, aneurysms) that interrupt the hypothalamic-hypophyseal portal venous system; conditions that cause intrathoracic or chest wall irritation that mimics breast suckling (eg, herpes zoster), the physiologic stimulus to prolactin release; hypothyroidism, in which thyrotropin-releasing hormone-mediated prolactin release is increased; and renal failure, in which both prolactin production and clearance are deranged.

A significant minority of women have no obvious cause for their hyperprolactinemia. Patients with idiopathic hyperprolactinemia are believed to have very small pituitary adenomas or lactotroph hyperplasia that cannot be seen radiographically. The amenorrhea caused by hyperprolactinemia is often associated with galactorrhea (nonpuerperal lactation); however, when a previously pregnant woman with regular menses develops galactorrhea, it is rarely a sign of disease.

Amenorrhea can also be caused by the inhibitory effects of excess circulating androgens on production of hypothalamic GnRH and pituitary luteinizing hormone (LH) and follicle-stimulating hormone (FSH). The ovaries and, less commonly, the adrenal glands can be sources of androgen overproduction in women. The most common of these disorders is the chronic anovulatory syndrome (also termed polycystic ovary syndrome). This syndrome probably results from a heterogeneous group of disorders that cause amenorrhea and lesser menstrual disturbances re-

Table 4.5–2. Common pathologic causes of hyperprolactinemia.

Causes	Clinical Clues
Central nervous system dopamine disturbances	
Tumor, granulomatous, or infiltrative disorders	Headache, seizures, diabetes insipidus, weight gain, somnolence, multisystem disease
Pituitary stalk section Meningitis	Tumor, surgery, trauma See Chapter 8.3
Prolactin-secreting pituitary tumors	Headache, visual field cut, extraocular muscle disturbances, gynecomastia
Primary hypothyroidism	Fatigue, cold intolerance, constipation, muscle cramps (see Chapter 4.4)
Pharmacologic agents	Treatment with phenothiazines, tricyclic antidepressants, metoclopramide, estrogens, verapamil, reserpine, α-methyldopa, opiates
Neurogenic	Spinal cord lesions, herpes zoster, chest wall trauma, breast disease
Chronic renal failure	See Chapter 5.5
Idiopathic	

flecting anovulation (oligomenorrhea, irregular menses, and infertility), along with hirsutism and often obesity.

The pathogenesis of the chronic anovulatory syndrome is incompletely understood. One hypothesis is that in genetically predisposed women, weight gain leads to insulin resistance in target tissues. To compensate, the pancreas produces more insulin. Hyperinsulinemia then stimulates ovarian production of androgens, which are converted in fat tissue to estrogens, chiefly estrone. These estrogens then feed back on the hypothalamus and pituitary to alter GnRH and gonadotropin secretory patterns. This alteration often, but not invariably, increases the ratio of LH:FSH serum concentrations to greater than 2.5:1. The abnormal gonadotropin patterns may further worsen ovarian androgen overproduction. This self-perpetuating cycle is believed to lead to chronic anovulation.

Some but not all patients with the chronic anovulatory syndrome have polycystic ovaries, presumably reflecting past cycles of incomplete follicle maturation. Although the initial cause of the increased androgen production in women with primary chronic anovulatory syndrome remains uncertain, excess androgens from any disorder (eg, Cushing's disease) can also lead to anovulation and polycystic ovaries.

Evaluation: Pregnancy should always be excluded first as a cause of amenorrhea, by screening of serum or urine for human chorionic gonadotropin (hCG). In nonpregnant women, the physician should then search for hypothalamic, pituitary, hyperandrogenemic, and primary ovarian disorders. The history often yields strong clues, such as weight loss, strenuous exercise, or previous chemotherapy. Physical examination can provide clues such as a vi-

sual field deficit, galactorrhea, hirsutism, or enlarged ovaries (see Table 4.5–1).

Laboratory studies should include a complete blood count, electrolyte values, and kidney, liver, and thyroid function tests (both free T_4 and thyroid-stimulating hormone [TSH]), to identify systemic diseases. A low estradiol level confirms estrogen deficiency, whereas serum FSH and LH concentrations indicate the type of derangement. For example, the gonadotropins are elevated during menopause, as in other causes of primary ovarian failure. Low or inappropriately normal gonadotropin levels are found in patients with hypothalamic or pituitary dysfunction. Although most women with low gonadotropins ultimately prove to have functional hypothalamic amenorrhea, they must undergo computed tomography (CT) or magnetic resonance imaging (MRI) of the hypothalamic-pituitary region to exclude tumors and other organic disease. A serum prolactin should always be part of the initial screen to detect hyperprolactinemia. In women with hirsutism or other signs of androgen excess, a test for serum testosterone level is useful to screen for androgen overproduction by the ovaries, and a test for serum dehydroepiandrosterone sulfate (DHEA-S) screens for overproduction by the adrenal glands (see "Evaluation" under "Hirsutism and Virilization" below). Women with physical findings suggesting hypercortisolism (Chapter 4.3) should have a 24-hour urine free cortisol determination.

These initial tests show a significant number of amenorrheic women to have normal estrogen and gonadotropin levels without elevated prolactin or androgen concentrations. In these patients, the main diagnostic possibilities remain hypothalamic amenorrhea, chronic anovulatory syndrome with very modest androgen excess, or uterine abnormalities that may be inapparent on routine pelvic exam. These possibilities can be differentiated with a progesterone challenge test, in which patients are given either an intramuscular injection of progesterone or a 5-day course of oral medroxyprogesterone. Patients with normal estrogen levels who do not develop vaginal bleeding within 1 week after the last progesterone dose probably have uterine disease. In patients who have vaginal bleeding, the diagnostic possibilities are then limited to hypothalamic amenorrhea and chronic anovulatory syndrome. Chronic anovulatory syndrome can often be confirmed with additional serum androgen determinations, including the free testosterone, taken on multiple occasions.

Management: Women with functional hypothalamic amenorrhea should be advised to avoid excessive exercise and to increase their caloric intake until they reach a normal body weight. Most patients with prolactin-secreting pituitary tumors are treated with the dopamine agonist bromocriptine (Chapter 4.2). Those with other types of pituitary tumors undergo surgical resection. Surgery can also correct some anatomic abnormalities of the uterus and genital outflow tract.

Other treatments are available for patients who cannot recover normal estrogen production. Patients who have responded to progesterone with withdrawal bleeding can be treated with intermittent progestin therapy; this induces periodic bleeding to prevent endometrial hyperplasia and carcinoma. Combined estrogen-progestin therapy induces monthly withdrawal bleeding in patients with severe estrogen deficiency and prevents osteoporosis and other complications of chronic estrogen deprivation. The most physiologic therapy for patients with GnRH deficiency is pulsatile parenteral administration of a synthetic GnRH analog, but this complex, expensive therapy is used primarily for women seeking fertility in addition to gonadal steroid replacement.

Clomiphene citrate can also stimulate ovulation and restore fertility in patients with hypothalamic amenorrhea or the chronic anovulatory syndrome; clomiphene's complex action mimics both positive and negative estrogen effects on the hypothalamus and pituitary. Another alternative for women with primary gonadotropin or GnRH deficiency is gonadotropin therapy. Few patients with primary ovarian failure become fertile, but occasional women have spontaneous remission or respond to clomiphene or gonadotropin stimulation of ovulation.

Hirsutism and Virilization

Hirsutism is the growth of androgen-dependent hair in areas of a woman's body where hair is not normally found. About 10% of normal women have hair growth on the face and periareolar regions, and 2% have hair on the sternum. The definition of abnormal androgen-dependent hair growth varies among ethnic groups: What may be entirely normal in a woman of Mediterranean ancestry could be an indication of significant underlying disease in a woman of Scandinavian descent. Virilization is more severe masculinization of women, with hirsutism, temporal balding, deepening of the voice, pectoral muscle development, and clitorimegaly.

Androgen disorders are caused by increased androgen action in patients with either normal or elevated androgen levels. Hirsutism can be a distressing cosmetic problem without severe medical ramifications. However, clinical evidence of marked hyperandrogenism in the form of a new, explosive onset of hirsutism or any degree of virilization demands evaluation for possible serious ovarian or adrenal disease.

The major circulating androgen in women is testosterone. It is secreted by the ovaries and adrenals and is also derived from weak precursor androgens (androstenedione, DHEA, and DHEA-S) in peripheral tissues. Only unbound circulating testosterone, 2% of the total, is biologically active. Within the skin, testosterone is converted by 5α-reductase to dihydrotestosterone, a potent androgen that regulates androgen-dependent hair growth.

Causes: Hirsutism can be caused by drugs or by pathologic conditions involving the ovaries, adrenals, or skin (Table 4.5–3). Women with so-called "idiopathic hirsutism" are otherwise normal, with regular menses, no virilization, and normal androgen levels. Some of these patients are

Table 4.5–3. Common causes of hirsutism.

Causes	Clinical Clues
Ovarian	
Idiopathic hirsutism	Pubertal onset, regular menses
Polycystic ovary syndrome	Pubertal onset, irregular menses, family history
Androgen-producing ovarian neoplasms	Explosive course, virilization, abdominal or pelvic pain
Insulin resistance syndromes	Diabetes, acanthosis nigricans, skin tags
Adrenal	
Nonclassic 21-hydroxylase deficiency	Family history, Ashkenazic Jews
Androgen-producing adrenal neoplasms	Explosive course, virilization, abdominal or flank pain
Cushing's syndrome	Hypertension, muscle weakness, easy bruisability
Hyperprolactinemia	See Table 4.5–2
Medications	
Anabolic steroids	Virilization
Phenytoin	
Minoxidil	Growth of fine, nonpigmented hair in androgen-independent areas
Cyclosporine	
Glucocorticoids	

thought to have augmented conversion of testosterone to dihydrotestosterone within the skin. The chronic anovulatory syndrome (see "Causes" under "Amenorrhea" above) is also commonly associated with hirsutism. Together, idiopathic hirsutism and chronic anovulatory syndrome account for 90% of patients with hirsutism.

In about 5% of patients, hirsutism is caused by nonclassic (also called late-onset) congenital adrenal hyperplasia, most often from 21-hydroxylase deficiency. Patients may present similarly to those with idiopathic hirsutism or chronic anovulatory syndrome. Nonclassic congenital adrenal hyperplasia is inherited as an autosomal recessive trait and is caused by partial deficiency of this adrenal enzyme, essential for cortisol synthesis. Since cortisol normally reduces adrenocorticotropic hormone (ACTH) by negative feedback control, the resulting elevated ACTH augments synthesis of adrenal steroid precursors such as 17-hydroxyprogesterone, which are shunted to form adrenal androgens.

A minority of patients with hirsutism and virilization have androgen-producing ovarian or adrenal neoplasms—benign or malignant. A few patients have Cushing's syndrome, caused by an ACTH-producing pituitary tumor, adrenal neoplasm, or ectopic ACTH secretion (Chapter 4.3). Other conditions associated with hirsutism include hyperprolactinemia, which can increase adrenal androgen production, and insulin resistance states, which are accompanied by hypersecretion of ovarian androgens. Drugs such as anabolic steroids, phenytoin, minoxidil, and cyclosporine can also cause excessive hair growth.

Evaluation: The history should define the onset of hirsutism and its rate of progression. Benign conditions such as chronic anovulatory syndrome and idiopathic hirsutism typically begin soon after puberty and progress gradually, whereas most serious disorders begin after age 20 and progress quickly. The physical exam should focus on the extent of hirsutism, signs of virilization, signs of hypercortisolism (Chapter 4.3), and possible pelvic or abdominal masses.

Laboratory testing should be used to seek serious underlying conditions and define the source of androgen excess, allowing the more common benign hyperandrogenemic disorders to be treated. Initial screening tests should include a plasma testosterone and DHEA-S. A high testosterone (over 150 ng/dL or 5 nM/L) suggests an ovarian neoplasm; a high DHEA-S (over 500 µg/dL or 13 µM/L) suggests an adrenal neoplasm. A few patients with tumors have less pronounced elevations of these hormones. Tumors should be promptly sought with abdominal CT or MRI and pelvic ultrasonography.

Modestly elevated levels of testosterone and DHEA-S suggest a benign cause for the hirsutism. Normal testosterone levels suggest idiopathic hirsutism; in patients with otherwise normal routine laboratory findings, this diagnosis can sometimes be confirmed by an elevated level of free testosterone, androstenedione, or 3α-androstanediol glucuronide, a metabolite of dihydrotestosterone.

A patient with clinical features of Cushing's syndrome should have a 24-hour urine collection to measure free cortisol. Nonclassic congenital adrenal hyperplasia caused by 21-hydroxylase deficiency is diagnosed by an elevated 17-hydroxyprogesterone, the metabolite proximal to the enzyme block, either on an early morning specimen or after ACTH stimulation. Serum prolactin should be measured, especially if menses are irregular. Insulin resistance in patients with hirsutism and hyperglycemia may be confirmed by measurement of insulin in the fasting state or during a glucose tolerance test.

Management: Androgen-secreting ovarian and adrenal tumors should be excised. Cushing's syndrome should be treated according to its etiology (Chapter 4.3). Congenital adrenal hyperplasia should be controlled with the lowest effective adrenal-suppressive dose of glucocorticoid. Whether idiopathic hirsutism and hirsutism associated with the chronic anovulatory syndrome should be treated medically or just cosmetically depends on its severity and how distressing it is to the patient. Effective local measures include shaving (which does not increase hair growth), bleaching, topical depilatories, and electrolysis, which is most useful when combined with medical therapy to prevent recruitment of new follicles. In obese patients, weight loss decreases hair growth by lowering insulin levels and insulin-mediated ovarian androgen production and by increasing serum protein binding of testosterone, thereby decreasing levels of the free hormone.

For more severely affected women who have no contraindications, drug treatments can include oral contraceptives, antiandrogens, and GnRH analogs. Oral contraceptives decrease ovarian and adrenal androgen synthesis, reducing hair growth in some patients with endogenous hirsutism. Birth control pills are especially useful for women with predominantly ovarian testosterone overproduction who are otherwise candidates for oral contraception. Preparations with the least androgenic progesterone should be used.

Successful treatment of moderate-to-severe hirsutism usually requires an antiandrogen drug such as spironolactone or flutamide. These drugs prevent androgen from binding to its receptor. They also accelerate androgen catabolism and may block conversion of testosterone to the more potent dihydrotestosterone. Finasteride, a 5α-reductase inhibitor used to treat men with prostatic enlargement, is potentially useful for managing hirsutism.

The response to medical therapy—both birth control pills and antiandrogens—tends to be slow, requiring 6–12 months to halt progression or bring noticeable improvement. Responses are typically best in younger patients with a shorter history of mild hirsutism. Patients taking antiandrogens must use contraception, because these agents may impair masculinization of the male fetus.

Long-acting GnRH analogs can also reduce ovarian androgen production, but they must be given with combination estrogen-progestin therapy to minimize the side effects of estrogen deficiency. In general, these agents' expense and side effects make them second- or third-line drugs for treatment of hirsutism.

Menopause

Menopause is the age-related depletion of ovarian follicles, resulting in cessation of ovarian estrogen production and amenorrhea at an average age of 51. Menopause comes slightly earlier in cigarette smokers. It is considered premature in women younger than 40. The most important medical consequences of the menopause are vasomotor instability, genital tissue atrophy, osteoporosis, and increased risk for cardiovascular disease (Table 4.5–4). Most women have vasomotor instability, hot flushes that are especially severe in early menopause. Hot flushes are described as a sudden feeling of warmth, often with sweats that usually affect the upper body. Vaginal atrophy, commonly developing 5–10 years after menopause, can cause vaginal dryness, pruritus, and dys-

Table 4.5–4. Consequences of the menopause.

Causes	Clinical Clues
Vasomotor symptoms	Hot flushes, insomnia
Psychological disturbances	Fatigue, irritability, moodiness, memory loss, depression
Urogenital atrophy	Vaginal dryness, dyspareunia, secondary loss of libido, dysuria, infection, urgency incontinence
Osteoporosis	Loss of height, thoracic kyphosis, spontaneous fractures
Atherosclerotic cardiovascular disease	See Chapter 1.3

pareunia. Atrophy of the urethral mucosa, also an estrogen-sensitive tissue, can lead to dysuria and infection.

Postmenopausal osteoporosis results from accelerated bone loss, primarily within the first 5–10 years after menopause (Chapter 4.6). Trabecular bone is affected more than cortical bone, potentially leading to vertebral crush fractures and distal fractures of the radius. Similar bone loss results from premature surgical menopause and from the amenorrhea associated with anorexia, excessive physical exercise, and hyperprolactinemia.

Atherosclerotic cardiovascular disease, a major consequence of menopause, is the principal cause of death in older women. Premenopausal women are relatively protected from atherosclerosis by estrogen, which keeps low-density lipoprotein (LDL) an average of 15% below that in postmenopausal women and high-density lipoprotein (HDL) comparably higher. Estrogen may also inhibit the prostaglandin-thromboxane system and enhance the activity of endothelium-derived nitric oxide, thereby dilating vessels and reducing the potential for thrombosis.

Treatment for Complications of Menopause: Estrogen replacement therapy controls all significant consequences of menopause. Estrogen prevents hot flushes and disturbing symptoms of gonadal steroid-dependent tissue atrophy. Most important, menopausal women taking estrogen suffer 50% fewer deaths from cardiovascular disease. Since progestin reduces some of the favorable actions of estrogen on serum lipoproteins, the effects of the widely used combined estrogen-progestin therapy on the risk of ischemic heart disease are less certain. Estrogen also prevents postmenopausal bone loss in most women if started soon after menopause and continued indefinitely.

Postmenopausal estrogen replacement therapy has some potential complications. Estrogen given alone increases the risk for uterine cancer three- to eightfold, but this excess risk is virtually eliminated by combining estrogen with progestin. (Women who have had a hysterectomy can be treated with estrogen alone.) Whether or not estrogen replacement increases the risk for breast cancer remains controversial. Estrogen may increase the risk in predisposed women (eg, those with a strong family history of breast cancer) and perhaps in normal women who take estrogen replacement for more than 10 years. However, epidemiologic studies suggest that the major benefits of estrogen replacement therapy, especially protection against heart disease, outweigh any increased cancer risk.

Many women are given oral estrogen with a progestin in a monthly pattern to mimic the menstrual cycle. But few women want the menstrual periods that this regimen induces. Coming into wider use is continuous combined estrogen-progestin, which usually causes menstruation for only the first several months. Transdermal estrogen is an alternative for women in whom oral estrogen causes gastrointestinal distress. Unfortunately, estrogen patches do not appear to have the beneficial effects on LDL and HDL metabolism reported with the oral form, which travels first to the liver via the portal circulation.

REPRODUCTIVE ENDOCRINE SYNDROMES IN MEN

Hypogonadism

The testes have two major functions: to form sperm and to synthesize testosterone. Male hypogonadism is a defect in one or both of these processes.

Causes: Male hypogonadism can stem from disturbances in the hypothalamus, pituitary, or testes. Hypothalamic GnRH deficiency can be either congenital or acquired. Autosomal dominant and recessive as well as X-linked inheritance patterns have been described for congenital GnRH deficiency, which is more common in boys than in girls. When associated with anosmia (no sense of smell), the disorder is called *Kallmann's syndrome,* a condition with midline deficits of both GnRH-secreting neurons and the olfactory bulb. The clinical presentation of congenital GnRH deficiency resembles that of simple delayed puberty, another familial disorder that is more common in boys than girls. In a boy with an intact sense of smell, it may be impossible to distinguish congenital GnRH deficiency from delayed puberty, even with sophisticated endocrine and radiographic testing. GnRH deficiency can also follow destruction of the hypothalamus by tumor or a granulomatous disease such as sarcoidosis.

Furthermore, hypogonadism can develop when gonadotropin-producing pituitary cells are destroyed by pituitary adenomas or other neoplasms around the sella turcica. Although hypersecretion of prolactin by pituitary tumors can impair GnRH production in men as it does in women, prolactinomas in men do much of their damage by directly compressing adjacent gonadotropic cells. Unfortunately, by the time most prolactinomas in men are discovered, they have grown into macroadenomas (diameter greater than 1 cm) (Chapter 4.2); this is probably because the first clues to hyperprolactinemia in men are impotence and decreased libido, complaints not often volunteered or elicited during a clinical exam. Gynecomastia is uncommon in men with hyperprolactinemia, and galactorrhea is rare.

Primary testicular diseases cause hypogonadism. In both congenital and acquired testicular disorders, spermatogenic cells may be affected even when the Leydig cells that synthesize testosterone are not. The most common congenital cause of primary testicular dysfunction is Klinefelter's syndrome, a disorder characterized by one or more extra X chromosomes, affecting 1 in 500 boys. Patients typically have small, firm testes plus gynecomastia and eunuchoid body proportions with abnormally long extremities. Hyalinization of the seminiferous tubules precludes significant spermatogenesis. Most patients have low testosterone levels, although some have normal levels (so their only abnormality is infertility). Some patients with Klinefelter's syndrome also have social and behavior problems.

Other inherited enzyme defects can prevent or limit testosterone production. Congenital abnormalities in androgen receptors can cause a partial or complete insensitivity to normal male levels of testosterone. Men with the Sertoli-cell-only syndrome are infertile because they are born with no germ cell elements.

Testicular dysfunction can be acquired in a number of ways. Mumps is the most common infectious disease affecting the testes. Radiation, chemotherapy, and certain pesticides can impair both testicular functions or damage only the seminiferous tubules. Alcohol and marijuana can inhibit testosterone as well as sperm production. Anabolic steroids can permanently impair spermatogenesis.

Evaluation: Sexual immaturity and eunuchoid proportions in men indicate androgen deficiency that began before puberty. Sexually mature men with recent-onset androgen deficiency may have not only decreased libido and impotence but decreased stamina and muscle strength. Chronic hypogonadism causes testicular atrophy (testes less than 5 × 3 cm), gynecomastia, diminished muscle mass, and reduction of body hair. Other consequences of long-term testosterone deficiency can include anemia and osteopenia. Some infertile men have testicular atrophy but maintain normal serum testosterone levels because 90% of the testicular mass is spermatogenic cells. Infertile men with obstructed ducts typically have normal genitalia.

Laboratory evaluation of the man with suspected hypogonadism should begin with a serum testosterone level. If the testosterone is low, serum gonadotropin measurements help to localize the abnormality. A high LH level is consistent with a primary decrease in testicular androgen production, whereas FSH is elevated in men with primary testicular impairment of spermatogenesis. In contrast, low or inappropriately normal gonadotropin values suggest a defect in the pituitary or hypothalamus. Patients with hypothalamic-pituitary dysfunction should have a serum prolactin and imaging of the hypothalamic-pituitary region by CT or MRI. A karyotype confirms a suspicion of Klinefelter's syndrome.

Semen is analyzed to evaluate germinal epithelial function. If a man with azoospermia but normal endocrine function has a normal testicular exam, testicular biopsy showing normal spermatogenesis is needed to confirm duct obstruction.

Management: Testosterone deficiency of any cause can be corrected by intramuscular injections of long-acting testosterone preparations every 2 weeks or transcutaneously by patches. Testosterone replacement restores libido and potency and prevents other consequences of androgen deficiency.

Testosterone alone cannot stimulate spermatogenesis. This can sometimes be promoted in other ways. Intramuscular hCG, which has LH-like effects, can stimulate testosterone production and spermatogenesis in men with gonadotropin or GnRH deficiency; patients who do not produce any gonadotropin also require FSH treatment to complete spermatogenesis. In men with GnRH deficiency,

daily pulsatile subcutaneous GnRH from a portable infusion pump stimulates normal testosterone synthesis and spermatogenesis. Men with hypogonadism from a prolactin-secreting tumor may become fertile with bromocriptine therapy.

It is difficult to restore fertility to men with primary testicular dysfunction. Surgical repair can be tried for potentially correctable urologic lesions like obstructed ducts or a large varicocele. Some oligospermic men are helped by clomiphene, which promotes endogenous GnRH and gonadotropin release.

Impotence

Impotence is the inability to achieve an erection sufficient to permit sexual intercourse. Impotence is more common in older men, affecting 50% of those over age 75. The basic requirements for erectile function are normal testosterone levels, an adequate penile blood supply, and intact parasympathetic autonomic nervous system function at the level of the sacral spinal cord. Finally, the man must be free of psychological disturbances that inhibit sexual performance (Table 4.5–5).

The causes of testosterone deficiency have been discussed (see "Causes" under "Hypogonadism" above). Vascular impotence, caused by compromised penile arterial blood flow, can accompany aorto-iliac atherosclerosis and is relatively common, especially in older men. Neurogenic disturbances causing impotence include diabetic and alcoholic neuropathy, surgical interruption during prostatic and other pelvic surgery, and central nervous system disturbances such as stroke. Psychological problems can be the fundamental cause of erectile dysfunction or can exacerbate preexisting organic impotence.

Drugs are an important cause of impotence. Two widely used drugs, cimetidine and spironolactone, act as antiandrogens. Other commonly used medications that can impair sexual performance by unknown mechanisms are antihypertensives (eg, diuretics, β-blockers), tranquilizers, and antidepressants. These drugs are unpredictable, causing impotence in some men but not others. Antihypertensives that rarely cause impotence are angiotensin-converting enzyme inhibitors and calcium channel blockers.

Evaluation: The physician should ask men about their libido and potency. Men who complain of impotence with intercourse should be asked about morning erections and ability to masturbate. Sleep-related erections may be objectively assessed by strain gauge technique in a sleep laboratory. Loss of all erectile function argues for an organic rather than a psychogenic cause.

A concomitant decrease in libido suggests testosterone deficiency. Suspected endocrine-related impotence should be tested by measuring the serum testosterone level and, if it is low, serum gonadotropins. The serum prolactin should be also measured in all impotent men, since for unclear reasons hyperprolactinemia can cause erectile

Table 4.5–5. Some causes of impotence.

Causes	Clinical Clues
Hypogonadism	
Hypothalamic-pituitary disease	
Kallmann's syndrome	Family history, anosmia
Functional hypogonadism	Systemic illness, anorexia, psychological stress
Hypothalamic sarcoidosis, vasculitis, or tumor	Headache, diabetes insipidus, weight gain, somnolence
Prolactin-secreting pituitary tumors	Headache, visual field cut, extraocular muscle dysfunction
Cranial radiation	
Obesity	
Testicular disease	
Klinefelter's syndrome	Eunuchoid body habitus, gynecomastia, small firm testes
Orchitis	Family history, other autoimmune endocrine disease, history of postpubertal mumps, chemotherapy, radiation
Androgen resistance syndromes	Abnormal genitalia, reduced virilization
Vascular disease	Cigarette smoking, hypertension, claudication, diminished femoral pulses, hypercholesterolemia
Neurogenic disturbances	Stroke, spinal injury, epilepsy, diabetes, pelvic surgery, voiding dysfunction
Psychological problems	Depression, loss of a partner, dysfunctional interpersonal relationships
Drugs and toxins	
Alcohol, marijuana, anabolic steroids	
Antihypertensives, antidepressants, tranquilizers, spironolactone, cimetidine	

dysfunction, even in men with a normal serum testosterone.

Impotence in a man with a history of claudication and diminished femoral pulses suggests aorto-iliac atherosclerosis. An accurate test for vascular insufficiency is injection of papaverine (a smooth muscle relaxant) into the corpora cavernosa. The normal response is an erection within 10 minutes. If the patient does not develop an erection, Doppler ultrasonography and plethysmography can further test for vascular patency.

Management: Most impotence caused by endocrine disease is readily reversed; treating nonendocrine impotence is more difficult. If possible, suspected medications should be stopped. Patients with an intact penile blood supply can produce erections sufficient for sexual intercourse by injecting their corpora cavernosa with papaverine (alone or with phentolamine, an α-adrenergic blocker) or prostaglandin E_1. Unfortunately, these injections can cause pain and priapism. Effective alternatives can be surgically implanted mechanical devices and negative suction apparatuses. Patients with psychogenic impotence may benefit from psychiatric or sex therapy. Physicians should resist the temptation to offer testosterone therapy to impotent men who already have normal testosterone levels. This treatment is no more effective than placebo and may increase risk for prostate disease.

Gynecomastia

Gynecomastia is an increase in the glandular tissue of a man's breasts. Estrogen is the major hormone responsible for breast tissue growth, and gynecomastia can often be explained by an increase in the ratio of estrogens to androgens (Table 4.5–6). However, in many patients the cause of gynecomastia is unknown.

Causes: Pubertal gynecomastia, which most boys have to some degree, has been attributed to increased testicular estrogen production associated with the pubertal LH rise. Pubertal gynecomastia usually resolves within 2–3 years. The prevalence of physiologic gynecomastia then increases with age, affecting nearly 50% of men over 60. Gynecomastia should be a source of alarm if it progresses quickly or is associated with marked tenderness, asymmetry, or a discrete mass.

Congenital disorders causing gynecomastia include Klinefelter's syndrome and androgen resistance syndromes. Men with decreased testosterone production can acquire gynecomastia from the underlying disorder or from increased estrogen production or decreased estrogen degradation. Gynecomastia may be the first sign of an

Table 4.5–6. Pathologic causes of gynecomastia.

Hypogonadism (see Table 4.5–5 and "Causes" under "Hypogonadism")
Tumors
  Estrogen-secreting (testes, adrenal)
  Human chorionic gonadotropin-producing (testes, lung, liver, kidney)
Liver disease
Renal failure
Hyperprolactinemia (see Table 4.5–2)
Hyperthyroidism
Recovery from starvation
Therapeutic drugs
  Hormones (estrogens, androgens)
  Antiandrogens (spironolactone, flutamide, cyproterone, cimetidine)
  Estrogen-like drugs (digitalis)
Abused drugs
  Alcohol, heroin, marijuana, anabolic steroids
Idiopathic

estrogen-secreting tumor of the testes or adrenals. hCG-producing tumors like seminoma and lung carcinoma increase testicular secretion of estradiol. Men with liver disease have impaired estrogen degradation, which can lead to gynecomastia; in men with renal insufficiency, gynecomastia can be caused by impaired estrogen clearance and associated hypogonadism. Hyperprolactinemia can cause gynecomastia. Hyperthyroidism can produce gynecomastia because of increased extragonadal aromatization of androgens to estrogens and an increase in circulating sex steroid binding globulin.

Numerous drugs and abused substances cause gynecomastia. Implicated are estrogens used to treat prostate cancer, compounds convertible to estrogens (eg, anabolic steroids), and agents containing trace amounts of estrogen (eg, hair tonics, skin creams). Other medications produce gynecomastia by mimicking the action of estrogen (eg, digitalis) or inhibiting androgen effects (eg, spironolactone, cimetidine).

Evaluation: On physical exam, it may be difficult to differentiate glandular from adipose causes of breast enlargement, especially in obese men. If there is no glandular tissue, the physician can usually palpate the rib and intercostal space when pressing on the nipple.

A pubertal boy with mild gynecomastia as his only abnormality may require no further evaluation. In contrast, a grown man with recent-onset or progressive gynecomastia needs extensive testing. Serum testosterone, gonadotropins, and prolactin levels should be measured if the patient has a history of impotence. Serum hCG, estradiol, and estrone should be measured to rule out an occult neoplasm. The physician should also test for systemic conditions like liver disease and hyperthyroidism because they are so common.

Management: Mild gynecomastia often resolves—spontaneously in pubertal boys, after treatment in older men. More advanced gynecomastia does not regress significantly; reductive plastic surgery is recommended to spare patients undue psychological harm. Some patients are helped by tamoxifen, an antiestrogen, or by testolactone, an inhibitor of testosterone-to-estrogen conversion.

SUMMARY

▶ Symptoms and signs of gonadal dysfunction are often overlooked, particularly in men, but may be important manifestations of underlying disease.

▶ Gonadal disorders that begin suddenly or severely (eg, hirsutism in women, gynecomastia in men) are especially likely to be caused by a serious systemic disorder.

▶ The most common causes of secondary amenorrhea, excluding pregnancy, are functional hypothalamic amenorrhea, chronic anovulatory syndrome, and hyperprolactinemia.

▶ The major consequences of menopause are vasomotor instability, genital tissue atrophy, osteoporosis, and increased risk for cardiovascular disease. Estrogen replacement therapy controls these problems, but may increase some women's risks of endometrial and breast cancer.

▶ Impotence can be caused by hypogonadism or vascular, neurologic, or psychological disorders. Most impotence caused by endocrine disease is readily reversed; treating nonendocrine impotence is more difficult.

SUGGESTED READING

Belchetz PE: Hormonal treatment of postmenopausal women. N Engl J Med 1994;330:1062.

Braunstein GD: Gynecomastia. N Engl J Med 1993;328:490.

Haseltine FP et al (editors): An NICHD Conference: Androgens and women's health. Am J Med 1995(Suppl 1A):98.

NIH Consensus Conference. Impotence. JAMA 1993;270:83.

Plymate S: Hypogonadism. Endocrinol Metab Clin North Am 1994;23:749.

Warren MP: Evaluation of secondary amenorrhea. J Clin Endocrinol Metab 1996;81:437.

Disorders of Mineral and Bone Metabolism

Michael A. Levine, MD

Patients commonly present with two types of disorders of calcium and phosphorus metabolism, and of bone metabolism and structure. First, most women are at risk for osteoporosis after menopause. Second, patients with many systemic diseases can have disordered mineral metabolism, for example, vitamin D deficiency caused by gastrointestinal malabsorption or chronic renal failure, or hypercalcemia of malignancy.

Internists generally recognize persons with disorders of mineral and bone metabolism in one of three ways: (1) Patients present with a complication of their underlying mineral or skeletal disorder, such as a seizure with hypocalcemia or a hip fracture with osteoporosis. (2) Before patients develop clinical features, their disorder is identified by laboratory or radiographic studies done routinely or to assess another condition. For example, the hypercalcemia of primary hyperparathyroidism may be found on multichannel laboratory screening; Paget's disease may be discovered as an incidental bone lesion on x-ray. (3) Alert physicians anticipate these disorders in characteristic settings, such as secondary hyperparathyroidism in patients with chronic renal insufficiency and osteoporosis in patients being treated with glucocorticoids.

HYPERCALCEMIA

Pathogenesis

The plasma calcium concentration reflects an equilibrium of calcium flux among the extracellular fluid and the skeleton, the gastrointestinal tract, and the kidney. Hypercalcemia is the result of more calcium being delivered to the extracellular fluid compartment than the kidney can remove. Clinicians must be aware that elevations of calcium-binding plasma proteins (eg, albumin), inappropriate

blood sampling technique (eg, prolonged tourniquet application), and laboratory errors all can cause apparent serum calcium elevations that are spurious or not physiologically relevant. After true hypercalcemia is identified, its cause must always be determined (Table 4.6–1).

Clinical Manifestations

The symptoms and signs of hypercalcemia depend on both the level and the rate of elevation of serum calcium concentration. Many patients suffer mental and behavioral disturbances, particularly when the serum calcium concentration exceeds 12 mg/dL; these abnormalities can range from mild confusion and depression to stupor and coma. Patients may also develop muscle weakness and depressed deep tendon reflexes.

Cardiovascular features can include hypertension and electrophysiologic effects—a decreased conduction velocity and shortened refractory period that are similar to and synergistic with the inotropic and toxic manifestations of digitalis. An electrogram (ECG) showing a prolonged QRS complex and a shortened QT interval implies a calcium above 13 mg/dL.

Renal symptoms of polyuria, polydipsia, and nocturia arise from distal tubule and collecting duct resistance to antidiuretic hormone (vasopressin) action. Resulting dehydration can further elevate the calcium level. Hypercalciuria is common and can be complicated by nephrolithiasis and nephrocalcinosis; the latter can lead to potassium wasting, albuminuria, hyposthenuria, and, eventually, azotemia.

Gastrointestinal symptoms can include constipation, dyspepsia, anorexia, nausea, and vomiting. A resulting decrease in fluid intake, along with polyuria, can cause severe dehydration and can worsen hypercalcemia. Abdominal pain may be nonspecific or may indicate pancreatitis or peptic ulcer disease.

Table 4.6–1. Important causes of hypercalcemia.

Primary hyperparathyroidism*
    Parathyroid adenoma
    Parathyroid hyperplasia (eg, multiple endocrine neoplasia
       syndrome [MEN] types I and IIa)
    Familial hypocalciuric hypercalcemia
Malignancy-associated hypercalcemia*
    Humoral hypercalcemia of malignancy
    Local tumor osteolysis
Granulomatous diseases
    Sarcoidosis
    Tuberculosis
    Fungal infections
Medications
    Vitamins A and D
    Thiazide diuretics
    Lithium
Endocrinopathies
    Hyperthyroidism
    Adrenal insufficiency
Immobilization with Paget's disease

*Most common causes.

Differential Diagnosis

The two most common causes of hypercalcemia are primary hyperparathyroidism and malignancy (see Table 4.6–1). The patient's history and a review of previous serum calcium values often suggest which of the two is more likely. Chronic mild hypercalcemia, often associated with kidney stones, is typical of primary hyperparathyroidism; moderate-to-severe hypercalcemia of recent onset, often with weight loss, suggests cancer.

The serum parathyroid hormone concentration is critical in establishing the cause of hypercalcemia. In hyperparathyroidism, the concentration is usually elevated; in malignancy, it is typically suppressed.

Causes

Primary Hyperparathyroidism: About six out of every seven patients with primary hyperparathyroidism have a solitary adenoma in one parathyroid gland. Almost all other patients have four-gland hyperplasia. Parathyroid hyperplasia is usually part of one of the autosomal dominant syndromes of multiple endocrine neoplasia (Chapter 4.1). In less than 1% of patients is primary hyperparathyroidism caused by parathyroid carcinoma.

Classically, primary hyperparathyroidism has been described as a syndrome of "stones, bones, abdominal groans, and psychic overtones," referring to the nephrolithiasis, metabolic bone disease, and nonspecific gastrointestinal and neuropsychiatric complaints of full-blown disease. Other nonspecific symptoms include fatigue, pruritus, metallic taste, dry skin, and joint pain from pseudogout or gout. Actually, because of earlier diagnosis and treatment, more than 50% of patients with primary hyperparathyroidism are now entirely asymptomatic at the time of diagnosis. Only 20% of current patients present with a history of nephrolithiasis or nephrocalcinosis. Less than 2% have marked skeletal disease—osteitis fibrosa cystica,

which causes bone pain; pathologic fracture (fracture without substantial trauma); or overt, radiographically evident loss of bone mass.

Most patients with primary hyperparathyroidism have no physical findings. When a neck mass is palpated, it is much more likely to be an incidental thyroid nodule than a parathyroid adenoma. Rarely, parathyroid carcinoma presents as a palpable neck mass. Hypertension is common and often continues despite correction of hyperparathyroidism. Only rare patients have band keratopathy, representing ectopic calcification of the cornea. Neuromuscular findings can include proximal muscle weakness, cranial nerve abnormalities (especially fasciculations of the tongue), and loss of pain and vibratory sensation.

Osteitis fibrosa cystica, the classic bone lesion in hyperparathyroidism, can cause diffuse bone pain or pathologic fracture. On x-ray, occasional patients have localized bone cysts, a "salt and pepper" appearance of the skull, loss of the lamina dura of the teeth, and subperiosteal erosion of the distal phalangeal tufts or the lateral ends of the clavicles. However, the most common radiographic manifestation of moderate primary hyperparathyroidism is osteopenia, with more bone loss from areas enriched in cortical bone (distal radius) than from sites enriched in cancellous bone (vertebral spine). Milder reductions in bone density can be measured with sensitive techniques like x-ray or dual photon absorptiometry and quantitative computed tomography (CT).

Diagnosis: Primary hyperparathyroidism is confirmed when the serum parathyroid hormone (PTH) concentration is elevated in a patient with hypercalcemia. More than 90% of patients have elevations of both PTH and calcium; the remaining 10% have hypercalcemia with an inappropriately normal PTH level. Although elevated serum PTH concentrations are relatively specific for hyperparathyroidism, increased PTH levels have been described in rare patients taking lithium and a few patients with lung or ovarian cancer.

Management: Surgical excision of the hyperfunctioning parathyroid gland or glands is curative, but not all patients require treatment. Surgery is generally indicated for (1) patients with a serum calcium level more than 1 mg/dL higher than the upper limit of normal; (2) patients with complications of primary hyperparathyroidism or hypercalcemia such as nephrocalcinosis, nephrolithiasis, reduced renal function, or overt bone disease; (3) patients at high risk for renal or skeletal complications, for example, patients with hypercalciuria (above 250 mg per day in women, above 300 mg per day in men) or substantial or progressive bone loss; and (4) young patients who face lifelong exposure to the risks of primary hyperparathyroidism and the expense of monitoring. Surgery should also be considered for patients who have neuromuscular, neuropsychiatric, or gastrointestinal manifestations or who may have difficulty with long-term monitoring.

Surgery for hyperparathyroidism entails identifying and excising the overactive parathyroid gland or glands. Preoperative imaging procedures such as sonography, radionuclide scanning, magnetic resonance imaging (MRI), and CT are imperfect predictors of the position and extent of diseased glands and are rarely indicated unless the patient has already had unsuccessful parathyroid surgery. Likewise, invasive procedures such as venous catheterization with PTH sampling and selective angiography should be reserved for patients who have already undergone surgery. Serum calcium levels generally fall 12–24 hours after successful surgery. Transient mild postoperative hypocalcemia is common. Patients with severe skeletal disease may develop profound hypocalcemia lasting for weeks, so-called "hungry bones."

Patients who do not need surgery should be monitored yearly for evidence of biochemical progression, deterioration of renal function, and progressive skeletal demineralization. They should be advised to maintain adequate hydration to reduce the risk of kidney stones and to remain physically active to limit bone loss. They should avoid thiazide diuretics, which can worsen hypercalcemia. Dietary calcium restriction is of little benefit.

Medical treatments for primary hyperparathyroidism are generally of limited value. Oral neutral phosphate often lowers serum and urinary calcium, but its effect is usually modest and limited by gastrointestinal side effects and the possibility of metastatic tissue calcification. In postmenopausal women, estrogen replacement may lower serum calcium levels and reduce urinary calcium excretion. Patients who present with hypercalcemia of more than 14 mg/dL, particularly if they also have mental deterioration or renal insufficiency, should be treated vigorously to reduce the serum calcium before surgery (see "Management" of hypercalcemia below).

Malignancy: Hypercalcemia is a common complication of many malignant tumors (see Chapter 12.2 and Table 4.6–2). Typically, hypercalcemia appears abruptly and late in the course, when the diagnosis of cancer is already known. In some patients, however, the tumor is occult and must be identified. Finally, physicians should remember that coexisting primary hyperparathyroidism can be responsible for hypercalcemia in a patient with a history of cancer and should not overlook this treatable disorder.

Table 4.6–2. Tumors commonly causing hypercalcemia.

Humoral hypercalcemia of malignancy
  PTHrP-mediated
    Squamous or epidermoid carcinomas (head and neck, lung, esophagus, cervix, vulva, skin)
    Breast cancer
    Bladder and kidney cancer
    Ovarian carcinoma
    Human T-cell leukemia virus (HTLV) I-associated leukemia and lymphoma
  $1,25(OH)_2D$-mediated
    Hodgkin's disease
    Lymphomas

Hypercalcemia caused by skeletal invasion by tumor
  Multiple myeloma
  Breast cancer
  Prostate cancer

Malignancy-associated hypercalcemia can develop in three ways. (1) Patients may have humoral hypercalcemia of malignancy, a syndrome in which the cancer produces a humoral factor, termed PTH-related protein (PTHrP), which increases bone resorption. (2) Lymphocytes from some patients with lymphoma can synthesize and secrete $1,25(OH)_2D$, which enhances intestinal absorption of calcium and accelerates bone resorption. (3) Patients with solid tumors may develop skeletal metastases in which malignant cells release cytokines that can activate osteoclasts (Chapter 12.2).

The diagnosis of malignancy-associated hypercalcemia is supported by serum PTH values that are suppressed or low in a patient with an elevated concentration of total calcium or ionized calcium. Humoral hypercalcemia of malignancy as the cause of hypercalcemia is confirmed by detection of elevated PTHrP levels in specific immunoassays. Serum $1,25(OH)_2D$ concentrations are elevated in many patients with lymphoma, but are normal or depressed in patients with elevated PTHrP levels. Some patients who have direct tumor invasion of bone may need radiographic evaluation of the skeleton and histologic exam of bone biopsy specimens to diagnose cancer as the basis for their hypercalcemia.

Vitamin D Intoxication and Granulomatous Disorders: Hypervitaminosis D is usually caused by excessive use of vitamin D preparations, but vitamin D intoxication has also been described in persons who drank milk that was excessively fortified with vitamin D. Vitamin D intoxication causes excessive gastrointestinal absorption of calcium and accelerated osteoclastic bone resorption. Hypercalciuria typically precedes hypercalcemia and not infrequently leads to renal insufficiency or kidney stones. Affected patients have suppressed serum PTH concentrations, decreased urinary phosphorus and bicarbonate excretion, and, when renal function deteriorates, hyperphosphatemia. Thus, the combination of hypercalcemia, hyperphosphatemia, azotemia, and mild alkalosis suggests vitamin D intoxication. Serum levels of 25(OH)D (25-hydroxyvitamin D) are typically elevated, but $1,25(OH)_2D$ (1,25-dihydroxyvitamin D) levels can be only modestly elevated or normal, because of suppression of PTH and lack of its enhancement of renal 1-hydroxylation activity. 25(OH)D is 25-hydroxyvitamin D, which includes both $25(OH)D_3$, made from cholecalciferol, synthesized in the skin in response to sunlight, and $25(OH)D_2$, made from diet-derived ergocalciferol. $1,25(OH)_2D$ is 1,25-dihydroxyvitamin D, which includes both $1,25(OH)_2D_2$ and $1,25(OH)_2D_3$ (calcitriol).

A form of endogenous vitamin D intoxication affects patients with sarcoidosis or other granulomatous diseases like tuberculosis. These patients commonly develop hypercalcemia, hypercalciuria, or both, as a consequence of elevated serum $1,25(OH)_2D$ levels. Activated pulmonary alveolar macrophages and lymphocytes convert dietary or sunlight-derived 25(OH)D to $1,25(OH)_2D$ in an unregulated fashion that depends on the serum concentration of 25(OH)D rather than the body's need for $1,25(OH)_2D$.

Glucocorticoid therapy ameliorates both exogenous and endogenous vitamin D intoxication. Glucocorticoids act by decreasing ectopic 1-hydroxylation, inhibiting vitamin D action in the small intestine and increasing renal clearance of calcium.

Medications: Thiazide diuretics often cause mild short-term hypercalcemia by contracting volume and enhancing renal conservation of calcium. Persistent hypercalcemia in a patient who is taking a thiazide diuretic suggests an underlying disorder of mineral metabolism, most likely primary hyperparathyroidism. Vitamin A, lithium, and theophylline are less often implicated as causing hypercalcemia.

Miscellaneous Causes: Hyperthyroidism, adrenal insufficiency, and pheochromocytoma are unusual endocrine causes of mild hypercalcemia. Estrogens and anti-estrogens can cause hypercalcemia in patients who have metastatic breast cancer.

Immobilization, as with prolonged bed rest, accelerates osteoclastic bone resorption and decreases osteoblastic bone formation. Hypercalciuria and hypercalcemia occasionally affect immobilized patients whose bone turnover is high, for example, growing children and adolescents and patients with primary hyperparathyroidism, hyperthyroidism, or extensive Paget's disease. Weightlessness, as during space flight, can also lead to decreased bone mass and hypercalciuria. An unusual cause of hypercalcemia is milk alkali syndrome, caused by ingestion of excessive quantities of alkaline calcium salts.

Familial hypocalciuric hypercalcemia (also called benign familial hypercalcemia) is an asymptomatic, benign autosomal dominant condition in which hypercalcemia begins before age 10. This condition is caused by mutations in the gene encoding a calcium receptor expressed on parathyroid and renal tubular cells. Renal clearance of calcium is markedly reduced, and the ratio of calcium clearance to creatinine clearance is typically less than 0.01, far below that in typical primary hyperparathyroidism. Patients with familial hypocalciuric hypercalcemia have mild hyperplasia of all parathyroid glands and normal or mildly elevated serum PTH concentrations. Complications of hypercalcemia are infrequent except in newborns, in whom the disease may manifest paradoxically as life-threatening hypercalcemia.

Management

Patients with mild hypercalcemia (serum calcium below 12 mg/dL) typically derive little benefit from a reduction in serum calcium concentration. By contrast, patients with a serum calcium above 12 mg/dL should be treated to reduce their risk for complications, and patients with severe hypercalcemia (above 14 mg/dL) should receive urgent treatment.

Treatment of hypercalcemia has three aims: to increase renal clearance of calcium, to decrease skeletal release of calcium, and to treat the underlying cause. The most important initial measure is volume expansion. Saline in-

creases glomerular filtration and inhibits tubular reabsorption of calcium, thus increasing calcium excretion. Calciuria can be further enhanced by a loop diuretic, given carefully to avoid dehydrating the patient. Patients who are refractory to volume expansion or have renal insufficiency may respond to peritoneal or hemodialysis with a low-calcium solution.

Patients who have severe hypercalcemia or whose serum calcium remains high after treatment with saline and loop diuretics should be treated so as to inhibit osteoclast-mediated bone resorption. The bisphosphonates etidronate and pamidronate are both highly effective in reducing bone resorption. Because bisphosphonates are poorly absorbed in the gastrointestinal tract, they must be given intravenously to treat hypercalcemia. Pamidronate is more potent than etidronate. After a single dose, 70–90% of patients have a normal serum calcium. The drug causes an initial decline within 2 days and a nadir within 7 days. Its duration of action ranges from 1 to several weeks.

Plicamycin (formerly called mithramycin) is another effective antiresorptive agent that is best suited for patients who do not respond to pamidronate; plicamycin can have significant toxicity. Another option for these patients is gallium nitrate. Clinical experience is still too limited to say whether gallium nitrate is more effective than other compounds, but it is known to be potentially nephrotoxic. Calcitonin is fast-acting—it can lower the serum calcium within a few hours—but it is a weak agent that rarely reduces the calcium to normal. Glucocorticoids are effective treatments for the hypercalcemia not only of adrenal insufficiency but also of vitamin D intoxication, sarcoidosis, milk alkali syndrome, lymphoma, breast cancer, and multiple myeloma. Finally, intravenous infusion of phosphate effectively and reliably reduces serum calcium, primarily by precipitating calcium into bone and soft tissue. However, because widespread metastatic calcification, life-threatening arrhythmias, and irreversible renal damage have been reported as complications of phosphate treatment, it should be used only as a last resort. Oral phosphate therapy has no role in the acute management of hypercalcemia, but it can be useful in the chronic management of mild hypercalcemia.

HYPOCALCEMIA

Hypocalcemia develops when either PTH or vitamin D is deficient or defective, or when target tissues fail to respond to either hormone. Serum albumin levels and pH can influence the calcium concentration; therefore, diagnosis by measurement of the ionized calcium concentration is preferred in patients with plasma protein or systemic acid-base abnormalities. The pathognomonic clinical feature of hypocalcemia is tetany, a condition characterized by muscle cramps that can progress to carpopedal spasm; few patients develop generalized muscle spasm, laryngospasm, or seizures. Patients with mild hypocalcemia typically have perioral or acral paresthesias. Patients with severe hypocalcemia may also experience emotional lability, anxiety, delirium, and frank psychosis.

An important sign of hypocalcemia is carpopedal spasm, which the physician can elicit by compressing nerves in the patient's upper arm with a sphygmomanometer inflated 20 mm Hg above the systolic pressure for 3 minutes (Trousseau's sign). The clinician may also glean evidence of increased neuromuscular irritability by tapping the patient's facial nerve anterior to the parotid gland and then observing contraction of facial muscles (Chvostek's sign); however, this sign can also be elicited in 10% of persons who have a normal serum calcium.

Patients with severe hypocalcemia have a prolonged QT interval on ECG. Rare patients have decreased cardiac contractility and heart failure. Some patients have papilledema, with or without a rise in cerebrospinal fluid pressure. Patients with chronic hypocalcemia and elevated serum phosphate levels may develop cataracts and calcification of the basal ganglia.

Causes

The causes of hypocalcemia can be divided into conditions associated with decreased and elevated serum PTH concentrations.

Hypoparathyroidism: The most common cause of hypoparathyroidism is destruction or damage to the parathyroid glands, typically a consequence of parathyroid, thyroid, or neck cancer surgery (Table 4.6–3). Less common causes of hypoparathyroidism are radiation-induced damage or infiltration of the parathyroid glands by metastatic cancer cells, by iron in hemochromatosis, or by

Table 4.6–3. Important causes of hypocalcemia.

Conditions with decreased parathyroid gland function
Hypoparathyroidism
  Idiopathic, familial, autoimmune hypoparathyroidism
  Surgical hypoparathyroidism
Depressed parathyroid gland function
  Infiltration with iron, copper, cancer
  Hypo- or hypermagnesemia

Conditions with increased parathyroid gland function
Inadequate vitamin D
  Dietary deficiency
  Malabsorption syndrome, gastric surgery
Impaired activation of vitamin D
  Liver diseases (eg, chronic active hepatitis, primary biliary
    cirrhosis)
  Kidney diseases
  Vitamin D-dependent rickets type I
Target organ resistance to $1,25(OH)_2D$
  Vitamin D-dependent rickets type II
Target organ resistance to parathyroid hormone
  Pseudohypoparathyroidism
  Magnesium deficiency
Acute pancreatitis
Acute rhabdomyolysis
Multiple transfusions of citrated blood

copper in Wilson's disease. Other uncommon causes are idiopathic, autoimmune, and familial hypoparathyroidism. These disorders are usually detected in childhood, but some patients are diagnosed as adults. Autoimmune hypoparathyroidism has been reported in siblings. It may also appear as a component of type I polyglandular autoimmune syndrome, in association with primary adrenal insufficiency, moniliasis, diabetes mellitus, hypothyroidism, pernicious anemia, chronic hepatitis, malabsorption, and hypogonadism. Familial hypoparathyroidism may result from an inactivating mutation in the structural gene for PTH or an activating mutation of the calcium sensing receptor gene. Congenital absence of the parathyroids and thymus, caused by maldevelopment of the third and fourth branchial pouches, is termed DiGeorge syndrome.

Markedly high or low serum concentrations of magnesium are uncommon causes of hypocalcemia. High magnesium levels can suppress PTH secretion and may possibly inhibit PTH action. Magnesium intoxication, unusual in patients who have normal renal function, is almost always caused by excessive intake of or treatment with magnesium salts. Paradoxically, severe hypomagnesemia can also cause hypocalcemia, through reversible interference with either parathyroid gland secretion or target tissue responsiveness to PTH.

Pseudohypoparathyroidism describes a group of diverse endocrine syndromes that share a resistance by the target organs—bone and kidney—to the biologic actions of PTH. Patients with pseudohypoparathyroidism display the biochemical features of hypoparathyroidism—hypocalcemia and hyperphosphatemia—despite generally high circulating PTH levels. Patients with pseudohypoparathyroidism type Ia have a genetic deficiency of the $G_s\alpha$ protein that couples hormone receptors to activation of adenylyl cyclase. These patients have generalized hormone resistance as well as a peculiar constellation of somatic characteristics including subcutaneous ossifications, brachydactyly (short metacarpals), obesity, round facies, and short stature.

Nonhypoparathyroid Hypocalcemia: Vitamin D deficiency, whether it is caused by dietary insufficiency, impaired vitamin D synthesis in the skin, or defective activation of $1,25(OH)_2D$ in the liver or kidney, leads to reduced gastrointestinal calcium absorption and impaired mobilization of calcium from the skeleton. Profound hypocalcemia is unusual in vitamin D-deficient disorders because patients develop secondary hyperparathyroidism. Laboratory findings suggesting vitamin D deficiency include low to low-normal serum calcium, high serum PTH, hypophosphatemia, and high serum alkaline phosphatase levels. This hypocalcemia and hypophosphatemia may lead to impaired mineralization of bone, conditions termed "osteomalacia" and "rickets" (see "Osteomalacia and Rickets" below).

Vitamin D deficiency is unusual in the United States and other countries where milk and other foods are fortified with vitamin D. In these countries, dietary vitamin D deficiency is found mainly in food faddists and people who have inadequate exposure to both sunshine and dietary vitamin D. Two groups at risk are breast-fed infants of dark-skinned mothers and confined elderly people who have a nutritionally restricted diet. In developed countries, vitamin D deficiency is more likely to affect patients who have a malabsorption syndrome or receive long-term treatment with drugs such as phenytoin or barbiturates, which accelerate hepatic catabolism of vitamin D. Impaired conversion of 25(OH)D to 1,25(OH)$_2$D, and secondary hyperparathyroidism, are central to the pathogenesis of renal osteodystrophy (Chapter 5.5). Vitamin D-dependent rickets is an uncommon autosomal recessive disorder in which children are unable to synthesize 1,25(OH)$_2$D (type I) or respond to it (type II).

Miscellaneous Causes: Hypocalcemia can accompany acute pancreatitis, fat embolism, rhabdomyolysis, sepsis, osteoblastic metastases, and liver failure. Systemic alkalosis can depress the ionized calcium concentration and produce tetany, as happens in the hyperventilation syndrome, alkali ingestion, and hypokalemia. Finally, hypocalcemia can be produced by hypocalcemic agents such as plicamycin, bisphosphonates, calcitonin, phosphate, and ethylenediaminetetra-acetic acid (EDTA), and by multiple transfusions of citrated blood. A careful history and measurement of serum electrolytes can usually identify these causes.

Management

The goals of treating hypocalcemia are to relieve symptoms and maintain serum calcium in the low-normal range (8.5–9.5 mg/dL). Patients with marked hypocalcemia or symptoms of tetany should be treated with intravenous calcium. Acute symptoms are quickly relieved by a single ampule of calcium gluconate given by slow intravenous injection. Thereafter, patients should be given calcium gluconate by continuous or repeated (eg, every 4–6 hours) intravenous infusion until symptoms of tetany have resolved and hypocalcemia has been corrected. Serum calcium levels should be closely monitored during intravenous therapy. Patients should be started on oral therapy with calcium and a vitamin D preparation if the clinician anticipates persistent hypocalcemia.

Most patients with nutritional vitamin D deficiency can be treated with multivitamin supplements; severe deficiency may require pharmacologic amounts of vitamin D. Chronic hypoparathyroidism should be treated with oral calcium combined with vitamin D or one of its metabolites. The choice of vitamin D preparation depends on cost (ergocalciferol is least expensive), duration of action (calcitriol has the shortest half-life), and underlying pathophysiology. Patients with renal failure cannot convert 25(OH)D to 1,25(OH)$_2$D, and so must be treated with calcitriol.

In the absence of PTH, tubular reabsorption of calcium is diminished, so patients who are treated too vigorously may develop hypercalciuria. In addition to calcium and vitamin D supplements, some patients with hypoparathyroidism require a thiazide diuretic plus a low-salt diet to maintain eucalcemia while avoiding hypercalciuria.

HYPOPHOSPHATEMIA

Although moderate hypophosphatemia (1–2.5 mg/dL) is common in hospitalized patients, these patients do not develop signs and symptoms of phosphate deficiency until the phosphate drops below 1 mg/dL. Because only 1% of total body phosphate is in extracellular fluids, hypophosphatemia does not necessarily indicate total body phosphate depletion. Conversely, a patient can suffer significant phosphate depletion despite normal serum phosphate concentrations.

Hypophosphatemia results from decreased gastrointestinal absorption of phosphorus, increased urinary loss of phosphorus, or a shift of phosphate from the extracellular to the intracellular compartment. Measurement of urinary phosphate excretion is helpful in distinguishing among these three general mechanisms. In alcohol abusers, severe hypophosphatemia can result from poor nutrition, vomiting, and increased urinary loss of phosphate. Chronic hypophosphatemia can be caused by abnormal proximal tubular reabsorption of phosphate, as in Fanconi's syndrome.

Phosphate depletion has widespread clinical consequences. Many patients experience muscle weakness or myalgia. Few have congestive heart failure or rhabdomyolysis. Patients with severe hypophosphatemia can develop metabolic encephalopathy or renal dysfunction. Hematologic consequences include red cell dysfunction and, rarely, hemolysis; impaired leukocyte function and a predisposition to infection; and shortened platelet survival.

Chronic hypophosphatemia may lead to rickets or osteomalacia (see "Osteomalacia and Rickets" below). Although the clinical and radiographic features of hypophosphatemic rickets are similar to those of calcium or vitamin D deficiency, patients with this form of hypophosphatemia do not develop hypocalcemia or secondary hyperparathyroidism.

A number of benign neoplasms, including giant cell, mesenchymal, angiomatous, and sarcomatous tumors, can produce a hypophosphatemic syndrome that has been termed *oncogenous osteomalacia.* Analogous disturbances afflict patients with extensive fibrous dysplasia of bone, neurofibromatosis, metastatic carcinoma of the breast or prostate, and multiple myeloma.

Patients with serum phosphorus concentrations below 2 mg/dL should receive supplemental phosphorus. Moderate hypophosphatemia may be treated with milk or other dairy products. An alternative is supplements of the neutral salt, given orally, intravenously, or rectally. Patients with oncogenous osteomalacia require aggressive therapy with pharmacologic doses of phosphorus and calcitriol.

METABOLIC BONE DISEASES

Metabolic bone diseases can be characterized by decreased bone mass (osteopenia) with normal (osteoporosis) or defective (rickets, osteomalacia) bone mineralization, and dysplastic bone formation (eg, Paget's disease, McCune-Albright syndrome). Osteoporosis, the most common cause of osteopenia in countries that fortify foods with vitamin D, increases patients' risk for fracture.

Osteomalacia and Rickets

Inadequate supplies of either calcium or phosphate impair mineralization of the bone matrix (osteoid) and lead to rickets in children, or its adult counterpart, osteomalacia. *Rickets,* a condition of defective mineralization in growing bone, can cause skeletal deformities. Adults with osteomalacia rarely develop skeletal deformities because their mineralization defect affects only mature bone. Osteomalacia causes subtle clinical manifestations of diffuse muscle weakness and bone pain. The most common radiographic manifestation of osteomalacia is a generalized decrease in bone density, although some patients develop pseudofractures ("Milkman's lines," also called "Looser's zones") on the concave sides of the shafts of the long bones, ribs, scapulae, and pubic rami.

Rickets and osteomalacia are diagnosed by examining nondecalcified sections of a bone biopsy specimen. Before the biopsy, patients should receive two 3-day pulses of tetracycline 10–14 days apart, to "label" the areas of active osteoid mineralization. The biopsy should be performed 1–2 days after the last tetracycline dose. Normally, mineralizing osteoid shows two fluorescent lines corresponding to tetracycline-labeled mineralization fronts. A widened noncalcified osteoid seam with diffuse or absent fluorescence is diagnostic of defective mineralization.

Rickets and osteomalacia most commonly arise from deficiencies of vitamin D, calcium, or phosphate, but other causes are possible, including inherited defects in vitamin D action or phosphate metabolism. Reduced intestinal calcium absorption in patients with vitamin D deficiency often causes secondary hyperparathyroidism, which then leads to decreased renal tubular reabsorption of phosphate and to hypophosphatemia and an increased skeletal alkaline phosphatase concentration. Serum levels of $25(OH)D$ and $1,25(OH)_2D$ may be normal, high, or low, depending on the pathophysiology.

Osteoporosis

Primary osteoporosis is often subclassified into two archetypal syndromes. Type I (postmenopausal) osteoporosis, which affects 25% of white women, characteristically appears 10–15 years after menopause. A lower percentage of hypogonadal men develop an equivalent disorder. It has been proposed that bone resorption and mobilization of skeletal calcium are increased by loss of the protective effects of gonadal hormones on the skeleton. Patients have accelerated and disproportionate loss of trabecular bone.

The most common clinical manifestations are vertebral crush fractures, distal wrist (Colles') fractures, and mandibular resorption with increased tooth loss. Typically, minimal trauma causes vertebral compression fractures, often with acute back pain and progressive loss of height. The most frequently affected vertebrae are those from T6 to L3; complete compression is more characteristic than anterior wedging.

Type II (senile) osteoporosis causes proportionate losses of trabecular and cortical bone. This disorder affects both women and men (female:male ratio = 2:1) aged 70 and older. The main complications are hip, pelvic, and vertebral fractures. Vertebral fractures are characteristically of the wedge type, leading to progressive dorsal kyphosis (dowager's hump). As with postmenopausal osteoporosis, the pathogenesis of senile osteoporosis is uncertain. One theory is age-related decreases in osteoblast function and renal production of $1,25(OH)_2D$, leading to reduced intestinal absorption of calcium and to mild secondary hyperparathyroidism.

Other features may play a role in the pathogenesis of both types of osteoporosis. Genetic and constitutional factors are important determinants of peak bone mass and may influence the rate of bone loss. In general, white and Asian women have a greater risk of osteoporosis than black women. Many patients with osteoporosis are less muscular, have a lower average body weight, and have a lighter frame with thinner bones than do unaffected people. A significant risk factor is cigarette smoking, which is linked to low circulating estrogen levels and early menopause. A high alcohol and caffeine intake contributes to excess bone loss. A sedentary lifestyle is a risk factor, as is immobilization. Conversely, weight-bearing exercise and physical activity increase bone formation and can reverse bone loss in some patients with osteoporosis. Studies of a role for dietary calcium deficiency in osteoporosis are incomplete or conflicting.

Osteoporosis can develop secondary to a number of systemic diseases, heritable conditions, and medications, all of which must be ruled out before primary osteoporosis can be established. Malignancies, particularly multiple myeloma, can also masquerade as primary osteoporosis.

If a patient does not have a typical fracture, osteopenia can be confirmed by a demonstration of reduced bone mass. Standard x-rays are a relatively insensitive indicator of bone loss because typically at least 30% of bone density must be lost before becoming noticeable on x-ray. Nonetheless, radiographic features of the osteoporotic vertebral body can include increasing prominence of both vertical striations and end plates as trabecular bone mass decreases—so-called "picture frame" vertebral bodies. The intervertebral disks often intrude on the weakened vertebral body, leading to biconcave "codfish" vertebrae.

Dual photon and dual energy x-ray absorptiometry and quantitative CT can establish whether a patient has lost enough bone mass to be at risk for fracture. Bone mass measurements are indicated for (1) estrogen-deficient women in whom a diagnosis of reduced bone mass would help the physician make decisions about hormone replacement therapy, (2) patients who have vertebral abnormalities or radiographic evidence of osteopenia, and (3) patients with asymptomatic primary hyperparathyroidism, in whom a low or decreasing bone mass would be an indication for surgery. Bone mass measurements should also be considered for patients who are to receive long-term treatment with glucocorticoids, thyroid hormone, or anticonvulsants. Otherwise, routine measurement of bone mass in asymptomatic patients is not clinically useful.

Blood studies in primary osteoporosis are nearly always normal. Some patients have mild hypercalciuria, but most have normal excretion rates of calcium and phosphorus. Measurement of urinary excretion of pyridinium cross-links or *N-telopeptides* (breakdown products of bone collagen) can identify patients who have accelerated bone resorption. The physician should exclude other causes of secondary osteoporosis such as Cushing's syndrome, hyperthyroidism, and occult malignancies like multiple myeloma.

Management: The cornerstone of osteoporosis management is prevention of further bone loss. Secondary osteoporosis should be managed with treatment of the underlying condition, for example, reducing excessive doses of thyroid hormone or glucocorticoids.

The most effective treatment for women with type I osteoporosis is estrogen. Estrogen decreases the rate of bone resorption and reduces risk for bone fracture. Estrogen replacement therapy appears to be of benefit in inhibiting bone turnover, no matter how long after menopause it is given. Although estrogen is primarily an antiresorptive agent, many patients experience a modest (2–4%/year) increase in bone mass during the first few years of therapy. In some studies, a combination of estrogen and progestin increases bone mass even more. Estrogen's effects persist as long as therapy continues, but bone loss begins again when treatment is stopped. Thus, most patients should receive long-term treatment, for 10–15 years.

Women with an intact uterus should be prescribed estrogen combined with a progestin to lower the risk of endometrial carcinoma. There is less consensus about risk for breast cancer in women who receive estrogen therapy. However, authorities agree that estrogen should not be routinely prescribed for postmenopausal women who have had breast cancer. These patients may benefit from tamoxifen, an estrogen antagonist that may also reduce bone loss and prevent osteoporosis.

All patients with osteoporosis who do not have hypercalciuria should maintain a calcium intake of 1000 mg/day; 1500 mg/day is indicated for postmenopausal women who are not taking estrogen replacement. Higher calcium intake than this has not been shown to be more effective, and it may cause hypercalciuria. Patients should receive the recommended daily allowance of vitamin D (400 IU). Higher doses of vitamin D, or therapy with any of its more active metabolites, may accelerate bone destruction and should be reserved for patients with specific disorders of vitamin D metabolism.

Several alternatives to estrogen are available to prevent and treat osteoporosis. In the United States, salmon calcitonin has been approved for treatment of osteoporosis, but has not yet been shown effective in prevention. Salmon calcitonin is also a reasonable treatment for young men and women who have high bone turnover, idiopathic osteoporosis, or glucocorticoid-induced osteoporosis. New bisphosphonates and sodium fluoride are being tested in the treatment of osteoporosis. Daily therapy with alendronate can significantly increase bone mass and reduce fractures.

Patients should be taken off unnecessary or excessive medications that increase bone loss or the tendency to fall and should be given common-sense advice to help avoid falls.

Paget's Disease

Paget's disease is a disorder of locally increased bone remodeling. Clinical manifestations depend on the lesions' location and extent. Most patients are asymptomatic; their lesions are detected during radiographic evaluation of unrelated illness. Local pain and joint stiffness are common complaints in the minority of patients who are symptomatic when diagnosed. Because the spine, pelvis, femur, and skull are the usual sites of involvement, common symptoms are hip pain, lower back pain, headaches, and tinnitus. Patients may present with pathologic fractures.

The most common neurologic complication in patients with Paget's disease is combined conductive and sensorineural hearing loss. In advanced disease, basilar skull invagination may compress the cerebellar tonsils and lead to progressive ataxia and quadriplegia. Paraplegia can be caused by concentric narrowing of the spinal canal or shunting of blood away from the spinal cord through hypervascular skin and bone.

Patients with extensive skeletal involvement may have markedly increased cardiac output because of augmented bone blood flow. This hyperkinetic circulation can aggravate preexisting cardiac dysfunction and hasten the development of congestive heart failure in the elderly.

Physical findings, when present, are an enlarged skull with prominent superficial veins, as well as impaired hearing, progressive kyphosis with shortening of stature, and deformity of long bones. The skin overlying a lesion may feel warm, and flow murmurs may be audible. Some patients have angioid streaks in the retina.

Paget's disease is more common in the elderly than is generally recognized. About 3% of all adults may be affected, and, by the ninth decade, as many as 5–11%. The basic pathologic process is excessive osteoclastic activity accelerating bone resorption, followed by osteoblastic regeneration and formation of new bone. But this new bone is defective and often deformed. Fortunately, less than 1% of patients suffer sarcomatous degeneration of their bone lesions. And most patients do not develop new lesions after they have been diagnosed with Paget's disease; rather, existing bone lesions tend to worsen and cause greater disability. The etiology of Paget's disease remains unknown; one possibility is a slow virus infection of the osteoclasts.

Serum calcium and phosphorus are usually normal. Hypercalciuria is common. However, when patients are immobilized with severe pain or fractures, their excessive bone resorption continues while new bone formation is diminished, potentially causing hypercalcemia.

Management: Evaluation of patients with Paget's disease entails localizing their lesions and defining the extent and severity of their disease activity. The anatomic evaluation can be made by conventional radiography and radioisotope scanning. About 85% of bone lesions can be detected by both radiography and scanning; 10% are visualized by x-ray alone and 5% by scan alone. Most lesions detected by bone scan are symptomatic. Measurements of urinary excretion of pyridinium crosslinks and hydroxyproline reflect the rate of osteoclastic bone resorption and are useful indices of disease activity, whereas serum alkaline phosphatase and osteocalcin concentrations reflect bone formation. These markers can be used to assess response to treatment.

Patients with mild Paget's disease can be treated symptomatically with nonsteroidal anti-inflammatory drugs or acetaminophen. Indications for more specific treatment include significant bone pain, hearing loss, neurologic compromise, high-output congestive heart failure, prevention of further deformity, preparation for joint replacement, and markedly elevated (greater than three times normal) levels of serum alkaline phosphatase.

Paget's disease is usually amenable to treatment with calcitonin, which restores normal bone remodeling. Salmon calcitonin, by virtue of its long half-life, has proved more potent than porcine or human calcitonin. However, in many patients the efficacy of salmon calcitonin may be limited by development of antibodies that neutralize the hormone. Human calcitonin often restores responsiveness in these patients.

Paget's disease can also be treated with bisphosphonates, which bind strongly to hydroxyapatite crystals to slow bone turnover. These agents are as effective as calcitonin. Oral etidronate should not be given for periods longer than 6 months because after this time it may impair bone mineralization. Even more useful than etidronate are newer drugs like pamidronate and alendronate.

Polyostotic Fibrous Dysplasia (McCune-Albright Syndrome)

McCune-Albright syndrome is the triad of polyostotic fibrous dysplasia, cutaneous hyperpigmentation, and endocrine dysfunction. Radiographically, the bone lesions look like cysts in the cortex or ground glass in expanded cortex. The skin lesions are café-au-lait spots with irregular ("coast of Maine") outlines, typically in a dermatomal distribution. Both bone and skin involvement is usually unilateral, often on the same side. Associated endocrine syndromes are precocious puberty, hyperthyroidism, hypercortisolism, growth hormone excess, and hyperprolactinemia.

Patients with the McCune-Albright syndrome have postzygotic somatic mutations in the $G_s\alpha$ gene that enhance activity of the protein $G_s\alpha$. In affected bone, skin, and endocrine tissues, these mutations lead to constitutive activation of adenylyl cyclase, resulting in the proliferation and autonomous hyperfunction of hormonally responsive cells. The mosaic distribution of cells containing the $G_s\alpha$-activating mutation no doubt accounts for the unusual distribution of skin, bone, and endocrine lesions.

The endocrine manifestations in McCune-Albright syndrome are managed according to the specific therapy for each endocrine disorder. Fibrous dysplasia may respond to treatment with new, powerful bisphosphonates such as pamidronate or alendronate.

SUMMARY

▶ Primary hyperparathyroidism and malignancy, the most common causes of hypercalcemia, can be distinguished by measuring the serum parathyroid hormone concentration.

▶ Surgical hypoparathyroidism and magnesium deficiency are the most common causes of hypocalcemia, which can cause paresthesias, tetany, and seizures.

▶ The common metabolic bone disease postmenopausal osteoporosis is most effectively treated by estrogen replacement.

▶ Most patients with Paget's disease are asymptomatic and require no specific therapy. Calcitonin or bisphosphonate therapy is indicated for patients with pain, progressive deformity, neurologic compression syndromes, or heart failure.

SUGGESTED READING

Bilezikian JP: Management of acute hypercalcemia. N Engl J Med 1992;326:1196.

Favus MJ et al (editors): *Primer on the Metabolic Bone Diseases and Disorders of Mineral Metabolism,* 2nd ed. Raven Press, 1993.

Liberman UA et al: Effect of oral alendronate on bone mineral density and the incidence of fractures in postmenopausal osteoporosis. N Engl J Med 1995;333:1437.

Slatopolsky E, Hruska K, Klahr S: Disorders of phosphorus, calcium, and magnesium metabolism. In: *Diseases of the Kidney,* 5th ed. Schrier RW, Gottschalk CW (editors). Little, Brown, 1993.

Diabetes Mellitus

Christopher D. Saudek, MD

Diabetes mellitus is defined by hyperglycemia. When people have blood glucose levels greater than about 200 mg/dL, they develop polydipsia (excessive thirst), polyuria (excessive urination), fatigue, and weight loss. Asymptomatic hyperglycemia is sometimes detected by blood glucose testing.

Diabetes has multiple etiologies, multiple metabolic abnormalities, and multisystem complications. The hyperglycemia is caused by insufficient circulating insulin, resulting from either absolute hormone deficiency or peripheral tissue resistance to its actions. Other metabolic aberrations, such as hypertriglyceridemia and ketosis, are also caused primarily by insufficient insulin secretion. Secondary complications of diabetes mellitus include a microangiopathy that principally affects the kidney and retina, as well as atherosclerotic vascular disease and several forms of neuropathy. The likelihood of developing these complications correlates with the severity of chronic hyperglycemia.

The physician's goal is to reduce acute and long-term diabetic complications by managing the insulin-glucose dynamics and controlling other risk factors. A person with inadequately treated diabetes may suffer severe acute and chronic complications, whereas most well-treated people can lead a long and healthy life.

GENERAL CONSIDERATIONS

Diabetes has an enormous impact on an individual and a family. Restrictions on diet and living patterns require self-discipline. Add to this the fear of complications, the sense of being different, widespread job and licensing discrimination, and difficulty obtaining affordable insurance, and it is clear that diabetes takes an emotional as well as a physical toll.

Diabetes affects 6% of the United States population—14 million people, 50% of them undiagnosed. The disease is especially prevalent in American blacks, Hispanics, and Pima Indians.

Diagnosis

The diagnosis of diabetes can be established or excluded with certainty. Even when diabetes has a gradual onset or its symptoms are subtle, it can be positively diagnosed by established blood glucose criteria (Table 4.7–1). Although few patients need it, the 75-g oral glucose tolerance test is the definitive way to establish the diagnosis or rule it out. Screening for diabetes with random or postprandial plasma glucose determinations is indicated in pregnant women and in persons at high risk for diabetes, for example, obese people, women who have borne large babies, and people with a strong family history or suggestive symptoms.

Classification

Since classification guides treatment, it is important to classify the patient correctly. The current categories are based on typical clinical features more than pathogenesis. The two common forms of primary diabetes are *insulin-dependent diabetes mellitus* (IDDM; type I) and *non-insulin-dependent diabetes mellitus* (NIDDM; type II) (Table 4.7–2). Type I diabetes most commonly develops in young persons of normal or low weight who have little or no endogenous insulin secretion. In contrast, type II diabetes typically presents in middle-aged or older persons who are overweight and have peripheral tissue resistance to a normal or high plasma insulin level. In the so-called secondary forms of diabetes, the cause is usually clear, for example, surgical pancreatectomy, pancreatitis, or corticosteroid use. *Gestational diabetes mellitus* is so common and carries such serious implications for the developing fetus that it merits a category of its own. Finally, *impaired glucose tolerance* is a diagnosis made when oral glucose tolerance tests results are abnormal but do not meet the criteria for diabetes (see Table 4.7–1).

Acute Complications

The acute complications of diabetes are those caused directly and immediately by lack of insulin in a person with a high blood glucose level (Table 4.7–3). These com-

Table 4.7–1. Glycemic criteria for diabetes mellitus and impaired glucose tolerance.

Normal glucose tolerance in nonpregnant adults
 Fasting plasma glucose <140 mg/dL *and*
 After 75 g oral glucose, plasma glucose:

at 30 min	60 min	90 min	120 min
<200	<200	<200	<140 mg/dL

 (A plasma glucose higher than these values but not meeting the criteria for impaired glucose tolerance or diabetes is considered nondiagnostic)

Diabetes mellitus in nonpregnant adults
 Random plasma glucose ≥200 mg/dL, with classic symptoms of hyperglycemia (polydipsia, polyuria, weight loss) *or*
 Fasting plasma glucose ≥140 mg/dL at least twice *or*
 After 75 g oral glucose, plasma glucose ≥200 mg/dL at 2 hr *and* at least once between 0 and 2 hr

Gestational diabetes mellitus (pregnant women)
 After 100 g oral glucose, two plasma glucose values:

Fasting	at 60 min	120 min	180 min
>105	>190	>165	>145 mg/dL

Impaired glucose tolerance in nonpregnant adults
 Fasting plasma glucose <140 mg/dL *and*
 After 75 g oral glucose, plasma glucose 140–200 mg/dL at 2 hr *and* ≥200 mg/dL at least once between 0 and 2 hr

plications resolve within hours to days after glycemic control improves. Polydipsia can be so severe that patients drink gallons of liquid each day; polydipsia is a response to the hyperosmolarity of high blood glucose, with each 100 mg/dL of blood glucose contributing 5.5 mOsm/L. Polyuria is caused both by increased fluid intake and by

Table 4.7–2. Clinical features of insulin-dependent diabetes mellitus (IDDM) and non-insulin-dependent diabetes mellitus (NIDDM).

Feature	IDDM (Type I)	NIDDM (Type II)
Age at onset	Usually <40 yr	Usually >40 yr (except MODY)
Body weight	Usually normal or low	Usually overweight
Family history of diabetes	Uncommon	Common
Residual endogenous insulin secretion	No	Yes
Peripheral insulin resistance	Sometimes	Yes
Labile glycemic control	Usually yes	Usually no
Sulfonylurea treatment required	No	Sometimes yes
Insulin treatment required	Yes	Sometimes yes
Tendency to diabetic ketoacidosis	Yes	No
Tendency to hyperosmolar coma	No	Yes
Tendency to long-term complications	Yes	Yes

MODY, maturity-onset diabetes of youth.

Dx: >140 mg/dl upon fasting (2x tested)

Table 4.7–3. Acute and long-term complications of diabetes mellitus.

Acute
 Polydipsia (excessive thirst)
 Polyuria (excessive urination)
 Weight loss
 Fatigue
 Poor wound healing
 Blurred vision
 Vaginitis
 Diabetic ketoacidosis
 Hyperosmolar nonketotic states

Long-term
 Small-vessel disease: retinopathy, nephropathy
 Large-vessel atherosclerosis: peripheral vascular disease, coronary artery disease, cerebrovascular accidents
 Neuropathy (see Table 4.7–7)
 Dermopathy: necrobiosis lipoidica diabeticorum, shin spots, lipid hypertrophy, lipoatrophy
 Dental caries, gingivitis

osmotic diuresis from glucosuria. Weight loss is caused predominantly by glucose spilling into the urine. Other acute complications, such as fatigue, blurred vision, poor wound healing, and vaginitis, are less specific but equally suggestive of poor glycemic control.

Two distinct syndromes caused by uncontrolled metabolic complications of diabetes are potentially fatal emergencies: diabetic ketoacidosis and nonketotic hyperosmolar states. Ketoacidosis is the hallmark of untreated IDDM; nonketotic hyperosmolar states can develop in NIDDM.

Long-Term Complications

The long-term complications of diabetes can develop after years to decades of disease (see Table 4.7–3). Typically, these complications do not reverse quickly or completely with improved glycemic control. The different forms of diabetes have differing patterns of complications, for example, more severe atherosclerosis in NIDDM. But patients with all types of diabetes can develop all the long-term complications.

TYPES

Insulin-Dependent Diabetes Mellitus (Type I)

IDDM is the form of diabetes that without insulin therapy leads to ketoacidosis. Clinical features usually make the diagnosis obvious (see Table 4.7–2). Typically, IDDM begins before age 40 in thin to normal-weight people, and blood glucose remains labile despite insulin treatment. Although IDDM represents only about 5% of all diabetes worldwide, it is the most alarming form of the disease.

IDDM is an autoimmune disease that damages the beta cells of susceptible individuals, producing overt hyperglycemia and symptoms after several years. Autoimmunity is indicated by circulating antibodies to islet cells, to insulin, and to glutamic acid decarboxylase. Each of these markers of the immune process diminishes with time; although all are specific, none is currently sensitive enough to be a practical defining characteristic of IDDM.

Few patients have a known family history of IDDM. One parent with IDDM confers only a 2–6% risk of IDDM in a child. Still, IDDM clearly has a genetic component, shown by associations with certain HLA haplotypes and by the fact that monozygotic twins have about a 35% concordance rate if one twin has IDDM. An occasional family has an autosomal dominant pattern of IDDM with high penetrance, often associated with other autoimmune endocrine deficiencies. An individual's genetic susceptibility to IDDM varies according to specific HLA haplotypes. Haplotypes DR3, DR4, DR1, and a variant of DQβ increase the risk of IDDM, whereas haplotypes DR2 and DR5 are protective.

The susceptibility to ketoacidosis that defines IDDM reflects its pathophysiology: complete or almost complete loss of pancreatic insulin secretion. Patients with IDDM who have been started on treatment may have a "honeymoon" period of 6–12 months during which their diabetes is relatively stable and they require little or no insulin. But, inevitably, their pancreatic beta cells are destroyed (alpha and delta cells remain intact) and their endogenous insulin secretion falls to nil. Patients' metabolic control then becomes unstable ("brittle" or "labile"), because the only available insulin is what has been injected. They have no remaining physiologic feedback control of insulin secretion.

Non-Insulin-Dependent Diabetes Mellitus (Type II)

NIDDM is the form of diabetes that, in the basal, unstressed state, does not require insulin to prevent ketoacidosis. The name can be confusing, because up to 30% of people with NIDDM require insulin, but NIDDM is usually easy to distinguish clinically from IDDM (see Table 4.7–2). NIDDM accounts for 90–95% of all diabetes. The risk of NIDDM in an individual and the prevalence in a population correlate closely with obesity.

An uncommon form of NIDDM is *maturity-onset diabetes of youth* (MODY). This diabetes behaves like NIDDM in most respects except age of onset, which is usually the teens. MODY has a strong hereditary component, with several specific gene mutations described, and appears to be especially common in American blacks.

The pathophysiology of NIDDM includes two distinct abnormalities: delayed pancreatic insulin secretion and peripheral insulin resistance. The two abnormalities are probably linked, but it is not clear which comes first. Patients with NIDDM do have some degree of residual endogenous insulin secretion, but markedly attenuated acute insulin release in response to a glucose challenge. This diminished responsiveness is evident in the early phases of glucose intolerance and may be caused by amyloid protein deposition in the pancreatic beta cells. All patients with NIDDM have peripheral insulin resistance. They have abnormally few insulin receptors, but this is probably secondary to hyperinsulinemia rather than a primary defect. The nature of a postreceptor defect causing insulin resistance is unknown.

NIDDM is strongly hereditary. Over 90% of monozygotic twins show concordance for NIDDM if one twin has it, and about 12–15% of children develop NIDDM if one parent has it. Therefore, many patients have a family history of NIDDM, although it is difficult to differentiate the inheritance of NIDDM from that of obesity.

Other Types

Other types of diabetes are secondary forms with well-defined causes. For example, surgical pancreatectomy, infiltrative diseases of the pancreas (eg, hemochromatosis), and chronic pancreatitis all cause diabetes by eliminating beta-cell secretory capacity. Diseases of excess counter-insulin hormones, such as acromegaly (growth hormone), Cushing's syndrome (glucocorticoids), and glucagonoma, tip a patient with borderline insulin reserve into frank diabetes. Drugs can precipitate diabetes in patients with limited pancreatic reserve; for example, thiazides can trigger diabetes by increasing these patients' tissue insulin resistance. The physician who recognizes and corrects an underlying endocrinopathy or takes a patient off an offending drug can often reverse the abnormal glucose tolerance.

Conditions that cause generalized islet cell destruction, such as infiltrative diseases, tumor, infection, and other inflammation of the pancreas, leave some patients with deficient glucagon as well as deficient insulin secretion, and thus with deficient glucose counterregulation. These patients may be especially susceptible to hypoglycemia if they take insulin or oral hypoglycemic agents.

Gestational Diabetes Mellitus: Diabetes first diagnosed during pregnancy is termed gestational diabetes mellitus. It develops in women whose insulin secretory reserve is borderline and begins in pregnancy because of the gestational counter–insulin hormones. In about 75% of patients, glucose tolerance normalizes quickly postpartum. But because gestational diabetes mellitus in essence is signaling patients' limited ability to secrete insulin, they are at high risk for later NIDDM. Maintaining normal weight can decrease the risk.

Gestational diabetes mellitus is important to recognize because it is dangerous to the developing fetus. Hyperglycemia during organogenesis in the early weeks of pregnancy causes a high rate of congenital anomalies. Later in pregnancy, maternal hyperglycemia causes fetal hyperglycemia, which leads to excessive fetal insulin secretion. The result is a large, fat baby who may nonetheless be immature, for example, in lung development, and is at high risk for hypoglycemia and other neonatal complications.

All pregnant women should be screened for gestational diabetes mellitus between weeks 24 and 28. Patients are given 40 g of oral glucose and then their plasma glucose is measured. If at 1 hour their plasma glucose exceeds 140 mg/dL, they should have a full 100-g oral glucose tolerance test (see Table 4.7–1).

To prevent fetal macrosomia, women with gestational diabetes should keep very tight glycemic control. Diet and exercise may suffice, at least at first, but patients may need to be started on insulin.

Impaired Glucose Tolerance: Impaired glucose tolerance is differentiated from diabetes by the oral glucose tolerance test (see Table 4.7–1). About 30–40% of people with impaired glucose tolerance eventually develop diabetes. Because of the social and personal liabilities of being labeled "diabetic," impaired glucose tolerance should *not* be called "chemical," "subclinical," or "pre-" diabetes. Measures such as weight loss and exercise decrease the risk of later NIDDM.

MANAGEMENT

Patients with diabetes must be partners in their own care. To be effective partners, they must understand their disease. Patient education is essential.

Ideally, the primary physician delivers care as one member of a team. The physician establishes the diagnosis, treats risk factors, and adjusts medications. Other team members can include diabetes educators, dietitians, ophthalmologists, podiatrists, pharmacists, psychologists, and social workers.

The minimum goal in treating diabetes is to keep the patient free of symptoms and free of ketoacidosis or hyperosmolar coma. But freedom from symptoms is no longer an adequate goal. Protracted severe hyperglycemia is now known to cause the long-term complications of diabetic retinopathy, nephropathy, and neuropathy. Excellent glycemic control can significantly reduce the development and progression of these complications.

Some long-term complications such as large vessel disease may be related less to diabetic control than to smoking, high blood pressure, and lipid abnormalities. These risk factors have strongly additive effects with hyperglycemia in causing complications. Reducing them depends on controlling both glycemia and other risk factors throughout the course of diabetes.

Patients want to know just how good their glycemic control must be to reduce their risk for complications. The answer seems to be that the better the control, the less frequent and serious are the complications. However, since better control of diabetes by insulin therapy increases the risk of severe hypoglycemia, a practical approach is to keep blood glucose as normal as possible, consistent with an acceptable lifestyle and an acceptable rate of treatment side effects such as hypoglycemia. Some patients can achieve very good glycemic control with minimal intervention. For others, blood glucose targets may be relaxed if hypoglycemia is especially dangerous, if life expectancy is limited, or they are not adequately motivated. The physician must exercise discretion and judgment within the context of keeping blood glucose as close to normal as possible.

When complications do occur, the goal becomes to reduce their impact. For example, even patients who have established peripheral neuropathy and arterial insufficiency can markedly reduce their risk of needing an amputation by taking care of their feet. Eye care, including properly timed laser photocoagulation, can reduce visual loss from diabetic retinopathy. Diet and blood pressure control can delay progression to end-stage renal disease.

Monitoring of Diabetic Control

Blood glucose varies widely throughout the day, particularly in people with diabetes. Continuous blood glucose monitoring is not available to document these fluxes, but glycemic control can be estimated accurately when patients monitor their own blood glucose (see "Self-Monitoring of Blood Glucose" below). A single blood glucose tells little about overall glycemic control (except in patients with stable NIDDM, whose fasting blood glucose is a fairly good index of diurnal control). Glycated hemoglobin and fructosamine are useful indices of chronic control. Urine glucose is less useful. When nothing is monitored, assessment of symptoms must suffice.

Self-Monitoring of Blood Glucose: Self-monitoring of blood glucose is a mainstay of modern diabetic care. Patients apply a drop of their blood to a glucose-oxidase-impregnated reagent strip that they may read or, preferably, have read by a meter. With careful technique, the results should be accurate to within 10–20% of actual blood glucose, although less accurate at the extremes of low and high. Recommendations vary on the frequency and timing with which patients should test their blood glucose in relation to meals. In general, glucose levels are determined in the fasting state, before meals, and at bedtime. Stable, reliable patients with NIDDM may need to test only once a day or even less; ideally, they should test at various times of the day rather than always in the fasting state. Labile, intensively treated patients with IDDM should check their blood glucose 3–5 times a day. The physician should help patients get insurance reimbursement for the expensive reagent strips and meters.

With the results of self-monitoring, the knowledgeable patient can immediately adjust insulin or food intake and can also note patterns of glycemia such as lows before lunch or highs after dinner. In some centers, data can be downloaded electronically from a meter into a personal computer, greatly facilitating analysis of self-monitoring results.

Glycated Hemoglobin and Other Glycated Proteins: Individual blood glucose measurements assess only one point in a continuously varying parameter. Assays of glycated hemoglobin (hemoglobin A_{1c}) or fructosamine (protein-bound glucose) assess the mean blood glucose over a longer period. Glycated hemoglobin, for example, reflects mean glycemia over the previous 8–12 weeks (more heavily weighted toward more recent weeks). Fructosamine measures glycemia over about 2 weeks. The assays are used to assess glycemia before a check-up and to assess progress in glycemic control.

Urine Glucose Testing: Glucosuria indicates a blood glucose level of at least 200 mg/dL. But relying on urine testing alone has serious limitations. It does not reveal hypoglycemia. It reflects glycemia over the previous several hours, not currently. And it is highly subject to dilution of urine, measuring concentration rather than absolute amount of glucose. For all these reasons, glucosuria is far less informative than self-monitoring of blood glucose.

Diet

Diet is part of all diabetes care, but simply handing patients a written diet or booklet is not enough. The successful diet is personalized for each patient, taking into account individual customs, likes, and dislikes. Certain features of the diabetic diet, however, stay relatively consistent.

First, total caloric intake should be adjusted to establish and maintain normal weight. One formula for establishing the daily caloric requirement is:

> 10 calories/lb of desirable weight
> plus
> 33% for sedentary lifestyle
> or
> 50% for moderate physical activity
> or
> 75% for heavy physical activity

An excess or deficit of 3500 calories, accumulated over whatever period of time, amounts to roughly a 1-lb change in weight. People who eat 500 calories per day less than their caloric requirement lose about 1 lb per week.

Patients with diabetes are generally advised to use artificial sweeteners rather than concentrated sweets. This issue is somewhat controversial, since, at least theoretically, patients should be able to "cover" concentrated sucrose with just the right amount of injected insulin. But since it is virtually impossible to know the sucrose content of various sweets, the best approach is to avoid them altogether.

The caloric distribution recommended for diabetes does not restrict carbohydrate. The recommendations are 55–60% carbohydrate, 30% fat, and 10–15% protein. Some have criticized this high carbohydrate intake as a cause of hypertriglyceridemia and insulin resistance. But it is agreed that in order to reduce plasma cholesterol, fat intake should be moderated and should be predominantly polyunsaturates and monounsaturates, with less than 10% of total caloric intake being saturated fat. In line with the anti-atherogenic diet, total cholesterol should be less than 300 mg per day. High-fiber foods smooth the absorption of carbohydrate. There is also mounting evidence that reducing dietary protein to less than 0.8 g/kg of desirable body weight each day can slow the deterioration of renal function in patients with established diabetic nephropathy.

How are these recommendations translated into reasonably normal eating patterns? Most people with diabetes benefit from consultation with a dietitian. Patients need not weigh foods or follow preplanned menus. Instead, most learn to recognize portions of various foods and consciously exchange items within a food group, for example, a small potato for an ear of corn or a teaspoon of margarine for a tablespoon of salad oil. Many patients use diabetic exchange lists—lists of foods that have equal nutritional content. Patients can integrate most desired foods into a balanced, attractive diet, and their families can probably eat more healthfully if they follow it as well.

Although few people with IDDM are calorie-restricted, diet is central to their management. Total caloric intake should be adequate to maintain normal weight; for many patients, gaining weight is harder than losing it. Patients must carefully match their portion sizes, particularly of carbohydrate, to the amount of insulin taken. People taking insulin are prone to hypoglycemia if they do not eat regularly. Not only should they eat on time, but they should always carry a concentrated sweet with them to eat if they become hypoglycemic.

Most people with NIDDM are overweight and should be on a low-calorie diet. There are innumerable approaches to losing weight, but several principles hold true: (1) Allowing diabetes to go uncontrolled causes weight loss, but is not an acceptable long-term way to control weight. (2) Very low-calorie diets produce rapid early weight loss, largely as a result of diuresis, but this rate levels out and long-term weight loss depends on how low-calorie the diet remains. (3) Glycemic control improves abruptly with very low-calorie diets, even before patients lose much weight. Patients with NIDDM should maintain a low-fat diet (less than 30% of calories), and those with high blood pressure, a low-sodium diet. In some patients with NIDDM, weight loss alone restores sufficient insulin responsiveness to control diabetes without drugs.

Exercise

There is mounting evidence that an active lifestyle with regular exercise helps prevent the long-term complications of diabetes and may even help prevent diabetes itself. But there are several pitfalls. Vigorous exercise potentiates insulin action, sometimes causing hypoglycemia as long as 6–12 hours later. Patients may have complication-specific reasons to modify exercise, for example, when cardiovascular disease limits exercise potential or peripheral neuropathy increases the danger of foot trauma. Nevertheless, sensible exercise—for many patients, vigorous exercise—is part of the optimal diabetes regimen.

Oral Hypoglycemic Agents

Until 1995, the only oral hypoglycemic agents available in the United States were sulfonylureas. All sulfonylureas act by the same mechanism: potentiation of insulin secretion. They increase basal, unstimulated insulin secretion, but they are especially potent enhancers of physiologic secretagogues. Thus, patients have a significantly greater rise in insulin levels after a meal when they are taking a sulfonylurea. Different sulfonylureas vary in their duration of action, mode of excretion, and side effects. The longest-acting oral hypoglycemic agent, chlorpropamide, causes free water retention, and some patients develop facial flushing whenever they drink alcohol. The two newer sulfonylureas, glyburide and glipizide, are given in much lower doses than the "first-generation" agents. It is not known whether any sulfonylureas have specific therapeutic advantages over others, but glyburide and glipizide are said to have fewer drug-drug interactions.

Metformin was released in the United States in 1995, although it has been in use around the world since the mid-1970's. Metformin is of particular use because its mechanism of action is different from that of the sulfonylureas. Rather than stimulating insulin secretion, metformin reduces hepatic glucose uptake and, at least to some extent, enhances glucose utilization in muscle. Therefore, metformin can be used not only as the first drug in treating NIDDM, but it can be effective when added to a sulfonylurea that is no longer controlling glycemia. A frequent side effect of metformin treatment is weight loss, obviously a benefit for many people with NIDDM. The major caution is not to give metformin to patients who are at particular risk for lactic acidosis, such as those with an elevated creatinine or unstable cardiovascular disease, or during surgery.

Insulin

Combined beef-pork and purified pork or beef were the only insulins available from 1922 until about 1982. Now, human insulin has increasingly replaced beef-pork, which is being gradually phased out of manufacture. Human insulin should be used in newly treated patients because it causes less antibody response than animal insulin, and thus lowers the risk of allergic reactions and insulin resistance. But patients who are doing well on beef-pork insulin may stay on it.

The formulation of insulin is more important than the species of origin (Table 4.7–4). Regular (crystalline zinc, soluble, or clear) insulin is unmodified, native insulin with a relatively rapid absorption and short duration of action. Regular insulin is used before meals to provide the peak

of insulin needed to metabolize ingested calories. Intermediate-acting insulins come in two forms: (1) NPH (neutral protamine Hagedorn) insulin, which has protamine to slow subcutaneous absorption, and (2) lente insulin, which retards absorption by its zinc-insulin crystal size. Ultralente, with larger zinc-insulin crystals, is the longest-acting preparation in common use. It maintains a relatively steady basal insulin tone, but most patients need an additional injection of regular insulin at each mealtime.

Figure 4.7–1 shows idealized curves of action of single and mixed insulin doses. Depth of injection, exercise of the area injected, and temperature cause considerable unpredictability in the glycemic response to subcutaneously delivered insulin, a variability that patients cannot practically avoid.

Insulin-Induced Hypoglycemia: By far the most common and potentially serious side effect of insulin therapy is hypoglycemia (an insulin reaction). Three issues are most important in evaluating hypoglycemia: frequency, severity, and timing. Occasional insulin reactions are usually insignificant unless severe; some people have mild symptoms of hypoglycemia almost daily. Severity is measured by the disruption of normal life: Do patients develop a drenching sweat, or simply hunger and tremulousness? Do they become confused (evidence of neuroglycopenia), requiring help from another person, or can they always treat their own reactions successfully? If patients are prone to confusion or coma without premonitory symptoms (hypoglycemic unawareness), the degree of glycemic control may need to be eased. If the timing of hypoglycemia follows a pattern, for example, predominantly before lunch or overnight, treatment can be adjusted.

Using Insulin in IDDM: Since patients with IDDM must completely replace pancreatic insulin secretion, many require complex insulin regimens, mixing short-acting with long-acting preparations given as 2–4 injections a day (see Figure 4.7–1). Intensive regimens try to mimic physiologic constant insulin levels between meals and the sharp peaks in insulin concentrations after meals. One such regimen uses ultralente insulin for the basal level, combined with pre-meal regular insulin. Another alternative is the external insulin infusion pump. Patients wear the external pump on their belt, and they control the rates at which the pump delivers insulin through a catheter to a needle inserted in the abdominal skin. External pumps have been well accepted by some patients eager to control their diabetes and willing to monitor their blood glucose regularly.

Using Insulin in NIDDM: Insulin therapy does not change the diagnosis of NIDDM, but may change its name to "insulin-requiring NIDDM." Many patients require 75–150 U of insulin daily, indicating a substantial level of insulin resistance. Despite needing this high dose, most patients have relatively stable glycemia, without the abrupt peaks and valleys seen in IDDM. Simple insulin regimens usually suffice.

Table 4.7–4. Insulin formulations.

Formulation	Timing of Bioactivity (hr)*		
	Onset	Peak	Duration
Short-acting			
Regular (native insulin)	0.5	2–4	5–7
Semilente (small zinc crystals)	0.5	2–4	5–8
Intermediate-acting			
NPH (protamine suspension)	1–2	6–12	18–24
Lente (mixture of 70% semilente and 30% ultralente)	1–2	6–12	18–24
Long-acting			
Ultralente (large zinc crystals)	4–6	8–16	24–36

NPH, neutral protamine Hagedorn.
*Timing of bioactivity is highly variable, depending, for example, on depth of injection, vascularity of tissue, and serum anti-insulin antibody titer.

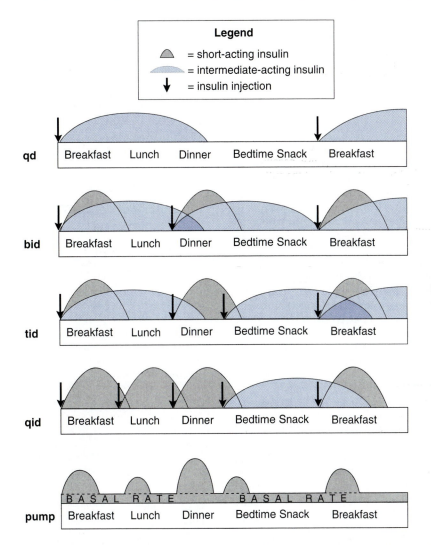

Figure 4.7–1. Idealized curves of action of subcutaneously delivered insulin. The regimens of one, two, three, and four doses per day use short-acting (regular or semilente) and intermediate-acting (NPH or lente) insulin, alone or in combination. The external insulin pump delivers a continuous basal rate of short-acting insulin, with increases before meals. The basal rate delivered by the pump can be simulated by once- or twice-daily injections of ultralente insulin. Actual curves of action for all regimens vary greatly from patient to patient and injection to injection. (Modified and reproduced, with permission, from Skyler J et al: Algorithms for adjustment of insulin dosage by patients who monitor blood glucose. Diabetes Care 1981;4:311. © 1981 by American Diabetes Association, Inc.)

Treating NIDDM with insulin has side effects. Beyond the obvious drawback of daily injections, patients' risk of hypoglycemia increases. Insulin therapy can stimulate appetite, so patients may gain weight. They have worsening of peripheral hyperinsulinism, which may be a risk factor for coronary heart disease. Therefore, diet, exercise, and oral hypoglycemic drugs should be optimized before the physician considers insulin treatment.

Combined Insulin and Oral Hypoglycemic Agents: There is growing interest in treating NIDDM by combining insulin with oral hypoglycemic agents. The sulfonylureas enhance endogenous insulin secretion in response to meals, whereas intermediate-acting insulin given at bedtime suppresses nocturnal hepatic gluconeogenesis. Small studies of combination therapy indicate that glycemia can be slightly improved, insulin dose reduced, or both.

Sequencing of Therapy in NIDDM: The principle of sequenced care applies particularly to NIDDM. Once treatment goals are established, patients are started on diet and exercise; these alone may be adequate to reach target plasma glucose levels. If not, the next step is oral hypoglycemic agents in graded doses. If these are not enough, the final step is insulin. Most patients have time to try each treatment for weeks or months. For many patients, a given stage of treatment is effective for years or even permanently. But glycemic control is not the only goal of treatment, and it is probably less important than control of other cardiovascular risk factors in preventing the major complication of NIDDM, premature cardiovascular disease.

Diabetic Ketoacidosis

Before the advent of insulin therapy in the early 1920's, diabetic ketoacidosis was the inevitable fatal outcome of IDDM. It still can be fatal if not adequately treated. Diabetic ketoacidosis results from complete insulin lack causing unrestrained lipolysis that raises circulating free fatty acid levels. In the absence of adequate tricarboxylic acid cycle activity, these fatty acid levels cause the liver to pour out ketone bodies (acetoacetate, β-hydroxybutyric acid, and acetone), which are products of fatty acid oxidation. As these metabolic acids accumulate in excess of the body's ability to metabolize or excrete them, patients develop the characteristic wide anion gap metabolic acidosis. With acidosis come hyperpnea (Kussmaul's respiration), nausea, vomiting, debilitation, and, ultimately, vascular collapse. Arterial pH reflects the severity of acidosis. Patients may have many other laboratory abnormalities. Electrolyte imbalances characteristically include hyperkalemia and hyperphosphatemia. Leukocytosis, often to 20,000/μL, is common even without infection. Prerenal azotemia reflects patients' poor hydration.

The physician should pursue the cause of diabetic ketoacidosis. Usually, the explanation is missed insulin doses or an illness-induced increase in insulin requirements. A common mistake is for patients to stop taking insulin if they eat less during an intercurrent illness, when in fact the stress of illness increases their need for insulin. The insulin requirement is increased particularly by infections—acute (eg, influenza) or chronic (eg, dental abscess)—which predictably raise levels of counterregulatory hormones such as cortisol and catecholamines.

The mainstays of treatment for diabetic ketoacidosis are rehydration and insulin (Table 4.7–5). Physicians must not lower the blood glucose too fast. Furthermore, they must anticipate and correct the rapid fall in serum potassium that occurs as acidosis is reversed and potassium enters insulin-responsive cells along with glucose. Intravenous bicarbonate is indicated only when the acidosis is severe, with arterial pH less than 7.00–7.10. Ketonuria often persists long after acidosis is corrected, since therapy converts β-hydroxybutyric acid to acetoacetate; only acetoacetate is measured by nitroprusside bedside tests of ketosis.

Hyperosmolar Nonketotic States

As untreated diabetic ketoacidosis can be fatal in IDDM; therefore, the hyperosmolar nonketotic states that result from severe hyperglycemia and dehydration can be fatal in NIDDM. If serum osmolarity exceeds about 380 mOsm/L, it can cause coma; more often, patients become lethargic and prostrated. Most patients have contributing conditions such as a concurrent illness, stroke, drug therapy (especially diuretics), or trauma. In patients with impaired renal function, limited renal excretion of glucose

Table 4.7–5. Guidelines: Treatment of diabetic ketoacidosis.*

Goals

Begin improving plasma glucose and reversing acidosis immediately

Correct plasma glucose concentration to <250 mg/dL over 6–12 hr

Correct acidosis to normal arterial pH over 12–24 hr

Prevent late hypoglycemia

Prevent hypokalemia during correction of acidosis

Identify and correct any contributing illness or behavior, eg, pneumonia, myocardial infarction, omission of prescribed insulin

Monitoring

Check clinical status frequently

Check blood glucose every 2 hr

Check acid-base status and electrolytes every 4–6 hr

Keep flow sheet

Specific treatments

Regular insulin	Give 6–12 U/hr, preferably by IV infusion Double dose if no response by 4 hr Decrease dose to 1–2 U/hr when plasma glucose is <250 mg/dL
Fluids	Give 0.9% saline unless significant hypernatremia or danger of sodium overload, in which case give 0.45% saline Change to 5% dextrose when plasma glucose is <250 mg/dL Give 2–3 L fluid in first 3 hr.
Potassium	Give 10–20 mEq/hr KCl (or KPO₄ if serum phosphate is low) when serum K+ is 3.5–6.0 mEq/L Give 40–80 mEq/hr when serum K+ is <2.5 mEq/L
Bicarbonate	Give only when acidosis is severe (pH <7.00), as an infusion of 100 mEq/L in 0.45% saline

*Actual treatment must be individualized for each patient.

further contributes to hyperglycemia. As many as one-third of patients with hyperosmolar nonketotic states were not previously aware of their diabetes.

Serum osmolarity (mOsm/L) can be measured directly or estimated by this formula:

$$\text{Serum osmolarity} = \frac{\text{Plasma glucose}}{18} + 2[\text{serum Na}^+ + \text{K}^+] + \frac{\text{blood urea nitrogen}}{2.8}$$

The plasma glucose, serum Na+ and K+, and blood urea nitrogen are all measured in mg/dL.

Osmolarity thus depends most on sodium concentration. So if total body hydration is adequate to dilute serum sodium in response to hyperglycemia (by extracellular shift of water), total osmolarity stays relatively normal. By contrast, hyperosmolarity reflects severe dehydration, with hypernatremia as well as hyperglycemia.

Treatment must include large volumes of fluid; both normal saline and half-normal saline have been advocated. Hypotonic saline may be given to patients with severe hypernatremia and those whose cardiovascular status dictates salt restriction. Otherwise, patients should be given normal saline to replace the sodium lost by diuresis and to restore vascular volume. Insulin may also be infused, but it is preferable to correct severe hyperglycemia gradually over 12–24 hours rather than abruptly, since too fast a fall in serum osmolarity may cause cerebral edema. The physician must seek concurrent illnesses and potentially responsible medications.

Hyperosmolar states and ketoacidosis often overlap. Under stress, even patients with NIDDM may develop ketoacidosis, and many patients with IDDM and ketoacidosis become dehydrated enough to have serious hyperosmolarity. The elements of treatment for both conditions are similar—fluid and insulin to lower plasma glucose gradually and to correct acidosis, plus careful attention to balancing serum electrolytes and seeking precipitating causes.

MANAGEMENT OF LONG-TERM COMPLICATIONS

Retinopathy

Diabetic retinopathy is the leading cause of blindness in Americans younger than 60, blinding an estimated 5000 people each year (Table 4.7–6). Much of this loss of vision can be prevented if patients are diagnosed and treated at the right moment. This requires an annual dilated fundus exam by an ophthalmologist.

Diabetic retinopathy appears about 7 years after the onset of diabetes. Onset is usually mild. The early manifestations (background retinopathy) are microaneurysms, blot hemorrhages, and hard exudates, which rarely impair vision. These lesions may or may not progress to more severe retinopathy over many years. During an intermediate phase, findings that signal high risk for later proliferative retinopathy are macular edema (see Color Plates) (often evidenced by perimacular hard exudates), cotton-wool spots (see Color Plates), venous beading, and intraretinal microvascular abnormalities. Proliferative retinopathy (new vessels growing into the vitreous) rarely develops before 10 years of diabetes (see Color Plates). Prolifera-

tive retinopathy poses a significant risk for bleeding into the vitreous, causing loss of vision. Vitreous hemorrhages may resolve several times, but they are the predominant cause of the scarring, fibrotic bands, and retinal detachments that cause blindness in diabetes.

Laser photocoagulation has enormously reduced the loss of vision. Photocoagulation is usually indicated for clinically significant macular edema and for proliferative disease. Lesions are difficult to detect, so for timely diagnosis patients should start seeing an ophthalmologist yearly when they have had diabetes for 5 years. Vitrectomy—the removal of vitreous with clotted blood or fibrous tissue bands—is late-stage surgery that may restore at least some vision.

Nephropathy

Diabetic nephropathy is now responsible for about one-third of all end-stage renal disease in the United States. Nephropathy manifests later in diabetes than does retinopathy. The early lesions can be detected only by biopsy. The first sign is microalbuminuria, typically appearing after 8–12 years of diabetes. Over about the next decade, at extremely variable rates, the nephropathy may progress to persistent gross proteinuria, azotemia, and end-stage renal disease. Remarkably, most people with diabetes never develop proteinuria or any manifestation of renal disease. Of people diagnosed with IDDM since the 1950's, only about 10% have had nephropathy after 20 years of disease. There is no explanation for this selective protection against nephropathy, but improved glycemic control seems to play a role. Patients who have not developed proteinuria by 20 years of diabetes probably never will.

Nephropathy is managed with blood pressure control and a low-protein diet. Progression of nephropathy can probably be slowed by very good control of blood pressure and blood glucose. Angiotensin-converting enzyme (ACE) inhibitors are particularly attractive antihypertensive drugs because their selective afferent arteriolar vasodilatation reduces glomerular filtration pressure. Indeed, ACE inhibitors have been advocated for use in normotensive diabetic patients with proteinuria.

Large-Vessel Atherosclerosis

Atherosclerosis is accelerated in diabetes, necessitating over 50% of the nontraumatic lower extremity amputations in the United States and increasing patients' risk for coronary artery disease and stroke. Epidemiologically, diabetes virtually eliminates the delay in atherosclerotic cardiovascular disease normally found in premenopausal women. But hyperglycemia may be a less important factor than lipid abnormalities, high blood pressure, smoking, and a family history of atherosclerotic disease. (The combination of insulin resistance, hyperglycemia, abdominal obesity, and hypertension has been called syndrome X; it is both common and dangerous in NIDDM.) Once patients with diabetes have clinically apparent vascular disease, it tends to be diffuse and less amenable to surgery than in patients without diabetes.

Table 4.7–6. Common causes of visual impairment in diabetes.

Cause	Comments
Lens stiffening	Causes blurred vision in patients with unstable diabetic control; not related to retinopathy; vision stabilizes as blood glucose is controlled
Macular edema	Rarely identified by direct ophthalmoscopy; usually found along with significant background or proliferative retinopathy; indication for laser photocoagulation
Vitreous bleed	Causes acute loss of vision in one eye over hours, usually because of bleeding from proliferative retinopathy; may resolve but may cause severe sequelae that impair vision
Fibrous bands	Caused by vitreous bleeding; can lead to traction retinal detachment and blindness
Glaucoma	Especially common in patients with diabetes
Cataracts	Probably especially common in patients with diabetes

Neuropathy

By far the most common form of diabetic neuropathy is peripheral symmetrical polyneuropathy, caused by a segmental demyelination of axons (Table 4.7–7; Chapter 13.11). This neuropathy develops gradually over many years and is difficult or impossible to reverse. It causes numbness, tingling, and sometimes severe discomfort in the toes and hands, with symptoms slowly progressing proximally.

The discomfort of peripheral symmetrical polyneuropathy may be improved by amitriptyline (which has a specific benefit, not only antidepressant action), desipramine, or carbamazepine. Topical capsaicin cream has also been reported to be useful. Most patients have progressive numbness, which is less uncomfortable but more dangerous, since it leaves the feet at higher risk for unrecognized trauma. Peripheral neuropathy and arteriosclerosis combine to put patients at extremely high risk for losing a limb. The route to amputation is well defined. Almost all patients begin with minor foot trauma, such as a blister or cut. They may be oblivious to the broken skin because the foot is insensate, but the wound becomes infected, poor circulation inhibits healing, and gangrene sets in. The keys to saving limbs are to prevent trauma, check regularly for painless trauma, and treat limbs early and vigorously.

Similar damage to nerves can affect autonomic function. Many men have impotence, sometimes aggravated by penile vascular insufficiency. Some patients have orthostatic hypotension, or urinary retention caused by an atonic bladder. Gastrointestinal involvement usually begins with alternating diarrhea and constipation (diabetic enteropathy) and can progress to gastric atonia. Difficulty emptying the stomach leads to nausea, vomiting, irregular absorption of meals (gastroparesis), and gastroesophageal reflux.

Finally, ischemic neuropathy is characterized by sudden onset and focal symptoms, caused by a vascular occlusion of the vasa nervorum. Mononeuropathy may cause pain in a nerve root distribution, or a motor palsy, sometimes of a cranial nerve, typically III, IV, or VI. Occasionally, several individual nerves are affected (mononeuropathy multiplex), or patients develop severe proximal lower extremity weakness, pain, and cachexia, a pattern that has been called "lumbar plexopathy," "diabetic amyotrophy," and "diabetic cachexia." Patients with ischemic neuropathy improve gradually over 2–6 months.

Diabetic Dermopathy

Slow healing of minor skin trauma is typical of poorly controlled diabetes, but several skin lesions are specific to diabetes. The most characteristic is necrobiosis lipoidica diabeticorum (see Color Plates), usually found on the anterior tibia; this violet lesion has a diameter of 2 cm or more, with thinned skin, fine superficial veins, and sometimes central ulceration. Also characteristic of diabetes are shin spots—hyperpigmented round lesions about 1 cm in diameter. Finally, the local skin response to insulin injections may be lipid hypertrophy, lipoatrophy, or both.

Table 4.7–7. Diabetic neuropathy.

Type	Signs and Symptoms
Peripheral symmetric polyneuropathy	Numbness, tingling, dysesthesias, pins and needles, starting in toes and fingers, progressing proximally
Autonomic neuropathy	
Penile	Partial or complete failure of erections
Neurogenic bladder	Residual urine, incomplete emptying, hydroureter
Vascular	Orthostatic hypotension
Enteropathy	Constipation, diarrhea
Gastroparesis	Nausea, vomiting, abdominal bloating
Impaired sympathetic response to hypoglycemia	Anhydrosis, tachycardia, tremulousness when hypoglycemic
Mononeuropathy	
Cranial nerve palsy	Ptosis, Bell's palsy, trigeminal neuralgia
Single sensory nerve	Nerve route pain (abdomen, back, leg)
Single motor nerve	Footdrop, other single-nerve symptoms
Nerve compression syndromes	Carpal tunnel syndrome, etc
Mononeuropathy multiplex	Multiple single nerves involved
Diabetic amyotrophy (lumbar plexopathy, neuropathic cachexia)	Severe proximal muscle weakness, especially in legs and pelvic distribution; pain, weight loss, depression

SUMMARY

▶ Diabetes is defined by hyperglycemia. Long-term complications include retinopathy, nephropathy, neuropathy, and premature arteriosclerosis.

▶ Insulin-dependent diabetes mellitus (type I) is an autoimmune endocrinopathy, with complete loss of endogenous insulin secretion. Patients are prone to diabetic ketoacidosis, require insulin therapy, and have a labile metabolic course that depends directly on their insulin regimen.

▶ Non-insulin-dependent diabetes mellitus (type II) is caused by delayed insulin secretion and peripheral insulin resistance, with some degree of residual endogenous insulin reserve. Treatment builds from diet and exercise to oral hypoglycemic agents to insulin. Hyperosmolar coma is its extreme and potentially fatal metabolic complication.

▶ Diabetes care requires both management of daily metabolic aberrations that can become life-threatening within hours and effort by patients working in partnership with health care providers to prevent or manage the long-term complications.

SUGGESTED READING

American Diabetes Association: Clinical practice recommendations 1996. *Diabetes Care* 1996;19(Suppl 1):S1.

DeFronzo RA, Bonadonna RC, Ferrannini E: Pathogenesis of NIDDM: A balanced overview. Diabetes Care 1992;15:318.

Diabetes Control and Complications Trial Research Group: The effect of intensive treatment of diabetes on the development and progression of long-term complications in insulin-dependent diabetes mellitus. N Engl J Med 1993;329:977.

Lebovitz HE, Melander A (editors): Sulfonylurea drugs: Basic and clinical considerations. Diabetes Care 1990;13(Suppl 3):1.

Physician's Guide to Insulin-Dependent (Type I) Diabetes Mellitus: Diagnosis and Treatment. American Diabetes Association, 1988. (Available from the American Diabetes Association, Inc, National Service Center, 1660 Duke Street, Alexandria, VA 22314. Phone (800) 232-3472; ask for order department.)

Physician's Guide to Non-Insulin-Dependent (Type II) Diabetes: Diagnosis and Treatment, 2nd ed. American Diabetes Association, 1989. (Available as above.)

Hypoglycemia

Simeon Margolis, MD, PhD, and Angeliki Georgopoulos, MD

Hypoglycemia is a potentially fatal metabolic disorder caused by several serious diseases—many quite treatable—and by numerous drugs. Clinicians must recognize hypoglycemia and determine its cause because prolonged, severe hypoglycemia can permanently damage the brain. They must consider hypoglycemia in many situations because it can masquerade as a wide spectrum of neurologic and psychiatric syndromes. Physicians can readily confirm hypoglycemia in the laboratory and easily reverse it by giving glucose.

It is useful to differentiate hypoglycemic disorders based on whether they appear during fasting (more than 10 hours after eating) or postprandially. Fasting hypoglycemia is a potentially life-threatening condition. It can be caused by excessive insulin action, from either exogenously administered insulin or endogenous overproduction by an insulinoma. Fasting hypoglycemia can also be caused by extrapancreatic tumors, certain drugs, severe liver disease, or lack of either of two counterregulatory hormones—cortisol or growth hormone—which normally stimulate hepatic synthesis of glucose (gluconeogenesis) during a prolonged fast.

Central nervous system symptoms predominate in fasting hypoglycemia because the brain requires a continuous supply of glucose to function normally. Although a rapid fall in blood glucose can trigger adrenergic symptoms even in the fasting state, these symptoms are more typical of postprandial hypoglycemia (see below). Manifestations of fasting hypoglycemia vary widely in different patients, but each individual tends to have a recurring pattern. Common symptoms include headache, diplopia, blurred vision, confusion, inappropriate affect or behavior, and motor incoordination. Signs of severe hypoglycemia are highly variable, but can include hypothermia, mental status changes from confusion to coma, seizures, extensor rigidity of the limbs, and, ultimately, death.

Patients with postprandial or reactive hypoglycemia present with symptoms 2–6 hours after a meal. Their low blood glucose level typically triggers release of the counterregulatory hormones—epinephrine, glucagon, and cortisol—which normally stimulate hepatic glycogen breakdown and quickly return blood glucose to normal. Epinephrine is responsible for most of the symptoms of postprandial hypoglycemia, which include sweating, palpitations, tremor, nervousness, hunger, acral and perioral numbness, faintness, and weakness. Symptoms may be blunted or absent in patients taking β-blockers and in some patients with longstanding diabetes mellitus who have autonomic neuropathy. The symptoms of postprandial hypoglycemia may be troublesome, but the condition is not dangerous. Because similar symptoms can accompany anxiety attacks, thyrotoxicosis, and pheochromocytoma, patients require rigorous evaluation to prove that their symptoms are from hypoglycemia.

Two errors are commonly made in the diagnosis of hypoglycemia: (1) holding hypoglycemia responsible for symptoms that it does not typically cause and (2) confusing chemical with symptomatic hypoglycemia. Hypoglycemia rarely causes lack of energy, chronic anxiety, lethargy, mental dullness, and similar complaints. Physicians perform a valuable service by proving to patients that such symptoms are not being caused by hypoglycemia. Chemical hypoglycemia, most often defined as a plasma glucose level below 50 mg/dL, is fairly common, particularly in women and patients with insulin-dependent diabetes. However, the degree of hypoglycemia required to produce symptoms varies widely. For a diagnosis of symptomatic hypoglycemia, a low plasma glucose, usually below 50 mg/dL, must be accompanied by characteristic symptoms during a spontaneous postprandial episode, after an overnight fast, or during a glucose tolerance test.

HYPOGLYCEMIA IN THE FASTING STATE

Because fasting hypoglycemia is often caused by serious disorders, the hypoglycemia and its cause must be identified (Table 4.8–1). A low blood glucose in the fasting state implies a derangement in either hepatic or hormonal regulation of glycogenolysis or gluconeogenesis.

Table 4.8–1. Differential diagnosis of hypoglycemia.

Fasting
  Hepatic
    Extensive liver disease*
    Enzyme defects (in children)
  Hormonal†
    Insulin excess
      Insulinoma*
      Autoimmune hypoglycemia
    Growth hormone deficiency
    Glucocorticoid deficiency
  Hypoglycemia associated with serious illness
    Renal disease
    Malnutrition
    Sepsis
    Congestive heart failure
  Extrapancreatic tumors*

Postprandial
  Reactive*
  Alimentary
  Hypoglycemia associated with glucose intolerance

Drug-induced
  Insulin*
  Sulfonylureas*
  Alcohol*
  Salicylates
  Propranolol
  Poisons (plants, hepatotoxic substances)

*Most common causes.
†Hormonal abnormalities occasionally cause postprandial hypoglycemia.

Overnight fasting plasma glucose levels taken on three different days are the most useful screening test for fasting hypoglycemia. A fasting glucose below 50 mg/dL on any of the 3 days should raise suspicion of significant hypoglycemia.

In emergencies, patients suspected of having severe hypoglycemia should have a blood sample drawn to measure glucose levels before treatment is started with an intravenous 50% glucose solution.

Endogenous Causes

Liver Diseases: Primary liver disorders are an important cause of symptomatic hypoglycemia because of the central role that hepatic gluconeogenesis plays in maintaining normal fasting glucose levels. Hypoglycemia can follow acute viral or toxin-induced fulminant hepatic necrosis or extensive surgical resection of the liver. Symptomatic hypoglycemia is seen in some patients with severe cirrhosis or a hepatoma. Most commonly, patients with a poorly differentiated hepatoma have severe anorexia and weight loss, with hypoglycemia as a late complication. In contrast, a few patients with well-differentiated hepatomas develop early hypoglycemia, losing appetite and weight only late in their illness. The hypoglycemia in these patients has not been explained, but it can develop even if tumor has not replaced massive amounts of normal liver.

Genetic Disorders: In patients with inborn enzyme defects such as glycogen storage diseases, galactosemia, and hereditary fructose intolerance, hypoglycemic symptoms usually begin in infancy and are less prominent in affected adults.

Insulinomas: Insulinomas are rare tumors that affect equal numbers of men and women. These tumors are diagnosed at all ages, but most often between 30 and 70. About 10% of insulinomas are malignant. Because the early features can be so nonspecific—malaise, profound fatigue, confusion, and morning headaches—most patients have symptoms for a long time before the tumor is diagnosed. Confusion and impaired judgment during a hypoglycemic episode can make it difficult for patients to give a reliable history. Hunger and compulsive eating occasionally lead to weight gain. Adrenergic symptoms after meals, the presenting complaint in 30% of patients, become more prominent as the tumor grows. Patients may develop reversible paralysis, seizures, or neuropsychiatric manifestations. In one series, neuropsychiatric symptoms persisted in 50% of patients after their insulinomas were removed.

The diagnosis of an insulinoma requires proof of inappropriate hyperinsulinism. A useful screening test measures both plasma insulin and glucose after a 12-hour overnight fast. Insulinoma is suspected when the plasma insulin is above 20 μU/mL and the plasma glucose is below 60 mg/dL. Insulinoma can be diagnosed in more than 90% of patients after a 24-hour fast, but some must fast for up to 72 hours to rule out the tumor. Because a tumor may secrete only intermittently and insulin's half-life is short, plasma insulin, C peptide, and glucose should be measured every 4–6 hours during the fast. Strong evidence for an insulinoma is an insulin:glucose ratio above 0.33 when the plasma glucose is below 60 mg/dL. C peptide has a longer half-life than insulin. C peptide levels, which reflect solely endogenous insulin production, are suppressed in factitious hypoglycemia in patients who surreptitiously inject themselves with insulin (Chapter 14.6). Exogenous insulin can produce circulating antibodies that interfere with accurate determinations of plasma insulin. In patients with an insulinoma, both plasma insulin and C peptide remain high while blood glucose falls. Insulinoma is strongly suggested if the glucose curve and the insulin or C peptide curve cross over time.

Another clue to insulinoma is an elevation of proinsulin out of proportion to insulin. Infrequently needed tests can give still more clues to insulinoma: a failure of administered insulin to suppress C peptide release and excessive insulin secretion after patients are given tolbutamide, glucagon, leucine, or calcium.

Before surgery, the physician tries to localize the insulinoma and determine whether it is malignant. Serum levels of chorionic gonadotropin or its alpha or beta subunits are elevated in about two-thirds of patients with functioning malignant insulinomas, but not in those with benign or inactive tumors. If a liver scan reveals metastases, only palliative surgery is considered. Tumors larger than 2–3 cm can be detected by ultrasonography or computed tomography, but angiography is more sensitive for smaller tumors. The tumor can almost always be localized by transhepatic percutaneous venous sampling—measuring insulin concentrations in veins draining different parts of the pancreas. A concentration gradient at only one site locates a single insulinoma; diffuse hyperinsulinism means multiple adenomas or diffuse islet cell hyperplasia.

When surgery fails to restore normoglycemia or when a malignant tumor has spread, some patients' hypoglycemic episodes can be controlled with frequent high-carbohydrate feedings, diazoxide, and thiazide diuretics. Streptozocin, which destroys beta cells, improves hypoglycemic symptoms and lengthens survival in about 50% of those treated. Zinc, glucagon, and glucocorticoids reduce hypoglycemic manifestations, but their actions are short-lived, and glucocorticoids cause serious side effects.

Insulinomas can coexist with nonpancreatic tumors as part of the syndrome of multiple endocrine neoplasia (MEN type I) (Chapter 4.1). Most commonly, islet cell tumors secrete either insulin or gastrin (which causes the Zollinger-Ellison syndrome) (Chapter 6.4). Patients may develop diarrheal syndromes (Chapter 6.8) when their tumor produces vasoactive intestinal peptide (VIP), gastrin, somatostatin, or prostaglandin E.

Other islet cell tumors produce hormones that cause further symptoms and signs (Table 4.8–2). Tumors that secrete glucagon, somatostatin, or VIP can cause mild hyperglycemia. Glucagonomas, which usually affect women, can also cause necrolytic migratory erythema, diarrhea, glossitis, weight loss, and psychiatric disturbances; about 80% of these tumors are malignant. In addition to hyperglycemia, somatostatinomas cause gallstones, steatorrhea, and dyspepsia. The major manifestation of VIP-producing tumors is watery diarrhea, along with hypokalemia and other electrolyte disturbances; many patients also have hyperglycemia and hypercalcemia.

Autoimmune Hypoglycemia: This condition occurs in rare patients who produce antibodies to insulin without ever having received exogenous insulin. Even rarer patients who produce autoantibodies to insulin receptors can develop overwhelming, refractory hypoglycemia.

Table 4.8–2. Hormones produced by functioning islet cell tumors.

Hormone Product	Cell Type	Clinical Manifestations
Insulin	Beta	Hypoglycemia
Gastrin		Peptic ulcer, diarrhea
Glucagon	Alpha	Necrolytic migratory erythema, hyperglycemia, diarrhea, weight loss, psychiatric disturbances
Somatostatin	D	Hyperglycemia, gallstones, steatorrhea, dyspepsia
Vasoactive intestinal peptide (VIP)		Secretory diarrhea, hypokalemia, hyperglycemia

Growth Hormone and ACTH Deficiency: These conditions can lead to hypoglycemia in patients with all types of acquired pituitary insufficiencies. Glucocorticoid replacement therapy prevents symptomatic hypoglycemia in about 90% of persons whose panhypopituitarism began in childhood.

Glucocorticoid Deficiency: In patients with glucocorticoid deficiency, symptomatic hypoglycemia commonly follows a prolonged fast. Occasionally, patients with glucocorticoid deficiency exhibit hypoglycemic symptoms late in the postprandial period. Adequate corticosteroid replacement, with increased doses during times of stress and pregnancy, completely prevents attacks of hypoglycemia.

Other Serious Illnesses: Illnesses such as chronic renal failure, sepsis, and falciparum malaria, can cause severe hypoglycemia. Hypoglycemia can follow hemodialysis and extreme malnourishment. Transient hypoglycemia, which on occasion complicates congestive heart failure, may not be recognized if the symptoms are misinterpreted as evidence of cerebral anoxia.

Extrapancreatic Tumors: Hypoglycemia can complicate all types of extrapancreatic tumors, most often mesenchymal tumors, massive fibromas, and sarcomas; the most common sites (in decreasing order of frequency) are the retroperitoneal, intrathoracic, and intra-abdominal spaces. Other tumors that can produce hypoglycemia include hepatomas, adrenocortical tumors, and gastrointestinal, bronchial, and exocrine pancreatic carcinomas.

The causes of tumor-related hypoglycemia are complex and only partially understood. These tumors do not synthesize or store insulin, and circulating insulin levels are low during hypoglycemic episodes. However, increased insulin-like action of insulin-like growth factor II (IGF-II) has been reported in most extrapancreatic tumors. The mechanism is complex: Elevated levels of high molecular weight IGF-II, along with increased binding of IGF-II to IGF receptors, result in greater tissue availability of IGF-II and increased peripheral glucose uptake. A concomitant suppression of growth hormone levels also contributes to the development of hypoglycemia.

Many extrapancreatic tumors are too large to resect. Patients' blood glucose levels are raised with frequent feedings, glucose infusions, drugs like diazoxide or prednisone, or high doses of growth hormone.

DRUG-INDUCED HYPOGLYCEMIA

Insulin Overdose

The most common cause of hypoglycemia is insulin overdose in patients with diabetes. Most patients learn to recognize their own symptoms and abort attacks by eating carbohydrates. However, patients who have longstanding insulin-requiring diabetes with severe autonomic neuropathy or recurrent hypoglycemic episodes may have defective glucagon and epinephrine responses to low blood sugar. The poor production of these hormones, together with continuous insulin absorption from subcutaneous depots, can lead to occult and prolonged hypoglycemia. These defective responses are a particular problem in patients with intensively treated insulin-dependent diabetes, whose counterregulatory response occurs at unusually low glucose levels because of a functional defect induced by frequent hypoglycemic episodes. The defect can be partially reversed by better glucose control.

Nonmedically indicated self-administration of insulin to produce recurrent hypoglycemia is most common in relatives of patients with insulin-dependent diabetes and in hospital personnel. The discovery of injection marks or hidden insulin and syringes can reveal the true cause. Detection of insulin antibodies supports a suspicion of self-administered insulin. Patients' serum and urinary C peptide levels are low relative to their serum insulin.

Oral Hypoglycemic Agents

All of the sulfonylureas (oral hypoglycemic agents) can produce hypoglycemia, but the longer-acting drugs, such as chlorpropamide, are more often to blame. Sulfonylurea-induced hypoglycemia can be protracted and severe. It is most likely to occur in the very young and very old and in patients who are eating little, are malnourished, or have impaired liver, kidney, or adrenal function. Concomitant use of ethanol or other drugs, especially high-dose salicylates, augments the sulfonylureas' hypoglycemic effect. Patients found to have sulfonylurea-induced hypoglycemia should immediately be given an intravenous injection of 50% glucose; they should be hospitalized and their plasma glucose levels maintained at over 100 mg/dL with continuous intravenous glucose until their plasma glucose is stable on an oral diet.

Alcohol

Drinking alcohol can cause hypoglycemia. The most common setting is chronically malnourished alcoholics, 10–20 hours after they stop drinking alcohol and eating. However, alcohol can cause hypoglycemia in people who have a normal liver and normal hepatic glycogen stores: Healthy children and adults have been known to develop hypoglycemia after a short drinking spree. Normal amounts of liver glycogen protect somewhat against alcoholic hypoglycemia, which is caused mainly by hepatic gluconeogenesis being blocked by high levels of the cofactor reduced nicotinamide adenine dinucleotide (NADH) in the liver. Alcohol usually produces fasting hypoglycemia, but some people develop postprandial symptoms after they drink alcohol with a meal, especially one containing simple sugars. Patients with reactive hypoglycemia and those taking insulin or a sulfonylurea for diabetes are especially susceptible to ethanol-induced hypoglycemia. Obese people are relatively insensitive.

Alcoholic hypoglycemia may be difficult to diagnose when the symptoms are attributed to drunkenness. The physician should therefore measure plasma glucose in all symptomatic patients who have had a lot to drink. Patients may need prolonged glucose infusions over hours or even days to prevent recurrent hypoglycemia.

Other Drugs and Poisons

Hypoglycemia can be caused by other drugs and poisons. Drug-induced hypoglycemia is most common in children, patients with diabetes who are taking insulin or a sulfonylurea, and patients with compromised renal function. β-Blockers and salicylates interfere with hepatic glucose metabolism. Hepatotoxins can cause fatal hypoglycemia. So can eating certain poisonous plants, such as mushrooms and unripe, uncooked Jamaican akee fruit.

POSTPRANDIAL HYPOGLYCEMIA

Lay publications have popularized the notion that hypoglycemia is a common disorder that produces a wide variety of often vague complaints. In contrast, some experts question the very existence of postprandial hypoglycemia. The truth lies somewhere in between. A few people do get hypoglycemic symptoms after eating, and a few adults whose usual diet is low in carbohydrate become hypoglycemic after eating any appreciable amount of carbohydrate.

Postprandial hypoglycemia rarely causes significant central nervous system symptoms. Adrenergic symptoms usually abate within 30 minutes, because release of glucagon and epinephrine quickly raises the plasma glucose.

Postprandial hypoglycemia is suggested by a recurrent pattern of symptoms that have a fairly constant relationship to eating and usually appear late in the morning or afternoon. The physician should take a careful diet history and determine how the timing of symptoms relates to patients' eating and drinking. It is important to ask patients about the sodas and juice that they drink, because many people do not consider these food.

Because adrenergic symptoms are so nonspecific, patients can be taught to test whether their symptoms are linked to a low blood glucose by using a glucose oxidase strip reagent to measure their blood glucose at the time of symptoms. Glucose levels higher than 80 mg/dL require no further workup. If the glucose is below 80 mg/dL, the diet should be modified, as described in "Management of Postprandial Hypoglycemia" below. Patients who have persistent symptoms with glucose values below 80 mg/dL should undergo a 5-hour glucose tolerance test.

Before this test, patients should avoid drugs such as β-blockers and thiazide diuretics that are known to affect glucose tolerance and should eat at least 250 g of carbohydrate each day for 3 days. In the test, patients take a drink containing 75 g of glucose; then blood samples are obtained every 30 minutes to monitor plasma glucose. The frequent samples are needed because the glucose nadir can be transient. Patients are told to notify the technician if they develop symptoms during the test, so that an immediate blood sample can be taken. A plasma glucose below 60 mg/dL with appropriate symptoms is generally accepted as confirming symptomatic hypoglycemia. Some normal people have values below 50 mg/dL without symptoms.

The history and the glucose tolerance test result usually enable the physician to distinguish among the three common types of postprandial hypoglycemia: reactive, alimentary, and hypoglycemia associated with glucose intolerance.

Reactive Hypoglycemia: Reactive (functional, idiopathic) hypoglycemia is the most common form of postprandial hypoglycemia, but its pathogenesis remains unclear. When patients with reactive hypoglycemia are tested with intravenous glucose, they do not develop symptoms. Their glucose tolerance is not impaired; in fact, many patients' glucose levels increase little or not at all after they take a glucose-containing drink. Their serum insulin response is usually delayed, but appropriate for the plasma glucose (Figure 4.8–1). Occasional patients have elevated serum insulin concentrations. Most patients become mildly anxious and restless 3–5 hours after a meal, but some have more blatant adrenergic symptoms. Although patients with reactive hypoglycemia were once thought to be especially tense, asthenic, hyperkinetic, emotionally labile, and obsessive-compulsive, psychological tests have shown similar personality profiles in patients with all types of postprandial symptoms.

Alimentary Hypoglycemia: Alimentary hypoglycemia is the most striking form of hypoglycemia, both clinically and on testing. The sudden entry of large amounts of glucose into the small intestine causes a precipitous rise in plasma glucose levels and provokes dramatic insulin secretion and hypoglycemia 1–2 hours later. The cause may be thyrotoxicosis or unexplained rapid gastric emptying, but the usual cause is rapid emptying of the stomach following gastric surgery. Alimentary hypoglycemia must be distinguished from the postgastrectomy dumping syndrome, another problem of rapid gastric emptying usually resulting from gastric resection. Patients with the dumping syndrome have symptoms such as epigastric fullness, a sensation of abdominal distention, nausea, sweating, and palpitations.

Late Postprandial Hypoglycemia Associated with Glucose Intolerance: Some patients with a normal fasting plasma glucose develop late postprandial hypoglycemia associated with glucose intolerance (see Figure 4.8–1). Only a small fraction of these patients later become diabetic, and people with overt diabetes do not have postprandial hypoglycemia. The hypoglycemia is attributed to a delayed but excessive insulin response to the glucose load: Insulin levels are high when plasma glucose is falling.

Management of Postprandial Hypoglycemia

Management of patients with postprandial hypoglycemia is hampered by a lack of controlled clinical trials and objective ways to measure the effectiveness of therapy. Management begins with diet changes, but may later

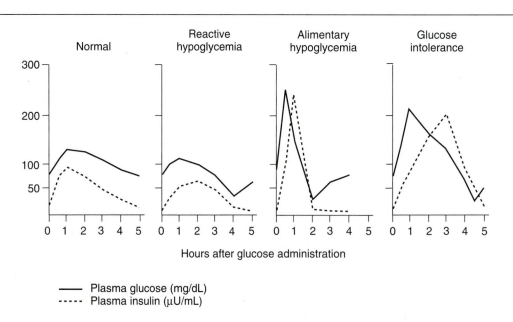

Figure 4.8–1. Comparison of glucose and insulin levels during a 5-hour glucose tolerance test: normal subjects and patients with three types of postprandial hypoglycemia.

include drugs. High-protein, carbohydrate-restricted diets are of little benefit. Instead, patients are instructed to eat complex, slowly digested carbohydrates rather than simple sugars and fruit drinks. Fiber and some fat should be included in every meal to delay gastric emptying. Fructose can be used as a sweetener because it increases blood glucose and insulin less than other sugars do. These measures, along with multiple small feedings throughout the day, may help patients with any type of postprandial hypoglycemia. Reduction to ideal body weight is an important goal for patients who have hypoglycemia with glucose intolerance.

If diet changes do not control hypoglycemic symptoms, patients may be helped by anticholinergic drugs that slow gastric emptying and intestinal motility and inhibit vagal stimulation of insulin release. Tincture of belladonna, atropine sulfate, or propantheline bromide taken 30 minutes before each meal may be effective, especially for patients with reactive hypoglycemia. In patients whose hypoglycemia is associated with glucose intolerance, a sulfonylurea hypoglycemic drug may relieve symptoms by stimulating early secretion of insulin. If symptoms still persist, patients may benefit from treatment for coexisting anxiety attacks.

SUMMARY

▶ The most important step in diagnosing symptomatic hypoglycemia is documenting that chemical hypoglycemia and typical symptoms coincide during a spontaneous attack or a provocative test.

▶ Fasting hypoglycemia, a potentially fatal metabolic derangement, causes manifestations of central nervous system glucose deprivation ranging from confusion and behavioral changes to seizures, coma, and death.

▶ The most common cause of hypoglycemia is insulin overdose in patients with diabetes. It is essential to identify other causes, for example, liver disease, insulinoma, hypopituitarism, adrenal insufficiency, extrapancreatic tumors, alcohol, and other drugs and toxins.

▶ The diagnosis of insulinoma requires proof of inappropriate hyperinsulinism.

▶ Adrenergic symptoms characterize postprandial hypoglycemia and can affect patients with fasting hypoglycemia.

SUGGESTED READING

Cherrington AD et al: Hypoglycemia, gluconeogenesis and the brain. Adv Exp Med Biol 1991;291:197.

Cryer PE: Hypoglycemia: The limiting factor in the management of IDDM. Diabetes 1994;43:1378.

Hofeldt FD: Reactive hypoglycemia. Endocrinol Metab Clin North Am 1989;18:185.

Mitrakou A et al: Hierarchy of glycemic thresholds for counterregulatory hormone secretion, symptoms, and cerebral dysfunction. Am J Physiol 1991;260:E67.

Vassilopoulou-Sellin R, Ajani J: Islet cell tumors of the pancreas. Endocrinol Metab Clin North Am 1994;23:53.

Disorders of Plasma Lipids and Lipoproteins

Simeon Margolis, MD, PhD

One in five adult Americans has hyperlipidemia, an elevation of plasma cholesterol, triglycerides, or both, resulting from an increased concentration of one or more of the plasma lipoproteins. Hyperlipidemia should be suspected in patients with premature atherosclerosis and is highly likely in those with xanthomas (accumulations of lipids in the skin or tendons). Most often, however, hyperlipidemia is first identified from the results of blood chemistries obtained routinely or for lipid screening.

Premature coronary artery disease is associated with high levels of LDL cholesterol, low levels of HDL cholesterol, and possibly high levels of lipoprotein(a) [Lp(a)] (for definitions, see "Lipoprotein Structure and Composition" below). Dietary changes and drugs are both effective in treating hyperlipidemia. Lowering plasma cholesterol levels reduces the incidence of myocardial infarctions, and, in persons with proven coronary artery disease, slows progression and causes regression of coronary artery lesions and decreases cardiovascular and overall mortality. In most studies, a triglyceride elevation is not an independent risk factor for coronary artery disease in men, but hypertriglyceridemia is usually accompanied by low levels of HDL cholesterol. In women and patients with diabetes mellitus, however, hypertriglyceridemia *is* a risk factor for coronary artery disease. Severe hypertriglyceridemia can also cause recurrent attacks of acute pancreatitis.

LIPOPROTEIN STRUCTURE AND COMPOSITION

The plasma lipids are transported on lipoproteins, spherical particles with a central core of apolar lipids (triglycerides and cholesterol esters) covered by a surface coat of proteins and more water-soluble lipids (cholesterol and phospholipids). The amount of lipid in the central core determines the size and density of each lipoprotein. Three major classes of lipoproteins are present during the fasting state: very low (VLDL), low (LDL), and high (HDL) density lipoproteins. Chylomicrons, the largest and least dense lipoproteins, carry absorbed fat from the intestine and are not found in normal individuals after an overnight fast.

Because the lipoproteins undergo extensive modifications in the circulation, the particles within each class are quite heterogeneous. Table 4.9–1 shows the average composition of lipids and proteins (called *apoproteins*) of each lipoprotein class. Triglycerides are the major component of chylomicrons (85–90%) and VLDL (55–65%). Cholesterol and cholesterol esters make up about 50% of LDL. Thus, an elevated plasma triglyceride is caused by an increased concentration of VLDL, chylomicrons, or both. When triglyceride levels are normal, hypercholesterolemia is caused by high LDL levels. The apoproteins (shortened to "apo") impart water solubility, mediate lipoprotein binding to cellular receptors, and activate enzymes that metabolize lipoprotein lipids.

Lp(a) is an LDL-like particle in which apo B_{100}, the sole apoprotein on LDL, is covalently linked to apo(a), a very large protein with structural features similar to a portion of plasminogen.

PHYSIOLOGY OF LIPID TRANSPORT

The major function of chylomicrons is transporting triglycerides from the intestine (Figure 4.9–1). Chylomicrons are formed within cells of the small intestine where the absorbed products of triglyceride digestion are resynthesized to triglycerides. In an American on a typical diet, chylomicrons also transport 200–350 mg of cholesterol

Table 4.9–1. Plasma lipoprotein classes.

Lipoprotein	Major Components	Apoproteins*	Important Features
Chylomicron	Triglycerides (85–90%) derived from dietary fat	B_{48}, C, (A)	Float in plasma after overnight refrigeration Synthesized in intestinal mucosal cells Not normally present after overnight fast
Chylomicron and VLDL remnants (β-VLDL)	Triglycerides (35%) Cholesterol esters (35%)	B_{48}, B_{100}, E	Quickly cleared after binding to apo E receptors in liver
Very low density (VLDL)	Triglycerides (55–65%) from endogenous synthesis	B_{100}, C, E, (A)	Synthesized in liver Apo C-II activates lipoprotein lipase
Low density (LDL)	Cholesterol (50%)	B_{100}	Formed mainly during metabolism of VLDL
High density (HDL)	Protein (50%)	A-I, A-II, (C, D, E)	Transport cholesterol from peripheral tissues to liver Apo A-I activates LCAT

*Minor apoprotein components are shown in parentheses.

per day from the intestine. VLDL carries triglycerides formed in the liver from fatty acids released from adipose tissue or synthesized from dietary carbohydrates. The enzyme lipoprotein lipase, located in the capillary endothelium of adipose tissue and muscle, removes triglycerides from chylomicrons and VLDL by splitting them into their constituent fatty acids plus glycerol. Lipoprotein lipase requires apo C-II for activation. The action of lipoprotein lipase produces both chylomicron and VLDL remnants (together referred to as "β-VLDL"), which are rich in cholesterol esters. Chylomicron remnants are quickly removed from the circulation after binding to apo E receptors in the liver. Further breakdown of triglycerides by a hepatic lipase converts VLDL remnants (also known as "intermediate density lipoprotein" or IDL) to LDL.

A major function of LDL is to transport cholesterol, an essential component of cell membranes and the precursor of steroid hormones. Dietary cholesterol is supplemented by endogenous synthesis in almost all cell types, especially in the liver and intestine. After binding to LDL receptors in the liver and peripheral tissues, LDL is carried into the cell and enters lysosomes where apo B_{100} and cholesterol esters are hydrolyzed. The rise in free cholesterol in liver cells stimulates cholesterol esterification, slows the formation of LDL receptors, and reduces cholesterol synthesis by decreasing the production of hydroxymethylglutaryl coenzyme A (HMG CoA) reductase, the rate-limiting enzyme in cholesterol formation. In this manner, the concentration of free cholesterol within liver cells controls cholesterol synthesis and the hepatic uptake of LDL.

HDL plays a pivotal role in the transport of cholesterol from peripheral tissues to the liver, which eliminates cholesterol from the body by secreting it into the bile directly or after converting it to bile acids. HDL is secreted from both liver and intestine as a disk-shaped, "nascent" lipoprotein composed primarily of apo A-I and phospholipids. Nascent HDL removes cholesterol from peripheral tissues. The enzyme lecithin:cholesterol acyltransferase (LCAT), released into the blood from the liver, forms cholesterol esters from cholesterol and lecithin. Apo A-I activates LCAT, and a cholesterol ester transfer protein shuttles some of the cholesterol esters to VLDL and LDL in exchange for triglycerides. The accumulation of cholesterol and its esterification by LCAT convert nascent HDL to a spherical particle called HDL_3. Cholesterol esters are returned to the liver either directly by HDL or after transfer to VLDL and LDL. During the metabolism of chylomicrons and VLDL, the transfer of cholesterol, phospholipids, and apoproteins to HDL_3 converts it to HDL_2.

EFFECTS OF LIPOPROTEINS ON THE ARTERIAL WALL

Elevated LDL levels have both chronic and acute effects. Long-term effects result from deposition of LDL into macrophages in the arterial wall. Acutely, elevated LDL levels promote vasoconstriction that may contribute to angina. The first step in atherogenesis is oxidation of the unsaturated fatty acids of LDL by free radicals formed within the intima of arteries. Following this oxidation, apo B_{100} is chemically modified and binds to scavenger receptors on the surface of macrophages within the arterial intima. Unregulated uptake of the cholesterol ester-rich, oxidized LDL results in the formation of foam cells and the development of fatty streaks that progress to form atherosclerotic plaques. Oxidized LDL also stimulates the entry of monocytes into the arterial wall, inhibits the egress of macrophages, and alters endothelial cell function to cause vasoconstriction. IDL, chylomicron remnants, and Lp(a) are also taken up by arterial macrophages. Because of its structural similarity to plasminogen, Lp(a) promotes thrombus formation by interfering with the conversion of plasminogen to plasmin and inhibiting plasmin-mediated thrombolysis. HDL helps prevent atherosclerosis by removing cholesterol from cells in the arterial wall and possibly by protecting LDL from oxidation.

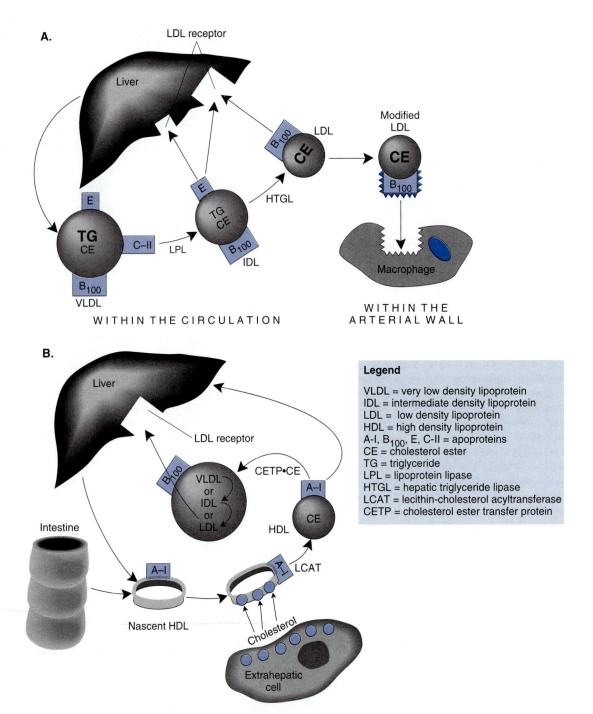

Figure 4.9–1. A: Basic mechanisms for endogenous fat transport. The liver releases triglyceride-rich VLDL. Apo C-II activates the enzyme LPL, which is bound to capillaries in adipose tissue and muscle, to split VLDL TG into glycerol and fatty acids (not shown). LPL's removal of TG from VLDL converts VLDL to the smaller lipoprotein IDL. IDL can be taken up by hepatic receptors for apo E, or HTGL can remove even more TG to convert IDL to LDL. LDL contains relatively little TG, but large amounts of CE. During the conversion of VLDL to LDL, all of the apoproteins on VLDL move to HDL (not shown), except for apo B_{100}, the only apoprotein of LDL. LDL is removed from the circulation by binding to LDL receptors in the liver and other tissues. Oxidation of the unsaturated fatty acids in LDL leads to modifications of the apo B_{100} on its surface; the modified LDL is then taken up by scavenger receptors on macrophages in the arterial wall. Engorgement of macrophages with CE produces foam cells, the first step in atherogenesis. **B:** Reverse cholesterol transport. The liver and intestine release nascent HDL, a disk-shaped particle containing primarily lecithin and apo A-I. Nascent HDL removes cholesterol from peripheral tissues, especially macrophages in the arterial wall. Apo A-I activates the enzyme LCAT to convert cholesterol to CE, which enters the center of the nascent HDL to form the spherical HDL particle. CE is carried back to the liver either on HDL itself, or by IDL or LDL after CETP transfers CE from HDL to VLDL, IDL, and LDL.

340

HYPERLIPIDEMIA

Classification

One classification delineates six phenotypic forms of hyperlipidemia (Table 4.9–2), based on an increased concentration of one or more of the plasma lipoproteins. An isolated elevation of chylomicrons is designated type I. LDL cholesterol concentrations are increased in both types IIA and IIB. In type IIA, only LDL cholesterol levels are increased; type IIB patients also have hypertriglyceridemia caused by elevated VLDL levels. Other forms of hypertriglyceridemia result from increased levels of VLDL (type IV), both VLDL and chylomicrons (type V), or chylomicron remnants and IDL (type III). In patients with type III, also known as dysbetalipoproteinemia or broad beta disease, plasma cholesterol and triglycerides are generally elevated to a similar degree.

Assignment of a specific type to each hyperlipidemic patient may aid in prognosis and management, but the typing scheme has serious deficiencies. Since distinctions are based entirely on phenotypic characteristics, the same type of hyperlipidemia may result from a primary genetic defect or environmental factors or may be a secondary manifestation of another disorder or may result from drug use. Moreover, treatment with diet or drugs may alter the lipoprotein pattern.

In most patients with type II or IV hyperlipidemia, the underlying cause is polygenic or involves factors such as obesity and a high-fat diet. Three common forms of hyperlipidemia are inherited as autosomal dominant traits. *Familial hypercholesterolemia* and *familial hypertriglyceridemia* each affect 0.1–0.2% of the US population. The most common monogenic form of hyperlipidemia is *familial combined hyperlipidemia.* Affected family members have type IIA, IIB, or IV patterns with about equal frequency.

Pathophysiology of Hyperlipidemia

Hyperlipidemia results from either increased synthesis or diminished removal of plasma lipoproteins and their constituent lipids. An abnormality in the enzymatic metabolism of the lipids or reduced binding of apoproteins to tissue receptors retards the removal of lipoproteins.

Primary Hyperlipidemia: Considerable progress has been made in the basic understanding of several genetic forms of hyperlipidemia. Type I results from defective formation of lipoprotein lipase. An inability to synthesize its activator, apo C-II, can cause type V. Patients with type III have abnormal forms of apo E, which bind poorly to apo E receptors in the liver; poor clearance of chylomicron remnants and IDL leads to their accumulation in the plasma. Some other factor must also be present for the expression of type III, since 1% of the population has abnor-

Table 4.9–2. Classification and clinical manifestations of hyperlipidemia.

Type	Prevalence	Appearance of Plasma After Overnight Refrigeration	Elevated Lipids and Lipoproteins	Signs and Symptoms	Risk for Coronary Artery Disease	Other Features
I	Rare	Creamy layer over clear infranatant	Triglycerides (chylomicrons)	Recurrent bouts of abdominal pain, eruptive xanthomas, and acute pancreatitis	Normal	Sensitive to dietary fat because of deficient lipoprotein lipase activity Symptoms begin in infancy or childhood
IIA IIB	Common Common	Clear Clear or cloudy	Cholesterol (LDL) Cholesterol and triglycerides (LDL and VLDL)	Tendinous and tuberous xanthomas; xanthelasma; corneal arcus	Very high	One autosomal dominant form, familial hypercholesterolemia, can be diagnosed at birth
III	Uncommon	Clear or cloudy	Cholesterol and triglycerides (β-VLDL)	Palmar and tuberoeruptive xanthomas High risk for peripheral vascular disease	Very high	Often associated with diabetes Abnormal forms of apo E lead to accumulation of β-VLDL
IV	Common	Clear or cloudy	Triglycerides (VLDL)	Tuberous xanthomas	Varies with genetic pattern	Often associated with diabetes In most patients, lipid abnormalities first manifest in early adulthood
V	Uncommon	Creamy layer over cloudy infranatant	Triglycerides (VLDL and chylomicrons)	Recurrent bouts of abdominal pain, eruptive xanthomas, and acute pancreatitis	Moderate	Sensitive to dietary fat Often associated with diabetes Symptoms begin in adulthood

mal forms of apo E, but the incidence of type III is far lower.

Homozygotes with familial hypercholesterolemia have absent or defective LDL receptors or an inability to internalize LDL. As a result, poor LDL uptake interferes with its degradation and leads to hepatic overproduction of cholesterol.

Familial hypertriglyceridemia results from both increased synthesis and reduced catabolism of VLDL. Familial combined hyperlipidemia is caused by overproduction of VLDL and apo B_{100}; the resulting elevation in plasma levels of apo B_{100} may account for the increased risk of premature coronary artery disease in patients with familial combined hyperlipidemia.

Secondary Hyperlipidemia: Hyperlipidemia can be caused by a number of disorders and by certain drugs (Table 4.9–3). Secondary hyperlipidemia may present as any of the phenotypes. An abnormal, cholesterol-rich lipoprotein (lipoprotein X) is found in patients with obstructive liver disease. Deficient activity of lipoprotein lipase in hypothyroidism or severe insulin deficiency can increase chylomicron levels. Insulin treatment quickly clears the chylomicronemia in insulin-deficient patients.

Many obese patients with non–insulin-dependent diabetes mellitus have syndrome X: abdominal obesity, insulin resistance, hyperinsulinemia, hypertension, hypertriglyceridemia, low HDL cholesterol, and high risk for coronary artery disease. Diabetics may also inherit a primary hyperlipidemia that raises triglycerides even further or causes hypercholesterolemia.

Both estrogens and alcohol can raise triglycerides to very high levels in patients with modest hypertriglyceridemia. HDL cholesterol levels may be lowered severely by anabolic steroids and modestly by β-blockers and the more androgenic progestational agents.

Although severe hyperlipidemia invariably results from a genetic abnormality or is secondary to some demonstrable disease, people who eat large amounts of animal fat

Table 4.9–3. Causes of secondary hyperlipidemia.

Diabetes mellitus
Hypothyroidism
Hypercortisolism
Acromegaly
Obesity
Nephrotic syndrome
Chronic renal failure
Acute intermittent porphyria
Glycogen storage disease
Macroglobulinemia associated with myeloma
Obstructive liver disease
Drugs
   Estrogens
   Thiazide diuretics
   β-blockers
   Vitamin A analogs
   Alcohol

may have modest elevations of their plasma LDL cholesterol. Such diet-induced hyperlipidemia generally responds well to diet modification.

Clinical Manifestations

Xanthomas (lipid accumulations in the skin or tendons; see Color Plates) are the only overt manifestations of hyperlipidemia. Xanthelasmas (slightly raised yellowish plaques along the eyelids; see Color Plates) are common in type II, but they do not correlate with the severity of the hypercholesterolemia; in fact, about 60% of patients with xanthelasmas have normal serum lipids. Patients with severe hypercholesterolemia may have corneal arcus before age 35. Tendon xanthomas (nodules or thickening of the tendons, caused by an accumulation of cholesterol esters) are almost always diagnostic of familial hypercholesterolemia, but they also appear in two rare hereditary conditions: Patients with sitosterolemia store plant sterols, and patients with cerebrotendinous xanthomatosis accumulate cholestanol, a breakdown product of cholesterol. Type III hyperlipidemia is characterized by xanthoma striatum palmare (planar, yellowish deposits of lipids in the palmar creases), tuberous xanthomas (nodular accumulations of lipids), and tuberoeruptive xanthomas (tuberous xanthomas with an inflammatory base). Tuberous xanthomas also occur in types II and IV. When extremely high plasma triglyceride levels are accompanied by chylomicronemia, patients may develop eruptive xanthomas (small yellowish papules) and lipemia retinalis (pink to whitish appearance of the retinal arteries and veins; see Color Plates).

Heterozygotes for familial hypercholesterolemia exhibit plasma cholesterol values of 300–500 mg/dL (either type IIA or IIB), tendon xanthomas, and premature coronary artery disease. Homozygotes may have plasma cholesterol levels exceeding 800 mg/dL. They develop tendon and planar xanthomas by age 10, and severe coronary atherosclerosis, often with aortic stenosis, by their teens; most die before age 20.

Dysbetalipoproteinemia causes both premature coronary and peripheral vascular disease. The risk of coronary artery disease is high in patients with familial combined hyperlipidemia, but not in familial hypertriglyceridemia. Extreme hypertriglyceridemia (over 1000 mg/dL) may produce eruptive xanthomas, hepatosplenomegaly, and severe abdominal pain from acute pancreatitis. Chylomicronemia can also cause arthralgias, dryness of eyes and mouth, emotional lability, and tingling in the extremities. Type I and apo C-II deficiency (manifest as type V) can be identified in childhood. Most often type V is first observed in adults; it is especially common in patients with diabetes. More than 50% of patients with hypertriglyceridemia have hyperuricemia.

Rationale for Treatment

The most important reasons for treating hyperlipidemia are to prevent the initial clinical manifestations of cardiovascular disease (primary prevention) and to reduce the likelihood of recurrent symptoms and events in patients with known cardiovascular disease (secondary prevention). Hypercholesterolemia is a major risk factor for coronary artery disease, because of LDL's atherogenic potency. Primary prevention trials have shown that lowering plasma LDL cholesterol reduces coronary events such as myocardial infarction and sudden death (a 2% decrease in events for every 1% fall in plasma cholesterol). In secondary prevention trials, a decrease in LDL cholesterol has slowed progression of lesions in the coronary arteries, caused lesions to regress, and decreased cardiovascular and total mortality.

Another reason for treating hyperlipidemia is to prevent attacks of acute pancreatitis provoked by severe hypertriglyceridemia, usually associated with the chylomicronemia of type I or V. Reducing fasting plasma triglycerides to below 500 mg/dL may completely prevent further attacks.

Concern about the possible dangers of lowering plasma cholesterol has been generated by several long-term trials of cholesterol-lowering drugs that showed a higher incidence of violent deaths (accidents, suicides, and murders) in the treatment group than the placebo group. In contrast, patients in one large study had a 30% decrease in overall mortality during $5^{1}/_{2}$ years when their LDL cholesterol was lowered with simvastatin, and there was no increase in noncardiovascular deaths. Other researchers have pointed out a *relatively* higher mortality from suicides, cirrhosis, and certain forms of cancer in persons with cholesterol levels below 160 mg/dL; however, the *absolute* overall mortality, especially from cardiovascular disease, rose progressively with increasing levels of cholesterol.

Guidelines for Detecting and Treating Hyperlipidemia

The use of these guidelines requires recognition of the biologic variability in plasma cholesterol and triglyceride levels, as well as the relative inaccuracy and imprecision of measurements of triglycerides and cholesterol, especially HDL cholesterol. Moreover, measurements can vary greatly from one laboratory to another. As a result, the diagnosis and treatment of any lipid disorder must be based on good agreement in at least two sets of baseline values obtained in the same laboratory over 10–14 days. Secondary hyperlipidemias are identified by history and blood tests for glucose, creatinine, thyroid-stimulating hormone, and liver function.

All types of hyperlipidemia may be genetically determined; therefore, first-degree relatives should be screened for abnormal plasma lipids so that the genetic disorder can be identified and patients can start treatment before they develop irreversible vascular changes. Familial hypercholesterolemia can be detected at birth; hypertriglyceridemia may not manifest until the late teens or early 20's.

Hypercholesterolemia: The following recommendations for the diagnosis and treatment of elevated LDL cholesterol levels were proposed by the Adult Panel of the

Table 4.9–4. Risk factors for coronary artery disease.

High risk (2 or more of the following)
Men older than 45
Women older than 55 or after premature menopause
Family history of premature coronary artery disease: myocardial infarction or sudden death in:
— Father or first-degree male relative before age 55
— Mother or first-degree female relative before age 65
Cigarette smoking
Hypertension or treatment for hypertension
HDL cholesterol <35 mg/dL

Very high risk (any 1 of the following)
Atherosclerotic disease: coronary artery, peripheral vascular, or cerebrovascular disease
Diabetes mellitus

"Negative" risk factor
If patients have an HDL cholesterol >60 mg/dL, 1 risk factor can be subtracted from their total

Modified and reproduced, with permission, from Summary of the Second Report of the National Cholesterol Education Program (NCEP) Expert Panel on Detection, Evaluation, and Treatment of High Blood Cholesterol in Adults (Adult Treatment Panel II). JAMA 1993;269:3015.

National Cholesterol Education Program, a group appointed by the National Institutes of Health. Screening tests, which do not require a fasting blood specimen, should measure total and HDL cholesterol. If the screening tests show a desirable cholesterol level (below 170 mg/dL in persons under 20; below 200 mg/dL in adults), the tests should be repeated in 5 years. Management decisions for other persons depend on a combination of their LDL cholesterol and risk status. "High" and "very high" risk are defined in Table 4.9–4. Low-risk adults with a cholesterol of 200–239 mg/dL should be instructed in proper eating habits and screened again in a year. Table 4.9–5 summarizes the recommendations for when to obtain a fasting lipid profile (cholesterol, triglycerides, and HDL cholesterol), so that the LDL cholesterol can be estimated according to this formula:

$$\text{LDL cholesterol} = \text{Total cholesterol} - \text{HDL cholesterol} - \frac{\text{triglycerides}}{5}$$

Measurements of Lp(a) may help the physician to decide whether to give medications to patients who have borderline cholesterol values and only one other risk factor.

Table 4.9–5. Indications for obtaining a lipid profile.

Total cholesterol
  Adults:
    200–239 mg/dL if at high risk, OR
    ≥240 mg/dL
  Children and teenagers:
    170–199 mg/dL if at high risk, OR
    ≥200 mg/dL
Very high-risk patients
HDL cholesterol <35 mg/dL

Measurements of apo B_{100} may help to distinguish between familial hypertriglyceridemia and familial combined hyperlipidemia. Measurement of other apoproteins is rarely needed.

Table 4.9–6 shows how the combination of risk status and LDL cholesterol values is used to make decisions on dietary and drug treatment.

Hypertriglyceridemia: The recent guidelines have suggested the following classification for plasma triglyceride levels in adults: below 200 mg/dL, normal; 200–399 mg/dL, borderline high; 400–999 mg/dL, high; and over 1000 mg/dL, very high. Patients with very high triglycerides require treatment with diet—and drugs, if necessary—to prevent attacks of acute pancreatitis. Management of patients with triglycerides of 200–1000 mg/dL is aimed at preventing premature vascular disease and is determined by individual circumstances. All patients should modify their diets. Drugs should be added if diet alone is insufficient for patients at high or very high risk.

Management of Hyperlipidemia

Management of any type of hyperlipidemia starts with dietary changes. When dietary measures are not followed or when they fail to lower lipid levels enough, five types of medications are available (Table 4.9–7). The HMG CoA reductase inhibitors are the most effective drugs for lowering total and LDL cholesterol. Niacin is the most effective agent for raising HDL cholesterol, and gemfibrozil is most effective for reducing triglycerides. With the possible exception of niacin, none of these agents lowers Lp(a) levels.

Elevated LDL Cholesterol:

Dietary treatment: Table 4.9–6 summarizes when dietary treatment should be started at various LDL cholesterol levels. The recommended diet for hypercholesterolemia has two stages. The Step 1 diet limits total fat to

Table 4.9–6. Management decisions based on LDL cholesterol.

Start diet when:

LDL cholesterol exceeds (mg/dL):	and Risk status is:
160	Low
130	High
100	Very high

Consider drug treatment when:

LDL cholesterol exceeds (mg/dL):	and Risk status is:
220	Low in men <35 and premenopausal women
190	Low in men >35 and postmenopausal women
160	High
100	Very high

Modified and reproduced, with permission, from Summary of the Second Report of the National Cholesterol Education Program (NCEP) Expert Panel on Detection, Evaluation, and Treatment of High Blood Cholesterol in Adults (Adult Treatment Panel II). JAMA 1993;269:3015.

Table 4.9–7. Effects of lipid-lowering drugs on serum lipids and lipoproteins.

Drug	LDL Cholesterol	Triglycerides	HDL Cholesterol
HMG CoA reductase inhibitors (statins)	↓↓↓↓	↓	↑
Bile acid sequestrants	↓↓↓	– or ↑	–
Niacin	↓↓	↓↓	↑↑
Probucol	↓	–	↓
Gemfibrozil	↓	↓↓↓	↑

30% of calories, saturated fat to below 10% of calories, and cholesterol to below 300 mg/day. If the LDL cholesterol remains too high after 3 months, the more restrictive Step 2 diet is recommended. This diet limits saturated fat to 7% of calories and cholesterol to below 200 mg per day. Patients may be taught the Step 1 diet by physicians or their staff, but an experienced dietician should give instructions for the Step 2 diet. Additional dietary measures include weight loss for obese patients and eating more of the water-soluble fiber found in oat bran, beans, legumes, and many fruits and vegetables. Although losing weight may not lower the LDL cholesterol, it lowers triglycerides and may raise the HDL cholesterol. Side effects (bloating and gas) often make it difficult to eat enough fiber to lower cholesterol levels. An alternative is taking products containing the water-soluble fiber of psyllium seeds.

Drug treatment: Table 4.9–6 lists recommendations for when to start drug treatment. Drugs are generally started only if 6 months of dietary management has not adequately controlled LDL cholesterol levels. Drugs can be started sooner in patients at very high risk or with extremely high LDL cholesterol levels. The HMG CoA reductase inhibitors are the first-choice drugs to treat an elevated LDL cholesterol. Bile acid sequestrants and niacin are also effective in lowering LDL cholesterol levels.

HMG CoA reductase inhibitors (statins). By blocking hepatic cholesterol synthesis, the HMG CoA reductase inhibitors (nicknamed "statins") increase production of LDL receptors and thereby increase removal of LDL from the circulation. They are the most effective drugs available to lower plasma cholesterol: Full doses can lower the LDL cholesterol by as much as 50%. Reductase inhibitors can also raise HDL cholesterol by 6–8% and lower triglycerides by 10%. Up to 2% of patients develop side effects, most often gastrointestinal symptoms, a rise in liver enzymes, and myositis. Despite the similarity in chemical structures among the four reductase inhibitors (lovastatin, pravastatin, simvastatin, and fluvastatin), many patients who develop side effects from one of them can tolerate another without any problem. Long-term risks remain a possibility, since these drugs have been in use for only a few years. Reductase inhibitors are most effective when given in the evening, because most cholesterol is synthesized at night.

Bile acid sequestrants. The bile acid sequestrants (cholestyramine and colestipol) work by binding bile acids in the intestine and removing them in the stool. The resultant increase in hepatic conversion of cholesterol to bile acids lowers the cholesterol content of liver cells and triggers an increase in the number of LDL receptors on their surface. Full doses of a sequestrant can lower LDL cholesterol by 25–30% and raise HDL cholesterol by 1–2%. Bile acid sequestrants may raise triglyceride levels, especially in hypertriglyceridemic patients. To minimize bloating and constipation, the major side effects of bile acid sequestrants, these drugs should be started in small doses and increased gradually over several weeks. Because these agents can bind and interfere with the absorption of many drugs, other medications should be taken 1 hour before or several hours after the sequestrants.

Niacin. Niacin blocks the liver's synthesis and release of VLDL. Thus, full doses of niacin can lower LDL cholesterol by 15–20% and triglycerides by 25–35%, while raising the HDL cholesterol by 10–20%. Common side effects of niacin are flushing episodes, abnormal liver enzymes, nausea, and epigastric pain. Flushing attacks can be ameliorated with aspirin. The slow-release forms of niacin most often appear to cause liver toxicity. Less common side effects include a decrease in glucose tolerance and a rise in uric acid levels that may lead to attacks of gout.

Probucol. Probucol becomes incorporated into the central apolar portion of LDL and speeds its removal from the blood. Unfortunately, probucol lowers both LDL cholesterol and HDL cholesterol by 10–20%. Despite these unfavorable effects on HDL cholesterol, probucol slows the oxidation of the unsaturated fatty acids of LDL and thereby apparently prevents an early step in the atherosclerotic process—LDL uptake by macrophages in the arterial wall. To date, no clinical trial has shown that this theoretical benefit of probucol translates into decreased coronary events or mortality. The drug is generally well tolerated. Mild diarrhea is the most common side effect.

Elevated Triglycerides:

Dietary treatment: The most effective measures for treating all forms of hypertriglyceridemia, except type I, are weight reduction and maintenance of ideal body weight. Weight goals are defined by weight gained after reaching full maturity. Alcohol intake is restricted because it can raise triglyceride levels in patients with hypertriglyceridemia. Other dietary measures are similar to the Step 1 diet described in "Dietary Treatment" above. However, when triglycerides exceed 1000 mg/dL, dietary fat intake must be reduced even further. Supplementation with medium-chain triglycerides, which contain fatty acids that are transported in the portal blood rather than as chylomicron triglycerides, can make severely fat-restricted diets more palatable.

Drug treatment: Niacin and gemfibrozil lower triglyceride levels in all forms of hypertriglyceridemia ex-

cept type I. The fall in triglycerides produced by gemfibrozil may be accompanied by a rise in LDL cholesterol levels. HMG CoA reductase inhibitors are effective in lowering both triglyceride and LDL cholesterol levels in patients with triglyceride levels below 350 mg/dL. Large doses of fish oil (up to 10 g/day) may be effective in patients with severe hypertriglyceridemia. When type V patients do not respond adequately to diet or other drugs, progestational agents (norethindrone acetate or medroxyprogesterone acetate) may be used in women, and the anabolic steroid oxandrolone in men.

Gemfibrozil. Gemfibrozil is the fibric acid derivative most widely used in the United States. Its major action is to enhance the conversion of VLDL to LDL. Gemfibrozil lowers LDL cholesterol by 10%, triglycerides by as much as 50%, and total cholesterol by about 10%, and it raises HDL cholesterol by about 10%. The main side effects—gastrointestinal complaints and a rise in liver enzymes—are not common. The drug causes a small, statistically insignificant increase in the incidence of gallstones. Gemfibrozil is cleared by the kidneys; therefore, the dose must be reduced in patients with renal insufficiency in order to avoid high blood levels that can cause myositis.

Drug combinations and other medications: Since each of the drug classes acts through different mechanisms, drug combinations have additive effects and may be useful when a single agent does not adequately control hyperlipidemia. The bile acid sequestrants can be used safely and effectively in combination with any of the other drugs. In some patients, combinations of HMG CoA reductase inhibitors with the lipid-lowering agents gemfibrozil or niacin, or with cyclosporine or erythromycin, cause severe myositis, which can lead to rhabdomyolysis and renal failure.

Although the benefits of adding antioxidants (vitamins E and C and beta carotene) have not yet been proven with prospective randomized trials, epidemiologic and animal data suggest their potential value in preventing the oxidation of LDL that leads to its deposition in macrophages of arterial walls. The incidence of coronary artery disease increases dramatically in postmenopausal women, and many studies have shown that estrogen replacement reduces their incidence of coronary events. Estrogen lowers LDL cholesterol and raises HDL cholesterol, but other, poorly defined effects of estrogen also contribute to the protection against coronary artery disease. Except in women who have had a hysterectomy, a progestational agent is added to prevent the increased risk of uterine cancer seen with estrogen replacement alone. Now under study are the effects of such combined hormone replacement on coronary events.

LOW HDL CHOLESTEROL LEVELS

In the United States, mean HDL cholesterol levels are 45 mg/dL in men and 55 mg/dL in women. An HDL cholesterol below 35 mg/dL is considered a risk factor in both men and women. It is difficult to make substantial increases in HDL cholesterol levels, which are largely under genetic control. However, the effort appears worthwhile because a 1% increase in HDL cholesterol reportedly decreases the incidence of coronary events by 2–4%. Lifestyle changes that may raise HDL cholesterol are more physical activity, quitting cigarette smoking, and weight loss in the obese. Many studies have shown that HDL cholesterol is increased by moderate alcohol intake. Diets rich in carbohydrates (low-fat diets), excessively high in polyunsaturated fats, or low in cholesterol content tend to lower the plasma HDL cholesterol at the same time that they lower LDL cholesterol levels.

Niacin is the most effective drug for raising HDL cholesterol. Less effective are gemfibrozil and HMG CoA reductase inhibitors. Although all these drugs are now approved only for treatment of elevated cholesterol or triglycerides, some authorities have recommended them for patients with proven coronary artery disease whose only lipid abnormality is a low HDL cholesterol.

OTHER FORMS OF DYSLIPOPROTEINEMIA

HDL Deficiency

Tangier disease results from failure to form mature apo A-I from secreted proapoprotein A-I (apo A-I Tangier), which associates poorly with lipoproteins. Thus, apo A-I and HDL constituents are catabolized quickly and their plasma levels fall to about 1% of normal. This autosomal recessive disorder is recognized by very low levels of HDL cholesterol, decreased LDL, and slightly increased VLDL. Cholesterol ester deposition in reticuloendothelial cells may produce hepatosplenomegaly and lymphadenopathy; the most dramatic clinical finding is grossly enlarged orange tonsils. Patients with Tangier disease have a moderate increase in coronary artery disease.

About 0.2% of the United States population is heterozygous for some kind of single amino acid substitution in apo A-I. Several of these mutants cause low HDL cholesterol and high triglyceride levels. A genetic defect causing an absence of apo A-I and C-III produces marked HDL deficiency, xanthomas, premature coronary artery disease, and mild corneal opacification. Patients with another genetic abnormality, *fish eye disease,* have striking corneal opacification and low HDL cholesterol levels; the defect has not been identified.

Apo B Deficiency

Apo B deficiency occurs in patients with familial hypobetalipoproteinemia (autosomal dominant) or abetalipoproteinemia (autosomal recessive). Patients with familial hypobetalipoproteinemia synthesize a truncated apo B protein; the defect in abetalipoproteinemia is absence of a microsomal triglyceride transfer protein. Homozygotes with either disorder have similar laboratory and clinical features. Their plasma cholesterol and triglyceride levels are below 50 mg/dL, and they have virtually no chylomicrons, LDL, or VLDL. The clinical manifestations are fat malabsorption with steatorrhea, growth retardation, ataxic neuropathy, acanthocytosis, and atypical retinitis pigmentosa. High doses of vitamin E can prevent further neurologic and retinal damage. Supplementary vitamins A and K may also be useful. Fat restriction reduces diarrhea. Heterozygotes have normal lipid and lipoprotein levels in abetalipoproteinemia and about half-normal levels in hypobetalipoproteinemia.

LCAT Deficiency

In patients with a deficiency of the enzyme LCAT, all plasma lipoproteins exhibit structural or compositional abnormalities because of an excess of cholesterol and phospholipids and a dearth of cholesterol esters. Hemolytic anemia seen in many of these patients may be caused by an increased cholesterol content in red blood cells. Deposition of lipids in the cornea causes marked corneal opacification; lipid deposits in the glomeruli cause proteinuria, and, ultimately, renal failure. Patients may benefit from a low-fat diet.

SUMMARY

▶ At least 20% of Americans have some plasma lipid or lipoprotein abnormality that increases their risk for cardiovascular disease.

▶ Lowering plasma LDL cholesterol levels reduces the initial incidence of coronary events (primary prevention). Lowering the LDL also slows progression and causes some regression of coronary artery lesions; it reduces cardiovascular and overall mortality in individuals with known coronary artery disease (secondary prevention).

▶ LDL is atherogenic: Uptake of oxidized LDL by macrophages in the intima begins atherosclerosis, and high LDL levels cause vasoconstriction. HDL is protective: It carries cholesterol from the arterial wall back to the liver for excretion.

▶ Hypertriglyceridemia is an independent risk factor for coronary artery disease in women and in patients with familial combined hyperlipidemia, dysbetalipoproteinemia, or diabetes mellitus. Severe hypertriglyceridemia (above 1000 mg/dL) can cause acute pancreatitis.

▶ Treatment decisions for hyperlipidemia are based on plasma lipid and lipoprotein levels and the patient's risk for coronary artery disease. Treatment begins with dietary changes—restricted intake of saturated fat and cholesterol and weight loss. If plasma lipids do not fall far enough, adding the right drug or drug combination usually controls them.

SUGGESTED READING

Breslow JL: Genetics of lipoprotein disorders. Circulation 1993;87:III-16.

Havel RJ, Rapaport E: Management of primary hyperlipidemia. N Engl J Med 1995;332:1491.

Levine GN, Keaney JF Jr, Vita JA: Cholesterol reduction in cardiovascular disease. N Engl J Med 1995;332:512.

Scandinavian Simvastatin Survival Study Group: Randomised trial of cholesterol lowering in 4444 patients with coronary heart disease: The Scandinavian Simvastatin Survival Study (4S). Lancet 1994;344:1383.

Summary of the second report of the National Cholesterol Education Program (NCEP) Expert Panel on Detection, Evaluation, and Treatment of High Blood Cholesterol in Adults (Adult Treatment Panel II). JAMA 1993;269:3015.

4.10

Nutritional Issues in Acute Illness

Ronenn Roubenoff, MD, MHS, and Rebecca A. Roubenoff, RD, MPH

WHY FEED PATIENTS?

Although all the body's systems need adequate nutrients, hospitalized patients are commonly kept NPO (*nil per os,* nothing by mouth) for days at a time, receiving only intravenous hypocaloric nonprotein fluids. Iatrogenic malnutrition is further compounded by liquid diets providing only 500 calories and 7–8 g protein/day. This nutritional inadequacy is an even greater problem for people who come to the hospital with a background of chronic illness that has already compromised their nutrition.

The most important reason to feed patients is to prevent the immunosuppression and impairment of physiologic organ functions that malnutrition causes. Immune system dysfunction is demonstrable when patients lose as little as 5% of lean body mass; this can happen after just a few days of severe illness.

Malnutrition can be prevented far more easily than it can be treated, and prevention should begin on hospital day 1. When a patient has become malnourished, prompt and effective intervention can halt and even reverse the physiologic and immunologic deterioration within 7–10 days, although full repletion of muscle and cell mass can take many months.

The Metabolic Stress Response

A healthy, nonstressed person who stops eating adapts to starvation over several days. Alterations in thyroid hormones and body composition lead to a reduced basal metabolic rate, whereas low insulin levels permit energy stores to be mobilized from body fat. Fatty acids are preferentially oxidized for energy, ketone bodies become the major energy substrate for the body, and body proteins are spared. Given adequate water, a healthy person can tolerate starvation-induced malnutrition for 4–6 weeks.

Acute conditions such as infection and burns cause the acute phase response, a state that prevents the normal adaptation to starvation. Cytokines, such as interleukin-1β, tumor necrosis factor-α, and interleukin-6, raise levels of both insulin and the insulin-antagonistic hormones glu-

cocorticoids, growth hormone, and catecholamines. The hyperinsulinemia prevents ketogenesis, making energy stores in fat relatively inaccessible. Muscle protein then becomes the body's chief energy source, providing amino acids for hepatic gluconeogenesis. This further impairs physical function. Cytokines also make acutely ill patients anorexic.

At the same time, the sick person needs extra energy and protein. Cytokines markedly increase the resting metabolic rate and production of acute phase proteins, and the immune response leads to clonal expansion of lymphocytes and increased production of phagocytes, immunoglobulin, and complement. All these energy- and protein-requiring processes increase demand for nutrients, even as the supply is falling.

The Impact of Disease-Induced Malnutrition

Virtually all patients with disease-induced malnutrition lose delayed cutaneous hypersensitivity when they become so malnourished that their serum albumin falls below 3 g/dL. Other immunologic functions become similarly deranged, as do the central nervous system, respiratory system, gastrointestinal tract, cardiovascular system, and kidneys (Table 4.10–1). All these impairments are prevented by adequate nutrition and can be reversed with nutritional intervention if they have not progressed so far that the patient can no longer take in and absorb nutrients.

When chronically ill patients, particularly older persons, come to the hospital with a superimposed acute illness, their metabolic reserves are already impaired by reduced protein and fat stores. Certain medications can also interfere with patients' food intake, digestion, or absorption. For example, captopril and bronchodilators may alter patients' sense of taste, nonsteroidal anti-inflammatory agents may cause dyspepsia, and chemotherapeutic agents often produce anorexia. Cholestyramine reduces bile acid activity, and aluminum-based antacids bind iron and phosphate.

Table 4.10–1. Effects of disease-induced malnutrition on organ function.

Organ or System	Impact
Central nervous system	Lethargy, ↓ alertness, confusion
Lungs	↓ Vital capacity, ↓ tidal volume, ↓ response to hypercapnia and hypoxia, ↓ cough
Stomach	Achlorhydria
Bowel	Mucosal atrophy, villus blunting, loss of brush border enzymes, ↓ peristalsis, malabsorption
Liver	↓ Mass, altered drug metabolism, ↓ protein synthesis
Cardiovascular system	↓ Mass, arrhythmias, potential for left ventricular failure with refeeding
Kidneys	↓ Excretion of titratable acid; hyposthenuria, impaired urine concentration with obligate diuresis
Immune system	↓ CD4/CD8 ratio, ↓ total lymphocyte count, ↓ delayed-type hypersensitivity, ↓ complement production, ↓ antibody production and affinity, ↓ polymorphonuclear cell chemotaxis and bacterial killing

Modified and reproduced, with permission, from Roubenoff RA, Roubenoff R: Nutritional support of the acutely and chronically ill patient. In: *Difficult Medical Management.* Taylor RB (editor). WB Saunders, 1991.

WHEN TO FEED PATIENTS

The sooner a person is fed adequately, the milder will be the consequences of malnutrition. As a rule of thumb, every week of nutritional depletion requires 3 weeks of nutritional rehabilitation. Patients' metabolic and clinical status defines the "demand" side of the body's metabolic equation, whereas their oral or intravenous intake plus their endogenous protein and fat reserves define the "supply" side.

Ideally, the physician and dietitian work as a team to evaluate the patient and the diet. This assessment should include estimates of patients' energy, protein, and micronutrient requirements and intake. Clinicians should plan both for current needs during the acute illness and for anticipated needs to meet long-term goals (eg, weight loss). However, acutely ill patients should never be put on a weight reduction diet; because their ketotic adaptation is impaired, they lose lean mass rather than fat.

Principles of Body Composition

The body can be divided into two major compartments: lean body mass and fat mass. Lean body mass accounts for 99% of the body's metabolically active mass; it includes the cell mass and intercellular connective tissue. A minimum cell mass is required to support physiologic functions. Loss of more than 40% of lean body mass is intrinsically fatal. Fat mass is the body's major energy depot, but is itself relatively inert metabolically. The amount of fat, its bodily distribution, and its fatty acid composition reflect the person's previous energy balance and hormonal status.

Assessing the Patient's Metabolic State

The clinician assesses the patient's metabolic state by answering three questions: (1) Is the acute phase response activated? If so, patients' energy and protein needs are increased, and protein can be depleted quickly. If not, patients' ad lib dietary intake may be adequate and they should not be overfed. (2) Do patients have cardiac, intestinal, hepatic, or renal dysfunction that may limit nutrient absorption or metabolism? If so, their intake of specific nutrients may need to be curtailed, as in the protein restriction required in hepatic encephalopathy or renal failure. (3) Do patients have physical evidence of malnutrition? Signs include temporal wasting, cheilosis, oral ulcers, abnormalities of the tongue (eg, beefy redness), brittle hair, thinned skin, pressure ulcers, and ridged, thinned, or dystrophic nails, as well as weakness, lassitude, and evidence of peripheral or cranial neuropathies.

Anthropometric assessment, an evaluation of the patient's size, weight, and body proportions, remains the standard method for clinical evaluation of body composition. The patient's weight and height should be measured on admission and before intravenous fluids are started and should be compared with previous records. Unintentional loss of more than 5% of usual weight during the past month, 7.5% over 3 months, or 10% over 6 months suggests major losses of protein, fat, and micronutrient reserves and an increased risk of death.

Skeletal protein mass can be further estimated. The physician can compare the patient's mid-arm circumference with published tables of norms for the person's age and sex (see Roubenoff and Roubenoff chapter in "Suggested Reading"), but should be aware that edema and obesity can spuriously increase arm circumference. A 24- or 72-hour urine collection can be used to measure creatinine excretion, which correlates roughly with amount of body muscle except in patients with renal insufficiency. This measure can be compared with healthy controls of the same height using the creatinine-height index (creatinine excretion in grams/height in meters), an index of muscle mass. A creatinine-height index of 60–80% of normal is considered mild muscle depletion; 40% or less is severe muscle depletion.

The protein content of the body's internal organs, termed the "visceral protein mass," can be estimated most readily by the serum albumin concentration. Because acute illness reduces albumin production, the drop in serum albumin with acute illness reflects both nutritional compromise and the severity of illness. A low serum albumin (less than 3.5 mg/dL) signals a poor prognosis and the need for prompt nutritional intervention. The clinician interpreting the albumin level must be aware of special factors. The albumin can be skewed by urinary loss in the nephrotic syndrome or by treatment with intravenous fluids or albumin. Furthermore, because albumin has a half-life of 18 days, it responds slowly to nutritional therapy.

Other circulating proteins used to assess visceral protein mass have included transferrin, retinol binding protein, prealbumin, and fibronectin. These proteins are less influenced by acute illness than is albumin. Furthermore, their shorter half-lives make them better indicators of patients' response to nutritional treatment.

The Quetelet body mass index, which is calculated as a patient's weight (in kilograms) divided by the square of the patient's height (in meters), is a crude measure of fat stores (see Roubenoff and Roubenoff chapter in "Suggested Reading"). However, more precise estimates are needed for nutritional assessment in the hospital. The most commonly used method is measurement of skinfold thickness with a caliper. The resulting estimate of subcutaneous fat correlates well with total body and percent fat, based on published tables (see Roubenoff and Roubenoff). Again, edema can render skinfold measurements less accurate.

A diet history also helps determine how long and how severely the patient has been nutritionally deprived. Patients with longstanding malnutrition have particular need for early, aggressive nutrition support.

Estimating the Patient's Energy and Protein Needs: The goals of nutrition support are to provide enough exogenous calories, vitamins, and minerals to meet the body's needs without overfeeding and to achieve and maintain a positive nitrogen balance. Total energy expenditure comprises the resting metabolic rate, the thermic effect of food (energy spent in its digestion, absorption, and metabolism), and the energy required for physical activity. In practice, clinicians can gauge total energy needs by estimating the basal metabolic rate using formulas based on body composition or by measuring resting energy expenditure using indirect calorimetry, and then multiplying by factors for illness and activity (see Roubenoff and Roubenoff chapter in "Suggested Reading").

In a normal diet, protein constitutes 16–20% of calories. Although a healthy adult needs only 0.8 g protein/kg body weight/day, patients generally need 1.5 or even 2.0 g/kg/day during a severe acute illness, and 1.1–1.2 g/kg/day as the illness improves and hypermetabolism abates. The amount of protein given may be limited by hepatic and renal insufficiency, which interfere with protein metabolism. Formal assessment of nitrogen balance may be based on simultaneous determination of creatinine and urea nitrogen in urine and blood, but requires familiarity with the technique (see Roubenoff and Roubenoff). Patients must also be given enough nonprotein calories to achieve and maintain a positive nitrogen balance, with a goal of +2 g/day. When the body lacks sufficient nonprotein energy, protein is used for gluconeogenesis.

Vitamin and Mineral Needs: A diet that provides enough energy and protein probably provides enough vitamin and mineral micronutrients. However, patients may need faster repletion of micronutrients if they are depleted of certain micronutrients or if there is reason to suspect that they digest or absorb certain nutrients poorly. Particularly in hospitalized patients, medications may disrupt normal micronutrient absorption, metabolism, activation, or elimination. Circulating levels of minerals such as iron, zinc, and selenium drop acutely during illness, but these changes reflect redistribution rather than true nutritional deficits. Supplementing these minerals beyond the amounts in food or standard enteral or parenteral formulas can be toxic and should be avoided unless patients have other evidence of deficiency.

HOW TO FEED PATIENTS

Choice of Feeding Route

Although there are exceptions, the rule for choosing enteral versus parenteral feeding is simple: "If the gut works, use it." Enteral nutrition, by mouth or feeding tube through the alimentary canal, has several advantages over parenteral nutrition. (1) Almost 100% of an enteral diet reaches the liver, via the portal circulation. The liver is a principal site of energy and protein metabolism. In contrast, with intravenous feeding into the superior vena cava, less than 30% of the formula reaches the liver. (2) Enteral nutrition maintains the height and brush border enzyme activity of villi in the gut. With parenteral nutrition, the intestinal mucosa atrophies; this allows bacteria to pass from the lumen to the serosal side of the intestine, a major route of gram-negative and anaerobic sepsis. (3) The bowel is an important source of glutamine, which is especially necessary for optimal function of immune cells and the gut itself. (4) Enteral nutrition has fewer side effects and is far less expensive.

If patients can receive enteral support, the clinician must decide whether they can eat real food or should be given an artificial formula. Food is preferable, both physiologically and psychologically. Many patients are given both regular food and a supplement, or even regular food combined with a nasoenteric feeding tube to deliver calories and protein that the patients cannot eat directly.

The clinician evaluating how much patients are taking in should not assume that patients who eat breakfast will also eat lunch and dinner. Patients generally do best with breakfast and falter on later meals. The best way to assess intake is for the dietitian to record a 72-hour calorie count. If this count shows that patients have not consumed enough, they must be fed directly into the gut. A small-bore nasoenteric tube is passed into the stomach and preferably beyond the ligament of Treitz into the jejunum. This more distal position reduces the risk of aspiration, which is the most common serious complication of enteral support. Feeding should begin only after x-rays confirm that the tube is in the stomach or beyond.

Patients who are expected to need prolonged enteral support should be considered for percutaneous endoscopic gastrostomy. This is a brief, safe procedure for which the only absolute contraindications are ascites, peritonitis, peritoneal dialysis, and gastric varices. After percutaneous endoscopic gastrostomy, a tube can be inserted into the jejunum. An alternative is surgical placement of a feeding tube directly into the jejunum. The feeding jejunostomy produced by either of these methods gives the best available protection against aspiration. This procedure is indicated for patients who have little or no gag reflex, have a tracheostomy, are comatose, or are otherwise unable to guard their airway.

When enteral therapy is impossible, parenteral nutrition can be given through a peripheral vein to patients who need less than 1000 kcal and 40 g protein per day for less than 1 week. Giving more nutrients than this may cause sclerosis of the vein. *Total parenteral nutrition* is provision of the patient's entire nutritional requirements through a central venous catheter. Total parenteral nutrition can deliver larger amounts of nutrients, but the clinician must take care not to give too much fluid or more glucose than the patient can metabolize (generally no more than 5.5 mg/kg/min). Because of the potential complications and expense of total parenteral nutrition, the clinician should periodically consider whether enteral feeding can be reinstated.

Choice of Enteral Formula

Clinicians should know the fundamentals of enteral formulas. Tailoring the formula to the individual, with the advice of a nutrition support team, can maximize the benefit to the patient while minimizing side effects such as diarrhea, hyperglycemia, hyponatremia, and fluid imbalance.

Enteral formulas are categorized by their complexity of nutrients, protein source, and energy density (calories/mL). Most current formulas are semisynthetic, that is, composed of food components rather than food itself. The most important distinction between types of formulas is protein composition. Intact nutrient formulas contain whole proteins and are appropriate for general use if the bowel has not atrophied from prolonged starvation. Addition of fiber to these formulas reduces the risk of diarrhea but can cause bloating. High-density formulas provide 1.5–2 kcal/mL instead of the standard 1 kcal/mL.

Predigested formulas, which provide protein primarily as di- and tripeptides, are best for patients with probable bowel atrophy. These include patients who are NPO and have been stressed for more than 7 days, patients with sepsis, and patients who cannot tolerate intact nutrients because of diarrhea or bloating. When no commercial formula is quite right, a nutritionist can blend nutrient modules that provide only fat, carbohydrate, or protein, to custom-make a formula.

Using Enteral Formulas

The choice of how much formula to give and how fast to give it requires balancing patients' nutritional goals with their gastrointestinal tolerance for the formula. Isotonic enteral feedings are tolerated best because they do not cause osmotic diarrhea. Since osmolality is determined by the number rather than the size of molecules in the formula, most predigested formulas that have many small molecules are hyperosmolar. However, most intact-nutrient formulas are close to isotonic.

Patients should be fed by continuous infusion. For most patients, formulas delivered to the stomach should be started at full strength. However, if the patient has delayed gastric emptying, has been off oral food for a long time, or is severely malnourished, the formula should be started at isotonic strength (300 mOsm/kg water). There is no need to dilute formula below isotonicity. A formula begun at isotonic strength can be increased in concentration or rate every 6–8 hours unless the patient has bloating, diarrhea, or high gastric residuals. In general, feeding into the stomach should not leave residual formula exceeding 1.5 times the hourly rate of the feeding. Higher residuals increase risk of aspiration.

Patients who need postpyloric (duodenal or jejunal) feedings should be given a fiber-containing formula at full strength, or a nonfiber formula begun at isotonic strength and increased to full strength as tolerated. Unlike gastric feedings, postpyloric feedings do not require checking of residuals.

Complications

Enteral Nutrition: Although many tube-fed patients develop diarrhea, the tube feeding is not usually at fault. The most common cause of this diarrhea is antibiotic-induced *Clostridium difficile* colitis, followed by other antibiotic-induced alterations in bowel motility or flora. These changes are especially common in patients receiving enteral support. Antibiotics can directly stimulate bowel motility and produce bowel edema and pseudomembranous colitis.

Another common problem is osmotic diarrhea caused by hypertonic medications given through the tube. For example, potassium chloride solution, with its osmolality of nearly 3000 mOsm/kg, is guaranteed to cause diarrhea in nearly all patients when given through a tube, especially if the tip of the feeding tube is below the ligament of Treitz.

Formula intolerance is actually an uncommon cause of diarrhea in tube-fed patients. Thus, rather than curtailing the feeding, clinicians should first test patients' stools for *Clostridium difficile* toxin, do routine stool cultures, consider sigmoidoscopy to confirm pseudomembranes, and review the patient's other medications for potential offenders. Switching from a semisynthetic formula to a predigested formula at isotonic strength can further reduce concern that the formula is causing the diarrhea.

Aspiration is the most serious complication of enteral support, affecting 1% of patients in intensive care units and 5% on regular wards. Aspiration of enteral formula, with its neutral pH, is potentially less harmful than aspiration of acid from an empty stomach. Risk of aspiration can be reduced by continuous rather than bolus feedings, by elevating the patient's head, and by minimizing gastric residuals. Because patients aspirate even without a feeding tube, fear of aspiration should not be a reason to avoid giving nutritional therapy. To prevent aspiration, jejunal feedings are indicated for patients whose gut works but who have an inadequate gag reflex or are not fully conscious. If the gut does not work, the only choice is parenteral nutrition.

In patients who cannot cooperate with the insertion because of altered mental status, the tube can be positioned by fluoroscopy or endoscopy or by use of serial portable x-rays.

Parenteral Nutrition: Adequate parenteral nutrition often means giving 1.5–3.0 L fluid/day in addition to other liquid medications. In patients with compromised cardiac or renal function, this can lead to fluid overload and heart failure. Patients' weights and input-output records must be monitored daily.

Likewise, the amounts of sodium, potassium, bicarbonate, magnesium, calcium, and trace minerals and vitamins that patients receive parenterally should be reconsidered daily in light of their changing metabolic status. Although the formula may not need to be changed, clinicians should approach each day as though it might. They should measure and record patients' serum electrolytes daily. Liver enzymes should be checked every 3 days at first, then weekly. Albumin and transferrin should be checked weekly. For acutely ill patients or those requiring long-term support, nitrogen balances can be calculated to optimize nutritional therapy; once a week is common practice in intensive care units. When discontinuing total parenteral nutrition, the clinician prevents hypoglycemia by giving an infusion of 10% dextrose for 6 hours to allow a gradual decline in glucose and insulin levels.

Insertion of central venous catheters for nutrition support leads to pneumothorax in 1–4% of patients. These catheters can also become sources of infection because (1) lines often stay in place for prolonged periods, allowing skin flora to migrate down the catheter and enter the blood; (2) the high glucose and lipid contents of parenteral formulas provide an excellent environment for bacterial and fungal growth; and (3) manipulation of the line to draw blood or give medications breaks the line's aseptic barrier and introduces organisms. Line sepsis is best prevented by dedicating the line solely to total parenteral nutrition, having a special team of nurses assigned to central line care, forbidding anyone to draw blood via the line, and relocating the line periodically. Patients who need prolonged total parenteral nutrition should be considered for a subcutaneous venous access such as a Hickman catheter.

SUMMARY

▶ The physician should consider the patient's nutritional status from the outset. Lost days can mean weeks of recovery, with greater risk of infection, muscle weakness, and skin breakdown.

▶ In acutely ill patients, accelerated energy use and protein catabolism increase nutritional requirements.

▶ When severely ill patients require nutrition support, the general rule for choosing between enteral and parenteral feeding is: "If the gut works, use it." Because of the potential complications and expense of total parenteral nutrition, the clinician should periodically consider whether enteral feeding can be reinstated.

▶ When a patient receiving an enteral formula develops diarrhea, the cause is more often an infection or drug than the formula itself. An isotonic predigested enteral formula can reduce the risk of diarrhea once other causes have been ruled out.

SUGGESTED READING

Hill GL: Body composition research: Implications for the practice of clinical nutrition. JPEN 1992;16:197.

Mullan H, Roubenoff RA, Roubenoff R: Risk of pulmonary aspiration among patients receiving enteral nutrition support. JPEN 1992;16:160.

Roubenoff R, Dallal GE, Wilson PWF: Predicting body fatness: The body mass index vs. estimation by bioelectrical impedance. Am J Public Health 1995;85:726.

Roubenoff RA, Roubenoff R: Nutritional support of the acutely and chronically ill patient. In: *Difficult Medical Management.* Taylor RB (editor). WB Saunders, 1991.

Young VR, Marchini JS, Cortiella J: Assessment of protein nutritional status. J Nutr 1990;120(Suppl 11):1496.

Section 5

Nephrology

Paul W. Ladenson, MD, Section Editor

Approach to the Patient with Kidney Disease

Andrew Whelton, MD

Kidney disease may manifest in several ways. Patients may have nonspecific complaints caused by renal insufficiency, such as fatigue, anorexia, or weakness. Symptoms may be caused by the specific renal insult, such as flank pain and hematuria with kidney stones or suprapubic pain and anuria with urethral obstruction. The physician may also suspect kidney disease based on nonspecific physical findings such as hypertension or edema or other findings that strongly implicate the renal system, such as enlarged kidneys in polycystic kidney disease. The first clue may be a routine blood test abnormality such as an elevated creatinine or blood urea nitrogen, or anemia, hyperkalemia, or hypocalcemia. The physician should also suspect renal impairment in patients who are receiving potentially nephrotoxic drugs and should confirm it with specific tests of kidney function—urinalysis, blood urea nitrogen, and serum creatinine.

Patients with kidney disease can have manifestations ranging from asymptomatic blood chemical changes to life-threatening catastrophes. Abnormal renal function may reflect an inherent kidney defect, a disease of the urinary tract, or the kidney's response to a pathophysiologic state elsewhere in the body, such as severe dehydration or heart failure. Symptoms of renal disease may arise from a single organ system, such as mild neurologic abnormalities, or from multiple systems.

Since the kidneys' heterogeneous functions include fluid-electrolyte and acid-base balance, endocrine modulation of mineral metabolism, erythropoiesis, contributions to systemic hemodynamic control, and elimination of drugs and toxins, the clinician faces a difficult task when developing a comprehensive approach to evaluating and managing patients with kidney disorders. Nonetheless, patients with known or previously unsuspected renal problems can be assessed systematically. Few physical signs pinpoint kidney disease, and the physical examination alone is unlikely to provide much guidance. Thus, the clinician needs to have formulated a differential diagnostic plan, or at least a diagnostic approach, by the end of taking the patient's history. The next step is a careful urinalysis and review of screening blood chemistry and hematologic studies, which should lead the physician toward a management plan.

This chapter outlines the first steps in detecting impaired kidney function or renal parenchymal disease, and the workup to characterize the problem and treat it.

HISTORY

Among the familial disorders that may cause kidney disease are diabetes mellitus, hypertension, collagen vascular diseases, and nephrolithiasis. The single most common autosomal dominant inherited disease manifesting in adults is polycystic kidney disease.

The kidney partially or completely eliminates most drugs from the body, but a great many drugs—both prescription agents and over-the-counter medicines whose dosing is unsupervised—can cause functional or structural nephrotoxicity (Table 5.1–1). A suspicious physician should cautiously ask patients whether they have taken illicit "street" drugs. All too common is kidney disease caused by parenteral drug abuse, often with intercurrent HIV infection (Chapters 5.6 and 8.10).

The occupational history is relevant if the patient has been exposed to volatile hydrocarbons, benzine, aniline, xylene, heavy metals, or ionizing radiation.

Renal Tract Pain

Kidney disorders infrequently cause pain, but pain may originate within the kidney in the calyces or renal pelvis, as well as in the ureter, bladder, urethra, and, in men, the prostate.

Table 5.1–1. Drugs with nephrotoxic potential.

Most prevalent
Aminoglycosides
Nonsteroidal anti-inflammatory drugs (NSAIDs)
Iodinated radiocontrast media
Angiotensin converting enzyme (ACE) inhibitors

Less prevalent
Other antibiotics
   Cephalosporins: cefoxitin, cephalexin, cephalothin
   Penicillins: amoxicillin, ampicillin, carbenicillin, methicillin,
    nafcillin, oxacillin, penicillin G
   Rifampin
   Sulfonamides
   Vancomycin
Amphotericin B
Chemotherapeutic agents: allopurinol, cisplatin, cyclosporine,
   mitomycin
Cocaine
H_2 receptor antagonists
Phenytoin
Sulfonamide diuretics: thiazides, bumetanide, furosemide,
   torsemide
Volatile hydrocarbons

In several acute forms of glomerular disease, kidney pain results from stretching of the kidney capsule by interstitial edema or from inflammation of the capsule itself. These disorders usually produce a constant dull achiness within the costovertebral angle areas. Pain in the pyelocalyceal region or ureters is usually caused by a dislodged kidney stone, often with infection; the patient may have gross hematuria (visible blood in the urine). Rarely, pain is produced within the calyces or ureters by the sloughing and passage of a renal papilla. When a stone has dislodged from its site of origin within a renal papillary tip protruding into a minor calyx, the stone's passage through the renal pelvis and the ureter typically causes colicky pain that often appears and disappears over several hours to days. However, a stone passing through the ureter can cause exquisite pain, which may radiate into the mid-abdomen and pelvis and into the testes and penis in men or the vaginal labia in women.

Bladder pain, typically felt in the suprapubic area, may be caused by outflow obstruction or by a tumor or stone in the bladder. This pain is most often produced by infection, which also causes urinary frequency and dysuria.

Prostate pain, sensed as perineal achiness, is usually caused by infection. When infection is severe, the patient may have diarrhea. Another cause of prostate pain is prostatic stones with associated infection.

Urethral pain usually signals infection and may produce a purulent discharge. Men perceive urethral infection as penile pain. In women, the pain is referred to the bladder.

Abnormal Micturition

The normal adult urinary bladder typically can expand comfortably to contain 300–500 mL of urine. Most healthy persons void urine four to five times a day, for a total excreted volume of about 1.5 L. The state of hydration influences this volume. Most do not need to urinate during the night unless they are well hydrated before going to bed, in which case they may need to void once during the night.

Polyuria and Nocturia: Polyuria is the excretion of more than 3 L/day of urine. Polyuria can be caused physiologically by excessive fluid ingestion. Alcohol causes polyuria by inhibiting antidiuretic hormone (ADH) production. Polyuria may be the presenting feature of excess solute excretion with obligatory water excretion, such as glycosuria in diabetes mellitus. Polyuria may be an early clinical clue to the progression of many forms of renal disease, because the kidneys lose their ability to concentrate urine. Diabetes insipidus manifests as polyuria; the cause may be an abnormality of central nervous system ADH production or nonresponsive renal tubules in nephrogenic diabetes insipidus.

Nocturia (frequent voiding at night) may be a component of any of the causes of polyuria. Nocturia may reflect posture-related (lying in bed) mobilization of edema fluid, as occurs in congestive heart failure, or may indicate primary bladder disease (eg, infection, stone, tumor) or prostate disease.

Hematuria and Pigment in the Urine: Blood can enter the urine at many sites in the renal outflow tract, from the nephron within the renal parenchyma through the pyelocalyceal system, ureter, bladder, urethra, and, in men, the prostate. Upper tract bleeding, in the glomeruli, may be caused by intrinsic glomerular disease or may reflect a systemic coagulopathy in a normal kidney. Blood that enters the upper tract is fully mixed with urine; blood entering the lower tract may appear chiefly at the start or end of micturition.

Hematuria can be gross or microscopic (Figure 5.1–1). Gross hematuria with pain is characteristic of the passage of a kidney stone or a sloughed renal papilla, either of which is often complicated by infection. Painless gross hematuria suggests an upper or lower tract tumor, systemic coagulopathy, excessive anticoagulant effect, or, less commonly, acute necrosis and sloughing of a papilla. Gross hematuria is often transient, as with the passing of a kidney stone, and the hematuria may then continue to be detected microscopically in the urine sediment. Red blood cell casts on microscopic urinalysis indicate a renal parenchymal source of blood, although there may be an additional bleeding source downstream.

Pigment added to the urine may be in the form of hemoglobin, derived from systemic red cell hemolysis; myoglobin from damaged muscle cells during rhabdomyolysis; vegetable pigment from foods, such as red beets; pigment from a drug, such as rifampin or phenazopyridine; or porphyrins, as produced in acute intermittent porphyria. The physician should be able to determine the cause of pigment in the urine by correlating the history with findings on urinalysis and blood chemistries. If hemoglobin or myoglobin is found, all patients who are clinically stable and can respond to fluid and diuretic administration should undergo a vigorous diuresis and al-

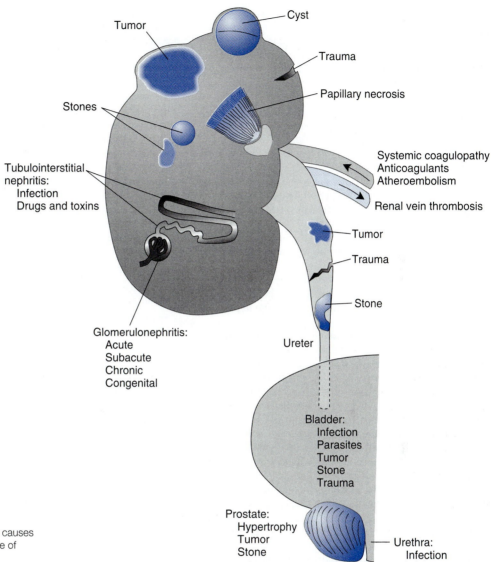

Figure 5.1–1. Common causes of hematuria and their site of origin.

kalinization of the urine to prevent renal tubular obstruction by hemoglobin and myoglobin casts and direct tubular injury by myoglobin (Chapter 5.4).

Incontinence and Obstruction: Most children have urinary incontinence until age 18–36 months. Thereafter, incontinence usually means a congenital anomaly of the outflow tract or trauma to the bladder sphincter. Many women complain of urinary incontinence, commonly caused by bladder sphincter trauma during labor and delivery. The incontinence is worsened by infection, abdominal strain, coughing, or sneezing, and it often progresses with age. The history directs work-up and management.

Sudden, persistent obstruction of the urinary outflow tract leads to acute renal failure, usually with pain. Com-

plete obstruction causes anuria; mechanical causes must be sought (Chapter 5.4). Slower development of obstruction is common in older men who have diseases that enlarge the prostate. Chronic obstruction is usually painless, but patients have difficulty in starting the stream of urine, slower release of urine, and dribbling after voiding. Workup should assess the mechanics of micturition and the patency of the prostatic urethra.

PHYSICAL EXAMINATION

A pale patient may have anemia caused by poor nutrition that reflects worsening chronic renal failure. Progression of severe chronic uremia may be marked by the skin turning yellowish to brown, but without scleral icterus. Chronic uremia also tends to make the skin dry and pruritic (Chapter 5.5). Renal disease can cause acute skin changes: rash in drug-induced tubulointerstitial nephritis, purpura in Henoch-Schönlein purpura or cryoglobulinemia involving the kidney, and livedo reticularis in atheroembolism within the kidney.

Abdominal distention may indicate ascites or fluid accumulation within the lumen of nonmotile or obstructed bowel. Pathologic accumulations of fluid in the abdomen or pleural space, or in the form of massive edema, are often called "third spacing" of fluid. Because the fluid accumulating within the third space is drawn from the extracellular fluid, the intravascular space contracts and organ perfusion is reduced. The reduction in blood flow to the kidney leads to renal failure.

Large polycystic kidneys may produce obvious abdominal distention, and a perinephric abscess may cause flank swelling and redness.

The external genitalia should be carefully examined for developmental anomalies. The eye exam should include funduscopic evaluation to look for damage from hypertension.

Typically, a healthy kidney cannot be palpated. The exception is in thin people, in whom the lower pole of the kidney may be palpable. As polycystic kidneys enlarge with age, they become readily palpable and cystic masses are easily detected. Splenic masses on the left side, or adrenal tumors on both sides, may be mistaken for an enlarged kidney. Most renal tumors, with the exception of Wilms' tumors in children, are detected by other means before they become palpable. Acute enlargement of the urinary bladder usually causes pain, which is worsened by palpation in the suprapubic region. Chronic distention of the bladder is more subtle, usually painless, and often difficult to confirm by palpation alone. Catheterization of the bladder is diagnostic. Tenderness in the suprapubic area, accentuated by palpation, may also reflect acute infection or cystitis in the lower urinary tract.

Men's external genitalia should be checked for tenderness and for masses reflecting infections such as tuberculosis or tumors such as seminoma. During the rectal exam, the prostate should be palpated to check for enlargement that might be obstructing urine flow and for tenderness indicating prostate infection and possible outflow obstruction. In women, vaginal and rectal exam helps to detect mechanical problems (cystoceles, infection) in the outflow tract.

Heart and lung conditions are often integrally linked with abnormalities in renal perfusion and function. Auscultation in the subcostal anterior abdomen of hypertensive patients may disclose a bruit that suggests a renovascular cause of the hypertension (Chapter 5.9).

URINALYSIS

Physical, chemical, and microscopic examination of the urine is the next best step to studying kidney tissue, which requires a biopsy. Urinalysis is crucial to directing further evaluation. The urinalysis is most valuable when well-informed clinicians perform it themselves, with careful microscopic analysis of the centrifuged urine sediment.

For accurate analysis, the urine specimen should be freshly voided (midstream collection) or a catheter specimen (although patients should not be routinely catheterized just to collect urine for urinalysis) to avoid including "contaminating" urethral cells (Chapter 8.8). Ideally, the specimen should be examined immediately or, with refrigeration, at least within 1–2 hours. After this time, cells in the urine may disintegrate. Routine chemical analysis can be performed reliably with impregnated dipsticks, but the protein analytic portion of the strips does not detect light chain proteins (Bence-Jones protein; Chapter 12.7). When the patient might have multiple myeloma or "trace" levels of proteinuria, the dipstick should be supplemented by 20% sulfosalicylic acid (SSA) testing for proteinuria.

Physical Characteristics

The urine should look clear and, depending on its concentration, yellow to straw-colored. Turbidity with a foul odor suggests infection. Turbidity developing as the urine cools indicates precipitation of phosphates in an alkaline urine or urates in an acid urine. These are benign findings. For the meaning of other color changes, see "Abnormal Micturition" above. Interpretation of the urine specific gravity depends on the patient's hydration. When patients have not consumed any fluid for 12–18 hours, determination of their urine specific gravity (or, preferably, osmotic concentration, determined in the chemistry laboratory) is an excellent screen of renal tubular function. After 18 hours of fluid deprivation, normal people have a high urine specific gravity (≥ 1.025) or osmolality (≥ 800 mOsm/kg). Similarly, interpretation of the urine pH depends on patients' acid-base status, level of hydration at the time of the urine collection, diet, and exposure to drugs that influence urine pH (eg, acetazolamide, which alkalinizes, or ammonium chloride, which acidifies).

Proteinuria

A healthy adult excretes a little protein (≤ 75 mg/day) in the urine. The protein is made up of albumin, light chains, and a high molecular weight glycoprotein called *Tamm-Horsfall protein*. This small amount of protein in the urine is not detected by dipstick or acid precipitation (20% sulfosalicylic acid), the usual laboratory urinalysis techniques. Proteinuria becomes detectable when the patient excretes about 150–300 mg/day. In such a patient, dipstick testing of a "spot" urine (voided during the office visit) discloses trace (10–20 mg/dL) levels of proteinuria. Progressively increasing protein excretions are usually reported as 1+ (30 mg/dL), 2+ (100 mg/dL), 3+ (300 mg/dL), or 4+ (500–1000 mg/dL). At 3+ to 4+ proteinuria, an adult is typically excreting 3 g or more per day and likely is manifesting signs of the nephrotic syndrome, including peripheral edema and ascites. Patients may also note that their urine has become "foamy" (Chapter 5.6). In patients with suspected plasma cell dyscrasias, dipstick testing for proteinuria does not reveal light chain polypeptides in the urine, but acid precipitation does.

The level of proteinuria, measured in a spot urinalysis or preferably in a 24-hour collection, is helpful—though not an absolute guide—in the differential diagnosis of the underlying renal abnormality (Table 5.1–2). Proteinuria may be of glomerular (Chapter 5.6) or tubular (Chapter 5.7) origin.

Glycosuria and Ketonuria

Glucose in the urine reflects either an elevated systemic serum glucose (usually >200 mg/dL) or, if serum glucose values are normal, proximal renal tubular damage. Ketones can be detected in the urine earlier than in the blood; they indicate conditions such as diabetic ketoacidosis or starvation.

Microscopic Examination

The microscopic sediment may disclose cells, tubular casts, crystals, infectious organisms, and artifacts. The sediment need not routinely be stained. The cells commonly detected are red blood cells, white blood cells, renal tubular epithelial cells, ureter and bladder transitional epithelial cells, and contaminating squamous epithelial cells. The finding of an abnormal number of cells, tubular casts, or crystals, or any infectious organisms, is called an *active sediment*.

Urine from a healthy person contains no cells or, at most, an occasional cell per high-power microscopic field. Tubular epithelial and transitional epithelial cells are found in healthy persons, but more than one per high-power field suggests damage to the tubules or bladder wall. More than one red cell per high-power field is abnormal, as are any white blood cells. It is sometimes difficult to distinguish tubular epithelial cells from white blood cells, but many tubular epithelial cells are not perfectly round, and a single nucleus resides at the edge of the cell. In general, the more cells per high-power field, the more active the renal disease.

As the name implies, tubular casts are casts of the lumen of the tubule. They are formed only in the distal portion of the nephron. The core of all casts is the high molecular weight glycoprotein Tamm-Horsfall protein. This protein tends to gel when the urine is both acid and concentrated. In alkaline urine, the protein dissolves over several hours—thus, the need for prompt microscopic evaluation of the urine.

An empty cast appears as a wispy, translucent, cylindrical replica of the tubular lumen and is called a *hyaline cast*. The addition of abnormal cells, protein, hemoglobin, myoglobin, or other debris to a cast helps characterize the form of renal disease. A red blood cell cast means that the hematuria originates at least in part within the kidney. The usual cause is glomerular damage, but another possibility is tubular damage, as from tubulointerstitial nephritis

Table 5.1–2. Protein excretion rate and underlying renal condition.

	Protein Excretion Rate (mg/day)			
	50–100	150–1000	1000–3000	>3000
Benign proteinuria				
Exercise proteinuria	+			
Febrile proteinuria	+			
"Isolated" proteinuria	+			
Tubulointerstitial nephritis				
Acute allergic drug toxicity	+	+		
Direct drug toxicity	+	+		
Radiation nephritis	+	+		
Infiltrative disease (eg, tumor)	+			
Pyelonephritis	+	+	+	
Primary glomerular diseases				
Minimal change glomerulonephritis			+	+
Focal segmental sclerosis			+	+
Membranous glomerulonephritis			+	+
Acute proliferative glomerulonephritis		+	+	+
Rapidly progressive glomerulonephritis		+	+	+
Systemic illness with glomerulonephritis				
Diabetic glomerulosclerosis			+	+
Systemic lupus erythematosus		+	+	+
IgA nephropathy	+	+	+	+
Goodpasture's syndrome			+	+
Polyarteritis		+	+	+
Wegener's granulomatosis		+	+	+
Multiple myeloma (plasma cell dyscrasias)		+	+	+
Amyloidosis			+	+
Subacute bacterial endocarditis		+	+	
Hypertensive nephrosclerosis		+	+	
Scleroderma		+	+	+

(Chapter 5.7). Correlating the sediment findings with the degree of proteinuria is most helpful, since glomerulopathies cause significant proteinuria whereas tubular disorders cause little. Fine granules within a cast reflect impacted filtered protein particles; coarse granules reflect degenerating cells within the cast. Tubular epithelial cell casts suggest tubular damage, and, when seen abundantly in a patient with trace to 1+ proteinuria, strongly suggest active tubulointerstitial nephritis. Hemoglobin casts represent systemic hemolysis, and myoglobin casts indicate systemic rhabdomyolysis.

Crystals in the urine may be benign or may signal disease. For example, calcium oxalate crystals or calcium-magnesium-ammonium phosphate crystals usually reflect the patient's diet, but calcium oxalate can also signal a kidney stone (Chapter 5.8) and calcium-magnesium-ammonium phosphate (the cause of struvite stones) is often seen in association with urinary tract infection (Chapter 8.8). Urine crystal interpretation charts are readily available.

Infectious organisms ranging from bacteria to fungi to trichomonads can be detected in urine.

Decisions to treat crystals or organisms should be based on the clinical setting.

Interpretation

The patient's degree of proteinuria usually allows the physician to distinguish tubular from glomerular sources of proteinuria (see Table 5.1–2). Proteinuria of tubular origin is invariably in the range of trace to 2+. In a patient with an active urine sediment, this finding suggests tubulointerstitial nephritis; a history of relevant drug or toxin exposure solidifies the diagnosis. Proteinuria of 3+ to 4+ (nephrotic range proteinuria) always has a glomerular component. By correlating the proteinuria level with the microscopic findings, the physician can often make a reasonable prediction of the tissue abnormalities that would be revealed by a renal biopsy.

When a patient has renal disease without evidence of multisystem problems, the decision to biopsy the kidney is based on the degree of proteinuria, activity of the urine sediment, the person's age, and likely response to prednisone. In contrast, when glomerulopathy is part of a systemic disease such as lupus nephritis, polyarteritis, or diabetes mellitus, the cause of the proteinuria is more apparent and fewer patients need biopsy.

LABORATORY TESTS AND IMAGING OF RENAL FUNCTION

Routine screening blood chemistry tests, done as part of the initial evaluation, may disclose several abnormalities in renal function: an elevated potassium, low bicarbonate, elevated creatinine, elevated blood urea nitrogen, low calcium, elevated phosphate, and elevated uric acid. Hematologic screening tests may reveal anemia reflecting chronic

renal failure, or hemolysis associated with acute renal failure. The screening results dictate the direction of further testing.

Tests of Glomerular Filtration

The blood urea nitrogen level, once the most used chemical marker for renal function, has fallen from favor because it is influenced by factors other than renal function; the level can rise during accelerated protein catabolism, gastrointestinal bleeding, and dehydration. A more accurate gauge of renal function is the serum creatinine level, which reflects the balance between creatinine production by muscle and excretion by the kidneys. The serum creatinine is a useful immediate guide to glomerular filtration, and serial determinations are helpful in following the progression of renal disease and the response to therapy (Figure 5.1–2). However, the serum creatinine does not become abnormal until the glomerular filtration rate has fallen by 50%.

A still more precise marker of glomerular filtration is the renal creatinine clearance. The test requires a timed collection of the patient's urine, usually for 24 hours; measurement of the urine creatinine concentration and the urine volume produced per minute; and simultaneous measurement of the serum creatinine, preferably at the midpoint of the urine collection. Calculation of the creatinine clearance (expressed as mL/min) is based on the formula:

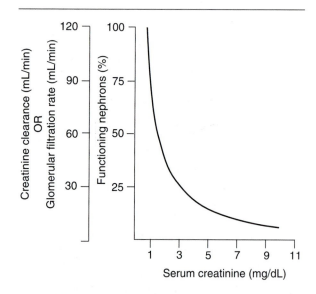

Figure 5.1–2. Relation between serum creatinine and creatinine clearance (glomerular filtration rate, which reflects the functioning nephron mass). This relation is especially important in assessing the progression of renal disease and response to therapy. In this graph, when all nephrons are functioning, the serum creatinine is 0.75 mg/dL. About 50% of renal function is lost before the serum creatinine doubles; 75% is lost by the time the serum creatinine passes 3 mg/dL.

$$\frac{U \times V}{P}$$

where U = the urine concentration of creatinine (mg/dL), V = the volume of urine produced per minute (mL), and P = the serum creatinine (mg/dL).

A normal adult's creatinine clearance fluctuates between 100 and 120 mL/min. Depending on their age, sex, and concomitant medical problems, some patients with glomerular filtration rates as low as 10–15 mL/min can perform their activities of daily living with little hindrance. But most patients need to begin dialysis when their creatinine clearance drops below 5–10 mL/min.

As renal function declines, creatinine clearance becomes a less reliable marker of the glomerular filtration rate because renal tubular secretion of creatinine makes up an increasing fraction of the total creatinine eliminated in the urine. In adults, the test becomes unreliable when glomerular filtration falls below about 30 mL/min. At this point, a more accurate test of glomerular filtration is measuring the clearance of a radiopharmaceutical agent such as technetium-labeled diethylene thiamine penta-acetic acid (Tc^{99} DTPA). However, because it is so much more expensive than the creatinine clearance, this test should be done only when the clinician must pinpoint the glomerular filtration rate and the response to treatment.

Tests of Tubular Function

The proximal tubule is responsible for reabsorption of two-thirds of the filtered load of salt and water, as well as reabsorption of glucose, amino acids, and small fractions of filtered proteins. Defects in proximal tubule function are reflected in the urine by glycosuria and a urine acidification defect that is reflected in the serum by hyperchloremic acidosis. Analysis of the urine for amino acid content and immunochemical protein analysis for short- or long-chain protein content further define a proximal tubular defect, such as Fanconi's syndrome.

The distal nephron concentrates urine and contributes to maintaining acid-base balance. Defects are clinically manifest when the tubule cannot fully concentrate or acidify the urine (Chapter 5.3).

Imaging the Kidney and Urine Outflow Tract

Selection of imaging technique depends on the site to be studied, the patient's clinical status, and the history.

Renal ultrasonography is the main noninvasive way to determine kidney size, location, contour, and cortical thickness, and to detect cysts and tumors. Ultrasound can also be used to evaluate the outflow tract for obstruction. Available and inexpensive, ultrasound has replaced flat plate abdominal x-ray for noninvasive evaluation of the kidneys.

Supplementing ultrasonography are computed tomography (CT) and magnetic resonance imaging (MRI), which provide detailed cross-sections of the kidney. These techniques are particularly useful in evaluating cysts, tumors, and large-vessel disease.

In intravenous excretion urography, an iodine-containing radiopaque compound is injected intravenously, filtered by the glomeruli, concentrated in the renal tubules, and excreted in highly concentrated form into the pyelocalyceal system, ureter, and bladder. The radiocontrast material provides excellent imaging of the pyelocalyceal and lower outflow tract and is particularly useful in locating radiolucent obstructions such as uric acid stones. Although the technique remains important in evaluating some acute stone obstructions, its use has declined dramatically because the radiocontrast can be nephrotoxic and can produce life-threatening systemic allergic reactions and arrhythmias.

In antegrade pyelography, a percutaneous catheter is introduced directly into the pyelocalyceal system, and radiocontrast is injected into the upper outflow tract. This technique is highly effective in defining obstructive lesions. It is particularly useful in patients with poorly functioning kidneys, because their glomeruli do not filter enough radiocontrast to permit visualization of an obstructive lesion. Further, if the percutaneous catheter is kept in place, it can be used to decompress an obstructed kidney, as when tumor blocks the lower urinary tract. Antegrade pyelography has largely supplanted retrograde pyelography. This older technique requires cystoscopy so that a catheter can be placed directly into the lower portion of the ureters; radiocontrast is then injected via the catheter to define the outflow tract.

Voiding cystourography assesses the patency of the penile urethra during voiding in boys and young men suspected of having congenitally obstructing valves in the urethra. In girls and young women, this test is particularly useful in assessing and measuring vesicoureteric reflux.

In renal angiography, the femoral or brachial artery is cannulated and radiocontrast is injected directly into the aorta, renal arteries, or both. This test is the only reliable way to assess obstructive lesions in the main renal arteries. When correlated with clinical features, the images may confirm a renal vascular cause of hypertension or may reveal vascular occlusion as causing progression of kidney failure. Many obstructive lesions are suitable for balloon angioplasty: A catheter is passed through the lumen of the obstructing lesion, and a balloon in the catheter's tip is inflated to force open the obstruction. Angioplasty may improve blood pressure and renal function. The intrarenal vascular images also help determine the acuteness or chronicity of renal vascular disease. Angiography has been made safer by new radiocontrast materials and computer enhancement that permits the use of smaller and hence less toxic amounts of radiocontrast.

In nuclear medicine imaging, a gamma-emitting radiopharmaceutical is injected intravenously, and detectors measure how fast it appears in both kidneys, disperses, and disappears into the ureters and bladder. The images tell much about bilateral flow and function. The glomeruli are best imaged with ^{99m}Tc DTPA. Renal tubular function can be assessed with the static imaging agent technetium-labeled dimercaptosuccinic acid (^{99m}Tc DMSA), which defines tubular lesions such as tumors and scarred areas of nonfunctioning tissue.

Renal Biopsy

Histologic evaluation of a sample of kidney tissue is the best study for renal parenchymal disease. Renal biopsy has been made much safer by ultrasonography or fluoroscopic guidance and by ensuring that all candidates have normal coagulation. Biopsy is indicated in most patients who have nephrotic range proteinuria with no obvious cause (eg, diabetes mellitus). Biopsy confirms tubulointerstitial nephritis and invariably clarifies the cause of persistent unexplained renal parenchymal hematuria. Biopsy is also indicated for patients with acute or advancing chronic renal failure that no other tests have been able to explain.

The most common complication of percutaneous renal biopsy, affecting less than 5% of patients, is bleeding serious enough to require transfusion. Less common is trauma to the liver, spleen, pancreas, or intestinal tract—injury that might require surgery. After a renal biopsy, patients should be advised to remain sedentary for at least 2 weeks, and not use anticoagulants, including salicylates, for at least 1 month.

SUMMARY

▶ Patients with acute or chronic renal failure can present with nonspecific symptoms such as fatigue, anorexia, and weakness. Specific renal complaints such as flank pain and hematuria may reflect a kidney stone or urinary tract infection.

▶ Kidney disease most often presents as asymptomatic blood chemical changes. Nonspecific physical findings are high blood pressure and edema; palpably enlarged kidneys reflect polycystic kidney disease.

▶ Crucial to guiding the evaluation is chemical and microscopic examination of the centrifuged urine sediment. "Trace" to 1+ proteinuria with an active urine sediment and a renal acidification defect likely means tubulointerstitial renal disease. Nephrotic range proteinuria (3–4+) indicates glomerular damage.

▶ Renal ultrasonography is the best first screen to define kidney size, contour, and outflow tract.

▶ Kidney biopsy is usually indicated to evaluate nephrotic range proteinuria without obvious cause, tubulointerstitial disease, or persistent hematuria. Biopsy should be considered for unexplained progression of renal insufficiency.

SUGGESTED READING

Corwin HL, Silverstein MD: Microscopic hematuria. Clin Lab Med 1988:8:601.

Geyer SJ: Urinalysis and urinary sediment in patients with renal disease. Clin Lab Med 1993;13:13.

Marcussen N et al: Analysis of cytodiagnostic urinalysis findings in 77 patients with concurrent renal biopsies. Am J Kidney Dis 1992;20:618.

Mariani AJ et al: The significance of adult hematuria: 1,000 hematuria evaluations including a risk-benefit and cost-effectiveness analysis. J Urol 1989;141:350.

Woolhandler S et al: Dipstick urinalysis screening of asymptomatic adults for urinary tract disorders. I. Hematuria and proteinuria. JAMA 1989:262:1214.

Disorders of Water and Electrolyte Balance

Christopher R. Burrow, MD, and Michael G. Kauffman, MD, PhD

Regulation of the chemical composition of the extracellular fluid is a complex task shared by many organs and hormones. These homeostatic mechanisms maintain body water, sodium, and potassium content within a narrow range despite potentially large changes in solute and water intake. Disorders of water and electrolyte balance commonly develop during many illnesses and are potential side effects of many widely used drugs. The clinical consequences of these imbalances can range from nonspecific symptoms like weakness and nausea to life-threatening derangements of cardiovascular and neurologic function like arrhythmias and coma.

One of the physician's first tasks is to determine whether the patient is among the majority whose fluid and electrolyte disorder has resulted from losses or gains of water, electrolytes, or both, which have overwhelmed the person's homeostatic responses, or whether the patient is among the relatively few with a specific disruption of one or more of the mechanisms that maintain water and electrolyte homeostasis. When patients' homeostatic responses have been overwhelmed, the condition is usually self-limited; once corrective measures have been taken, few patients need further work-up. But when patients have a disruption of homeostasis (eg, the syndrome of inappropriate antidiuretic hormone [SIADH] or hyperaldosteronism), simple correction of the presenting water (eg, hyponatremia) or electrolyte (eg, hyperkalemia) derangements is ineffective in the long run. Further studies are needed to define the patient's underlying disorder, find its fundamental cause, and plan how to cure or control it (Figure 5.2–1).

At the simplest level, most fluid and electrolyte disorders present as abnormalities in the volume, osmolality, or potassium concentration of the extracellular fluid compartment. It follows that the proper evaluation of patients with these disorders is (1) clinical observations (eg, skin turgor) and measurements (eg, body weight, venous pressures) that permit estimation of extracellular and intracellular fluid volumes, and (2) serum sodium and potassium levels, along with other routine chemical measures such as

blood urea nitrogen, creatinine, and glucose. Accurate diagnosis depends on physicians integrating both sets of findings in a logical and comprehensive way. Taken alone, patients' symptoms and signs (eg, obtundation, hypotension) or their laboratory abnormalities (eg, hypernatremia, hyperosmolality) typically leave a broad differential diagnosis, including conditions for which different and sometimes opposite treatments would be indicated. But when the two classes of information are considered together in light of the clinical history, the most probable explanation and best treatment are usually obvious.

DISORDERS OF EXTRACELLULAR FLUID VOLUME

The total body water normally accounts for about 60% of body weight, but can vary between 45% and 70%, depending on the person's age and percent body fat. Two-thirds of this water is inside cells; one-third is distributed between the interstitial and intravascular fluid spaces (normally in a ratio of 3:1), depending on their relative hydrostatic and oncotic pressures and capillary permeability. Sodium, the principal extracellular cation, is maintained at a concentration of 135–145 mEq/L in the extracellular fluid compartment, whereas potassium, the major intracellular cation, is largely restricted to the intracellular fluid compartment. Edema, an expansion of the interstitial compartment, develops when capillary hydraulic pressure rises (from local factors such as venous obstruction, or from an overall increase in the extracellular fluid volume), plasma oncotic pressure falls, capillary permeability increases, or lymphatic flow of interstitial fluid and protein to the plasma compartment is impeded.

The extracellular fluid compartment volume depends on the total body sodium content, which is maintained by homeostatic mechanisms that match daily urine sodium excretion to daily sodium intake. The serum sodium con-

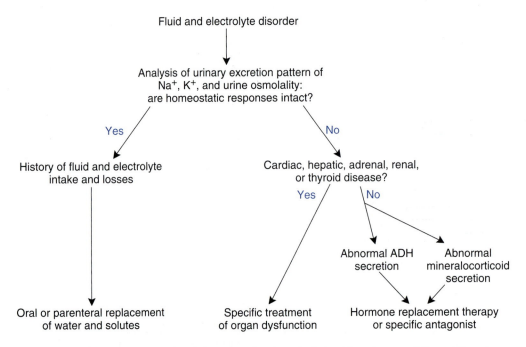

Figure 5.2–1. Evaluation and treatment of fluid and electrolyte disorders. Analysis of the urine osmolality and the urine excretion patterns of sodium and potassium establishes whether the patient's homeostatic responses are intact. If water and electrolyte homeostasis is defective, the patient has cardiac, hepatic, adrenal, renal, or thyroid (CHART) disease or a primary abnormality in secretion of antidiuretic hormone (ADH) or aldosterone.

centration is regulated independently from the total body sodium content by the thirst response and by pituitary release of appropriate amounts of antidiuretic hormone (ADH) (Figure 5.2–2). The homeostatic mechanisms that maintain total body sodium content and extracellular fluid volume in a normal range (Figure 5.2–3) are principally the secretion of renin and atrial natriuretic peptide, and the renin-mediated generation of angiotensin II, which itself controls adrenal aldosterone biosynthesis and secretion. The extracellular fluid volume cannot be reliably gauged from the extracellular sodium concentration, but must be estimated by physical examination.

Clinical features useful in assessing patients with extracellular fluid volume derangements are summarized in Table 5.2–1. Although changes in body weight in acutely ill patients accurately mirror changes in total body water and must be monitored in patients with fluid and electrolyte disorders, these changes do not indicate which fluid compartment or compartments are affected and alone are an unreliable measure of changes in extracellular fluid volume. Conversely, large amounts of water can shift between compartments (eg, with the development of edema or ascites) without a revealing change in body weight. It is therefore crucial that the physician independently catalogue changes in the patient's total body water as reflected by acute changes in body weight, changes in the interstitial compartment, and changes in the blood (intravascular) volume.

Disorders Causing Edema

Generalized pitting edema is a cardinal sign of expanded interstitial volume, usually by more than 3 L, and often indicates an expansion of the extracellular fluid volume and a commensurate increase in total body sodium (see Figure 5.2–3). The edema is less prominent in the morning, after overnight recumbency. Edema localizes to the legs in ambulatory patients and may be best detected over the sacrum in bed-bound patients. Edema fluid can be displaced with sustained local pressure, so-called "pitting." Uncomplicated edema caused by an increase in interstitial volume does not make the overlying skin ulcerated, hyperpigmented, warm, or tender; these features suggest localized edema caused by venous disease or soft tissue infection. Lymphedema, which produces brawny nonpitting edema, results from lymphatic obstruction caused by trauma, infection (eg, filariasis), neoplasm, or congenital malformation.

Generalized edema is commonly caused by heart disease, hepatic cirrhosis, renal dysfunction with sodium retention, and severe reductions in plasma albumin (less than 2 g/dL) such as those in the nephrotic syndrome and severe liver disease. All these states share abnormal sodium retention and expanded interstitial volume with or without increased plasma volume. However, plasma (intravascular) volume may be low in patients with cirrhosis and ascites and in patients with edema secondary to hypoalbuminemia. Furthermore, generalized edema in pa-

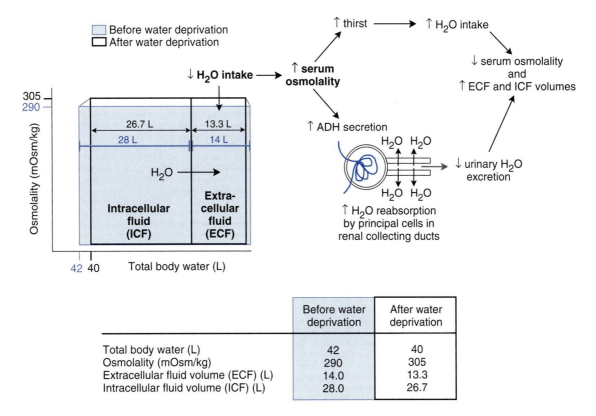

Figure 5.2–2. Water homeostasis: physiologic responses to water deprivation. The body fluid compartments in a 70-kg man can be estimated as: Total body water = 0.6 L/kg × 70 kg = 42 L. Extracellular fluid = 1/3 total body water = 14 L. Intracellular fluid = 2/3 total body water = 28 L. Water restriction increases serum osmolality in the extracellular fluid compartment, causing water to shift out of the intracellular fluid compartment to maintain osmotic equilibrium. The increased serum osmolality (1) triggers antidiuretic hormone (ADH) secretion, which limits water excretion by promoting water reabsorption by collecting duct principal cells, and (2) induces thirst, which spurs a compensatory increase in water intake to restore total body water to normal. In a person who lacks a normal thirst response, a 2 L water contraction causes the serum osmolality to rise to 305 mOsm/kg and the intracellular and extracellular fluid compartment volumes to fall as shown.

tients with sepsis or extensive burns may be caused primarily by changes in capillary permeability, and these patients may also have a subnormal plasma volume.

Optimal medical management of patients with edema depends on its cause and severity and on a skilled assessment of the relative volume of the interstitial and plasma compartments. The physician can judge patients' plasma volume from the physical exam, for example, by orthostatic blood pressure changes, a determination of central venous pressure, skin turgor, and cardiac exam (see Table 5.2–1). Therapy often combines a low-sodium diet with a diuretic to enhance renal sodium excretion. Available options are thiazides with distal tubular activity (hydrochlorothiazide, chlorthalidone); metolazone, which has activity in both the proximal and distal tubules; furosemide and bumetanide, so-called loop diuretics, which act on the loop of Henle; and the potassium-sparing diuretics triamterene, amiloride, and spironolactone. For refractory edema with extracellular fluid volume overload

(often associated with severe renal dysfunction), patients may need combined diuretics, such as a loop diuretic and a thiazide.

Patients must be carefully monitored during diuresis because the desired reduction in interstitial volume may also cause excessive plasma volume depletion, reduced tissue perfusion, and changes in water, sodium, potassium, and magnesium balances. In practice, the physician can monitor tissue perfusion by following the blood urea nitrogen and serum creatinine; when plasma volume is excessively depleted, the ratio of blood urea nitrogen to creatinine rises to more than 15:1, followed by a rise in the serum creatinine as glomerular filtration falls further. This is a common development, as when diuretic treatment of severe heart failure improves pulmonary congestion but precipitates reduced tissue perfusion. Treatment of edema in cirrhosis can likewise be hazardous and carries the risk of precipitating hepatic encephalopathy or the hepatorenal syndrome (Chapter 7.5).

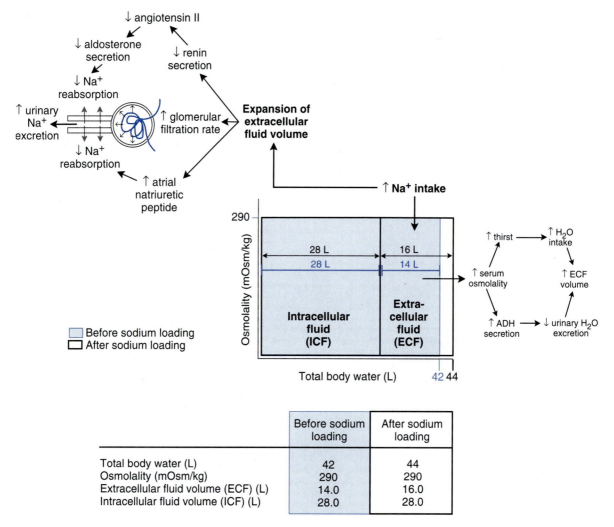

Figure 5.2–3. Sodium homeostasis: physiologic responses to an increase in sodium intake. The body fluid compartments were calculated as in Figure 5.2–2. Sodium loading leads to an increase in serum osmolality, an ADH-mediated compensatory decrease in water excretion, and a thirst response that increases water intake. The result is an isotonic expansion of the extracellular fluid compartment. Without a compensatory increase in sodium excretion, a net retention of 280 mEq of sodium chloride leads to a 2 L expansion of the extracellular fluid compartment without changing the osmolality. Physiologic suppression of renin secretion by the juxtaglomerular apparatus reduces blood angiotensin II levels and suppresses aldosterone secretion by the zona glomerulosa of the adrenal cortex. In concert with stimulation of atrial natriuretic peptide, these alterations increase the glomerular filtration rate, reduce sodium reabsorption and increase sodium excretion, and restore total body sodium to normal.

DISORDERS OF WATER HOMEOSTASIS

Hyponatremia (serum sodium less than 130 mEq/L, usually caused by abnormal water retention) and hypernatremia (serum sodium more than 145 mEq/L, caused by abnormal water depletion) are the laboratory manifestations that usually signify abnormal water homeostasis. The serum sodium concentration allows assessment of the total body water osmolality, since all body fluid compartments are in osmotic equilibrium. It is also worth restating

that the serum sodium concentration may not reflect a patient's actual total body sodium *content* or extracellular fluid volume. For example, hyponatremia can reflect plasma and extravascular fluid volume depletion in a patient with a compensatory pituitary ADH response to blood loss, or plasma and extravascular fluid volume expansion in a patient with SIADH, or discordant plasma volume depletion and extravascular fluid volume expansion in a patient with liver disease and ascites.

The most significant manifestations of hypo- and hy-

Table 5.2–1. Clinical features of patients with extracellular volume abnormalities.

Volume Depletion	Volume Expansion
History and symptoms	
Decreased fluid intake	Heart, liver, or kidney disease
Vomiting, diarrhea	Polyuria, oliguria, anuria
Fever, sweating	Edema
Polyuria ± polydipsia	Shortness of breath
	Weight gain
Signs	
Dry mucous membranes	Hypertension
No axillary sweat	Tachypnea
Lengthened capillary refill time	Jugular venous distention
Poor skin turgor	S3 gallop
Low urine output	Ascites
Tachycardia	Pulmonary rales
Resting or orthostatic hypotension	
Laboratory findings	
Normal, low, or high serum sodium	Normal or low serum sodium
High blood urea nitrogen, high uric acid	Low blood urea nitrogen
Blood urea nitrogen:creatinine ratio >15–20	Variable urine sodium
Low urine sodium	Hemodilution*
Fractional urine sodium excretion <1%	
Hemoconcentration*	

S3, third heart sound.
*Based on hematocrit and serum albumin, calcium, and uric acid.

pernatremia are confined to the central nervous system, and range from mild confusion and lethargy to seizure, coma, irreversible central nervous system injury, and death. These neurologic manifestations can be caused by cerebral edema in hyponatremia or by the correction of hypernatremia if extracellular fluid osmolality falls quickly. They can also be caused by cerebral dehydration in hypernatremia or by overly rapid correction of hyponatremia if extracellular fluid osmolality rises quickly.

Normal Regulation of Serum Osmolality

The osmolality of a solution is defined as the total number of dissolved solutes, expressed as millimoles per kilogram (mmol/kg) of solvent. This value correlates directly with the osmotic pressure exerted by such a solution across a water-permeable, solute-impermeable membrane. In a healthy person, the osmolality of all body fluid compartments stays equal at about 280–290 mOsm/kg, through the integrated actions of thirst and pituitary ADH secretion (see Figure 5.2–1). Serum osmolality can be measured directly or estimated by the following equation:

$$\text{Serum osmolality} = (2 \times [\text{serum sodium}]) + ([\text{blood urea nitrogen}])/2.8 + ([\text{serum glucose}])/18$$

Serum sodium is measured in mEq/L; blood urea nitrogen and serum glucose in mg/dL.

Although the serum sodium concentration usually re-lates directly to the serum osmolality, the rule has important exceptions. In certain disorders, the serum sodium concentration is reduced, whereas the serum osmolality is actually elevated. For instance, when severe hyperglycemia (eg, blood glucose over 300 mg/dL) causes elevated plasma osmolality, water shifts from the intracellular to the extracellular fluid compartment. Several other substances can similarly increase serum osmolality while lowering the serum sodium. Patients given radiocontrast agents or mannitol may develop this pattern, as may desperate alcohol abusers who drink methanol or ethylene glycol. In each of these patients, the serum osmolality measured by an osmometer exceeds the calculated osmolality by an amount equal to the concentration of the osmole in the serum. The finding of such an "osmolar gap" between the estimated and measured osmolalities suggests one of these unusual circulating osmolytes.

Hyponatremia with Low Serum Osmolality: It is difficult to produce hyponatremia in normal individuals by giving them large quantities of water. Healthy people can quickly suppress ADH secretion and increase their urine excretion to over 10 L per day in compensation for increases in water intake. However, hyponatremia is easy to produce in patients who have defective ability either to suppress ADH secretion or to dilute their urine because of parenchymal renal disease. Hyponatremia can develop in patients who have total body sodium depletion or sodium overload and in persons whose total body sodium content is normal. Thus, to determine the probable underlying cause of hyponatremia, the physician must estimate the extracellular fluid volume through clinical assessment of patients' volume status (see Table 5.2–1).

Hyponatremia with hypovolemia: When severe body sodium and fluid volume depletion compromises cardiac output, baroreceptor-mediated ADH release prompts renal water retention, even when serum osmolality falls. Patients may be thirsty; when they drink water or other hypotonic fluids, they become hyponatremic.

Clinical clues to hypovolemia in a patient with hyponatremia include static or postural hypotension, tachycardia, poor skin turgor, and dry mucous membranes. Common clinical settings are gastrointestinal disorders like diarrhea or repeated emesis, intestinal obstruction with accumulation of solute and water in distended loops of bowel, renal sodium wasting caused by chronic renal disease or overzealous diuretic therapy, and mineralocorticoid deficiency (Table 5.2–2). When the sodium loss is extrarenal and the kidneys retain sodium normally, the urine sodium concentration is less than 15 mmol/L. When renal sodium conservation is disrupted, the urine sodium concentration is over 20 mmol/L. Regardless of the cause, patients with hyponatremia from volume depletion should be treated by correcting the deficit with isotonic saline. Water retention then corrects itself as restoration of intravascular volume suppresses ADH secretion, and a water diuresis ensues.

Hyponatremia with normovolemic secretion of ADH: When a patient with hyponatremia has no clinical

Table 5.2–2. Differentiating among causes of hyponatremia.

Low extracellular fluid volume

Urine sodium concentration <20 mmol/L	Urine sodium concentration >20 mmol/L
(extrarenal sodium loss)	(renal sodium loss)
Gastrointestinal disorders	Diuretics
Burns	Salt-wasting nephritis
Pancreatitis	Adrenal insufficiency
Muscle crush injury	Osmotic diuresis
	Severe renal tubular acidosis with bicarbonaturia

Normal extracellular fluid volume

Urine sodium concentration <20 or >20 mmol/L
  Syndrome of inappropriate secretion of ADH (SIADH)
  Hypothyroidism
  Psychogenic polydipsia

Expanded extracellular fluid volume

Urine sodium concentration <20 mmol/L	Urine sodium concentration >20 mmol/L
Nephrotic syndrome	Acute renal failure
Congestive heart failure	Chronic renal failure
Cirrhosis	

The physician should also consider the possibility of pseudo-hyponatremia, which can be caused by hypertriglyceridemia, hyperglycemia, hyperproteinemia, or radiocontrast material.

evidence of extracellular fluid volume contraction or expansion, the differential diagnosis includes the syndrome of inappropriate SIADH, hypothyroidism, glucocorticoid deficiency, and psychogenic polydipsia.

SIADH is caused by persistent secretion of ADH despite a low plasma osmolality, resulting in inappropriate renal water retention and body fluid dilution. Causes include central nervous system tumors, hemorrhage, trauma, and infections like encephalitis and meningitis. SIADH can also be caused by tumors that produce ADH ectopically, particularly small cell lung carcinoma, and by other intrathoracic processes like pneumonia. Drugs such as oral hypoglycemics, trycyclic antidepressants, and carbamazepine can increase ADH release and cause SIADH. Some patients have completely autonomous ADH secretion at or above a normal level, whereas in others the hypothalamic osmostat is reset to defend an abnormally low plasma osmolality. Most persons with SIADH have a normal extracellular fluid volume and an only slightly reduced total body sodium.

SIADH should be considered in patients with hyponatremia who are clinically euvolemic, especially if, despite a hypo-osmolar serum, their urine osmolality is over 300 mOsm/kg. The urine sodium is usually over 20 mmol/L, but reflects recent sodium intake and can be below 20 mmol/L if sodium intake is low. Plasma dilution in SIADH is often associated with a low blood urea nitrogen and low serum uric acid, whereas hyponatremia associated with a reduced extracellular fluid volume most often produces elevations in blood urea nitrogen and uric acid (see Table 5.2–1).

To confirm that ADH secretion and a concentrated urine are truly inappropriate, the physician should rule out medical conditions in which effective plasma volume is low, such as heart failure, liver disease, and renal insufficiency. In this regard, SIADH alone does not cause edema, so edema suggests another process. The physician should exclude other conditions that can impair the kidney's ability to excrete free water: intrinsic renal disease and deficiencies of glucocorticoid (Chapter 4.3) or thyroid hormone (Chapter 4.4). Although the ultimate proof of SIADH is a detectable plasma ADH level in a patient with a serum osmolality less than 270 mOsm/kg, diagnosis and treatment need not await the result of an ADH assay.

Patients with SIADH can be treated just with water restriction if their hypo-osmolality is mild or its cause is transient. Patients with more severe or chronic SIADH can also be given demeclocycline, which inhibits ADH's action on the renal distal tubule and collecting duct. However, the usefulness of demeclocycline is limited by its potential hepatic toxicity. Patients who have hyponatremia and glucocorticoid deficiency respond to hormone replacement therapy within hours; those with thyroid hormone deficiency respond within days.

Hyponatremia with hypervolemia: Severe heart failure, liver disease, or the nephrotic syndrome can limit patients' capacity to excrete both water and sodium. Despite excessive total body retention of water and sodium, patients with these conditions have essentially an inadequate or ineffective circulating blood volume because of poor cardiac pump function or fluid sequestration in extravascular spaces (the interstitial, pleural, and peritoneal spaces). In all these patients, baroreceptor-mediated ADH secretion overrides the hypothalamic osmostat that ordinarily governs ADH secretion. Patients with renal insufficiency can also develop hyponatremia with expanded fluid volume, because of their kidneys' intrinsic inability to excrete a water load. Edema and collection of fluid in transcellular compartments (the pleural and peritoneal spaces) are clinical signs of an expanded extracellular fluid volume common to hyponatremic patients with hypervolemia; most also have other obvious signs of primary organ dysfunction. Thus, significant hyponatremia is seen in advanced—not mild—heart failure, advanced—not subtle—liver disease, and full-fledged nephrotic syndrome with hypoalbuminemia, edema, and marked proteinuria.

Hyponatremic patients with total body sodium and fluid overload should usually be treated with salt and water restriction. Some patients also benefit from the judicious use of potent diuretics (to control the sodium-dependent expansion of the extracellular volume) in combination with water restriction (to prevent progressive hyponatremia). Organ dysfunction is often severe enough to require drug treatment (eg, inotropic agents for heart failure) or transplant.

Management of acute hyponatremia: The urgency of treating patients with hyponatremia and the speed with which their serum sodium should be increased depend on three factors: (1) whether patients have symptoms or signs of the neurologic consequences of hyponatremia and a reduced serum osmolality, (2) the magnitude of the reduction in serum sodium concentration, and (3) how long it took their hyponatremia to develop.

Since physicians may not have serial laboratory data to help them pinpoint the course of a patient's serum sodium decline, they must determine the duration of hyponatremia clinically through the history. For example, in a previously healthy young woman who has hyponatremia after surgical anesthesia, the hyponatremia has almost certainly developed over hours; in the diuretic-treated patient with heart failure, the hyponatremia has probably progressed slowly over days or weeks.

Patients with symptomatic, severe, acutely developed hyponatremia require emergency treatment. As the osmolality of the extracellular fluid falls, movement of water into relatively hypertonic brain neurons can cause cerebral edema. In patients with progressive hyponatremia whose serum sodium concentration is dropping by more than 1 mmol/L/hr, cerebral edema can cause obtundation, coma, and cerebral herniation. These patients should be given hypertonic saline and loop diuretics to raise the serum sodium concentration by 1–2 mmol/L/hr, with the increment not to exceed 20 mEq/L/day. This treatment can be life-saving.

In contrast, patients with chronic hyponatremia that is causing few or no symptoms must be treated more conservatively. The serum osmolality in these patients has declined slowly enough to allow a compensatory decrease in brain solute content and avoid cerebral edema. Aggressive restoration of a normal serum sodium can lead to cerebral dehydration with devastating consequences, including cerebral demyelination with severe, permanent neurologic injury. Even with severe hyponatremia and an entirely normal neurologic exam, the safest course may be fluid restriction, to restore the serum sodium slowly to normal over a number of days (see article by Sterns in "Suggested Reading").

Hypernatremia

There is a good reason why hypernatremia, and hyperosmolar syndromes in general, are less common than hyponatremia: The body's defenses against dehydration—secretion of ADH coupled with the thirst mechanism—are very potent. Even the complete absence of ADH secretion in central diabetes insipidus leads to only mild hypernatremia, because patients who are otherwise well can increase their water intake to as much as 10 L/day, enough to prevent even moderate hyperosmolality. A person with significant hypernatremia is virtually sure to have been denied access to water through illness, intoxication, neglect, or environmental exposure. The exception to this rule is a patient who has a neural defect (eg, from a stroke) affecting the hypothalamic thirst center.

When confronted with a patient who has hypernatremia, the physician can first confirm that the renal tubular concentrating mechanism is intact and that ADH secretion and action are appropriately increased—all by

simply measuring the urine osmolality, or, when it is the only test readily available, the urine specific gravity. Either test can show that the urine is markedly concentrated in a person with an intact posterior pituitary and normal renal antidiuretic response.

For stable patients who have no obvious cause for their hypernatremia, the physician should measure the plasma osmolality and plasma ADH concentration during a water deprivation test. The results permit distinction among the potentially responsible disorders: central (neurogenic) diabetes insipidus, nephrogenic diabetes insipidus, and psychogenic polydypsia (Chapter 4.2).

Nephrogenic diabetes insipidus is a resistance to the renal effects of ADH. This disorder is commonly seen in patients receiving lithium, which inhibits ADH action in the collecting duct. Nephrogenic diabetes insipidus can also result from renal tubular dysfunction caused by amyloidosis, pyelonephritis, sarcoidosis, sickle cell anemia, ureteral obstruction, autosomal dominant polycystic kidney disease, and, rarely, an X-linked familial syndrome.

An under-recognized cause of polyuric hypernatremia is a sustained osmotic diuresis, for example, from hyperglycemia or administration of mannitol or radiocontrast dye. Many affected patients are thought to have primary nephrogenic diabetes insipidus when their real problem is a functional renal unresponsiveness to ADH brought about by washout of the normal renal medullary hypertonicity by extremely high urine flow rates. These patients have more than twice the normal daily osmole excretion rate of 600–800 mOsm, and a urine osmolality of about 300 mOsm/L. Treatment consists in lowering the rate at which solute is given and gradually reducing water intake, as guided by the need to prevent hypernatremia.

Hypernatremia rarely develops in people who have an expanded extracellular fluid volume, but it can happen in patients in intensive care units who have received large quantities of hypertonic sodium bicarbonate in misguided attempts to correct metabolic acidosis. In these patients, hyperosmolality can develop so quickly and become so severe that it causes significant cerebral dehydration. This can be prevented by judicious use of isotonic rather than hypertonic sodium bicarbonate (Chapter 5.3).

If oral rehydration is not possible, hypernatremia is treated with intravenous 5% dextrose to reduce the serum sodium concentration to 145 mmol/L. To ensure that the large dextrose infusion does not cause hyperglycemia, glucosuria, and osmotic diuresis, patients require careful monitoring and may need insulin. To prevent cerebral edema, the physician should lower the sodium toward 145 mEq/L by no more than 1 mmol/L/hr. The total water deficit can be estimated with this equation:

$$\text{Water deficit [L]} =$$
$$\text{Current total body water [L]} \times ([\text{sodium}]/140 - 1)$$

where total body water [L] = 0.6 × body weight [kg] and [sodium] = serum sodium concentration [mEq/L].

DISORDERS OF POTASSIUM BALANCE

Hypokalemia and hyperkalemia are relatively common in clinical practice and can have serious effects, particularly on the cardiac conducting system and muscle. Disorders of potassium balance arise either when potassium is abnormally distributed between the intracellular and extracellular compartments or when the patient has a sustained imbalance between potassium intake and excretion. The concentration of potassium in the extracellular fluid is tightly controlled between 3.5 and 5.0 mEq/L. The total body content of potassium is about 40–60 mEq/kg, of which 98% is intracellular. Potassium influx into cells is promoted by alkalemia, insulin, and β-adrenergic agonists; potassium efflux from cells is stimulated by exercise, acidemia, and β-adrenergic blocking agents. The external balance of potassium intake and excretion is regulated by adrenal aldosterone secretion, which governs the rate of potassium secretion in the renal collecting ducts and depends on an adequate glomerular filtration rate (Figure 5.2–4).

The serum potassium concentration does not reflect whether a person has a total body potassium deficit or excess. Although direct measurement of total body potassium stores is not clinically practical, the physician can often reliably estimate total body potassium by analyzing the patient's medical history, urine potassium values, and response to therapy.

Hypokalemia

Manifestations of hypokalemia are restricted to the heart and to skeletal and smooth muscle. Cardiac effects include repolarization abnormalities and ventricular arrhythmias. Skeletal muscle dysfunction can include weak-

ness, cramps, and, when the hypokalemia is severe, rhabdomyolysis. Another complication of hypokalemia is intestinal ileus caused by smooth muscle dysfunction.

Hypokalemia commonly results from excessive urinary excretion of potassium. The cause can be the pharmacologic effects of thiazide or loop diuretics, or the toxic effects on the renal epithelium of other drugs such as amphotericin and aminoglycosides. Tubulointerstitial diseases, especially pyelonephritis, chronic obstructive nephropathy, and magnesium deficiency, can cause renal potassium wasting and hypokalemia. When a patient has both hypokalemia and metabolic acidosis, the physician should consider renal tubular acidosis.

Another common cause of potassium depletion is gastrointestinal loss of potassium-rich fluids during infectious diarrheal diseases or in association with villous adenomas or with pancreatic islet cell tumors that secrete vasoactive intestinal peptide or gastrin. Hypokalemia can also develop when gastrointestinal secretions are lost by nasogastric suction, biliary drainage, or intestinal fistula. The physician should consider surreptitious use of enemas and laxatives as a cause of obscure hypokalemia.

The cause of potassium depletion is often obvious from the patient's medical and drug history. If not, a urine potassium concentration and 24-hour excretion rate can distinguish patients with renal potassium wasting syndromes (over 30 mEq/24 hr) from those with gastrointestinal potassium losses. An inversion in the ratio of urine sodium to potassium (normally 3:1 to 4:1) can be a clue to hyperaldosteronism. Hyperaldosteronism is established by a high plasma aldosterone concentration or high 24-hour urine aldosterone in a patient with suppressed plasma renin activity (Chapter 4.3). In contrast, high renin values are found in patients with secondary hyperaldosteronism caused by renovascular disease (Chapter 5.9), many in-

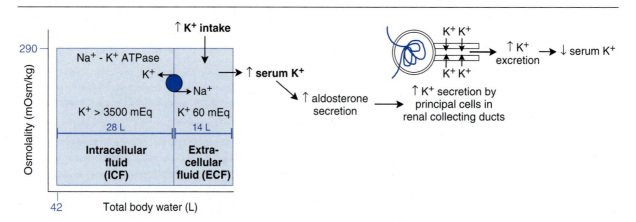

Figure 5.2–4. Potassium homeostasis: physiologic responses to an increase in potassium intake. The body fluid compartments were calculated as in Figure 5.2–2. In this example, the serum potassium is 4.3 mEq/L. The extracellular fluid potassium of 60 mEq is calculated by multiplying the extracellular fluid potassium concentration by the extracellular fluid volume (14 L × 4.3 mEq/L). Potassium loading results in intracellular transport of potassium by sodium-potassium ATPase and in stimulation of aldosterone biosynthesis and secretion by the adrenal cortex. Aldosterone directly stimulates sodium reabsorption and potassium secretion in the collecting duct principal cells. This kaliuretic response restores total body potassium to normal.

trinsic renal diseases, renin-secreting juxtaglomerular cell tumors, and Bartter's syndrome.

Rare patients have hypokalemia and renal potassium wasting secondary to the secretion of other mineralocorticoids (eg, deoxycorticosterone secretion by adrenal tumors) or Cushing's syndrome. Eating licorice that contains glycyrrhizic acid inhibits the enzyme 11-hydroxysteroid dehydrogenase, which normally prevents physiologic glucocorticoid concentrations in collecting duct cells from exerting mineralocorticoid action; the consequence is excessive mineralocorticoid activity, leading to hypertension and hypokalemia. Despite an abnormal urine sodium-to-potassium ratio, plasma renin and aldosterone levels both are low.

Redistribution of potassium to the intracellular compartment is much less common than potassium loss as a cause of hypokalemia. This happens in patients with metabolic or respiratory alkalosis, in which hydrogen ions shift out of cells in exchange for potassium. Potassium also moves into cells after a carbohydrate meal, through the action of insulin and catecholamines.

Hypokalemic periodic paralysis is an autosomal dominant disorder characterized by episodic weakness and hypokalemia; the cause is excessive potassium flux into cells, often after a carbohydrate meal or during rest after exercise. A similar disorder is seen in thyrotoxicosis, especially in Asians; the problem resolves after the hyperthyroidism has been controlled.

The best treatment for most patients with hypokalemia is oral potassium chloride, taken as a solution, a slow-release tablet, or a substitute for table salt. Taking 40–60 mEq of potassium chloride typically raises the serum potassium by 1.0–1.5 mmol/L, but the response varies considerably, depending on the intracellular potassium deficit. If done with caution, potassium chloride can also be given intravenously, at a rate not exceeding 10 mEq/hr, in a non-glucose-containing fluid. Especially in patients with renal insufficiency, overly vigorous potassium repletion runs the risk of triggering hyperkalemia and its arrhythmic consequences. Other potassium formulations (eg, potassium citrate, potassium bicarbonate) may be indicated to manage the hypokalemia and metabolic acidosis in patients with diarrhea and renal tubular acidosis.

Hyperkalemia

The most common and dangerous clinical manifestation of hyperkalemia is cardiac arrhythmia. Hyperkalemia interferes with the propagation of the action potential through the cardiac conduction system, as evidenced by prolongation of the PR interval and QRS duration. An early finding is a peaked T wave, reflecting altered ventricular repolarization. Hyperkalemia also increases ventricular irritability and automaticity. Because this combination of effects is potentially lethal, all patients with severe hyperkalemia require prompt, effective treatment.

Chronic hyperkalemia is a common finding when the glomerular filtration rate falls lower than 15 mL/min, especially if the patient's dietary potassium and protein have not been restricted. Patients with even milder renal insufficiency can develop hyperkalemia if they acquire hypoaldosteronism, either isolated as a result of hyporeninemia or as a component of primary adrenal insufficiency. A plasma aldosterone determination, plasma renin activity measurement, ACTH stimulation test, and exclusion of pseudohyperkalemia (see below) reveal the abnormality.

Drug-related hyperkalemia is seen in many patients with renovascular disease or renal insufficiency who have taken angiotensin converting enzyme (ACE) inhibitors that diminish their adrenal aldosterone secretion. "Potassium-sparing" diuretics like triamterene, amiloride, and spironolactone can also provoke hyperkalemia. Nonsteroidal anti-inflammatory drugs can worsen hyperkalemia in patients with diabetes mellitus, who may have impaired secretion of potassium in the distal nephron because of hyporeninemic hypoaldosteronism.

Hyperkalemia is most difficult to manage in patients whose potassium has been redistributed from the intracellular to the extracellular compartment. Many kinds of tissue and cell injuries (eg, rhabdomyolysis, crush injury, bowel infarction, and tumor lysis from chemotherapy) can release enough intracellular potassium to cause hyperkalemia, which, untreated, can be lethal within hours. Many patients with these injuries have compromised renal function, which heightens the danger by limiting renal potassium excretion; many patients require emergency hemodialysis.

Several circumstances can cause spurious laboratory results suggesting hyperkalemia, so-called pseudohyperkalemia. In vitro lysis of formed elements of the blood can result in a misleadingly high potassium report. This should be considered when patients have had prolonged hemostasis before venipuncture, when the analysis of the blood sample has been delayed, or when patients have severe leukocytosis or thrombocytosis. False potassium elevations are excluded by measuring plasma potassium promptly in a blood sample drawn without venous stasis.

Management of hyperkalemia depends on how quickly the serum potassium rose, its absolute level, and the severity of the patient's cardiac manifestations as assessed by electrocardiogram. Mild or moderate chronic hyperkalemia (serum potassium less than 6.0 mEq/L) can be managed with a low-potassium diet, discontinuation of drugs that interfere with potassium excretion (eg, ACE inhibitors, potassium-sparing diuretics), and correction of sodium and water deficits in volume-contracted patients, to optimize their renal function.

When the cardiac complications of severe hyperkalemia require emergency treatment, when the serum potassium is extremely high (greater than 7.0 mEq/L), or when the serum potassium is rising quickly because of release from intracellular stores, the first line of therapy is intravenous calcium. Calcium increases the action potential threshold, negating the membrane depolarization produced by hyperkalemia. Its effect is immediate but short-lasting. Emergency treatment of hyperkalemia also includes redistributing potassium from the extracellular to the intracellular compartment, by giving either (1) intravenous insulin and dextrose or (2) parenteral sodium bicarbonate to raise the pH of the extracellular fluid compartment. Preventing reaccumulation of potassium in the extracellular compartment requires correction of body sodium and water deficits, kaliuretic diuretic such as furosemide or bumetanide, the oral potassium-binding agent polystyrene sulfonate, and hemodialysis for patients with renal failure.

SUMMARY

▶ Abnormalities in total body sodium content can be detected only by clinical assessment of the extracellular fluid compartment volume, not by the serum sodium concentration.

▶ In hyponatremia with a low serum osmolality, the extracellular fluid volume can be low, normal, or high. Increased antidiuretic hormone (ADH) secretion accounts for water retention in patients with volume depletion or the syndrome of inappropriate ADH (SIADH); most patients with high extracellular fluid volumes and hypo-osmolar syndromes have advanced liver, heart, or kidney disease.

▶ Treatment with hypertonic sodium chloride solutions can cause severe neurologic complications in patients with chronic severe hyponatremia, but may be life-saving for patients with acute severe hyponatremia and cerebral edema.

▶ Hypo- and hyperkalemia require prompt correction to prevent cardiac arrhythmias and disturbances of skeletal muscle function, including life-threatening paralysis.

SUGGESTED READING

DeFronzo RA: Hyperkalemia and hyporeninemic hypoaldosteronism (clinical conference). Kidney Int 1980;17;118.

Funder JW et al: Mineralocorticoid action: Target tissue specificity is enzyme, not receptor, mediated. Science 1988;242:583.

Musch W et al: Combined fractional excretion of sodium and urea better predicts response to saline in hyponatremia than do usual clinical and biochemical parameters. Am J Med 1995; 99:348.

Robertson GL, Berl T: Pathophysiology of water metabolism. In: *The Kidney,* 4th ed. Brenner BM, Rector FC (editors). WB Saunders, 1991.

Sterns RH: Severe symptomatic hyponatremia: Treatment and outcome. A study of 64 cases. Ann Intern Med 1987; 107:656.

5.3

Acid-Base Disturbances

Andrew Whelton, MD, and Daniel G. Sapir, MD

Acid-base balance can be deranged by many illnesses, either diseases that afflict the lungs and kidneys—the organs responsible for acid-base balance—or disorders that alter tissue perfusion or metabolism. Defining the pathophysiology of a patient's acid-base disturbance helps physicians in several ways as they organize their clinical approach. First, knowing the pathophysiology narrows the differential diagnosis in a patient whose presentation can be nonspecific, for example, obtundation in a person with diabetic ketoacidosis. Second, the pathophysiology predicts a set of compensatory biochemical consequences and potential complications, such as hypokalemia with potential cardiac arrhythmias in metabolic alkalosis. Third, defining a patient's acid-base disturbance often makes clear what treatment is needed to reverse the metabolic derangement and eliminate its cause.

REGULATION OF SYSTEMIC pH

For clinical purposes, pH is used to represent the hydrogen ion (H^+) concentration in body fluids. The pH is the negative log of the hydrogen ion concentration: $1/\log[H^+]$. The pH of body fluids is maintained in a tightly controlled range. The normal range for arterial pH is 7.36–7.44. The extreme range of pH compatible with life is about 6.75–7.90. Any deviation of pH from the normal range causes clinically relevant acid-base disturbances. An abnormal drop in body pH is acidosis; an abnormal rise is alkalosis. (Because pH is typically measured in arterial blood, a reduction is termed "acidemia" and an elevation is termed "alkalemia.") Acidosis and alkalosis are further subdivided into problems of a metabolic origin and problems of a respiratory origin.

In healthy adults, production of acids from metabolic processes amounts to more than 12,000 mEq/day of H^+, or 12 L of 1N hydrochloric acid (Figure 5.3–1). To minimize changes in the H^+ concentration of body fluids, this prodigious amount of acid must be buffered in blood and in interstitial and intracellular fluids, then excreted from the body by the lungs and kidneys. The lungs normally deal

with 99% of this H^+ load by excreting CO_2 generated by breakdown of the volatile acid, carbonic acid (H_2CO_3), to CO_2 and H_2O. (A volatile acid is an acid that can be eliminated by the lungs.) This reaction is catalyzed by carbonic anhydrase, the enzyme system that regulates both the breakdown and formation of carbonic acid. Although the kidneys excrete much less H^+ (80–100 mEq/day), they are vital in eliminating nonvolatile acids (acids that cannot be eliminated by the lung, since they do not generate CO_2), thereby restoring the body fluids' buffering capacities. Nonvolatile phosphoric and sulfuric acids, which are generated by the metabolism of phospholipids and proteins, can be eliminated only by the kidneys.

The buffers in body fluids pick up H^+ from the tissues where they are produced and transport them to the lungs and kidneys for excretion. Buffers are pairs of weak, poorly dissociated acids and their highly ionized salts. The buffers minimize pH changes in body fluids by converting a strong, highly dissociated acid to a weak, poorly dissociated acid, (H_2CO_3), thereby reducing the concentration of H^+ and producing an acid that can be eliminated immediately by the lungs. In the extracellular fluid compartment, from which clinicians draw arterial blood samples for analysis, the dominant buffer pair is carbonic acid (H_2CO_3) and sodium bicarbonate ($NaHCO_3$). The ratio of this buffer pair is the crucial factor in determining a patient's extracellular pH. The H^+ concentration in the extracellular fluid is defined by the Henderson-Hasselbalch equation:

$$pH = pK + \log \frac{NaHCO_3}{H_2CO_3}$$

The pK, the constant for this buffer pair, is 6.1. This number is the pH at which this pair buffers most effectively, that is, the point at which the pH changes least when a given quantity of H^+ is added. Although this constant is low relative to the normal pH for body fluids, the relationship works well because H_2CO_3 is so quickly removed from the body, thus maintaining a 20:1 ratio of $NaHCO_3$

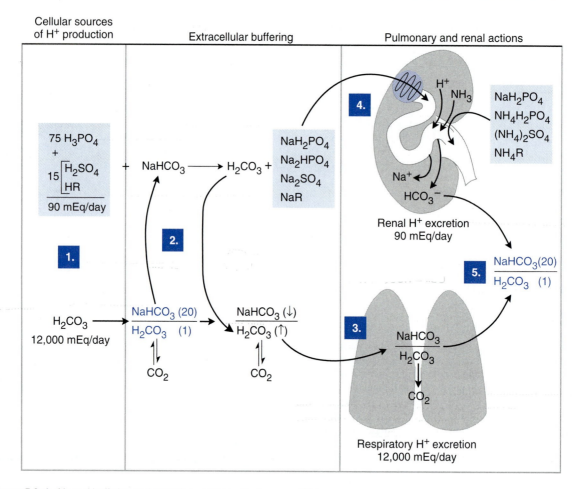

Figure 5.3–1. Normal buffering and excretion of acid by the lungs and kidneys.

1. Cell metabolism produces acid, almost all as carbonic acid (H_2CO_3). H_2CO_3 is quickly removed by the lungs as CO_2. Only about 90 mEq of all the acid generated per day is in the form of strong, nonvolatile acids. These strong acids cannot exist at physiologic pH; hence, they require immediate buffering. R = the anion of any nonvolatile acid besides H_3PO_4 and H_2SO_4 (eg, citrate).
2. When strong acids enter the extracellular fluid, they immediately lower the bicarbonate (HCO_3^-) concentration by producing H_2CO_3 and sodium salts of the acids.
3. The H_2CO_3 is excreted by the lungs as CO_2, thus lowering the H_2CO_3 concentration.
4. The nonvolatile anion portion of the sodium salts can be excreted by the kidney along with hydrogen ion (H^+) or with ammonium ion (NH_4^+). Secretion of H^+ or NH_4^+ leads to reabsorption of an equimolar quantity of sodium bicarbonate ($NaHCO_3$).
5. This $NaHCO_3$ is returned to the blood and restores the $NaHCO_3$:H_2CO_3 ratio to the normal 20:1, thereby restoring the buffering capacity of body fluids.

to H_2CO_3. Since the log of 20 = 1.3, the physiologic pH = 6.1 + 1.3 = 7.4.

As already noted, the concentration of H_2CO_3 is related to CO_2 by the reaction

$$H_2CO_3 = CO_2 + H_2O$$

Since the CO_2 concentration is about 700 times greater than the H_2CO_3 concentration at equilibrium, dissolved CO_2 represents virtually all the H_2CO_3 available. Hence, the CO_2 concentration can be considered a reasonable ap-

proximation of the H_2CO_3 concentration. Because the CO_2 concentration in body fluids can also be defined by its partial pressure (PCO_2), a more clinically useful form of the Henderson-Hasselbalch equation is

$$pH = pK + \log \frac{[HCO_3^-]}{PCO_2}$$

In clinical practice, the HCO_3^-, PCO_2, and pH can all be quickly measured in an arterial blood sample to determine the nature of an acid-base disturbance. At least two of these three determinations are always needed in defining an acid-base problem; the third can be calculated. Finding the cause of an acid-base disorder rests on analyzing the degree of change from the normal 20:1 $NaHCO_3:H_2CO_3$ ratio, in the context of the patient's history.

The other important body fluid buffers are proteins, hemoglobins, and the phosphate buffer system, but none of these is routinely measured in diagnosing acid-base disorders.

Role of the Lungs

Acid, as reflected by the generation of H_2CO_3, is produced at a rate of 10 mEq/min and is excreted by the lungs at the same rate. The effect of CO_2 on the H^+ concentration is determined by the following reactions:

$$CO_2 + H_2O = H_2CO_3 = HCO_3^- + H^+$$

The concentration of CO_2 (or H_2CO_3) in body fluids is determined by the balance between CO_2 production by the tissues and excretion by the lungs. The responsiveness of the H_2CO_3 concentration to changes in ventilatory rate allows the respiratory system to regulate the pH of body fluids. A drop in body pH normally stimulates an increase in alveolar ventilation, which increases the excretion rate of CO_2. This decrease in PCO_2 (H_2CO_3) moves the $NaHCO_3:H_2CO_3$ back toward the normal 20:1 ratio, thus moving the pH up toward normal. If body pH rises, the alveolar ventilation rate normally drops so as to restore the 20:1 $NaHCO_3:H_2CO_3$ ratio. If CO_2 is permitted to accumulate, the H^+ concentration will rise and pH will fall.

Role of the Kidneys

Although the lung excretes about 100 to 150 times more H^+ from the body than does the kidney, only the kidney can eliminate nonvolatile acids. Examples of nonvolatile acids in healthy people are phosphoric acid, produced by metabolism of proteins and phospholipids, and sulfuric acid, produced by metabolism of proteins. In the disease-state diabetic ketoacidosis, lipid metabolism produces the nonvolatile acids β-hydroxybutyric acid and acetoacetic acid. With the toxic ingestion of salicylate (aspirin), metabolism produces the nonvolatile acid salicylic acid.

When a nonvolatile acid is produced systemically, it is immediately buffered by the $NaHCO_3:H_2CO_3$ buffer system. This produces H_2CO_3, which the lung eliminates as CO_2. The resulting sodium salt of the nonvolatile acid (eg, sodium acetoacetate) is eliminated by the kidney. During its elimination, the distal tubule reclaims Na^+ in the form of $NaHCO_3$, to restore systemic HCO_3^- levels to normal.

Following glomerular filtration, HCO_3^- is reabsorbed or, more correctly, regenerated in the proximal tubule. Typically, by the end of the proximal tubule, virtually all filtered HCO_3^- has been reabsorbed, thereby restoring plasma HCO_3^- to the level entering the kidneys. However,

the kidney must also restore the HCO_3^- fraction spent in buffering the nonvolatile acids. This is done by H^+, which is derived from H_2CO_3 in distal tubular cells and then secreted into the tubular lumen. The H^+ is retained in the lumen bound both by phosphate buffers and by ammonia (NH_3^-) produced by the tubule.

As H^+ is secreted from a distal tubular cell, HCO_3^- remains within the cell. Na^+, which moves into the cell in exchange for the secreted H^+, may be derived from phosphate buffers or from a sodium salt such as NaCl or the sodium salt of a nonvolatile acid (eg, Na_2SO_4). Inside the cell, Na^+ from any of these sources joins with HCO_3^-, forming $NaHCO_3$. This $NaHCO_3$ diffuses out of the cell and replaces the $NaHCO_3$ lost in buffering nonvolatile acids.

When Na^+ is derived from a filtered salt such as NaCl, the movement of Na^+ into the cell in exchange for H^+ triggers production of the strong acid HCl in the tubular lumen. This HCl must be buffered immediately by NH_3. Within the terminal portions of the proximal tubule and in the distal tubule, NH_3 is readily made from glutamic acid and quickly diffuses into the lumen to link with free H^+, producing NH_4^+. NH_4^+ join with Cl^- to form the salt NH_4Cl, which is eliminated in the urine. NH_4^+ can also be exchanged for Na^+ in the sodium salts of all nonvolatile acids: One reabsorbed $NaHCO_3$ is produced for each eliminated NH_4^+.

CLINICAL AND LABORATORY CLASSIFICATION OF ACID-BASE DISORDERS

Both systemic acidosis and alkalosis can result from either primary metabolic or primary respiratory disorders. Metabolic disorders first disturb the HCO_3^- concentration, whereas respiratory disorders first disturb the PCO_2 and hence the H_2CO_3 concentration. In both metabolic and respiratory disorders, the ratio of the $HCO_3^-:H_2CO_3$ buffer components is altered from its normal 20:1 thus altering the pH of body fluids.

Table 5.3–1 shows the primary chemical and clinical changes in each of these fundamental disorders, along with the principal clinical features of acidosis and alkalosis. The clinical details are covered in chapters dealing with the diseases that cause acid-base disturbances.

When approaching a patient with a suspected acid-base disturbance, the physician should first confirm it and gauge its severity, by measuring the patient's arterial blood gases (Figure 5.3–2). For interpretation, the clinician needs at least two of the three following values: arterial pH, PCO_2, and HCO_3^-. The first task is to check the pH. This value shows whether the patient has acidemia (below 7.4) or alkalemia (above 7.4). Comparing the pH with the PCO_2 or HCO_3^- concentration shows whether the defect is of primary respiratory origin or represents compensation for a metabolic defect (see Table 5.3–1). Some patients have a single disturbance, such as respiratory aci-

Table 5.3–1. Primary or single disturbances of acid-base balance: Clinical and laboratory characteristics.

Primary Disturbance	Acute Primary Change	Partial Compensatory Response	Arterial pH	Serum K^+	Unmeasured Anions (Anion Gap)	Clinical Features
Respiratory						
Acidosis	↑CO_2 retention	↑HCO_3^-	↓	↑	Normal	Dyspnea, respiratory outflow obstruction, ↑ anteroposterior diameter of chest, rales, wheezes; in severe cases, disorientation, stupor, coma
Alkalosis	↓CO_2 depletion	↓HCO_3^-	↑	↓	Normal	Anxiety, occasional complaint of breathlessness, frequent sighing, lungs usually clear to exam, positive Chvostek's and Trousseau's signs
Metabolic						
Acidosis	↓HCO_3^- depletion	↓PCO_2	↓	↑ or ↓	Normal or ↑	Weakness, air hunger, Kussmaul respiration, dry skin and mucous membranes, poor skin turgor; in severe cases, coma, hypotension, death
Alkalosis	↑HCO_3^- retention	↑PCO_2	↑	↓	Normal	Weakness, positive Chvostek's and Trousseau's signs, hyporeflexia

dosis from acute ventilatory failure. But many have mixed acid-base disorders, such as a primary metabolic acidosis from hypovolemic shock superimposed on metabolic alkalosis due to preexisting recurrent vomiting. When the patient's blood gas values are determined, serum electrolytes are also routinely measured to define further the acid-base defect, for example, hypochloremic hypokalemic metabolic alkalosis.

The normal range of arterial pH is 7.36–7.44. The normal range for PCO_2 in arterial blood is 36–44 mm Hg. The normal range for HCO_3^- in arterial blood is 24–26 mEq/L, but in practice the HCO_3^- is usually measured in venous blood serum, where the level is slightly higher, 26.5–28.5 mEq/L.

Serum Electrolytes and the Anion Gap

The major intracellular cation, K^+, plays an important role in maintaining electroneutrality across the cell membrane. Movement of H^+ into a cell, or excess production of H^+ within the cell, prompts K^+ to move out of the cell to maintain electroneutrality. Conversely, when H^+ moves out of the cell to compensate for extracellular alkalosis, a comparable net amount of K^+ shifts into the cell. Hence, alkalosis—either respiratory or metabolic—usually results in a low serum K^+ level. In patients with acidosis, in whom K^+ leaves cells as H^+ enters, the situation can be more complex: The serum K^+ concentration may be high or low, depending on how fast the kidneys have been excreting the K^+ that has been added to extracellular fluid.

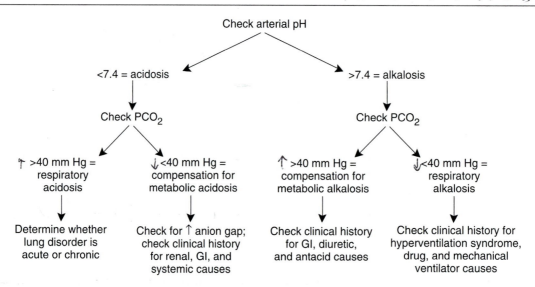

Check arterial pH

<7.4 = acidosis   >7.4 = alkalosis

Check PCO_2 Check PCO_2

↑ >40 mm Hg = respiratory acidosis

↓ <40 mm Hg = compensation for metabolic acidosis

↑ >40 mm Hg = compensation for metabolic alkalosis

↓ <40 mm Hg = respiratory alkalosis

Determine whether lung disorder is acute or chronic

Check for ↑ anion gap; check clinical history for renal, GI, and systemic causes

Check clinical history for GI, diuretic, and antacid causes

Check clinical history for hyperventilation syndrome, drug, and mechanical ventilator causes

Figure 5.3–2. Evaluation of acid-base disorders.

For example, in renal tubular acidosis, the serum K⁺ concentration is usually low because of increased urinary losses. In contrast, acute diabetic ketoacidosis, much more K⁺ leaves tissues and renal function is often compromised, so that many patients become hyperkalemic, even though their total body stores of K⁺ have been drastically depleted.

The anion gap (unmeasured anions in the serum) is useful in determining the cause of metabolic acidosis. The anion gap can be calculated from the following equation, which defines the electrical neutrality of serum:

$$\text{Anion gap} = ([Na^+] + [K^+]) - ([Cl^-] + [HCO_3^-])$$

A normal anion gap is 12–18 mEq/L. Any result above normal means an excess of some anionic serum constituent other than Cl^- or HCO_3^-. Possible explanations for an increased anion gap include lactate, as in patients with shock or tissue necrosis; acetoacetate and β-OH butyrate, as in patients with ketoacidosis; or phosphate and sulfate, as in patients with renal failure. The anion gap may also be increased by exogenous anions derived from drugs such as penicillin or cephalosporin analogues or from substances ingested accidentally or deliberately as in suicide attempts (eg, overdose of salicylate derived from aspirin) or from desperate substitutes for ethanol (eg, formate derived from the metabolism of methanol [wood alcohol] or oxalate derived from ethylene glycol [antifreeze]).

Clinical acid-base disturbances in which the anion gap remains normal (eg, renal tubular acidosis, chronic HCO_3^- loss in diarrheal fluid) are termed "nonanion gap" acidoses.

ACIDOSIS

Three alterations increase the H⁺ concentration: (1) addition of H⁺ from endogenous or exogenous sources (metabolic acidosis), (2) removal of HCO_3^- from body fluids (metabolic acidosis), and (3) addition of H_2CO_3 (that is, an elevation of PCO_2) as a result of alveolar hypoventilation (respiratory acidosis). It is useful to classify acidosis as metabolic or respiratory, since the cause influences management.

Metabolic Acidosis

Increased H⁺ production shifts the equilibrium reaction toward H_2CO_3, reducing the normal 20:1 ratio of $HCO_3^-:H_2CO_3$. The accompanying decrease in pH stimulates ventilation and leads to a drop in the H_2CO_3 (the PCO_2). These changes produce the laboratory hallmarks of a metabolic acidosis: decreased pH, decreased HCO_3^-, and decreased H_2CO_3 (measured as decreased arterial PCO_2) representing compensation for the drop in pH.

Table 5.3–1 and the steady-state acid-base nomogram in Figure 5.3–3 show the relationships among pH, PCO_2, and HCO_3^- in metabolic acidosis when metabolic and res-

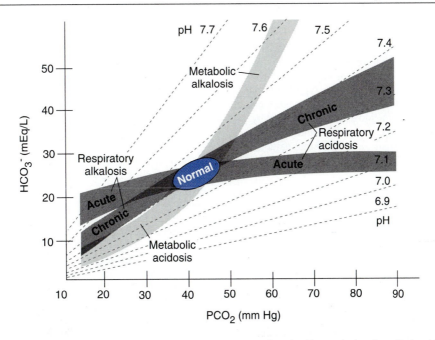

Figure 5.3–3. Nomogram for mixed acid-base disorders. (Modified and reproduced, with permission, from Graber M: Kidney Kard. Division of Nephrology, SUNY at Stony Brook, and the VA Medical Center, Northport, NY, © 1990.)

piratory compensations are complete. The kidneys respond to metabolic acidosis much more slowly than the lungs, but over hours the kidneys retard the drop in pH by adding HCO_3^- to body fluids.

Metabolic acidosis can be caused by endogenous or exogenous sources of H^+ (Table 5.3–2). Among the common endogenous causes are lactic acidosis from impaired tissue perfusion (eg, in hypovolemic shock or tissue infarction), as well as diabetic ketoacidosis. Another major endogenous cause is a decrease in H^+ excretion by the kidneys when the nephrons have suffered acute or chronic damage. Protein metabolism normally yields phosphoric and sulfuric acids, which react with the body's buffers to increase H_2CO_3 and decrease HCO_3^-. The resulting nonvolatile anions, existing as neutral salts of strong acids at physiologic pH, must be excreted by the kidneys and a comparable quantity of HCO_3^- regenerated and returned to the blood to restore the normal pH of the body fluids. This requires an intact renal tubular mechanism for H^+ secretion. In patients with renal failure, the kidneys' limited ability to secrete H^+ leads to acidosis with widening of the anion gap from retained sulfate and phosphate anions.

Normally, the kidneys reabsorb all the filtered HCO_3^- and regenerate an amount equal to that used systemically in the buffering of nonvolatile acids. In some forms of tubular disease, these functions are impaired; patients excrete excessive amounts of HCO_3^- in the urine despite worsening systemic acidosis. This urinary HCO_3^- wasting is accompanied by retention of Cl^-, so the anion gap characteristic of renal failure is missing. This "hyperchloremic acidosis" reflects the tubular damage. Exogenous administration of acetazolamide (a carbonic anhydrase-inhibiting diuretic) can also lead to acidosis by inhibiting tubular reabsorption of HCO_3^-.

Renal Tubular Acidosis: Renal tubular acidosis is the term given to disorders that result from defective H^+ transport in one or more segments of the tubule (Chapter 5.7). Two basic defects are recognized, type I involving the distal segment, type II the proximal segment. Classic (distal, type I) renal tubular acidosis is characterized by an abnormally high urine pH, hyperchloremia causing a normal anion gap, and usually mild systemic acidosis in a patient with a normal or only moderately reduced

glomerular filtration rate. Restoring the plasma HCO_3^- to normal by giving oral HCO_3^- (most often in the form of citrate to prevent direct interaction between HCO_3^- and gastric acid) usually produces only a mild increase in urinary HCO_3^- excretion.

Proximal (type II) renal tubular acidosis is characterized by more severe systemic acidosis. Most untreated patients have a low serum HCO_3^-, below 15 mEq/L. Untreated patients also have hyperchloremia. Most have a urine pH within the normal range (5.0 or below), since the distal tubule can acidify the urine adequately as long as large amounts of HCO_3^- are not being "dumped" from the proximal tubule. Returning the serum HCO_3^- to normal by infusing $NaHCO_3^-$ causes profound urinary HCO_3^- loss.

Either type of renal tubular acidosis can be incomplete or mild, and the distal and proximal types can coexist.

A hyperkalemic form of renal tubular acidosis (type IV) is almost always caused by diabetic renal disease. The plasma K^+ rises because of inadequate production of renin by the kidney, leading to reduced aldosterone production and impaired renal K^+ excretion. Most patients have only a mild defect in urine acidification.

Gastrointestinal Loss of Bicarbonate: Gastrointestinal loss of HCO_3^- leads to metabolic acidosis in pathologic conditions involving the small or large bowel. The HCO_3^- lost from the gut comes from secretions added to the small bowel lumen anywhere from the pancreatic duct through the lower third of the ileum. In the lower portion of the ileum, net secretion of fluid and electrolytes into the gut lumen begins to change to net reabsorption, a process completed within the large bowel. If reabsorption is impaired by disease or drugs, the resulting diarrheal fluid contains some amount of HCO_3^-. The more severe the diarrhea (the most severe diarrhea being in cholera or severe colitis), the greater the loss of HCO_3^-.

Other gastrointestinal conditions causing HCO_3^- wasting are biliary, pancreatic, and small bowel fistulas. Ileal loops used as urinary bladder replacements can produce HCO_3^- loss when they malfunction (eg, because of obstruction) and exchange urinary Cl^- for systemic HCO_3^- across the loop membrane.

In all these forms of gastrointestinal HCO_3^- loss, the kidneys cannot produce enough HCO_3^- to compensate fully, but they can easily retain NaCl and H_2O to prevent systemic volume contraction. The HCO_3^- loss combined with NaCl retention is reflected systemically as hyperchloremic acidosis.

Exogenous Intake of Acid: Increased exogenous intake of H^+ can produce metabolic acidosis. The most common drug to cause metabolic acidosis is salicylate. An infrequent cause is ammonium chloride, given as a test drug to evaluate renal tubular acidification disorders. Methanol and ethylene glycol are rare causes of severe metabolic acidosis. Table 5.3–2 lists the acids derived from the metabolism of all these compounds.

Table 5.3–2. Causes of metabolic acidosis.

	Exogenous	Endogenous
Gain of H^+	Aspirin (salicylic acid) Methanol (formic acid) Ethylene glycol (oxalic acid) Ammonium chloride* (hydrochloric acid)	Renal failure Renal tubular acidosis* Diabetic ketoacidosis Lactic acidosis
Loss of HCO_3^-	Carbonic anhydrase-inhibiting diuretics*	Diarrhea* Biliary or pancreatic fistulae* Ureteroileostomy*

*Normal anion gap.

Diagnosis: The clinical features of metabolic acidosis are always similar, regardless of etiology. Signs and symptoms relate to the severity of the pH disturbance rather than to the specific cause of the acidosis. Mild acidosis may cause no more than an increased ventilatory rate. More severe acidosis produces deep, rapid respirations (Kussmaul breathing, reflecting major respiratory compensation) as well as dryness of mucous membranes (caused by tachypnea with dehydration), somnolence, stupor, and coma. The cause of the acidosis can be suspected from the history. Preexisting diabetes, kidney disease, and recurrent kidney stones all should raise suspicion of renal failure as the cause of acidosis. In a patient who has metabolic acidosis along with primary liver, pulmonary, neoplastic, or cardiac disease, the most probable cause is lactic acidosis. A clear-cut history can be difficult to obtain when a patient presents with acidosis caused by a toxic ingestion. Clues to the cause may come from the patient's relatives and friends or from rescuers.

Management: In general, management of metabolic acidosis takes two forms: generic treatments for a particular category of acid-base derangement (eg, HCO_3^- for metabolic acidosis) and treatments directed at the specific cause (eg, insulin for diabetic ketoacidosis).

Acute metabolic acidosis accompanies many medical and surgical catastrophes, for example, cardiogenic or septic shock, or infarction of body tissues. In patients with these disorders, acidosis can further compromise circulatory function by blunting the normal peripheral vascular response to vasoconstrictive stimuli. When this happens, the physician may need to give intravenous fluids, pressor drugs, and HCO_3^- while managing the underlying disease. HCO_3^- should be given judiciously because it can lead to extracellular fluid volume overload, heart failure, and pulmonary edema.

Many patients with chronic renal failure or renal tubular acidosis have chronic, stable metabolic acidosis caused by H^+ retention, HCO_3^- wasting, or both. Systemic buffers, including calcium carbonate derived from bone, are called on to maintain acid-base balance. The chronic demand placed on bone buffers plays a major role in the development of renal osteodystrophy. Although the decline in pH is usually not severe enough to produce symptoms, the need to prevent renal osteodystrophy justifies treating patients who have chronic metabolic acidosis.

The aim of therapy for chronic metabolic acidosis should be a gradual restoration of normal pH over several days to weeks. Patients should not initially be given large quantities of HCO_3^-, because this may cause metabolic alkalosis with features ranging from paresthesias to tetany to seizures. The underlying nerve conduction abnormalities are caused by an alkalosis-induced reduction in extracellular ionized calcium (Ca^{2+}). Treatment can also precipitate acute hypokalemia, since many patients, particularly those with renal tubular acidosis, have latent or overt potassium deficiency. Management recommendations include dietary protein restriction, oral phosphate binders, attention to the underlying disorder, and judicious use of oral HCO_3^-, given as a sodium citrate-citric acid mixture (Chapter 5.5).

Respiratory Acidosis

By definition, respiratory acidosis is caused by impaired alveolar ventilation. Alveolar ventilation can be hampered by any condition that interferes with the functions of the lung, tracheobronchial tree, chest wall, or central nervous system control of respiration. Failure of pulmonary ventilation leads to CO_2 retention and, in response to the increased arterial PCO_2, an elevation of H_2CO_3.

Acute Respiratory Acidosis: Most patients appear acutely ill, complaining of dyspnea and making a greater than normal respiratory effort to increase alveolar ventilation. Many patients have hypoxemia, manifested as cyanosis. When the PCO_2 is very high (approaching 80 mm Hg), patients may have disorientation, stupor, and finally coma and death.

Treatment of uncomplicated acute respiratory acidosis is directed toward the cause, for example, airway obstruction, chest wall trauma, or cardiorespiratory arrest. When initial measures such as bronchodilators or chest tube placement do not correct the CO_2 retention, the patient may require mechanically assisted ventilation. Often the patient's respiratory distress is severe enough to require treatment before the blood pH and PCO_2 are measured. These levels may be obtained later to assess the adequacy of therapy.

Chronic Respiratory Acidosis: Longstanding obstructive pulmonary disease causes acid-base changes beyond those seen with acute CO_2 retention. Within several hours to a few days after the arterial PCO_2 rises, the kidneys begin to excrete more acid and reabsorb more HCO_3^-. This increase in circulating HCO_3^- partially compensates for the respiratory acidosis caused by CO_2 retention.

The goal of therapy is the same for both acute and chronic respiratory acidosis: to relieve CO_2 retention by improving ventilation. The difference is that in uncomplicated acute respiratory acidosis, removing the underlying cause allows the PCO_2 to return to normal, whereas in patients with chronic lung disease, treatment may not overcome the underlying structural damage, so the therapeutic end point is a chronic, stable state of partially compensated respiratory acidosis. When patients with chronic lung disease develop a superimposed acute impairment of ventilation, they typically have a combined acute and chronic respiratory acidosis. For these patients, therapy is dictated as much by their clinical state as by blood gas abnormalities.

In respiratory acidosis, the compensation produced by HCO_3^- retention is never sufficient to return the arterial pH to normal. Apparent total compensation, with arterial pH above 7.44, always means a mixed pH disturbance, with the secondary alteration being a metabolic alkalosis.

This may happen, for instance, when diuretic therapy has led to superimposition of a hypokalemic hypochloremic metabolic alkalosis.

ALKALOSIS

Alkalosis means a decrease in the H^+ concentration of the extracellular fluid. Increased alveolar ventilation decreases PCO_2, which decreases H_2CO_3 and leads to an increase in the $NaHCO_3:H_2CO_3$ ratio (greater than 20:1); this is known as respiratory alkalosis. Metabolic alkalosis is caused by loss of H^+, a gain of HCO_3^-, or both. The two most common causes of metabolic alkalosis are vomiting with loss of hydrochloric acid, and diuretic therapy that produces excessive loss of Cl^- and K^+ with retention of HCO_3^- (Table 5.3–3).

The respiratory compensation for metabolic alkalosis is alveolar hypoventilation with a resulting rise in PCO_2. Thus, a steady-state metabolic alkalosis is characterized by a low arterial H^+ concentration (increased pH), a high HCO_3^- concentration, and a high PCO_2.

The pH change in alkalosis is minimized by an immediate release of H^+ from intracellular buffers. As H^+ moves out from intracellular stores, Na^+ and K^+ move in. In severe states of alkalosis, this sudden shift in K^+ may acutely lower the plasma K^+, leading to the cardiac arrhythmias. This shift is particularly likely in patients who have a preexisting K^+ deficit from some other cause.

The kidneys' response to alkalosis is not simply HCO_3^- loss and concomitant H^+ retention. Most patients with alkalosis (eg, diuretic-induced) have a decrease in Na^+ stores, losing Na^+ and Cl^- from the extracellular fluid but not losing any HCO_3^-. The extracellular fluid volume contracts around the unchanged HCO_3^- stores, thereby increasing the HCO_3^- concentration and producing alkalosis. Renal compensation, the removal of HCO_3^- in the urine, ordinarily requires significant loss of Na^+. When intravascular hypovolemia develops, the stimulus to retain Na^+ is maximal, so virtually all filtered Na^+ is reabsorbed. Since the available Cl^- in the glomerular filtrate is limited (decreased extracellular fluid Cl^-), more Na^+ must be re-

absorbed than that retained with the filtered Cl^-. In this instance, Na^+ is reabsorbed with filtered HCO_3^- to maintain extracellular volume, and as a result the systemic HCO_3^- stays high, and the alkalosis is perpetuated. Because of the increased exchange of H^+ into the tubular lumen for Na^+, many patients with systemic metabolic alkalosis have a paradoxically acid urine. The hypokalemia commonly seen in alkalosis is caused by increased urinary K^+ loss from tubular exchange of K^+ for Na^+, often with additional extrarenal potassium losses, such as due to persistent vomiting.

Metabolic Alkalosis

Alkalosis produces few symptoms and signs, and many patients with alkalosis manifest mainly the symptoms of other electrolyte disorders. An acute increase in blood pH can cause tetany (see "Management" in "Metabolic Acidosis" section above), but few other clinical features can be attributed to alkalosis per se. Metabolic alkalosis is almost always accompanied by some degree of Na^+, Cl^-, and K^+ depletion, which often dominate the clinical picture. Rarely, ingestion of excessive amounts of HCO_3^- (in the form of baking soda, used as an antacid) can lead to metabolic alkalosis.

Metabolic alkalosis usually develops over several days or weeks, and most patients tolerate it relatively well. Thus, they can be given Na^+, Cl^-, and K^+ repletion over several days and be spared the dangers of receiving large quantities acutely.

Respiratory Alkalosis

Respiratory alkalosis is caused by alveolar hyperventilation, which reduces the blood's H_2CO_3 concentration (PCO_2).

The two initial compensatory mechanisms in acute respiratory alkalosis are reduction of extracellular fluid HCO_3^-, when it combines with H^+ released from body buffers, and a modest diuresis of HCO_3^-, a response limited by the need to maintain extracellular volume. If alveolar hyperventilation continues for several days, a new steady state of chronic respiratory alkalosis develops, with the HCO_3^- further lowered by a reduction in renal H^+ excretion and by retention of Na^+ with Cl^-. This state of hyperchloremia with a low plasma HCO_3^- may be mistaken for renal tubular acidosis unless the arterial blood gases are measured. Such a situation underscores the need to measure at least two of the pH, PCO_2, and HCO_3^- before characterizing an acid-base disorder.

Two types of patients with respiratory alkalosis require treatment. The more common setting is the patient on mechanically assisted ventilation. Their pH disturbance is severe and requires immediate control by adjustment of the respirator (Chapter 2.7). Either the minute volume can be reduced, or the dead space can be increased if a high rate of mechanical ventilation is needed to provide adequate oxygenation. The type of patient requiring treatment is the individual having an anxiety attack who hyperventilates,

Table 5.3–3. Causes of alkalosis.

Metabolic
Vomiting of gastric contents
Diuretics that cause virtually equal losses of Na and Cl
   (thiazides, loop diuretics)
Hyperaldosteronism
Hyperadrenocorticism
Bicarbonate compounds, excessive antacids
Posthyperventilation (posthypercapnic) alkalosis

Respiratory
Vigorous respirator therapy
Hyperventilation syndrome
Diffuse liver disease
Diffuse central nervous system disease
Salicylate drugs causing central nervous system stimulation

raising the blood pH, and developing paresthesias that can progress to tetany from the pH-related reduction in their extracellular Ca^{2+}. Rebreathing into a paper bag or breath-holding usually suffices to raise the PCO_2 high enough to correct the disturbance.

Milder forms of respiratory alkalosis, seen in liver and central nervous system disease, rarely require intervention. Unless the arterial pH and PCO_2 are measured, the compensatory decrease in these patients' serum HCO_3^- may be misinterpreted as a mild metabolic acidosis.

MIXED ACID-BASE DISORDERS

Many patients have more than one acid-base disorder at a time. For example, a person with chronic obstructive airway disease may develop both an acute respiratory acidosis and a superimposed metabolic acidosis or alkalosis. Conversely, a person who has developed an acute respiratory alkalosis from a salicylate overdose may develop a superimposed metabolic acidosis. Patients whose arterial pH, PCO_2, and HCO_3^- intersect at points outside the 95% confidence limits of the primary acid-base disorder shown in the nomogram (see Figure 5.3–3) either have a mixed acid-base disorder or were tested before enough time had elapsed to allow full compensation in a primary acid-base disorder. Typically, compensation is achieved within minutes in the lungs and several hours to days in the kidneys.

The essential step in evaluating acid-base measurements of single and mixed disorders is to confirm the accuracy of the laboratory findings and decide whether the data fit the patient's clinical picture. If the physician suspects that the results are at odds with the patient's presentation, the accuracy of the tests must be rechecked.

SUMMARY

▶ An acid-base disturbance may be the first manifestation of a systemic metabolic disorder or of a functional abnormality in the kidneys, lungs, gastrointestinal tract, or skin.

▶ Of the three arterial blood gas determinants—pH, PCO_2, and HCO_3^-—at least two are essential for accurate diagnosis of an acid-base disturbance.

▶ First, check the arterial pH: The patient with a pH below 7.4 has acidosis; above 7.4, alkalosis. To determine whether the disorder is metabolic or respiratory, measure the PCO_2; to determine the cause of metabolic acidosis, assess whether there is an anion gap and correlate with the clinical history.

▶ Correlate the history with the degree of blood gas abnormality to determine whether the acid-base disorder is life-threatening and how quickly it should be corrected.

▶ When the laboratory results are at variance with the patient's clinical presentation, the lab tests must be rechecked.

SUGGESTED READING

Bank N, Better OS: Acid-base balance and acute renal failure. Miner Electrolyte Metab 1991;17:116.

Goldberger E: *A Primer of Water, Electrolyte and Acid-Base Syndromes,* 7th ed. Lea & Febiger, 1986.

McLaughlin ML, Kassirer JP: Rational treatment of acid-base disorders. Drugs 1990;39;841.

Preuss HG: Fundamentals of clinical acid-base evaluation. Clin Lab Med 1993;13:103.

von Planta M et al: Pathophysiologic and therapeutic implications of acid-base changes during CPR. Ann Emerg Med 1993;22:404.

5.4

Acute Renal Failure

Andrew Whelton, MD, and Alan J. Watson, MRCPI

Acute renal failure, the abrupt decline in renal function occurring over hours or days, results in the systemic retention of nitrogenous wastes and the development of fluid, electrolyte, and acid-base disturbances. The syndrome represents a common response to many types of insults to the kidney, ranging from mild entities, such as transient drug nephrotoxicity, to the often fatal forms of acute renal failure seen with multisystem organ failure, such as may occur after surgery or trauma.

Physicians must recognize the often nonspecific clinical features of acute renal failure for several reasons. First, patients with acute renal failure can present as one of several potentially life-threatening states, such as profound obtundation, pulmonary edema, and hyperkalemia with its attendant cardiac arrhythmias. Second, the physician can often determine the cause of the acute renal failure logically, based on knowledge of how renal function has become deranged. Third, if acute renal failure is promptly recognized and carefully managed, it is usually reversible.

The pathophysiology of acute renal failure is categorized as prenatal, postrenal, or intrinsic to the kidney itself (Table 5.4–1). Prerenal failure is caused by conditions that decrease renal plasma flow and glomerular filtration rate. Postrenal failure is caused by disorders that obstruct the urinary outflow tract. Intrinsic acute renal failure varies in its presentation, depending on the major site of injury within the kidney, such as the glomeruli in acute glomerulonephritis and the renal tubules in acute tubular necrosis. Anuria (no urine output) usually signals obstructive renal failure. Otherwise, the degree of urine output associated with the three classes of renal injury depends on the cause, extent, and duration of the insult. Urine output of less than 500 mL/24 hours is considered oliguric renal failure; however, in current clinical practice, nonoliguric renal failure is the most typical initial presentation, which can then progress to oliguria.

PATHOPHYSIOLOGY

Prerenal Acute Renal Failure

Prerenal disorders cause acute renal failure by decreasing renal plasma flow. The usual trigger is a drop in circulating blood volume, such as that caused by hemorrhage,

septicemic shock, or profound loss of fluid and electrolytes. Heart conditions that markedly reduce cardiac output can lead to renal hypoperfusion and renal failure; among these conditions are cardiac tamponade and severe left ventricular failure after myocardial infarction or heart surgery. Profound reductions in intravascular protein concentration, such as those in patients with end-stage liver disease, extensive burns, or severe nephrotic syndrome, may contract intravascular volume to such an extent that patients develop acute renal failure. Furthermore, if renal hypoperfusion is severe and prolonged, prerenal failure can actually cause ischemic damage to nephrons (see below). Patients with severe liver failure may also hypoperfuse the kidney, resulting in acute renal failure; this is called the *hepatorenal syndrome*.

Vascular disease obstructing the renal arteries must be severe and bilateral to cause acute renal failure. Most patients with renal artery stenoses present with secondary hypertension (Chapter 5.9). Only when both renal arteries have stenoses of at least 95% is renal function impaired. When partial obstructions are present, renal function can be suddenly worsened by thrombosis or embolism at the site of stenosis or when angiotensin converting enzyme (ACE) inhibitors are started to treat hypertension.

Although not "prerenal," obstruction of the renal venous outflow can also precipitate acute renal failure. This is most commonly caused by rapidly developing, extensive thromboses in large renal veins. Hypercoagulable states (Chapter 11.10), such as the nephrotic syndrome and conditions that increase plasma viscosity, contribute to renal vein thrombosis. When renal vein thrombosis begins slowly, typically over several weeks, enough collateral outflow develops that the kidneys continue to function adequately.

Causes of Intrinsic Acute Renal Failure

Glomerulonephritis: Acute glomerulonephritis may be a primary kidney disorder or a component of a multisystem disease (Chapter 5.6). Many forms of acute primary glomerulopathy are caused by damage from infections, such as streptococcal or viral infections, and from the immunologic responses to them. Acute glomerulonephritis can develop secondary to systemic vasculitis, as in sys-

Table 5.4–1. Acute renal failure: Etiologic and differential diagnostic features.

Prerenal	Renal	Postrenal
History		
Dehydration (eg, skin, gut, or renal loss of fluid and electrolytes)	Prolonged renal ischemia	Prostate disease
Acute blood loss	Acute glomerulonephritis	Pelvic tumors
Extensive burns with plasma loss	Drug use (eg, aminoglycosides, NSAIDs, radiocontrast dyes)	Kidney stones
Low cardiac output	Thromboembolism	Blood clots in urine
Fluid retention with heart disease	Hypercoagulable state	Recent pelvic surgery
Increased thirst	Atheroembolism (vascular surgery, angiography)	
Physical examination		
Weight loss, or weight gain in heart disease	Weight gain	Weight gain
Poor skin and muscle turgor	Obtundation	Bladder distention
Orthostatic changes	Hypotension changing over days to hypertension	Pelvic mass
Segregated fluid accumulations (eg, ascites, ileus)	Increased jugular venous pressure and pulmonary congestion	Enlarged prostate
Weight gain with congestive heart failure	Muscle trauma or ischemia	
	Infected sites of, eg, venous or arterial catheters, surgical incisions	
	Livedo reticularis	
Laboratory findings		
Increased ratio of blood urea nitrogen: serum creatinine (>30:1)	Evolving oliguria with urine osmolality = serum osmolality	Stone or blood clot in urine
Low, normal, or high serum sodium	Urine sodium >40 mEq/L	Anuria
Concentrated urine	Hyperkalemia	Hydronephrosis with hydroureter and evidence of obstruction
Low urine sodium (<20 mEq/L), high osmolality (>500 mOsm/kg), high specific gravity (>1.030)	Acute hemolysis	
Low central venous pressure and pulmonary capillary wedge pressure, except in congestive heart failure	4+ proteinuria with glomerulonephritis	
	1+ proteinuria with nephrotoxicity	
	Pigment-containing tubular casts	
	Arterial or venous occlusions	
	Increased central venous pressure and pulmonary capillary wedge pressure	

NSAIDs, nonsteroidal anti-inflammatory drugs.

temic lupus erythematosus, drug-induced or idiopathic vasculitis, Wegener's granulomatosis, and Goodpasture's syndrome. Patients with these diseases develop acute renal failure when damage to the filtering surface of the glomerular capillaries becomes severe enough to reduce glomerular filtration.

Diagnosis of acute glomerulonephritis requires a thorough clinical evaluation, urinalysis, blood chemistry, and hematologic and serologic tests. The urine typically has significant proteinuria; microscopic evaluation shows red blood cells and tubular casts made of proteinaceous debris, disintegrating cells, or intact red blood cells. Although few patients need the diagnosis confirmed with a renal biopsy, it may be needed when the clinical evaluation and laboratory findings are not clear-cut, such as when the kidney is only one of several organ systems damaged by an autoimmune process. Although renal biopsy is an invasive procedure sometimes complicated by bleeding, it can nonetheless be performed safely, provided that the patient has normal coagulation and that a guidance technique such as ultrasonography or fluoroscopy is used.

The renal biopsy in patients with primary glomerular injury, such as with poststreptococcal glomerulonephritis, shows diffuse epithelial cell proliferation, which usually heals within days to weeks as the acute renal failure resolves. Secondary glomerulopathies often show histologic features of the underlying systemic disease. In Goodpasture's syndrome, for example, antibody-mediated damage to the glomerular basement membrane manifests as a proliferation of all cell types in the glomerulus, with epithelial crescents and a distinctive linear deposition of immunoglobulins within the lining of the glomerular capillary loops (see Figure 5.6–1).

Acute Tubular Damage, Including Ischemic Acute Renal Failure: The most common cause of renal tubular damage is ischemia, often associated either with precipitation of pigment such as myoglobin in the tubular lumen or with exposure to nephrotoxic drugs, chemicals, or radiocontrast dyes (Chapter 5.7). Ischemic acute renal failure can develop in any of the situations that cause prerenal insufficiency, but the ischemic insult is typically more severe and prolonged. Ischemic renal damage can develop after as little as 20 minutes of total or partial compromise of blood flow to the kidney, as during cardiopulmonary bypass. Although the damage is called "acute tubular necrosis," few necrotic tubular cells are seen on renal biopsy. The primary insult in ischemic acute renal failure is redistribution of the reduced blood flow from the renal cortex to the juxtamedullary region.

As might be expected in a disease with so little histologic disruption, ischemic acute renal failure can be completely reversible. The insufficiency typically lasts 10–20 days before renal function begins to recover. During this time, most patients need aggressive dialysis, nutrition support, careful management of fluid and electrolyte balance, and monitoring for and treatment of superimposed infections.

Pigment-Associated Acute Renal Failure: Filtered myoglobin released from injured muscle often contributes to post-traumatic, postsurgical, and even some nontraumatic causes of acute renal failure. Myoglobin promotes the formation of obstructive casts and is directly toxic to the tubules because of its metabolism in acidic urine. Thus, in patients with known or suspected myoglobinuria, prompt attention should be given to forcing diuresis and alkalinizing the urine—measures that can limit myoglobin-related tubular injury.

Hemoglobin can also contribute to the production of obstructive tubular casts, as in patients with intravascular hemolysis. If the hemolysis occurs in a patient with adequate renal plasma flow, it is unlikely to cause acute renal failure. However, if the patient also has hypotension, as from an anaphylactoid reaction to the transfusion of mismatched blood, the combination of ischemia and hemoglobinuria can cause acute renal failure.

Nephrotoxic Acute Renal Failure: Direct tubular toxicity most often follows exposure to radiocontrast dye or to drugs, especially aminoglycosides. Other causes are industrial solvents or salts of heavy metals such as lead, mercury, and cadmium. These forms of nephrotoxic acute renal failure account for 20–40% of all acute elevations of serum creatinine in hospitalized patients. The severity of injury ranges from mild, transient, or clinically insignificant acute renal insufficiency to complete renal failure, requiring dialysis.

Aminoglycoside antibiotics are the most commonly implicated nephrotoxic drugs. Their direct damage to the proximal tubules is related to the dose and duration of therapy. Aminoglycoside nephrotoxicity can usually be prevented by keeping the dose as low as possible, limiting therapy to 7–10 days, not repeating courses of therapy in close succession, and monitoring drug levels in the blood. In addition, patients must be monitored for dehydration, hypokalemia, and liver failure, and they should not be concurrently exposed to other nephrotoxins like radiocontrast dye. Finally, the dose must be adjusted for lean body weight in obese patients, decreased for elderly patients, and adjusted based on serum levels, which should be checked every 2–3 days during therapy in high-risk patients.

Other antimicrobials, such as amphotericin B, are also direct tubulotoxins. Cyclosporine commonly produces dose- and duration-related nephrotoxicity that limits the drug's use in transplant recipients. Cisplatin and some other antineoplastic drugs are also nephrotoxic.

In susceptible persons, nonsteroidal anti-inflammatory drugs (NSAIDs) precipitate acute renal failure. Patients with a pre-existing reduction in renal perfusion produce vasodilatory prostaglandins within the kidney as a compensatory mechanism to preserve renal function. When NSAIDs inhibit prostaglandin production by removing the compensatory hemodynamic response, patients may de-

velop some degree of acute renal failure, which is reversible when the drug is stopped.

Radiocontrast dyes induce acute renal failure by decreasing renal perfusion as a result of immediate and intense renal vasospasm, by increasing intratubular osmotic concentrations, and by directly harming tubules in distal segments of the nephron. At particular risk for radiocontrast-induced acute renal failure are the elderly, people with renovascular disease, and people with preexisting renal impairment from diabetes mellitus or multiple myeloma. When radiocontrast nephrotoxicity develops, the serum creatinine peaks 3–5 days after patients have received the dye, and then, for most patients, quickly falls to normal. The best ways to avoid radiocontrast nephrotoxicity are to hydrate patients adequately before and after the radiographic study, to use a nonhypertonic dye, and to give the smallest amount possible.

ACE inhibitor antihypertensive drugs can cause acute deterioration of renal function in patients with bilateral renal artery stenosis or unilateral stenosis with a nonfunctioning other kidney. Patients with preexisting chronic renal impairment, such as diabetic nephropathy, may show deterioration of function after several days or weeks of ACE inhibitor therapy. ACE inhibitors decrease the resistance to efferent capillary blood flow from the glomeruli, leading to a reduction in glomerular filtration pressure.

Interstitial Nephritis: An inflammatory reaction of the interstitium surrounding the renal tubules occurs as an acute allergic reaction to drugs such as the penicillins, cephalosporins, and sulfonamides (Chapter 5.7). Many other drugs or chemicals produce this form of acute renal failure, but only rarely. In some patients, no obvious etiologic exposure can be identified. Clues to interstitial nephritis are arthralgia, papillary rash, peripheral eosinophilia, and eosinophils in the microscopic urine sediment. A definitive diagnosis can be made only by renal biopsy.

If the inciting agent can be identified and the exposure stopped, the acute renal failure tends to resolve spontaneously. However, in most patients a brief 7–10-day course of corticosteroids hastens the recovery of renal function.

Fulminant bacterial pyelonephritis may present as acute renal failure. This is most likely to happen to patients with pre-existing renal impairment, such as recurrent kidney stones or diabetic nephropathy.

Atheroembolism: Atheroembolism of the renal parenchyma, typically following invasive vascular surgery or extensive angiographic exploration, can cause entrapment of an atheroma or cholesterol crystal within glomeruli. The functional consequences of extensive embolisms may lead to acute renal failure. The key to management is to prevent further atheroembolism.

Postrenal Acute Renal Failure

Obstruction to outflow from the pyelocalyceal system of the kidney to the urethral drainage tract of the urinary bladder causes postrenal failure. If the obstruction is complete and if acute infection—particularly bacterial—

develops proximal to the obstruction, rapid destruction of the renal parenchyma leads to irreversible renal failure within days. Correct diagnosis is urgently needed.

A patient who presents with acute renal failure and no urine output (anuria) may well have an acute obstruction of the urinary outflow tract. Such a patient may need renal ultrasonography, intravenous pyelography, radioisotopic flow studies, or a retrograde or percutaneous antegrade pyelographic study of the outflow tract. Although anuria usually signals obstructive acute renal failure, it may also be a presenting feature of renal cortical necrosis, as seen in patients with hemolytic uremic syndrome or complete thromboembolism of the renal arteries, or in some women with obstetric renal failure induced by amniotic fluid embolization or postpartum hemorrhage; however, all these patients have a patent urinary outflow tract. Several clinical and laboratory features permit ready differentiation of these conditions. Patients with the hemolytic uremic syndrome present with thrombocytopenia, and the peripheral blood smear shows red cell hemolysis. Patients with renal artery thromboembolism will likely present in a postvascular surgery setting or with clinical evidence of a disseminated thromboembolic process. In patients with obstetric renal failure, the history of concurrent abortion or delivery distinguishes cortical necrosis from complete obstruction of the urinary outflow tract.

It is also important to remember that obstructive uropathy can lead to renal insufficiency without causing complete anuria. For example, prostatic disease can lead to partial obstruction, in which urine volumes may be normal. Furthermore, when only one kidney is obstructed, the patient may not be anuric.

EVALUATION

History

Many patients with acute renal failure have an obvious predisposing factor—most often recent surgery, trauma, or a nephrotoxic exposure. When the cause is less obvious, the differential diagnosis can be challenging. Important clues are a history of jaundice, the presence of infection, or an active systemic process such as a collagen vascular disease or diabetes mellitus. Whenever possible, the physician should determine when the serum creatinine first rose and carefully review the patient's circumstances at that time. The clinician should review all medications that the patient received in the days and weeks before becoming ill and should assess exposures to other potential nephrotoxins such as radiocontrast dyes, chemicals, and environmental toxins. A history of drug allergy and rash suggests acute tubulointerstitial nephritis, while livedo reticularis suggests atheroembolism. A history of streptococcal sore throat followed by dark urine indicates post-streptococcal acute glomerulonephritis.

Physical Examination

The examination should focus on assessing the patient's volume status. Hypovolemia suggests prerenal acute renal failure, whereas hypervolemia suggests acute renal failure

resulting from intrinsic renal factors or outflow obstruction. Tachycardia, acute weight loss, and poor muscle and skin turgor indicate dehydration, whereas a high jugular venous pressure, basilar pulmonary rales, a third heart sound, and peripheral edema indicate salt and water accumulation from abrupt loss of excretory function. The duration of these features can help the physician to distinguish prerenal renal failure from established ischemic forms of intrinsic acute renal failure.

Patients with severe renal failure may have pericarditis, evidenced by elevated pulsus paradoxus, elevated jugular venous pressure, soft heart tones, or a precordial friction rub. Cardiac arrhythmias, a common complication of uremia, are usually related to hyperkalemia or other electrolyte disturbances.

Possible neurologic disturbances are lethargy, disorientation, progressive loss of reflexes, tremulousness, asterixis, seizures, and coma. Overly aggressive dialysis can produce similar neurologic features by causing a rapid fall in extracellular osmolality that follows faster removal of extracellular than intracellular urea. This drop in osmolality transiently promotes water influx into cells, leading to cerebral edema. It reverses within several hours after dialysis is stopped.

Urine Evaluation

All patients with acute renal failure should have a complete urinalysis. The severity of proteinuria varies with the responsible disease, but most prerenal and postrenal causes of acute renal failure produce only minimal proteinuria. Acute glomerular disorders typically cause 4+ proteinuria (at least 200 mg/dL), whereas tubular disorders usually cause only 1–2+ proteinuria (25–100 mg/dL). Microscopic examination of the urine sediment can give clues to the etiology. In prerenal acute renal failure, urinalysis is unremarkable, although it may show an abundance of hyaline casts. Red cells and red cell casts indicate active glomerulonephritis, and eosinophils suggest allergic tubulointerstitial nephritis. In acute tubular necrosis induced by nephrotoxins, the urine often contains renal tubular epithelial cells and debris. In contrast to hemoglobin, myoglobin is suggested by a positive reaction for heme by dipstick urine testing, when no red blood cells are seen on microscopy. This finding, together with abundant darkly pigmented casts in the microscopic urine sediment, provides solid evidence of rhabdomyolysis.

Urine volume assessment is useful. Prerenal acute renal failure is typically associated with oliguria (less than 400 mL/24 hr). However, patients who have some degree of preexisting renal impairment such as diabetes insipidus or diabetes mellitus are likely to present with polyuria (more than 2.5 L/24 hr). Partial obstruction of the urinary outflow tract may also lead to polyuria, because the increased tubular pressure damages proximal and distal segments of the nephron and induces a concentrating defect. As stated earlier, true anuria usually signifies total obstruction of the urinary outflow tract, renal cortical necrosis from fulminant glomerulonephritis, or a vascular catastrophe such as bilateral thromboembolism of the renal arteries.

Analyses of urine electrolytes and osmolality are useful in distinguishing prerenal from intrinsic causes of acute renal failure. In prerenal failure, inadequate perfusion of the glomerulus limits the production of filtrate. The tubular network, which is intact, responds as it would to profound dehydration by generating small volumes of urine that has virtually no sodium. A typical urine sodium is less than 10 mEq/L, and a typical osmolality is above 500 mOsm/kg. Glomerulonephritis and renal vascular accidents can produce a similar pattern, provided that the renal tubules remain functional. By contrast, in acute tubular necrosis the damaged tubular network is less able to modify the filtrate. Urine sodium levels tend to be above 40 mEq/L, and urine osmolality is near the isotonic range of 300–350 mOsm/kg.

The urine-to-plasma ratios of urea nitrogen and creatinine may also provide some clue to the nature of the underlying renal problem. A urine-to-plasma urea ratio above 8 or a urine-to-plasma creatinine ratio above 40 suggests urine concentration and a prerenal state. Ratios below 3 for urea and 20 for creatinine suggest established acute tubular necrosis. A urine-to-plasma osmolality ratio of less than 1 suggests established intrinsic renal failure, and a ratio more than 1.2 indicates prerenal failure.

Blood tests can also give clues to how long the patient has had renal failure. A uremic patient who does not have anemia or hypocalcemia probably has acute renal insufficiency.

Imaging Tests

The first imaging test should be ultrasonography to define the size of the kidneys and the outflow pyelocalyceal-ureteric tract. An increase in the size of the kidney and outflow tract indicates obstruction. If sonography suggests obstruction, the lesion may be further defined by retrograde or percutaneous antegrade pyelography. Intravenous pyelography should be used only in those with suspected partial outflow obstruction and a relatively normal serum creatinine. Radionuclide studies may help establish the patency of renal vessels, but angiography is the definitive test. Angiography will be required before undertaking vascular surgical or angioplasty procedures.

A renal biopsy should be considered if the acute renal failure remains unexplained, if the patient does not improve, or if the physician suspects a systemic disease like vasculitis.

MANAGEMENT

The physician must assess how the abrupt loss of renal function has affected the patient's electrolyte and volume status, acid-base balance, organ function, and nutrition.

Electrolytes

Sodium and Water: Many patients with acute renal failure have hyponatremia. Signs of volume expansion indicate an excess of total body salt and water. In patients

with these physical findings (noted above), hyponatremia suggests an even greater excess of water, the usual source of which is continued water intake. In the hospital, the problem is often that patients have been given hypotonic intravenous fluids. For most patients, the hyponatremia is mild, but a sudden drop in serum sodium and osmolality can cause neurotoxicity. The physician assessing a hyponatremic patient should exclude hyperproteinemia and hyperlipidemia, which can cause pseudohyponatremia. Particularly when the serum sodium is less than 120 mEq/L, hyponatremia can lead to cerebral edema, a medical emergency. Early symptoms are lethargy, confusion, nausea, and vomiting. The condition quickly progresses to seizures and coma. The physician must improve serum osmolality and alleviate brain swelling. The first task is to restrict free water intake. The second is to estimate the patient's excess free water, with the following formula:

$$\text{Excess} = \text{Current TBW (L)} - \left[\frac{\text{current serum Na}^+ \text{[mEq/L]} \times \text{current TBW [L]}}{\text{desired serum Na}^+} \right]$$

where TBW = total body water. To estimate the TBW, use body weight in kg $\times$ 0.6. When the excess body water has been calculated, it provides a therapeutic goal in fluid restriction.

The best rate at which to correct the serum sodium is controversial. In patients with chronic hyponatremia, the serum sodium should rise no more than 1–2 mEq/L/hr. Hyponatremia that has developed quickly, for example, after general anesthesia and surgery, must be at least partially reversed faster. When the serum sodium is restored to at least 125 mEq/L, the risk of further irreversible central nervous system injury is ameliorated. Patients with no kidney function may need dialysis to remove excess water.

As glomerular filtration improves after an episode of intrinsic renal failure, patients may have a water and electrolyte diuresis that causes dehydration and hypernatremia, the so-called polyuric phase of acute tubular necrosis. When an outflow tract obstruction is relieved, patients may have an osmotic diuresis as the glomeruli filter large quantities of urea, creatinine, and other solutes accumulated during the obstruction. During this osmotic "postobstructive" diuretic phase, the physician must pay careful attention to daily weights and volume intake and output to determine whether patients need fluid and electrolyte replacement.

Potassium: Hyperkalemia is a common electrolyte complication of acute renal failure, reflecting the kidney's key role in maintaining potassium balance. Hyperkalemia is most likely to accompany severe acidosis: As hydrogen ions move into cells, potassium moves out to the extracellular fluid. Hyperkalemia is also commonly associated with tissue destruction (eg, rhabdomyolysis), hematoma formation, and absorption of blood from the gut. Because the cardiotoxic effects of hyperkalemia can be fatal to patients with acute renal failure, serum potassium levels must be monitored frequently. Electrocardiographic changes often accompany hyperkalemia, including prolongation of the PR interval and QRS, with prominent peaking of the T wave and subsequent AV conduction defects and ventricular tachycardia. The physician should monitor both the absolute serum potassium level and the rate at which the potassium concentration rises.

Treatment of hyperkalemia has three steps: (1) minute-to-minute management of severe cardiotoxicity, (2) moving potassium back into cells, and (3) removing potassium from the extracellular fluid. In patients with severe cardiotoxicity, an intravenous infusion of calcium gluconate stabilizes cardiac muscle membranes and buys time for the serum potassium to be reduced by more definitive measures. Potassium can be moved back into cells either by increasing the pH in the extracellular fluid with infusion of sodium bicarbonate or by infusion of insulin with dextrose. The serum potassium begins to fall within 20–30 minutes, but it typically stops falling after 3–4 hours. Many patients need repeated treatments. Only dialysis or sodium polystyrene sulfonate resin, given by mouth or by retention enema, actually removes potassium from the extracellular fluid. Extracorporeal hemodialysis is much better than peritoneal dialysis at removing potassium.

Acid-Base Balance: Most patients in acute renal failure have metabolic acidosis, reflecting accumulation of acids that are by-products of metabolism and normally excreted by the kidney (Chapter 5.3). These retained acids, primarily sulfuric and phosphoric acid, are then buffered in the extracellular space by sodium bicarbonate. The increase in the anion gap seen in this type of metabolic acidosis is caused by the retention of sulfates and phosphates. The anion gap is calculated with this formula:

$$\text{Anion gap} = ([Na^+] + [K^+]) - ([Cl^-] + [HCO_3^-])$$

Normal range = 12–18 mEq/L.

The anion gap is a measurement of anions that are not counted in standard blood chemistries. In a noncatabolic person with renal failure, with basal rates of hydrogen production, the serum bicarbonate level falls about 1–2 mEq/L/24 hr. However, a patient with an infection, tissue trauma, or poor tissue perfusion has a much faster drop in bicarbonate. In such a patient, superimposed diabetic ketoacidosis or lactic acidosis must be considered. Treatment for the fall in bicarbonate is determined by the severity of the reduction and the adequacy of respiratory compensation. Another factor is the risk of further decreases in bicarbonate, as expected in patients with ongoing lactic acidosis. Treatment with bicarbonate solutions can lead to salt and water overload, hypokalemia, and possible worsening of cardiac function. The physician giving bicarbonate should use this formula in gauging the base deficit:

$$\text{HCO}_3^- \text{ deficit} = (\text{Desired serum HCO}_3^- \text{ [mEq/L]} - \text{actual serum HCO}_3^-) \times 0.35 \text{ body wt [kg]}$$

Dialysis can correct abnormal serum bicarbonate concentrations and protect against volume overload.

Mineral Balance: Hypocalcemia develops relatively early in the course of acute renal failure. The initial cause is systemic phosphate retention as renal function is lost. Another factor is reduced production and inhibited function of 1,25-dihydroxycholecalciferol, which normally stimulates gut absorption of calcium. The decrease in serum calcium promotes secondary hyperparathyroidism. Patients with rhabdomyolysis can develop severe hypocalcemia when phosphate released from damaged muscle cells accumulates systemically and when calcium and phosphate precipitate in the damaged muscle tissue. Therapy with phosphate binders ultimately restores a normal calcium level. Patients with a high serum phosphate and secondary hyperparathyroidism should not be given calcium, because it can trigger acute metastatic calcification.

Other Organs: In addition to controlling electrolyte, acid-base, and mineral disturbances in acute renal failure, physicians must manage the metabolic effects on all the body's systems. Acute renal failure reduces immunologic capacity; infection is the most common fatal complication. Indwelling venous catheters and urinary catheters should be placed with strict attention to asepsis and used as briefly as possible. Prophylactic antibiotics are not routinely recommended. However, patients with suspected bowel perforation or trauma should be treated for polymicrobial infection, pending further evaluation. Anemia tends to develop early in acute renal failure. Several factors contribute. Diminished production of erythropoietin leads to a hypoproliferative bone marrow. The anemia is further aggravated by low-grade hemolysis and blood loss from gastrointestinal bleeding or during hemodialysis. Red cell transfusion has been the mainstay of therapy, although recombinant human erythropoietin may prove to be of benefit. Uremia may impair coagulation, either from an acquired platelet defect or as a complication of the underlying disease, such as the disseminated intravascular coagulation seen with infection. Platelet transfusions are of little benefit, but dDAVP (desmopressin) or cryoprecipitate infusions improve platelet function and coagulation by releasing or providing procoagulant serum proteins.

Many problems in acute renal failure relate to uremia—accumulation in the blood of excessive amounts of urea and other toxins, typically with fluid and electrolyte abnormalities. To help counteract uremia, patients should be limited in their intake of protein, sodium, water, potassium, phosphate, and fluids. The degree of restriction depends on the severity and duration of the renal impairment.

Patients whose uremia does not improve with fluid, electrolyte, and dietary restrictions need dialysis. Extracorporeal hemodialysis requires vascular access, but effectively controls uremia and its complications. Hemodialysis should be started early in the course and repeated frequently, typically every other day except in hypercatabolic patients, in whom it may be needed on a daily basis used often. Peritoneal dialysis is equally effective, but takes four to five times longer to perform. Since peritoneal dialysis is continuous, it may be considered for hemodynamically unstable patients. These patients may also benefit from newer techniques of continuous arteriovenous or venovenous hemofiltration dialysis.

Specific Renal Therapies

In prerenal acute renal failure, increasing renal plasma flow improves overall kidney function. In postrenal failure, the goal is to relieve obstruction. In intrinsic failure, the definition of an effective treatment begins with a determination of the site of injury; subsequently, other tests may be required, such as renal biopsy in glomerulonephritis. In certain diseases, immunosuppression with corticosteroids and cytotoxic agents may retard the inflammatory process and improve function. In patients with allergic interstitial nephritis, withdrawing the offending agent may be enough to restore renal function, although some patients need corticosteroids.

The value of loop diuretics and mannitol in oliguric acute renal failure has not been proved. Mannitol should not be overused because accumulations can cause a syndrome of volume expansion with acute pulmonary edema, hyperkalemia, hyponatremia, and cerebral dehydration. Prevention and improvement of acute tubular necrosis are being studied with drugs such as calcium channel blockers, atrial natriuretic peptide, and prostaglandin analogs.

Nutrition

The diet for a patient with acute renal failure must be adjusted by the type of acute renal failure, degree of catabolism, and specific metabolic abnormalities. Patients need adequate calories and nitrogen in minimal volumes of fluid, along with restricted intake of sodium, potassium, phosphorus, and magnesium. Some patients require enteral or parenteral nutritional supplements.

Most patients with mild nonoliguric acute renal failure can continue to eat regularly. Patients who develop acute renal failure from an infection, tissue trauma, or prolonged surgery require nutritional support. Since this is often given parenterally in large volumes of fluid (1.5–2 L/day), frequent hemodialysis with fluid removal simplifies management. Patients with severe catabolism due, for example, to systemic infection resulting from large bowel damage in a post-traumatic acute renal failure patient, have high requirements for calories and other nutrients. Most of these patients need daily hemodialysis to maintain an acceptable level of blood urea nitrogen and fluid balance, and few of them survive long.

PROGNOSIS

Full recovery of kidney function is the rule for mild, nonoliguric acute renal failure and for essentially all forms of nephrotoxic acute renal failure, provided that the patient had normal baseline renal function. The outlook is not as good for the elderly or for patients with preexisting vascular disease. When these patients develop otherwise uncomplicated acute renal failure serious enough to warrant dialysis, most get back only 50–75% of their baseline kidney function.

Post-traumatic or postoperative acute renal failure is often fatal, despite aggressive dialysis and intensive hospital care. Important prognostic factors are the severity of the acute renal failure, as reflected by the increase in serum creatinine and blood urea nitrogen; intercurrent infection; old age; and multi-organ failure. Also predictive of poor outcome are jaundice, severe cardiovascular disease, and pulmonary disease.

SUMMARY

▶ Acute renal failure develops over hours to days and is signaled by an abrupt increase in serum creatinine and blood urea nitrogen.

▶ The severity of acute renal failure ranges from transient episodes caused by drug toxicity to fatal forms associated with multi-organ failure.

▶ Although anuria implies severe renal or urinary tract dysfunction, urine output is not always a reliable marker of renal function.

▶ The cause of renal failure can be determined by the history, clinical evaluation of prerenal perfusion status, sonographic examination for postrenal obstruction, and clues to intrinsic sites of damage through the urinalysis.

▶ The prognosis is generally good in nonsurgical, nontraumatic, and nephrotoxic forms of renal failure that are promptly diagnosed and treated, and poor in a post-traumatic or postoperative setting associated with multi-organ failure.

SUGGESTED READING

Bellomo R et al: Use of continuous hemodiafiltration: An approach to the management of acute renal failure in the critically ill. Am J Nephrol 1992;12:240.

Brezis M, Epstein FH: Cellular mechanisms of acute ischemic injury in the kidney. Ann Rev Med 1993;44:27.

Toback FG: Regeneration after acute tubular necrosis. Kidney Int 1992;41:226.

Chronic Renal Failure

Alan J. Watson, MRCPI, and Luis F. Gimenez, MD

Chronic renal failure is the slow, relentless, and usually irreversible loss of renal function. It is accompanied by a constellation of clinical features and laboratory abnormalities that are the shared end stage of numerous kidney disorders (Table 5.5–1). The syndrome reflects widespread disturbances caused by (1) accumulation of substances that are normally excreted by the kidneys (eg, urea, sodium, potassium, protein-derived acids) and their deleterious effects on the cardiovascular, nervous, skeletal, and hematologic systems; and (2) hormonal deficiencies resulting from renal damage (eg, erythropoietin, 1,25-dihydroxyvitamin D_3) and consequent hormonal adaptations (eg, secondary hyperparathyroidism).

These derangements can present as constitutional complaints, hypertension, edema, symptomatic pulmonary vascular congestion, or a spectrum of neurologic problems ranging from subtly altered mentation to seizures and coma. Any of these nonspecific features may suggest chronic renal failure in its early stages. But in most patients, the signs and symptoms appear only when the glomerular filtration rate has fallen to 10% of normal, that is, a creatinine clearance of less than 10–15 mL/min. Thus, the condition is often discovered serendipitously when uremia (an elevated serum urea nitrogen level) or one of its common clinical manifestations—anemia, hyperkalemia, hyperphosphatemia, or hypocalcemia—is found on blood tests done for other reasons.

Chronic renal failure presents several challenges to physicians. First, clinicians must consider the possibility that relatively nonspecific constitutional symptoms (eg, fatigue, anorexia, weakness) can be caused by renal insufficiency. Once considered, the diagnosis can be readily established or excluded by measuring the blood urea nitrogen (BUN) and creatinine.

Chronic renal insufficiency, caused by irreversible kidney damage, must be differentiated from acute renal failure for which the physician must seek a specific etiology and potential treatment (Chapter 5.4). A history of slowly progressive symptoms or a longstanding disorder that commonly causes renal failure (eg, hypertension, diabetes, polycystic renal disease) suggests that a patient's renal failure may be longstanding. Also suggestive are certain laboratory findings such as anemia, hyperphosphatemia, and hypocalcemia, as well as the finding of small kidneys by sonography.

Clinicians must be able to recognize and manage the serious complications (eg, heart failure, seizures, coagulopathy) that arise in a patient with chronic renal failure and must be prepared to preserve residual renal function whenever possible.

CLINICAL FEATURES

The onset of symptoms in patients with chronic renal failure is typically insidious. They include fatigue, malaise, anorexia, nausea, generalized pruritus, and decreased cognitive function. As uremia progresses, patients develop symptoms and signs referable to virtually every organ system (Table 5.5–2).

LABORATORY TESTS

Laboratory assessment of these patients begins with a biochemical and hematologic profile to determine the extent and severity of electrolyte, acid-base disturbances, and the anemia that usually accompanies them. BUN and creatinine levels provide an estimate of the degree of renal insufficiency, but do not reveal whether it is acute or chronic or its prognosis. When available, past laboratory data usually show a slow but relentless rise in BUN and creatinine over years (Chapter 5.1).

Progression of Renal Insufficiency

When both kidneys suffer a sustained and irreversible insult, chronic renal failure inevitably leads to end-stage renal disease (Table 5.5–3). However, the rate at which patients lose renal function can be variable. Progression of renal failure can be monitored by measuring and plotting the serum creatinine or the glomerular filtration rate over time. A less sensitive but clinically useful estimate is ser-

Table 5.5–1. Differential diagnosis of chronic renal failure.

Glomerular disease
Postinfectious (including poststreptococcal) glomerulonephritis
Rapidly progressive glomerulonephritis
Connective tissue disease
Diabetes mellitus
Drug abuse
Amyloidosis
Hereditary nephritis (Alport's syndrome)

Vascular disease
Chronic vasculitis
Hypertension
Renovascular disease

Tubulointerstitial disease
Chronic pyelonephritis
Analgesic nephropathy
Heavy metals
Drugs (lithium)

Congenital and obstructive disease
Renal cystic diseases
Obstructive and reflux uropathies

Table 5.5–3. Factors that can cause progression of chronic renal failure.

Poorly controlled hypertension
Chronic obstructive uropathy
Hyperfiltration
Nephrocalcinosis
Nephrotoxic drugs
Recurrent infections of the urinary tract

potentially reversible factors that may be hastening the loss of renal function.

This search should include a careful drug history looking for exposure to potentially nephrotoxic agents, checking for poorly controlled hypertension, assessing the patient's extracellular fluid volume for dehydration, obtaining urine cultures to search for infection, and getting a urinary tract sonogram to look for obstruction of the urinary tract.

ial plotting of the reciprocal of the serum creatinine (1/serum creatinine), over time. This graph assists the physician in making a rough estimate of whether the patient is likely to need dialysis; more important, if the slope of the curve shows an acute and unexplained change for the worse, the clinician should be prompted to look for

ORGAN SYSTEM COMPLICATIONS

Cardiovascular and Pulmonary Systems

About 90% of the patients with chronic renal failure who begin dialysis are hypertensive. The hypertension is usually caused by intravascular volume expansion, because the diseased kidneys cannot efficiently excrete ingested sodium and water. Many patients also develop heart failure, which may be caused by extracellular volume overload, alone or with ischemic or hypertensive heart disease. Other contributing factors can include anemia, infection, acidosis, unidentified uremic toxins, poor nutrition, and when present, the arteriovenous fistula used for chronic dialysis. Cardiac arrhythmias can be a complication of renal failure, particularly when impaired renal potassium excretion leads to hyperkalemia and when patients have coexisting hypocalcemia. Most patients with advanced untreated uremia develop pericarditis, the precise cause of which is unknown. The coagulopathy of uremia can cause a hemorrhagic pericardial effusion with hemodynamic compromise, particularly during dialysis.

Pulmonary dysfunction in chronic renal failure is usually caused by extracellular fluid overload and pulmonary congestion or edema. Pleural effusions are commonly seen on chest x-ray, but are seldom clinically important. Calcification of lung parenchyma may be seen when hyperphosphatemia leads to $CaPO_4$ precipitation in soft tissues.

Gastrointestinal Tract

Many patients with uremia have functional and structural abnormalities of the bowel manifested by anorexia, malnutrition, and weight loss. The mucosal membrane of the gastrointestinal tract can become inflamed at any level from mouth (stomatitis) to rectum (proctitis). Upper gas-

Table 5.5–2. Signs and symptoms of chronic renal failure.

Organ System	Symptoms	Signs
General	Malaise Asthenia	Listlessness
Cardiovascular	Chest pain Dyspnea Orthopnea	Pericardial rub Hypertension Edema
Gastrointestinal	Dysgeusia Anorexia Nausea and vomiting	Uremic fetor Melena
Musculoskeletal	Weakness Bone pain	Proximal myopathy
Neurologic	Restlessness Insomnia Cognitive impairment Cramps Paresthesias	Asterixis Myoclonus Seizures Coma
Pulmonary	Dyspnea Pleuritic pain	Tachypnea Rales Pleural rub
Skin	Pruritus Dryness Easy bruising	Excoriations Hyperpigmentation Pallor Purpura
Urinary and gonadal	Nocturia Irregular menses Decreased libido	Gynecomastia Amenorrhea Small testes

trointestinal lesions range from mild edema to chronic ulceration, usually complicated by protracted bleeding facilitated by uremic coagulopathy. Upper gastrointestinal hemorrhage is responsible for 5–10% of deaths in patients with chronic renal failure. Such hemorrhages are most often caused by peptic ulcer disease or gastric telangiectasia, whereas angiodysplasia of the ascending colon and cecum is usually responsible for lower gastrointestinal hemorrhage.

Musculoskeletal System

Muscle weakness, bone pain, fractures, and soft tissue and metastatic calcification all can accompany renal insufficiency (Chapter 4.6). Renal osteodystrophy is the result of the pathologic alterations in mineral and bone metabolism in patients with chronic renal failure. The primary event is retention of phosphate because of impaired renal excretion of this ion. Hyperphosphatemia in turn causes hypocalcemia because (1) the solubility product of phosphorus and calcium is exceeded in extracellular fluids, prompting their precipitation, and (2) an elevated tissue phosphate concentration down-regulates renal activation of 25-hydroxyvitamin D (1-hydroxylation), which in turn decreases calcium absorption by the gut. The progressive decrease in renal function also is associated with an intrinsic drop in the rate of 1,25-dihydroxyvitamin D_3 synthesis leading to a profound deficit of this hormone. Hypocalcemia in patients with advanced uremia then leads to secondary hyperparathyroidism with its characteristic radiographic features of subperiosteal bone resorption, osteitis fibrosa cystica, and decreased bone density. Bone biopsy may be indicated in patients with bone pain or progressive osteopenia; common histopathologic findings include (1) an increase in osteoclastic activity caused by hyperparathyroidism and (2) an increase in noncalcified osteoid matrix caused by defective mineralization from 1,25-dihydroxyvitamin D_3 deficiency.

Marked elevation of the calcium-phosphorus product, particularly in patients with secondary hyperparathyroidism, can cause metastatic calcification of blood vessels and solid organs such as the heart, lungs, pericorneal space, tendons, and kidneys; the skin may also be affected. Calciphylaxis is a painful ischemic gangrene of the fingers and toes caused by small vessel calcification; in many patients, the affected digits have to be amputated. Metastatic calcification may warrant parathyroidectomy if the calcium-phosphorus product cannot be controlled medically.

Aluminum has been implicated as another cause of renal osteodystrophy. Formerly, the most common cause of aluminum accumulation was exposure to inadequately treated water during dialysis. Now, the usual cause is the use of aluminum-containing antacids prescribed to control the serum phosphorus level. Aluminum deposits in the osteoid seam impair bone mineralization. Aluminum excess has also been implicated in causing central nervous system dysfunction and in the genesis of microcytic anemia in uremic patients.

Blood

All blood cell lines are adversely affected by uremia. Red cell production is reduced early in renal failure, and most patients become anemic by the time the serum creatinine has risen to 4 mg/dL. The anemia is typically a normochromic, normocytic hypoproliferative disorder caused by a combination of decreased erythropoietin production by the diseased kidney, circulating inhibitors of hematopoiesis (eg, polyamines), and low-grade chronic hemolysis. Recombinant human erythropoietin almost always improves the hematocrit of patients with chronic renal failure, whether on or off dialysis.

Platelet dysfunction and impaired factor VIII activity in patients with uremia cause a bleeding diathesis. Clinical manifestations can include epistaxis, purpura, intracranial hemorrhage, gastrointestinal hemorrhage, and hemorrhagic pericarditis. This coagulopathy may make surgical or biopsy procedures riskier. The bleeding time is the best predictor of the likelihood of significant hemorrhage. Treatments for this bleeding diathesis include dialysis and the use of cryoprecipitate, blood transfusions, deamino D-arginine vasopressin (dDAVP), recombinant human erythropoietin, and estrogens.

Although white cell counts are normal, cell-mediated and humoral immunity may be impaired. In part, this may account for uremic patients' vulnerability to both commonly acquired and certain opportunistic infections, such as upper respiratory tract infections and tuberculosis.

Nervous System

Uremia causes two major neurologic disturbances: encephalopathy and peripheral neuropathy. Mild encephalopathy is manifested by insomnia, fatigue, shortened attention span, and depression. More advanced disease can cause lethargy, seizures, and stupor progressing to coma. Patients may also have asterixis, myoclonus, and signs of neuromuscular irritability.

The peripheral neuropathy of uremia is a sensorimotor neuropathy similar to that of diabetes mellitus, usually involving the lower extremities. The sensory defect may be subtle or extreme; an extreme form is "burning feet syndrome," in which even light touch causes severe pain. Patients may also develop "restless legs syndrome" (akathisia), an aching and restlessness that often interfere with sleep. Some patients have single nerve involvement, such as carpal tunnel syndrome or footdrop. Carpal tunnel syndrome is also a feature of dialysis-related amyloidosis, which is caused by abnormal deposition of B_2-microglobulin. Autonomic neuropathy can impair cardiovascular reflexes, predisposing patients to postural hypotension, especially when hemodialysis causes changes in extracellular fluid volume. Occasional patients also have abnormal autonomic control of gastrointestinal function and sweating.

Dialysis dementia is a rapidly fatal syndrome of dementia, myoclonus, asterixis, and dysphasia that has been related to aluminum toxicity. The incidence of this disorder has been lowered by better means of removing aluminum from the water used in dialysate and by avoidance of aluminum-containing antacids, whenever possible.

Endocrine Glands

Chronic renal failure reduces the kidneys' ability to produce erythropoietin. Reduced activation of vitamin D contributes to the development of secondary hyperparathyroidism and renal osteodystrophy. Prolactin, gastrin, and growth hormone are normally cleared by the kidney and thus accumulate in renal failure. Hyperprolactinemia is especially common in uremic women; it is caused by increased pituitary secretion of prolactin, as well as by impaired renal clearance. Along with direct uremic effects on gonadotropin-releasing hormone (GnRH) and gonadotropin secretion, hyperprolactinemia contributes to the amenorrhea and infertility in women with chronic renal failure and to hypogonadism and gynecomastia with galactorrhea in men.

Uremia can disturb thyroid function at several levels: decreased thyroid-stimulating hormone (TSH) secretion, decreased extrathyroidal T_4-to-T_3 conversion, and accelerated clearance of thyroid hormones. Although thyroid function test abnormalities are common, actual hypothyroidism—evidenced by a high serum TSH level—is unusual.

Many patients with uremia have impaired glucose tolerance; some have frank hyperglycemia. Patients with type I or type II diabetes mellitus and chronic renal failure who are taking insulin often develop hypoglycemia because of decreased insulin clearance by the failing kidneys. To prevent this, most patients need a reduction in insulin dosage. Many patients with advanced uremia have elevated triglyceride levels, reflecting an increase in very low-density lipoprotein (VLDL) that is thought to be caused by decreased lipoprotein lipase and hepatic lipase activities.

Skin

Pruritus is often a troublesome feature of renal failure (Chapter 9.2). The etiology is multifactorial. Secondary hyperparathyroidism and an increase in the calcium-phosphorus product have been implicated. An increase in mast cell concentration in the skin has also been noted, suggesting a histamine-related disorder; however, histamine receptor blockade is usually ineffective. Dry skin itself may predispose to pruritus, and moisturizing lotions may provide some relief. The yellowish skin pigmentation seen in many patients with end-stage renal disease results from accumulation of retained urochromes, increased melanin secretion, or both.

Genitourinary Tract

Sustained nocturia is an early marker of progressive renal failure. The cause is impairment of the kidneys' ability to concentrate urine at night. This may be aggravated by the mobilization of edema in patients who have developed fluid retention. Patients with chronic renal failure can develop secondary renal cystic disease, manifested as hematuria and flank pain.

In patients with end-stage chronic renal failure, urinalysis is usually remarkable only for broad casts and proteinuria on dipstick. Less often, the urine sediment reflects the underlying disease, such as red blood cell casts in patients with glomerulonephritis.

BIOCHEMICAL FEATURES

Sodium and Water

In patients with mild-to-moderate chronic renal failure, diminished reabsorption of filtered sodium by the surviving tubules is an adaptive response that maintains sodium balance. However, when the glomerular filtration rate falls below 10 mL/min, unrestricted sodium intake can cause progressive sodium retention that may lead to peripheral edema, hypertension, and ultimately extracellular volume overload with pulmonary edema and anasarca.

As renal failure worsens, patients may develop defects in urine concentration and dilution. These defects are explained in part by the increased solute load being excreted, but also by the anatomic and functional loss of nephron segments responsible for concentrating and diluting the urine (ie, loop of Henle and collecting ducts). Most patients with severe renal failure have mild hyponatremia (serum sodium, 130–135 mEq/L), particularly if they take in too much free water. However, hypernatremia can also develop if free water intake is limited, particularly when patients become unresponsive to antidiuretic hormone.

Potassium

The proportion of filtered potassium excreted by each nephron rises, so that most patients with mild-to-moderate uremia maintain a reasonably normal potassium balance. The major adaptive mechanisms are an aldosterone-mediated increase in distal tubular secretion of potassium and an increase in sodium potassium ATPase (adenosine triphosphatase) activity. A similar exchange occurs in the colon when fecal potassium rises as the glomerular filtration rate falls. However, drugs that impair these adaptive mechanisms can precipitate severe hyperkalemia, as when beta-adrenergic blockers inhibit renin production, angiotensin converting enzyme (ACE) inhibitors decrease angiotensin converting enzyme activity, or spironolactone blocks aldosterone action.

Acid-Base Metabolism

The hydrogen ion balance is maintained by reclamation of filtered bicarbonate and excretion of titratable acid in the form of ammonia and organic acids such as sulfates and phosphates (Chapter 5.3). Ammonia is produced by the distal and proximal tubular cells, primarily from the metabolism of glutamine. Then the ammonia is titrated with hydrogen ions in the tubular lumen, forming ammonium, thereby trapping the hydrogen ions, which ultimately are excreted into the urine. The rate at which the tubular cells synthesize ammonia can be upregulated, depending on the requirement for hydrogen ion excretion.

This mechanism is effective, both disposing of the hydrogen ions produced by protein catabolism and generating additional bicarbonate.

Bicarbonate is reclaimed primarily in the proximal nephron, allowing the maintenance of a stable pool of readily available bicarbonate in the extracellular fluid to buffer newly generated hydrogen ions. Reclamation of filtered bicarbonate decreases as the glomerular filtration rate declines, leading to a chronic base deficit. Finally, the excretion of titratable organic anions such as sulfates and phosphates also makes a lesser contribution to net acid excretion.

In the early stages of renal failure, as the glomerular filtration falls, the hydrogen ion balance is maintained predominantly by an increase in tubular synthesis of ammonia. However, there is a point (glomerular filtration rate falls below 22 mL/min) when this mechanism can be upregulated no further, resulting in hydrogen ion accumulation. The result is development of an anion gap acidosis because of the retention of organic acids (sulfates and phosphates within the extracellular fluid compartment). It is important to address this problem in patients with chronic renal disease because chronic metabolic acidosis impairs vital organ functions (eg, the myocardium) and contributes to bone decalcification. A therapeutic goal is to maintain serum bicarbonate levels above 18 mEq/L to minimize the effects of the chronic acidotic state. To this end, sodium bicarbonate can be given as tablets or as liquid sodium citrate. It is important to bear in mind that both agents represent an increase in sodium intake, which may precipitate extracellular fluid volume overload.

Phosphorus, Calcium, and Magnesium

Phosphate retention is a relatively early consequence of declining glomerular filtration rate (usually when it falls below 70 mL/min). This leads to a reciprocal drop in serum calcium, which in turn stimulates secretion of parathyroid hormone. Hypocalcemia is also a result of decreased production of 1,25-dihydroxyvitamin D by the kidneys. Maintenance of a normal serum phosphorus level helps to normalize serum calcium levels and minimize renal osteodystrophy. This is accomplished by restricting dietary intake of phosphorus and giving oral phosphate binders. Once serum phosphorus is normal, the patient's diet can be supplemented with extra calcium in the form of calcium carbonate or acetate (which also happens to be a good phosphate binder). If the serum calcium does not correct with this maneuver, the next step is to add vitamin D supplements in the form of oral calcitriol, which can be adjusted every 2–4 weeks, depending on the serum calcium levels.

Since the only route of magnesium excretion is the kidney, it follows that as the glomerular filtration rate declines, levels of serum magnesium can increase, especially if dietary intake of magnesium remains unrestricted. For this reason, it is recommended that the patient abstain from ingesting magnesium-containing medications such as laxatives or antacids.

MANAGEMENT

Nutritional Therapy

A daily protein intake of between 0.7 g/kg and 0.9 g/kg of body weight is usually recommended to strike a balance between adequate nutrition and excessive generation of nitrogenous metabolites, which may accelerate the development of uremic symptoms. Unrestricted dietary protein intake has also been associated with accelerated degeneration of residual renal function. Patients whose protein intake is limited need adequate caloric intake in the form of carbohydrates to prevent malnutrition. Patients must also restrict their intake of salt, water, and dietary potassium and phosphorus.

Drug Therapy

All patients with anemia of renal failure should be treated with recombinant human erythropoietin and iron supplements after the physician makes sure that there is no occult gastrointestinal blood loss. Supplemental 1,25-dihydroxyvitamin D_3 may be given orally or intravenously to correct the deficiency of this vitamin. Calcium-based phosphate binders should be preferred over aluminum-containing binders because patients with severe renal impairment accumulate aluminum. This aluminum may eventually deposit in the bones, further contributing to metabolic bone disease, or in the brain, leading to impaired cognitive and neurologic functions. However, patients with severe hyperphosphatemia (serum phosphorus at least 8.0 mg/dL) may require a short course of aluminum-containing binders, which are more effective than calcium-containing PO_4 binders for the management of severe hyperphosphatemia.

Because hypertension can hasten the progression of renal failure, particularly in patients with diabetes, the physician must aggressively control patients' blood pressure. Hypertension caused by fluid accumulation may be treated with a loop diuretic if salt restriction proves ineffective. ACE inhibitors and calcium channel blockers are commonly used and are effective and well tolerated. For patients who do not yet need dialysis, these agents may also slow progression of renal disease, especially in patients with diabetes.

Patients with severe renal insufficiency must be taught to avoid potentially nephrotoxic agents, such as nonsteroidal anti-inflammatory drugs. Many drug doses need to be adjusted to accommodate the degree of reduction in glomerular filtration rate, especially if the drugs are excreted mainly through the kidney.

Dialysis

Once a patient's glomerular filtration rate falls below 10–15 mL/min, medical management is usually ineffective in overcoming the problems caused by fluid and electrolyte imbalance. Dialysis then becomes necessary to sustain the patient's life until a kidney transplant becomes available (see "Kidney Transplantation" below).

Certain clinical indications should alert the physician to

start dialysis; the most urgent are acute uremic pericarditis and hyperkalemia. Refractory fluid overload, worsening uremic syndrome, or severe malnutrition should also be considered a relatively urgent indication for dialysis, especially in patients who have a relentless deterioration of their overall medical condition. Dialysis can also be effectively used to treat drug overdose.

Hemodialysis: Hemodialysis is the removal of solutes from blood by diffusion through a semipermeable membrane. Blood is removed from the patient's body, then circulates through an "artificial kidney" (usually a hollow fiber dialyzer) and is returned to the body. As blood flows through small capillary tubes in the dialyzer, a dialysate solution flows in the opposite direction in the space between the tubes. The composition of the dialysate solution is designed to allow diffusion of solutes (ie, creatinine, BUN, PO_4, and so on) from blood to dialysate down a concentration gradient. Fluid is removed by manipulating the hydrostatic pressure gradient between the blood and the dialysate compartments.

Before dialysis can be started, the patient needs to have a suitable vascular access created. An arteriovenous fistula is surgically constructed in one of the patient's forearms by anastomosing an artery and vein side-to-side or end-to-side. Sometimes this anastomosis needs to be created artificially with a plastic tube (Gore-Tex graft), especially in patients who have significant peripheral atherosclerotic or diabetic vascular disease. Most patients require 3–4 hours of treatment three times per week. Complications of hemodialysis include hypotension, air embolism, systemic infections, and thrombotic and infectious problems within the vascular access.

All patients on dialysis need regular biochemical monitoring. Iron stores and availability are assessed by serum ferritin levels and percentage of transferrin saturation. Parathyroid hormone levels are measured twice yearly or more frequently, if necessary, to detect hyperparathyroidism. Liver function tests are done regularly, usually monthly, with hepatitis serologies as indicated, because patients are at risk for contracting viral hepatitis.

Peritoneal Dialysis: Here, the peritoneal membrane acts as the dialyzing membrane. The peritoneal capillaries provide the blood flow, and the dialysate is instilled into the abdominal space through a permanent abdominal catheter. By exchanging 1.5–2 L of dialysate four to six times per day, most patients have adequate solute clearance and ultrafiltration. This regimen is called *continuous ambulatory peritoneal dialysis* (CAPD). Like hemodialysis, peritoneal dialysis requires the prior creation of a suitable peritoneal access. This is done by inserting a special double-cuff Silastic catheter called a Tenckhoff catheter, which is left in place indefinitely and through which the peritoneal dialysis exchanges are done. The dialysate solution contains glucose as an osmotic agent to facilitate the removal of fluid. The concentration of this compound can be changed to minimize or maximize the ultrafiltration rate, thereby regulating extracellular fluid volume as clinically necessary.

Kidney Transplantation

Kidney transplantation is the best treatment for end-stage renal failure; it makes sense both clinically and economically. However, patients must be carefully selected to minimize the operative risks and long-term complications related to other medical problems, such as cardiovascular disease or diabetes. Better understanding of immunology and histocompatibility issues in transplantation has led to the development of better and more powerful immunosuppressant drugs, such as FK-506, cyclosporine, prednisone, and azathioprine. Monoclonal antibody (OKT3) and intravenous methylprednisolone are used to treat acute rejection. Drug regimens developed by combining these medications have significantly lengthened graft and patient survival. It is important to select a donor and recipient by properly matching their histocompatibility (HLA-B, C, D, or DR) antigens. The more antigens shared by donor and recipient, the better the long-term outlook and survival rate for allograft and patient.

In general, patients with a history of malignancy or chronic infections (such as tuberculosis refractory to usual therapy), cirrhosis of the liver, or severe intractable cardiomyopathy are not considered for kidney transplantation. Although old age is also an important factor to consider, it is rarely an absolute contraindication; many older patients who are in excellent physical condition apart from their kidney disease do as well as younger transplantation candidates.

Surgical complications of kidney transplantation include postoperative leaks and vascular problems that can impair the blood supply to the allograft. Medical complications are of two types: those related to long-term immunosuppression (eg, opportunistic infection, malignancy) and those related to corticosteroid side effects. Finally, patients risk a recurrence of certain original renal diseases (eg, diabetes, amyloidosis, IgA nephropathy, and membranoproliferative glomerulonephritis) in the transplanted kidney.

SUMMARY

▶ Patients with chronic renal failure, the shared end stage of a number of kidney diseases, can present with nonspecific constitutional complaints or with manifestations of its major complications, such as hypertension, heart failure, and seizures.

▶ The variable progression of chronic renal failure should be monitored by serial determinations of glomerular filtration rate. Accelerated deterioration should prompt a search for such reversible factors as dehydration, hypertension, infection, urinary tract obstruction, and exposure to nephrotoxic drugs.

▶ Heart failure, renal osteodystrophy, anemia, and other organ system complications of chronic renal failure should be anticipated, treated, and, when possible, prevented.

▶ Patients require dialysis or a kidney transplant when the glomerular filtration rate falls below 5–10 mL/min. Both treatments pose risks such as infection and accelerated atherosclerosis.

SUGGESTED READING

Alfrey AC, Chan L: Chronic renal failure: Manifestations and pathogenesis. In: *Renal and Electrolyte Disorders,* 4th ed. Schrier RW (editor). Little, Brown & Co, 1992.

Malangone JM et al: Clinical and laboratory features of patients with chronic renal disease at the start of dialysis. Clin Nephrol 1981;31:77.

Slatopolsky E et al: Parathyroid-calcitriol axis in health and chronic renal failure. Kidney Int 1990;29(Suppl):S41.

Watson AJ, Gimenez LFG: Bleeding in uremia. Semin Dial 1991;4:86.

Glomerular Diseases

Barbara J. Ballermann, MD, and Jean L. Olson, MD

In some patients, glomerular disease begins dramatically, with massive edema, renal failure, gross hematuria, or reduced urine flow. In others, glomerular injury produces no obvious symptoms and is detected only by routine urinalysis or blood biochemistry. The physician must recognize those glomerular diseases for which timely intervention can prevent or delay renal failure and those that are the first indication of multisystem disease.

Renal glomeruli are particularly vulnerable to immunologically mediated injury. It can be restricted solely to the kidney or can reflect multisystem disease. Immunoglobulin deposition with complement activation triggers an influx of inflammatory cells, release of inflammatory mediators, and proliferation of glomerular cells, leading to structural damage. Vasculitis, which is immune injury to blood vessels with little or no immunoglobulin deposition, destroys endothelium and vessel walls and often involves renal arterioles and glomeruli.

Not all glomerular injury is immunologically mediated. For instance, in diabetic nephropathy and focal segmental glomerulosclerosis, normal glomerular tissue is replaced with excess collagen and other matrix proteins. In a small subset of diseases termed *thrombotic microangiopathies,* the glomeruli are damaged by intravascular coagulation and fibrin deposition. A final source of injury is extrarenal overproduction of abnormal immunoglobulin-related paraproteins and their deposition within the glomerulus.

Glomerular disease without evident extrarenal abnormalities (primary) is generally distinguished from glomerular injury complicating systemic diseases (secondary). However, since the mechanisms of injury often overlap, this chapter replaces these older terms with the more accurate concepts of "kidney-limited" and multisystem disease (Figure 5.6–1).

CLINICAL MANIFESTATIONS OF GLOMERULAR DISEASE

The cardinal manifestations of glomerular disease are proteinuria, hematuria, and reduction in the glomerular filtration rate. Glomerular diseases fall into two broad groups, those dominated by proteinuria or the nephrotic syndrome and those dominated by hematuria and hypertension. The degree and pace of reduction in glomerular filtration rate help to further define the underlying disease.

Proteinuria

Filtration across the glomerular capillary wall delivers enormous quantities of fluid to the renal tubules for processing, 150–180 L/day in adults. Despite the rapid rate of fluid flux, plasma proteins are retained in the vascular space. Plasma albumin is restricted primarily because its net negative charge hinders passage through the negatively charged glomerular capillary wall; immunoglobulins and other large proteins are restricted primarily by their size. This normal barrier to protein filtration is disturbed in glomerular disease, causing albumin and other plasma proteins to appear in the urine. In *minimal change disease* (see "Minimal Change Disease" below), the negative charges of the glomerular capillary wall are lost, causing large quantities of albumin—but not larger proteins—to appear in the urine. This is *selective proteinuria.* In most other diseases, the size-selective property of the glomerular capillary wall is disrupted, resulting in nonselective proteinuria, in which all plasma proteins, including albumin, pass the glomerular barrier.

Examining the urine for protein is central to the evaluation of patients with potential glomerular injury. Chemically impregnated test strips (dipsticks) detect urinary albumin with a sensitivity of 10–20 mg/dL. However, they are relatively insensitive to immunoglobulins and immunoglobulin light chains. Furthermore, because of the physiologic variation in urine concentration, they can underestimate significant albuminuria in dilute urine and overestimate albuminuria in concentrated urine.

Proteinuria can also be detected by precipitating the urine proteins with acid. These methods detect all proteins, including immunoglobulins, to a sensitivity of about 5–10 mg/dL. Sulfosalicylic acid (SSA) is added to urine in a 1:20 (SSA:urine) ratio, or the urine is heated to boiling and then glacial acetic acid is added, also in a 1:20 ratio. If protein is present, the urine becomes cloudy with the protein precipitate. Bence Jones proteins (immunoglobulin light

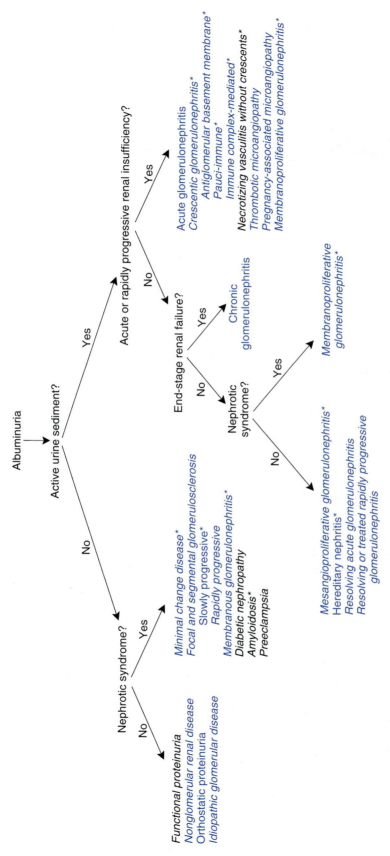

Figure 5.6–1. Evaluation of suspected glomerular disease.

Albuminuria

Active urine sediment?

No → Nephrotic syndrome?

No → *Functional proteinuria*
Nonglomerular renal disease
Orthostatic proteinuria
Idiopathic glomerular disease

Yes → *Minimal change disease**
Focal and segmental glomerulosclerosis
  Slowly progressive
  Rapidly progressive
*Membranous glomerulonephritis**
Diabetic nephropathy
*Amyloidosis**
Preeclampsia

Yes → Acute or rapidly progressive renal insufficiency?

No → End-stage renal failure?

Yes → *Chronic glomerulonephritis*

No → Nephrotic syndrome?

Yes → *Membranoproliferative glomerulonephritis**

No → *Mesangioproliferative glomerulonephritis**
*Hereditary nephritis**
Resolving acute glomerulonephritis
Resolving or treated rapidly progressive glomerulonephritis

Yes → *Acute glomerulonephritis*
*Crescentic glomerulonephritis**
*Antiglomerular basement membrane**
  *Pauci-immune**
  *Immune complex-mediated**
Necrotizing vasculitis without crescents*
Thrombotic microangiopathy
Pregnancy-associated microangiopathy
*Membranoproliferative glomerulonephritis**

Legend

Kidney-limited disease
Associated with systemic disease
Either kidney-limited or associated with systemic disease

*Biopsy usually required for diagnosis

397

chains produced by myeloma cells) precipitate at 40–60° C (104–140° F) and redissolve at 100° C (212° F) in acetic acid (Chapter 12.7).

If albuminuria is detected, the amount of protein excreted per day helps to define the severity of the glomerular capillary wall defect. Usually, the urine volume and protein concentration in a 24-hour urine collection are measured. Protein excretion rates exceeding 125–150 mg/day are abnormal, and nephrotic-range proteinuria is defined as protein excretion greater than 3.0–3.5 g/day. Because the dipstick cannot detect early diabetic nephropathy, patients with diabetes have their albumin excretion measured rather than their total protein; microalbuminuria is defined as albumin excretion of 40–300 mg/day.

Urine protein electrophoresis is performed to identify the proteins. In patients with glomerular lesions caused by loss of negative charges, albumin forms the predominant peak and larger plasma proteins are not seen. Patients with glomerular lesions caused by disruption of the size barrier show all plasma proteins. Proteinuria of tubular origin contains mostly β_2 microglobulin and little or no albumin. If the patient has no glomerular capillary wall damage (no urinary albumin), the only immunoglobulin components freely filtered are immunoglobulin light chains. These light chains are found in patients with light chain-producing myeloma. Light chains also appear in the urine of patients with primary amyloidosis, but these patients have glomerular capillary wall damage, so they show albumin as well as larger plasma proteins.

Patients with the nephrotic syndrome also have lipid in their urine. This lipid is seen in the urine sediment as free fat droplets, in cells laden with fat (oval fat bodies), and in casts. Lipid in any form is best recognized under polarized light, where it takes on the appearance of Maltese crosses.

Hematuria

Examining the urine for blood and the urine sediment to see whether it is "active" helps to determine whether the glomerular lesion has an inflammatory component. An active urine sediment contains red blood cells, white blood cells, and cellular casts. Casts are aggregates of cells, cell debris, precipitated plasma proteins, and sometimes fat droplets embedded in Tamm-Horsfall protein, a mucoprotein secreted by tubules. Since these materials aggregate in renal tubules, they produce casts of the tubules. Casts that contain easily recognizable cellular components have formed very recently and indicate active inflammation.

A normal urine sediment contains no more than one to two red blood cells and one to two white blood cells per high-power field (× 400). When red blood cell casts are seen, the cause is almost always glomerular bleeding. Excessive white blood cells are found most commonly with urinary tract infection, but casts containing white blood cells without bacteriuria are often seen with glomerular inflammation. Cellular elements embedded in urinary casts can be in various stages of disintegration, causing the casts to look granular. If they were formed by red blood cells, they take on a reddish tint. Granular casts in the urine are

consistent with glomerular inflammation, although they can be seen with any renal parenchymal disease. Patients with longstanding renal parenchymal disease of either glomerular or nonglomerular origin may show waxy casts, which are dense, homogeneous, and birefringent. Broad casts form in dilated tubules with any chronic renal parenchymal disease, including glomerular disease.

Reduction in Glomerular Filtration Rate

Glomerular diseases often lead to a reduction in the glomerular filtration rate (GFR). A low GFR is not usually symptomatic until it falls below 15–20 mL/min. The cause can be intrarenal vasoconstriction, loss of filtration surface area because of accumulation of inflammatory cells, proliferation of intrinsic glomerular cells, or obliteration of glomerular structure by scarring. A reduction in GFR caused by vasoconstriction or acute inflammation is often reversible, but glomerular scarring is not. The physician should also keep in mind that nonsteroidal anti-inflammatory drugs (NSAIDs) inhibit the vasodilatory prostaglandins needed to counteract vasoconstrictor mediators in glomerulonephritis. Therefore, patients with glomerulonephritis should not be given NSAIDs, because they can precipitate acute renal failure.

A reduced GFR causes the serum creatinine and urea concentrations to rise. These provide the most convenient estimates of GFR, although the following limitations must be noted. The steady-state serum creatinine concentration doubles with each 50% drop in GFR. With renal failure, therefore, the serum creatinine rises exponentially. In women, the serum creatinine is normally around 0.6–0.8 mg/dL; a 30–50% drop in GFR raises the serum creatinine only to around 1.2–1.4 mg/dL, which many physicians incorrectly interpret as normal. In contrast, when the baseline serum creatinine is much higher—for example, in patients with chronic renal failure—an increment of 0.6 mg/dL reflects a much smaller drop in GFR. The absolute serum creatinine value can also be misleading if the GFR falls acutely, because the serum creatinine must reach its new steady state before it reflects the GFR.

When renal function falls gradually, the creatinine clearance is a useful measure of GFR. Normal creatinine clearances (GFR) are 100–125 mL/min in men and 85–105 mL/min in women. As the GFR falls below 30 mL/min, the creatinine clearance reflects GFR less and less accurately, because the fraction of creatinine secreted by tubules increases. The GFR can be determined more precisely with the radioisotope filtration marker ^{125}I-iothalamate or ^{99m}Tc DTPA (Chapter 5.1).

When a patient has a severely depressed GFR and either significant proteinuria or an active urine sediment with red blood cells and casts or both, the physician should determine whether the glomerular damage is acute or chronic. Two clues to chronic disease are an ultrasonogram showing small, shrunken kidneys, explained by gradual replacement of renal parenchyma with scar tissue, and a normochromic, normocytic anemia, caused by reduced renal erythropoietin production.

In all patients with glomerular disease, loss of GFR can be markedly accelerated by hypertension. Thus, one critical component of management is excellent blood pressure control.

GLOMERULAR DISEASES PRESENTING WITH PROTEINURIA

The physician who finds proteinuria must determine whether it reflects significant glomerular disease and needs further evaluation, whether it is caused by tubular dysfunction, or whether it represents functional or postural proteinuria.

Isolated Proteinuria

This is mild proteinuria of 1.5 g/day or less, with a normal urine sediment and no overt systemic disease that could damage the glomeruli. Fever, congestive heart failure, and heavy exercise all can give rise to proteinuria, usually less than 1 g/day; this functional proteinuria abates with resolution of the underlying problem. Mild proteinuria can also be found in patients with renal diseases not primarily involving the glomeruli, such as hypertensive nephrosclerosis, chronic interstitial nephritis, polycystic kidney disease, and obstructive uropathy. Mild isolated proteinuria is not further evaluated if the patient has any of these disorders with a normal urine sediment.

Isolated postural proteinuria is defined as normal protein excretion during recumbency but excessive protein excretion during ambulation. About 30–50% of patients with this condition have normal renal biopsies; the rest have only mild mesangial changes. Renal function almost always remains normal, and the proteinuria usually resolves with time. Patients with isolated postural proteinuria can be reassured and followed up without biopsy or treatment.

Most other patients with mild isolated proteinuria have a glomerular lesion. Nevertheless, if their GFR is normal, few of these patients need biopsy unless their proteinuria worsens or they develop an active urine sediment, signaling glomerular inflammation. Patients who do not need biopsy are followed up once or twice a year with urinalysis and measurement of their serum creatinine and protein excretion rates.

The Nephrotic Syndrome

The nephrotic syndrome is defined as urinary protein loss in excess of 3–3.5 g/day, accompanied by decreased serum albumin and total protein concentrations, increased serum cholesterol and lipoprotein concentrations, and edema formation.

In patients who do not have an active urine sediment, the nephrotic syndrome suggests a limited number of diagnoses, including minimal change disease, focal and segmental glomerulosclerosis, membranous nephropathy, diabetic nephropathy, amyloidosis, and, in pregnant women, preeclampsia. Among these, diabetic and HIV nephropathy (a form of focal and segmental glomerulosclerosis) and preeclampsia can usually be diagnosed without renal biopsy. In patients with amyloidosis, biopsy of nonrenal tissue is often sufficient to make a diagnosis. Most other adults with the nephrotic syndrome need a renal biopsy to determine the cause and to define treatment.

As outlined below for each diagnostic possibility, glomerular diseases that cause the nephrotic syndrome can result from chronic infection, malignancies, drugs, autoimmune disease, and metabolic disorders. Before biopsy, therefore, serologic tests are done for syphilis, hepatitis B, and HIV, and a skin test is performed to rule out tuberculosis. Patients are also tested for antinuclear antibodies, which are found in more than 90% of persons with systemic lupus erythematosus and in many persons with other connective tissue disorders. Patients also undergo limited screening for solid tumors, including chest x-ray, stool tests for occult blood, and, in women, mammography and Papanicolaou smear.

Minimal Change Disease: The minimal change lesion accounts for the nephrotic syndrome in about 30% of adults (Table 5.6–1). The glomeruli are normal by light

Table 5.6–1. Clinical clues to "kidney-limited" glomerular diseases.

Glomerular Histology	Level of Proteinuria	Activity of Urine Sediment	Age	Response to Corticosteroid Treatment
Minimal change	4+	0–1+	Children	Excellent
Focal segmental sclerosis	4+	0–1+	All ages	Usually poor
Membranous	4+	0–1+	Adults	Usually poor
Postinfectious diffuse proliferative	4+ → 1+	4+	All ages	Corticosteroids not indicated
Diffuse crescentic	1+–2+	4+	All ages	Usually good (may also need cyclophosphamide ± plasmapheresis)
Membranoproliferative	2+–4+	4+	Adults	Poor
Mesangial proliferative	1+–2+	2+	Adults	Corticosteroids not indicated
Hereditary nephritis	0–1+	1+–2+	All ages	Corticosteroids not indicated

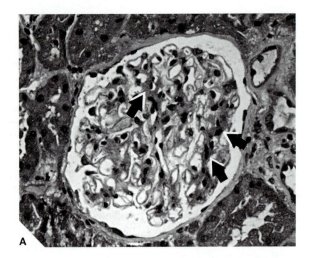

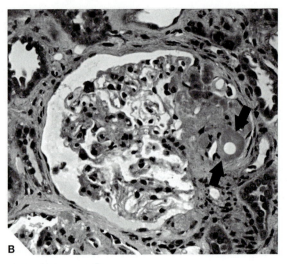

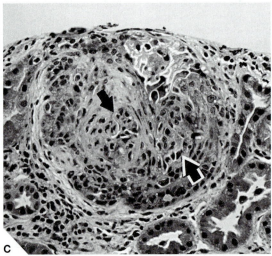

Figure 5.6–2. Light micrographs of glomeruli. **A:** Normal glomerulus has thin, delicate capillary walls with usual mesangial matrix (arrows) containing fewer than four nuclei per mesangial area (H&E, × 250). **B:** Glomerulus from a patient with focal and segmental glomerular sclerosis shows two areas of sclerosis. The larger of these contains a hyalinosis lesion (arrows) and has formed an adhesion to Bowman's capsule (H&E, × 240). **C:** A crescent nearly obscures the glomerular tuft (arrows) (H&E, × 240).

microscopy (Figure 5.6–2A), but electron microscopy shows injury to glomerular podocytes, with loss of their normal interdigitating foot processes. These changes are believed to be caused by a circulating cytokine derived from T lymphocytes. Glomerular podocyte injury and loss of negative charge lead to selective proteinuria, with albumin excretion rates often as high as 10–20 g/day. The typical presenting symptom of minimal change disease is edema, with an often rapid and dramatic onset; GFR and blood pressure are usually normal. Corticosteroids are highly effective in reducing protein excretion rates, usually to normal. Patients who do not improve on corticosteroids or who relapse when they are withdrawn should

be suspected of having focal and segmental glomerular sclerosis.

Although usually limited to the kidney, minimal change nephropathy has been described as a complication of non-Hodgkin's and Hodgkin's lymphomas. The glomerular lesion resolves when the underlying lymphoma is treated.

Focal and Segmental Glomerular Sclerosis with Hyalinosis: Two forms of focal and segmental glomerular sclerosis with hyalinosis have been recognized: slowly progressive and rapidly progressive. "Sclerosis" is an increase in glomerular matrix, and "hyalinosis" is accumulation of plasma proteins in the capillary lumen (see Figure 5.6–2B). "Focal" signifies that only some glomeruli contain lesions, and "segmental" means that only a portion of any glomerular tuft is involved. Visceral epithelial cell injury is evident on light and electron microscopy.

Slowly progressive focal and segmental glomerular sclerosis can be a late complication of childhood reflux nephropathy, but most patients have no identifiable underlying disease. The nephrotic syndrome in these patients tends to develop slowly; many have hypertension and an increase in urinary red blood cell excretion. The GFR declines progressively and most patients eventually require dialysis or kidney transplantation. Nevertheless, recent studies suggest that as many as 30–40% of adults with idiopathic focal and segmental glomerular sclerosis can achieve a complete remission from the nephrotic syndrome when treated with corticosteroids either alone or in combination with cyclophosphamide or chlorambucil, and patients who go into remission have an excellent prognosis. By comparison, only 5–10% of untreated patients have remissions. Given the poor prognosis without remission, immunosuppressive therapy is a logical treatment option.

A more fulminant (also called "collapsing" or "malignant") form of focal and segmental glomerular sclerosis is found in rare patients with the idiopathic nephrotic syndrome and in many patients with HIV infection. In patients with fulminant disease, the nephrotic syndrome develops abruptly and renal function declines quickly over weeks to months. Whether corticosteroids help these patients is still unclear.

Membranous Glomerulonephritis: Membranous glomerulonephritis is caused by immune complex deposition on the epithelial side of the glomerular basement membrane. By light microscopy, all the glomeruli show thickened capillary walls without significant increases in mesangial matrix or cellularity. Silver stain shows classic "spikes," which represent extension of glomerular basement membrane between the immune deposits. Immunofluorescence shows granular capillary loop staining for IgG and the C3 component of complement, and electron microscopy shows subepithelial deposits. Membranous nephropathy often develops in patients who have underlying disease; if none can be found, the condition is called *idiopathic membranous nephropathy.* Causes of membranous nephropathy include chronic infections like secondary syphilis, hepatitis B, leprosy, and schistosomiasis; solid tumors; drugs like D-penicillamine and gold; and connective tissue disorders like systemic lupus erythematosus, rheumatoid arthritis, mixed connective tissue disease, Sjögren's syndrome, and sarcoidosis. Patients with infection, tumor, or drug-induced membranous nephropathy should have the underlying disorder treated or the offending drug stopped. Most patients with disease secondary to connective tissue disorders should be given corticosteroids.

Idiopathic membranous glomerulonephritis resolves spontaneously in about 30% of patients. In contrast, a poor prognosis is suggested by hypertension, proteinuria greater than 10 g/day, or a reduced GFR. The prognosis may be improved by treatment combining corticosteroids with a cytotoxic drug such as cyclophosphamide or chlorambucil. Even with treatment, many patients with idiopathic membranous glomerulonephritis continue to lose renal function and eventually require dialysis or kidney transplantation.

Diabetic Nephropathy: In patients with diabetes mellitus, the nephrotic syndrome is almost always a sign of diabetic nephropathy (Chapter 4.7). Overall, 30–40% of patients with diabetes develop diabetic nephropathy. Patients with either insulin-dependent or non–insulin-dependent diabetes are at risk. The first clue, microalbuminuria (40–300 mg albumin/day), predicts significant glomerular disease with about 90% accuracy. Microalbuminuria begins 5–10 years after the onset of diabetes and is followed 2–5 years later by overt nephropathy. Additional risk factors for diabetic nephropathy are poor long-term glycemic control, hypertension, and an abnormally high GFR early in the course of diabetes caused by glomerular capillary hypertension (even without systemic hypertension) and glomerular hypertrophy.

Diabetic nephropathy is a devastating disease that progresses relentlessly from overt proteinuria to end-stage renal failure. Even when treated with dialysis or kidney transplantation, patients with diabetic nephropathy have a much poorer prognosis than those with end-stage renal disease caused by other conditions. Therefore, timely preventive therapy is crucial.

The risk of diabetic nephropathy can be significantly lessened by meticulous blood glucose control and by reduced protein intake early in the disease. All patients with diabetes should be taught how to maintain their blood glucose concentrations as close to normal as can be safely achieved. Urinary albumin excretion rates and GFR should be measured at least yearly, and patients who develop microalbuminuria or hypertension should be started on an angiotensin converting enzyme (ACE) inhibitor. These drugs dramatically lower the incidence of progressive loss of GFR and renal failure in patients with early diabetic nephropathy. ACE inhibitors are more effective than other antihypertensive drugs because ACE inhibitors reduce glomerular capillary hypertension and probably also inhibit glomerular hypertrophy. Patients with microalbuminuria should take an ACE inhibitor even if their blood pressure is normal.

After patients have developed the nephrotic syndrome, strict blood glucose control does not seem to reverse or slow the progressive glomerular damage. Nonetheless, patients with a serum creatinine below 2.5 mg/dL (GFR above 30 mL/min) still benefit from ACE inhibitors. When the GFR is 25–30 mL/min or less, the risk increases that ACE inhibitors will cause acute renal failure or hyperkalemia. But even at this late stage, excellent blood pressure control slows the loss of renal function. Therefore, patients should be tried on ACE inhibitors and followed up carefully; if they develop complications, other antihypertensive drugs should be substituted.

Renal biopsy is not usually needed to diagnose diabetic nephropathy. However, if a patient with diabetes develops the nephrotic syndrome without accompanying systemic diabetic vascular disease, if heavy proteinuria begins within 5 years after onset of diabetes, or if the urine sediment contains red blood cells and casts, the physician should suspect another glomerular lesion and should consider a biopsy.

Amyloidosis: Primary amyloidosis is a diffuse infiltrative disorder in which N-terminal fragments of the variable region of immunoglobulin light chains (the AL variety of amyloid) are deposited in renal glomeruli and interstitium as well as in heart, gastrointestinal tract, tongue, and other organs. Many patients also have carpal tunnel syndrome and autonomic neuropathy. Primary amyloidosis usually signals a plasma cell dyscrasia with an overproduction of light chains. This diagnosis should be considered in patients who develop the nephrotic syndrome after age 50, particularly if ultrasonography shows large kidneys. Since amyloid deposition injures the glomerular capillary wall, urine protein electrophoresis shows both albumin and immunoglobulin light chains. Abdominal fat pad biopsy yields the diagnosis in 90% of patients with primary amyloidosis; biopsy of rectal mucosa is almost as sensitive.

Secondary amyloidosis is caused by the deposition of another protein (the AA variety of amyloid) in the kidney and other organs. This form of amyloidosis often begins before age 50. The underlying causes are systemic diseases such as chronic suppurative infections (eg, osteomyelitis and bronchiectasis), chronic inflammatory diseases (eg, rheumatoid arthritis and ankylosing spondylitis), and malignancies. Secondary amyloidosis is also seen in many paraplegics, presumably because of chronic urinary tract infection, and in patients with familial Mediterranean fever.

Neither primary nor secondary amyloidosis can be effectively treated apart from therapy for the underlying disease. The renal failure is usually progressive, and most patients develop end-stage renal disease.

Managing Complications of the Nephrotic Syndrome: The most obvious manifestation of the nephrotic syndrome is edema. Edema results from reduced renal salt excretion relative to dietary salt intake, leading to an increase in the extracellular fluid volume. Most patients with the nephrotic syndrome retain salt because of a primary increase in renal tubular sodium reabsorption. In a small subset of patients, circulating plasma volume is diminished because the low plasma oncotic pressure allows water and solutes to escape into the interstitium; volume depletion, in turn, activates the renin-angiotensin-aldosterone axis and other neurohumoral mechanisms that increase renal sodium reabsorption.

Since edema always results from an imbalance between sodium intake and excretion, the most effective management combines reduced dietary salt intake with diuretics. Indeed, diuretics succeed in removing excess extracellular fluid volume only when salt intake is also restricted. Overly aggressive diuretic treatment, giving insufficient time for the edema fluid to move from the interstitium into the vascular space, can cause significant plasma volume depletion. Plasma volume depletion, recognized on physical examination by orthostatic hypotension and tachycardia, in turn can precipitate acute renal failure. Thus, edema should be mobilized gradually so that patients lose no more than 1 kg/day.

Another cardinal feature of the nephrotic syndrome is hyperlipidemia (Chapter 4.9). The reduction in serum albumin and immunoglobulin concentrations, caused by both urinary protein loss and degradation of up to 20 g/day of filtered protein by tubule cells, in turn stimulates hepatic protein synthesis. Elevated serum lipids reflect, at least in part, increased synthesis of lipoproteins, particularly those containing apoprotein B, which have more oncotic activity than other apoproteins. Catabolism of lipoproteins may also be decreased. Since patients may have the nephrotic syndrome for years, they are at significant risk for developing cardiovascular complications from hyperlipidemia. Furthermore, hyperlipidemia increases the rate at which patients lose renal function.

Reducing dietary cholesterol and fat intake has limited efficacy in bringing down lipid levels in patients with the nephrotic syndrome. But hydroxymethylglutaryl-CoA reductase inhibitor therapy can reduce patients' serum cholesterol and triglyceride concentrations by 30–40%. Still, any long-term reduction in risk from coronary heart disease remains to be proved.

The nephrotic syndrome is often complicated by a hypercoagulable state (Chapter 11.10), caused by a combination of increased synthesis of various clotting factors, loss of antithrombin III, and increased platelet aggregation. A serious complication of the hypercoagulable state in the nephrotic syndrome is renal vein thrombosis, which most often affects patients with membranous glomerulonephritis; about 10% of patients with renal venous thrombosis suffer potentially life-threatening acute pulmonary embolism and thrombosis. Renal venous thrombosis manifests with flank pain, a sudden increase in the urinary protein excretion rate, an abrupt drop in GFR, hematuria, and renal swelling, which ultrasonography may show to be unilateral. Magnetic resonance imaging or venography is used to make the diagnosis. Treatment requires anticoagulation.

Patients with the nephrotic syndrome are also unusually susceptible to infection because of immune system dysfunction caused by loss of components of the alternate complement pathway and of immunoglobulins. Protein malnutrition and deficiencies in trace metals and vitamins have also been reported. Thyroxine-binding globulin is lost, reducing the total but not the free thyroxine concentration without clinical consequences.

INFLAMMATORY AND PROLIFERATIVE GLOMERULAR DISEASES

This group of diseases is characterized by glomerular injury caused by inflammatory cell infiltration or glomerular cell proliferation. Patients present with hematuria, active urine sediment, proteinuria, and reduced GFR. Volume retention usually manifests as hypertension with little or no edema. Hypertension can also reflect primary activation of the renin-angiotensin system because of reduced renal blood flow.

Acute Glomerulonephritis

Acute glomerulonephritis is a complication of infectious or autoimmune diseases usually caused by glomerular deposition of immune complexes, which produce diffuse proliferative glomerular lesions. "Diffuse" refers to the involvement of all glomeruli; "proliferative" to glomerular hypercellularity. Included in the differential diagnosis are rapidly progressive glomerulonephritis, systemic vasculitis (Chapter 3.5), thrombotic microangiopathies, and nonglomerular causes of acute renal failure.

Acute Postinfectious Glomerulonephritis: Acute poststreptococcal glomerulonephritis, the most common form of postinfectious glomerulonephritis, presents with hematuria, extracellular fluid volume expansion with pulmonary congestion, hypertension, and peripheral and periorbital edema. Oliguric acute renal failure is common, although some patients have only mild renal insufficiency. Patients may report bloody or cola-colored urine. Urinalysis shows red blood cells, red cell casts, and proteinuria. The urine sodium is below 20 mEq/L, reflecting renal vasoconstriction with avid renal sodium retention.

Acute postinfectious glomerulonephritis is most often a complication of skin or pharyngeal infection with group A (β-hemolytic) streptococci. Serologic studies show a depressed C3 and a high titer of antistreptolysin O antibodies. Renal biopsy is not necessary in patients with a typical presentation and positive serology. The typical pathologic finding is hypercellularity in all glomeruli, with increased numbers of both intrinsic glomerular cells and inflammatory cells. Immunofluorescence shows scattered large granular deposits of both IgG and C3, chiefly on capillary loops. Electron microscopy shows large "humps" of immune complexes on the subepithelial side of the glomerular basement membrane, with occasional mesangial deposits as well.

Milder forms of postinfectious glomerulonephritis can develop after almost any other bacterial or viral infection. Such patients present with hematuria, active urine sediment, proteinuria, variable degrees of hypertension, and loss of GFR. In addition, an immune complex-mediated acute glomerulonephritis can be caused by some chronic bacterial infections, most prominent among them subacute bacterial endocarditis, infection of ventriculo-atrial shunts, and visceral abscess.

Management of acute postinfectious glomerulonephritis, including poststreptococcal glomerulonephritis, is supportive, with salt and fluid restriction as well as diuretics, antihypertensive drugs, and dialysis as necessary. Immunosuppressive drugs are not normally given. If the cause of glomerulonephritis is a chronic bacterial infection, the infection must be treated. The lesions of acute postinfectious glomerulonephritis generally resolve spontaneously over weeks to months.

Autoimmune-Mediated Diffuse Proliferative Glomerulonephritis: Patients with acute glomerulonephritis caused by autoimmune disease (eg, systemic lupus erythematosus) present with hematuria, an active urine sediment, proteinuria, and often some degree of renal insufficiency and hypertension; very few present with acute renal failure. Patients may also have signs and symptoms of their systemic disease. Most patients with lupus nephritis test positive for antinuclear antibodies and double-stranded DNA and have low levels of C3 and C4. Biopsy can show three types of changes: diffuse proliferative glomerulonephritis with polymorphonuclear leukocyte infiltration, areas of glomerular necrosis, and crescents. Immunofluorescence studies show staining for C3 and C1$_q$, as well as IgG, IgA, and IgM. Electron microscopy shows immune deposits in the mesangium and the subendothelial space, and occasionally in the subepithelial location of the capillary basement membrane.

Even when a diagnosis of lupus nephritis seems secure, most nephrologists favor renal biopsy, because clinical clues correlate poorly with the severity of the glomerular disease and pathology can show patterns other than diffuse proliferative glomerulonephritis, such as mesangial proliferative, focal proliferative, membranous, and a mixture of these.

Diffuse proliferative glomerulonephritis caused by systemic lupus erythematosus is usually treated with immunosuppressive drugs. If the condition is left untreated, renal function is not likely to recover.

Rapidly Progressive Glomerulonephritis

Rapidly progressive glomerulonephritis is a clinical pattern associated with crescentic glomerulonephritis on biopsy. Many patients present with only vague fatigue at a time when their renal function is already impaired. Some patients give a history of hematuria. If the disease is caused by a systemic disorder, patients may have complaints related to other organ systems. The urine shows proteinuria and hematuria with an active sediment. Many patients have hypertension and a rapidly progressive fall in GFR, often over weeks. Untreated crescentic glomerulonephritis destroys glomeruli quickly and irreversibly, and even a 1- or 2-day delay in diagnosis can significantly worsen the prognosis, as can incorrect treatment. Therefore, patients need urgent diagnostic renal biopsy, and their prognosis can improve markedly with appropriate immunosuppressive therapy.

The common pathologic finding in all forms of rapidly

progressive glomerulonephritis is crescentic glomerulonephritis. Under light microscopy, biopsy specimens show crescents in more than 80% of glomeruli (see Figure 5.6–2C). Crescents are located in Bowman's space surrounding the glomerular capillary tuft; they consist of proliferating epithelial cells and invading macrophages and other chronic inflammatory cells. The glomeruli often have segmental necrotizing lesions. Silver stain shows breaks in the glomerular basement membrane.

Diseases that cause rapidly progressive glomerulonephritis fall into three groups, distinguished by immunofluorescence patterns: antiglomerular basement membrane disease, pauci-immune diseases, and immune complex-mediated diseases. Disorders in all three groups can be caused by multisystem disease or disease limited to the kidney.

Antiglomerular Basement Membrane Disease: Antiglomerular basement membrane disease is characterized by linear immunofluorescent staining of the capillary wall for IgG. The disorder is called *Goodpasture's syndrome* if the patient has associated pulmonary hemorrhage, and *antiglomerular basement membrane antibody-mediated idiopathic crescentic glomerulonephritis* if it is limited to the kidney. Patients with either form have circulating antiglomerular basement membrane antibodies. Treatment includes plasmapheresis, corticosteroids, and cytotoxic drugs.

Pauci-Immune Crescentic Glomerulonephritis: Crescentic glomerulonephritis with little or no immunoglobulin deposition is called pauci-immune glomerulonephritis. Therefore, the glomeruli do not stain by immunofluorescence. Pauci-immune crescentic glomerulonephritis is termed *Wegener's granulomatosis* if it is associated with necrotizing upper respiratory tract or pulmonary lesions, and *pauci-immune idiopathic crescentic glomerulonephritis* if it is limited to the kidney. Both forms are identified by circulating antineutrophil cytoplasmic antibodies (C-ANCA). Both respond to corticosteroids and cyclophosphamide; plasmapheresis has not been shown to be effective.

Pauci-immune crescentic glomerulonephritis can also be seen in patients with vasculitis. These patients have a different antineutrophil cytoplasmic antibody, P-ANCA. Again, treatment is a combination of corticosteroids and cytotoxic drugs.

Immune Complex-Mediated Crescentic Glomerulonephritis: By immunofluorescence, the immune complex-mediated diseases show granular capillary loop and mesangial staining for at least IgG and C3 and often for other immunoglobulins and complement components. Immune complex-mediated crescentic glomerulonephritis can be caused by multisystem diseases like systemic lupus erythematosus and Henoch-Schönlein purpura. When the disease is limited to the kidney, it is called *immune complex-mediated idiopathic crescentic glomerulonephritis.* Both kidney-limited disease and disease complicating lupus are usually treated with corticosteroids and cytotoxic drugs; patients' renal function generally improves. However, this treatment has been reported to benefit only isolated patients with Henoch-Schönlein purpura and crescentic glomerulonephritis.

Hematuria with the Nephrotic Syndrome

The clinical pattern of hematuria with nephrotic syndrome differs from acute and rapidly progressive glomerulonephritis in that renal failure is not usually a presenting problem. Instead, patients have an active urine sediment with cellular and occasional red blood cell casts, and proteinuria is in the nephrotic range. Many patients have hypertension. The GFR may be normal at first, but it usually declines slowly over months to years.

Hematuria with the nephrotic syndrome most often predicts membranoproliferative glomerulonephritis on biopsy. This glomerular lesion is seen with several systemic diseases, including systemic lupus erythematosus, essential mixed cryoglobulinemia, and Henoch-Schönlein purpura. Among diseases limited to the kidney, this pattern is seen in types I and II idiopathic membranoproliferative glomerulonephritis and rarely in IgA nephropathy.

The first step in evaluation is to seek multisystem disease. Systemic lupus erythematosus classically presents with serositis, dermatitis, arthritis, and hematologic abnormalities; mixed essential cryoglobulinemia with Raynaud's phenomenon; and Henoch-Schönlein purpura with raised purpuric lesions on the legs and buttocks, plus gastrointestinal symptoms. Serologic tests that help define the diagnosis include antinuclear antibodies, C3, and C4. Serum cryoglobulins and hepatitis C antibodies are found in more than 90% of patients with mixed essential cryoglobulinemia. In patients with idiopathic membranoproliferative glomerulonephritis, which usually manifests before age 30, the C3 is often severely and persistently depressed.

Most patients with hematuria and the nephrotic syndrome undergo diagnostic renal biopsy. The characteristic pattern on light microscopy is diffuse involvement of the glomeruli, with hypercellularity affecting all glomerular components, as well as increased mesangial matrix and thickened capillary walls. Silver stain may show apparent duplication of the basement membrane. Electron microscopy often shows large subendothelial and mesangial deposits; type II membranoproliferative glomerulonephritis is characterized by an electron-dense transformation of the glomerular and tubular basement membranes.

Although treatment with anticoagulants, immunosuppressive drugs, and plasmapheresis has been tried in patients with idiopathic membranoproliferative glomerulonephritis, effectiveness has not been proven. Henoch-Schönlein purpura also tends not to respond to immunosuppressive therapy. By contrast, immunosuppressive treatment is effective against membranoproliferative glomerulonephritis in patients with systemic lupus.

The membranoproliferative glomerulonephritis of hepatitis C-induced mixed essential cryoglobulinemia responds to interferon-α.

Hematuria with Non-Nephrotic Proteinuria

Hematuria without other symptoms or signs is often seen in patients with mild glomerular proliferation or inflammation. These patients typically present with episodes of painless gross hematuria or with microscopic hematuria discovered by routine urinalysis. They may have hypertension and a slowly progressive reduction in GFR. Proteinuria is mild.

Biopsy usually reveals the mesangial proliferative pattern: Light microscopy shows an increase in the mesangial matrix and mesangial cell hypercellularity without abnormalities in the capillary wall. IgA or IgM deposits, found by immunofluorescence in the mesangium, are diagnostic for IgA and IgM nephropathy, respectively. Deposition of all immunoglobulin classes as well as C3, $C1_q$, and C4 is consistent with systemic lupus erythematosus.

Hereditary forms of nephritis also present with hematuria and little proteinuria. Mild mesangial hypercellularity without immune deposits, but with widespread splitting and lamination of the glomerular basement membrane, suggests Alport's syndrome. The lack of mesangial hypercellularity, with a thinner than normal basement membrane on electron microscopy, supports thin basement membrane disease.

Immune Complex-Mediated Mesangial Proliferative Glomerulonephritis:

The most common disorder presenting with this clinical pattern, IgA nephropathy, is limited to the kidney. The cause is glomerular IgA deposition. Occasionally, a similar disease is caused by IgM deposition. IgA and IgM nephropathy infrequently progress to end-stage renal disease. Neither disorder is treated with immunosuppressive drugs.

Many patients with systemic lupus erythematosus also present with this pathologic picture. These patients have a better prognosis than those with diffuse proliferative or membranoproliferative lupus glomerulonephritis. Systemic lupus with mesangial proliferative glomerulonephritis is usually treated with corticosteroids.

Hereditary Nephritis:

Patients with Alport's syndrome, an X-linked hereditary disease with abnormal type IV basement membrane collagen, present with clinical features that are indistinguishable from IgA nephropathy except for a family history of males going on to end-stage renal failure. Many patients also suffer from sensorineural hearing loss. In affected males, Alport's syndrome commonly progresses to terminal renal failure. Homozygous females, although rare, exhibit the same progression to end-stage renal failure; heterozygous females often have hematuria but no loss of GFR. As expected for a primary defect in basement membrane collagen, immunosuppressive therapy is not effective.

Patients with thin basement membrane disease also present with hematuria and minimal proteinuria. As with Alport's syndrome, they have a family history of hematuria, but without renal failure, sensorineural hearing loss, or a male preponderance. Unlike patients with Alport's syndrome, individuals with thin basement membrane disease have an excellent prognosis.

Chronic Glomerulonephritis

Chronic glomerulonephritis is a term reserved for glomerular diseases that cannot be defined more specifically. Patients present with already small, contracted kidneys and end-stage renal failure. Pathologic examination of the kidney does not usually reveal the underlying disease process because most of the glomeruli have already become sclerotic, the tubules have atrophied, and the renal interstitium has fibrosed. Many patients present with lassitude and exercise intolerance caused by the anemia associated with chronic renal failure. Most patients have hematuria, proteinuria, and hypertension, and their urine contains casts suggestive of chronic disease. When patients present with established end-stage renal failure and small, contracted kidneys, their only treatment options are dialysis and transplantation.

THROMBOTIC MICROANGIOPATHIES

The principal mechanism in thrombotic microangiopathic disorders is endothelial cell injury leading to platelet activation and fibrin deposition in small blood vessels and hemolysis caused by shearing of red blood cells by the microvascular thrombi. Clinically, thrombotic microangiopathies can mimic other forms of glomerular disease: Patients present with a decreased GFR, often to the point of oliguria or anuria, as well as hematuria with red blood cell casts, and proteinuria that may be in the nephrotic range.

The most prominent thrombotic microangiopathies are the hemolytic-uremic syndrome and thrombotic thrombocytopenic purpura. Thrombotic microangiopathy with renal failure can also complicate treatment with cyclosporine, mitomycin, and other chemotherapeutic agents. Diagnosis is made by detection of purpura, thrombocytopenia, and hemolysis with signs of fragmented red cells on the blood smear.

Scleroderma crisis and malignant hypertension can also produce oliguric renal failure, with proteinuria and an active urine sediment caused by microvascular injury and fibrin deposition in renal vessels. The most serious clinical problem is usually severe hypertension; the hematologic abnormalities are not prominent. Biopsy is not usually needed to make the diagnosis. Indeed, renal biopsy is extremely dangerous for patients with severe thrombocytopenia or malignant hypertension and should be done only if the diagnosis is in doubt—and then only after platelet transfusion and pharmacologic correction of hypertension.

The hemolytic-uremic syndrome responds best to

plasma exchange and corticosteroid therapy. This treatment is less effective for patients with thrombotic thrombocytopenic purpura. Scleroderma crisis is best treated with an ACE inhibitor, and a number of antihypertensive drugs can reverse malignant hypertension. Recovery of renal function is variable.

GLOMERULAR DISEASE DURING PREGNANCY

Preeclampsia develops in about 3–4% of all pregnant women and is most prevalent in primiparas. The disease is characterized by proteinuria, edema, and hypertension, usually beginning in the third trimester. The urine sediment is not active, and the GFR is usually only mildly depressed. Proteinuria is often in the nephrotic range. Preeclampsia may progress to produce central nervous system deficits with convulsions or coma; the condition is then called *eclampsia*. Some women develop frank disseminated intravascular coagulation, with a decreased platelet count, hemolysis, a microangiopathic blood smear, and abnormal liver function, with or without acute renal failure caused by cortical necrosis. Treatment centers on controlling the blood pressure and delivering the fetus.

Pregnancy not uncommonly uncovers or worsens preexisting glomerular disease, most notably glomerulonephritis caused by systemic lupus erythematosus, and focal and segmental glomerular sclerosis. During pregnancy, these disorders may be difficult to distinguish from preeclampsia. Biopsy is almost always deferred until after delivery, unless the physician suspects rapidly progressive glomerulonephritis that could respond to immunosuppressive drugs. If patients with presumed preeclampsia still have proteinuria and hypertension for longer than 4–6 weeks after delivery, the physician should suspect a different disease.

SUMMARY

▶ Glomerular injury leads to albuminuria with or without an active urine sediment and often with a reduction in the glomerular filtration rate.

▶ With crescentic glomerulonephritis and glomerular diseases complicating systemic lupus erythematosus or systemic vasculitis, prompt diagnosis and treatment can make the difference between continued renal function and life on dialysis.

▶ Patients with chronic, progressive loss of renal function require control of hypertension, avoidance of nonsteroidal anti-inflammatory drugs, and appropriate use of immunosuppressive drugs.

▶ Diagnostic renal biopsy is urgently needed to guide therapy in patients with rapidly progressive glomerulonephritis. The only glomerular diseases that can usually be diagnosed without biopsy are minimal change disease, diabetic nephropathy, HIV nephropathy, amyloidosis, and acute poststreptococcal glomerulonephritis.

▶ Patients with systemic lupus erythematosus can develop diffuse proliferative (with or without crescents), mesangial proliferative, membranous, or a mixed pattern of glomerulonephritis. The type and severity of disease are best determined by renal biopsy.

SUGGESTED READING

Agnello V, Chung RT, Kaplan LM: A role for hepatitis C virus infection in type II cryoglobulinemia. N Engl J Med 1992; 327:1490.

Cortes L, Tejani A: Dilemma of focal glomerular sclerosis. Kidney Int 1996;49(Suppl):557.

Couser WG: Pathogenesis of glomerulonephritis. Kidney Int 1993;42(Suppl):S19.

Detwiler RK et al: Collapsing glomerulopathy: A clinically and pathologically distinct variant of focal segmental glomerulosclerosis. Kidney Int 1994;45:1416.

Galla JH: IgA nephropathy. Kidney Int 1995;47:377.

Harris RC, Ismail N: Extrarenal complications of the nephrotic syndrome. Am J Kidney Dis 1994;23:477.

Lewis EJ et al: The effect of angiotensin-converting-enzyme inhibition on diabetic nephropathy: The Collaborative Study Group. N Engl J Med 1993;329:1456.

Rao TK: Human immunodeficiency virus (HIV) associated nephropathy. Annu Rev Med 1991;42:391.

5.7

Tubulointerstitial Disease

Andrew Whelton, MD, and Alan J. Watson, MRCPI

Tubulointerstitial nephritis is a class of renal disorders that primarily affect the tubular portion of the nephron, including the tubules themselves, renal interstitial tissue, and the extensive surrounding vascular network. Patients with these kidney diseases can have widely varied presentations, ranging from rapidly progressive renal failure to chronic asymptomatic renal dysfunction that slowly advances over years. Tubulointerstitial kidney diseases are responsible for about 20% of cases of end-stage renal failure. They are also important because if diagnosed and treated promptly, tubulointerstitial nephritis is often reversible, as in drug-induced nephritis.

Physicians can recognize that renal dysfunction is due to tubulointerstitial renal disease based on the urine sediment, which is characterized by minimal proteinuria and tubular casts that (unlike glomerulnephritis) are rarely composed of red cells, and on changes in the urine and serum that reflect tubular cell dysfunction, such as renal tubular acidosis, aminoaciduria, and abnormal urine concentrating ability. Patients with tubulointerstitial nephritis should be classified as having either acute or chronic disease, based on clinical circumstances and features of the urinary sediment. This is important because the most likely causes, most appropriate management, and prognosis all differ for patients with acute tubulointerstitial nephritis from those with chronic disease (Table 5.7–1).

When renal biopsies are performed, acute tubulointerstitial nephritis is characterized pathologically by interstitial edema, an inflammatory infiltrate, and tubular damage with sparing of the glomeruli. In chronic tubulointerstitial nephritis, there is interstitial fibrosis, a chronic cellular infiltrate, and variable tubular loss that includes the glomeruli serving the fibrosed tubules.

Cystic diseases of the kidney, which are also covered in this chapter, are a distinct group of inherited and acquired diseases of the tubulointerstitial network.

CLINICAL FEATURES SUGGESTING TUBULOINTERSTITIAL NEPHRITIS

Patients with tubulointerstitial diseases have specific clinical features that enable the clinician to distinguish these diseases from those that dominantly involve the glomerular portion of the nephron. The patient's clinical history often reveals one of the specific causes of tubulointerstitial nephritis. However, the urinalysis may provide the most compelling indication of tubulointerstitial nephritis. Although glomerular disorders are reflected by abundant (4+) urine protein, tubulointerstitial disorders typically cause only trace to 1+ levels of protein. This is because only a small amount of protein, mainly albumin and β_2-microglobulin, is normally filtered and reabsorbed by action of the proximal tubule. As tubular damage develops and progresses, reabsorption of these proteins is impaired and they appear in the urine.

Microscopic evaluation of urine sediment from patients with tubulointerstitial nephritis reflects the acuteness or chronicity of the disorder. In acute tubulointerstitial nephritis, abundant tubular casts are composed of sloughed tubular epithelial cells, white blood cells, or both. Rarely, when red cell casts are present, they signify profound acute tubular damage. The urine also contains individual tubular epithelial cells, white blood cells, and red blood cells. Urine eosinophils, which are detectable by Wright's or Hansel's stain, are indicative of allergic tubulointerstitial nephritis, but are detectable in only 25% of such patients. In chronic tubulointerstitial nephritis, there are minimal urine microscopic findings such as chronic lead nephropathy.

Urine acidification defects in patients with tubular function also provide an early indicator of tubulointerstitial nephritis. In established tubulointerstitial nephritis, the urine pH is typically less than maximally acid (pH 5.0 or higher), whereas the blood chemistries reflect a hyperchloremic acidosis (Cl^- above 105 mEq/L; HCO_3^- below

407

Table 5.7–1. Common causes of tubulointerstitial nephritis.

Causes	Important Examples
Acute	
Drug hypersensitivity	Antibiotics, eg, penicillin; diuretics; nonsteroidal anti-inflammatory agents
Infections	*Escherichia coli*, Hantavirus, *Leptospira*
Systemic diseases	Sjögren's syndrome, amyloidosis
Miscellaneous	Xylene, toluene
Chronic	
Obstruction	Benign prostatic hypertrophy
Reflux nephropathy	Congenital urethral valves
Toxic nephropathy	Heavy metals: cadmium, lead
Metabolic disorders	Gout, primary and secondary oxalosis
Ischemic nephritis	Sickle cell disease
Autoimmune disease	Sjögren's syndrome, kidney transplant rejection
Neoplastic and hematologic disorders	Lymphoma
Granulomatous nephritis	Sarcoidosis, tuberculosis, phenytoin
Endemic disease	Environmental toxins and viruses

Table 5.7–3. Common causes of large kidneys.

Obstructive hydronephrosis
Cystic kidney disease
Acute tubulointerstitial nephritis
Renal cell carcinoma
Invasive infiltrates of tumor or amyloid
Granulomatous disease
Renal vein thrombosis
Nephrotic syndrome

24 mEq/L) without an increase in the anion gap. These acidification tubular defects and criteria for their differentiation into proximal and distal tubular types are presented in Table 5.7–2 and are reviewed in more detail in Chapter 5.3.

Additional Laboratory Tests

Several additional studies may be useful in the diagnosis and differential diagnosis of tubulointerstitial nephritis. Renal biopsy is definitive. Serial determinations of serum creatinine and, as needed, creatinine clearance studies provide useful markers of the progression or stability of the patient's overall renal functional status. Progression of renal impairment, if it occurs, also manifests by conversion of the patient's hyperchloremic nonanion gap acidosis to an increasing anion gap acidosis, a reflection of retained systemic acids.

When indicated by the appearance of kidney disease, renal size and urinary outflow tract patency can be assessed by ultrasonography. In acute tubulointerstitial nephritis, the kidneys are often slightly enlarged (Table 5.7–3). Ultrasound studies are particularly helpful in identifying cysts within the kidney; magnetic resonance imaging (MRI) or computed tomography (CT) can further define the size and extent of cystic abnormalities. Intravenous pyelographic study should usually be avoided, since radiocontrast may further impair renal function.

Isotopic gallium scanning of the kidney may provide additional evidence of a diffuse inflammatory infiltrate. Gallium is taken up by the inflammatory cells within the renal parenchyma, and its presence in the kidney 72 hours after administration is evidence of renal parenchymal inflammation. However, isotopic gallium scanning is a nonspecific test and may be positive in other clinical circumstances, such as in nephrotic syndrome.

When the diagnosis of tubulointerstitial nephritis is not apparent based on the clinical setting and urinary sediment, kidney biopsy study should be considered, especially if the patient's renal function is deteriorating or failing to improve. Therapeutic decisions, such as the appropriateness of corticosteroid therapy, can also be made, based on evaluation of the histopathology of renal biopsy tissue.

ACUTE TUBULOINTERSTITIAL NEPHRITIS

Acute tubulointerstitial nephritis can be caused by drug hypersensitivity and toxicity; kidney infections; and systemic infectious, autoimmune, and neoplastic diseases (see Table 5.7–1).

Table 5.7–2. Clinical and laboratory consequences of chronic tubulointerstitial nephritis.

Site	Diseases	Tubular Defect	Clinical Features
Proximal tubule	Multiple myeloma Toxic nephropathy (eg, cadmium)	↓ reabsorption of HCO_3^- PO_4^{2-} Uric acid Amino acids Glucose	Proximal renal tubular acidosis Glycosuria Fanconi's syndrome
Distal tubule	Sjögren's syndrome Obstructive uropathy	↓ excretion of K^+, H^+ ↓ reabsorption of Na^+	Distal renal tubular acidosis Hyperkalemia Volume contraction
Collecting duct	Analgesic nephropathy Sickle cell disease Lithium	↓ maximal concentration and dilution of urine	Nephrogenic diabetes insipidus

Drug-Induced Tubulointerstitial Nephritis

Many drugs can cause acute renal failure as a part of a systemic hypersensitivity reaction that also includes fever, arthralgia, rash, and eosinophilia. In the kidney, the characteristic features of acute tubulointerstitial nephritis are present. Antibiotics are the usual offenders. One antibiotic, the penicillin analogue methicillin, is no longer used because of its propensity to induce acute tubulointerstitial nephritis.

When a patient presents with features suggesting acute tubulointerstitial nephritis but no obvious kidney infection, the clinician should have a high index of suspicion that the problem is caused by a drug or toxin and should get a comprehensive history of such exposures. Often, this requires requestioning the patient or family contacts. The possibility that interstitial nephritis is a drug-induced disease is further suggested by associated fever and arthralgia and by the findings of eosinophilia and eosinophils in the urine. The microscopic urine sediment is active, as described earlier, and occasionally gross hematuria may be present. If necessary, the diagnosis may be confirmed by a renal biopsy, which typically shows infiltration with macrophages, eosinophils, and lymphocytes, predominantly cytotoxic suppressor T cells. Immunofluorescent staining of the tubular network may show deposition of immunoglobulins, such as with penicillin hypersensitivity.

The first step in treatment is obviously withdrawing the offending antigen. If renal function does not improve within 1–2 weeks, patients should be given a 2-week course of corticosteroids. Virtually all patients recover, but a few go on to develop chronic renal failure, particularly if their nephritis has gone unrecognized for some time.

Infectious Tubulointerstitial Nephritis

Infection-induced tubulointerstitial nephritis rarely causes overt acute renal failure, except when a susceptible individual, such as a patient with diabetes mellitus, has involvement of both kidneys. The development of acute renal failure in a septic patient should prompt a search for papillary necrosis. Renal papillae have a tenuous blood supply in comparison with the renal cortical blood flow. In the presence of conditions that further compromise the vascular system, such as diabetes mellitus, the papillae become prone to infarction with acute infection. The infarcted papillae slough off and can cause acute ureteric outflow obstruction with acute deterioration of renal function.

Patients with bacterial pyelonephritis typically present with flank pain, fever, and chills. Microscopic urinalysis shows bacteria, white blood cells, tubular epithelial cells, and occasionally white cell casts. Urine cultures are always positive, and blood cultures are often also positive. *Escherichia coli* is the usual offending organism. *Staphylococcus aureus* predominates when infection is spread through the blood, as typically happens in the elderly and in immunocompromised persons. Many other infections can cause acute tubulointerstitial nephritis (see Table 5.7–1).

Systemic Disease

Acute tubulointerstitial nephritis can affect patients with systemic diseases, such as Sjögren's syndrome (Chapter 3.4) and systemic lupus erythematosus (Chapter 3.2), although these more commonly affect the renal glomerulus. It is also a prominent feature of renal transplant rejection. In these settings, an immune-mediated pathogenesis appears likely. Leukemias and lymphomas can involve the kidney, producing interstitial edema and an infiltrative inflammatory response; functional renal impairment resolves when the malignancy is treated. Myeloma kidney, amyloidosis, and light chain nephropathy associated with plasma cell dyscrasias often manifest as tubulointerstitial nephritis.

Idiopathic Disease

In some patients, no cause for tubulointerstitial nephritis can be found. Many such patients also have uveitis, suggesting an underlying systemic process. Their renal failure may be severe enough to warrant transient dialysis, although most recover or improve spontaneously after a course of corticosteroids.

CHRONIC TUBULOINTERSTITIAL NEPHRITIS

Although chronic tubulointerstitial nephritis can arise from progression of unrecognized acute tubulointerstitial nephritis, it more commonly is caused by a relatviely distinct set of disorders (see Table 5.7–1). These include renovascular disease (Chapter 5.9), glomerulonephritis, and chronic heavy metal toxicity. Chronic tubulointerstitial nephritis is responsible for 15–20% of cases of end-stage renal disease, some of which were previously assumed to be chronic pyelonephritis.

Patients with chronic tubulointerstitial nephritis characteristically develop defects in tubular cell functions, followed by slow progression of renal dysfunction. In the early stages, renal tubular dysfunction is manifested as renal tubular acidosis and an inability to regulate urinary sodium loss. The precise clinical and biochemical abnormalities resulting from tubular dysfunction depend on which part of the tubular network is most affected (see Table 5.7–2).

Obstructive Uropathy

Patients with chronic obstruction to urinary outflow develop tubular dilatation, interstitial inflammation, and ultimately widespread fibrosis of the interstitium. The most common causes of obstructive uropathy in men are benign prostatic hypertrophy and prostatic and rectal carcinomas. The most common cause in women is cervical carcinoma obstructing the ureters. In both sexes, tubulointerstitial nephritis can also be caused by obstructing urinary stones.

Obstructive uropathy may be symptomless, although patients with benign prostatic hypertrophy or partial obstruction may have altered urinary flow patterns, such as alternating anuria and polyuria. Physical examination may identify prostate enlargement, pelvic masses, or a distended bladder. A sonogram of the urinary tract is usually diagnostic, showing hydronephrosis and hydroureter. The physician who is suspicious of obstructive uropathy based on one or more of the above findings must then consider more definitive studies such as antegrade or retrograde pyelography to confirm the diagnosis.

Reflux Nephropathy

Reflux nephropathy is characterized by cortical scarring and susceptibility to infection. It is usually encountered in children and adolescents. The basic problem is congenital incompetence of the vesicoureteric valves. A straight insertion of the ureter into the bladder, in contrast to the usual oblique insertion, allows reflux of urine during micturition. Ureteric reflux may also be secondary to increased intravesical pressure in patients with bladder outlet obstruction or in young males born with congenital urethral obstructive valves.

Recurrent urinary tract infections in young children should raise suspicion of reflux nephropathy. A voiding cystourethrogram will document reflux. Cystoscopy may also help in the diagnosis. Patients need early prolonged antibiotic therapy to prevent irreversible interstitial fibrosis. Patients with persistent hydroureter require surgical reimplantation of the ureters.

Analgesic Nephropathy and Toxic Nephropathy

Analgesic abuse was first recognized as a cause of chronic tubulointerstitial nephritis in the 1950's. In the United States now, only 1–2% of end-stage renal disease in dialysis patients is caused by analgesic abuse. The common offending agents are phenacetin, acetaminophen, and aspirin taken in combination. Phenacetin is now no longer available for clinical use in the United States, and there is no solid evidence that acetaminophen or aspirin, when taken on their own on a long-term basis using usual therapeutic regimens produces this form of nephropathy. The nephrotoxic effect of the analgesic combination is dose-related, with the minimum toxic cumulative dose estimated as 3 kg or more over 3–5 years or more.

Analgesic abuse nephropathy presents with an insidious loss of renal function. Early in the process, only tests of urine concentration and dilution may be abnormal. Many patients also have anemia, peptic ulcer, and transitional cell carcinomas that are probably secondary to the prolonged excretion of toxic analgesic metabolites. The treatment is to stop taking the analgesic combination, which may require intense psychological support. In its early phases, renal dysfunction may be reversible.

Other toxins can cause interstitial inflammation and scarring. Industrial exposure to heavy metals such as lead or cadmium primarily affects the proximal tubules with manifestations of tubular dysfunction. Patients with this form of tubulointerstitial fibrosis present with impaired concentration and dilution of urine. Many have associated hypertension and, in the case of lead exposure, gout.

About one-third of patients who take lithium carbonate for manic depression develop tubular dysfunction in the form of nephrogenic diabetes insipidus, and unresponsiveness to vasopressin, as a direct tubular effect of lithium carbonate. This form of nephrogenic diabetes insipidus is also caused by other toxins and diseases (Chapter 4.2). The lithium-induced unresponsiveness of the collecting duct to circulating antidiuretic hormone is usually reversible when lithium is discontinued. Chemotherapeutic agents such as cisplatin, methyl-CCNU (lomustine), BCNU (carmustine), and possibly cyclosporine may also cause chronic tubulointerstitial nephritis.

Hereditary Nephritis

Hereditary nephritis consists of a group of genetic disorders characterized principally by interstitial involvement of the kidney. The nephritis may occur alone or may be accompanied by sensorineural deafness, in which case it is known as Alport's syndrome. Alport's syndrome usually afflicts boys and typically leads to end-stage renal failure in the late teens.

Metabolic Disorders

In patients with prolonged hypercalcemia of any cause, calcium in the form of hydroxyapatite or calcium oxalate, can precipitate in the renal interstitium, with associated tubular cell necrosis and interstitial fibrosis on renal biopsy. If renal function is to be preserved, the underlying cause of hypercalcemia must be recognized and the metabolic disturbance promptly corrected. Progressive tubulointerstitial nephritis may also be associated with chronic hyperuricemia (Chapter 3.8). However, the role of uric acid as the proximate offender is not clear, since many patients with hyperuricemia and chronic gout do not develop tubulointerstitial nephritis. Those who do develop nephritis may have other underlying conditions.

Primary hyperoxaluria is a rare inherited disorder due to an abnormality in the enzymatic metabolism of glyoxylic acid. However, secondary hyperoxaluria is more common, caused by increased oxalate absorption from the gastrointestinal tract in patients with inflammatory bowel disease or patients who have an intact colon after small bowel resection. In these patients, fat malabsorption is present. In the bowel lumen, calcium binds to fatty acids rather than precipitating with dietary oxalate, and excess oxalate is absorbed from the colon. Increased urinary excretion of oxalate or urate may lead to crystal formation and aggravate underlying chronic tubulointerstitial nephritis by superimposing an obstructive component on the nephropathy. Therapy of these disorders consists of dietary restrictions designed to reduce the intake of purines and oxalates and, when necessary, pharmacologic allopurinol to reduce the filtered load of uric acid (Chapter 3.8).

Ischemic Nephritis

Sickle cell disease can affect many parts of the kidneys, including the interstitium. Intracapillary sickling of red blood cells causes ischemic lesions in the renal medulla, leading to scarring and fibrosis. Necrosis of the renal papillae usually progresses slowly, but patients with acute sloughing of a papilla may present with gross hematuria or ureteric obstruction. Distal tubular function tends to be most affected, resulting in a distal renal tubular acidosis with hyperkalemia. Chronic interstitial nephritis may also develop in patients with sickle cell trait and sickle cell thalassemia.

Vascular diseases, including forms of renovascular disease and arteriolar nephrosclerosis, can produce an interstitial ischemic nephropathy. Recognition and treatment of the primary disease can slow progression of renal failure.

Radiation Nephritis

Radiation nephritis can cause ischemic tubulointerstitial nephritis after patients' kidneys are exposed to more than 2500 cGy. Acute postradiation tubulointerstitial nephritis may progressively resolve only to be followed by chronic tubulointerstitial disease some 10–20 years later. Patients invariably develop hypertension, which is usually severe. Postradiation ureteric or retroperitoneal fibrosis may aggravate chronic renal failure by producing an obstructive uropathy. Radiation-related disorders are better prevented than treated, and their incidence has greatly decreased in recent years.

Autoimmune Disorders

A wide variety of renal lesions can develop in patients with Sjögren's syndrome (Chapter 3.4), but the most common renal manifestation of the syndrome is tubulointerstitial nephritis, usually of a chronic nature. Prominent clinical features are distal renal tubular acidosis and nephrogenic diabetes insipidus. The concept of an autoimmune etiology is supported by immune complex deposition on biopsy, along with frequent findings of circulating autoantibodies (Chapter 3.1). Corticosteroids are indicated for the management of overt renal disease in patients with Sjögren's syndrome. Immunosuppressant therapy is typically associated with a good outcome.

Chronic rejection of a kidney transplant is generally an insidious process developing over months or years, with narrowing of arterioles and chronic interstitial scarring. Antitubular basement membrane antibodies are often detectable in biopsy specimens. The stimulus for the production of these antibodies is presumably antigens within the transplanted kidney. Immunosuppression therapy may slow the process, but rarely prevents progression to advanced renal disease.

Plasma Cell Disorders

Renal failure is a common feature of multiple myeloma and other paraproteinemias because of immunoglobulin light chain toxicity. Other contributing factors include hypercalcemia, hyperuricemia, and an increased susceptibility to infections. The initial manifestations are those of proximal tubular dysfunction: aminoaciduria (urine chemical analysis) and renal tubular acidosis. As the disorder progresses, renal failure develops and may pursue a precipitous course, necessitating dialysis. Pathologic features revealed by renal biopsy include proteinaceous casts, tubular atrophy, and a peritubular inflammatory reaction, with glomerular and peritubular light chain deposits on immunofluorescent staining. Renal amyloid deposition is also frequently detected in myeloma renal disease. The renal failure is usually irreversible, but many patients enjoy a good quality of life on maintenance dialysis.

Granulomatous Nephritis

Sarcoidosis can produce granulomatous tubulointerstitial disease with widespread defects of tubular function. Hypercalcemia and nephrocalcinosis, which may develop in association with sarcoidosis, are further risk factors for tubulointerstitial disease. Corticosteroids have proved useful in reversing this form of renal failure.

Unrecognized tuberculosis of the kidney causes progressive loss of renal parenchyma due to granulomatous replacement of renal tissue. Typical clinical features include flank pain, sterile pyuria, and hematuria. Many patients have an abnormal pyelogram, positive urine cultures, and signs of tuberculosis elsewhere. Prolonged therapy for tuberculosis is required to clear the infection. Granulomatous tubulointerstitial nephritis can also occur in patients with Wegener's granulomatosis and berylliosis and with phenytoin therapy.

Renal Papillary Necrosis

The most common cause of papillary necrosis is diabetes mellitus, particularly when renal parenchymal infection is superimposed. As noted previously, other causes are analgesic nephropathy, sickle cell disease, and obstructive nephropathy.

The vascular supply to the papilla from the vasa recta and the calyceal arteries is tenuous, predisposing to tissue necrosis. Clinical features are varied, ranging from an insidious onset of progressive chronic renal failure to severe flank pain, gross hematuria, and acute renal failure. On occasion, the presenting feature is renal colic, when a sloughed papilla obstructs a ureter. The diagnosis is confirmed by pathognomonic abnormalities on pyelography. The recovery of a sloughed papilla from strained urine samples is also diagnostic.

CYSTIC DISEASES OF THE KIDNEY

Renal cysts occur in several forms of renal disease, some of which are hereditary. Cystic diseases are classified as polycystic, medullary, and acquired. Single cysts within the kidney are often noted as an incidental finding and have been present from birth. They are invariably benign, but enlargement occasionally causes mechanical problems.

Polycystic Kidney Disease

There are two genetically distinct types of polycystic kidney disease. The first, usually presenting in children, is an autosomal recessive disorder occurring in 1 in 14,000 live births. Concomitant cystic disease of the liver is very common, and most patients die in childhood of kidney or liver failure.

The second and much more common type of polycystic kidney disease is an autosomal dominant disorder affecting about 1 in 1000 adults. Men and women are affected equally as often. The genetic defect is on chromosome 16. Clinical manifestations tend not to emerge until adulthood, and in many patients they do not become significant until middle age. The renal cysts are derived from either proximal or distal tubular segments of the nephron and in essence represent a diverticulum along the nephron. Current concepts on the genesis of these cysts indicate that two dominant factors are involved: (1) the epithelial cells forming the wall of the tubule possess an increased capacity to proliferate, and (2) there is a reversed membrane polarity of Na^+K^+-ATPase. These factors in concert lead to cystic tubular dilatation with progressive intracystic fluid and electrolyte accumulation.

Complications of autosomal dominant polycystic kidney disease include episodic flank pain and hematuria from cyst rupture, and cyst infection, hypertension, and renal failure. Cysts may develop in other organs such as the liver, pancreas, and reproductive organs. Various gastrointestinal symptoms may be caused by massive enlargement of the kidneys, which are easily palpable. About 10% of patients with adult polycystic kidney disease have intracranial vascular aneurysms and are at increased risk of intracerebral hemorrhage. Other complications are aortic aneurysms, diverticular disease in the gastrointestinal tract, and cardiac valve regurgitation. Ultrasonography is the best simple screening test for patients and their immediate relatives. It is wise to wait until children are in their late teen or adult years so that kidney growth will make the cystic abnormalities more obvious.

Treatment is directed against complications of the cysts and toward retarding the progression of renal failure by controlling blood pressure and promptly treating parenchymal infections. Many patients ultimately require dialysis. About 10% of all patients undergoing chronic dialysis management have autosomal dominant polycystic kidney disease as their underlying form of renal disease. Renal transplantation is particularly useful in acceptable candidates, although most patients must have their native kidneys removed as a preparatory measure.

Medullary Cystic Kidney Disease

Medullary cystic kidney disease is a heterogeneous group of disorders, the common feature of which is progressive chronic renal failure. Tubular dysfunction often manifests as a salt-wasting syndrome or as an inability to concentrate the urine. Patients can become quickly dehydrated if deprived of adequate fluid or salt intake and can suffer a precipitous decline in renal function. Most patients reach end-stage renal disease as teenagers or young adults. Treatment is with dialysis and renal transplantation after end-stage renal disease has developed.

Acquired Cystic Kidney Disease

Acquired cystic kidney disease is a recently recognized form of renal cystic disease. Most patients who have been on maintenance dialysis for more than 3 years have multiple cysts throughout the kidney, primarily in the cortex. The cysts are probably caused by scars obstructing remnant functioning nephrons, leading to cystic dilatation. Clinical consequences include flank pain, infection, hematuria, retroperitoneal bleeding, and the formation of adenoma or even adenocarcinoma. CT or MRI appears to be more sensitive than sonography in screening for cystic changes in patients on dialysis. These evaluation steps are used only when the patient develops symptoms (flank pain) or signs (gross hematuria) of kidney complications.

SUMMARY

▶ Suspect acute tubulointerstitial nephritis when a patient's renal function deteriorates following infection or drug or toxin exposure or when there is minimal proteinuria and a microscopic urine sediment principally composed of tubular or white cell casts.

▶ Renal function can be restored in patients with acute tubulointerstitial nephritis if the inciting agent is removed promptly; some patients also need short-term corticosteroids.

▶ Suspect chronic tubulointerstitial nephritis in patients with chronic renal failure who have minimal proteinuria and a nonactive microscopic urine sediment or who have renal tubular acidosis. Management includes treating reversible defects and controlling underlying systemic disorders.

▶ Autosomal dominant polycystic disease affects 1 in 1000 adults, often manifesting as end-stage renal disease, typically at age 30–60. Control of hypertension and urinary tract infections can delay the progression of renal impairment.

SUGGESTED READING

Gabow PA: Autosomal dominant polycystic kidney disease (review). N Engl J Med 1993;329:332.

Jones CL, Eddy AA: Tubulointerstitial nephritis (review). Pediatr Nephrol 1992;6:572.

Meeus F, Rossert J, Druet P: Cellular immunity in interstitial nephropathy (review). Ren Fail 1993;15:325.

Wilson PD, Burrow CR: Autosomal dominant polycystic kidney disease: Cellular and molecular mechanisms of cyst formation. Adv Nephrol 1992;21:125.

Kidney Stones

Patricia A. Thomas, MD

Few illnesses present as distinctively and dramatically as renal colic. Managing the patient with kidney stones requires not only acute care for renal colic, but also a careful metabolic assessment and prescription to prevent future stones.

ACUTE MANAGEMENT OF KIDNEY STONES

Clinical Features and Diagnosis

The patient is often a healthy young adult who suddenly develops severe pain, beginning in the flank of the involved side. The pain increases over 15–30 minutes, becoming steady and so excruciating that it can cause nausea and vomiting and can be controlled only by narcotic analgesics. Pain that migrates in a typical pattern, anteriorly along the dermatome into the groin, implies that the stone is moving into the lower third of the ureter. When the stone enters the bladder, the patient may have urgency, frequency, dysuria, and gross hematuria. If the stone has obstructed and infected the urinary tract, the patient may have symptoms of sepsis—fever, shock, and altered mental status.

Urinalysis of a patient with an "active" kidney stone confirms microscopic hematuria and may reveal white blood cells. Examining the urine with a polarizing microscope, the physician may be able to identify crystals of calcium oxalate, uric acid, or brushite. The complete blood count may show a leukocytosis with a left shift, consistent with acute stress or infection. Although gross hematuria presents dramatically, only in rare patients is it severe enough to cause a drop in the hematocrit. Depending on the stone's etiology, the biochemistry panel may show abnormalities of electrolytes, serum calcium, or uric acid. A normal panel does not exclude kidney stones.

The differential diagnosis of acute flank pain includes other causes of visceral pain. Right-sided pain suggests gallbladder disease, appendicitis, and inflammatory bowel disease. Diverticulitis can present with acute left lower quadrant pain. Pelvic inflammatory disease and ectopic pregnancy can present acutely with low pelvic pain on either side. However, patients with all these conditions have voluntary guarding and other physical findings of an "acute abdomen," which are not seen in patients with renal colic. Microscopic hematuria also helps to differentiate stone disease. Other renal conditions such as pyelonephritis and abscess may present with costovertebral angle and flank pain, but the onset of pain is usually more insidious than the sudden pain of stone disease. Unlike renal colic, acute muscular low back pain improves with rest.

Since more than 80% of kidney stones contain calcium, many stones can be visualized with a plain abdominal x-ray, the so-called KUB (kidney, ureter, bladder). The plain film should be followed by an emergency intravenous pyelogram (IVP). The IVP documents the stone's size and location, shows any urinary obstruction, identifies radiolucent stones, and gives an indication of renal function. Renal ultrasonography is less sensitive than IVP for smaller stones. Computed tomography (CT) is sensitive and specific for stones. CT can distinguish radiolucent uric acid stones from blood and other tissue; attenuation numbers from CT may give more information about the type of stone. The major drawbacks of CT are its expense and limited availability.

Treatment

Once a kidney stone is shown to be causing the patient's symptoms, the next question is whether the stone must be removed surgically. If it appears likely that the stone will pass spontaneously, the patient should be made comfortable with analgesia and treated with vigorous hydration. Spontaneous passage is least likely with stones larger than 7 mm, stones that remain in the renal pelvis or upper one-third of the ureter, and calcium oxalate stones, which tend to be spicular. Surgery is indicated if the patient presents with sepsis, intractable pain, or renal obstruction, which after 72 hours can cause permanent nephron loss.

Acknowledgment: Michael A. Levine, MD, consulted in the preparation of this chapter.

Several nonsurgical techniques are available to remove stones. Fewer than 5% of all patients now require open surgery. A stone's location and size determine how it is removed. Stones lodged in the upper two-thirds of the ureter are best treated with extracorporeal shock-wave lithotripsy (see below). Stones lodged above the pelvic brim are pushed back into the renal pelvis by an endoscope and then treated with lithotripsy. Most stones in the lower third of the ureter can be retrieved with an endoscopic basket.

Lithotripsy succeeds in fragmenting 80% of stones that are less than 2 cm in diameter. Larger stones require a combination of lithotripsy and removal by percutaneous nephrolithotomy. It is important to remove all fragments of infected stones. Large staghorn calculi, which involve the renal pelvis, require open surgical removal.

Introduced in 1984, the extracorporeal shock-wave lithotriptor focuses high-intensity shock waves on the kidney to break stones into smaller fragments that are easier to pass. Although it obviates open surgery, lithotripsy does require sedation or anesthesia and can cause significant complications, including pain, perinephric hematoma, pancreatitis, urosepsis, and a rise in blood pressure. Stone fragments from lithotripsy sometimes form an obstructive column in the ureter (*steinstrasse*). As much as 20% of patients receiving lithotripsy need an additional procedure, such as a second lithotripsy or percutaneous nephrolithotomy.

Once a stone is gone—either passing spontaneously or removed—most patients' renal colic disappears, although some patients continue to have vague flank pain for days to weeks. However, kidney stone disease is a chronic illness: Fifty percent of first-time stone formers will pass another stone within 5 years. Thus, the next phase of management is prevention. To prescribe appropriate preventive treatment, the physician must identify the metabolic disorder that led to the patient's stone.

PATHOGENESIS OF KIDNEY STONES

Theories of Stone Formation

Kidney stones are the end point of several metabolic pathways that result in various salts crystallizing in urine. Altering the urine alters the ease with which a salt remains dissolved. For example, changing the pH affects dissociation of ions, changing the volume of solute affects the salt's concentration, and adding a "seed" can anchor and promote the formation of crystals.

The urine of most healthy people is supersaturated with calcium oxalate, so it is not surprising that calcium oxalate is the most common type of stone. People who do not form stones are believed to be protected by natural properties of the urine and the lining of the urine collecting system.

Several theories of stone formation have been suggested. The most common is the nucleation theory, which supposes that a foreign body or another crystal serves as a nucleus around which a crystal lattice grows in urine that is supersaturated with the salt of the second crystal. In supersaturated solutions, calcium oxalate can form clusters that eventually become the nidus of a crystal. Uric acid is often thought to be the nucleus for calcium oxalate crystals; for this reason, recurrent formers of calcium stones may be successfully treated with uric acid-lowering therapy.

Another proposed mechanism of stone formation suggests that an organic matrix of proteins, such as abnormal Tamm-Horsfall urinary proteins, aggregates and becomes the framework for crystal formation.

Lastly, stones may form when the urine has abnormally low levels of such natural inhibitors of crystallization as citrate and magnesium and of such kidney proteins as nephrocalcin and uropontin. Low concentrations of these inhibitors—for example, the hypocitraturia that accompanies acidotic states—promotes stone formation.

Types of Stones

Calcium-Containing Stones: The most common stones are made of calcium oxalate (Table 5.8–1). Many patients with calcium oxalate stone disease have hypercalciuria from any of a number of causes (Table 5.8–2). Between 30% and 60% of patients with calcium oxalate stones have hypercalciuria but a normal serum calcium. Hypercalciuria (greater than 200 mg per day) promotes stones not only by increasing the calcium concentration in the urine, but also by reducing natural inhibitors of stone formation.

The most common form of hypercalciuria is absorptive hypercalciuria, found in 50% of patients with calcium oxalate stones. Absorptive hypercalciuria affects men and

Table 5.8–1. Composition of kidney stones.

Composition	% of Patients	Causes
Calcium stones		
Calcium oxalate	60	Hypercalciuria, hypocitraturia, hyperoxaluria, hyperuricosuria, acid urine
Hydroxyapatite	20	Hypercalciuria, hypocitraturia, hyperuricosuria
Brushite	2	Hypercalciuria, hypocitraturia, hyperuricosuria
Non-calcium stones		
Uric acid	7	Hyperuricosuria, acid urine
Struvite	7	Infection with urea-splitting organism
Cystine	3	Cystinuria
Triamterene	<1	Triamterene therapy
2,8-dihydroxyadenine	<1	2,8-dihydroxyadeninuria
Silica	<1	Trisilicate therapy

Modified and reproduced, with permission, from Pak CYC: Etiology and treatment of urolithiasis. Am J Kidney Dis 1991;18:624.

Table 5.8–2. Causes of hypercalciuria, and laboratory findings in patients with no dietary calcium restriction.

Cause	Parathyroid hormone	Calcitriol	% of Patients
Idiopathic hypercalciuria			
Absorptive hypercalciuria	Normal/↓	↑	80
Renal calcium leak	↑	↑	5–10
Primary hyperparathyroidism	↑	↑	5–10
Renal tubular acidosis	Normal	Normal	2–5
Other diseases	Normal/↓	Variable	<10

women equally. Many of the patients have a family history of stones, usually with autosomal dominant inheritance. The mechanism of absorptive hypercalciuria is abnormally high absorption of calcium from the intestine, particularly after meals. In normal people, calcium is absorbed primarily in the duodenum and jejunum via a vitamin D-dependent mechanism. Most patients with idiopathic hypercalciuria have elevated levels of calcitriol (1,25-dihydroxyvitamin D), the active form of vitamin D, which increases intestinal calcium absorption and suppresses parathyroid hormone secretion. Patients with absorptive hypercalciuria type I show a marked increase in urinary calcium (greater than 0.20 mg of urinary calcium per mg of urinary creatinine) when they increase their calcium intake; patients with type II show normal urinary calcium (less than 200 mg per day) on a restricted diet.

A second type of hypercalciuria is renal hypercalciuria, caused by a so-called "renal calcium leak," which is a renal tubular defect in the reabsorption of urinary calcium. This loss of calcium causes increased secretion of parathyroid hormone, which can lead to hypophosphatemia and increased synthesis of calcitriol. More calcium is absorbed from the intestine, and bone resorption may be accelerated. Many patients give a history of preceding urinary tract infection, which may damage the renal parenchyma, leading to the tubular defect. The urinary calcium in these patients is elevated both in the fasting state and on a calcium-restricted diet; their serum parathyroid hormone and calcitriol levels may be elevated.

Primary hyperparathyroidism (Chapter 4.6) also causes hypercalciuria, but accounts for only about 5% of stone disease. Increased serum parathyroid hormone increases calcium absorption in the intestine, increases calcium resorption from bone, and thereby increases the filtered load of urinary calcium. Serum parathyroid hormone also increases renal tubular reabsorption of calcium, but this effect is overcome by the increased filtered load of calcium. Patients with primary hyperparathyroidism have a high urinary calcium despite fasting and restricted calcium intake. Their serum calcium should be high, their serum phosphate may be low, and their serum parathyroid hormone is high.

About 10% of patients with hypercalciuria have another metabolic disorder identified as causative. This might be sarcoidosis, thyrotoxicosis, metastatic cancer, Paget's disease, lymphoma, multiple myeloma, immobilization, or milk-alkali syndrome. Other risk factors for hypercalciuria are high intake of sodium, protein, or glucose, and low phosphate levels.

Another cause of calcium stones is hyperuricosuria, found in 20% of calcium stone formers. Increased uric acid in the urine can come from eating purines (in poultry, meat, and fish) or from increased endogenous production, as is found in gouty patients (Chapter 3.8). The pKa of uric acid is 5.75. In acid urine, uric acid is primarily undissociated; thus, it is less soluble than the salt and contributes to stone formation. Urine is more acid than normal in renal tubular acidosis and chronic diarrheal states, but patients may have normal serum uric acid levels.

Hyperoxaluria (greater than 44 mg per day) can be caused by congenital disease that presents in childhood or can be acquired by eating too much oxalate (in tea, chocolate, nuts, citrus fruits, and certain green leafy vegetables) and oxalate precursors such as ascorbic acid (more than 500 mg/day of vitamin C). Oxalate absorption from the large bowel is increased in inflammatory bowel disease, jejunoileal bypass, and chronic biliary disease. The mechanism for this enteric hyperoxaluria is fat malabsorption; free fatty acids bind calcium in the gut, decrease calcium absorption, and increase the free oxalate available for intestinal absorption.

Hypocitraturia (below 320 mg per day), another important cause of calcium stone formation, occurs in acidosis. Acidosis increases renal tubular absorption of citrate and impairs citrate production. Hypocitraturia is seen in patients with renal tubular acidosis or intestinal malabsorption syndromes, in patients with low urine volume, and in patients taking diuretics or eating large amounts of red meat.

Non-Calcium-Containing Stones: The most common type of noncalcium stone is the uric acid stone. It can be caused by increased uric acid in the urine or by increased urinary acidity (pH below 5.5), which promotes crystal formation. About 10–25% of gouty patients form uric acid stones. Although some patients with gout are hyperuricemic because of decreased urate clearance, the gouty patients who form stones are overproducers and overexcreters of uric acid. These patients typically have an acidic urine of unknown etiology and urate overproduction, with a 24-hour urinary uric acid level above 1000 mg. The rate at which gouty patients form stones relates to their serum uric acid level. As noted above, normouricemic patients with increased urine acidity can also develop uric acid stones.

Struvite stones, a complex of magnesium-ammonium phosphate and carbonate apatite, have been identified in patients who have chronic urinary tract infections with urea-splitting bacteria, commonly *Proteus,* but also *Pseudomonas, Klebsiella,* and some staphylococci. The hallmark of struvite stones is urine that has been made alkaline by these organisms' urea metabolism. Many patients with struvite stones have other metabolic abnormalities that promote stone formation, and the stones may trigger the chronic urinary tract infection. These patients should be fully evaluated for a metabolic cause of their stones. Staghorn calculi, with their typical "ginger root" appearance, are usually made of struvite.

About 3% of noncalcareous stones are cystine, resulting from an autosomal recessive disorder that causes defective renal tubular reabsorption of cystine, ornithine, lysine, and arginine. Healthy people do not excrete any cystine. Heterozygotes for the inherited disorder, usually presenting in adulthood, excrete 0–300 mg of cystine/24 hr; homozygotes, usually presenting as children, excrete over 600 mg/24 hr. Another rare metabolic disorder, 2,8-dihydroxyadeninuria, causes stones of 2,8-dihydroxyadenine. The diuretic triamterene can produce triamterene stones, and antacids containing trisilicate can produce silica stones.

DETERMINING RISK FOR FUTURE STONES

How to evaluate a patient with kidney stones depends on how the patient presents (Table 5.8–3). A basic metabolic evaluation is recommended for all first-time stone formers. A more extensive evaluation is recommended for patients with multiple stones or recurrent stones despite therapy, as well as for patients at increased risk, for example, because of having only one kidney.

The basic evaluation for first-time stone formers begins in the emergency room or doctor's office with a comprehensive history, which may reveal predisposing factors such as gouty arthritis, chronic diarrhea, or a family history of stones. The physical exam may reveal endocrinopathy, skeletal disease, malignancy, or infection. Laboratory tests include serum electrolytes, creatinine, calcium, phosphorus, uric acid, urinalysis, and urine culture. If cystine crystals are found on urinalysis, a qualitative cystine screen may be indicated, although the yield is low. Every effort should be made to retrieve and analyze stones that have been passed. The IVP should be used to determine the anatomy of the collecting system, search for

Table 5.8–3. Metabolic evaluation of the stone former.

Simple evaluation
  Biochemical screen
  Urinalysis and culture
  Qualitative cystine screen
  Stone analysis, if available
  Intravenous pyelogram

Extensive evaluation
  Two 24-hour urine collections for volume, pH, calcium,
    phosphorus, sodium, uric acid, oxalate, citrate, creatinine
  Third collection on restricted calcium (400 mg), sodium
    (100 mEq), and oxalate diet
  Serial measurement of urine pH

Modified and reproduced, with permission, from Pak CYC: Etiology and treatment of urolithiasis. Am J Kidney Dis 1991;18:624.

other stones, and document that both kidneys are functioning.

This evaluation identifies a cause in about 40–50% of stone formers. Hypercalcemia suggests primary hyperparathyroidism, which should be confirmed by parathyroid hormone assay. Abnormal electrolytes suggest renal tubular acidosis. A gouty diathesis presents with arthropathy and hyperuricemia. The remainder of stone formers have some form of hypercalciuria, the specific etiology of which requires further testing.

Children with stones, and adults who have multiple stones or suffer a second stone within 1 year, should undergo a more extensive metabolic evaluation. In addition to the basic tests listed above, patients should have two 24-hour urine collections made while on a free diet and free fluid intake, preferably at least 4 weeks after the stone is removed. Each collection should be tested for volume, pH, calcium, phosphorus, sodium, uric acid, oxalate, citrate, and creatinine. If the initial urine pH was above 5.5, the physician should exclude renal tubular acidosis by giving the patient a roll of nitrazine paper with which to record serial urine pH values. Once hypercalciuria is documented, only patients who are not responding to secondary treatments (see "Secondary Prevention" below) need more sophisticated urine tests while on restricted and 1-g calcium diets.

SECONDARY PREVENTION

Secondary prevention reduces the need for later invasive treatment. One general recommendation is to drink more fluids, generally to double urine output or increase it to 3 L/day. However, no controlled studies have been done to support this recommendation, and the threshold of hydration that prevents stones may be much lower. Sodium restriction to 100 mEq/day is also recommended, since high sodium intake can increase urinary calcium excretion.

More specific preventive treatments are based on the presumed cause of the stone. Prevention of calcium oxalate stones caused by metabolic disease relies on treatment of the underlying disorder. Patients with primary hyperparathyroidism and kidney stones should undergo parathyroidectomy. Idiopathic calcium stone disease is treated by decreasing the urine calcium concentration or increasing calcium solubility. Efforts to decrease intestinal calcium absorption in patients with absorptive hypercalciuria have focused on a low-calcium diet and giving sodium cellulose phosphate to bind calcium in the gut. But there are no controlled trials of these treatments. Sodium cellulose phosphate increases urinary oxalate excretion and may worsen bone mineral loss in patients who are already in negative calcium balance. Since sodium cellulose phosphate works only if it is taken with every meal, this drug has not been widely used.

Thiazide diuretics are a more practical treatment for hypercalciuria, whether the increased urine calcium excretion results from intestinal hyperabsorption or renal tubular loss. Thiazides decrease intestinal calcium absorption and markedly reduce renal calcium excretion. If necessary, thiazides may be given with potassium citrate to treat hypocitraturia and the hypokalemia that the thiazide causes. Patients who cannot tolerate thiazides may respond to orthophosphate, which reduces intestinal calcium absorption and calcitriol synthesis.

Treatment for enteric hyperoxaluria is to reduce dietary fat and oxalate, increase fluid intake, and take oral citrate supplements, calcium supplements to precipitate oxalate in the intestinal lumen, and cholestyramine to bind fatty acids, bile acids, and oxalate.

Renal tubular acidosis and hypocitraturia are treated with potassium citrate, which corrects the acidosis as well as hypokalemia and low urinary citrate. The result is a mild increase in urine pH, increased urinary citrate, and decreased urinary calcium.

Hyperuricosuria has been linked to both calcium stones and uric acid stones. The goals of treatment for hyperuricosuria are to decrease the urinary uric acid concentration by increasing hydration and to increase the ratio of urate to uric acid load with allopurinol, which inhibits formation of uric acid from purine degradation. In calcium stone formers, allopurinol has been shown to reduce the recurrence of stones. Potassium citrate is used to alkalinize the urine. Patients should also be instructed to eat less meat, fish, and poultry, which are rich in purines. This regimen may prevent pure uric acid stones. Increasing the urine pH can also be effective treatment for already-formed uric acid stones. Potassium citrate raises the urine pH to over 6.8 and leads to the formation of potassium urate, which is far more soluble than uric acid or sodium urate. Uric acid stones, unlike calcium oxalate stones, readily dissolve in this alkaline urine.

Because it is difficult to decrease dietary intake of cystine precursors, initial treatment for cystinuria is high fluid intake and use of an alkalinizing agents like potassium citrate to raise the urinary pH above 7.0 and increase solubility. If this regimen does not work, penicillamine can be added. Penicillamine works by complexing with cysteine, a precursor of cystine. The product is more soluble than cystine. *N*-acetylcysteine given by percutaneous nephrostomy can directly bathe a stone and cause chemolysis.

Recurrent infectious stones can be prevented if infection is controlled, but this requires removing the initial stones with either lithotripsy or percutaneous nephrolithotomy. If possible, other foreign bodies in the urinary tract (eg, catheters) should also be removed. Acetohydroxamic acid, a urease inhibitor, has been shown to prevent stone growth and may cause dissolution of existing stones. However, this agent can cause significant complications, including hemolytic anemia, deep vein thrombosis, and tremor.

Preventive treatment is lifelong. Physicians should monitor patients every 4–6 months for adherence with and response to treatment.

SUMMARY

▶ Managing a patient with kidney stones requires removing the stone that is currently causing symptoms, determining the risk of recurrence, and treating to prevent more stones.

▶ Whether a stone will pass spontaneously or need removal depends on its size, location, and chemical composition, best determined by intravenous pyelography.

▶ To prevent future stones, the physician should analyze passed stones and should test and treat patients for metabolic disorders such as hypercalciuria, primary hyperparathyroidism, renal tubular acidosis, and gout.

SUGGESTED READING

Coe FL, Parks JH, Asplin JR: The pathogenesis and treatment of kidney stones. N Engl J Med 1992;327:1141.

Consensus Conference: Prevention and treatment of kidney stones. JAMA 1988;260:977.

Levy FL, Adams-Huet B, Pak CYC: Ambulatory evaluation of nephrolithiasis: An update of a 1980 protocol. Am J Med 1995;98:50.

Pak CYC: Etiology and treatment of urolithiasis. Am J Kidney Dis 1991;18:624.

Renovascular Hypertension

Paul K. Whelton, MD, MSc, and Michael J. Klag, MD, MPH

Renovascular hypertension differs from essential hypertension in its rarity, cause, and potential for cure. Renovascular hypertension arises from adaptive hormonal responses to a stenosis-induced decrease in blood flow to the kidneys. In patients who have a stenosis of a renal artery, the reduced renal blood flow triggers renin release, which in turn leads to an excess of circulating angiotensin II. The clinical consequences are vasoconstriction, hyperaldosteronism, volume expansion, and hypertension.

CLINICAL PRESENTATION

Several features in the history and physical examination suggest that hypertension is renovascular, but no finding is definitive (Table 5.9–1). Renovascular disease is more likely when hypertension begins unusually early (before age 35) or late (after 60). It is also more likely in patients who have no family history of hypertension and in those whose hypertension is severe, abrupt in onset, recently worsened, or difficult to control. In two-thirds of patients, renal artery disease is caused by atherosclerosis; in the remaining one-third, the cause is fibromuscular disease. Atherosclerotic lesions are more common in men, especially older men and those with other risk factors for atherosclerosis. In contrast, fibromuscular lesions are more common in women and often manifest during the third and fourth decades. Fibromuscular disease is rare in blacks.

The most specific finding on physical examination is an abdominal bruit, particularly a high-pitched, continuous (systolic and diastolic) bruit that radiates from the mid-abdomen to the flank or back. Such a bruit can be heard in at least one-third of patients with renovascular hypertension, but is rare in those with essential hypertension. For this reason, the physician should always auscultate the abdomen when examining patients with hypertension. Carotid and femoral bruits suggest widespread atherosclerosis, a common accompaniment of renovascular hypertension. Funduscopic abnormalities and a left ventricular

heave may also be found, especially in patients who present with severe or poorly controlled hypertension.

Suggestive laboratory features include hypokalemia from secondary aldosteronism, and proteinuria or an elevated serum creatinine level from kidney damage. The physician should also be suspicious when a patient starts taking an angiotensin converting enzyme inhibitor and has an abrupt increase in serum creatinine.

Types of Renovascular Disease

Renovascular hypertension arises from renal ischemia caused by either an atherosclerotic or a fibromuscular stenosis in one or both renal arteries. Stenoses are more common in the right kidney than the left. About 25% of patients have bilateral lesions. Disease confined to small branch vessels is usually caused by fibromuscular dysplasia, whereas most atherosclerotic lesions are in the proximal third of the main renal artery. Many atherosclerotic plaques begin in the aorta but encroach on the orifice of the renal artery (Figure 5.9–1).

Fibromuscular stenoses, which are usually found in the mid to distal part of the main renal artery, can be divided into four subtypes that have different natural histories. (1) About 70% of patients with fibromuscular disease have medial fibroplasia (Figure 5.9–2). On angiography, it resembles a string of beads. Medial fibroplasia rarely progresses to complete occlusion of the vessel. (2) Perimedial fibroplasia, which accounts for about 20% of cases, is also bead-like but more severely narrows the lumen, on occasion completely occluding the vessel. Two rarer forms of renal artery disease, (3) medial hyperplasia and (4) intimal fibroplasia, usually present as ring-like stenoses. They can follow a progressive course complicated by intimal dissection and renal thrombosis or embolism.

CONFIRMING THE DIAGNOSIS

Most patients who have any of the features listed in Table 5.9–1 should be evaluated for renovascular hypertension, provided that they are candidates for renal revas-

Table 5.9–1. Routine clinical and laboratory features suggesting renovascular hypertension.

History
  Onset of hypertension before age 35 or after 60
  No family history of hypertension
  Severe hypertension of recent onset
  Worsening of previously controlled hypertension

Physical examination
  Abdominal bruit
  Retinopathy

Laboratory findings
  Hypokalemia
  Proteinuria
  Elevated serum creatinine after starting treatment with an
    angiotensin converting enzyme inhibitor

cularization. Traditionally, noninvasive tests have been used for screening, and more invasive tests have been reserved for patients who screen positive. Today, many physicians skip the noninvasive tests and go right to invasive renal vascular studies because some of them can now be done safely in outpatients.

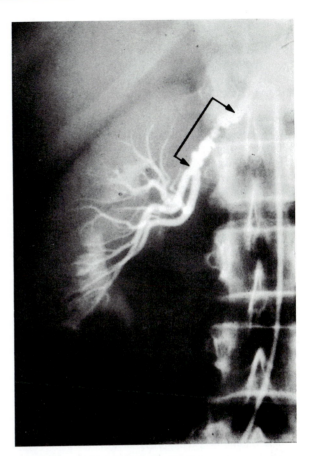

Figure 5.9–2. Renal arteriographic appearance of the medial fibroplasia form of renal fibromuscular disease. The stenosis (arrows) looks like an irregular string of beads in the mid to distal part of the right renal artery.

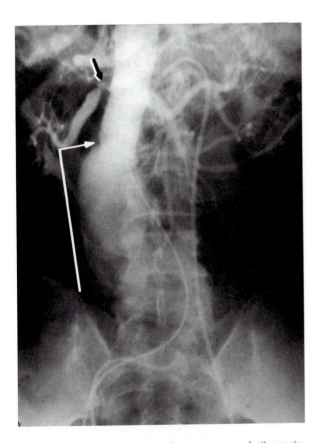

Figure 5.9–1. Renal arteriographic appearance of atherosclerotic stenosis (short black arrow) in the orifice of the right renal artery. The left renal artery is not visible at all, indicating total occlusion. Irregularity in the aortic wall is compatible with atherosclerosis. The long white arrow points to a distal aortic aneurysm.

Noninvasive tests include hypertensive pyelography, isotope renography, and the captopril test. In the hypertensive (rapid sequence) pyelogram, findings consistent with renovascular hypertension are a delay in the appearance or excretion of dye in one kidney, and a discrepancy of at least 2 cm between the lengths of the kidneys. The sensitivity and specificity of hypertensive pyelography are only about 60–70%. Isotope renography is no more accurate; this procedure is probably best reserved for patients who are not candidates for a contrast study. Lastly, a decline in plasma renin and blood pressure after administration of captopril has been advocated as a noninvasive test for renovascular hypertension, but this procedure is time-consuming and also probably no better than a hypertensive pyelogram.

The three invasive options are renal arteriography and arterial and venous digital subtraction angiography. Blood pressure should be controlled before patients undergo any of these tests. Renal arteriography is the gold standard for diagnosing renal artery stenosis. In this test, a cannula is advanced into the renal artery, and serial x-rays are taken of the renal arteries as they fill with radiocontrast dye. Renal arteriography is the best way to detect stenosis in branch vessels, but it can miss disease at the renal artery orifice. Although the procedure does not require much dye, it is the most invasive diagnostic option and requires hospital admission. This method is most useful for young patients with suspected fibromuscular disease.

Arterial subtraction angiography and venous digital subtraction angiography are two alternatives that do not require insertion of a catheter into the renal artery and that can be done in outpatients. In these tests, the dye is usually injected into the femoral artery or vein. Vascular anatomy is highlighted by elimination of background radiographic images. Digital subtraction angiography is good at detecting stenosis near the renal artery orifice, but not as good at detecting disease in branch vessels. Arterial digital angiography is the procedure of choice for most elderly patients with atherosclerosis. Although arterial angiography is more invasive than corresponding venous studies, it requires less dye and provides better x-rays. Typically, arterial angiography is almost as accurate as renal arteriography, with less morbidity; in some reports, its sensitivity and specificity have exceeded 90%. Venous digital angiography is the least sensitive and specific method; the x-rays do not always have adequate resolution and they may miss lesions in branch vessels. Furthermore, venous angiography requires so much dye as to pose concern for older patients and those with renal insufficiency.

The finding of a renal artery stenosis does not definitively answer the question, "Is this patient's hypertension caused by renal ischemia?" This can be clarified by concurrent sampling of peripheral and renal venous blood at the time of angiography to measure plasma renin activity. Higher plasma renin activity in renal than in peripheral veins implies that the renal artery stenosis is affecting kidney function. Such higher plasma renin activity levels in renal veins are most prominent early in the disease. Later, ischemic damage to the kidneys leads to salt and water retention, expansion of intravascular volume, and a compensatory decline in plasma renin levels. Ischemic renal artery stenosis is strongly suggested when the plasma renin level is more than 50% higher in the vein draining the involved kidney than in the lower inferior vena cava or in the vein of the uninvolved kidney. The greater the discrepancy between renin levels in the affected and unaffected kidneys, the greater the chance of renal artery ischemia. The diagnosis is even more certain when the patient's peripheral vein plasma renin activity level is also high. Stimulating the renin-angiotensin system with a diuretic may accentuate the difference in renal vein plasma renin activity levels and improve the test's accuracy.

A diagnosis of renovascular hypertension can usually be confirmed by the combination of digital subtraction angiography and renal vein renin measurements, but these tests are not foolproof. In a few patients, one or both tests are negative despite suspicious clinical findings. Patients with renovascular hypertension may benefit from a repeat study with diuretic preparation; those with a high-grade stenosis and renal insufficiency deserve special scrutiny. Rarely, even though renovascular hypertension cannot be established preoperatively, revascularization is warranted to preserve renal function.

MANAGEMENT

An antihypertensive drug regimen that includes an angiotensin converting enzyme (ACE) inhibitor normalizes the blood pressure in most patients with renovascular hypertension. Most patients with uncomplicated unilateral renal artery stenosis tolerate ACE inhibitors well, but an occasional patient suffers a rapid deterioration in kidney function. For this reason, patients' renal function should be checked before they start ACE inhibitor therapy and again 1 and 7 days after. The drug-related decline in renal function reverses quickly when the drug is stopped. Beta-blockers are less effective inhibitors of the renin-angiotensin system, but they are the best alternative for patients in whom ACE inhibitors are contraindicated or poorly tolerated.

After the diagnosis of renovascular hypertension has been confirmed and the patient's blood pressure has been controlled, the physician should consider revascularizing the ischemic kidney by percutaneous transluminal angioplasty or surgery. Revascularization cures most patients with fibromuscular lesions and improves the hypertension in most patients with atherosclerotic lesions. Angioplasty is preferred because it is as effective as surgery but less invasive. Angioplasty can be performed under local anesthesia. A catheter is threaded through the artery across the stenosis, and an intraluminal balloon is inflated to open the vessel. Most lesions in the main renal artery can be dilated satisfactorily. Lesions at the orifice of the renal artery are often extensions of a larger aortic plaque and tend to recur soon after angioplasty. A vascular surgeon should be consulted before angioplasty and should be available to operate, if needed. In occasional patients, the catheter damages the renal or femoral arteries, which must be repaired surgically.

Surgery is the treatment of choice for relatively healthy patients in whom angioplasty has been unsuccessful or is technically infeasible. During surgery, every effort should be made to preserve renal mass. However, final decisions about whether to perform a revascularization procedure, segmental resection, or nephrectomy can be made only at the operating table.

When both angioplasty and surgery are impracticable or not completely successful, patients require long-term treatment with antihypertensive drugs. The goal in these patients should be to normalize blood pressure and ensure stability of renal function.

SUMMARY

▶ Atherosclerotic or fibromuscular narrowing of the renal arteries often causes a severe but potentially reversible form of hypertension.

▶ Clinical features suggesting renovascular hypertension include abrupt onset of severe or worsened hypertension in white women younger than 35 years and in men older than 60, and a bruit over the abdomen, flank, or back.

▶ The diagnosis of renal artery stenosis can be usually confirmed with a digital subtraction angiogram and measurements of renal vein plasma renin activity.

▶ After the blood pressure is controlled, most patients with renovascular hypertension can be cured by percutaneous transluminal angioplasty or surgery to open the stenosis.

SUGGESTED READING

Davidson RA, Wilcox CS: Newer tests for the diagnosis of renovascular disease. JAMA 1992;268:3353.

Kaplan NM: Renal vascular hypertension. In: *Clinical Hypertension,* 5th ed. Kaplan NM (editor). Williams & Wilkins, 1990.

Rimmer JM, Gennari FJ: Atherosclerotic renovascular disease and progressive renal failure. Ann Intern Med 1993;118:712.

Vidt DG: The diagnosis of renovascular hypertension: A clinician's viewpoint. Am J Hypertens 1991;4:663S.

Working Group on Renovascular Hypertension: Detection, evaluation, and treatment of renovascular hypertension: Final report. Arch Intern Med 1987;147:820.

Section 6

Gastroenterology

John D. Stobo, MD, Section Editor

6.1

Approach to the Patient
With a Gastrointestinal Disorder

Theodore M. Bayless, MD

Most digestive tract disorders are successfully managed by primary care physicians. A gastroenterologist can help direct the diagnostic work-up of patients with complex symptoms of gastrointestinal disease, since many of these features are nonspecific and can be worsened or otherwise changed by environmental or psychological factors. A gastroenterologist may also advise on management of complex illnesses like ulcerative colitis and difficult-to-treat problems like gastroesophageal reflux that does not respond to the usual antacid or H_2-receptor antagonist (H_2 blocker) therapy. For some complicated illnesses such as Crohn's disease and advanced liver disease, the gastroenterologist may best serve as the primary physician, bringing specialized knowledge and experience to the timing and use of expensive medications and institutional resources.

Six principles describe the evaluation and management of most digestive tract disorders:

1. Approach the differential diagnosis recognizing that the gastrointestinal tract has a limited repertoire of symptoms with which to react to many types of dysfunction.
2. Determine the organ of origin and the pathophysiologic derangements causing the patient's symptoms.
3. Establish a specific diagnosis whenever possible.
4. Be alert to the difficulty of distinguishing organic from "functional" digestive tract disease.
5. Set reasonable long-term therapeutic goals. Treat as specifically as possible, and consider the role of surgical as well as medical treatment.
6. Build a partnership with the patient. Many gastrointestinal disorders are chronic; continued communication and patient education are important to successful management.

This chapter elaborates on the six principles, drawing examples from later chapters of the "Gastroenterology" section. Because some gastrointestinal symptoms overlap disease boundaries, this section is organized primarily around the evaluation of some symptoms and signs: swallowing disorders, abdominal pain (including peptic ulcer and dyspepsia), gastrointestinal bleeding, infections, and diarrhea (see also Chapters 6.7 and 8.7). Other chapters are devoted to gastrointestinal cancers, malabsorption, and inflammatory bowel disease (Crohn's disease and ulcerative colitis). Each chapter tries to outline a logical, direct approach to diagnosis, with the goals of minimizing patient discomfort and expense, treating specifically, and managing these often chronic diseases over the long term.

DIFFERENTIATE AMONG THE MANY DISORDERS PRODUCING THE LIMITED RANGE OF GASTROINTESTINAL SYMPTOMS

In approaching the differential diagnosis, the physician must recognize that the gastrointestinal tract has a limited repertoire of symptoms with which to respond to dysfunction: pain, difficulty swallowing, bleeding, nausea, vomiting, anorexia, weight loss, bloating, and diarrhea. Differentiating among the many possible causes of these symptoms is challenging, and the task is made more difficult by the nongastrointestinal disorders that can also cause many of these symptoms. For example, the pain of diffuse esophageal spasm is often mistaken for that of myocardial infarction. Furthermore, pain can be "referred" to a site distant from the actual source of disease. For example, at least 25% of patients with dysphagia (difficulty swallowing) who point to the upper neck as the site where their food sticks are found to have a lesion in the lower esophagus. A carcinoma originating in the sigmoid colon may cause distention of the splenic flexure area of the colon and pain under the ribs in the left upper quadrant, leading the patient and the unwary physician to suspect an upper gastrointestinal or even cardiac problem.

DETERMINE THE ORGAN OF ORIGIN AND THE PATHOPHYSIOLOGIC DERANGEMENT CAUSING SYMPTOMS

With some disorders, such as cancer of the colon or pancreas, symptoms appear only late in the course. With other disorders, such as gastroesophageal reflux, symptoms begin early in the course.

Often the physician can ask a series of questions in the history and physical examination to help determine which organ is involved and what the dysfunction might be. The skilled physician helps patients describe the nature, location, and course of their symptoms—often a much more valuable diagnostic tool than a series of invasive, expensive tests.

For example, when patients have lost weight, the physician should ask about their appetite and what they are eating. Weight loss despite a "normal" appetite raises the possibility of hypermetabolism such as hyperthyroidism or the disordered metabolism of diabetes mellitus or intestinal malabsorption. Not eating enough calories may be obvious, or may require questioning or, for inpatients, observation of food trays by someone attuned to nutritional requirements. Patients who have repeatedly lost and regained large amounts of weight may be depressed or have another psychological condition.

As another example, dysphagia is usually caused by an organic disorder that should be diagnosable. If liquid regurgitates through the nose or the patient chokes (aspirates) while swallowing, the physician should suspect cranial nerve dysfunction, as might follow a cerebrovascular accident. The occasional transient sticking of a piece of meat in the esophagus suggests esophageal spasm or perhaps a borderline obstruction secondary to a peptic stricture or lower esophageal ring. Cold liquids seem to aggravate esophageal spasm, whereas warm liquids may give temporary relief. Progressive worsening of dysphagia—beginning with difficulty in swallowing solids, later soft foods, and eventually liquids—suggests gradual narrowing of the lumen, as by a cancer or a benign peptic stricture. Patients with achalasia may have trouble with both liquids and solids; they may also describe undigested food or liquid on their pillow in the morning. Other patients tell of "always" eating slowly or of learning to drink carbonated beverages so they can force the esophageal contents through an incompletely relaxing lower esophageal sphincter. Extremely painful swallowing (odynophagia) suggests that the esophageal lining is ulcerated, as might happen with drug-induced esophagitis (caused, for example, by tetracycline, quinidine, or nonsteroidal anti-

inflammatory drugs) or with an ulcerating infection (eg, *Candida,* and herpetic esophagitis).

The diagnostic search can be aided by the family history. Whenever a patient's close relative has a history of a gastrointestinal disorder, that disorder should be considered in the patient and other family members, who should be sought and evaluated. Potentially lethal but treatable inherited gastrointestinal conditions include colon cancer, familial polyposis, hemochromatosis, Wilson's disease, and the multiple endocrine neoplasia (MEN) syndromes. Likewise, about 20% of patients with Crohn's disease or ulcerative colitis seem to have an inherited tendency to the disease. The physician should suspect Crohn's disease after eliciting a family history of the disease from a young patient with arthritis, unexplained fever, or perianal disease. Some patients may also inherit a tendency to peptic ulcer, especially in a virulent form.

A medication history and a dietary history are also important. For example, medications such as nonsteroidal anti-inflammatory drugs can aggravate both upper gastrointestinal problems such as gastroesophageal reflux or peptic ulcer and colonic problems, most often ulcerative colitis. Undigested food components such as lactose and fructose may worsen the symptoms of irritable bowel or cause symptoms on their own.

ESTABLISH A SPECIFIC DIAGNOSIS WHENEVER POSSIBLE

Physicians are often able to put together the puzzle of the patient's symptoms by confirming their clinical suspicions with judicious use of tests. One of the satisfying aspects of managing gastrointestinal disease is learning the pathophysiologic basis for the patient's complaints, then confirming a clinical diagnosis using endoscopy, radiography, and pathology.

The means available to establish a specific diagnosis have increased dramatically since the late 1970's. Fiberoptic endoscopy permits visualization and biopsy of the esophagus, stomach, duodenum, terminal ileum, and colon. Enteroscopes almost complete the tour of the gastrointestinal tract by allowing visualization of at least 50% of the small intestine, including most of the jejunum and varying amounts of the ileum. Endoscopic ultrasonography allows direct evaluation and staging of distal esophageal, duodenal, pancreatic, and perirectal lesions.

Radiographic contrast studies of the upper and lower gastrointestinal tract can help identify early mucosal lesions, often at a treatable or curable stage. Cine barium swallows permit detailed analysis of complex dysphagia problems, such as those involving both cranial nerve defects and organic pharyngeal lesions. Sonography of the gallbladder is now the standard study for gallstones. High-resolution sonography can also detect acute appendicitis with high sensitivity and specificity. Nuclear medicine gastric emptying studies have become the standard for evaluating delayed gastric emptying and gastroparesis, as well as for studying esophageal and bile duct emptying. Nucleotide-tagged red blood cells can be used to mark an otherwise obscure site of gastrointestinal bleeding.

Imaging studies such as computed tomography (CT) are sensitive and effective for detecting pancreatic tumors, intra-abdominal masses, and small bowel and colonic thickening, as in Crohn's disease. Magnetic resonance imaging (MRI) is quickly becoming the standard in some pancreatic and liver disorders.

The physician caring for patients with digestive tract or liver disorders can deliver excellent diagnostic and management services only with the help of an experienced and communicative pathologist. For example, identification of Barrett's esophagus, a premalignant condition in the lower esophagus of patients with chronic gastroesophageal reflux, depends on the pathologist identifying Barrett's epithelium—cells arising from metaplasia of the columnar epithelium of the stomach as it extends upward into the damaged esophagus. Since patients with Barrett's esophagus are at high risk for developing adenocarcinoma of the esophagus, the gastroenterologist and pathologist form a team, searching yearly biopsies of Barrett's epithelium for dysplasia, a premalignant neoplastic lesion that increases cancer risk at least 30-fold. Confirmed dysplasia is usually an indication for surgical removal of part of the esophagus. The pathologist plays a similar pivotal role in providing surveillance for dysplasia in patients with longstanding ulcerative pancolitis; these patients have a 20- to 30-fold increased risk of colon cancer.

The pathologist also plays an important role in nonmalignant conditions. For example, pathologic identification of *Helicobacter pylori,* now known to be the most common cause of gastric and duodenal ulcers, allows the physician to cure most infections with antibiotics. This usually prevents ulcer recurrence, which had been a major problem before pathologists confirmed the role of *H pylori* in ulcer disease.

DISTINGUISH ORGANIC FROM "FUNCTIONAL" DISEASE

About 30–50% of patients seen by a gastroenterologist have complaints with some functional component (symptoms without known organic basis). It is generally accepted that stress affects the gastrointestinal tract; for example, the patient may say, "my stomach is tied in knots," or may have the urgent diarrhea that can precede a final exam, big game, or job interview. But both patients and physicians often fail to recognize or evaluate the environment's role in their gastrointestinal problems. The digestive tract is easily affected by both central and enteric nervous system stimuli like anxiety, stress, and depression. These effects can worsen the symptoms of both organic illnesses and so-called "functional illnesses" like the irritable bowel syndrome.

The challenge to the physician—whether primary care doctor or specialist—is to recognize both the organic and functional components of a person's illness. Some patients have only organic disease, others have mainly functional problems, and still others have a combination.

It is an error to attribute all of a patient's problems to functional disease. For example, although irritable bowel syndrome is a functional disease, patients with what appears to be irritable bowel may have features that a label of "functional disease" cannot explain. Findings inconsistent with irritable bowel include weight loss (unless the patient has frank depression), occult gastrointestinal bleeding, anemia, onset in the elderly (irritable bowel syndrome usually appears in the teens or early 20's), and night-time diarrhea (patients with functional bowel disease usually sleep peacefully through the night, since gastrointestinal motility decreases with sleep).

Another common error is the doctor's failure to take the time to explain functional gastrointestinal disease to the patient. After adequate but not exhaustive screening, the doctor should reassure patients and explain that they have a specific though poorly understood illness for which there is symptomatic therapy. Unfortunately, as pointed out by the fine clinician Philip A. Tumulty (see "Suggested Reading"), many physicians find it faster and easier to send patients for another test—usually a more expensive and perhaps riskier test—than to spend time questioning them thoroughly about their symptoms and explaining to them and their worried families the physical and environmental factors affecting their condition.

Other pitfalls include handing the patient a prescription as a way to shorten a difficult visit and giving the patient an iatrogenic "crutch" such as a flattened T wave, asymptomatic hiatal hernia, silent gallstone, or small uterine cyst, rather than a real explanation. In this era of great and expensive technologic advances, the restraints of managed health care, and the threat of malpractice suits, a good doctor takes the time needed to get an accurate history, perform a complete physical exam, and order a minimum of well-selected screening tests. The doctor then has the courage to arrive at a diagnosis of functional disease when it is appropriate. Both the patient and the health care system benefit.

SET LONG-TERM THERAPEUTIC GOALS AND TREAT SPECIFICALLY

The physician should formulate an individual treatment plan for every patient. This plan should define what will be considered an adequate response to reasonable therapy and should outline a sequence of alternative measures if the patient does not respond adequately. The physician should know the indications for and expected benefits of surgery and should discuss the risk-benefit ratio with the patient and others involved in the patient's care.

A good illustration of the value of a long-term plan is in

the management of gastroesophageal reflux of gastric acid. Informed physicians begin by prescribing the optimum dose of the indicated medication, such as an H_2 blocker to lessen acid secretion. They inform the patient of expected or possible complications of reflux, as well as side effects of the medication. They instruct the patient in mechanical measures to lessen reflux and to enhance emptying of the acid load from the stomach. They explain the goals of reducing the acid sensitivity of the lower esophagus and correcting aggravating factors such as nonsteroidal anti-inflammatory drugs and excessive weight gain (which puts more pressure on the stomach and increases reflux).

The treatment plan might state that if the patient's symptoms do not improve significantly within 2 weeks, more effective acid blockade should be added. This might be the sodium-hydrogen pump blocker omeprazole, plus medications such as cisapride to enhance gastric emptying of the acid contents. If the patient's reflux is still not controlled despite optimum medical therapy, the physician should be prepared to discuss with the patient the indications for the very effective surgical procedures for reducing reflux.

Surgery and therapeutic endoscopy of the alimentary tract continue to improve as better understanding of pathophysiology is combined with more accurate preoperative diagnosis. Biliary tract surgery has improved with better imaging and the development of percutaneous laparoscopic techniques. More knowledge of the symptoms and natural history of Crohn's disease has helped patients benefit from better use of medical therapy and of properly timed and planned surgery, including laparoscopy-assisted ileocolonic resections. Ileoanal pouch surgery has become a well-accepted alternative to standard ileostomy for patients with familial adenomatous polyposis or ulcerative colitis.

Another of the satisfactions of managing patients with gastrointestinal diseases is the ability to treat an increasing number of gastrointestinal disorders with specific therapies. For example, as mentioned in the above section, "Establish a Specific Diagnosis," most patients with duodenal ulcer caused by *H pylori* infection can now be cured by a 1- or 2-week course of antibiotics and are thus spared multiple relapses or long-term H_2-blocker therapy to reduce acid secretion. As another example, most patients who present with dysphagia caused by achalasia are relieved of their symptoms by procedures, such as esophageal dilatation or perhaps botulinum toxin injection into the lower esophageal sphincter, which allow the hypertensive sphincter to relax with swallowing. Patients who present with acute bleeding and vomiting of blood from a duodenal ulcer may recover after endoscopic cauterization of a "visible" vessel in the ulcer's base. Patients who present with jaundice may have a common bile duct stone removed by endoscopic sphincterotomy. Patients who present with steatorrhea and weight loss may be diagnosed with celiac disease and may respond dramatically to a gluten-free diet. Patients who present with 4

L/day of secretory diarrhea may recover after resection of a pancreatic VIP (vasoactive intestinal polypeptide) secreting tumor.

BUILD A PATIENT-DOCTOR RELATIONSHIP

Since many digestive diseases are chronic but not fatal, effective long-term care depends on a strong patient-doctor relationship. This starts with the thorough history during the first interview. Then physicians should explain to the patient why they have chosen particular screening and diagnostic tests, what are the potential results, and, most important, how those results will influence the patient's care. A thorough but not exhaustive initial evaluation should serve to reassure both patient and doctor. Many patients with gastrointestinal complaints are anxious, worried, or depressed; a calm, helpful discussion of the findings and the recommendations is in part a form of psychotherapy. The physician continues to earn the patient's trust during return appointments and by being available on the telephone between visits.

Another part of successful care is patient education. The physician and allied health professionals should give patients and their families a thorough explanation of the diagnosis and its management, including possible side effects of medications. Clinicians can supplement their explanations with print and audiovisual materials, and patients and their families can benefit from support groups such as the Crohn's Colitis Foundation. Still, patients should be able to ask follow-up questions of an informed source, usually their physician.

SUMMARY

▶ Approach the differential diagnosis recognizing that the gastrointestinal tract has a limited repertoire of symptoms with which to react to many types of dysfunction.

▶ Determine the organ of origin and the pathophysiologic derangements causing the patient's symptoms. Establish a specific diagnosis whenever possible.

▶ Be alert to the difficulty of distinguishing organic from "functional" digestive tract disease.

▶ Set reasonable long-term therapeutic goals. Treat as specifically as possible, and consider the role of surgical as well as medical treatment.

▶ Build a partnership with the patient. Many gastrointestinal disorders are chronic; continued communication and patient education are important to successful management.

SUGGESTED READING

Davies GJ et al: Bowel function measurements of individuals with different eating patterns. Gut 1986;27:164.

Drossman DA et al: Psychological factors in the irritable bowel syndrome: A multivariate study of patients and nonpatients with irritable bowel syndrome. Gastroenterology 1988; 95:701.

Hanson JS, McCallum RW: The diagnosis and management of nausea and vomiting: A review. Am J Gastroenterol 1985;80:210.

Harvey RF, Salih SY, Read AE: Organic and functional disorders in 2000 gastroenterology outpatients. Lancet 1983;1:632.

Tumulty PA: Functional illness. In: Bayless TM (editor): *Current Therapy in Gastroenterology and Liver Disease—2*. BC Decker, 1986.

6.2

Disorders of Swallowing

William J. Ravich, MD, and Thomas R. Hendrix, MD

Dysphagia (difficulty swallowing) may be classified by the level (oropharyngeal versus esophageal) or type (neuromuscular versus structural) of the patient's impairment. Oropharyngeal dysphagia is most often caused by neurologic or neuromuscular disease. Esophageal dysphagia is more likely than oropharyngeal dysphagia to be caused by structural lesions narrowing the lumen (Table 6.2–1).

The patient's own sensation of the level at which food gets stuck is not always accurate. However, by carefully analyzing the patient's complaints, the clinician can often predict the level of dysfunction and the underlying pathophysiology. For example, a patient who reports regurgitation, coughing while eating, and a weak voice should be suspected of having an abnormality in the oropharynx. In contrast, a patient who complains of regurgitation without airway symptoms, and who has chest pain while eating or coughs after eating, should be suspected of having an esophageal lesion (Table 6.2–2).

Although many patients with dysphagia are anxious, anxiety is usually a consequence rather than a cause of dysphagia. Pure psychogenic dysphagia, if it exists at all, is rare.

PHYSIOLOGY OF SWALLOWING

Between swallows, the pharynx is open to the larynx to permit breathing; the entrance to the esophagus is closed by a tonically contracted muscle, the upper esophageal sphincter, to prevent the esophagus from filling with air. At the lower end of the esophagus, another tonically contracted muscle, the lower esophageal sphincter, separates esophagus and stomach to prevent reflux of gastric contents into the esophagus.

As the tongue forces a bolus of food into the pharynx, the nasopharynx is closed by elevation of the soft palate and contraction of the superior pharyngeal constrictor muscles. At the same time, inhibition of neural stimulation relaxes the upper esophageal sphincter, permitting a wave of contraction (pharyngeal peristalsis) to push the swallowed bolus into the esophagus unimpeded. The peri-

staltic wave continues down the length of the esophagus (esophageal peristalsis). Before the bolus arrives in the distal esophagus, cessation of firing of vagal excitatory nerves and activation of vagal inhibitory nerves relax the lower esophageal sphincter, permitting easy passage into the stomach.

Four mechanisms prevent swallowed material from entering the airway: Respiration is inhibited, the larynx elevates, the vocal cords move together, and the epiglottis covers the larynx. The fact that there are four ways to close off the airway during swallowing points to the importance of protecting the airway. Even if one mechanism fails—for example, after epiglottectomy for cancer—the swallowed bolus rarely penetrates the airway.

EVALUATION

History

Dysphagia occurring only with solid foods suggests a structural lesion narrowing the pharynx or esophagus. Conversely, dysphagia occurring with both solids and liquids indicates a motor disorder. As mentioned, patients are not always accurate in identifying the level of obstruction. Many patients feel the food sticking above the actual site of obstruction. For example, one-third of patients with an obstruction at the lower end of the esophagus complain that food is sticking in their neck. Dysphagia that patients think is in the neck can be caused by disorders anywhere in the pharynx or esophagus. In contrast, few patients complain of food sticking at a site distal to the actual lesion.

Regurgitation of undigested food during a meal can result from dysphagia of any cause. Regurgitation during swallowing, especially when associated with airway distress, suggests a pharyngeal disorder; delayed regurgitation without coughing suggests an esophageal disorder. Regurgitation of recognizable food hours after eating limits the diagnostic possibilities, primarily to a pharyngeal or esophageal diverticulum or to achalasia. Regurgitation of sour- or bitter-tasting food or liquid indicates that the

Table 6.2–1. Common causes of dysphagia.

Neuromuscular Dysfunction	Structural Lesion
Oropharynx	
Brain-stem infarcts	Pharyngeal pouches (eg,
Amyotrophic lateral sclerosis	Zenker's diverticulum)
Head trauma	Pharyngeal webs (eg,
Bulbar poliomyelitis	Plummer-Vinson syndrome)
Cranial neuropathies	Head and neck neoplasms
(eg, diabetes)	Surgical resection
Myasthenia gravis	Thyromegaly
Polymyositis	
Hyper- or hypothyroidism	
Upper esophageal sphincter	
dysfunction	
Esophagus	
Achalasia	Inflammation (eg, reflux,
Paresis (eg, scleroderma,	candidiasis, virus)
Raynaud's phenomenon)	Extrinsic compression
Spastic disorders	Esophageal cancer
	Inflammatory stricture
	Esophageal web (eg,
	Schatzki's ring)

regurgitated material is coming from the stomach rather than the esophagus.

Coughing during eating usually reflects a problem with the oral or pharyngeal phase of swallowing, although some patients cough with esophageal disease. Coughing after meals suggests an esophageal disorder. Some patients with swallowing disorders present with complaints of coughing or recurrent pneumonia. In these people, recognizing that aspiration underlies chronic or recurrent pulmonary symptoms requires a high index of suspicion.

Chest pain is a common symptom that may derive not only from the esophagus but from the heart, aorta, chest wall, gallbladder, and peripheral nervous system (Chapters 1.2, 1.4, 1.10, 2.10, 6.3). Chest pain of esophageal origin may be sharp or squeezing. It is usually retrosternal and often radiates into the back. The pain can mimic that of myocardial ischemia in both description and distribu-

Table 6.2–2. Differentiating oropharyngeal from esophageal swallowing disorders.

Oropharyngeal
Nasal regurgitation
Airway obstruction while eating
Coughing while swallowing
Regurgitation during or immediately after swallowing
Weak or hoarse voice
Abnormalities on examination of the oropharynx

Esophageal
No airway distress during dysphagia
Regurgitation after swallowing
Meal-related chest pain
Coughing after eating
Frequent heartburn
Systemic findings suggesting scleroderma or other collagen
vascular disease
Left supraclavicular adenopathy indicating metastatic
carcinoma of the esophagus

tion. Chest pain in patients with dysphagia strongly suggests an esophageal cause. Unfortunately, esophageal chest pain is not always associated with swallowing. All too often, physicians consider an esophageal cause of chest pain only after coronary angiography shows no abnormality. However, coronary and esophageal disease are both common and can coexist.

Heartburn is the characteristic symptom of gastroesophageal reflux. Heartburn is usually described as a burning sensation behind the sternum, often radiating to the neck. This, too, is a very common symptom, often provoked by dietary indiscretion in otherwise normal people and does not necessarily imply significant disease.

Odynophagia is pain during swallowing, felt in either the throat or the chest. Odynophagia strongly suggests mucosal inflammation such as pharyngitis or erosive esophagitis.

The globus sensation is a persistent feeling of a lump or fullness in the throat, not usually associated with dysphagia. Indeed, many patients with globus say that swallowing momentarily relieves the sensation. Although many physicians consider globus to be hysterical in origin (globus hystericus), studies have failed to show hysterical tendencies in most patients. The symptom has been attributed to a variety of causes, including chronic sinusitis, upper esophageal sphincter dysfunction, and gastroesophageal reflux. If patients also have dysphagia, the dysphagia should be evaluated first. Even patients without dysphagia should be worked up to rule out serious conditions like neoplasms.

Physical Examination

The physician should carefully examine the patient's oral cavity for evidence of cancer or inflammatory disease. Because chewing is vital to allow proper transit, the physician should note the patient's dental hygiene and the presence and fit of dentures. It is also important to evaluate oral muscle strength and tone, and oral sensation. Clues to a neurologic disorder are loss of tongue mass, asymmetry of oropharyngeal structures, fasciculations of the tongue, poor touch awareness on the tongue or soft palate, and no gag reflex. The physician should assess voice quality: A nasal tone, weak voice, or hoarseness suggests vocal cord dysfunction. The rest of the neurologic exam may reveal specific neurologic disease causing oropharyngeal motor involvement (see "Neurogenic Dysphagia" below). However, many patients with neurologically impaired oropharyngeal function have a normal peripheral neurologic exam.

The physical exam is less helpful in evaluating esophageal dysphagia, but it can provide several clues to esophageal disease. One is the uncommon and late appearance of left supraclavicular lymphadenopathy (Virchow's node), which is associated with esophageal, gastric, and pancreatic cancer. Another is the skin changes of Raynaud's phenomenon and scleroderma; many patients with these disorders have dysfunction of the smooth muscle in the lower esophagus.

Laboratory Tests

The evaluation of swallowing disorders depends on both the predominant symptom and any associated symptoms. The major discriminating factors are whether the underlying disorder is thought to be oropharyngeal or esophageal and whether it is more likely structural or motor (see Table 6.2–1).

Contrast Radiography: In general, contrast (barium) radiography is the first test to order for a patient with dysphagia. Barium studies are equivalent or superior to endoscopy for detecting structural abnormalities of the pharynx and esophagus and far superior for detecting motor abnormalities of both pharynx and esophagus.

Most esophageal disorders can be evaluated adequately with a standard barium swallow, in which the examiner observes the transit of barium through the esophagus under fluoroscopy and shoots spot films to document important findings. However, the oropharyngeal phases of swallowing happen so quickly that it is easy to miss motor dysfunction and even significant structural lesions of the pharynx and upper esophagus. For this reason, the physician who suspects an abnormality in the oral or pharyngeal phases of swallowing should use cine- or videoradiography. These dynamic imaging techniques permit slow-motion and stop-action review of the events of swallowing.

Pharyngoscopy and Esophagoscopy: If symptoms such as neck pain or voice changes suggest a pharyngeal process or if the barium study shows a structural abnormality of the oropharynx, the pharynx should be evaluated directly by pharyngoscopy. This exam is performed without sedation, usually by an otolaryngologist. Pharyngoscopy reveals most structural disorders of the throat. Neurologic disorders present as wasting, muscle weakness, or pooling of secretions in the oral cavity or pharynx. The physician should recognize that pharyngoscopy is limited to the oral cavity, pharynx, and larynx and does not enable visualization of the pharyngoesophageal segment or below.

Esophagoscopy is the most effective way to define anatomic abnormalities observed in the esophagus on barium studies, and it occasionally allows detection of structural abnormalities missed by x-ray. Esophagoscopy is generally safe and well tolerated when performed with flexible instruments on a patient under light intravenous sedation. Esophagoscopy is essential for any patient whose dysphagia is not explained by barium studies, especially if predominantly solid food dysphagia suggests a structural obstruction.

Esophageal Manometry: Manometric studies (studies of esophageal pressure) assess the strength and coordination of the peristaltic wave, as well as the resting pressure and relaxation function of the upper and lower esophageal sphincters. Manometry is often used to clarify the findings of barium studies.

Manometric studies may help patients with dysphagia in whom no abnormality is found on barium studies or esophagoscopy. Manometry offers a second chance to look for dysmotility, without requiring additional radiation. In addition, certain types of esophageal dysmotility produce contractions of very high amplitude, but with normal progression of the peristaltic wave down the esophagus (nutcracker esophagus). The role of manometry in the evaluation of pharyngeal function is not well established.

For patients who present with chest pain without dysphagia, esophageal manometry combined with acid reflux studies (see "Reflux Testing" below) may be the first tests, in place of barium studies.

Reflux Testing: A patient who has the classic symptoms of reflux—frequent heartburn and regurgitation of sour or bitter liquid—may not need any confirming tests. When testing is desired, the current "gold standard" is continuous pH monitoring, in which an intraesophageal pH electrode records esophageal pH. This study assesses the presence, frequency, and severity of reflux and can determine the temporal relationship between symptoms and reflux events. Continuous pH monitoring has largely replaced older tests to confirm gastroesophageal reflux.

EXAMPLES OF SWALLOWING DISORDERS

Oropharyngeal Dysphagia

Neurogenic Dysphagia: The "swallowing center" in the brain stem provides central neurologic control of swallowing. Sensory input is transmitted to this center via cranial nerves V, IX, and X, as well as from cortical centers, while motor function is transmitted via cranial nerves V, VII, IX, X, and XII. Damage to any component of this transmission and integration system can interfere with swallowing.

Neurogenic dysphagia describes any condition—neurologic, neuromuscular, or myogenic—affecting oral or pharyngeal motor function. Patients report dysphagia in the throat, often with nasal regurgitation and coughing during swallowing. Dysphagia usually is for both liquids and solids and may be particularly severe with thin liquids. Coughing and pulmonary infection from aspiration may dominate the clinical picture.

Patients need a general neurologic exam and a careful assessment of oropharyngeal sensation and oral muscle strength and function. To confirm oropharyngeal dysfunction and determine the specific pattern of dysfunction, they require a detailed cine- or videoradiographic study of swallowing. Barium studies rarely permit a specific etiologic diagnosis. Even if a barium swallow shows neurogenic dysfunction, definitive diagnosis may require further evaluation under the direction of a neurologist.

The most common causes of neurogenic dysphagia are brain-stem infarcts, head trauma, and amyotrophic lateral sclerosis (ALS). Other neurologic and myopathic disorders that can cause dysphagia include Parkinson's disease, Huntington's disease, myasthenia gravis, hyper- and hypothyroidism, certain muscular dystrophies, and polymyositis. Prognosis and therapy depend on the underlying disease. It is particularly important to diagnose potentially treatable disorders such as Parkinson's disease, myasthenia gravis, thyroid dysfunction, and polymyositis. When these conditions are treated correctly, most patients have dramatic improvement or complete resolution of their swallowing disorder.

Upper Esophageal Sphincter Dysfunction and Zenker's Diverticulum: An isolated abnormality of upper esophageal sphincter function (often called "cricopharyngeal achalasia") is occasionally diagnosed by barium studies when the pharyngoesophageal segment opens incompletely or closes prematurely. Careful review of a dynamic barium study usually reveals associated pharyngeal weakness (neurogenic dysphagia). Truly isolated upper esophageal sphincter dysfunction is rare.

Zenker's diverticulum is an outpouching of the posterior wall of the hypopharynx just above the upper esophageal sphincter (Figure 6.2–1). Patients with Zenker's diverticulum typically are elderly and have dysphagia for both liquids and solids. Patients may regurgitate undigested food and liquid into the pharynx many hours after eating; this often causes paroxysms of coughing. Aspiration may be particularly severe at night. Although it is commonly held that upper esophageal sphincter dysfunction increases pharyngeal pressure, which in turn is responsible for development of the diverticulum, this is often not confirmed manometrically. Obstruction further downstream in the esophagus may also create conditions conducive to formation of diverticula.

Esophageal Dysphagia

Esophageal Stenosis: The swallowing channel can be narrowed by many benign and malignant processes (Figure 6.2–2). The most common benign causes of stenosis are webs, rings, and benign strictures. The most common malignant causes are squamous cell carcinoma and adenocarcinoma of the esophagus. Rare malignancies are metastatic cancer and lymphoma. An extrinsic mediastinal mass, whether benign or malignant, may compress the esophagus enough to cause dysphagia.

Patients with esophageal stenosis present with dysphagia for solid food. Symptoms tend to be worst with tough, difficult-to-chew foods, especially if the patient is rushed or distracted during meals. Patients may report particular problems with soft foods like pasta and bread, which may form a gluey mass in spite of chewing.

Patients develop dysphagia when a swallowed bolus, too large to pass easily through the narrowed segment, becomes impacted. The food may ultimately pass spontaneously or with a liquid chaser or may be regurgitated back to the mouth. As long as dysphagia persists, patients may have trouble swallowing even liquids. Some patients

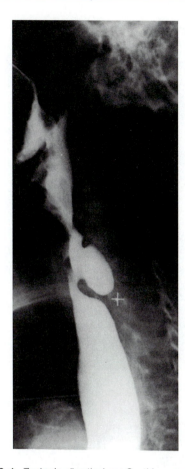

Figure 6.2–1. Zenker's diverticulum. On this x-ray, a barium-filled pouch protrudes from the posterior wall of the hypopharynx and extends behind the pharyngoesophageal junction. The diverticulum remains filled after the rest of the barium has passed into the esophagus. Many authorities believe that the narrow pharyngoesophageal segment represents a nonrelaxing upper esophageal sphincter, but manometric studies to confirm this interpretation have given mixed results.

have learned to induce regurgitation to clear the obstruction. The diagnosis is usually made by barium x-rays. However, the distinction between benign and malignant strictures requires endoscopy with biopsies for tissue confirmation, since malignant strictures can appear benign radiographically and vice versa.

The frequency and severity of symptoms depend on the degree of luminal narrowing, how fast the cause of stenosis worsens, and the patient's eating habits. Few patients complain of dysphagia until the lumen has narrowed by at least 50%. Webs and rings, which tend to remain unchanged over years, usually produce intermittent episodes of dysphagia separated by asymptomatic periods of irregular duration. Benign strictures may produce intermittent symptoms at first. Over time, the patient notices symptoms more often, and with foods that had not previously

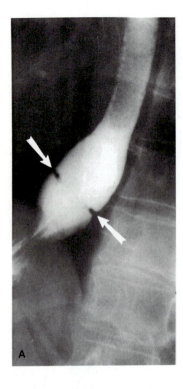
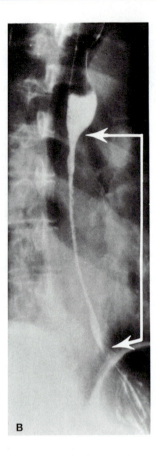
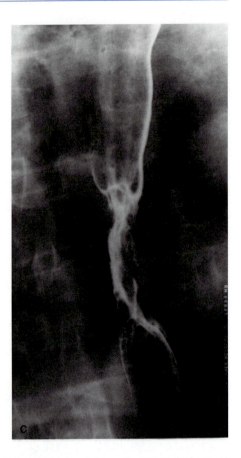

Figure 6.2–2. Three types of esophageal stenosis, seen on barium esophagogram. **A:** Schatzki's ring. A thin web narrows the lumen at the esophagogastric junction. A hiatal hernia with longitudinal gastric folds extends up to the bottom of the ring. **B:** Benign stricture. A long, gradually tapering, smooth-walled stenosis with a central lumen is seen in the midesophagus. **C:** Malignant stricture. This stenosis produces an asymmetrically located and nodular lumen. Small erosions are seen en face at the top of the stricture as tiny dots of pooled barium. Erosions within the stricture are seen in silhouette as tiny spokes extending out from the lumen. (Panels A and B reproduced, with permission, from Ravich WJ: Esophageal dysphagia. In: *Dysphagia: Diagnosis and Management,* 2nd ed. Groher ME [editor]. Butterworth-Heinemann, 1992.)

caused difficulty. Attempts to minimize the problem (cutting food into small pieces, careful chewing, modifying diet) become more restrictive and less successful. With malignant strictures, symptoms usually worsen faster, evolving over a few months from pure solid food dysphagia to dysphagia for liquids and solids.

Benign stenosis can be managed by dilation. Although many patients with esophageal webs and rings enjoy permanent relief of symptoms, symptoms of benign stricture often recur, especially if the underlying cause of inflammation is not removed or controlled. Patients with a stricture caused by reflux disease should have the reflux treated vigorously to prevent ongoing mucosal injury.

Esophageal cancer that appears to be restricted to the distal esophagus is usually treated by resection. Unfortunately, the surgical cure rate is only about 10%. Computed tomographic scanning or endoscopic ultrasonography appears helpful in selecting patients with a higher potential

for cure. Even without cure, surgery may be appropriate palliation.

For those who are deemed inoperable, radiation may provide palliation. Endoscopic therapy—with dilatation, stent placement, or laser therapy—is useful for palliation in patients who are not candidates for, or whose disease recurs after, surgery or radiation therapy.

Disorders of Esophageal Motility

Achalasia: Achalasia is a disorder of esophageal motor function in which the resting lower esophageal sphincter pressure is elevated and fails to relax normally after swallowing and in which peristalsis is lost in the body of the esophagus. The result is a functional obstruction at the esophagogastric junction. Achalasia is caused by an unexplained degeneration of ganglion cells in the myenteric plexus of the esophagus.

Most patients with achalasia are middle-aged, with a history of slowly progressive dysphagia, episodes of regurgitation, chest pain during eating, or aspiration pneumonia. Untreated, the obstruction causes retention of food and liquid; late in the disease, the esophagus can become massively dilated and tortuous (sigmoid esophagus). Many patients lose weight. Most regurgitate food from the esophagus, often hours after eating it. If patients regurgitate at night, they may awaken from sleep with paroxysms of coughing from aspiration.

The diagnosis of achalasia is suggested by the radiographic finding of a dilated esophagus with a column of barium supported above a tight esophagogastric junction (Figure 6.2–3). Because a stricture can look similar on x-ray, the diagnosis must be confirmed by upper endoscopy. If a standard endoscope (9.5–11.4-mm diameter) can pass into the stomach, the patient probably has achalasia rather than a stricture. The examiner must obtain a retroflexed view of the gastric fundus to rule out a carcinoma, which can also mimic achalasia.

At manometry, the lower esophageal sphincter pressure in achalasia is usually but not always elevated and fails to relax completely with swallowing (Figure 6.2–4). The body of the esophagus shows no peristalsis. Although

manometry is of pathophysiologic interest, it is generally not essential for a diagnosis of achalasia.

Because there is no way to reestablish normal esophageal function, therapy for achalasia aims at weakening the lower esophageal sphincter, thereby decreasing the barrier to gravity-assisted flow of food from esophagus to stomach. Although drugs like long-acting nitrates and calcium channel blockers have been reported effective, they are best used to buy time while arranging more definitive treatment. Sphincter tone is reduced by forceful dilation of the lower esophageal sphincter with large-diameter balloon dilators or surgical myotomy. Dilation is preferred because it causes the least morbidity, the hospitalization is shorter, and only rare patients develop gastroesophageal reflux with esophagitis, a common sequela of surgical myotomy. An alternative means of treating achalasia is by reducing lower esophageal sphincter pressure with endoscopic intrasphincteric injection of botulinum toxin.

Diffuse Esophageal Spasm and Related Disorders:
Diffuse esophageal spasm is an esophageal motility disorder characterized by intermittent chest pain, dysphagia, or both, along with abnormal, nonperistaltic contractions of the body of the esophagus. Many patients report that eat-

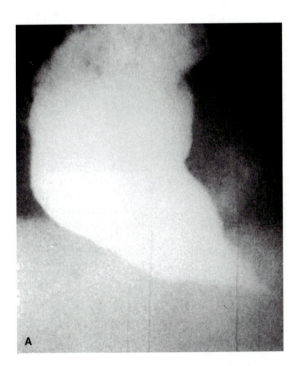 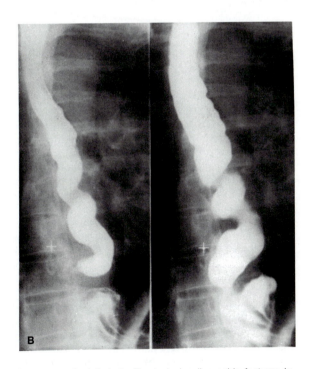

Figure 6.2–3. Achalasia and esophageal spasm, seen on barium esophagogram. **A:** Achalasia. The typical radiographic features include a dilated esophagus with a column of barium retained above the esophagogastric junction, and a smoothly tapering obstruction of the distal esophagus, giving a "bird-beaked" or "parrot-beaked" appearance. Most patients have no peristalsis, but some have forceful segmental contractions, a variant called *vigorous achalasia.* **B:** Esophageal spasm. The normal smooth silhouette and proximal squeezing action of the peristaltic wave are replaced by simultaneous indentations at multiple points along the barium column. These simultaneous contractions may be so prominent as to segment the barium, producing an appearance of multiple large pseudodiverticula, or the corkscrew appearance seen here. (Reproduced, with permission, from Ravich WJ: Esophageal dysphagia. In: *Dysphagia: Diagnosis and Management,* 2nd ed. Groher ME [editor]. Butterworth-Heinemann, 1992.)

Figure 6.2–4. Manometric tracings: normal, achalasia, and diffuse esophageal spasm. Intraluminal pressure is shown for the lower esophageal sphincter (bottom tracings) and from 5 cm (middle) and 10 cm (top) above it. When a normal person takes a swallow of water, the lower esophageal sphincter relaxes, and then the esophagus is swept clear by a peristaltic wave followed by contraction of the sphincter. In achalasia, lower esophageal sphincter resting pressure is usually elevated and fails to relax to intragastric baseline in response to swallowing. There is no peristalsis within the esophagus. In diffuse esophageal spasm, the manometric findings are variable and can include high-amplitude, long-duration, repetitive, and simultaneous contractions in any combination and with irregular frequency. Interspersed with these abnormal contractions may be normal progressive peristaltic waves.

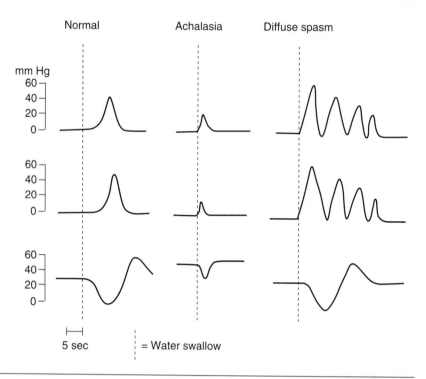

ing gives them pain. When the pain is not related to eating, the physician may mistakenly suspect angina pectoris.

The physician must confirm a clinical impression of diffuse esophageal spasm by showing abnormal esophageal motility on barium swallow or manometry. On barium swallow, normal peristalsis is replaced by simultaneous contractions throughout the esophagus (see Figure 6.2–3). Manometric findings often fluctuate, changing from swallow to swallow or on tests performed at different times. Findings can include any combination of high-amplitude, long-duration, repetitive, and simultaneous contractions (see Figure 6.2–4), sometimes interspersed with normal progressive peristaltic waves. Some patients with a history of chest pain or dysphagia have high-amplitude, prolonged, but nonetheless peristaltic contractions (nutcracker esophagus). The role of manometry in evaluating pharyngeal function is not well-established.

Esophageal dysmotility can develop secondary to a number of conditions, primarily esophageal inflammation and distal obstruction. Primary (idiopathic) esophageal spasm is actually relatively rare. Thus, the physician considering a diagnosis of esophageal spasm must always look for underlying causes. Probably the most common cause is gastroesophageal reflux. The physician must rule out reflux-induced spasm because the drugs used to treat idiopathic spasm can exacerbate reflux.

Idiopathic esophageal spasm is managed with reassurance and instruction to eat slowly and chew food well. Since there is no cure, patients are best encouraged to live with their discomfort if they can tolerate it. Some patients who find their symptoms intolerable are helped by drugs that relax esophageal smooth muscle, such as nitrates or calcium channel blockers. However, these drugs give many normotensive patients headaches, dizziness, and other distressing side effects, which may be as bad as the symptoms they are intended to treat.

Many asymptomatic people are shown by barium studies and manometry to have some degree of esophageal motor abnormalities. An incidental finding of esophageal dysmotility on an upper GI series does not warrant further evaluation or treatment. There is evidence that both the presence and severity of chest pain in patients with esophageal spasm may relate to an unusual sensitivity to esophageal distention.

Scleroderma: The esophagus is second only to the skin as a site of involvement in scleroderma (Chapter 3.10). The typical motility findings include little or no lower esophageal sphincter pressure and no contractions in the body of the esophagus. These motility abnormalities predispose patients to severe reflux and its complications, such as esophagitis and stricture. Physicians should assume all patients with scleroderma to be at risk for reflux and its sequelae and should consider tests of esophageal involvement (by barium studies or manometry) and reflux (by pH probe studies). Prophylactic reflux therapy should be started in those with characteristic motility abnormalities or severe reflux, even if they have no symptoms or evidence of esophageal inflammation.

Gastroesophageal Reflux and Nonreflux Esophagitis

Gastroesophageal Reflux Disease: Heartburn, especially when associated with sour or bitter regurgitation, is virtually pathognomonic of gastroesophageal reflux. However, heartburn is a common symptom, experienced by up to 10% of apparently normal people at least once a week. Although reflux is the most common cause of esophagitis, only a minority of patients with reflux symptoms have esophageal inflammation. For most patients, reflux is a nuisance without serious ramifications.

Three mechanisms protect the esophagus from damage by gastroesophageal reflux: (1) an antireflux barrier attributed to a combination of the strength of the lower esophageal sphincter and the anatomy of the esophagogastric junction, (2) the ability of esophageal peristalsis to return gastric contents to the stomach, and (3) the acid-neutralizing effect of swallowed saliva.

The approach to diagnosis depends on how the patient presents. Patients with typical symptoms can be started on treatment without objective confirmation. Patients require further evaluation when they have severe heartburn that cannot be controlled by changes in diet and lifestyle (see below). The best test to document reflux and assess its severity is continuous pH monitoring. If dysphagia is a major symptom, the patient should undergo a barium esophagogram.

Because only a minority of patients with documented gastroesophageal reflux disease have esophageal inflammation, not all patients who complain of heartburn require endoscopy. However, in patients with suspected esophagitis, endoscopy with biopsies is the only reliable way to assess the presence and severity of esophageal mucosal damage. Endoscopy is indicated when symptoms are severe and unresponsive to medical therapy, when the patient has odynophagia, when continuous pH monitoring shows severe reflux, or when barium studies suggest a stricture or erosions.

Severe reflux can lead to erosions and ulceration. If the esophagus does not heal quickly, a stricture may form. Furthermore, the destroyed squamous epithelium may be replaced by a more acid-resistant columnar epithelium (Barrett's esophagus). The significance of Barrett's esophagus is its predisposition to undergo malignant transformation in perhaps 10% of patients. Dysplasia increases the risk that Barrett's esophagus will progress to cancer.

Medical treatment for reflux depends on its severity. Most patients are first told to modify their diet and lifestyle—eating many small meals instead of three large ones; avoiding coffee, alcohol, and smoking; not eating within an hour of bedtime; and losing weight. Patients should put 6-inch blocks under the head of their bed so gravity will help keep gastric contents from refluxing at night. Many patients who use these measures require only occasional antacids to control their symptoms.

If symptoms are more frequent or fail to abate with this regimen or if reflux esophagitis is documented, patients should be started on drug treatment. The drugs most commonly used to treat reflux disease are H_2-blockers (cimetidine, ranitidine, nizatidine, famotidine), which decrease gastric acid secretion. If these drugs do not control patients' symptoms or esophagitis, the physician can increase the H_2-blocker dose, add a prokinetic drug (bethanechol, metoclopramide, cisapride) to enhance upper gastrointestinal motility, or substitute a powerful acid-suppressant proton pump inhibitor (omeprazole, lansoprazole).

If medical therapy for reflux is unsuccessful, the physician may consider surgery to reestablish or reinforce the antireflux barrier. In general, surgery should be restricted to patients with evidence of reflux-induced esophageal damage that has failed to heal with dietary and lifestyle changes combined with drug therapy. With currently available gastric acid-lowering drugs, most patients' symptoms can be satisfactorily controlled without surgery. However, some patients who would require long-term, high-dose drugs elect surgery instead. Especially when there is no evidence of esophageal damage, debilitating symptoms that fail to respond to intensive medical therapy should prompt the physician to question the diagnosis. Less than 5% of patients with significant reflux symptoms should require surgery.

Pill-Induced Esophagitis: Reflux is not the only cause of esophageal inflammation. A detailed drug history is important in all patients presenting with esophageal symptoms. Certain medications—most often tetracycline, iron, potassium, quinidine, and nonsteroidal anti-inflammatory drugs—can produce caustic injury to the esophageal mucosa. Enteric-coated formulations of these agents are particularly likely to cause esophageal injury because their larger size predisposes to sticking in the esophagus; the enteric coating does not prevent the pill from dissolving in the nonacidic esophagus. Patients should be cautioned to be upright when they take pills and to wash them down with plenty of water. Patients with underlying esophageal disorders may be at particular risk for retaining pills.

Odynophagia is more common in drug- than reflux-induced esophageal injury because drug-induced disease is often erosive. Drug-induced esophagitis can provoke formation of strictures and fistulas.

Infectious Esophagitis: Esophageal infections are rare in the immunocompetent host. However, HIV infection and aggressive cancer chemotherapy have put many patients at risk for infectious esophagitis. The predominant organisms involved are *Candida* species (usually *C albicans*), cytomegalovirus, and herpes simplex.

As with drug-induced esophagitis, odynophagia is common. Patients with known immunodeficiency who present with dysphagia or odynophagia should undergo endoscopy with biopsies, brushings, and viral cultures. Treatment with antiviral and antifungal agents is usually effective.

SUMMARY

▶ Swallowing disorders can be characterized by the location of the abnormality—oropharyngeal or esophageal. However, the site where patients feel the food sticking does not reliably correspond to the site of the lesion.

▶ Oropharyngeal dysphagia is most often caused by neurologic or neuromuscular disorders such as brainstem infarcts or amyotrophic lateral sclerosis.

▶ Esophageal dysphagia may be caused by structural lesions or motility abnormalities.

▶ The first test to order in evaluating dysphagia is a barium x-ray. A standard barium swallow is usually adequate for detecting esophageal lesions, but dynamic imaging such as a cine- or videoesophagogram is needed to evaluate oropharyngeal lesions.

▶ The best test for diagnosing gastroesophageal reflux disease is continuous pH monitoring.

SUGGESTED READING

DeMeester TR et al: Patterns of gastroesophageal reflux in health and disease. Ann Surg 1976;184:459.

Edwards DAW: Diagnostic procedures: History and symptoms of esophageal disease. In: *Diseases of the Esophagus.* Vantrappen G, Hellemans J (editors). Springer-Verlag, 1974.

Katz PO et al: Esophageal testing of patients with noncardiac chest pain or dysphagia: Results of three years' experience with 1161 patients. Ann Intern Med 1987;106:593.

Richter JE et al: Esophageal manometry in 95 healthy adult volunteers: Variability of pressures with age and frequency of "abnormal" contractions. Dig Dis Sci 1987;32:583.

Vantrappen G et al: Achalasia, diffuse esophageal spasm, and related motility disorders. Gastroenterology 1979;76:450.

6.3

Abdominal Pain

Thomas R. Hendrix, MD, Gregory B. Bulkley, MD, and Marvin M. Schuster, MD

Only a minority of patients presenting with acute abdominal pain are found to have a problem that requires surgical treatment. In an analysis of 1000 consecutive patients presenting to a university hospital emergency room with acute abdominal pain (see Brewer reference in "Suggested Reading"), almost 50% had no identifiable cause. In the remainder, the most common diagnoses were conditions that required medical, not surgical, treatment: gastroenteritis, pelvic inflammatory disease, urinary tract infection, and ureteral stone. Surgical conditions—appendicitis, acute cholecystitis, intestinal obstruction, complications of duodenal ulcer, pancreatitis, and abdominal aneurysm—altogether accounted for less than 15% of cases.

In some conditions for which surgery is indicated, the prognosis worsens if surgery is delayed. Common examples are a perforated viscus (duodenal ulcer), a bowel with compromised blood supply (strangulated obstruction), and inflammatory disease that is apt to lead to necrosis and perforation (appendicitis). Therefore, the physician must determine promptly whether the patient has a surgical condition.

The diagnosis usually rests on physical examination. Diagnosis of an "acute surgical abdomen" depends on peritoneal signs, that is, signs of parietal peritoneal inflammation. One sign is rebound tenderness—pain elicited by sudden release of gentle pressure over an area of the abdomen remote from the area of pain. However, this sign is notoriously unreliable. The most accurate indicator of peritonitis is involuntary guarding—reflex spasm of the abdominal wall muscles during gentle superficial palpation, which does not abate when the patient relaxes the abdominal wall. In addition to peritoneal signs, most patients with a "surgical abdomen" have markedly decreased or absent bowel sounds. The following findings correlate closely with diagnoses requiring prompt surgery: involuntary guarding, pain for less than 48 hours and pain followed by vomiting, advanced age, and prior surgery. The single most valuable test for a possible acute surgical abdomen is repeated physical exams by the same physician over an extended period.

Laboratory data can support the clinical suspicion, but rarely does the decision to operate rest on a laboratory value. Leukocytosis (white blood cell count greater than 10,000/μL) is found in 90% of patients with appendicitis, 80% with acute cholecystitis, and 60% with intestinal obstruction, but it is also found in 30% of patients in whom no cause is found for the attack of acute abdominal pain.

The physician who decides that the patient does not need immediate surgery must consider the many diagnoses that require medical intervention. These diverse conditions include pelvic inflammatory disease, acute pyelonephritis, hepatitis, acute hepatic congestion caused by congestive heart failure, abdominal crisis in sickle cell anemia, tabes dorsalis, diabetic ketosis, lactic acidosis, familial Mediterranean fever, and acute porphyria.

ORIGIN OF ABDOMINAL PAIN

Knowing the origin of abdominal pain is useful in understanding its differential diagnosis. Although 80–90% of the nerve fibers in the vagus nerves are afferent, all visceral pain stimuli reach the central nervous system via the splanchnic nerves.

The alimentary tract, from the esophagus to the anal canal, is insensitive to many stimuli that produce pain in structures innervated by the peripheral (somatic) nervous system. Mucosal biopsies of the alimentary tract produce acute ulcers but never cause pain at the time of biopsy nor during healing, while similar lesions in the buccal mucosa are very painful. The intestine can be cut or crushed without pain. However, if the intestine is distended or its muscle coat contracts with spasm, pain may be severe. As a general rule, only three processes are capable of producing pain in the alimentary tract: tension in the wall (caused by intense muscle contraction or distention), ischemia, and inflammation of the serosa (peritoneum).

Pain Caused by Tension

Colic, the wave-like pain associated with forceful peristaltic contractions, is the most characteristic type of pain arising from the viscera. Powerful peristalsis can be started by an irritant substance (eg, the oxalic acid from green apples), infection with a virus or bacteria, or the gut's attempt to force its luminal contents through an obstruction. Other conditions, such as inflammation and ischemia, cause pain that is steady and continuous.

Pain is also caused by tension on the mesentery and by acute stretching of the capsule of an organ such as the liver, spleen, or kidney. Serosal stretch receptors similar to those in muscle are the presumed source of these impulses, which are sensed as pain.

Pain Caused by Ischemia

Ischemia of skeletal, cardiac, or visceral muscle produces intense, continuous pain. The most common cause of intestinal ischemia is strangulation of the bowel from obstruction by an adhesion, hernia, or volvulus. Less often, ischemic pain is caused by mesenteric vascular occlusion.

Pain Caused by Peritoneal Inflammation

Inflammation of the peritoneum is the third major source of abdominal pain. At first, the inflammation is usually limited to the serosa covering the inflamed organ (eg, appendix or gallbladder), that is, a visceral peritonitis. As the inflammatory process extends to the adjacent parietal peritoneum, it produces localized peritonitis; the pain becomes more severe and is experienced in the corresponding area of the abdominal wall. Parietal peritonitis causes reflex spasm of the overlying muscles, resulting in involuntary rigidity (involuntary guarding) as well as pain and tenderness of the abdominal wall. Generalized peritonitis is often sterile when gastric juice, pancreatic juice, or bile leaks into the peritoneal cavity; it is septic when the cavity becomes contaminated with contents of the colon or an abscess.

LOCATION OF ABDOMINAL PAIN

Distention of the stomach or duodenum usually produces pain between the xiphoid and umbilicus in the midline. The nearer the stimulus is to the third portion of the duodenum, the nearer the pain is to the umbilicus.

Stimulation of the small intestine typically leads to periumbilical pain.

Pain originating in the colon is usually referred to the midline between the umbilicus and the pubic symphysis. Pain from the ascending or descending colon or from the hepatic and splenic flexures may also be localized to the side involved, presumably because of pressure on adjacent structures.

Rectosigmoid distention characteristically produces suprapubic pain, and distention of the rectum usually leads to pain in the area of the sacrum and perineum. Bladder distention also produces suprapubic pain.

Gallbladder distention or inflammation produces mid-epigastric pain radiating to the right upper quadrant or to the right scapular area as the distention increases. With common bile duct distention, pain is often felt in the mid-epigastrium, sometimes radiating to the shoulders.

Pancreatic pain is typically mid-epigastric. The pain often radiates laterally and to the back, especially when the posterior wall of the abdomen becomes involved.

HISTORY

A careful history that documents the onset, characteristics, and course of abdominal pain is most important in determining its cause.

Sudden onset is most often caused by the perforation of a viscus, such as a peptic ulcer. Acute intestinal ischemia, such as that caused by a superior mesenteric artery embolus, can also produce sudden pain. In conditions that cause obstruction of a hollow viscus or inflammation of its walls—such as bowel obstruction, appendicitis, cholecystitis, and diverticulitis—pain begins more gradually, usually taking several hours to reach its peak.

Colic, the most characteristic type of abdominal pain, is often a manifestation of increased peristalsis proximal to an obstruction of a hollow viscus. Colic, an intermittent wave-like pain, should be distinguished from the continuous, steady pain produced by ischemia, inflammation, or peritoneal irritation. This distinction is often critical. Patients should be asked whether their pain has an intermittent, cramp-like component.

Patients may have pleuritic pain when the inflammatory process involves the diaphragm or when movement of the diaphragm brings an inflamed organ against the peritoneum. Patients may also describe their abdominal pain as sharp, dull, burning, tearing, or aching. Unfortunately, these terms usually offer little insight into the underlying disorder.

Vomiting is a common accompaniment of abdominal pain. It may be a manifestation of intestinal obstruction or a visceral reflex caused by pain. Patients with intestinal blockage may have early vomiting if the obstruction is high, but late vomiting or none at all if the obstruction is low. Vomiting does not often help define the specific cause of abdominal pain, but it is a good (not infallible) indicator that the pain is of visceral origin.

PHYSICAL EXAMINATION

Observing the Patient

When evaluating acutely ill patients, the physician must always observe, question, and examine carefully. The first task is to observe patients so as to assess the gravity of their illness. Do they have evidence of impending shock or vascular collapse? Are they restless, as is commonly seen with colic, or do they lie immobile in bed, as is commonly seen with peritonitis or advanced ischemia of the bowel? The initial examination rarely establishes the diagnosis of a surgical abdomen with enough certainty to proceed with laparotomy. The answer is more often provided by repeating the exam at regular intervals, because the evolution of clinical findings is usually more important than the signs themselves.

Abdominal Examination

The abdominal exam should provide answers to these questions:

1. Are there signs of peritonitis? If so, is the peritonitis localized or diffuse? The single most reliable indicator of parietal peritonitis is involuntary guarding. This must be carefully distinguished from voluntary guarding because of the pain or, more often, because of the patient's fear that the examiner will worsen the pain by a too abrupt palpation. Guarding is determined by *gentle* palpation of the abdominal wall, not by deep palpation of the underlying organs. It is essential that the physician palpate the abdomen slowly and very gently.
2. What is the character of the bowel sounds? Are they hyperactive and coming in rushes, as is typical of intestinal obstruction? Or, are there no sounds, as is characteristic of peritonitis, advanced ischemia, and strangulation of the bowel? The physician should allow enough time—up to 3–5 minutes—to determine the bowel sounds. For example, patients with mechanical small bowel obstruction may have high-pitched, hyperactive sounds interposed with periods of silence. Bowel sounds may be present early in the course of ischemia and strangulation, but may disappear as the process evolves.
3. Can any masses be seen or felt? Occasionally, a dilated loop of bowel, visible peristalsis, or a distended gallbladder is more clearly seen than felt. The physician should exclude inguinal and femoral hernias by specifically looking for them.
4. Is there evidence of free fluid in the abdomen, as determined by examining for shifting dullness or a fluid wave? If there is free fluid, the physician may be wise to obtain a sample by direct needle aspiration or with ultrasonographic guidance. For example, fat droplets or a high amylase content in the aspirate usually indicates pancreatitis, but also may accompany perforation of a duodenal ulcer. Gross blood suggests a ruptured aneurysm or spleen, or an ectopic pregnancy. Cloudy, dirty fluid is found after the bowel perforates.

Pelvic and Rectal Examinations

The pelvic and rectal exams help to differentiate disorders of the female reproductive tract from inflammatory diseases of the bowel. In occasional patients with appendicitis or diverticulitis, the rectal exam reveals a tender localized mass even though the abdominal exam is normal. In addition, a bimanual pelvic and rectal exam allows direct palpation of the uterus and adjacent peritoneum. It is particularly important to exclude pelvic inflammatory disease, which is usually managed without surgery, from causes of the acute surgical abdomen.

Other Important Observations

Fever makes the diagnosis of an acute inflammatory condition more likely. On the other hand, a rectal temperature above 39°C (102°F) is less often found with abdominal than with pulmonary and renal infections. When a patient with abdominal pain has a fever this high, the physician should consider whether the pain is being referred from an extra-abdominal site.

Pulses in all four extremities should be checked to look for evidence of a dissecting abdominal aneurysm.

LABORATORY STUDIES

Blood Tests

The hematocrit provides important information in patients with acute abdominal pain. When elevated, it suggests hemoconcentration and hypovolemia; when low, it suggests intra-abdominal hemorrhage. But a normal hematocrit does not exclude an acute, massive hemorrhage for which the body has not yet compensated. Leukocytosis indicates acute inflammation and often accompanies disorders that require surgery.

Urinalysis

In addition to providing evidence of urinary tract infections, stones, and acute glomerulonephritis, urinalysis may give the first indication of diabetes mellitus, which can present with a tender acute fatty liver. Bilirubinuria can be the first clue to hepatobiliary disease. Finally, examining the urine for porphobilinogen is the simplest way to diagnose porphyria.

Stool Examination

Blood in the stool suggests that abdominal pain originates in the gut. Blood is usually seen with intussusception, late mesenteric vascular occlusion, and obstructing neoplastic or inflammatory lesions.

Serum Chemistries

Serum levels of amylase, bilirubin, and alkaline phosphatase should be obtained if the pancreas or biliary tract may be involved. To interpret the results, the physician must know when in the course of the illness the blood sample was obtained. For example, serum bilirubin and alkaline phosphatase levels may be normal early in acute biliary tract obstruction but later rise to abnormal levels. For another example, the serum amylase level may fall to normal as early as 48 hours after the onset of pain in patients with pancreatitis, even though they still have pain.

Hyperlipidemic serum is found in up to 20% of patients with acute pancreatitis. Hyperlipidemia may obscure the diagnosis because many patients with it have a normal serum amylase level due to the fact that amylase is distributed only to the serum water. If 20% of the serum is lipid, an elevated concentration of amylase in serum water may be near normal when reported as amylase concentration per unit volume of serum. Serum electrolytes and blood urea nitrogen should also be determined so that abnormalities can be corrected, particularly if the patient may need surgery.

Imaging Studies

All patients being evaluated for an acute abdomen should have a supine and upright x-ray of the abdomen and a chest x-ray. Findings that may explain the abdominal pain include lower lobe pneumonia, free air under the diaphragm (indicating a perforated viscus), absent psoas shadows (suggesting retroperitoneal bleeding or inflammation), displaced stomach, fluid in the bowel or peritoneal cavity, small bowel air fluid levels (suggesting paralytic or mechanical ileus), large bowel gas or air fluid levels (suggesting an ileus, volvulus, or obstruction), and pancreatic, biliary, or urinary calcifications.

If an emergency barium enema is performed to define the site and nature of a colonic obstruction, the full amount of barium is not necessary because the goal is to locate the obstructing lesion, not to study details of the mucosa. A water-soluble contrast medium should be used when perforation is a possibility. Barium should not be given by mouth when colonic obstruction is suspected, but barium by mouth to confirm small bowel obstruction is perfectly safe and preferable to water-soluble contrast media.

Ultrasonography, which does not expose patients to x-rays, is the best way of screening for cholelithiasis. It is also ideal for identifying cystic lesions throughout the abdomen, evaluating the intrahepatic and extrahepatic biliary tract and urinary tract, and looking for pancreatic enlargement. Ultrasonography is particularly useful in the pelvis, an area less well visualized by conventional x-rays. Furthermore, guided-needle aspiration or biopsy under sonographic control often permits the definitive diagnosis of mass lesions in the liver, pancreas, kidney, and retroperitoneum.

Computed tomography (CT) provides the best imaging of soft tissue structures throughout the abdominal cavity. In the retroperitoneum, CT is especially useful in delineating the pancreas. With or without contrast material, CT greatly increases diagnostic capability. The technique is best used to confirm a suspected diagnosis.

Esophogastroduodenoscopy

Upper abdominal symptoms should be investigated by esophogastroduodenoscopy (EGD). It is the most definitive and risk-free way to establish whether chronic abdominal pain is being caused by structural abnormality, such as unrecognized peptic ulcer disease, inflammation, or gastric neoplasia, or by a functional abnormality.

Sigmoidoscopy

Lower abdominal symptoms should be evaluated by fiberoptic sigmoidoscopy. This test should be done in preference to a barium enema because (1) it is simpler to perform and more easily tolerated, (2) the endoscope used in sigmoidoscopy produces more sensitive results in ex-amining the rectum than the barium enema, and (3) if a lesion is found, the examiner can take biopsy specimens for tissue diagnosis.

COMMON CAUSES OF ACUTE ABDOMINAL PAIN

The most common causes of acute abdominal pain, discussed here, are appendicitis, acute diverticulitis, acute cholecystitis, acute pancreatitis, perforated peptic ulcer, intestinal obstruction, paralytic ileus, and acute mesenteric ischemia (Table 6.3–1). A large number of disorders simulate an acute surgical abdomen on presentation but can be identified as not requiring surgical treatment by serial examination (Table 6.3–2).

Appendicitis

Early and accurate diagnosis of acute appendicitis is paramount. Delay greatly increases the risk of perforation, complications, and death. The clinical course of appendicitis illustrates the importance of serial observation of the patient. For many patients, the first symptom of acute appendicitis is epigastric discomfort attributed to indigestion; the right lower quadrant may not be tender. For other patients, the first symptom is colicky periumbilical pain; if these patients also have diarrhea, they and their physician will probably conclude that their problem is gastroenteritis. Anorexia, nausea, and vomiting are also common at this stage.

Within hours, the pain shifts to the right lower quadrant. Often, but by no means always, the physician can elicit tenderness on deep palpation of the right lower quadrant at McBurney's point. Patients develop a temperature elevation of 1° or 2°, together with leukocytosis. If patients are not treated, the appendix may perforate, causing generalized peritonitis or a periappendicular abscess.

Appendicitis would not be so difficult to diagnose if it always developed this way, but probably no more than 20% of patients follow the pattern. The variable clinical picture seen in acute appendicitis is caused in part by the mobility of the cecum and appendix and in part by the consequent lack of contact between the inflamed appendix and the parietal peritoneum in the right lower quadrant.

The most common sign of acute appendicitis is localized abdominal tenderness, which is not sufficiently specific. The physical signs of appendicitis evolve slowly and are frequently atypical, thus making early diagnosis difficult. When the cecum resides high in the midabdomen, appendicitis can simulate cholecystitis or pyelonephritis. When the appendix lies deep in the right lower quadrant, appendicitis can mimic Crohn's disease, psoas abscess, ureteral stone, or even hip disease. In the pelvis, an inflamed appendix may produce bladder symptoms or, in women, symptoms suggesting disease of the right fallopian tube or ovary. A particularly difficult distinction is that between acute appendicitis and pelvic peritonitis of

Table 6.3–1. Common causes of acute abdominal pain.

Condition	Location of Pain	Interval Between Onset and Peak Intensity	Important Features
Appendicitis	Epigastrium or periumbilical, later shifting to right lower quadrant	Several hours	Localized right lower quadrant tenderness, fever, leukocytosis
Acute diverticulitis	Left lower quadrant	Several hours	Localized left lower quadrant tenderness, fever, leukocytosis; CT useful in defining extent of process
Acute cholecystitis	Epigastrium, right upper quadrant, or both	1 to several hours	Pain may radiate to right scapula; gallstone on ultrasound; positive HIDA scan
Acute pancreatitis	Epigastrium, radiating to the back	30 minutes to several hours	Nausea and vomiting usually prominent; elevated amylase; CT useful
Perforated peptic ulcer	Epigastrium	1 to several minutes	Rigid abdomen, free air under diaphragm
Acute intestinal obstruction	Periumbilical or hypogastric colic	30 minutes to several hours	Vomiting if obstruction high, distention if low
Acute mesenteric ischemia: Arterial occlusion	Periumbilical	Minutes to 1 hour	Pain out of proportion to physical findings; white blood cell count <20,000/μL
Venous occlusion	Periumbilical	Days	Polycythemia
Ruptured abdominal aneurysm	Periumbilical, radiating to the back	1 to several minutes	In some patients, unequal pulses in the extremities
Ureteral stone	Colic in flank, radiating to groin	1 to several minutes	Red blood cells in urine
Ruptured ectopic pregnancy	Hypogastrium	1 to several minutes	Missed menstrual period

HIDA, hepato-iminodiacetic acid (for hepatobiliary imaging).

pelvic inflammatory disease. Gynecologic disease accounts for 20% of all disorders mimicking appendicitis. Most of this confusion can be resolved by careful serial examinations, including rectal, pelvic, and urinary exams.

Acute Diverticulitis

Diverticula are outpouchings of the mucosa through muscular defects in the intestinal wall. Diverticulosis refers to asymptomatic diverticula. Diverticular disease (abdominal pain associated with diverticula) is seen when muscle spasm accompanies diverticulosis. Diverticulosis

Table 6.3–2. Disorders that may mimic an acute surgical abdomen.

Cardiac	Myocardial infarction, pericarditis, congestive heart failure (acute congestion of the liver)
Pulmonary	Pneumonia, pulmonary embolus, pneumothorax, pleurodynia
Gastrointestinal	Viral gastroenteritis, "food poisoning," typhoid fever, pancreatitis
Urologic	Ureterolithiasis, pyelonephritis
Gynecologic	Pelvic inflammatory disease, mittelschmerz, ovarian cyst
Neurologic	Herpes zoster, tabes dorsalis, spinal nerve compression
Metabolic and toxic	Diabetic ketoacidosis, addisonian crisis, lead poisoning, hyperlipidemia, arachnoidism, narcotic withdrawal
Hematologic	Hemolytic crisis (sickle cell crisis), acute leukemia
Miscellaneous	Acute porphyria, familial Mediterranean fever, vasculitis, psychiatric disorders

of the entire colon is not associated with circular muscle spasm and hypertrophy, whereas sigmoid diverticulosis usually is. Diverticulitis occurs when diverticula become inflamed.

Acute diverticulitis most often involves the sigmoid colon. It may appear with no premonitory symptoms or may be superimposed on longstanding constipation and left lower quadrant pain. The pathologic process is a microperforation of the mucosa of a single diverticulum leading to peridiverticulitis, rather than diffuse inflammation of the wall of the diverticulum. The symptoms are pain in the left lower quadrant, with severe constipation, nausea, and, uncommonly, vomiting. Patients develop fever and leukocytosis. It is not surprising that this condition has been called "left-sided appendicitis." Frequently, the stool sample obtained by rectal exam shows occult blood, but diverticulitis rarely causes gross bleeding. Most attacks subside in a few days.

The diagnosis of acute diverticulitis should be suspected in elderly patients with left lower quadrant pain, fever, and leukocytosis. If peritoneal signs suggest a perforation or abscess, an abdominal CT scan should be obtained to determine the extent and nature of the pericolic inflammation. After the attack subsides, fiberoptic sigmoidoscopy should be done to ensure that the wall thickening seen on the CT is not caused by carcinoma. If the attack does not subside promptly with medical treatment, the patient may need early surgery.

Treatment for acute attacks is broad-spectrum antibiotics and intravenous fluids. Most patients should not be allowed anything by mouth. Nasogastric aspiration may be useful for several days. After the attack subsides, the bulk in the diet should be increased by supplements of bran or a bulk laxative to produce soft stools and prevent constipation. If patients suffer recurrent attacks with fever and leukocytosis, or if pericolic abscess complicates the picture, resection is indicated. Ultimately, 10–20% of patients need surgery.

Acute Cholecystitis

Signs and Symptoms: Patients with acute cholecystitis characteristically have pain in the epigastrium and the right upper quadrant of the abdomen. At first, the pain may be colicky; then it becomes steady and increases in intensity for several hours. The attack is usually caused by a stone obstructing the cystic duct. As the stone passes through the duct, patients may also feel pain at the inferior angle of the right scapula and at times on top of the shoulder. Many patients also develop nausea, vomiting, and a low-grade fever. Later, signs of irritation of the parietal peritoneum appear in the right upper quadrant. Leukocytosis is usual, and mild hyperbilirubinemia and bilirubinuria may be found after 24 hours. Many patients have constipation as well as mild paralytic ileus (see "Intestinal Obstruction" below) with an air-filled jejunal loop (sentinel loop) seen on abdominal x-ray.

Gallstones are found in 95% of patients with cholecystitis. Although less than 20% of gallstones are radiopaque, most are visible by abdominal sonography. Cholecystitis was once thought to be caused by primary infection of the gallbladder. The precipitating factor is now believed to be cystic duct obstruction, usually by a gallstone. If the obstruction interferes with gallbladder emptying, the distention, consequent ischemia, and chemical irritation cause acute cholecystitis. Bacterial infection is a secondary phenomenon, rarely appearing in less than 48 hours.

Diagnosis: The diagnosis of acute cholecystitis is supported by gallstones and a dilated gallbladder, demonstrated by ultrasonography. When the sonogram shows a thickened gallbladder wall surrounded by a "halo" of edema, it is diagnostic. Cholecystitis may also be confirmed by hepatobiliary imaging (HIDA scan) using one of several technetium Tc99m iminodiacetic (HIDA) derivatives, when the hepatobiliary tract but not the gallbladder is visualized. In HIDA scanning, soon after the labeled iminoacetic acid derivative is injected intravenously, it is taken up by the liver and excreted into the bile, thus visualizing the biliary tract. However, if a stone occludes the cystic duct, the gallbladder cannot be seen.

Management: Prompt cholecystectomy is the treatment of choice for acute cholecystitis. With surgery, patients avoid the small risk of perforation, a somewhat larger risk of sepsis, and a second hospitalization for elective cholecystectomy. Most important, surgery decreases the risk of sepsis and septic cholangitis. If the gallbladder does perforate, it is often contained in a well-localized abscess. But occasionally this leads to bile peritonitis or to a rare complication, such as a large stone passing from the gallbladder into the intestine and obstructing the ileocecal sphincter (gallstone ileus) or a permanent fistula caused by a stone eroding into the adjacent duodenum or colon (cholecyst-duodenal or cholecyst-colonic) with a chronic retrograde infection of the biliary tract in the case of the latter. Cholecystectomy is usually performed laparoscopically, even in cases of acute cholecystitis. However, experienced laparoscopic surgeons do not hesitate to convert the procedure to conventional cholecystectomy when inflammation obscures the anatomic landmarks, thereby reducing the risks of injury to the common and hepatic bile ducts and associated hepatobiliary blood vessels.

Acute Pancreatitis

Signs and Symptoms: The clinical presentation of pancreatitis is as variable as the setting in which it occurs. It can range from a sudden acute abdominal catastrophe with shock and cyanosis, to mild episodes of deep epigastric pain and vomiting, which, if seen in an alcoholic patient, may be attributed to "alcoholic gastritis." The patient's first several attacks may be recorded in the emergency room as gastritis; the diagnosis changes only when an elevated serum amylase level is found during an acute attack.

No specific clinical feature allows the clinician to diagnose pancreatitis. Measuring serum amylase is the most specific aid to the diagnosis, but often it is only transiently elevated, and it may return to normal in 48–72 hours despite continuing symptoms. In addition, as much as 20% of patients with acute pancreatitis have either normal or only borderline elevation of amylase. Striking elevations (greater than 1000 U/dL) are almost always caused by pancreatitis or acute obstruction of the pancreatic duct by a gallstone in the ampulla, if mumps can be excluded. But mild-to-moderate elevations of amylase are seen in many situations, such as a perforated viscus, strangulated bowel, mesenteric thrombosis, renal insufficiency, and Sjögren's syndrome. Differentiation from pancreatitis is difficult in 5% of patients. Morphine can also mildly elevate the serum amylase level.

An enlarged pancreas on ultrasonography or CT increases the likelihood that pancreatitis is the cause of an attack of acute abdominal pain. Unfortunately, early in an attack when the patient most needs help, the pancreas probably has not enlarged enough to be diagnostic. Ultrasonography and CT are extremely accurate in diagnosing late complications, primarily pseudocysts and abscesses.

Other manifestations of pancreatitis are mild hyperbilirubinemia and bilirubinuria (about 20% of patients), hyperglycemia (about 25%), and hypocalcemia. With severe disease, the serum calcium level falls at some point between the third and tenth days, occasionally low enough to cause tetany.

Acute pancreatitis simulates the complete picture of an

acute surgical abdomen, with fever, leukocytosis, severe pain, sterile peritonitis, and, in many patients, cardiovascular collapse. Acute pancreatitis and acute pelvic inflammatory disease are the only conditions with this presentation that do not require immediate surgery. Thus, recognizing pancreatitis is critical to management. When the diagnosis is unclear, it is safest to explore the patient surgically, to exclude other causes of an acute abdomen. If pancreatitis is found, the abdomen may be closed and the patient treated medically.

Pathogenesis: The pathogenesis of pancreatitis is not known. A single mechanism is unlikely. Pancreatitis, like pneumonia, can be caused by many conditions. By far the most common cause is alcohol abuse, followed by cholelithiasis, hyperlipidemia, trauma, drugs, hypercalcemia, penetrating peptic ulcer, and distention of pancreatic ducts during endoscopic retrograde cholangiopancreatography (ERCP). Potentially remediable causes should be given careful consideration.

Regardless of antecedent factors, the final common pathway in the pathogenesis of pancreatitis is the liberation of activated pancreatic juice into the tissues of the pancreas. In the mildest form of pancreatitis, patients develop only edema, which clears without causing residual changes in the structure or function of the pancreas. In the most severe form, tissue destruction extends to the blood vessels, leading to hemorrhagic pancreatitis, a disease with a mortality rate of 50–85%. With severe disease, and especially with repeated attacks, patients lose acinar tissue and islets of Langerhans, and they develop pancreatic insufficiency with steatorrhea, diabetes, or both.

Management: The treatment of acute pancreatitis is supportive. Since hypovolemia may be severe, blood volume must be restored. Elderly patients and patients with signs of a serious or grave prognosis (leukocyte count above 16,000/μL, blood glucose above 200 mg/dL, tachycardia above 130 bpm, adult respiratory distress syndrome, low urine output, falling hematocrit, falling serum calcium) should be admitted to the intensive care unit for central venous pressure monitoring, aggressive fluid replacement, administration of oxygen, and liberal analgesia. Continued secretion of pancreatic juice into the substance of the pancreas increases tissue damage; oral intake should be withheld in an effort to suppress pancreatic secretion.

A host of treatments (eg, glucagon, antitrypsins, anticholinergic agents, nasogastric suction, somatostatin, corticosteroids, antibiotics, peritoneal dialysis) have been tried, but in controlled trials these treatments have not clearly increased patients' chance of survival. Because severe pancreatitis precludes oral caloric intake, many patients have nutritional deficiencies, with striking protein loss and catabolism; parenteral hyperalimentation should be started early. Patients should be followed closely to detect other possible causes of the acute abdominal pain, as well as complications of the pancreatitis. Among the many complications of acute pancreatitis are pseudocyst formation, renal failure, massive pleural effusion, hypocalcemia, pancreatic abscess, and pancreatic ascites.

Perforated Peptic Ulcer

About 5–10% of patients with duodenal ulcer have a perforation. Perforation of a gastric ulcer is much less common. Most patients, especially those with duodenal ulcer, give a history of periodic dyspepsia compatible with peptic ulcer, antedating the perforation. But in a few patients, the sudden, severe, prostrating pain of perforation is the first indication of peptic ulcer disease (Chapter 6.4).

The escape of gastric contents into the peritoneal cavity causes immediate chemical peritonitis, which produces severe pain, first in the epigastrium, then quickly spreading over the entire abdomen. Patients appear critically ill, with shallow thoracic respirations. They have a rigid, board-like abdomen and are reluctant to move. As fluid pours out from the peritoneal surface, the pain may diminish, but this should not be misinterpreted as a sign of recovery. Fluid becomes detectable in the flanks, and liver dullness may be lost on physical exam if a large amount of air escapes into the peritoneal cavity; this is more likely with the perforation of a gastric than with that of a duodenal ulcer.

On x-ray, about 80% of patients with perforations have free air in the peritoneal cavity. An upright chest x-ray is most likely to show free air under the diaphragm. If the patient cannot stand, a left lateral decubitus film of the abdomen usually demonstrates free air. Free air in the abdomen may come from other causes, such as spontaneous or traumatic perforation of the bowel. Air is regularly found for several days after laparotomy. Finally, pneumatosis cystoides intestinalis can cause a benign asymptomatic pneumoperitoneum. The diagnosis of pneumatosis cystoides intestinalis may be suspected by a finding of localized collections of air along segments of the bowel wall.

A patient suspected of having a perforated peptic ulcer should immediately be readied for laparotomy. This entails aggressive replacement of fluid lost from the intravascular space into the peritoneal cavity. Recurrence rates as high as 60–70% have been reported after simple ulcer closure, even in patients who do not have a history suggesting chronic ulcer. Therefore, patients should be given definitive surgery, such as a highly selective vagotomy. The only patients who should have simple closure are those who have had the perforation for an excessive period (longer than 12 hours) or are elderly or extremely ill.

Intestinal Obstruction

Symptoms and Classification: The hallmarks of intestinal obstruction are abdominal pain, distention, vomiting, and obstipation (inability to pass gas or stool) (Table 6.3–3). Not every patient has all four symptoms, and the severity of each varies with the level and type of obstruction. When an obstruction is high in the small intestine,

Table 6.3–3. Causes of intestinal obstruction.

Mechanical intestinal obstruction
Intraluminal lesions: intussusception, gallstones, food impaction
Intramural lesions: congenital (Hirschsprung's disease, stenosis, duplication), inflammatory (Crohn's disease, diverticulitis, actinomycosis, tuberculosis), neoplasms, trauma, hematoma
Extrinsic lesions: adhesions, hernias, neoplasms

Paralytic ileus
Postoperative ileus
Infection: peritonitis, pneumonia
Inflammation: pancreatitis
Metabolic disorders: hypokalemia, uremia
Drugs: narcotics, anticholinergics, ganglion-blocking drugs
Mesenteric vascular occlusion
Neuromuscular diseases: diabetic visceral neuropathy, scleroderma, pseudo-obstruction

vomiting characteristically appears early and may be copious; distention may be minimal. Patients with a colonic obstruction may have marked distention but no vomiting. Intractable constipation may be overlooked because the patient has two or three bowel movements early in the obstruction, until the bowel distal to the obstruction has been evacuated. On physical exam, the abdomen is usually distended and bowel sounds typically are high-pitched and occur in rushes.

Intestinal obstruction is most usefully classified into small or large bowel obstruction. The obstruction may be (1) simple obstruction, in which the lumen of the bowel is obstructed but the blood supply is intact; (2) strangulated obstruction, with both the lumen blocked and the blood supply to the intestine interrupted; and (3) closed-loop obstruction, in which the blood supply may or may not be interfered with, but egress of the intestinal contents is blocked both proximally and distally, causing rapid distention of the loop and risk of both strangulation and perforation.

Etiology: Intestinal obstruction has many causes, including extrinsic lesions, such as adhesions or an intra-abdominal abscess; intrinsic lesions, such as inflammation (eg, Crohn's disease) and neoplasms of the bowel wall; and intraluminal masses, such as a bezoar, gallstone, or fecal impaction. In the past, incarcerated inguinal hernias constituted the most common cause of small bowel obstruction. However, with ready access to hernia repair and with the increasing amount of abdominal and pelvic surgery being done, 80% of small bowel obstructions are recently caused by postoperative adhesions. Incarcerated hernias probably remain the second most common cause, followed by such conditions as Crohn's disease, intussusception, volvulus, internal hernias, and small bowel neoplasms. The predominant cause of large bowel obstruction is carcinoma, followed by diverticulitis, cecal or sigmoid volvulus, and Crohn's disease.

Differential Diagnosis: Differentiating a mechanical bowel obstruction from paralytic ileus (failure of propulsive motor activity) requires careful serial observations.

Typically, patients with paralytic ileus have no bowel sounds, but feeble sounds may be heard early in the episode. In contrast, patients in the early stage of a mechanical obstruction have strong, high-pitched, active bowel sounds; later, bowel sounds may decrease or disappear as the bowel becomes dilated or strangulated, or peritonitis develops. Paralytic ileus can be caused by any severe disease and is regularly seen temporarily after anesthesia and abdominal surgery. Common causes are peritonitis and severe electrolyte disturbances, especially potassium deficiency. Drugs such as narcotics, anticholinergics, and ganglion-blocking drugs may increase the severity of the ileus. Treatment of paralytic ileus is supportive: intestinal decompression and restoration of fluid and electrolyte balance. If the primary disorder is correctable, the ileus is self-limiting.

Management: Large bowel obstruction should always be treated as an urgent situation because of the danger of cecal distention and perforation. This is particularly true when the patient has a competent ileocecal valve, producing a closed-loop obstruction. The indicated procedure is early surgical decompression with a colostomy. Small bowel obstruction is a less urgent situation, and more time can be taken to prepare the patient for surgery, with the passage of a long intestinal tube and administration of intravenous fluids. However, unless there are extenuating circumstances, surgery should not be delayed beyond 12–24 hours. This is because of the 30% risk of strangulation. Strangulation cannot be reliably differentiated from simple obstruction on the basis of symptoms, physical signs, and laboratory studies. Therefore, the physician should not decide that a patient with complete small bowel obstruction can be managed nonoperatively, based on the clinical impression that the obstruction is not strangulated. Such an impression is wrong about one-third of the time.

Acute Mesenteric Ischemia

Acute mesenteric ischemia is an uncommon cause of abdominal pain. Sudden occlusion of the mesenteric blood supply leads to ischemic injury and then to infarction of the intestine. If intestinal necrosis is to be avoided and the patient's life saved, early diagnosis and surgical correction are vital. Miraculous recoveries are possible, and patients who lose a large percentage of the small intestine may do surprisingly well.

Arterial Occlusion: Infarction of the bowel can be caused by either arterial or venous occlusion. With acute arterial occlusion, often from an embolus or thrombosis of an arteriosclerotic plaque, the symptoms usually begin acutely. Pain is characteristically colicky at first, soon progressing to a steady, severe ache as tissue is damaged. On physical exam, bowel sounds are initially hyperactive, but then diminish or disappear. Patients may have only mild abdominal tenderness, if any, and their pain is much more severe than the tenderness would suggest. Many patients have hemoconcentration and a striking leukocytosis. With supportive care, some patients may deceptively appear to stabilize for 2–4 days, then develop necrosis, perforation, peritonitis, sepsis, and acidosis. If patients are to survive, the diagnosis must be made early, often on clinical findings alone. Only in a minority of cases is there the time or opportunity to confirm the diagnosis by mesenteric arteriography. The patient should be explored and, if possible, revascularized. Nonviable bowel should be resected within hours of the occlusion if the patient is to survive. Most superior mesenteric artery occlusions are caused by emboli in patients with atrial fibrillation or a recent myocardial infarction. If surgery is performed early, embolectomy or revascularization may be possible; otherwise, patients often require massive bowel resection to remove the compromised bowel prior to development of gangrene and perforation.

Venous Occlusion: The symptoms of mesenteric venous occlusion are usually subtler and slower to evolve, often continuing for days or even weeks. Because the clinical picture is less dramatic, diagnosis may be more difficult. The cause of venous occlusion is not usually determined. Many patients have polycythemia. The extent of bowel involvement may be more limited than with arterial occlusion, but postoperative extension is frequent and anastomotic disruption common.

Nonocclusive Mesenteric Ischemia: Intestinal infarction can be caused by reflex vasospasm of the mesenteric resistance vessels. This condition is called *nonocclusive mesenteric ischemia.* Infarction can be an endogenous response to severe physiologic stress or to exogenous administration of splanchnic vasoconstrictive agents—most often sympathomimetics or digitalis glycosides. Nonocclusive mesenteric ischemia is usually seen in severely ill patients after a hypotensive episode related to sepsis, myocardial infarction, major surgery, respiratory insufficiency, or hypovolemic shock. Unlike occlusive mesenteric ischemia, the first symptoms and signs are often mild, nonspecific (distention and malaise) and obscured by obtundation. Early in the disease, when the ischemic damage to the intestine is still reversible, patients do not have specific physical or laboratory signs. The diagnosis can be made only by angiography, obtained at this stage only if the physician has a high index of suspicion in vulnerable patients. Treatment is pharmacologic reversal of the vasospasm with intra-arterial vasodilators. Surgery is reserved for later resection of infarcted bowel and therefore is preferably done only after angiography and vasodilator therapy (see Table 6.10–1).

COMMON CAUSES OF CHRONIC AND RECURRENT ABDOMINAL PAIN

The most important causes of chronic and recurrent abdominal pain are irritable bowel syndrome, peptic ulcer, chronic cholecystitis and cholelithiasis, chronic relapsing pancreatitis, intermittent and chronic intestinal obstruction, chronic peritonitis, carcinoma of the stomach and pancreas, and some systemic diseases and intoxications (Table 6.3–4). With the exception of peptic ulcer (see Chapter 6.4), all these conditions are discussed in the text that follows.

Irritable Bowel Syndrome

"Irritable bowel syndrome," "functional bowel disorder," and "spastic colon" all are terms used to designate the most common cause of chronic or recurrent abdominal pain. The pain is most often localized to the left lower quadrant of the abdomen or to the hypogastrium. When located in the left upper quadrant, the condition is often called "splenic flexure syndrome"; when in the right upper quadrant, "hepatic flexure syndrome." Distention and localized spasm are thought to result from gas collecting in these two areas. Splenic flexure symptoms are sometimes confused with the pain of coronary artery disease, but they are relieved by the passing of flatus. Hepatic flexure symptoms may mimic symptoms of gallbladder dysfunction, and pain in the left lower quadrant may be attributed to diverticulitis. Patients with irrita-

Table 6.3–4. Common causes of chronic abdominal pain.

Condition	Most Frequent Location of Pain	Important Features
Irritable bowel syndrome	Hypogastrium or left lower quadrant, but can be anywhere	Onset difficult to date; patients are not awakened by pain; association with altered bowel pattern: constipation, diarrhea, or both
Chronic cholecystitis and cholelithiasis	Epigastrium, radiating to right upper quadrant and right subscapular region	Pain most prominent after meals; range: nonspecific dyspepsia to biliary colic
Chronic relapsing pancreatitis	Epigastrium, radiating to the back	Triad of pancreatic calcification, diabetes, and steatorrhea in only 20% of patients; alcohol abuse most common factor, but least amenable to treatment
Intermittent or chronic intestinal obstruction	Periumbilical or hypogastrium	May be difficult to differentiate from irritable bowel syndrome unless plain films of abdomen taken when asymptomatic are compared with films taken at height of symptoms; can coexist with irritable bowel syndrome

ble bowel syndrome are specifically sensitive to stimuli that induce intestinal pain, but are no more sensitive to somatic pain than people without irritable bowel.

Signs and Symptoms: Upper gastrointestinal tract symptoms of dyspepsia, bloating, belching, aerophagia, and anorexia may be part of the clinical picture, but vomiting is rare. Significant weight loss is unusual and cannot be attributed to this functional disorder unless accompanied by severe depression. Rarely are patients awakened at night by their symptoms; in the past, this was thought to imply a psychogenic origin, but it has been shown that when people sleep, their fasting intestinal motor pattern becomes more regular. Patients generally appear healthy, and the physical exam is normal except for a tender, cord-like sigmoid colon and hyperresonance over areas of the abdomen. A palpable sigmoid colon itself is not significant, but notable tenderness is meaningful.

Irritable bowel syndrome usually appears in early adulthood and rarely begins in a person older than 55. The condition is more common in women than men. Symptoms are often precipitated by meals or stress, and they are attributed to spastic and uncoordinated muscle contractions of the colon. Although irritable bowel syndrome has been perceived as a psychosomatic disorder, it is a disorder of intestinal motility that can be influenced by a number of stimuli, of which stress is but one. Both the symptoms and abnormal motility patterns also can be precipitated by meals, neurohumoral agents such as neostigmine, gastrointestinal peptides such as cholecystokinin, and intestinal distention. Furthermore, distention of the colon in one quadrant of the abdomen can produce pain that is perceived in a different quadrant.

An acute attack of diarrhea from a bacterial or viral infection, parasitic infestation, or antibiotic use may trigger symptoms of irritable bowel syndrome, probably in patients who have a predisposition to the disorder and are barely compensated when these precipitating factors supervene.

Diagnosis: The diagnosis of irritable bowel syndrome is based on abdominal pain with altered bowel habits but no detectable structural changes. The altered bowel habit may be constipation or diarrhea, or, more often, alternating constipation and diarrhea. Although a definition of irritable bowel syndrome based on abdominal pain and altered bowel habits suffices for most clinical purposes, more restrictive criteria have been proposed for clinical research purposes. Many patients have increased mucus with the stools. Abdominal bloating and distention are common complaints, and hyperresonance to percussion is a frequent finding. Eating often aggravates the pain. Defecation may provide some relief, but many patients feel that their defecation is incomplete.

Proctoscopy may reveal spasm and sometimes increased mucus on the mucosa, but bleeding is never found and mucosal biopsies are always normal. Patients also have normal complete blood cell count, erythrocyte sedi-

mentation rate, and blood chemistries, and stool examinations are negative for occult blood, white blood cells, ova, and parasites. Colonoscopy and barium enema, if obtained, are also normal.

Management: Management of irritable bowel syndrome begins with reassurance, conveyed by the physician's attitude, a relaxed and detailed interview, and negative diagnostic tests. The physician should describe the syndrome to the patient as a specific entity, a motility disorder usually involving the colon and more proximal gastrointestinal tract, caused by intestinal spasm triggered by a number of stimuli, most often stress, fatigue, or meals. Management also includes a high-fiber diet or bulk agents, such as psyllium hydrophilic mucilloid, to interrupt the constipation-diarrhea cycle and reestablish regular bowel habits. Anticholinergic drugs sometimes help relieve painful spasm. Agents such as loperamide or diphenoxylate may be used to control diarrhea. Antidiarrheal agents are used only for severe diarrhea and must be prescribed with caution so that they do not induce constipation in patients who tend to develop alternating diarrhea and constipation.

Diet restriction and manipulation have been grossly overemphasized in the management of irritable bowel syndrome. However, lactose intolerance should be ruled out as a contributing factor whenever the diagnosis is suspected, since lactose intolerance can completely mimic or aggravate the symptoms.

Chronic Cholecystitis and Cholelithiasis

Gallstones are formed from precipitated bile pigment (bilirubin) or cholesterol. Pigment stones develop in patients who have increased bilirubin excretion, as in hemolytic disorders like sickle cell disease. Cholesterol gallstones form from lithogenic bile. In lithogenic bile, the concentrations of bile acids and lecithin are not sufficient to maintain cholesterol in solution, especially when the bile is concentrated in the gallbladder. Stasis and changes in the gallbladder epithelium also appear to play a role. Gallstones can intermittently obstruct the cystic duct and produce biliary colic and cholecystitis.

Signs and Symptoms: The symptoms attributed to chronic cholecystitis and gallstones range from nonspecific symptoms that are indistinguishable from functional dyspepsia, to recurrent attacks of biliary colic, fever, and jaundice.

Typical biliary colic appears in the epigastrium, radiating to the right upper quadrant and subscapular regions. In about 25% of patients, the pain also radiates to the left upper quadrant or left subscapular area; in occasional patients, left-sided discomfort is the most prominent feature. Not all clinically significant gallbladder disease is associated with biliary colic, however. Because the gallbladder is stimulated to contract by humoral (cholecystokinin) and neural (vagus) stimuli released by eating, biliary colic often appears after meals. The suspicion of chronic cholecystitis is often based on a history of pain or dyspepsia after meals, especially fatty meals, and on the demonstration of gallstones. But there are several flaws in this formulation:

1. Gallstones and inflammation of the wall of the gallbladder are increasingly common with advancing age. Autopsy reveals gallbladder disease in up to 50% of all persons in their 60's. These pathologic changes cannot regularly be equated with a clinical syndrome.
2. The dyspepsia and belching caused by eating fatty foods, cabbage, and so on, have traditionally been considered characteristic of chronic cholecystitis. But these symptoms are not specific. More patients with fatty food intolerance have functional gastrointestinal disease than gallbladder disease.
3. Some patients who have had cholecystectomy for dyspeptic symptoms return later with complaints similar to their preoperative symptoms. Although often labeled *postcholecystectomy syndrome,* these patients' symptoms are usually caused by one of the following conditions: (a) unrecognized peptic or functional gastrointestinal disease, with symptoms erroneously attributed to gallbladder disease; (b) stones remaining in the common duct or cystic duct; (c) partial obstruction of the common duct; or (d) pancreatitis. Before advising surgery for chronic cholecystitis, the physician should seriously consider whether the patient's symptoms might be caused by one of these other conditions.

Diagnosis: Since clinically significant chronic cholecystitis is almost always caused by gallstones, the physician should prove the presence of gallstones before seriously considering the diagnosis. Ultrasonography is the most accurate way to detect gallstones in the gallbladder, but it does not readily detect common duct stones.

The physician can be more confident that gallbladder disease is causing the patient's symptoms if the patient has a history of biliary colic, fever, jaundice, or an elevated alkaline phosphatase. The jaundice and elevated alkaline phosphatase develop when stones being passed out of the gallbladder transiently obstruct the common bile duct. If the physician suspects gallbladder disease based on the patient's symptoms, and then excludes other diseases that mimic gallbladder disease and finds evidence of gallstones, the treatment is cholecystectomy, which can often be performed laparoscopically.

Management: Cholecystectomy as treatment for asymptomatic gallstones remains controversial. The risks from an elective cholecystectomy are small, and the likelihood of the patient's developing symptomatic gallbladder disease is said to be 3–20%. But the patient faces the surgical risk immediately, whereas the "silent" stone is unlikely ever to become symptomatic, and if it does, it may take 5–20 years. On the other hand, if surgery is delayed until the patient develops a complication such as common duct

stones with jaundice, the operation carries a much greater risk than if it had been performed electively. Much of the past interest in nonoperative treatment of cholelithiasis by gallstone dissolution therapy or lithotripsy has disappeared with the demonstration of the low morbidity, safety, and efficacy of laparoscopic cholecystectomy. In addition, many patients treated nonoperatively get recurrent gallstones unless they continue to take supplemental bile salts, such as ursodeoxycholic acid, to decrease the lithogenicity of bile. Cholecystectomy, on the other hand, decreases the lithogenicity of bile by increasing cycling of the bile salt pool and eliminating the normal stasis and concentration of bile in the gallbladder. As a consequence, gallstones only rarely recur following cholecystectomy.

Chronic Relapsing Pancreatitis

In the United States, over 90% of chronic relapsing pancreatitis is caused by alcohol abuse. Each episode of pancreatitis further damages acinar cells and distorts the pancreatic ducts. The patient may have an elevated serum amylase, especially in a blood sample drawn early in the attack. But with each succeeding episode, pancreatic exocrine function decreases and the likelihood of finding an elevated amylase diminishes. The precise pathogenesis of the progressive destruction of the pancreas is unclear, but the obstruction of the ducts by proteinaceous plugs sets the stage for extravasation of enzymes into the pancreatic parenchyma, causing further damage.

Patients who have lost 90% of their pancreatic acinar function develop fat malabsorption (Chapter 6.9). Late in the disease, the proteinaceous plugs calcify; calcification seen on plain abdominal x-ray indicates the diagnosis of chronic pancreatitis in 20% of patients.

Although chronic pancreatitis is characterized by the triad of pancreatic calcification, diabetes mellitus, and steatorrhea, no more than 20% of patients have the complete syndrome. In patients who do not have diagnostic pancreatic calcifications, several imaging techniques can show the characteristic anatomic changes: dilated ducts, pseudocysts, early calcification, and enlargement of the pancreas. Ultrasonography is useful to screen for these changes, but abdominal CT gives the most detailed views of the pancreas. Endoscopic retrograde cholangiopancreatography (ERCP), which shows details of the pancreatic ducts (strictures, rupture, and pseudocysts), is useful in planning surgery.

Management: Many surgical procedures have been advocated for chronic relapsing pancreatitis. Those currently used include sphincteroplasty, longitudinal pancreaticojejunostomy, 95% pancreatectomy, and resection of the head of the pancreas by means of a pancreatoduodenectomy (Whipple's operation). The main purpose of these procedures is to control pain, but their results are inconsistent. For this reason, some add destruction of the celiac plexus to interrupt the major pain pathway. The major reason for failure is that many patients with recurrent pancreatitis are unreformed alcoholics, and no operation has been devised that will permit these patients to drink with impunity.

In some patients, pancreatitis is associated with cholelithiasis, peptic ulcer, hyperparathyroidism, or hyperlipidemia. When these conditions are corrected, the attacks of pancreatitis often lessen or cease if the pancreatitis has not advanced to the point that it is autonomous of the original stimulus.

Intermittent or Chronic Intestinal Obstruction

Postoperative adhesions are often blamed for chronic or recurrent abdominal pain. Adhesions cause pain by partially or completely obstructing the intestine. Before a patient undergoes an operation to lyse the adhesions, partial intestinal obstruction should be demonstrated. An intermittent incomplete volvulus is occasionally the cause of recurrent abdominal pain, but it can be diagnosed only if abdominal x-rays are taken during an attack. The inflammatory bowel lesion that most often produces partial intestinal obstruction and chronic abdominal pain is Crohn's disease (Chapter 6.10).

Neoplastic lesions commonly cause chronic obstructive symptoms. The most common is carcinoma of the colon, especially on the left side. Lymphoma of the small bowel also produces symptoms of progressive obstruction. Intestinal polyps, such as those found in Peutz-Jeghers syndrome, and carcinoid of the small intestine may give rise to intermittent obstructive symptoms, usually by causing intussusception.

In addition to causing acute abdominal pain, intestinal ischemia can produce symptoms of obstruction when a short ischemic segment of bowel in the process of healing becomes narrowed and fibrotic.

Intestinal pseudo-obstruction is a rare intestinal motor abnormality that causes chronic or episodic abdominal distention and pain. Abdominal x-rays showing dilated intestinal loops with air-fluid levels are interpreted as demonstrating a mechanical obstruction, but at laparotomy no obstructing lesion is found. If a site of obstruction is not clear, careful small bowel contrast studies should be done to prevent an unnecessary operation.

Chronic Peritonitis

Chronic tuberculous peritonitis causes chronic diffuse abdominal pain, minimal tenderness, low-grade fever, and sometimes ascites. When associated with cirrhosis and ascites, tuberculous peritonitis is difficult to diagnose, and it is often overlooked or found unexpectedly at laparotomy.

Carcinoma of the Stomach

In the 1930s, carcinoma of the stomach (Chapter 6.6) was the most common cause of cancer death in the United States; today it ranks eighth. The decrease is explained not by earlier diagnosis or improved treatment, but by a lower incidence. The clinical manifestations of gastric carcinoma can be so vague that the tumor may progress to the point of inoperability while the patient is being carefully followed up by a physician. Weight loss, anorexia, vomiting, and pain are the most common symptoms, but unfortunately not early ones. The presenting complaint may also be symptoms of chronic blood loss anemia. A mass is palpable in only one-third of patients and often is a sign of advanced disease. The first test to be ordered in patients with suspected gastric carcinoma is fiberoptic gastroscopy with endoscopic biopsies and cytologic brushings. The treatment is surgery, but the 5-year survival rate is 10% overall, and only 25% if the lesion appears to have been completely resected.

Carcinoma of the Pancreas

Although the incidence of gastric cancer is decreasing, cancer of the pancreas (Chapter 6.6) is increasing and is now the fifth most common cause of cancer death. To make matters worse, early diagnosis is usually made only by accident. The 5-year survival rate is no more than 1%. Even when the tumor is in the head of the pancreas and jaundice is an early symptom, the survival rate is less than 10%. Pain is the most common presenting symptom, reported by 75% of patients with carcinoma of the head of the pancreas and by practically all patients with involvement of the body and tail of the pancreas. Usually, the pain is a dull ache in the epigastrium; the pain may radiate to the right upper quadrant of the abdomen if the tumor is in the head, and to the left if it is in the body and tail. Many patients have crampy lower abdominal pain with constipation and are initially thought to have irritable bowel syndrome. Twenty percent of patients have steady pain in the back or in the lower lumbar region.

Jaundice is found in 70% of patients with carcinoma of the head of the pancreas, but in less than 15% of those with involvement of the body. The only two tests that show any promise of permitting early diagnosis and a better chance of survival are CT scanning and endoscopic cannulation of the pancreatic duct by ERCP. Isolated examples of early diagnosis have been reported, but the overall grim picture of pancreatic cancer is not improving. A modified Whipple's operation can be performed in those without metastases or involvement of a major vessel such as the superior mesenteric vessels; all of these patients received useful palliation, and about 20% of patients are alive after 5 years. Patients with unresectable disease often can be palliated by bypassing the obstruction to the gastric outlet and biliary tree. Radiation treatment or alcohol injection of the celiac ganglia controls some patients' pain. The tumor is poorly responsive to chemotherapy or radiation therapy.

Systemic Diseases and Intoxications With Recurrent Abdominal Pain

Chronic or recurrent abdominal pain can be part of a number of systemic diseases and intoxications, among them polyarteritis nodosa, systemic lupus erythematosus, lead poisoning, hypercalcemia, diabetic neuropathy, ketoacidosis, porphyria, familial Mediterranean fever, and tabes dorsalis. Unfortunately, the pain does not have any special characteristics that allow the physician to decide which disease is the cause. A specific diagnosis rests with each disease's extra-abdominal signs and symptoms.

SUMMARY

▶ Only a minority of patients with acute abdominal pain are found to have a condition that requires surgical treatment.

▶ Only three processes are capable of producing pain in the alimentary tract: tension in the wall (caused by intense muscle contraction or distention), ischemia, and inflammation of the serosa (peritonitis).

▶ The single most valuable test for a possible "acute surgical abdomen" is repeated physical exams by a physician over an extended period.

▶ The diagnosis of irritable bowel syndrome is based on abdominal pain with altered bowel habits but no detectable structural changes.

SUGGESTED READING

Brewer BJ et al: Abdominal pain: An analysis of 1,000 consecutive cases in a university hospital emergency room. Am J Surg 1976;131:219.

Glambek I, Arnesjo B, Soreide O: Correlation between gallstones and abdominal symptoms in a random population: Results from a screening study. Scand J Gastroenterol 1989;24:277.

Klein KB, Mellinkoff SM: Approach to patient with abdominal pain. In: *Textbook of Gastroenterology,* 2nd ed. Yamada T (editor). JB Lippincott, 1995.

Schuster MM: Irritable bowel syndrome. In: *Gastrointestinal Disease,* 5th ed. Sleisenger MH, Fordtran JS (editors). WB Saunders, 1993.

Silen W (editor): *Copes' Early Diagnosis of the Acute Abdomen,* 19th ed. Oxford University Press, 1995.

Peptic Ulcer and Dyspepsia

Anthony N. Kalloo, MD, and Thomas R. Hendrix, MD

Peptic ulcer disease is one of several disorders of the upper gastrointestinal tract mucosa, caused at least in part by gastric acid. Ulcers can develop in the esophagus, stomach, or duodenum; at the margin of a gastroenterostomy; in the jejunum, as may be seen in Zollinger-Ellison syndrome; and in association with a Meckel's diverticulum containing ectopic gastric mucosa. Patients with peptic ulcer disease can present with mild abdominal discomfort or with catastrophic bleeding or perforation.

Dyspepsia is abdominal discomfort, pain, or nausea, usually either relieved or worsened by meals. Peptic ulcer patients can present with dyspepsia, and dyspepsia can signal peptic ulcer, but each can exist independently. Dyspepsia occurring alone is called "non-ulcer dyspepsia."

PEPTIC ULCER DISEASE

Pathogenesis

The old dictum, "no gastric acid, no peptic ulcer," does not tell the whole story. Excessive secretion of gastric acid is but one factor in the pathogenesis of ulcers. The other is decreased mucosal defense against gastric acid, particularly from nonsteroidal anti-inflammatory drugs (NSAIDs) or infection with *Helicobacter pylori*.

The integrity of the upper gastrointestinal tract mucosa depends on the balance between "hostile" factors (gastric acid, pepsin) and "protective" factors (prostaglandins) affecting the mucosa (Table 6.4–1). The mucosa can be damaged when increased gastric acid secretion overwhelms normal mucosal protection. For example, in Zollinger-Ellison syndrome, the sole cause of gastric acid hypersecretion is a gastrin-secreting tumor. The role that gastric acid plays in mediating inflammation and ulceration is supported by the fact that agents that reduce or neutralize acid allow peptic ulcers to heal and limit their recurrences.

Pepsin is often overlooked as a hostile agent. The precursor of pepsin is pepsinogen, produced by the chief cells in the gastric glands in the fundus and body of the stomach. Pepsin, like other acid proteases, is most active at a pH below 4.0 and is inactivated at a pH above 6.0. This is why pepsin's effect can be controlled by reducing or neutralizing acid.

The mucosa can also be damaged by a decrease in mucosal defense. Two factors protect the gastroduodenal mucosa: secretion of mucus and bicarbonate, and integrity of mucosal blood flow. Both depend on the production of prostaglandins. When prostaglandin synthesis is inhibited, as by NSAIDs, patients are at risk for developing peptic ulcer even if they do not have gastric hypersecretion. The importance of mucosal defense is proved by occasional patients with gastrinomas who have massive acid hypersecretion but no ulcers.

About 20% of patients taking a course of NSAIDs develop at least endoscopic evidence of peptic ulcer disease. Gastrointestinal bleeding and perforation are well-recognized complications of long-term NSAIDs, especially in the elderly. Oral NSAIDs damage the gastric mucosa both by local irritation and systemically by inhibiting mucosal prostaglandin synthesis. Even enteric-coated preparations injure the mucosa, although they do less damage because the drug has less topical effect. Intravenous NSAIDs damage the mucosa, also by inhibiting prostaglandin synthesis. Aspirin, even when taken in low doses to prevent coronary artery disease, injures the mucosa, though usually without causing symptoms.

Helicobacter pylori is a gram-negative rod that has been implicated in the pathogenesis of peptic ulcer disease. *H pylori* is found in the gastric antrum of almost all patients with duodenal ulcers, and if *H pylori* is eliminated, the ulcers do not recur. *H pylori* is also associated with gastric ulcers. But, like gastric acid, *H pylori* is only one factor contributing to the pathogenesis of peptic ulcer disease: In industrialized countries, 50% of people over age 50 are infected with *H pylori,* but no more than 10% have ever had a peptic ulcer.

The mechanism by which *H pylori* injures the gastric mucosa is complex. The organism produces virulent factors (eg, proteases, urease, cytotoxins) and increases gastrin secretion. Although duodenal ulcers heal on standard acid-reducing regimens that do not eliminate *H pylori*, 80% of patients have recurrent ulcers within 1 year unless they continue on maintenance acid suppressant therapy.

Table 6.4–1. Factors responsible for maintaining gastrointestinal mucosal integrity.

Factor	Mechanism
Mucus production	Provides barrier from hostile factors
Bicarbonate secretion	Neutralizes acid
Specialized acid-resistant apical surface membrane	Resists diffusion of acid into the mucosa
Blood flow to the mucosa	Delivers bicarbonate to surface epithelium
Prostaglandin production	Maintains mucosal blood flow and stimulates secretion of mucus and bicarbonate

The role of *H pylori* in causing non-ulcer dyspepsia is less clear. Some randomized trials of non-ulcer dyspepsia have shown slight clinical improvement when the organism is eradicated, but most studies have not shown any benefit. Cigarette smoking, another important risk factor for peptic ulcer disease, also impairs mucosal defense by inhibiting prostaglandin synthesis. Although increased acid secretion has been touted as important in the pathophysiology of peptic ulcer disease in cigarette smokers, several studies have shown that smokers have unchanged or even reduced acid secretion.

Clinical Presentation

Most patients with peptic ulcer disease present with abdominal discomfort, pain, or nausea. The pain is in the epigastrium and usually does not radiate. Pain radiating to the back suggests that an ulcer has penetrated posteriorly, or the pain might be from the pancreas. Pain radiating to the right upper quadrant suggests disease of the gallbladder or bile ducts.

Patients may describe the pain of peptic ulcer as burning or gnawing, or as hunger pain building slowly for up to 1–2 hours and then gradually going away. To varying degrees, the pain is relieved by antacids. Classically, the pain of gastric ulcers is aggravated by meals, whereas the pain of duodenal ulcers is relieved by meals (Table 6.4–2). Hence, patients with gastric ulcers tend to avoid food and present with weight loss, but few patients with duodenal ulcers lose weight. It is important to remember that although these patterns are typical, they are not pathognomonic.

Diagnosis

Patients with peptic ulcer disease most commonly present with abdominal pain or discomfort (Chapter 6.3), but these symptoms are not specific. They may be the presenting symptoms of other disorders such as gastric and pancreatic malignancies, mesenteric ischemia, gallstones, irritable bowel syndrome, pancreatitis, and depression. Anorexia, significant weight loss, and lack of response to conventional treatment for peptic ulcer disease should suggest conditions other than benign peptic ulcer, warranting endoscopy and abdominal imaging.

Endoscopic and Radiographic Studies: Peptic ulcer disease is best defined by upper gastrointestinal esophagogastroduodenoscopy (EGD). The endoscopist can detect subtle mucosal lesions and biopsy lesions to establish their histopathologic basis (see Color Plates). For example, the endoscopist might suspect malignancy in a gastric ulcer that has heaped-up, irregular margins (see Figure 6.6–3); fewer than 5% of malignant ulcers look completely benign. Endoscopic biopsies are indicated for all gastric ulcers at the time of diagnosis. Duodenal ulcers are always benign, so no biopsies are needed.

Barium x-ray is widely available and less expensive than endoscopy, but limited by being less sensitive and less accurate at defining mucosal disease (gastritis) or distinguishing benign from malignant ulcers. The x-ray can be difficult to interpret in patients who have anatomic deformity from previous gastric surgery or from scarring caused by chronic inflammation. X-rays have up to a 30% false-negative and a 10% false-positive rate.

Laboratory Tests: Patients with uncomplicated peptic ulcer disease do not need specialized testing. Patients with refractory (not healed after 8 weeks of optimal therapy) or recurrent disease should have their serum gastrin and serum calcium measured to screen for gastrinoma and multiple endocrine neoplasia (MEN) (Chapter 4.1). They should also undergo gastric acid analysis to determine whether the ulcer is caused by gastric acid hypersecretion (a basal acid output exceeding 10 mEq/hr) or decreased mucosal protection.

Patients with recurrent peptic ulcers may have an underlying *H pylori* infection. The gold standard for diagnosing *H pylori* is histologic examination of biopsies of the gastric antrum, usually obtained at endoscopy. *H py-*

Table 6.4–2. Distinguishing clinical features of gastric and duodenal ulcers.

	Gastric Ulcer	Duodenal Ulcer
Effect of meals	Pain usually worsened; weight loss common	Pain usually relieved; weight loss uncommon
Causes	Decreased mucosal protection from gastric acid, caused by, eg, *H pylori* gastritis, NSAIDs, intestinal metaplasia	Decreased duodenal mucosal protection from gastric acid, caused by, eg, peptic duodenitis (gastric metaplasia + *H pylori*), gastric hypersecretion
Helicobacter pylori	Often	Usually
Chance of malignancy	Yes	No
Follow-up	Prove healing endoscopically	Follow symptoms

lori is not routinely cultured because the organism is difficult to grow. Serologic tests for *H pylori* are available, but unfortunately a positive test indicates only past exposure and is not useful for determining that the infection has been cured. *H pylori* produces large quantities of the enzyme urease; this property is used in developing "urea breath tests" to diagnose current infections. Breath tests have the potential to be very useful because they are simple and noninvasive.

Management

The principle of medical therapy for peptic ulcer disease is either to reduce the hostile factors or to augment the protective factors (see Table 6.4–1). Antacids, histamine H_2-receptor antagonists (H_2 blockers), proton pump inhibitors (eg, omeprazole, lansoprazole), and surgery work primarily by neutralizing gastric acid or reducing acid production. Agents such as sucralfate and prostaglandins enhance mucosal protection. Eradication of *H pylori* infection not only restores normal mucosal resistance, but, unlike other treatments, does not require maintenance therapy to prevent ulcer recurrence. Patients should avoid factors known to contribute to peptic ulcer disease, such as NSAIDs, smoking, and alcohol.

Medical Treatment: Antacids neutralize gastric acid and are more effective than placebo in healing both duodenal and gastric ulcers. However, antacids have to be taken in relatively large doses 1 and 3 hours after meals and at bedtime, and they cause side effects. The major side effect of magnesium-containing antacids is diarrhea.

Histamine H_2-receptor antagonists reduce gastric acid production by blocking the H_2 receptor on the parietal cell (Figure 6.4–1). The available H_2 blockers, used to treat both gastric and duodenal ulcers, are cimetidine, ranitidine, famotidine, and nizatidine. Choice of drug should be dictated by cost, convenience of dosing schedule, and possible drug interactions.

The proton pump inhibitors—omeprazole and lansoprazole—are substituted benzimidazoles that inactivate the parietal cell's hydrogen-potassium ATPase. These enzymes act as a proton pump and constitute the final common pathway in the secretion of hydrogen ions. Increasing the omeprazole or lansoprazole dose can reduce acid secretion to the point of making patients achlorhydric—something that H_2 blockade cannot do. Thus, the proton pump inhibitors are primary treatment when gastric hypersecretion is resistant to other therapy, as in patients with Zollinger-Ellison syndrome (see "Gastrinoma" below).

Sucralfate is the aluminum salt of a sulfated disaccharide. The drug forms a barrier over the ulcer crater, stimulates prostaglandin synthesis, and binds to noxious agents such as bile salts. Sucralfate is as effective as H_2 blockers in healing duodenal and gastric ulcers, but patients are less likely to follow a sucralfate regimen because it requires multiple doses a day. Since sucralfate is not absorbed systemically, its only notable side effect is constipation.

Misoprostol is a prostaglandin E_1 analog that increases mucosal resistance and, to a minor degree, inhibits acid secretion. Misoprostol has been advocated for prophylaxis of NSAID-induced mucosal injury. But the drug has significant side effects, primarily mild-to-moderate diarrhea, and is too expensive to be used by most patients taking NSAIDs long-term.

H pylori is not effectively treated by single-drug therapy because the organism quickly becomes resistant to

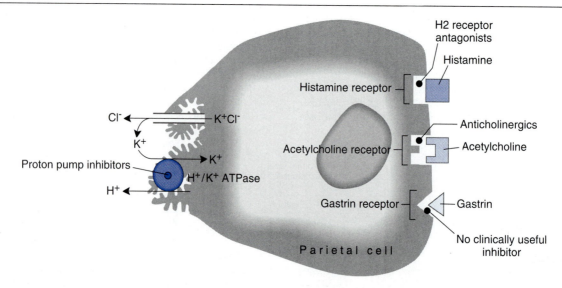

Figure 6.4–1. Parietal cell, showing receptors for stimuli of gastric acid secretion, and sites of action of inhibitory drugs.

antibiotics. A 2-week course of triple therapy with amoxicillin (or tetracycline), metronidazole, and bismuth clears the organism in about 90% of patients, but causes side effects in 20% of patients. Newer and simpler regimens are being developed. A promising combination is omeprazole with an antibiotic such as amoxicillin or clarithromycin.

Treatment recommendations for *H pylori* are still evolving. Patients with recurrent ulcers who are found to harbor *H pylori* should have it treated; during this treatment, patients need not take an H_2 blocker to suppress acid. Until simpler regimens for *H pylori* become available, many patients' first peptic ulcer episode will continue to be treated by a once-a-day H_2 blocker. However, the physician should always offer patients with peptic ulcer disease the option of curative anti-*H pylori* therapy.

Surgery: In the United States, the past few decades have seen a declining need for elective surgery for peptic ulcer. This decline probably has several explanations, primary among them the widespread use of H_2 blockers. The major indication for surgery is complications such as gastrointestinal hemorrhage, perforation, and gastric outlet obstruction.

Since duodenal ulcers are always benign, the physician can usually monitor patients' response to medical therapy by following their symptoms, without needing to confirm healing by endoscopy. When patients with duodenal ulcers need surgery, the principal procedure is vagotomy. However, truncal vagotomy causes delayed gastric emptying and necessitates a concurrent drainage procedure such as antrectomy, pyloroplasty, or gastroenterostomy. A more selective vagotomy (proximal gastric vagotomy) does not necessitate a drainage procedure.

Gastric ulcers that have not healed by 8 weeks of conventional medical therapy must be reevaluated by multiple endoscopic biopsies and cytology to ensure that a gastric carcinoma has not been missed. If no malignancy is seen on biopsy, patients are given 6 weeks of aggressive therapy to eradicate *H pylori*, suppress acid with full doses of omeprazole, or do both in turn. A gastric ulcer that does not heal after this second course of medical therapy may suggest underlying malignancy, even if repeat biopsies are negative. Besides, any unhealed gastric ulcer, benign or malignant, keeps patients at risk. For all these reasons, nonhealing gastric ulcers should be resected surgically. The most common reason for surgery for benign gastric ulcers is the patient's inability to comply with treatment recommendations.

The usual surgery for gastric ulcer is wedge resection with vagotomy and a drainage procedure. Vagotomy may not be necessary in patients with gastric acid hyposecretion, since the primary mechanism of their ulcer disease is decreased mucosal defense.

Complications

The complications of peptic ulcer disease are hemorrhage, perforation, and gastric outlet obstruction. Gastrointestinal hemorrhage affects 5–20% of patients, more often those with duodenal than gastric ulcers. Management of gastrointestinal bleeding is discussed in Chapter 6.5. About 5–10% of patients with peptic ulcer suffer a perforation. Perforations are especially likely in elderly patients on NSAIDs. Surgery remains the only treatment.

Fewer than 5% of patients develop gastric outlet obstruction from pyloric stenosis. Varying degrees of obstruction are seen in acute peptic ulcer disease, caused by inflammatory swelling involving the pyloric channel. The physician may be able to elicit a succussion splash; this is a technique for detecting excess fluid in the stomach, resulting from obstruction of the gastric outlet. Patients should be managed with nasogastric aspiration, a parenteral H_2 blocker, and intravenous hydration. Whether the obstruction has opened may be determined by the saline load test: 750 mL of normal saline is instilled into the stomach, and the residue is measured after 30 minutes; recovery of 400 mL or more suggests persistent gastric outlet obstruction. Obstruction caused by a fibrotic stricture can sometimes be opened by endoscopic balloon dilatation of the pyloric channel. Surgical resection of refractory strictures is effective.

GASTRINOMA (ZOLLINGER-ELLISON SYNDROME)

The classic triad of Zollinger-Ellison syndrome is peptic ulcers in unusual locations (eg, the jejunum), massive gastric acid hypersecretion, and a gastrin-producing islet cell tumor of the pancreas (gastrinoma). But only 50% of patients have their gastrinoma in the pancreas. Another 20% have it in the duodenum, and others have it in the stomach, peripancreatic lymph nodes, liver, ovary, or small bowel mesentery.

Zollinger-Ellison syndrome accounts for only about 0.1% of all duodenal ulcer disease. One-fourth of patients have Zollinger-Ellison as part of the multiple endocrine neoplasia syndrome type I (MEN I) (Chapter 4.1).

Patients with gastrinoma tend to have intractable ulcer disease. Since gastrin is trophic to the gastric mucosa, endoscopy or x-ray may show hypertrophy of the gastric rugae. Patients may also have diarrhea (including steatorrhea from acid inactivation of lipase) and gastroesophageal reflux. In 75% of patients, the symptoms are episodic.

The physician should suspect gastrinoma when a patient with gastric acid hypersecretion has an elevated fasting serum gastrin. The fasting serum gastrin should be measured in patients who have ulcers in atypical locations such as the second and third portions of the duodenum and in patients who have recurrent ulcers, ulcers with diarrhea, or ulcers with complications such as perforation or hemorrhage. Serum gastrin levels higher than 1000 pg/mL are considered diagnostic for gastrinoma. The physician should also measure gastric acid output, because patients with achlorhydria have a compensatory elevation of the serum gastrin, usually to over 1000 pg/mL. Patients with a

Table 6.4–3. Conditions associated with gastric acid hypersecretion (basal acid output exceeding 10 mEq/hr).

With elevated gastrin
  Gastrin-producing tumor (Zollinger-Ellison syndrome)
  Hyperplasia of antral G cells
  Retained antrum (since antral G cells left in with the duodenum
    after gastrectomy are not exposed to acid, their gastrin
    secretion is not inhibited)

With normal gastrin
  Normal individuals (5% of healthy people have a normal gastrin
    but gastric acid hypersecretion)
  Duodenal ulcers (40% of patients have gastric acid
    hypersecretion)
  Malignant carcinoid, systemic mastocytosis, and basophilic
    leukemia (in these conditions, gastric acid hypersecretion is
    caused by hyperhistaminemia)
  Pyloric obstruction
  Hypercalcemia
  Small bowel resection
  Conditions caused by stress, eg, brain injury, multiple burns

Table 6.4–4. Common causes of dyspepsia.

Gastrointestinal conditions
  Peptic ulcer disease
  Gastritis, duodenitis, esophagitis
  Delayed gastric emptying
  Gastric cancer
  Chronic pancreatitis
  Pancreatic cancer
  Colorectal cancer

Nongastrointestinal conditions
  Ischemic heart disease
  Metabolic diseases (eg, diabetes mellitus, electrolyte disorders)
  Drugs (eg, NSAIDs, digitalis)
  Nongastrointestinal intra-abdominal malignancies (eg, renal cell
    carcinoma, ovarian cancer)

NSAIDs, nonsteroidal anti-inflammatory drugs.

serum gastrin of 200–1000 pg/mL require provocation testing to distinguish benign causes of hypergastrinemia (Table 6.4–3). A commonly used provocation test is the secretin test: After the patient is given secretin, a rise of at least 200 pg/mL in the serum gastrin is considered diagnostic for gastrinoma.

Management of gastrinoma begins with controlling gastric acid hypersecretion. Most patients' hypersecretion can be controlled with high doses of omeprazole. Efforts should be made to localize the gastrinoma, and, if possible, resect it. Useful preoperative tests to localize a gastrinoma are abdominal ultrasonography, computed tomography, arteriography and venous sampling for gastrin, and endoscopic ultrasonography. No test is completely accurate.

In patients who have MEN I without gastrinoma, gastric acid secretion may be controlled by correcting hypercalcemia, which is a common result of parathyroid hyperplasia. In most patients, subtotal parathyroidectomy normalizes serum calcium levels and decreases acid secretion, gastrin levels, and medication requirements.

DYSPEPSIA

Dyspepsia is abdominal discomfort, pain, or nausea made better or worse by meals. Peptic ulcer disease causes these symptoms, but not all dyspepsia is caused by peptic ulcer (non-ulcer dyspepsia). Non-ulcer dyspepsia is at least as common as peptic ulcer disease (Table 6.4–4). Inflammatory conditions of the upper gastrointestinal tract, such as esophagitis, gastritis, and duodenitis, can present as dyspepsia and can be accurately diagnosed only by endoscopic biopsy. Dyspepsia can be associated with the irritable bowel syndrome and with delayed gastric emptying. The latter may be identified by scintigraphic measurement of gastric emptying.

The main issue in evaluating dyspepsia is determining whether the patient has serious underlying disease. Some

gastroenterologists recommend starting empiric treatment with antacids or an H₂ blocker; patients who do not respond to this treatment after 6 weeks need endoscopy or barium x-ray to rule out significant pathology, especially cancer (Chapter 6.6). However, H₂ blockers can reduce the inflammation of malignant gastric ulcers and temporarily mask their symptoms. A better approach is early endoscopic evaluation of patients over age 40 with recent onset of dyspepsia, especially if they have weight loss, anorexia, or other evidence of underlying disease. In younger patients who have no evidence of underlying disease and no family history of peptic ulcer, a reasonable first step is reassurance, antacids, and limiting environmental factors like alcohol, cigarette smoking, and NSAIDs. Patients who do not improve after 2 weeks need further evaluation.

SUMMARY

▶ Peptic ulcer presents with pain, perforation, or bleeding. The most common causes are *Helicobacter pylori* infection and nonsteroidal anti-inflammatory drugs (NSAIDs).

▶ The goal of medical therapy is to heal the peptic ulcer by decreasing gastric acid secretion (eg, with an H₂ blocker) or increasing mucosal protection (eg, with eradication of *H pylori*, or, if the patient does not have *H pylori*, with sucralfate and avoidance of NSAIDs).

▶ Relapse of duodenal ulcers can be prevented by eradicating *H pylori*.

▶ Healing of gastric ulcers should always be documented, because nonhealing may mean underlying malignancy.

▶ Dyspepsia is abdominal discomfort, pain, or nausea, usually made better or worse by meals. Dyspepsia should be evaluated with endoscopy in patients over age 40, patients with anorexia or weight loss, and patients whose dyspepsia persists despite conventional medical therapy.

SUGGESTED READING

Barbara L et al: Definition and investigation of dyspepsia: Consensus of an international *ad hoc* working party. Dig Dis Sci 1989;34:1272.

Graham DY, Agrawal NM, Roth SH: Prevention of NSAID-induced gastric ulcer with misoprostol: Multicentre, double-blind, placebo-controlled trial. Lancet 1988;2:1277.

Meier RF et al: Endoscopy as final arbiter in controlled clinical trials in peptic disorders. Clin Gastroenterol 1986;15:377.

Walsh JH, Peterson WL: The treatment of *Helicobacter pylori* infection in the management of peptic ulcer disease. N Engl J Med 1995;333:984.

6.5

Gastrointestinal Bleeding

Thomas R. Hendrix, MD, Francis M. Giardiello, MD, and H. Franklin Herlong, MD

The patient with gastrointestinal bleeding may have a life-threatening emergency with hematemesis (vomiting blood), hematochezia (passage of blood from the rectum), or melena (passage of black, tarry stools). At the other extreme, gastrointestinal bleeding may be occult and chronic and discovered only in a search for the cause of anemia. In recent decades, mortality rate from acute gastrointestinal bleeding has remained at an average of 10%, despite more accurate diagnosis and new therapies. This continuing high mortality rate is explained primarily by physicians' failure to determine how much blood the patient has lost and the inadequacy of volume replacement. Successful management of an acute gastrointestinal hemorrhage often requires close cooperation between internist and surgeon.

ACUTE GASTROINTESTINAL BLEEDING

The evaluation and management of acute gastrointestinal bleeding can be divided into three overlapping phases. The first and most crucial phase is support—estimating blood loss and providing adequate volume replacement. The second is diagnosis—establishing the source of the bleeding (Table 6.5–1) and assessing the risk of further bleeding. The third is treatment—giving specific and nonspecific treatment for the bleeding lesion.

Supportive Management

Estimate of Blood Volume Deficit: The lack of a simple, reliable test to provide serial measurements of functional blood volume (blood still available to perfuse tissues) forces the clinician to use indirect observations to estimate blood volume deficit (Table 6.5–2). From this estimate, the physician determines the type, rate, and volume of initial fluid replacement.

Hematemesis, melena, and hematochezia: The greater the rate of bleeding and the higher the lesion is in the gastrointestinal tract, the more likely that the patient will vomit blood. If patients have had hematemesis in which the emesis is all blood and if they have vomited more than once, they should be considered to have lost one-third to one-half of their blood volume. Basing blood replacement on this assumption minimizes the chances of underestimating the blood loss and of suddenly finding it necessary to combat vascular collapse.

As little as 50–80 mL of blood introduced into the upper gastrointestinal tract can turn the stools black. Thus, in evaluating a patient with melena, the physician must use other signs to estimate the volume of blood lost. Hematochezia also does not provide a useful estimate of the volume of blood lost, since a much larger hemorrhage is required to produce red blood through the rectum from a upper gastrointestinal source than from a lower source.

Blood pressure and pulse: Recumbent patients with hypotension (systolic blood pressure below 90 mm Hg, diastolic below 60 mm Hg) and tachycardia (pulse above 110/min) have probably lost at least 50% of their normal blood volume. Fifty percent of patients with systolic blood pressure below 100 mm Hg on admission have had a massive hemorrhage requiring more than 2.5 L blood replacement, while only 13% of patients requiring less than 2.5 L have an admission blood pressure below 100 mm Hg. Comparing supine and standing blood pressure and pulse also gives valuable indications of the volume of blood loss. A drop of more than 15 mm Hg in systolic blood pressure from recumbency to standing, together with a rise in pulse rate of greater than 20 bpm, is a reliable indicator of blood loss of more than 20% of normal blood volume.

Most gastrointestinal hemorrhages, especially those of arterial or variceal origin, occur in episodes lasting about 30 minutes. After each bleeding episode the patient's blood pressure and pulse stabilize, and the physician may be lulled into a false sense of security. Each recurrent episode of bleeding, however, depletes the patient's reserve, and if blood replacement is inadequate, further bleeding leads to vascular collapse.

Urine output: One of the early indications of a decrease in blood volume is a fall in urine output. With a 20% decrease in functional blood volume, urine output falls from the normal level of 50 mL/hr to 20–30 mL/hr.

Table 6.5–1. The most common causes of gastrointestinal bleeding.

Upper GI Tract	Lower GI Tract
Acute bleeding	
Duodenal and gastric ulcer	Diverticulosis
Gastric erosions	Angiodysplasia
Congestive gastropathy and	Colitis
gastroesophageal varices	Neoplasms
Mallory-Weiss tear	Undetermined
Chronic bleeding	
Angiodysplasia	Inflammatory bowel disease
Congestive gastropathy and	Meckel's diverticulum
gastroesophageal varices	Neoplasms
Neoplasms	Anal and rectal lesions
Duodenal and gastric ulcer	(hemorrhoids, anal fissure)
Undetermined	Undetermined

With greater deficits, there is a further fall in urine output (eg, urine output of 5–15 mL/hr is associated with a 30% deficit, and little or no urine output with a 40–50% deficit). When volume replacement is adequate, output rises to 50 mL/hr.

Central venous pressure: Central venous pressure is the most accurate indicator of functional blood volume but requires the insertion of a catheter into the superior vena cava. Because the largest fraction of the blood volume is in the venous compartment, one of the first indications of decompensation is a falling central venous pressure. In a study of gastroduodenal hemorrhage, rapidly falling pressure (2 cm H_2O/min, with an overall fall of 5 cm H_2O) was always found to be associated with arterial bleeding. This event should alert the clinician to the likelihood that emergency surgery may be required. Since the range of normal central venous pressure is wide—5–12 cm—the direction and rate of change are more significant than the initial pressure. Monitoring the central venous pressure also helps guard against overtransfusion, because the pressure rises before pulmonary congestion and edema occur. Overtransfusion, especially in patients with portal hypertension, leads to further increase in portal pressure and may induce more bleeding from esophageal varices. Blood volume is usually replaced in such patients to bring the central venous pressure to 6–8 cm H_2O. In general, central venous pressure is

Table 6.5–2. Evaluating volume of blood loss in patients with acute gastrointestinal bleeding.

Reliable signs
   Massive hematemesis (gross blood with clots)
   Orthostatic hypotension
   Recumbent hypotension (systolic blood pressure <100 mm Hg)
      or recumbent tachycardia (pulse >100/min)
   Urine output <30 mL/hr
   Central venous pressure <5 cm H_2O

Unreliable signs
   Melena
   Hematochezia
   Normal blood pressure
   Normal hematocrit

used to monitor blood volume in patients estimated to have lost more than 20% of blood volume and in patients bleeding from esophageal varices.

Hematocrit: The hematocrit is not a useful index of the extent of acute gastrointestinal bleeding. It tells only the percentage of red cells and is not an accurate measure of blood volume in the bleeding patient. In fact, the hematocrit determined soon after the initial hemorrhage is near normal, since a period of 24–72 hours or more is required after a hemorrhage for hemodilution to be complete.

Volume Replacement: The first priority in the management of gastrointestinal hemorrhage is rapid restoration of the blood volume to a level that will preclude shock if additional bleeding occurs. A large-caliber intravenous line should be placed immediately and a rapid infusion of Ringer's lactate or saline solution started. If the patient is in shock, fluid should be given through two lines. Since crystalloid-containing fluids rapidly equilibrate with the extravascular spaces, the volume infused needs to exceed the estimated deficit two- to threefold. To avoid fluid overload, as soon as the initial hypovolemia is stabilized the physician should change the infusion fluid to a colloid (plasma protein fraction or albumin), which retains fluid in the vascular compartment. If the hematocrit is below 30%, packed red blood cells should be added. It is not necessary to raise the hematocrit above 30%, because tissue hypoxia in hemorrhage is primarily due to decreased perfusion (hypovolemia) and not to insufficient oxygen carrying capacity of the blood. Patients in shock should receive oxygen by nasal catheter at a flow rate of 4–6 L/min to improve oxygenation until volume replacement produces adequate tissue perfusion.

Flowchart: All clinical data should be recorded on a flowchart at the patient's bedside (Table 6.5–3). Included should be pulse, blood pressure, urine output, central venous pressure if a catheter is in place, volume and type of fluid infused, and loss of blood as manifested by hematemesis or the passage of blood-containing stools. Each set of observations should lead to an estimate of volume deficit. It should be remembered that melena and hematochezia do not give an accurate assessment of blood loss, and a normal blood pressure and normal hematocrit do not exclude massive gastrointestinal bleeding.

Diagnosis

The aim of diagnostic procedures in the bleeding patient is to ascertain three factors: (1) site of bleeding (upper or lower gastrointestinal tract), (2) type of bleeding vessel (arterial, venous or capillary, or variceal), and (3) nature of the bleeding lesion (eg, ulcer, vascular anomaly, or neoplasm).

Site of Bleeding: The first step is to determine whether the bleeding originates in the upper or lower gastrointestinal tract, so that appropriate diagnostic and therapeutic procedures can be used (Table 6.5–4). If the patient vom-

Table 6.5–3. Sample bedside flowchart for tracking status of patients with gastrointestinal bleeding.

Time*	Pulse (Supine or Sitting)	Blood Pressure (Supine or Sitting)	Central Venous Pressure	Urine Output	Volume Replaced (Crystalloid, Colloid, or Packed RBC's)	Hematemesis	Stool (Black or Red)
3:30 pm	96 supine 110 sitting	120/80 supine 110/65 sitting	3 cm H₂0	30 cc/hr	300 cc PRBC	none	black
4:00 pm	74 supine 74 sitting	128/76 supine 125/70 sitting	7 cm H₂0	50 cc/hr	none	none	black

*Until the patient is stabilized, clinical data should be measured and recorded at 15-minute intervals, then at 30-minute, and finally at 60-minute intervals.

its blood, the bleeding lesion is almost always proximal to the ligament of Treitz. If the patient has not vomited blood, a tube should be passed into the stomach. If the gastric aspirate contains blood, the bleeding site is above the ligament of Treitz. If the stomach is free of blood, there are three possibilities: (1) the site of bleeding is below the ligament of Treitz, (2) bleeding has stopped and all the blood has passed into the intestine, or, (3) rarely, the site of bleeding is distal to the pylorus and proximal to the ligament of Treitz (eg, duodenal ulcer) but at the time of intubation the bleeding was not brisk enough to cause reflux of blood into the stomach.

Rectal examination should be done in all patients with gastrointestinal bleeding to assess the stool color and document the presence of blood. If a tarry stool is passed, the lesion is probably at or above the ileocecal sphincter. Passage of red blood by rectum usually indicates a bleeding site within the colon. However, with massive hemorrhage and rapid intestinal transit, red blood passed through the rectum can emanate from a bleeding lesion as high as the esophagus. Thus, the color of the blood passed is as much a function of the rate of bleeding and passage through the gastrointestinal tract as it is an indication of the site of bleeding. In general, the larger the hemorrhage, the more rapid is the passage through the gut.

Table 6.5–4. Localizing gastrointestinal bleeding to an upper or lower tract source.

Features of upper GI bleeding
  Hematemesis
  Melena
  Positive nasogastric aspirate (not necessary in patients with hematemesis)
  History of peptic ulcer disease, NSAID use, anticoagulant therapy, previous GI bleeding, chronic liver disease
  Physical findings of chronic liver disease, portal hypertension, changes in skin or mucous membranes associated with rare vascular lesions of the GI tract

Features of lower GI bleeding
  Hematochezia (red blood per rectum) (note: the larger the volume and more frequent the movement, the less certain that the source is within the colon)
  Absence of history of disorders associated with upper GI bleeding

NSAID, nonsteroidal anti-inflammatory drug.

History: The history should answer several questions. First, are there recent or remote symptoms of peptic ulcer disease? Peptic ulcer is the most common cause of massive upper gastrointestinal tract hemorrhage.

Second, is there a history of recent heavy intake of alcohol or drugs, especially aspirin, other nonsteroidal anti-inflammatory drugs, corticosteroids, or anticoagulants? The recent ingestion of any of these substances suggests diffuse gastric erosions, an acute peptic ulcer, or an iatrogenic bleeding disorder aggravated by the medication effect. A history of blood appearing only after vomiting, especially after an alcoholic binge, should lead to a consideration of the Mallory-Weiss syndrome, in which retching leads to a longitudinal mucosal tear at the gastroesophageal junction.

Third, is there historical evidence of liver disease? Not every alcoholic patient has cirrhosis, not everyone with cirrhosis has varices, and not every cirrhotic patient with varices bleeds from them. Indeed, in patients with demonstrated varices and upper gastrointestinal tract bleeding, up to 50% are found to be bleeding from lesions other than the varices.

Physical examination: Signs of chronic liver disease (eg, spider angiomata, palmar erythema, splenomegaly, jaundice, and ascites) should be sought (Chapter 7.4). Many of the rare causes of hemorrhage from both the upper and lower gastrointestinal tracts have characteristic physical findings: (1) Melanin spots on the lips and buccal mucosa, found in patients with Peutz-Jeghers syndrome, may raise suspicion of bleeding from intestinal polyps. (2) Telangiectatic lesions of Osler-Weber-Rendu disease (hereditary hemorrhagic telangiectasia), seen on fingers, face, lips, and mucous membranes, may raise suspicion of bleeding from similar vascular lesions in the gastrointestinal tract. (3) The characteristic "plucked chicken" skin changes of pseudoxanthoma elasticum are associated with vascular lesions that can bleed; these are most often found in the stomach. (4) Less commonly, café-au-lait spots may suggest that intestinal neurofibromas of the intestinal tract are the source of the bleeding. (5) Cutaneous "caviar" vascular lesions, "pinch" purpura with amyloidosis, and hyperextension of joints with Ehlers-Danlos syndrome all may indicate a bleeding gastrointestinal vascular anomaly. Finding manifestations of any of these rare diseases, however, cannot be taken as proof that they are the cause of gastrointestinal hemorrhage. (6) Purpura, ecchymoses, or bleeding gums, which can be overlooked easily if not specifically sought, are evidence of a bleeding diathesis.

Acute Upper Gastrointestinal Tract Hemorrhage:

Peptic ulcer, erosive gastritis, and esophageal varices are the most common causes of upper gastrointestinal tract hemorrhage. Because these disorders may have radically different treatments, it is important to make a specific diagnosis. For example, patients with persistent arterial bleeding from a gastric or duodenal ulcer can be treated promptly and effectively by surgery, whereas surgery has little to offer in the care of patients with gastric erosions. Although variceal bleeding may be controlled by surgical portosystemic shunting, the combined stress of hemorrhage and surgery is often more than the diseased liver can tolerate.

Endoscopy: If the clinical evidence favors an upper gastrointestinal source of the bleeding, endoscopy should be performed after hypovolemia has been corrected. Fiberoptic endoscopes make it possible to examine the esophagus, stomach, and first part of the duodenum with ease and safety. To ensure that the lesion is visualized, blood is removed by gastric lavage through a large-bore gastric tube. Endoscopy identifies that the bleeding site in over 90% of patients with upper gastrointestinal tract bleeding and is the only way to diagnose Dieulafoy's arterial anomaly, a rare but potential fatal source of hemorrhage in which a small artery penetrates to the mucosal surface. Even if a clear diagnosis cannot be made at endoscopy, certain diagnoses should be excluded, if possible, particularly bleeding from esophageal varices, diffuse erosive gastritis, and peptic ulcer.

Angiography: If endoscopy has failed to identify the source of bleeding or if bleeding is so rapid that the stomach cannot be cleared of blood sufficiently for endoscopy and brisk bleeding continues, angiography should be considered. Selective visceral arteriography of the celiac artery not only localizes the site of upper gastrointestinal bleeding but may be used to control hemorrhage by the infusion of vasoconstricting drugs or embolic occlusion of the bleeding vessel. The rate of bleeding must be greater than 0.5 mL/min for consistent identification of the source. Arterial bleeding is episodic, and it slows or stops as hypovolemia occurs. If the likelihood of identifying the source of bleeding by angiography is to be maximized, it is important to do the study when the blood volume deficit has been restored.

Barium studies: Barium studies have (no role) in the evaluation of massive gastrointestinal hemorrhage because they rarely provide a definitive diagnosis and until the barium is cleared from the gastrointestinal tract preclude the more accurate techniques of endoscopy and angiography.

Lower Intestinal Tract Hemorrhage:

Lower intestinal tract hemorrhage is most frequently attributed to an eroded artery in a colonic diverticulum or to angiodysplasia (arteriovenous malformation), although definitive proof is found in only 10–30% of hemorrhages believed to be of colonic origin.

Anoscopy and proctoscopy: If the patient is passing bright red blood, the first diagnostic procedures should be anoscopy and proctoscopy. These procedures are performed with the patient in the head-down position and permit better visualization of the mucosa of the rectum than does fiberoptic endoscopy because blood can be cleared from the rectum more effectively. It can thus be determined whether the bleeding is from the rectum or anal canal or from the more proximal bowel. Bleeding lesions commonly identified are diffuse mucosal lesions, such as ulcerative and ischemic colitis; local vascular lesions, including hemorrhoids; an arterial bleeding point; and tumors, such as polyps or cancer.

Colonoscopy: If the anal and rectal examination does not reveal the source of bleeding, if clinical findings suggest that the lower bowel is the source, and if the patient's blood volume has been restored, colonoscopy after lavage given by mouth or nasogastric tube is the most productive diagnostic procedure. Fiberoptic endoscopy makes it possible to visualize angiodysplastic lesions, diverticula, and neoplastic and inflammatory lesions of the colon. Colonoscopy should not be attempted if fulminant colitis or colonic perforation is suspected. If ischemic bowel disease is the most likely diagnosis, endoscopy should be carried out with caution because distending the bowel with air may add to the vascular compromise.

Angiography: If colonoscopy fails to identify the source of bleeding and bleeding continues at a rapid rate, angiography of the superior and inferior mesenteric arteries is the most effective method of localizing the source of the bleeding. With more frequent use of angiography in patients with colonic hemorrhage, the necessity for emergency surgery has diminished, because local infusion of vasoconstrictor agents through the angiographic catheter controls the bleeding in most patients. Angiography has shown vascular ectasia or angiodysplasia of the colon to be commonly associated with massive as well as chronic colonic bleeding.

Radionuclide scintigraphy: For a solution to the problem of identifying the location of acute intermittently bleeding lesions, radionuclide scintigraphy has been advocated. The patient's red blood cells are labeled in vivo and returned by intravenous infusion. Abdominal scintiscans then are obtained at regular intervals during the following 24–48 hours. When investigation of a previous bleeding episode was unproductive, starting with a radionuclide study when the patient is admitted with a subsequent hemorrhage may localize the bleeding site.

If the patient is younger than 30, the possibility of bleeding ectopic gastric mucosa in a Meckel's diverticulum should be tested by scintigraphy after injection of technetium Tc 99m pertechnetate. This is the most common cause of massive lower intestinal tract hemorrhage in younger persons.

Barium studies: Barium studies are not performed in the acute phase of lower intestinal tract bleeding because they are not capable of demonstrating the most common cause (ie, vascular ectasias) and they make it impossible to perform more definitive studies such as angiography or endoscopy.

MANAGEMENT

Upper Gastrointestinal Tract Bleeding

The source of gastrointestinal hemorrhage should be sought vigorously, so that if bleeding continues or recurs, definitive therapy can be promptly instituted (Table 6.5–5). In addition, the definitive therapy for an arterial bleeding lesion (eg, duodenal or gastric ulcer) is different from that for bleeding from esophageal varices or gastric erosions. Patients at high risk for a poor outcome (ie, cardiac failure, stroke, renal failure, or death) should be identified to ensure optimal supportive care and prompt definitive therapy. Predictors of poor outcome in acute upper gastrointestinal tract hemorrhage are age over 75; concurrent disease, especially liver, heart, lung, or kidney disease; blood pressure 100 mm Hg or lower during the first hour in the hospital; fresh blood in the gastric aspirate during the first hour in the hospital; ascites; an abnormal prothrombin time; a "visible vessel" (actually, a clot protruding from the bleeding vessel) seen during endoscopy; and arterial bleeding seen during endoscopy.

Arterial Bleeding

Arterial lesions bleed rapidly for 15–30 minutes; then, as the blood volume is depleted, intense vasoconstriction of the splanchnic vessels allows a clot to form. Over the next 1–4 hours, the blood volume is replenished by fluid absorbed from the intestine and drawn from the extravascular spaces. As splanchnic blood flow and pressure rise with increasing blood volume, another episode of arterial bleeding will occur if the clot in the artery does not hold. Rarely does exsanguination occur with the first episode of arterial bleeding, even with an aortoduodenal fistula. Usually, two or more bleeding episodes occur before signs of shock appear.

Peptic (gastric and duodenal) ulcer is the most common cause of severe upper gastrointestinal tract arterial bleeding. Nevertheless, 60–70% of bleeding peptic ulcers do not bleed again after the patient has been admitted to the hospital. Such patients require no treatment other than that designed to heal the ulcer (Chapter 6.4). Two endoscopic findings are predictive of recurrent bleeding in peptic ulcer disease: a spurting arterial lesion and a visible vessel. Treating these lesions with endoscopic hemostasis (laser, epinephrine injection, electrocautery, or thermal probe) has been shown to decrease the frequency of recurrent bleeding, the need for emergency surgery, and mortality. Recurrent bleeding of a peptic ulcer after attempted endoscopic hemostasis is an indication for surgical treatment. In poor-risk patients, angiographically directed embolization of the bleeding vessel may be tried before resorting to surgery.

Bleeding from Mallory-Weiss tears may be arterial but usually stops spontaneously. If bleeding continues, several techniques have been used to stop hemorrhage, including endoscopic electrocautery or laser coagulation, angiographic infusion of vasopressin or embolization, and surgery.

Variceal bleeding: The most common cause of death in patients with chronic liver disease is esophageal variceal hemorrhage. Varices develop when portal blood is rerouted to the systemic circulation through collateral vessels as a result of increased resistance to blood flow to or through the liver (Chapter 7.4). This obstruction may occur at the level of the hepatic veins (in Budd-Chiari syndrome, veno-occlusive disease), the hepatic sinusoids (in cirrhosis, granulomatous hepatitis), or the portal veins (in schistosomiasis, portal vein thrombosis). Isolated gastric varices, in the absence of esophageal varices, are most often caused by thrombosis of the splenic vein.

Although only about 25% of patients with varices bleed from them, once they do, half of these will have recurrent bleeding within the following 6 months. The risk of death from a variceal hemorrhage is related to the stage of the underlying liver disease. About 50% of patients with decompensated cirrhosis die from the bleed; only about 1 in 10 patients with well-compensated liver disease dies because of the hemorrhage. Patients who bleed from varices caused by portal vein thrombosis with intact hepatocellular function have an excellent prognosis even with multiple bleeding episodes.

The usual presenting symptom in variceal hemorrhage is hematemesis, but occasional patients have only melena. With severe bleeding, hematochezia may be the initial

Table 6.5–5. Treatment of acute gastrointestinal bleeding according to type of bleeding vessel.

Bleeding Vessel	Common Lesion	Treatment
Artery	Peptic ulcer	Endoscopic hemostasis Angiographic vasoconstriction or embolization Surgical ligation of bleeding vessel
	Diverticulum or angiodysplasia	Angiographic vasoconstriction Segmental colon resection
Vein	Esophageal varices	Sclerotherapy or banding Vasopressin TIPS Urgent surgery
Capillary	Erosive gastritis	Antacids Sucralfate

TIPS, transjugular intrahepatic portosystemic shunt.

symptom. Very rarely, occult iron deficiency anemia is the only manifestation of variceal hemorrhage.

Endoscopy is the most reliable way of diagnosing esophageal variceal hemorrhage. Barium studies should not be used, since they can identify varices but cannot establish whether varices are the source of the hemorrhage.

Therapy for esophageal variceal hemorrhage includes controlling the acute bleeding and reducing the risk of later bleeding. Volume replacement should maintain the central venous pressure between 5 and 8 cm H_2O. Somatostatin or vasopressin infusion and endoscopic sclerotherapy (injection of a sclerosing agent into the varix) are the two methods most commonly used to control acute bleeding. An alternative endoscopic approach to controlling acute esophageal variceal hemorrhage is placing small rubber bands around the varices. For patients who continue to bleed despite endoscopic and pharmacologic attempts at control, tamponade of the varices by the insertion of a Sengstaken-Blakemore tube or emergency shunt surgery was once the only alternative. However, these approaches have fallen into disfavor because of their high morbidity and mortality. Transjugular intrahepatic portosystemic shunt (TIPS), a nonsurgical technique for producing a portosystemic shunt, is more effective than balloon tamponade and is associated with less morbidity and mortality than surgery. By means of an angiographic catheter, an expandable metal stent is placed to produce an intrahepatic shunt between a portal vein and hepatic vein.

Capillary bleeding: Erosions of the gastroduodenal mucosa, by definition, do not penetrate below the muscularis mucosae. The most clearly recognized clinical associations are with drug ingestion, hypoperfusion of the gastric mucosa caused by heart failure or sepsis, extensive burns (Curling's ulcer), and intracranial operations (Cushing's ulcer). Erosions with the latter three associations are often referred to as "stress ulcers" and may at times lead to a true ulcer when necrosis extends through the muscularis mucosae and into the submucosa or deeper (Chapter 6.4).

Bleeding from erosions associated with drugs is usually self-limited if the offending agent is discontinued. Maintaining gastric pH above 4.0 with the frequent use of antacids or of antacids in combination with H_2-receptor antagonists decreases the frequency of stress ulcer. If bleeding does not stop with hourly administration of antacids, selective infusion of vasopressin into the left gastric artery stops bleeding in over 75% of patients. Endoscopic cauterization of erosions is usually impractical because they are so numerous, but if the bleeding seems to be primarily from one or several erosions, cautery should be tried. Surgery should be avoided because the mortality rate is as high as 40%. Most surgical deaths are attributable, however, to the underlying disorders that set the stage for stress ulcers.

Lower Intestinal Tract Bleeding

Most lower intestinal tract hemorrhages cease spontaneously; if not, angiography of the superior and inferior mesenteric arteries not only may identify the source of bleeding but also may provide an opportunity to control the bleeding by infusion of vasoconstrictors such as vasopressin. When active bleeding slows or stops, colonoscopy should be performed in an attempt to locate the site of bleeding. It also provides a means of treating localized lesions such as angiodysplasia, which are usually found in the right colon, with electrocautery or laser. Bleeding associated with diverticula is arterial. If bleeding cannot be controlled by infusion of vasoconstrictors into the mesenteric artery, resection of the segment containing the bleeding diverticulum may be necessary. Unfortunately, in patients with massive lower bowel bleeding requiring surgery, the site of bleeding usually is not established despite the use of all diagnostic procedures. As a consequence, major bowel resection may have to be performed in an attempt to ensure that the bleeding site has been removed. It is common, unfortunately, that such resections fail to prevent recurrent bleeding.

CHRONIC GASTROINTESTINAL BLEEDING

Chronic gastrointestinal bleeding may be intermittent or continuous. The rate of bleeding may be so slow that no change is visible in the stools but the blood loss exceeds the capacity of iron absorption to maintain body stores. The resultant anemia often provides the first indication of gastrointestinal bleeding. The lesions responsible range from the simple, such as hemorrhoids or anal fissures, to the ominous, such as carcinoma of the colon. But the most common are anal lesions, inflammatory bowel disease, colonic neoplasms, and, in young people, Meckel's diverticulum.

Site of Bleeding

If the first evidence of chronic gastrointestinal bleeding is blood in the stool, in the toilet bowl, or on the toilet paper, prompt examination of the patient gives the greatest chance of identifying the source. The first examination should be a rectal examination, followed by standard proctoscopy without preparatory enemas or cathartics. If no mucosal lesion such as colitis is seen, if the patient has seen blood with the passage of a stool, and if stool sampled from the upper part of the rectum or the sigmoid colon is negative for occult blood, the source of bleeding is almost certainly in the anal canal. In these circumstances, bleeding may be demonstrated by leaving a large cotton swab in the rectum as the proctoscope is removed and then withdrawing the swab to simulate the passage of a stool. A telltale streak of blood often appears on the swab. With this information it is easy to locate the source of bleeding by anoscopy.

Because most lesions that cause chronic occult gastrointestinal bleeding are in the colon, colonoscopy should be performed if proctoscopy fails to demonstrate an anorectal source of bleeding. Colonoscopy not only enables the examiner to visualize vascular lesions such as angiodysplasia, but also may provide treatment of the bleeding lesion by excision (endoscopic polypectomy) or by cautery.

If colonoscopy fails to reveal a source of bleeding and if examination of the upper gastrointestinal tract is negative and the patient continues to have occult blood in the stools, a "bleeder tube" (a mercury-weighted small-caliber tube that is swallowed and allowed to pass to the cecum) should be used to identify the site of bleeding. Intestinal fluid is aspirated every 4 hours and tested for blood. When the level of bleeding has been identified, contrast material may be injected through the tube to determine whether a gross lesion is present.

Finally, the upper intestinal tract may be the source of chronic bleeding. The common lesions are esophagitis, drug-induced gastritis, and carcinoma of the stomach.

Management

The treatment of chronic gastrointestinal bleeding is the treatment of the primary lesion if one is found. In all patients, particularly elderly ones, in whom no lesion is found, oral iron replacement should be instituted and supplemented by parenteral iron if necessary. In patients with striking anemia and limited cardiovascular reserve, it may be necessary to give transfusions with packed red blood cells.

SUMMARY

▶ Survival of patients with a gastrointestinal hemorrhage depends on accurate serial estimates of hypovolemia and prompt volume replacement.

▶ Acute massive (more than 50%) blood loss is indicated by hematemesis, recumbent hypotension (less than 100 mm Hg systolic), recumbent tachycardia (more than 100/min), urine output less than 30 mL/hr, or central venous pressure less than 5 mm H_2O. Signs that do not give accurate information about the amount of blood lost are melena, hematochezia, a normal blood pressure, and a normal hematocrit.

▶ Endoscopy is the best diagnostic procedure for bleeding from above the ligament of Treitz, whereas anoscopy, proctoscopy, or colonoscopy is best at detecting the source of bleeding in the colon.

▶ In the treatment of gastrointestinal hemorrhage, first and most important is the prompt restoration of blood volume to protect the patient from the complications of hypovolemia.

SUGGESTED READING

Dudnick R, Martin P, Friedman LS: Management of bleeding ulcers. Med Clin North Am 1991;75:947.

Groszmann RJ, Atterbury CE: The pathophysiology of portal hypertension: a basis for classification. Semin Liver Dis 1982; 2:177.

Jensen DM, Machicado GA: Diagnosis and treatment of severe hematochezia: the role of urgent colonoscopy after purge. Gastroenterology 1988;95:1569.

Kovacs TOG, Jensen DM: Endoscopic control of gastroduodenal hemorrhage. Ann Rev Med 1987;267.

Spechler SJ, Schimmel EM: Gastrointestinal tract bleeding of unknown origin. Arch Intern Med 1982;142:236.

6.6

Gastrointestinal Cancer

Francis M. Giardiello, MD, and Stanley R. Hamilton, MD

People are diagnosed with gastrointestinal cancer either when it is detected through screening or when they present with symptoms of advanced disease. Since most gastrointestinal cancers remain asymptomatic until they are advanced, the chance of curing a symptomatic patient is small. Gastrointestinal malignancies account for 21% of all cancer in the United States and cause 25% of cancer deaths. This chapter covers the common gastrointestinal cancers. Small bowel tumors, which are rare, are not discussed.

COLORECTAL CANCER

Cancer of the colon and rectum is second only to lung cancer in causing cancer deaths in the United States. The development of colorectal cancer is influenced by environmental, dietary, and genetic factors. The importance of environmental factors is shown when populations such as the Japanese, who normally have low rates of colon cancer, move to a country with a higher rate, and their incidence quickly rises to that of their adopted country. Dietary factors predisposing to colorectal cancer include low-fiber diet (which prolongs colorectal fecal transit time, allowing the colorectal mucosa more contact with higher concentrations of putative fecal carcinogens), and high meat and animal fat intake, particularly saturated fat and cholesterol.

A predisposition to colorectal cancer can be inherited as familial adenomatous polyposis, an autosomal dominant disorder with almost 100% penetrance. Patients develop hundreds of adenomatous polyps in the colorectum during late childhood or young adulthood. The cause of familial adenomatous polyposis is a mutation in the APC (adenomatous polyposis coli) gene on the long arm of chromosome 5. Individuals at risk can now be genotyped for the mutation. Unless patients have prophylactic colectomy, they develop colorectal adenocarcinoma, usually in the left colon, by their 40's.

"Hereditary nonpolyposis colorectal cancer" (also known as the Lynch syndromes) is the autosomal dominant disease in families that have multiple members with colorectal and certain other cancers, but not adenomatous polyposis coli. At least four mutated genes have been associated with hereditary nonpolyposis colorectal cancer: human MutS homolog 2 gene (hMSH2), MutL homolog 1 gene (hMLH1), human PMS homolog 1 gene (hPMS1), and human PMS homolog 2 gene (hPMS2). A working definition of hereditary nonpolyposis colorectal cancer is that (1) a family has at least three members with colorectal cancer and one of the relatives is a first-degree relative of the other two; (2) at least two successive generations are affected; and (3) one relative is diagnosed with colorectal cancer before age 50. The syndrome causes predominantly right-sided colon cancer and produces primary cancers in other sites.

Other individuals who have a first-degree relative with colorectal cancer are at a two- to fourfold higher risk for colorectal cancer than the general population. Some studies have suggested that this susceptibility to colorectal cancer has autosomal dominant inheritance with moderate penetrance. However, many patients with colorectal cancer have no family history of the condition; their cancer is termed "sporadic."

Persons with ulcerative colitis are also at high risk for colorectal cancer. Risk increases with longer duration and greater extent of colitis. The risk is low for the first 7–8 years after diagnosis, but increases to 8–30% after 25 years of pancolitis. The risk appears to warrant surveillance for epithelial dysplasia, the precursor to cancer in these patients; they should have a colonoscopy with biopsies every 1–2 years. Persons with Crohn's disease have a smaller increased risk of colorectal cancer.

Other rare conditions that cause polyposis increase patients' risk for colorectal cancer to three to six times that of the general population. Peutz-Jeghers syndrome is characterized by hamartomatous polyps in the gastrointestinal tract and pigmentation on the lips and mucocutaneous membranes. Juvenile polyposis presents with polyps primarily in the colon.

Pathology

The molecular biology of colorectal cancer has been studied intensively and is evolving quickly. As normal mucosa progresses to an adenomatous polyp and then to colorectal cancer, multiple genetic changes take place within the tissue. These include the activation of at least one dominantly acting oncogene (eg, the *ras* gene), and the loss of several recessive tumor suppressor genes, whose job is to suppress tumor growth. The identified suppressor genes include the APC (Adenomatous Polyposis Coli) gene for familial adenomatous polyposis and the MCC (Mutated in Colorectal Cancer) gene, both on the long arm of chromosome 5; the p53 gene on the short arm of chromosome 17; and the DCC (Deleted in Colorectal Carcinoma) gene on the long arm of chromosome 18.

About 75% of large bowel adenocarcinomas are located in the colon, and 25% are in the rectum (Figure 6.6–1). Most large bowel cancers are moderately well-differentiated gland-forming adenocarcinomas.

Risk factors for carcinoma developing in an adenoma include diameter greater than 1 cm, extensive villous pattern (similar to the finger-like mucosal projections of the small intestine), high-grade dysplasia, other adenomas or colorectal cancer, and increasing patient age. It has been estimated that of 1000 colonic polyps, only 100 are neoplastic; of these, 10 are large adenomatous polyps and 2–3 are invasive carcinoma. Because of the malignant potential of colorectal adenomas, they should be removed, preferably by colonoscopic polypectomy, but if necessary by surgery. Colorectal cancer can spread by direct extension into contiguous structures or the peritoneal cavity; invasion of lymph vessels, leading to lymph node metastases; invasion of veins, leading to liver metastasis via portal vein tributaries; and seeding during surgery.

Clinical Features

The symptoms of colorectal cancer depend on tumor location. Right-sided lesions typically present with abdominal pain or lower gastrointestinal tract bleeding as bright red blood, occult bleeding, or melena. Melena is usually a sign of bleeding above the ligament of Treitz, but can occur with bleeding below the ligament of Treitz (eg, in the cecum or right colon) if transit time to the anus is prolonged.

Tumors of the cecum are likely to present as palpable abdominal masses because the cecum is so capacious that tumors can grow large without being otherwise detected. Intestinal obstruction is a late sign, since the liquid stool in the right side of the colon can maneuver around the tumor, causing watery bowel movements.

Tumors of the left colon usually cause partial colonic obstruction with colicky abdominal pain and a change in bowel habits. Many patients have occult or gross blood in the stool.

Rectal tumors can present with rectal bleeding, rectal pain, and the feeling of incomplete evacuation of stool.

Most adenomatous polyps are asymptomatic, but as they grow they can bleed. Villous adenomas occasionally cause severe diarrhea that depletes serum potassium and other electrolytes.

Diagnosis and Screening

Persons with suspected colorectal cancer should have the entire colorectum evaluated, either by colonoscopy, which examines the complete length of the large intestinal lumen, or by a combination of barium air contrast enema and sigmoidoscopy. A classic radiographic finding is the "napkin ring" or "apple core," marking partial obstruction in the distal colon (Figure 6.6–2). Patients with symptoms localized to the rectum may undergo a more limited endoscopic exam with flexible sigmoidoscopy. Endoscopy has several advantages over radiographic exam: greater sensitivity and specificity, and the ability to remove or biopsy the lesions encountered. The disadvantages of colonoscopy are cost, the risk of perforating the colon, and the need for sedating medications. Nonetheless, endoscopic evaluation of the colon is generally preferred for working up the symptoms of colorectal cancer.

By the time they develop symptoms, 25% of patients with colorectal cancer already have widespread metastasis and a poor prognosis. Fortunately, colorectal cancer is amenable to screening (Table 6.6–1). The precursor lesion (the adenoma) is detectable, and the surgical cure rate is higher with earlier stage of malignancy. Routine screening for the general population should include an annual digital rectal exam starting at age 40. Annual stool occult blood slide tests are recommended beginning at 50. Also beginning at 50, sigmoidoscopy is recommended every 3–5 years after two initial negative sigmoidoscopies 1 year apart. Persons with above-average risk for colorectal cancer need more frequent and extensive screening.

The guaiac test for occult blood in the stool is currently used to detect colorectal cancer in asymptomatic persons. This inexpensive and easy-to-perform test uses the peroxidase activity of hemoglobin to cause a change in reagent. But since an intestinal lesion can bleed intermittently, the false-negative rate is high. When the test is used as part of population screening, about 50% of patients with a

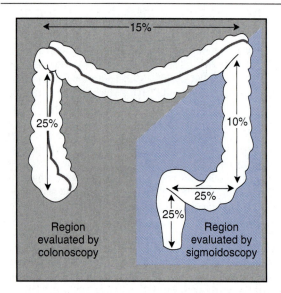

Figure 6.6–1. Distribution of colorectal cancer.

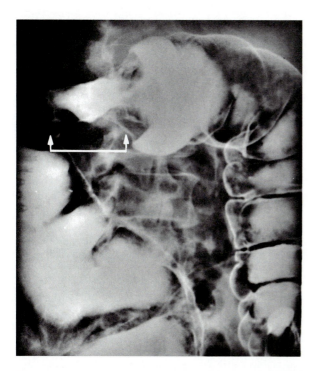

Figure 6.6–2. Adenocarcinoma of the colon. Barium enema study shows a 10-cm ulcerating annular lesion (arrows) at the hepatic flexure–the classic "apple core" lesion of carcinoma. (Reproduced, with permission, from Jones B, Braver JM: *Essentials of Gastrointestinal Radiology.* WB Saunders, 1982.)

Table 6.6–1. Colorectal cancer screening recommendations.

Persons at average risk (no family history, no previous colorectal cancer)
- Digital rectal exam yearly, starting at age 40
- Fecal occult blood tests yearly, starting at age 50
- Sigmoidoscopy at age 50; if negative, repeat in 1 yr, then every 3–5 yr

Persons at above-average risk
If two first-degree relatives have had colorectal cancer:
- Fecal occult blood tests yearly and colonoscopy every 3–5 yr, starting at age 35–40 or 5–10 yr before age at which relatives' earliest cancer was diagnosed

If patient has had a colorectal adenoma:
- If no polyps, colonoscopy every 3 yr
- If polyps found, colonoscopy every 6–12 mo until colon is free of polyps, then every 3 yr

If patient has had colorectal cancer:
- Colonoscopy in 6–12 mo, then 1 and 2 yr later, then every 3 yr
- Fecal occult blood tests yearly
- Carcinoembryonic antigen (CEA) at 6, 12, and 18 mo, then every year for 5 yr

If patient has Crohn's disease; ureterosigmoidostomy; history of endometrial cancer, Peutz-Jeghers syndrome, or juvenile polyposis; or first-degree relative with colorectal cancer:
- Individualized endoscopic screening

Persons at high risk
If patient has a parent with familial adenomatous polyposis:
- Flexible sigmoidoscopy yearly, starting at age 10–12
- Genotypic testing
    If positive, flexible sigmoidoscopy every 1–2 yr
    If negative, flexible sigmoidoscopy at ages 18 and 35

If patient is at risk for hereditary nonpolyposis colon cancer syndrome or family cancer syndrome:
- Fecal occult blood tests yearly and colonoscopy every 2–3 yr, starting at age 20–25 or 5–10 yr before age at which relatives' earliest cancer was diagnosed
- Endometrial surveillance every 6 mo
- Genotypic testing, when available

If patient has ulcerative colitis:
- Colonoscopy with multiple biopsies every 1–2 yr, starting after 8–10 yr of disease

positive result are later found to have a colorectal neoplasm—either an adenomatous polyp or colorectal adenocarcinoma. Patients are instructed to eat a high-fiber diet free of red meat and nonsteroidal anti-inflammatory drugs for at least 48 hours before testing. Two samples are taken from each of three stool specimens, and the slides are developed within 3 days. If any of the six slides are positive, the patient should have a complete exam of the colon.

Another screening test is flexible sigmoidoscopy with a fiberoptic tube that allows the physician to inspect the lumen for polyps and cancers from the anus through the descending colon. About 60% of all neoplasms are found in this distribution. Through the sigmoidoscope, the physician can take biopsies of suspicious lesions for histologic exam.

Management

Complete surgical resection of colorectal adenocarcinoma gives the best chance for cure. But before receiving any treatment, patients must be evaluated for metastatic disease with physical exam, chest x-ray, biochemical tests of liver function, computed tomography (CT) of the abdomen, and a plasma carcinoembryonic antigen (CEA) test to establish a baseline CEA level. Another colorectal polyp or cancer is found in about 10% of patients with

colorectal cancer. Since an additional lesion may alter the surgical approach, the entire colon should be inspected, preferably by colonoscopy. Patients with metastases may require palliative surgical resection to relieve colonic obstruction or bleeding. Surgical removal of metastases to the liver may lengthen survival.

The prognosis for colorectal cancer patients depends on the extent of spread and the adequacy of resection. Prognosis worsens with distant metastasis, lymph node metastasis, deep local extension, poor differentiation, and invasion of blood and lymphatic vessels in perirectal or pericolic soft tissue. For patients who undergo resection for colorectal cancer, several staging systems are available (Table 6.6–2).

After resection, patients should be monitored by physician exam, liver function tests, and plasma CEA. A rise in CEA can signal recurrent tumor. Because colorectal cancer occasionally recurs at the site of surgical anastomosis and because patients are at increased risk for additional

Table 6.6–2. Dukes-Turnbull classification of colorectal cancer.

Stage	Depth of Invasion	Cancer-Free 5-Year Survival (% of Patients)
Carcinoma in situ	Noninvasive	100
A	Invades submucosa but extends no further than muscularis propria	99
B	Penetrates muscularis mucosa and may extend through the serosa into pericolic fat B_1 = into muscularis B_2 = through serosa	85
C	Regional lymph node metastases C_1 = ≤4 involved nodes C_2 = >4 involved nodes	67
D	Distant metastases	14

colorectal adenomas and cancers, colonoscopic surveillance is advisable, starting yearly and then at longer intervals.

Treatment of colorectal adenomas should not be overlooked, since removing polyps decreases risk for colorectal cancer. An adenomatous polyp 1–2 cm in diameter has about a 10% chance of already harboring adenocarcinoma, and a polyp larger than 2 cm has a 40% chance. Most adenomatous polyps can be removed by colonoscopic polypectomy, without major surgery. The adequacy of polypectomy can be assessed by histopathologic review of the specimen: When carcinoma or residual parts of large polyps are found, the patient may need surgery to remove segments of large bowel.

GASTRIC CANCER

Adenocarcinoma of the stomach accounts for about 3% of all cancers in the United States. Worldwide migration studies reveal a lower incidence of gastric cancer as people move from areas of high to low gastric cancer incidence, suggesting that, as with colorectal cancer, environment plays a role in prevalence. Foods and food additives have received the greatest attention as risk factors. An association has been noted between gastric cancer and starch, specifically hot rice, rice wine, salted fish and meat, smoked foods, and pickled vegetables. Many of these foods are eaten by the Japanese, who have one of the world's highest rates of gastric cancer. In contrast, gastric cancer correlates inversely with the ingestion of whole milk, fresh vegetables, citrus fruits, vitamin C, and refrigerated foods. Nitrates, eaten in dried, smoked, and cured foods, may also be involved in the pathogenesis of gastric cancer. Gastric bacteria can convert nitrates to nitrosamines and nitrosoamides, which are gastric carcinogens in animal models.

Persons with hypochlorhydria or achlorhydria from per-

nicious anemia and partial gastrectomy may be predisposed to gastric cancer by carcinogens generated from bacterial overgrowth. Also at risk are patients with gastric adenomas, as well as patients with chronic atrophic gastritis in whom stomach mucosa has been replaced by intestinalized mucosa. It has been suggested that infection of the stomach with the bacterium *Helicobacter pylori* (Chapter 6.4) increases risk for gastric adenocarcinoma and for lymphoma.

Pathology

About 90% of neoplasms of the stomach are adenocarcinomas. Most of the other 10% are non-Hodgkin's lymphomas, leiomyosarcomas, and carcinoid tumors of the stomach.

Most gastric adenocarcinomas are in the antrum. Although the tumors have a broad spectrum of histopathologic appearances, most can be assigned to one of two main groups: intestinal type or diffuse type. An intestinal-type tumor is more likely to appear in the antrum and lesser curvature and often presents as an ulcer (see Color Plates); this type predominates in high incidence areas. Diffuse-type tumor is found more often in younger patents. It infiltrates throughout the layers of the stomach, causing a loss of gastric pliability (called linitis plastica, or "water bottle stomach" from its radiographic appearance), and carries a poor prognosis.

Clinical Features

The most common presenting complaint in patients with gastric carcinoma is intermittent, often nondescript, epigastric discomfort. By the time of diagnosis, about 85% of patients have abdominal pain. The pain may resemble that of peptic ulcer, being either relieved by food or antacids or worsened by eating. Patients may also suffer from early satiety or complain of abdominal fullness, often an indication that the tumor has involved the muscular wall of the stomach. Other symptoms include weight loss, anorexia, weakness, and belching.

Physical exam is often unrevealing. However, 30% of patients with advanced disease have a palpable abdominal mass. Physical signs of metastasis include sentinel (Virchow's) node (an enlarged left-sided supraclavicular node), Irish's node (an enlarged left anterior axillary node), rectal shelf of Blumer (a mass in the cul de sac), Sister Mary Joseph's node (infiltration of the umbilicus), or Krukenberg's tumor (ovary enlarged by metastasis).

Diagnosis

Upper endoscopy is the preferred test for diagnosing gastric cancer. Often, the question of malignancy arises during evaluation of a gastric ulcer. Malignancy is more likely if an ulcer is larger than 1 cm and on barium x-ray has mucosal folds that do not radiate toward the center of the crater (Figure 6.6–3). If the ulcer looks benign radiographically, most gastroenterologists recommend upper endoscopy 4–8 weeks later to document healing. Suspi-

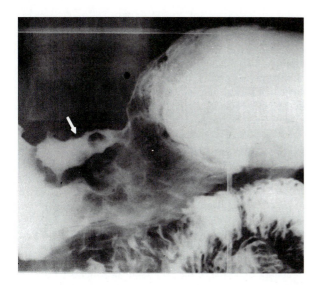

Figure 6.6–3. Adenocarcinoma of the stomach. Upper gastrointestinal series shows an irregular ulcerating mass (arrow) on the lesser curve of the stomach. Within the ulceration is a nodule of cancerous tissue. (Reproduced, with permission, from Jones B, Braver JM: *Essentials of Gastrointestinal Radiology.* WB Saunders, 1982.)

cious lesions should immediately be evaluated by biopsies and brushings. Highly suspect are gastric ulcers that fail to heal on conventional medical therapy within 3–4 months, even though biopsy and brushings have not shown cancer. These ulcers should be resected surgically.

Patients who have undergone partial gastrectomy for benign disease such as peptic ulcer have an increased risk of cancer in the gastric remnant, beginning about 20 years after surgery.

Management

In the United States, the overall 5-year survival rate for patients with gastric adenocarcinoma is a dismal 10–15%. By contrast, in high-risk countries like Japan, where endoscopic surveillance for gastric cancer is justifiable, a high percentage of cancer is detected early in asymptomatic patients, and their 5-year survival rate is almost 90%.

Once gastric cancer is diagnosed, the extent of disease should be determined by physical exam, routine blood tests to seek liver metastases, and abdominal CT to determine the extent of metastases.

Since surgical resection offers the only chance for cure, surgery should be considered for all patients who do not have metastatic disease, who are good surgical risks, and whose primary tumor is resectable. In the United States, only one-third of patients qualify. Patients who are found at surgery to have regional tumor spread should be considered for palliative radiation therapy or chemotherapy. Those with disseminated disease should receive supportive treatment.

PANCREATIC CANCER

Over the past 50 years, the incidence of pancreatic cancer in the United States has increased steadily, now accounting for 13% of all gastrointestinal malignancies.

The cause of pancreatic cancer is unknown. Risk factors include age over 60, male gender, cigarette smoking, inherited colorectal cancer and polyposis syndromes, hereditary pancreatitis, chronic pancreatitis, and diabetes mellitus. Often mentioned but unlikely precipitants include coffee, alcohol, and prior cholecystectomy or gastrectomy.

Over 80% of adenocarcinomas of the pancreas originate in the epithelium of the pancreatic ducts and about 15% in acinar cells; 5% are anaplastic. About 70% of pancreatic tumors develop in the head of the pancreas. Tumors in this critical area can obstruct the common bile duct and pancreatic duct or invade the portal and superior mesenteric veins. This is why pancreatic head tumors are recognized earlier than tumors of the body or tail. Cancer of the head of the pancreas often causes weight loss and progressive jaundice, with or without abdominal pain. In contrast, many cancers in the body (20% of tumors) or tail (10%) of the pancreas grow silently for long periods and can present as palpable masses, often invading the stomach and the splenic artery and vein.

About 90% of patients with pancreatic cancer have abdominal pain in the left upper quadrant or epigastrium. The discomfort is most often described as persistent, relentless, aching, boring pain that penetrates through to the back. Patients can sometimes relieve the pain by bending forward, lying on their side, and drawing their knees to their chest or chin.

On physical exam, a palpable gallbladder (Courvoisier's sign) in a patient with jaundice should raise suspicion of cancer in the head of the pancreas. Tumors in the body and tail of the pancreas may present as palpable abdominal masses or as ascites from tumor seeding of the peritoneum. A rare sign of pancreatic cancer is passage of stool that looks silver because of blood and acholia from bile duct obstruction.

Rarely, patients present with paraneoplastic syndromes, particularly Trousseau's syndrome of recurrent venous and arterial thrombosis (Chapter 12.2). Also uncommon is gastrointestinal bleeding from direct extension of tumor into the intestinal lumen.

CT scan of the abdomen is the best first test for suspected pancreatic cancer (Figure 6.6–4). CT has about 80% sensitivity and specificity. The diagnosis can be confirmed with cytology obtained by CT-guided needle biopsy of the mass. If the diagnosis is still in doubt, another option is endoscopic retrograde cholangiopancreatography (ERCP). Occasionally, before surgery, angiography is done to look for tumor invading blood vessels. (Islet cell tumors of the pancreas are discussed in Chapter 4.8.)

Adenocarcinoma of the pancreas is almost always fatal. Only surgical resection by pancreaticoduodenectomy (Whipple's operation) offers a chance of cure, but its 5-year survival rate is 4%. Most patients undergo palliative

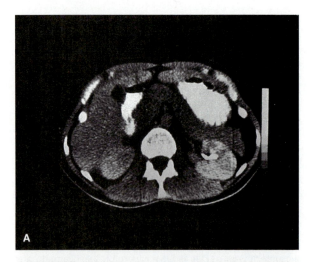

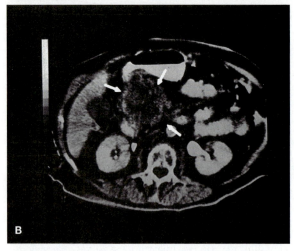

Figure 6.6–4. A: Normal CT scan of the abdomen. **B:** Carcinoma of the head of the pancreas (arrows). (Reproduced, with permission, from Siegelman SS: CT scanning of the abdomen. In: *Patient Care and Digestive Disease: An Update in Gastroenterology* [slide-tape program]. Bayless TM [editor]. The Johns Hopkins University School of Medicine, 1979.)

procedures to control symptoms. Biliary or duodenal obstruction can be relieved by surgery or by endoscopic or percutaneous stent placement. Pain is usually treated with generous doses of narcotics and less often by neurolytic celiac plexus blocks. Malabsorption can be controlled with pancreatic enzymes.

ESOPHAGEAL CANCER

In the United States, esophageal cancer accounts for about 1% of cancers; most patients are elderly black men in urban areas. Worldwide, the incidence of esophageal cancer varies dramatically. High rates are found in an "esophageal cancer belt," which extends from northeast China to north central Asia, through Afghanistan and northern Iran. Other high-risk groups include the white population in parts of South Africa and residents in some areas of Finland, Iceland, and France. Factors implicated in the pathogenesis of esophageal cancer include alcohol, tobacco, and Barrett's esophagus (see below).

About 90% of esophageal cancers are squamous carcinomas arising from squamous epithelium that lines most of the esophagus. The other 10% are adenocarcinomas, usually arising in the distal third of the esophagus or at the esophagogastric junction.

Barrett's esophagus is the precursor to most adenocarcinomas of the esophagus (Chapter 6.2). Barrett's esophagus is the replacement of squamous by columnar epithelium in the lower esophagus, usually because of chronic gastroesophageal reflux. Although the incidence of adenocarcinoma of the esophagus in patients with Barrett's esophagus is only about 1 per 200 patient-years, surveillance by endoscopic biopsies and brush cytology is currently recommended every 1–2 years.

Esophageal cancer is lethal. It presents as quickly progressive dysphagia, first for solids, and over the next several weeks to months, for liquids. Since patients begin to have trouble swallowing only when the esophageal lumen has narrowed significantly, most symptomatic patients have advanced, incurable disease. Other symptoms can include weight loss, chest pain, odynophagia, gastrointestinal bleeding, and aspiration of retained food and secretions. Extension of the cancer into periesophageal soft tissues, facilitated by the lack of serosa covering the esophagus, can cause laryngeal paralysis from recurrent laryngeal nerve involvement, as well as superior vena cava obstruction and Horner's syndrome. Spread of cancer into the mediastinum and intrathoracic structures (tracheobronchial tree, aorta, lung) can cause tracheoesophageal or aortoesophageal fistula.

Esophageal cancer is diagnosed by barium contrast studies of the esophagus (see Figure 6.2–2C). In most patients, the esophageal lumen is markedly narrowed and the mucosa has an irregular ragged pattern. However, the differential diagnosis of esophageal narrowing can include benign peptic strictures, motility disorders such as achalasia, benign tumors of the esophagus (eg, leiomyomas), and extrinsic compression of the esophagus by mediastinal structures. The exact nature of the radiographic esophageal abnormality should be pursued by esophagoscopy. Biopsies and cytologic brushings taken through the esophagoscope permit the diagnosis of more than 98% of esophageal cancers, and the endoscopist can determine the location and extent of tumor.

Only about 5% of patients are alive 5 years after a diagnosis of esophageal cancer. The mainstay of attempts at cure is surgical resection, sometimes combined with chemotherapy and radiation. Over one-third of tumors are inoperable because they involve mediastinal structures or have metastasized widely. Furthermore, cancers in the cervical and proximal thoracic area of the esophagus pose surgical difficulties, so most patients with these tumors are treated with radiation.

Most patients ultimately receive palliative treatment. The focus should be on general supportive care, treatment of complications, and nutrition. If patients are to be able to swallow saliva and food, the stenotic esophageal lumen must be opened by peroral dilatation or radiation therapy.

CARCINOID TUMORS

Carcinoid tumors have characteristics of enterochromaffin or enterochromaffin-like cells that can synthesize many hormones and autocoids (substances that act on the cell that secretes them) and can therefore cause systemic as well as local disease. More than 90% of carcinoid tumors originate in the gastrointestinal tract, representing 1.5% of gastrointestinal neoplasms.

Carcinoid tumors can arise throughout the gastrointestinal tract, but most develop in the appendix (50%), ileum (30%), and rectum (15%). Carcinoids of the proximal colon (appendix and ileum) can present (1) with local invasion; (2) by stimulating a desmoplastic reaction in the retroperitoneum or mesentery, leading to mechanical obstruction; or (3) by metastasizing to the liver, allowing systemic symptoms to emerge (see below). In contrast, most patients with rectal carcinoids present with rectal bleeding.

When a carcinoid tumor is localized to the gastrointestinal tract, the secretions that can produce systemic manifestations are inactivated as they pass through the liver in the portal venous system. With metastatic disease, this detoxifying mechanism is lost. Thus, patients with metastatic carcinoid tumor can present with the "carcinoid syndrome" of diarrhea, abdominal cramps, borborygmi, episodic flushing, telangiectasias, cyanosis, pellagra-like skin lesions, bronchospasm with wheezing, dyspnea, and endocardial fibrosis. The characteristic flushing seen in about two-thirds of patients involves repeated episodes of cyanotic, red, or tricolored (white, blue, then red) flushes over the face, upper extremities, and chest. Carcinoid causes paroxysms of flushing and diarrhea; in contrast, pheochromocytoma causes paroxysms of hypertension, pallor, and sweating. The typical cardiac findings of carcinoid are tricuspid regurgitation and pulmonic stenosis, which can cause right heart failure.

The carcinoid syndrome has been attributed to release by carcinoid cells of pharmacologically and physiologically active substances including 5-hydroxytryptamine (serotonin), 5-hydroxytryptophan (5-HTP), kinin peptides, histamine, catecholamines, and prostaglandins.

The carcinoid syndrome is diagnosed by a finding of increased urinary excretion of 5-HIAA, the metabolic product of serotonin. The blood serotonin level confirms the diagnosis in rare patients with the syndrome who have normal urinary 5-HIAA levels. The diagnosis can be reinforced by CT scan of the abdomen and confirmed by histopathologic exam of tissue obtained by laparotomy or liver biopsy.

The prognosis for patients with metastatic carcinoid is highly variable. Some are alive more than 20 years after diagnosis. Surgery is rarely curative and can provoke the release of vasoactive substances, inducing a crisis of carcinoid symptoms. Symptomatic patients can be treated medically. Among the drugs used are H_1 and H_2 blockers, corticosteroids, and prochlorperazine. Somatostatin analogue (octreotide) suppresses many carcinoid symptoms, especially the watery diarrhea. Combination chemotherapy is reserved for patients with late-stage metastatic disease.

SUMMARY

▶ Most cancers of the gastrointestinal tract are asymptomatic until they are large or metastatic.

▶ Stool tests for occult blood and flexible sigmoidoscopy are recommended for colorectal cancer screening in average-risk persons after age 50.

▶ Gastric ulcers should be evaluated endoscopically to ensure that they do not harbor a malignancy.

▶ Carcinomas of the pancreas and esophagus are usually widespread by the time that patients present. The exception is tumors of the head of the pancreas, which can show early with signs and symptoms of bile duct obstruction.

▶ Gastrointestinal carcinoid is a rare intestinal tumor found primarily in the appendix and ileum. When the tumor metastasizes, it releases systemically active substances that can cause paroxysms of flushing, diarrhea, abdominal cramps, and wheezing.

SUGGESTED READING

Basson MD et al: Biology and management of the midgut carcinoid. Am J Surg 1993;165:288.

Ellis P, Cunningham D: Management of carcinomas of the upper gastrointestinal tract. BMJ 1994;308:834.

Hamilton SR: The molecular genetics of colorectal neoplasia. Gastroenterology 1993;105:3.

Jessup JM, Posner M, Huberman M: Influence of multimodality therapy on the management of pancreas carcinoma. Semin Surg Oncol 1993;9:27.

Lynch HT et al: Genetics, natural history, tumor spectrum, and pathology of hereditary nonpolyposis colorectal cancer: An updated review. Gastroenterology 1993;104:1535.

Acute Infectious Diarrhea

John G. Bartlett, MD

Acute diarrhea caused by a viral, bacterial, or parasitic infection is one of the most common complaints managed in general medical practice. Adults in the United States average almost two gastrointestinal infections each year. Most of these illnesses are not serious and resolve quickly without antimicrobial treatment. But in mortality worldwide, diarrheal diseases rank second only to cardiovascular disease and constitute the leading cause of childhood death in developing countries, killing 4.6–6 million children per year in Asia, Africa, and Latin America. Decisions about the diagnosis and treatment of infection-induced diarrhea are thus an important part of both the art and science of medicine.

Diarrheal diseases almost always cause an increase in stool water and usually an increase in the frequency of bowel movements. Normal daily stool water on an American diet averages 130 mL, and normal stool is 65–85% water. Diarrheal diseases can be objectively defined as daily stool weights of greater than 200 g. More practically, diarrhea is diagnosed when a patient has three or more liquid or semisolid stools a day for an arbitrary period, usually at least 2 or 3 consecutive days. Diarrhea is classified as acute (symptoms begin suddenly and typically last less than 1 week) or chronic (symptoms usually begin insidiously and last longer than 4 weeks) (Chapter 6.8).

Diarrhea has four general pathophysiologic categories (Table 6.7–1):

1. Osmotic diarrhea results from ingestion of poorly absorbed solutes or maldigestion, as with the short bowel syndrome or disaccharidase or lactase deficiency. Osmotic diarrhea generally responds to fasting and shows a large solute gap (greater than 50 mOsm/L), defined as:

   Solute gap = plasma osmolality – [2 × (stool Na⁺ + K⁺)]

2. Secretory diarrhea produces large volumes of watery diarrhea and persists despite fasting. The stool osmolality is close to the plasma osmolality. Causes include laxative abuse, bacterial enterotoxins (see "Bacteria"

below), and hormonal causes such as the pancreatic cholera syndrome.

3. Abnormal morphology of the intestine can cause diarrhea, as with viral gastroenteritis, invasive bacteria or parasites, idiopathic inflammatory bowel disease, intestinal ischemia, and eosinophilic or collagenous colitis.

4. Abnormal motility can cause diarrhea from bacterial overgrowth, diabetic neuropathy, or postgastrectomy dumping syndrome.

Table 6.7–1 gives some sense of the array of both infectious and noninfectious causes that the physician must consider, depending on the features of an individual patient's diarrhea.

The physician should suspect that an infection is the cause of diarrhea when a previously healthy person develops otherwise unexplained diarrhea. The probability of infection increases if the patient has fever or stools showing blood or polymorphonuclear cells, if the person has recently traveled to an underdeveloped country (traveler's diarrhea), and during outbreaks.

Infectious diarrhea is caused by enteric viruses, bacteria, and parasites. Most people acquire the infection by ingesting the agent. The likelihood of developing disease and the severity of disease are described by the formula (Chapter 8.1):

$$\text{Disease severity} = \frac{(\text{virulence of microbe}) \times (\text{number of organisms})}{\text{host resistance}}$$

DEFENSE MECHANISMS

The body has four major defenses against gastrointestinal infection:

1. Gastric acidity: The pH of the stomach is usually below 2, which creates a hostile environment for most

Table 6.7–1. Differential diagnosis of diarrhea.

Osmotic diarrhea (responds to fasting)
Ingestion of poorly absorbed solutes: $MgSO_4$, laxatives, some antacids (eg, $MgOH_2$), mannitol, sorbitol
Maldigestion: disaccharidase deficiency, short bowel syndrome, postgastrectomy syndrome, intestinal ischemia, lactase deficiency
Mucosal transport defects

Secretory diarrhea (large-volume, watery diarrhea)
Caffeine, laxatives, laxative abuse
Enterotoxins (eg, enterotoxigenic *Escherichia coli, Vibrio cholerae*)
Pancreatic cholera syndrome
Carcinoid syndrome
Zollinger-Ellison syndrome

Morphologic changes in intestine
Viral gastroenteritis
Bacterial or parasitic invasion (*Shigella, Entamoeba histolytica*) or toxin (*Clostridium difficile, E coli* 0157:H7)
Sprue
Idiopathic inflammatory bowel disease
Lymphoma
Ischemia
Whipple's disease
Radiation enteritis
Collagen vascular disease
Eosinophilic colitis or enteritis
AIDS enteropathy

Abnormal motility
Irritable bowel syndrome
Diabetic neuropathy
Postvagotomy or postgastrectomy dumping syndrome
Small bowel overgrowth

microbes. This "gastric barrier" protects the small bowel and colon from most ingested pathogens, except when the microbes are resistant to gastric acidity or when drugs or disease reduce acidity.

2. Small bowel motility: The small bowel's constant peristaltic movement prevents bacteria from colonizing it. Needle aspiration of the small bowel during intestinal surgery reveals a few bacteria that are simply passing through. But if the patient develops stasis from an obstruction, blind loop, or diverticulum, the stagnant segment acquires a large flora of bacteria. This "small bowel overgrowth" is defined as more than 100,000 bacteria/mL of small bowel contents.

3. Normal colonic flora: The colon is a relatively stagnant segment of the intestine and contains about 1 billion bacteria/g of lumen contents, a concentration that approaches the geometric limits with which bacteria can occupy space. Thus, stool is composed almost exclusively of water and bacteria. These microbes defend against foreign intruders by consuming available nutrients, occupying space, and producing by-products that create an environment inhospitable to other microbes.

4. Intestinal immunity: The gastrointestinal tract produces specific immunoglobulins against invading organisms. Immunoglobulins may protect against future infection with the homologous species. A crucial component is IgA, a secretory immunoglobulin that is considered especially important in defending against organisms that invade through the mucosa.

ENTERIC PATHOGENS

Viruses

The viruses that cause infectious diarrhea are legion, but two are especially prevalent: the Norwalk agent and rotavirus. The Norwalk agent is a cube-shaped viral particle that has at least seven antigenically related variants. It causes diseases that most people call "viral gastroenteritis." The agent attacks primarily adults and older children worldwide and can cause large epidemics through contaminated water. The incubation period is 18–48 hours. Most patients have vomiting, diarrhea, and low-grade fever lasting 48–72 hours. Biopsies of the small bowel show villous flattening, epithelial cell disorganization, and a mononuclear cell infiltrate in the lamina propria. The organism is not seen in the mucosa; detection requires electron microscopy or immune electron microscopy of stool. Physicians rarely bother to confirm the diagnosis because the tests are so expensive and the disease is self-limited and not treatable. Establishing the diagnosis of infection with a Norwalk virus is most important in epidemiologic studies.

Rotavirus is an RNA virus with at least four antigenic serotypes. Rotavirus infection is unusual in neonates, presumably because of maternal antibody; babies become susceptible at 3–4 months of age, and the incidence peaks at 6–24 months. Few adults become infected because almost everyone has been exposed and has developed immunity.

Parasites

Parasites of the gut are classified as protozoa (single-cell eukaryotes) and helminths (worms). Worms (*Ascaris, Enterobius, Trichuris,* and hookworm) are commonly found in the colon, especially in migrant farm workers and refugees from developing countries, but worms are not common causes of diarrhea. Important intestinal protozoa in the United States are *Giardia lamblia, Entamoeba histolytica,* and *Cryptosporidium.* About 4% of healthy, asymptomatic US citizens harbor *G lamblia,* and 0.6% harbor *E histolytica.*

Most people who harbor protozoan parasites are asymptomatic. The clinical spectrum of giardiasis ranges from nonspecific complaints such as bloating, flatulence, and some degree of change in bowel habits, through chronic diarrhea with malabsorption, to acute gastroenteritis. In symptomatic patients, *G lamblia* targets the small bowel and can be found attached to the mucosal surface. *E histolytica* has tropism for the colon. Most patients are asymptomatic "cyst passers," but some develop amebic colitis (called "amebic dysentery"), characterized by colonic inflammation and passage of bloody stools; sometimes the organism invades the liver, causing an amebic abscess. The difference between asymptomatic carriage and disease seems to be explained by whether the infecting trophozoite makes a surface lectin that is needed to adhere to target cells.

Cryptosporidium is an enteric protozoan parasite that invades the small bowel and is located just beneath the basement membrane. The parasite can cause two distinct syndromes. Immunocompetent hosts get acute gastroenteritis, with watery diarrhea lasting 7–14 days. Immunosuppressed hosts, primarily patients with AIDS, get bouts of watery diarrhea that may continue over several months, sometimes with fluid losses of 5–10 L/day. *Cryptosporidium* can cause outbreaks of diarrhea (see "Foodborne and Waterborne Outbreaks" below).

Bacteria

Bacteria often cause infectious diarrhea, usually by one of two mechanisms. Bacteria cause secretory diarrhea by producing enterotoxin in the small bowel, and inflammatory diarrhea by either invading the colon or disrupting it by producing toxin.

Enterotoxigenic *Escherichia coli* (ETEC): Enterotoxigenic *E coli* is responsible for the prototypical secretory diarrhea from enterotoxin production and is the most common cause of traveler's diarrhea. Cholera, a devastating disease in the developing world, has an almost identical mechanism. The sequence of events is the following: The patient ingests a sufficient inoculum (usually estimated at about 100 million bacteria). The organisms adhere to the mucosal surface of the small bowel, colonize it, and produce an enterotoxin that inhibits sodium absorption from the gut and induces chloride secretion into the gut lumen. To maintain osmotic equilibrium, water shifts into the gut lumen. The volume of fluid in the small bowel exceeds the colon's absorptive capacity, and the result is watery diarrhea.

An enterotoxin can cause this fluid flux into the gut lumen without producing an inflammatory reaction. Thus, biopsies of the small bowel—and even electron microscopic exams—are entirely normal. Patients have large volumes of watery diarrhea that does not contain blood or fecal leukocytes. *E coli* produces at least two enterotoxins, referred to as heat stable (ST) and heat labile (LT). The LT toxin's A subunit is closely related to cholera toxin.

Cholera is easily detected with stool cultures, since any finding of *Vibrio cholerae* is abnormal. But virtually all adults harbor *E coli,* so diagnosing enterotoxigenic *E coli* requires recognizing the strains that produce the toxin. This can be done in several ways, but all require culturing several strains of *E coli* and testing each for toxin production with a number of assays that are not generally available in diagnostic microbiology laboratories.

Enterotoxigenic *E coli* is just one of at least five mechanisms by which *E coli* can produce diarrhea. But this microbe is particularly important because it contaminates the food and water in developing countries, and travelers to these places are almost sure to be exposed.

Shigella: *Shigella* causes the prototypical diarrhea characterized by inflammation of the colonic mucosa. Only about 10 *Shigella* organisms are needed to cause disease—the fewest of any enteric pathogen. Even a fly can carry an infecting dose of *Shigella* on its feet. The sequence of events is complicated: After a patient ingests the organisms, they must survive the gastric barrier, reach the small intestine, attach to the mucosal surface, and produce an enterotoxin that causes watery diarrhea. Then the organisms continue on to the colon, where they attach to and invade the colonic mucosa (with or without producing a toxin that is sometimes called "Shiga toxin") and cause colonic inflammation with micro-ulcerations.

In the United States, shigellosis is spread mainly by person-to-person fecal-oral transmission. Transmission rates increase with crowding and poor personal hygiene. Other mechanisms of exposure are contaminated water and food and exposure in the microbiology laboratory. The clinical features are fever, abdominal pain, and diarrhea. Early in the infection, the diarrhea is large-volume and watery, presumably caused by enterotoxin production in the small bowel. After 24–48 hours, the character of the stool often changes: The volume drops (fractional stools), and blood and mucus appear (dysentery). Patients may start to complain of fecal urgency and painful defecation.

Many or most strains of *Shigella* produce the same enterotoxin or Shiga toxin. In the small bowel, it causes watery diarrhea; in the colon, it causes inflammation and bloody diarrhea. *Shigella* is easy to detect with stool cultures, since the organism is never part of the normal colonic flora. *Shigella* can cause disease in both adults and children, but children are far more often affected, presumably because they have greater exposure to fecal-oral contamination and because they are immunologically naive.

Three other clinically important "invasive bacterial enteric pathogens" are *Campylobacter jejuni, E coli* 0157:H7, and *Clostridium difficile*. *C jejuni* is the most common agent of invasive diarrhea in the United States and can cause outbreaks. But this organism is treatable and easily detected with stool cultures. *E coli* 0157:H7 is a serotype of *E coli* that produces the Shiga toxin and can cause bloody diarrhea. Exposure is often through hamburgers from fast food restaurants (see "Foodborne and Waterborne Outbreaks" below). Diagnosis requires that stool assays detect either this serotype of *E coli* or the Shiga toxin. *C difficile* usually lies dormant in the colon and causes diarrhea only when the patient has been treated with antibiotics that eliminate competing bacteria. Then *C difficile* produces a toxin that causes diarrhea or colitis (see "Antibiotic Treatment" below).

Salmonellosis: Salmonellosis works by a third—unique—mechanism of enteric disease. When the patient ingests the organism, it penetrates the small bowel, travels the mesenteric lymph nodes, crosses to the thoracic duct, and eventually reaches the bloodstream to cause bacteremia. In contrast, bacteremia does not complicate enterotoxic *E coli,* because the organism is contained in the small bowel mucosa; bacteremia is seen only rarely with shigellosis, because *Shigella* usually remains confined to the colonic mucosa. Bacteremia is characteristic of typhoid fever, which is caused by *Salmonella typhi.*

Other species of *Salmonella* (often called "nontyphoid *Salmonella*") produce a similar syndrome called "enteric fever." The organisms circulate, then get sequestered in the reticuloendothelial system and are eventually returned to the gut lumen, where they cause diarrhea. Thus, fever and toxicity without diarrhea are prominent early in the infection, reflecting rapid involvement of the gastrointestinal lymphatics and bacteremia, but minimal inflammation in the gut. Diarrhea and abdominal cramps appear late, presumably reflecting secondary involvement of Peyer's patches or organisms delivered to the intestine via the biliary tract. Nontyphoid *Salmonella* is usually carried asymptomatically or causes a nonspecific gastroenteritis syndrome resembling viral gastroenteritis. Enteric fever is relatively unusual, but important to recognize because it is the form that requires antibiotic treatment.

Typhoid fever is a major systemic disease in the developing world, but is rare in the United States. Salmonellosis caused by nontyphoid *Salmonella* is now a major problem throughout the world, the United States included. These organisms are often responsible for large outbreaks of infectious diarrhea. One of the biggest took place in the Chicago area in 1985, when *Salmonella typhimurium* contamination of milk affected about 180,000 people. Since 1988, transovarial passage of *Salmonella enteritidis* in chickens has caused epidemic contamination of grade A eggs. Public health measures to interrupt this epidemic include attempts to control spread in farms and the recommendation for longer cooking of eggs. Because *Salmonella* has more than 1400 serotypes and immunity is serotype-specific, people continue to be susceptible when exposed to different strains.

Diagnosis and Management

Tests for patients with suspected infectious diarrhea fall into two categories: tests to detect anatomic changes and tests for pathogens. The methods for seeking anatomic changes are endoscopy, x-rays with contrast material, and computed tomography. These studies often determine the site of infection and characteristic pathophysiologic changes and are usually not needed to determine the pathogen; they are all expensive, and many are painful.

The favored way to establish the cause of infectious diarrhea is to detect the pathogen. Microscopic examination of stool for fecal leukocytes is a simple and inexpensive way of distinguishing inflammatory from secretory causes of diarrhea (Table 6.7–2). This generally works best with the stool lactoferrin test. The standard tests for detecting microbes are stool cultures for bacteria, antigen assays for *C difficile* toxin and rotavirus, and microscopic exam for parasites. Because the colon is populated by a huge number of bacteria from more than 400 species, stool cultures must be done with selective media that inhibit the normal flora while promoting growth of specific pathogens. This is easily done for *Salmonella, Shigella,* and *C jejuni;* it can also be done for *Aeromonas, Plesiomonas,* enterohemorrhagic *E coli* 0157:H7, *V cholerae,* and other noncholera vibrios. Antigen detection is available for the toxin produced by *C difficile,* the major identifiable cause of antibiotic-associated colitis, as well as for rotavirus and for the toxin produced by enterohemorrhagic *E coli.* Protozoan parasites are large enough to identify under the microscope; the major pathogens are *E histolytica, G lamblia,* and, with acid-fast stain, *Cryptosporidium, Isospora,* and *cyclospora.* Nonpathogenic commensals that are commonly found in the stool of healthy persons include *Blastocystis hominis, Endolimax nana, Entamoeba hartmanni,* and *Entamoeba coli.*

Most patients with diarrhea either do not have any infectious cause or have a self-limited disease caused by a microbe that should not or cannot be treated. Thus, routine

Table 6.7–2. Fecal polymorphonuclear leukocytes (PMNs) in infectious diarrhea.

PMNs Common	PMNs Sometimes Seen	No PMNs

Campylobacter jejuni
Shigella
Exacerbations of inflammatory
  bowel disease
	Salmonella
	Yersinia
	Vibrio parahaemolyticus
	Clostridium difficile
	Aeromonas
	Plesiomonas
	Enterohemorrhagic
	  Escherichia coli 0157:H7*
		Vibrio cholerae
		Enterotoxigenic *E coli*
		Food poisoning
		  Staphylococcus aureus
		  Bacillus cereus
		  Clostridium perfringens
		Viral gastroenteritis
		  Adenovirus
		  Rotavirus
		  Norwalk agent
		Parasitic infection
		  Giardia
		  *Entamoeba histolytica**
		  Cryptosporidium
		  Isospora
		Small bowel overgrowth
		AIDS enteropathy

*Often associated with bloody diarrhea.

Table 6.7–3. Causes of infectious diarrhea, by epidemiologic setting (percentage of patients).*

	Traveler's Diarrhea†	Adults in United States		Adults in Bangladesh	Outbreaks in US	Patients with AIDS in US
		All Patients	Blood and Pus in Stools			
Enterotoxigenic *Escherichia coli*	40	–	–	30	–	–
Salmonella	10	2	8	1	33	10
Shigella	10	1	7	5	8	2
Campylobacter	1	5	31	–	–	2
Vibrio cholerae + noncholera vibrios	–	–	–	25	–	–
Clostridium perfringens	–	–	–	–	14	–
Staphylococcus aureus	–	–	–	–	26	–
Rotavirus	–	–	–	–	1	1
Giardia	–	–	–	–	3	1
Cryptosporidium	–	–	–	–	–	20
Microsporidia	–	–	–	–	–	20

*Categories marked by a dash have virtually no cases, or the organism was not sought in most studies.
†Diarrhea in adults from developed countries who visit developing countries in Central and South America, Africa, India, and Asia. Patterns of microbes vary by geographic area; the data shown are for Mexico.

stool microbiology is one of the least cost-effective of tests. Stool cultures cost about $30 per specimen, but over $1000 per *positive* specimen because of the low yield. In the average clinical microbiologic laboratory, only about 5–10% of stool samples are positive by bacterial culture, *C difficile* assay, or parasite exam. The low yield has two explanations: Most laboratories can detect only a limited number of enteric pathogens, and most diarrhea is caused by noninfectious conditions or agents that are either not detectable or not important to detect. Research laboratories using all available tests for agents of diarrhea identify a likely cause in 70–80% of carefully selected patients. The organisms implicated vary greatly by epidemiologic setting (Table 6.7–3).

The message is that laboratory evaluation should usually be confined to patients who have devastating diarrhea, chronic diarrhea, fecal leukocytes, diarrhea complicating antibiotic treatment or immunodeficiency, or infectious diarrhea during an outbreak. The standard workup is stool exam for ova and parasites (including acid-fast stain), culture for bacterial pathogens, and *C difficile* toxin assay. Patients with negative stool exams but with severe or persistent symptoms usually undergo endoscopy.

Therapy is directed against the microbial cause. Many patients with devastating diarrhea need supportive care, which includes hydration and electrolyte replenishment.

HOST CATEGORIES OF INFECTIOUS DIARRHEA

Inflammatory Diarrhea

Patients with inflammatory diarrhea are more likely than average to have serious disease and are far more likely to have a treatable cause. Clinical features that suggest inflammatory diarrhea include fever, abdominal cramps, painful defecation, and small-volume stools that show blood or mucus. Inflammatory diarrhea is usually confirmed by a finding of fecal leukocytes (see Table 6.7–2).

Traveler's Diarrhea

Most studies show that 30–40% of persons from industrialized countries who visit developing countries get traveler's diarrhea. The most common cause is enterotoxigenic *E coli* (see "Enterotoxigenic *E coli*" above). This is usually a mild, self-limited form of diarrhea involving a pathogen that clinical laboratories cannot detect. To help travelers minimize their risk, most physicians give them antimicrobial drugs to take empirically if they get symptoms, and advise strict sanitary precautions to limit exposure (Chapter 8.15): Travelers should eat only freshly prepared food that is steaming hot, fruit that must be peeled, vegetables that have been washed in previously boiled or bottled water, and syrups, jellies, bread, hot tea or coffee, and bottled carbonated and alcoholic beverages. Although enterotoxigenic *E coli* is the most common cause of traveler's diarrhea, other likely agents are *Shigella, Salmonella, Aeromonas* (especially in Thailand), noncholera vibrios (coastal areas of Asia), *Cryptosporidium* (especially St. Petersburg), *Giardia* (North America and Russia), Norwalk agent, and rotavirus (especially Mexico).

Foodborne and Waterborne Outbreaks

About 400–600 outbreaks of foodborne and waterborne illnesses are reported in the United States each year, but far more go unreported. Current estimates are about 6 million cases of waterborne and foodborne illnesses a year.

Most food poisoning is caused by bacteria, especially *Salmonella*. Less common are toxin-producing bacteria (*Clostridium perfringens* type A, *Staphylococcus aureus*, and *Bacillus cereus*), enterotoxigenic *E coli*, enterohemorrhagic *E coli* 0157:H7, *V cholerae, Yersinia, Aeromonas,* and *Vibrio parahaemolyticus*. Parasites that can cause outbreaks include *G lamblia, E histolytica, Diphyllobothrium latum,* and *Cryptosporidium.*

Waterborne outbreaks most often involve *G lamblia* or *Cryptosporidium*; both have been implicated in epidemics caused by drinking of chlorinated but inadequately filtered water.

The cause of food or water poisoning is traced through the symptoms, possible source, and incubation period. The tests to do depend largely on the suspected pathogen. Often, these tests are done primarily in the interest of public health, since most of the conditions are brief and self-limited with minimum morbidity and most patients cannot be treated. An exception was a 1993 outbreak of entero-hemorrhagic *E coli* infection from fast-food restaurant hamburgers in the northwest United States: Patients got bloody diarrhea, some had severe complications such as the hemolytic-uremic syndrome, and some died. The epidemic was interrupted by having people cook beef longer and improving control of the animal source. A 1993 waterborne epidemic of cryptosporidiosis in Milwaukee was notable because it made so many people (419,000) sick for so long (1–2 weeks or more) and because the source, an inadequately decontaminated municipal water supply, had to be purified. *Salmonella* has also caused epidemics that are important because of their size and frequency and because of the potential implications of antibiotic-resistant strains appearing in food animals that have been given antibiotics to promote growth. In summation, an epidemic of diarrhea may be important because it causes serious disease, treatable disease, large-scale disease, preventable disease, or the need to interrupt the epidemic.

Antibiotic Treatment

Diarrhea is a common complication of antibiotic treatment, reported in 15–25% of patients receiving clindamycin, 5–15% on ampicillin, 5–10% on oral cephalosporins, and 5–8% on tetracyclines. The organism implicated in most patients is *Clostridium difficile.* This bacterium may be responsible for a spectrum of diarrheal conditions ranging from simple diarrhea to colitis and pseudomembranous colitis. *C difficile* produces one toxin (toxin A) that causes the diarrhea and another toxin (toxin B) that is cytopathic in tissue-cultured cells and is commonly used to detect the organism. *C difficile* is the only commonly identifiable cause of antibiotic-associated diarrhea and by far the most common identifiable cause of hospital-acquired infectious diarrhea. The diarrhea develops after patients acquire the organism in a hospital or nursing home, antibiotics disrupt the normal colonic mucosa, and the *C difficile* produces toxins whose vegetative forms grow quickly. *C difficile* is a relatively frequent, potentially serious, and treatable form of infectious diarrhea.

The Compromised Host

Diarrhea in the immunocompromised host can be caused by any of a number of enteric pathogens. The defect tends to dictate the pathogen. (1) Impaired humoral immunity predisposes to giardiasis and, to a lesser extent, cryptosporidiosis. (2) Neutropenia does not clearly predispose to any specific microbe. (3) Antimicrobial drug treatment predisposes to diarrhea caused by *Clostridium difficile.* (4) Defective cell-mediated immunity is associated with the enteric pathogens *Salmonella,* cytomegalovirus, *Cryptosporidium, Microsporidia, Mycobacterium avium,* and *Isospora.* Many of these enteric infections are particularly severe or persistent in immunosuppressed hosts.

SUMMARY

▶ Infection should be suspected as the cause of diarrhea when a previously healthy person develops unexplained diarrhea, especially with fever or stools showing blood or polymorphonuclear cells, after travel to an underdeveloped country or during an outbreak.

▶ The major enteric pathogens are viruses (Norwalk agent, rotaviruses), bacteria (*Escherichia coli, Salmonella, Shigella, Clostridium difficile, Campylobacter jejuni*), and protozoan parasites (*Giardia, Entamoeba histolytica, Cryptosporidium*).

▶ Routine diagnostic microbiology is of limited use because common pathogens are not detectable or not treatable or because they cause only self-limited diarrhea.

▶ Laboratory evaluation should usually be confined to patients who have devastating diarrhea, chronic diarrhea, fecal leukocytes, diarrhea complicating antibiotic treatment or immunodeficiency, or infectious diarrhea during an outbreak.

SUGGESTED READING

Almroth S, Latham MC: Rational home management of diarrhoea. Lancet 1995;345:709.

Bartlett JG: *Clostridium difficile:* Clinical considerations. Rev Infect Dis 1990;12(Suppl 2):S243.

DuPont HL, Ericsson CD: Prevention and treatment of traveler's diarrhea. N Engl J Med 1993;328:1821.

Guerrant RL: Lessons from diarrheal diseases: Demography to molecular pharmacology. J Infect Dis 1994;169:1206.

Siegel DL, Edelstein PH, Nachamkin I: Inappropriate testing for diarrheal diseases in the hospital. JAMA 1990;263:979.

6.8

Chronic Diarrhea

Freddy T. Kokke, MD, Roxan F. Saidi, MD, Alastair J.M. Watson, MD, and Mark Donowitz, MD

Diarrheal diseases almost always cause an increase in stool water and usually an increase in the frequency or fluidity of bowel movements. Normal daily stool water on an American diet averages 130 mL, and normal stool is 65–85% water. Diarrheal diseases can be objectively defined as conditions associated with daily stool weights greater than 200 g. It is more difficult to say how many bowel movements would be considered diarrhea, since a change in bowel habits is part of the definition. Three bowel movements a day is probably the upper limit of normal on an American diet. Patients who have diarrhea for longer than 4 weeks are classified as having chronic diarrhea, since most forms of infectious enteritis and other causes of acute diarrhea (Chapter 6.7) resolve spontaneously within 4 weeks.

Patients with chronic diarrhea must be approached differently from those with acute diarrhea because of the following: (1) Diagnostic possibilities are more heterogeneous. Infections, the predominant cause of important acute diarrhea, are less likely to cause chronic diarrhea, although some infections (more often parasites than bacteria) can elude detection for weeks. (2) Factitious and functional diseases, secretory problems, and malignancies are more common with chronic than with acute diarrhea. (3) Dehydration is less of a problem with chronic diarrhea, since most patients can drink. (4) Chronic diarrhea must be evaluated. Since most acute diarrhea resolves within 1–2 weeks, it is neither necessary nor cost-effective to evaluate all patients with acute diarrhea.

CLASSIFICATION OF DIARRHEAL DISEASES

Diarrhea can be classified as "secretory" or "osmotic," according to the underlying mechanism.

Secretory Diarrhea

Many diarrheal diseases increase active Cl^- secretion, decrease active Na^+ absorption (usually by inhibiting neutral NaCl absorption), or do both. The causes of secretory diarrhea can be categorized as (1) microorganisms and their toxins and other products, (2) inflammation in the bowel wall, (3) hormone-secreting tumors, (4) damage to villus cells, and (5) hypermotility. A feature common to all five categories is activation of intestinal cell intracellular second messengers: the adenylate cyclase-cyclic AMP (cAMP) system, the guanylate cyclase-cyclic GMP (cGMP) system, and elevated intracellular calcium and the diacylglycerol-protein kinase C system. These intracellular messengers activate specific protein kinases, which then either directly or indirectly affect ion transport proteins in the enterocyte. In crypt enterocytes, the result is stimulated Cl^- secretion. In villus enterocytes, NaCl absorption is inhibited. Stimulated Cl^- secretion, inhibited Na^+ absorption, or both lead to fluid and electrolyte loss into the intestinal lumen.

Osmotic Diarrhea

In conditions that increase luminal osmolality, water flows passively from the capillaries below the epithelial cells through the tight junctions to enter the lumen, producing diarrhea. The disaccharide deficiencies, particularly lactase deficiency, constitute the most common cause of osmotic diarrhea. Lactose (glucose-galactose disaccharide) is normally broken down in the jejunum to glucose and galactose. This causes a slight increase in osmolality, producing a slight, transient water secretion, but is followed by rapid absorption of glucose and galactose since lactase is in close proximity to the Na^+/glucose-galactose co-transporter.

Lactase deficiency largely produces colonic diarrhea. The lactose is not broken down in the small intestine, and the intraluminal lactose holds water isosmotically. As the lactose passes into the colon, bacteria break the glucose-galactose bond. This increases the osmolality, and because there is no colonic Na^+/substrate cotransport sys-

Acknowledgment: This chapter is adapted, with permission, from Donowitz M, Kokke FT, Saidi R: Evaluation of patients with chronic diarrhea. N Engl J Med 1995;332:725.

tem, the increased osmolality pulls water into the lumen. The prominent abdominal cramps of lactase deficiency develop because the water secretion distends the colon and because bacterial metabolism of the glucose and galactose generates CO_2.

Lactase deficiency is one of the most common causes of diarrheal disease worldwide. Far less common are other disaccharidase deficiencies, including sucrase-isomaltase deficiency and trehalase deficiency (patients with this disorder get diarrhea when they eat mushrooms that contain trehalose).

The diarrhea related to steatorrhea or malabsorption of fat has only a small osmotic component. The colonic luminal contents contain relatively few molecules of nonabsorbed fatty acids, since they have limited solubility and precipitate, or they associate to form micelles. Since the number of free molecules in solution determines the osmotic force, the number of micelles is what matters, not the number of fat molecules; therefore, a much smaller osmotic force is exerted. The diarrhea of steatorrhea is not osmotic, but is explained by decreased Na^+ absorption and stimulated Cl^- secretion. The fatty acids that are not absorbed by the small intestine are converted by colonic bacteria to form OH-fatty acids. Both fatty acids and OH-fatty acids cause colonic Cl^- secretion and decreased Na^+ absorption.

DIFFERENTIAL DIAGNOSIS

Common causes of chronic diarrhea are listed in Table 6.8–1. The initial history and physical examination and a limited, directed laboratory evaluation often point to the cause. Some of the causes of chronic diarrhea have distinguishing characteristics:

In *giardiasis,* organisms are found predominantly in the duodenum and proximal jejunum. The diarrhea is often a "frothy stool" associated with upper abdominal cramps. Initial evaluation should be only a single, fixed, concentrated stool specimen for ova and parasites; this test is cheap and has a sensitivity of 50–75%. If this test does not turn up the cause of the chronic diarrhea, second and third stool specimens should be examined, followed by a stool specimen for *Giardia* antigen; all these tests are quite sensitive and specific. Only then should the physician consider a therapeutic trial with metronidazole or quinacrine hydrochloride. There is no evidence that biopsy of the small intestine, study of the attached mucus from the biopsy, or a swallowed string capsule has a higher diagnostic yield.

Amebic diarrhea can be either watery or bloody and can last for many years. The best screen for amebiasis is examination of fixed specimens of stools. The stool for this test must be collected directly into fixative or first into a dry container and then fixative, rather than being recovered from the toilet bowl, since urine and water destroy the parasite and it deteriorates quickly on its own. Barium in the gastrointestinal tract also hampers detection of ame-

Table 6.8–1. Common causes of chronic diarrhea in non-HIV-infected patients.*

Chronic or relapsing gastrointestinal infection: amebiasis, giardiasis, *Clostridium difficile*
Inflammatory bowel diseases
Steatorrhea
• Carbohydrate malabsorption: disaccharidase deficiency (lactase, sucrase), poorly absorbed substances (fiber, lactulose, sorbitol, fructose)
Drugs and food additives: antibiotics, antihypertensives, antiarrhythmics (quinidine, digitalis), antineoplastics, magnesium-containing antacids, sweeteners (sorbitol, fructose), ethanol, caffeine
Previous surgery: gastrectomy, vagotomy, cholecystectomy, intestinal resection
Endocrine disorders: adrenal insufficiency, hyper- or hypothyroidism, diabetes
Laxative abuse
• Ischemic bowel disease
Radiation enteritis or colitis
Paradoxical diarrhea in colon cancer
Hormone-producing tumors: gastrinoma, VIPoma, villous adenoma, medullary thyroid carcinoma, ganglioneuroma, pheochromocytoma, carcinoid tumor, mastocytosis
Infiltrative disorders: scleroderma, amyloidosis, diffuse gut lymphoma
Epidemic chronic diarrhea caused by an infectious agent in raw milk or untreated water, and possibly related chronic self-limited idiopathic diarrhea
Fecal incontinence masquerading as diarrhea
Food allergy
Functional diarrhea: irritable bowel syndrome

VIP, vasoactive intestinal polypeptide.
*Listed from most to least common.
Adapted and reproduced, with permission, from Donowitz M et al: Evaluation of patients with chronic diarrhea. N Engl J Med 1995; 332:725.

bae for an undefined period, although not permanently. Thus, ova and parasite tests must be performed before barium studies. Culturing of amebae is so time-consuming and expensive that it is not clinically justified. Indirect hemagglutination and ELISA (enzyme-linked immunosorbent assay) are preferred. They are readily available, and have about 85–100% sensitivity for amebic liver abscess and 50–95% sensitivity for severe amebic dysentery. Their sensitivity for the watery diarrhea of amebiasis is not known.

Early *Crohn's disease* of the small bowel is often difficult to diagnose radiographically and is not ruled out by a negative small bowel x-ray. The physician who suspects Crohn's disease despite a negative small bowel series should do enteroclysis (an air-barium distention study of the small bowel, with the barium given through a small nasogastric tube) to distend the small bowel and show more mucosal detail.

Half of patients with *steatorrhea* complain of watery diarrhea. Floating stools indicate bacterial production of gases, including methane, but not steatorrhea. Indicators of steatorrhea are a history of weight loss, greasy or bulky stools that are difficult to flush down, bad odor that cohabitants complain about, and oil that sticks to the toilet bowl and requires a brush to remove.

The diarrhea of *carbohydrate malabsorption* can be intermittent. The diarrhea is usually accompanied by bloating, flatus, and cramping, since less carbohydrate is needed to produce excessive gas than to cause diarrhea. This type of diarrhea can be secondary to another insult such as viral enteritis or antibiotic therapy. Antibiotics alter the balance or number of colonic bacteria. These bacteria metabolize the 30 g of ingested carbohydrate that enters the colon of normal people each day, converting it into efficiently absorbed short-chain fatty acids. The drop in colonic bacteria can impair this conversion and lead to a colonic osmotic diarrhea. Stool pH below 5.3 is diagnostic of carbohydrate intolerance; acid stools can cause excoriation and perianal pain.

Primary lactase deficiency can present as chronic diarrhea in adulthood, and secondary lactase deficiency can accompany virtually all causes of small bowel-related diarrhea. Patients whose acute diarrhea seems to persist should be tried on a nutritionist-supervised lactose-free diet before undergoing more tests.

As much as 4% of chronic diarrheas are caused by *medications and food additives* (see Table 6.8–1). One such additive is sorbitol, used as a nonabsorbable sweetener in diet foods. One sugar-free mint or one stick of sugar-free chewing gum can contain up to 2 g of sorbitol. In one study, 50% of subjects ingesting 10 g of sorbitol developed diarrhea, abdominal pain, and bloating. Sorbitol has also been used in elixir formulations of theophylline, sucralfate, isoniazid, acetaminophen, trimethoprim-sulfamethoxazole, and cimetidine.

Long *resections of the ileum and right colon* can cause diarrhea because of inadequate absorptive surface, shortened transit time, malabsorption of bile acids, and a smaller bile acid pool, leading to steatorrhea. Shorter intestinal resections (less than 100 cm) can lead to bile acid diarrhea (*cholerrheic enteropathy*), since malabsorbed bile acids cause colonic secretion of water and electrolytes. This diarrhea follows meals and stops with fasting. The stool volume is usually about 300 g per 24 hours, with less than 15–20 g fat and a pH above 6.8. After *cholecystectomy*, about 10% of patients develop diarrhea of unknown mechanism, often with impaired bile acid absorption. Diarrhea caused by intestinal resections can worsen any other diarrheal disease. In occasional postcholecystectomy patients, the diarrhea responds to cholestyramine.

About 1 in 20 patients presenting to a gastroenterology clinic for evaluation of chronic diarrhea is eventually found to be abusing *laxatives*. Virtually all of these patients deny using laxatives, and the only clinical clues are psychiatric disease and macroscopic melanosis coli (a dark pigment seen at colonoscopy). Five stereotypes have been described for people with laxative-induced factitious diarrhea: younger patients with an eating disorder (anorexia nervosa or bulimia nervosa) (Chapter 14.5), middle-aged hysterical patients, patients driven by desire for secondary gain, patients with Munchausen syndrome (Chapter 14.6), and children who have been given laxa-

tives as a form of abuse (called Polle syndrome). Women laxative abusers exceed men by about 10:1. A disproportionate number of abusers are medical workers. Many laxative abusers have major metabolic derangements and clinical features that can be confused with other chronic diarrheal diseases: hypokalemia (with or without nephropathy), clubbing, hyperpigmentation of skin, steatorrhea, colonic inflammation, uric acid kidney stones, osteomalacia, and protein-losing enteropathy.

Physicians should be more aggressive about screening for laxative abuse in patients with chronic diarrhea. Several good tests are available (Table 6.8–2). One is alkalinization of stool, urine, or both for diphenolic laxatives (phenolphthalein and some anthraquinones). Alkalinization above pH 9 turns the acid-base indicator phenolphthalein red, but elevating the pH further makes the dye colorless again. Rhubarb in the stool also turns red with alkalinization. Therefore, red stool on alkalinization should be confirmed with thin-layer chromatography or spectrophotometry. Screening of urine or stool by thin-layer chromatography specifically for anthraquinones, phenolphthalein, bisacodyl, and dioctyl sodium sulfosuccinate has been a major diagnostic advance. Since laxative abuse may be intermittent, patients should be screened more than once. Urine specimens have the highest yield; patients should be asked to submit several first-morning specimens, including a Monday sample to detect weekend purge. Anthraquinones are detectable by thin-layer chromatography for at least 32 hours after a single dose.

Ischemic bowel disease, specifically chronic mesenteric vascular ischemia, may manifest as watery diarrhea with patchy inflammation and may be mistaken histologically for an inflammatory bowel disease.

Many years after patients undergo *abdominal radiation,* many develop diarrhea from chronic enterocolitis caused by progressive small-vessel disease. Increased bowel movements and diarrhea are much more common than suspected in these patients.

Colon cancer and fecal impaction can cause secretion proximal to partial bowel obstruction and can present as watery diarrhea, so-called "*paradoxical diarrhea.*"

Table 6.8–2. Laboratory evaluation for laxative abuse.

Barium enema showing cathartic colon (including ahaustral right colon)
Rectal biopsy showing gross melanosis coli (microscopic form can be a normal variant)
Alkalinization of stool, urine, or both
Thin-layer chromatography of urine or stool water for anthraquinones, bisacodyl, phenolphthalein, dioctyl sodium sulfosuccinate
Stool and serum osmolality
Stool sodium, potassium, sulfate, phosphate
Stool osmotic gap (if >50 mOsm/L, measure stool magnesium)

Adapted and reproduced, with permission, from Donowitz M et al: Evaluation of patients with chronic diarrhea. N Engl J Med 1995; 332:725.

Hormone-producing tumors such as pancreatic cholera cause a dramatic diarrhea from the outset and are often quickly diagnosed. All patients have more than 0.7 L stool per 24 hours, 70% have more than 3 L, and volumes of 10–21 L have been reported. Hypokalemia is also a sensitive but nonspecific test for pancreatic cholera, since all patients have a low potassium level, almost always below 2.5 mEq/L.

Patients with *villous adenomas* can present with diarrhea and electrolyte losses from an as yet unidentified secretagogue or from prostaglandin E_2 production. Most of these tumors are in the distal colon or rectum and are more than 3–4 cm in diameter. Water can be seen pouring from their surface, although water and electrolytes can also be secreted in other parts of the gut.

Epidemic chronic diarrhea was reported in Brainerd, Minnesota, in people drinking raw milk (1983–1984) and in Henderson County, Illinois, in people drinking untreated water (1987–1989). No pathogen was identified in these epidemics and the patients did not respond to antibiotics; the diarrhea was self-limited, but for most patients lasted for at least 1 year. Somewhat similar in description, although without the epidemiologic clustering, was a study in which about 10% of patients tested for chronic diarrhea at a tertiary referral center had a negative evaluation and no systemic illness. As in the epidemics, these patients' diarrhea began suddenly, persisted on fasting, caused weight loss, did not respond to antibiotics, and resolved on its own after a mean of 15 months (range 7–31 months). In more than 50% of the patients, the diarrhea began 1–4 weeks after travel within the United States.

Perhaps most important is that as many as 30–60% of patients with protracted diarrhea are not found to have any organic abnormality. These patients are classified as having *functional diarrhea*. If they also have abdominal pain, they are said to have a diarrhea-predominant form of irritable bowel syndrome. However, so many patients with apparent functional diarrhea turn out to have occult organic disorders that all patients with chronic diarrhea deserve a thorough evaluation.

A full diarrheal disease workup misses only a few conditions, primarily Crohn's disease, some parasitic diseases, lymphoma, and laxative abuse. (Because so few disorders are missed, repeating the full evaluation every few years is not recommended.) Almost certainly, some functional diarrhea is caused by still undefined organic conditions.

No current screening test is sensitive enough to predict that a patient's chronic diarrhea has an organic cause. But there are clues that a problem is organic rather than functional: sudden onset of symptoms, a shorter duration of diarrhea (2–24 months), continual rather than intermittent diarrhea, prominent nocturnal diarrhea, weight loss of more than 5 kg, high erythrocyte sedimentation rate, low hemoglobin, low albumin, and average daily fecal weight greater than 400 g.

DIAGNOSIS

Outpatient Evaluation

If the cause of chronic diarrhea is not obvious after the history, physical exam, and directed laboratory studies, patients should have a step-wise evaluation (Table 6.8–3). The initial tests help to classify the diarrhea by characterizing the stool and intestinal anatomy and by detecting some infectious causes. Since most patients can function outside the hospital, these tests are usually done as outpatient procedures over several weeks. If the initial evaluation does not turn up the cause, patients should undergo a second series of more costly and invasive tests, also over a short period. If patients are referred after evaluation elsewhere, the physician should review not just the results but also the quality of the tests.

In-Hospital Evaluation

If no cause for chronic diarrhea is found after an outpatient evaluation, patients are considered to have *diarrhea of unknown origin* (Table 6.8–4). They are then offered further evaluation, especially if they are having trouble maintaining hydration. Nearly all patients want a definitive explanation for their diarrhea. Diarrhea of unknown origin should be evaluated in-hospital because many causes that have eluded diagnosis are those missed by poor-quality tests or inadequate outpatient stool collections (Table 6.8–5). In-hospital evaluation allows more precise and detailed evaluation of several aspects of chronic diarrhea.

The physician's first task is to confirm that all tests in the outpatient evaluation (see Table 6.8–3) have been done and are of adequate quality. This is particularly important because the increasing reliance on outpatient testing required by managed care may prolong the initial evaluation to the point that it is difficult to keep track of which tests have been done.

Measuring stool weight reveals whether the patient has true diarrhea. On admission, patients are placed on their usual home diet, even if they need to bring in snacks from home, and a 24-hour stool weight is determined. This test is done immediately, because the prolonged bed rest of hospitalization tends to decrease stool output—both normal and abnormal. If stool output is more than 1 kg/24 hours, secretory diarrhea is likely. If stool output is more than 0.5 kg/24 hours, the cause of the diarrhea is unlikely to be irritable bowel syndrome. If stool output is less than 0.2 kg/24 hours, the patient does not have true diarrhea; more likely, the diagnosis is fecal incontinence, irritable bowel syndrome (its abdominal pain not having been recognized during the outpatient evaluation), or rectal disease.

An important part of evaluating chronic diarrhea is determining whether patients have fecal incontinence, and, if so, how severely. About 50% of patients with chronic diarrhea also have at least intermittent incontinence. Incontinence can be so devastating that patients would

Table 6.8–3. Outpatient evaluation of patients with chronic diarrhea.

Initial Tests	Further Tests*
Stool tests	
White blood cells	*Giardia* antigen by ELISA
Ova and parasites × 3 (done before barium studies)	Alkalinization (for phenolphthalein)
Clostridium difficile toxin	Sodium
pH	Potassium
Stool weight/24 hr (must be requested specifically)	Sulfate
72-hr stool fat while on a 75–100 g fat/24-hr diet	Phosphate
	Magnesium
	Osmolality
Blood tests	
Fasting gastrin	Ameba hemagglutination or ELISA
Thyroid-stimulating hormone (TSH)	
Thyroxine (T_4)	
Complete blood count with differential	
Erythrocyte sedimentation rate	
Electrolytes	
Blood urea nitrogen	
Creatinine	
Urine tests	
None	Thin-layer chromatography for bisacodyl, phenolphthalein, anthraquinones, dioctyl sodium sulfosuccinate
Radiographic tests	
Plain abdominal x-ray for pancreatic calcification	Enteroclysis
High-quality barium studies of the upper GI tract, small bowel, colon	Abdominal CT
Endoscopic tests	
Sigmoidoscopy and biopsy (done before barium studies and without hyperosmotic preparation)	Colonoscopy and ileoscopy (for right-sided colitis, amebiasis, Crohn's disease)
	Upper endoscopy, including small-bowel biopsy
Other tests	
Bile acid breath test	Nutritionist-supervised lactose-free diet for 3–5 days
If large-volume diarrhea (>1 L/day), especially with hypokalemia: VIP, substance P, calcitonin, histamine	
If diarrhea with flushing: urine 5-HIAA	

ELISA, enzyme-linked immunosorbent assay; VIP, vasoactive intestinal polypeptide; 5-HIAA, 5-hydroxyindoleacetic acid.
*Further tests should be done only when the initial tests do not produce a diagnosis.
Adapted and reproduced, with permission, from Donowitz M et al: Evaluation of patients with chronic diarrhea. N Engl J Med 1995; 332:725.

rather become homebound than risk the embarrassment of having a public accident. Many incontinent people who have no significant diarrhea get all the way to an in-hospital evaluation for diarrhea of unknown origin without volunteering that incontinence is their main problem. Therefore, the physician must ask about it directly. Incontinence most often affects the elderly and women after

Table 6.8–4. Underlying causes of diarrhea of unknown origin.

Laxative abuse (factitious diarrhea)
Fecal incontinence
Inflammatory bowel diseases, especially microscopic (lymphocytic) and collagenous colitis
Any of the other causes in Table 6.8–1, missed on initial evaluation, especially steatorrhea, medications, food additives, bacterial overgrowth of the small bowel

Adapted and reproduced, with permission, from Donowitz M et al: Evaluation of patients with chronic diarrhea. N Engl J Med 1995; 332:725.

vaginal delivery. Up to about one in eight primiparous women and one in four multiparous women have urgency or frank incontinence 6 weeks postpartum, most in association with anal sphincter defects.

Laxative abuse causing factitious diarrhea is the most common cause of diarrhea of unknown origin, eventually being found in one-third of patients. In hospital, laxative abusers may stop taking laxatives or use them only intermittently, although surprisingly many patients continue them at full doses. Thus, urine should be screened for laxatives by thin-layer chromatography and alkalinization (see Table 6.8–2) on hospital admission and several more times during the hospitalization.

Next in the evaluation of diarrhea is determining daily stool weights during a 72-hour fast, but with enough intravenous hydration to keep the patient out of danger. This study differentiates chronic secretory diarrhea from nonsecretory diarrhea (Tables 6.8–6 and 6.8–7). In secretory diarrheal diseases, diarrhea persists after 48 hours of fasting; stool electrolytes account for most of the stool osmo-

Table 6.8–5. Evaluation of hospitalized patients with diarrhea of unknown origin.

Review and confirm results of outpatient evaluation	
Day 1	Measure stool weight or volume on normal diet Screen for laxatives by urine thin-layer chromatography and stool or urine alkalinization Measure stool sodium, potassium, sulfate, phosphate Determine stool and serum osmolality Calculate stool osmotic gap
Days 2–4	72-hr fast with IV hydration Determine daily stool weights
Days 5–8	75–100-g fat/24-hr diet Measure stool weight and fat content on days 6, 7, 8

Adapted and reproduced, with permission, from Donowitz M et al: Evaluation of patients with chronic diarrhea. N Engl J Med 1995; 332:725.

Table 6.8–7. Causes of chronic nonsecretory diarrhea.

Incontinence
Bile acid diarrhea
Steatorrhea
Osmotic diarrhea:
  Carbohydrate malabsorption
  Excessive carbohydrate ingestion
  Laxatives (containing poorly absorbable anions: sodium
    sulfate, sodium phosphate, or sodium citrate), magnesium

Adapted and reproduced, with permission, from Donowitz M et al: Evaluation of patients with chronic diarrhea. N Engl J Med 1995; 332:725.

lality, resulting in a fecal osmotic gap below 50 mOsm/L. By contrast, in nonsecretory diseases, the diarrhea always ceases by 48 to 72 hours (if the diarrhea stops before 72 hours, the patient need not continue fasting) and the fecal osmotic gap is above 50 mOsm/L.

The formula to determine the fecal osmotic gap is:

$$\text{Fecal osmotic gap} =$$
$$\text{plasma osmolality} - \{2 \times [\text{stool } (Na^+) + (K^+)]\}$$

There is some debate about whether the plasma osmolality used in this calculation should be assumed to be a normal value of 290 mOsm/L rather than a value determined for each patient by freezing point depression. Actual stool osmolality cannot be used in this calculation because fecal osmolality usually is elevated (from bacterial metabolism), thus falsely increasing the osmotic gap. The major reason for measuring actual stool osmolality is to search for laxative abuse and factitious diarrhea. If stool osmolality is significantly less than 290 mOsm/L, water or dilute urine has been added to the stool. Water is

Table 6.8–6. Causes of chronic secretory diarrhea.

Laxatives, diuretics
Inflammatory bowel diseases
Celiac sprue
Intestinal lymphoma
Villous adenoma of the rectum
Zollinger-Ellison syndrome
Pancreatic cholera
Carcinoid tumor
Medullary carcinoma of the thyroid
Chronic infections (eg, tuberculosis, giardiasis, amebiasis)
Hyperthyroidism
Congenital diarrhea (chloride-bicarbonate exchange deficiency,
  sodium-hydrogen exchange deficiency, microvillus inclusion
  disease)
Intestinal resection
Bacterial overgrowth

Adapted and reproduced, with permission, from Donowitz M et al: Evaluation of patients with chronic diarrhea. N Engl J Med 1995; 332:725.

most likely to have been added by patients with factitious diarrhea. Urine can also be detected by finding creatinine in the stool.

Most of the diseases known to cause chronic secretory diarrhea are usually diagnosed during the initial outpatient evaluation (see Table 6.8–6). Diarrhea that stops during a fast is caused directly or indirectly by a dietary substance. Foremost among nonsecretory diseases (Table 6.8–7) are the osmotic diarrheas. Most are caused by either laxative abuse (including magnesium, citrate, or phosphate laxatives) or carbohydrate malabsorption. Stool pH can discriminate between the two, since pH is below 5.3 only in carbohydrate malabsorption. A patient with a stool osmotic gap (above 50 mOsm/L) may be abusing magnesium laxatives, so the stool magnesium should be measured. A normal stool magnesium is less than 45 mM (90 mEq/L), with a daily stool excretion of less than 30 mEq.

Next, the physician tests the patient for steatorrhea. A nutritionist should monitor how much fat the patient consumes during the 3-day collection. There is a linear relationship between the amount of long-chain fatty acids consumed and the amount excreted in the stool. Normal people who ingest even up to 300 g of fat a day absorb about 95%. At zero fat intake, people still excrete about 2 g of fat in stool, as measured by van de Kamer analysis. This fat comes from epithelial cell turnover and bacterial cell wall loss. On a normal American diet of 75–100 g fat, fecal fat is up to 7 g/24 hours $(100-[100 \times 0.95] + 2)$. However, patients with steatorrhea may consume much less fat, to self-treat their diarrhea. Although patients are instructed to consume 75–100 g of fat/24 hours for the outpatient test, they may eat less, thus giving a falsely low fecal fat in the stool collection. In addition, diarrhea itself can decrease the efficiency of fat absorption. Experimental osmotic diarrhea can cause loss of up to 13 g of fat/24 hours. Therefore, inpatients who produce at least 14 g of fat/24 hours have significant steatorrhea. If stool fat is 7–14 g/24 hours, the steatorrhea may be secondary to the diarrhea.

The success of outpatient evaluation for chronic diarrhea is not known, but inpatient evaluation for diarrhea of unknown origin yields a definite diagnosis in at least two-thirds of patients. After both comprehensive outpatient and inpatient evaluations, around 90% of patients have a diagnosis: About 20–40% have an organic disorder, up to

33% are taking laxatives or diuretics surreptitiously, and 30–60% have functional diarrhea. The remaining 4–15% of patients are said to have "chronic idiopathic diarrhea"; fortunately, this is often self-limited.

MANAGEMENT

A crucial part of management is maintaining patients' hydration. The most reliable means is chronic use of oral rehydration solutions. These solutions are remarkably underused in the United States.

Thorough evaluation of patients with chronic diarrhea should enable the physician to diagnose the source and treat it specifically, whether it be bacterial overgrowth, lymphoma, celiac sprue, inflammatory bowel disease, or another condition. If no specific cause is found, the physician should try to control the diarrhea, usually with an opiate agonist such as codeine or loperamide.

SUMMARY

► Patients who have diarrhea for longer than 4 weeks should be evaluated for chronic diarrheal diseases. Thorough stepwise evaluation yields a diagnosis in about 90% of patients.

► The most common currently diagnosable causes of chronic diarrhea are chronic or relapsing gastrointestinal infection, inflammatory bowel diseases, steatorrhea, carbohydrate malabsorption, and drugs and food additives.

► Pitfalls in the evaluation include surreptitious laxative use, difficulty in diagnosing Crohn's disease, steatorrhea as a result rather than a cause of chronic diarrhea, and fecal incontinence.

► As yet unrecognized organic disorders probably cause much of the chronic diarrhea that is now labeled as "functional diarrhea."

SUGGESTED READING

Donowitz M: Pathophysiology of diarrhea. In: *Core Textbook of Gastroenterology.* Eastwood GL (editor). JB Lippincott, 1984.

Fine KD, Krejs GJ, Fordtran JS: Diarrhea. In: *Gastrointestinal Disease: Pathophysiology, Diagnosis, Management,* 5th ed. Sleisenger MH, Fordtran JS (editors). WB Saunders, 1993.

Powell DW: Approach to the patient with diarrhea. In: *Textbook of Gastroenterology.* Yamada T et al (editors). JB Lippincott, 1995.

Read NW et al: Chronic diarrhea of unknown origin. Gastroenterology 1980;78:264.

Schiller LR: Chronic diarrhea of obscure origin. In: *Diarrheal Diseases.* Field M (editor). Elsevier, 1991.

Malabsorption

Theodore M. Bayless, MD, and Thomas R. Hendrix, MD

Like other essential organ systems, the gastrointestinal tract has excess functional capacity to safeguard against extensive but subtotal injury or loss. For example, over 90% of carbohydrates and proteins are absorbed by the time a meal passes the first few loops of jejunum. Furthermore, the gastrointestinal tract adapts after injury or loss through epithelial cell hypertrophy and hyperplasia and gut lengthening. This efficiency enables humans to survive on oral feeding even after they lose 80% of their 24 feet of small intestine. They have some malabsorption of nutrients and fluid, but they can survive. Likewise, people must lose more than 90% of their pancreatic exocrine function before decreased fat digestion leads to malabsorption.

Malabsorption can involve the intestinal absorption of a single compound, such as lactose in lactase deficiency or vitamin B_{12} in pernicious anemia, or it can involve all elements of the diet, as in a diffuse mucosal abnormality like celiac disease or AIDS enteropathy. Generalized malabsorption, that is, of many nutrients, can cause serious dysfunction through both loss of unabsorbed food substances and secondary deficiencies of specific vitamins and minerals. The most common clinical manifestation of generalized malabsorption, seen in more than two-thirds of patients, is weight loss from caloric deficiency even though the patients consume seemingly normal amounts of nutrients. The second most prominent manifestation is steatorrhea (increased fat and hydroxy fatty acids in the stool). The sign of steatorrhea is pale, bulky, floating, foul-smelling stools; major symptoms are diarrhea and abdominal bloating. Because bacterial metabolism of unabsorbed dietary fatty acids produces excessive hydroxy fatty acids, a small percentage of patients complain of watery diarrhea rather than the classic steatorrhea. Most patients with any form of generalized malabsorption have a change in stool character, but less than 10% have obvious steatorrhea. Most present with less obvious symptoms such as anemia, bone fragility, or easy bruising—consequences of deficiencies in essential nutrients like vitamin B_{12} (cobalamin), vitamin D and calcium, or vitamin K.

The clinician who recognizes that a patient has malabsorption can provide a systematic evaluation that usually uncovers a treatable cause. Prompt diagnosis and effective management depend on identifying which steps in the digestive-absorptive process are deranged: (1) the intraluminal phase, during which the physical and chemical states of nutrients are altered in preparation for absorption; (2) the epithelial phase, with surface hydrolysis at the brush border, followed by uptake and preparation for extrusion into the lamina propria; or (3) the transit phase, during which absorbed material is removed from the lamina propria by lymph and blood flow.

This chapter explains how pathophysiologic alterations in digestion and absorption produce the signs and symptoms of generalized malabsorption. These alterations explain both the classification of malabsorptive disorders and the steps in evaluating patients with suspected malabsorption. The goal of evaluation is to reach a specific diagnosis because very effective therapies exist for most of the common causes of malabsorption.

PHYSIOLOGY OF DIGESTION AND ABSORPTION

Preparation of food for absorption begins in the mouth, where salivary amylase partially converts starch to dextrins and maltose. In the stomach, food is homogenized and emulsified, and pepsin exerts its proteolytic action by cleaving proteins to peptides.

The arrival of acidified chyme from the stomach causes the duodenum to release the hormones cholecystokinin and secretin. These, in turn, stimulate the gallbladder to contract and empty bile into the duodenum. At almost the same time, the hormones stimulate the pancreas to release digestive enzymes and bicarbonate. Conjugated bile salts form micelles, which carry the products of lipolysis, cholesterol, and lipid-soluble vitamins in micellar solution to the absorbing surface of the intestine. The lipids pass into the epithelial cells, whereas the bile salts remain in the lumen to continue transporting lipids. Finally, the bile salts are absorbed by the ileum and carried in the portal blood to the liver to be excreted again into the bile. This enterohepatic circulation of bile salts is 95% efficient, so that each day the liver has to synthesize only enough bile acid to replace the 5% lost into the colon. In the process of absorbing a meal, the bile salt pool completes two or more enterohepatic cycles.

Pancreatic amylase continues the hydrolysis of polysaccharides to disaccharides. Disaccharides are hydrolyzed to monosaccharides by enzymes (disaccharidases) on the brush border of the small intestinal epithelium. Glucose absorption releases gastric inhibitory peptide from the intestinal mucosa; this peptide stimulates insulin release and inhibits gastric acid secretion. The pancreatic proteolytic enzymes are secreted in an inactive form. An intestinal enzyme, enterokinase, converts trypsinogen into active trypsin, which in turn converts the other proteolytic proenzymes into their active forms—chymotrypsin, elastase, carboxypeptidases, and so on. The major products of intraluminal protein digestion are small polypeptides and amino acids. Brush border peptidases hydrolyze large peptides to dipeptides and tripeptides, which are actively absorbed by a peptide transport carrier. There are also amino acid transport carriers.

The small intestine's motor activity mixes and churns the chyme and digestive enzymes and brings the products of digestion into contact with the intestine's absorbing surfaces to facilitate the second phase of absorption, the transfer to the surface epithelium. The small intestine's normal propulsive activity prevents stasis of the intestinal contents and thus prevents multiplication of bacteria that could interfere with absorption. Bacterial overgrowth both deconjugates bile salts and interferes with absorption of vitamin B_{12}; the bacteria consume the vitamin before it reaches its site of absorption in the ileum.

The third phase of the absorptive process is the actual transfer of the products of digestion from the intestinal lumen to the blood and lymph. Nutrients are absorbed chiefly in the duodenum and jejunum, whereas bile salts and vitamin B_{12} are absorbed in the ileum.

The epithelial cells of the villi are the functional units in intestinal absorption, with cells at the tips playing the major role. Materials such as most water-soluble vitamins, nucleic acid derivatives, and urea pass through the intestinal cells by simple diffusion. Lipids enter the cells by nonionic diffusion. But most foodstuffs are absorbed by more efficient and often highly specialized active transport processes. For example, glucose and galactose share the same sodium-coupled active transport mechanism; fructose enters by carrier-facilitated diffusion. Although there are at least four specific amino acid transport mechanisms, amino acids are also absorbed as peptides, with hydrolysis to amino acids being completed within the absorbing cell. Intestinal absorption of materials such as iron, copper, calcium, and magnesium involves specific and complex regulatory systems.

The portal blood is the primary route for all absorbed materials except lipids. The absorbed fatty acids and monoglycerides are reesterified within the absorbing cells. These triglycerides, along with other absorbed lipids, are packaged in a protein coat and extruded from the cell as chylomicrons, which are carried from the intestine by the lymphatic vessels.

PATHOPHYSIOLOGY OF MALABSORPTION

Diseases causing malabsorption can be grouped according to the alterations that they cause in digestive and absorptive physiology (Table 6.9–1). Defects in intraluminal digestion are classified as "failure of digestion" (maldigestion), whereas defects in mucosal absorption are "failures of absorption" (malabsorption). "Impairment in lymph and blood flow" is the classification for defects in the transit phase of absorption. Later in this chapter, the section "Specific Disorders Causing Intestinal Malabsorption" covers the most common disorders in each category and their therapeutic import.

The most common causes of maldigestion are inadequate pancreatic secretion of lipase for fat digestion and of bicarbonate for neutralizing gastric acid in the duodenum; acid must be neutralized to permit optimum intraluminal activity of lipase and other digestive enzymes. Pancreatic insufficiency can result from chronic pancreatitis with damage to the pancreatic acini and ducts. Oral replacement of pancreatic enzymes can markedly improve patients' fat digestion.

Another mechanism for maldigestion is excessive gastric acid secretion, as stimulated by a gastrin-secreting tumor (Zollinger-Ellison syndrome). Hypersecretion of acid interferes with duodenal neutralization and with normal bile salt and enzyme activity.

Even if pancreatic secretion and acid neutralization are adequate, deficiency or changes in the conjugation of bile acids can cause maldigestion. For example, bile acid deficiencies result from decreased reabsorption of bile acids secondary to either extensive ileal disease, such as Crohn's disease, or surgical resection of several feet of small bowel. Bile acid concentrations in the duodenum are then inadequate to form normal micelles with fatty acids, and fatty acid absorption is impaired. Similarly, fatty acids are malabsorbed if bile acids, even in adequate concentration, are deconjugated by bacterial overgrowth in the usually bacteria-free environment of the upper small intestine.

Malabsorption of normally digested food constituents results from an inadequate small bowel surface for absorption. At least 2 feet of small bowel is needed to sustain life without parenteral alimentation or a small bowel transplant. But people develop malabsorption when they lose 75% of small intestinal function, as do some patients who must have most of the bowel removed because of extensive ischemic injury. If more than 80–100 cm of ileum is resected, as happens to about 20% of patients with extensive Crohn's disease in the ileum, bile salt reabsorption is inadequate for micelle formation and fat absorption. Damage to the absorbing epithelial cells of the duodenum and jejunum, as in celiac disease (see "Celiac Disease" below), causes malabsorption of normally digested nutrients; if the apparent antigen, wheat gliadin, is removed

Table 6.9–1. Pathophysiologic classification of malabsorption.

Failure of digestion (intraluminal phase)
Decreased pancreatic enzymes
　Pancreatic insufficiency (pancreatitis, pancreatic resection, cystic fibrosis, protein deficiency, pancreatic cancer)
　Inactivation of pancreatic enzymes by gastric hypersecretion (Zollinger-Ellison syndrome, ileal resection)
　Failure to convert proenzyme to active form (enterokinase and trypsinogen deficiencies)
Impaired bile acid micelle formation
　Impaired bile acid synthesis (severe hepatocellular disease)
　Interrupted enterohepatic circulation (ileal resection, cholestasis, bile duct obstruction, biliary cirrhosis)
　Bile acid deconjugation (bacterial overgrowth)
　　Stasis caused by a motor abnormality (scleroderma, intestinal obstruction, diabetic visceral neuropathy)
　　Stasis caused by anatomic abnormalities (multiple diverticula; strictures; blind loops, including long afferent loop of a
　　　gastrojejunostomy)
　　Small bowel contamination (gastrocolic or jejunocolic fistula)
Inadequate mixing of food, bile, and pancreatic enzymes, eg, with gastrojejunostomy

Failure of absorption (mucosal phase)
Inadequate absorptive surface (intestinal resection, intestinal bypass for obesity, inadvertent gastroileostomy)
Damaged absorbing surface (celiac disease, tropical sprue, giardiasis, *Cryptosporidium* sp, *Microsporidium* sp, AIDS "enteropathy,"
　cancer chemotherapy, radiation therapy)
Biochemical defect without anatomic alteration
　Disaccharidase deficiency (lactase and sucrase deficiencies)
　Transport deficiency
　　Carbohydrate (glucose-galactose malabsorption)
　　Lipid (α-β-lipoproteinemia)
　　Amino acids (cystinuria, Hartnup disease, methionine malabsorption)
　　Vitamin B_{12} malabsorption
Infiltration of intestinal wall (Whipple's disease, lymphoma, amyloidosis, Crohn's disease, *Mycobacterium avium-intracellulare*)

Impaired lymph and blood flow (transit phase)
Developmental abnormality (intestinal lymphangiectasia, Milroy's disease [congenital lymphedema])
Lymphatic obstruction (lymphoma, Whipple's disease, tuberculosis)
Mesenteric vascular insufficiency (rare, if ever)

from the diet, the absorbing cells promptly return to normal. Lymphatic flow of digested and absorbed nutrients in the circulation can be blocked if the lymphatic channels are obstructed by tumor, as with an extensive intra-abdominal lymphoma.

CLINICAL MANIFESTATIONS OF MALABSORPTION

Regardless of the cause of maldigestion or malabsorption, the clinical manifestations result from (1) unabsorbed food substances affecting other intestinal functions, for example, fats and fatty acids producing foul-smelling bulky or watery diarrhea, and (2) secondary deficiencies of specific nutrients that are eaten but not absorbed, for example, osteoporosis secondary to fat-soluble vitamin D and calcium malabsorption.

Diarrhea

Diarrhea is usually a major complaint of patients with malabsorption, but some with mild steatorrhea do not mention any change in their stools. Since the colon's reservoir capacity is intact and there is no rectal disease to cause urgency or tenesmus, the only complaints of patients with celiac disease or pancreatic insufficiency may be several bowel movements per day or even constipation because their stools are so bulky. Because eating can worsen bloating (caused by unabsorbed gas and liquid) and diarrhea, some patients avoid discomfort by eating less.

Unabsorbed fats and fatty acids cause stools to be bulky and voluminous. In addition, particularly after bacterial hydroxylation, fatty acids stimulate colonic fluid secretion, thus increasing the stools' water content and producing diarrhea. If excess bile salts enter the colon because of ileal dysfunction or resection, they further increase fecal water by stimulating colonic fluid secretion. Rancid fats impart a particularly offensive odor to flatus and feces. In patients with disaccharidase deficiencies, unabsorbed carbohydrates act as an osmotic load that interferes with fluid reabsorption in the ileum and colon (Chapter 6.8).

If a patient's description of the stools is inadequate, the physician must inspect the stool.

Weight Loss

Weight loss and weakness are often the patient's chief complaints. The weight loss is explained in part by loss of calories, especially from fats, but also by the anorexia that accompanies malabsorption in celiac disease and some other conditions. Prolonged, severe malabsorption states like Whipple's disease, intestinal fistulas, and celiac disease can present as advanced malnutrition, and, in women, amenorrhea. Such cachectic patients can be mistakenly thought to have cancer or AIDS.

Edema

Hypoalbuminemia and peripheral edema result from prolonged malabsorption of protein and from loss of serum proteins into the intestinal lumen. Serum proteins are lost when lymphatic or venous flow is blocked, as in intestinal lymphangiectasia, Whipple's disease (see "Whipple's Disease" below), constrictive pericarditis (Chapter 1.10), or portal hypertension (Chapter 7.5). Excessive protein is also lost into the gastrointestinal tract with ulcerating mucosal diseases like gastric cancer, ulcerative colitis, and Crohn's disease (Chapter 6.10); with gastric hyperplasia, as in Ménétrier's disease (giant hypertrophic gastritis); and with colonic neoplasia, as in a villous adenoma.

Bone Demineralization and Tetany

Osteoporosis and osteomalacia can be presenting features of celiac disease, postgastrectomy steatorrhea, and chronic obstructive jaundice. Patients have bone pain and pathologic fractures secondary to malabsorption of dietary calcium, albumin, and vitamin D (which is fat-soluble). Secondary hyperparathyroidism can complicate chronic hypocalcemia, further depleting the bone matrix. A few patients with prolonged malabsorption of vitamin D, calcium, and magnesium develop tetany (carpopedal spasm, muscle twitches, cramps, and convulsions). These patients are likely to have Trousseau's sign (putting pressure on a nerve causing spasmodic contractions in its accompanying muscle) and Chvostek's sign (tapping the facial nerve near the parotid gland causing spasm of the facial muscles).

Bleeding

Patients with malabsorption of fat-soluble vitamin K and resultant hypoprothrombinemia may have a bleeding diathesis, usually manifested by ecchymoses but occasionally by melena or hematuria. Parenteral vitamin K corrects a prothrombin deficiency caused by malabsorption. Patients with any form of malabsorption should have their prothrombin time checked before dental work or elective surgery.

Anemia

In patients with malabsorption, anemia may be caused by impaired absorption of iron, folic acid, or vitamin B_{12}, singly or in combination.

Kidney Stones

Many patients with malabsorption or diarrhea of any cause have concentrated urine, which contributes to a greater-than-expected incidence of kidney stones in patients with steatorrhea. In addition, patients with malabsorption tend to have hyperoxaluria because their colon absorbs an unusually high proportion of dietary oxalate. Normally, most dietary oxalates are precipitated in the lumen as calcium oxalate, but patients with steatorrhea form calcium soaps, leaving oxalate in solution to be absorbed by the intact colon. This problem is most prominent in the patient with ileal disease, such as Crohn's disease or ileal resection, whose colon is still functioning. Patients with oxalate stones are managed by lowering dietary oxalate intake and reducing steatorrhea so that less calcium is bound to fat.

Other Manifestations

Patients with malabsorption may also have peripheral neuropathy, presumably a result of vitamin deficiency; night blindness, caused by a lack of vitamin A; and nocturia, caused by delayed absorption of water.

Milk (lactose) intolerance (see "Lactase Deficiency and Milk Intolerance" below) is characterized by bloating, flatulence, and cramps. Some patients also develop watery, frothy diarrhea after consuming 1–2 glasses of milk, especially on an empty stomach. Lactose intolerance is caused by lactase deficiency, which is either inherited or the result of small bowel mucosal damage, as from celiac disease or tropical sprue.

Historical Clues to Malabsorption

Other items in a patient's history that should alert the physician to the possibility of malabsorption include: AIDS or risk factors for HIV infection, since the low helper T4 cell count increases susceptibility to small bowel bacterial and parasitic infestations; chronic cholestatic liver disease, which interferes with bile flow; chronic alcoholism or recurrent upper or midabdominal pain, which suggests recurrent pancreatitis; diabetes (with or without peripheral neuropathy), which suggests pancreatitis or bacterial overgrowth in the small bowel; previous surgery, especially gastrectomy, gastroenterostomy, vagotomy, or intestinal resection; severe peptic ulcer diathesis with watery diarrhea, as with a gastrin-secreting tumor; sudden onset of diarrhea and weight loss after prolonged peptic ulcer activity, resulting from a gastrocolic fistula; a childhood history of diarrhea, anemia, potbelly, or failure to thrive, as with celiac disease; previous residence or travel in a tropical area where sprue or giardiasis is endemic; and previously effective antibiotic therapy, especially broad-spectrum antibiotics, as for Whipple's disease, multiple jejunal diverticula, or any cause of stasis and bacterial overgrowth in the small bowel.

DIAGNOSIS OF MALABSORPTION

Symptoms, stool appearance, evidence of secondary deficiencies, or an abnormal small bowel x-ray should make the physician suspect malabsorption, but the diagnosis must be confirmed with laboratory tests (Figure 6.9–1). The usual first step is proving fat malabsorption; then come tests to distinguish maldigestion from malabsorption. Having determined the pathophysiologic alteration, the clinician establishes a specific diagnosis and, whenever possible, starts specific therapy.

Radiographic Examination of the Small Bowel

An abnormal small bowel pattern discovered on x-ray of the upper gastrointestinal tract may be the first clue that malabsorption is the basis for the patient's symptoms. A small bowel barium x-ray series may suggest which category of disorders is the most likely cause. For example, dilated small bowel loops are common in both celiac disease (Figure 6.9–2) and scleroderma (Chapter 3.10), but

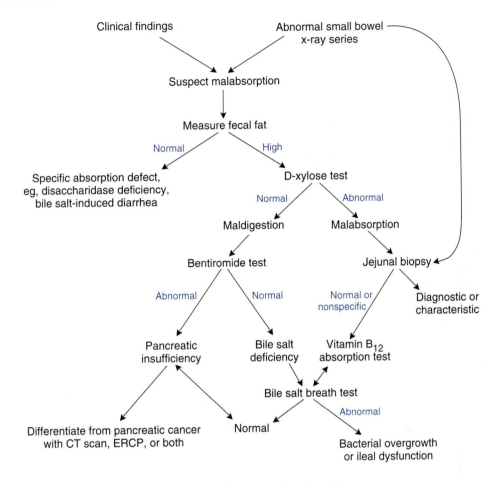

Figure 6.9–1. Evaluation of malabsorption.

additional esophageal and duodenal dilatation favor scleroderma. Nodular thickened mucosal folds are common in infiltrative disorders like Whipple's disease, amyloidosis, intestinal lymphoma, granulomatous diseases, and *Mycobacterium avium-intracellulare* infection.

A normal small bowel series in a patient with proven steatorrhea suggests but does not prove pancreatic insufficiency or some other cause of intraluminal maldigestion. An astute observer may notice pancreatic calcification on plain abdominal films or computed tomography (CT), reflecting chronic relapsing pancreatitis that underlies maldigestion. Pancreatic atrophy or lipoid replacement on CT, or an abnormal endoscopic retrograde pancreatogram, also points toward pancreas-related maldigestion.

Proving Malabsorption

Since dietary fat is one of the most difficult materials to digest and absorb, the adequacy of fat absorption is used as a marker of normal or abnormal intestinal absorption. Microscopic examination for stool fat is an easy, fast, convenient in-office test for steatorrhea. In many patients, this test can also distinguish pancreatic insufficiency from other causes of steatorrhea: Neutral fats, indicating pan-

creatic steatorrhea, are detected by Sudan III-stained fat globules that appear when a stool sample is warmed on a microscope slide. Split fats, indicating nonpancreatic steatorrhea, can be detected only when the stool sample is acidified with acetic acid. False-negatives can occur when the patient has watery diarrhea or has recently had a barium x-ray study. False-positives can occur after a patient eats poorly absorbed fats like mineral oil.

For an accurate assessment of fat absorption or of the success of a therapeutic trial, all stools are collected for 3 days and the average daily fecal fat excretion is determined. The patient should eat a normal amount of fat (70–120 g/day) before and during the collection period. On this intake, normal fecal fat is less than 6 g per day.

Less commonly used and more elaborate tests of fat absorption include measurements of radioactive tracer in the breath, serum, or stool after the patient ingests ^{14}C-labeled fat.

A helpful screening test of fat absorption is measurement of blood levels of fat-soluble materials like carotene. About 90% of patients with steatorrhea have subnormal carotene levels. A low level of serum carotene does not prove malabsorption, because low levels are also found in

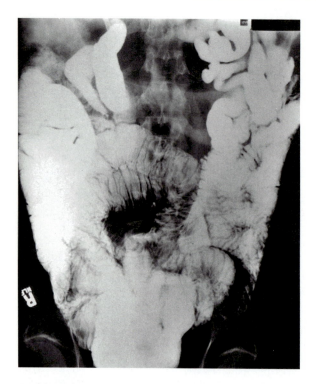

Figure 6.9–2. Celiac disease. Characteristic x-ray from small bowel series shows that the normal pattern of folds is reversed: Folds in the jejunum are effaced ("moulage" or "toothpaste" appearance), while folds in the ileum resemble those usually seen in the jejunum. The ileum is dilated. (Courtesy of Bronwyn Jones, MD.)

mal liver and kidney function and no delay in gastric emptying, urinary excretion of D-xylose is an adequate clinical measure of the absorbing capacity of the upper part of the small intestine.

A normal person who takes 25 g of D-xylose has a 5-hour urinary excretion exceeding 4.5 g. Urinary excretion and blood levels are low in more than 90% of patients with malabsorption caused by diffuse mucosal disease of the duodenum and jejunum, such as celiac disease or tropical sprue. In contrast, levels are normal in 95% of patients whose defect is in intraluminal digestion, as in chronic pancreatitis with pancreatic insufficiency. Urinary excretion of D-xylose may be decreased in patients with stasis of the small bowel contents and subsequent bacterial overgrowth, because the excessive intraluminal bacteria metabolize the D-xylose before it can be absorbed.

As previously mentioned (see "Radiographic Examination of the Small Bowel" above), a small bowel series may suggest a mucosal malabsorptive disease such as celiac disease (see Figure 6.9–2) or a maldigestive disorder such as chronic pancreatitis. In the latter category, a finding of multiple jejunal diverticula may explain bacterial overgrowth, bile salt deconjugation, and maldigestion.

Establishing a Specific Diagnosis

Pancreatic Insufficiency: Bentiromide Test: Bentiromide (NBT-PABA; N-benzoyl-L-tyrosyl-p-aminobenzoic acid), a synthetic tripeptide when taken orally, is specifically cleaved by the pancreatic enzyme chymotrypsin. The released p-aminobenzoic acid (PABA) is quickly absorbed from the small intestine, conjugated by the liver, and excreted in the urine. The amount of PABA recovered in the urine reflects the amount and activity of pancreatic chymotrypsin in the intestinal lumen, and so provides a measure of pancreatic exocrine function. An oral dose of 500 mg and a 6-hour urine collection provide optimal sensitivity.

The bentiromide test is 60–90% sensitive and up to 60% specific. It is most sensitive in patients with severe pancreatic insufficiency. The test is simple, noninvasive, inexpensive, and widely available. Results compare favorably with older tests of pancreatic exocrine function—the Lundh test, which was based on the duodenal trypsin concentration after a test meal, and the secretin stimulation test of duodenal bicarbonate concentration—both of which have fallen from clinical use.

Disturbed Bile Acid Metabolism: Bile Acid Breath Test: The second intraluminal step in lipid assimilation is micellar solubilization. If the intestinal concentration of conjugated bile acids is below the critical micellar concentration (2–3 mmol/L), lipids are not solubilized and diffusion to the absorbing surface is severely limited.

The bile salt breath test is a way to assess the role of interrupted enterohepatic circulation of bile salts in the pathogenesis of steatorrhea. Patients are given oral glycocholate with the glycine moiety labeled with ^{14}C, and then $^{14}CO_2$ is measured in expired air. If the enterohepatic cir-

patients who do not eat enough carotene-containing foods (vegetables). Levels may be normal in patients with pancreatic insufficiency who have a good appetite and eat large amounts of fat, absorbing enough to maintain normal carotene levels. Also suggesting malabsorption can be subnormal blood levels of other fat-soluble substances, like vitamin A, cholesterol, and vitamin K (as measured by prothrombin time), as well as low serum levels of calcium, phosphorus, albumin, iron, folic acid, and vitamin B_{12}.

Distinguishing Maldigestion From Malabsorption: D-Xylose Test and Small Bowel X-Rays

Maldigestion can be differentiated from malabsorption by testing the intestine's ability to absorb a substance that does not require preliminary digestion. The clinician can measure the amount of a quickly absorbed oral test substance that appears in the blood or urine. If a patient with generalized malabsorption has a normal level of the test material, the cause is likely maldigestion. A low level points toward a mucosal absorptive defect.

The pentose D-xylose is used most often as the test material because it does not require digestion before absorption and because a large portion of the absorbed sugar is excreted unmetabolized in the urine. If the patient has nor-

culation is intact, less than 5% of the bile salt escapes reabsorption and enters the colon. There, bacteria remove the glycine and convert it to labeled CO_2, which is absorbed and then excreted in the breath. However, labeled CO_2 is also released if the labeled bile acid is exposed to colonic bacteria that have overgrown the small bowel, as in patients with scleroderma or multiple jejunal diverticula. Therefore, if a patient has ileal dysfunction or bacterial overgrowth in the small intestine, the increased deconjugation of glycocholate is manifested by higher $^{14}CO_2$ concentrations in the breath. To detect bacterial overgrowth, some laboratories do the ^{14}C-xylose breath test or measure elevation of fasting breath hydrogen levels by a gas chromatogram.

Diagnosis of Mucosal Disease: Peroral Small Bowel Biopsy:

The late 1950's brought a major advance in diagnosing causes of malabsorption: the development of peroral techniques to obtain superficial biopsies of the small intestinal mucosa (stopping at the submucosa) with a spring-loaded biopsy capsule. The procedures, which are well tolerated, do not cause perforations. Most gastroenterologists now obtain small bowel biopsies through an endoscope with small biopsy forceps.

A distal duodenal or jejunal biopsy has pathognomonic histologic features in a number of treatable disorders, including Whipple's disease, giardiasis, and *M avium-intracellulare* (Table 6.9–2). Diagnostic abnormalities may be missed in conditions like intestinal lymphoma, amyloidosis, and Crohn's disease, because the lesion does not involve the intestine uniformly.

Although not diagnostic, the small bowel biopsy findings in celiac disease are characteristic: a flattened mucosa and chronic inflammation with damage to the absorbing epithelial surface (Figure 6.9–3). In temperate regions, more than 90% of patients with these features respond to a gluten-free diet, confirming celiac disease.

A normal jejunal biopsy in a patient with steatorrhea

Table 6.9–2. Interpretation of jejunal biopsies.

Diagnostic findings
  Whipple's disease
  Giardiasis
  Mycobacterium avium-intracellulare
  Amyloidosis
  α-β-lipoproteinemia
  Lymphoma
  Coccidiosis
  Mast cell disease
  Lymphangiectasia
  Macroglobulinemia

Characteristic findings
  Celiac disease
  Tropical sprue
  Eosinophilic gastroenteritis
  Dermatitis herpetiformis
  Dysglobulinemia

Nonspecific abnormalities
  Crohn's disease
  Bacterial overgrowth

Normal
  Pancreatic insufficiency
  Bacterial overgrowth
  Bile salt deficiency

rules out celiac disease, and, if the small bowel x-ray is normal, often implicates one of the intraluminal steps such as pancreatic lipid digestion or micelle formation by conjugated bile acids.

Therapeutic Trial

The development of specific therapies for many of the diseases causing malabsorption has increased the importance of making a definitive diagnosis. The therapeutic trial, such as a gluten-free diet for celiac disease, pancreatic enzyme replacement for pancreatic insufficiency, or tetracycline for bacterial overgrowth, is used to confirm the specific cause of malabsorption and should be the culmination of a logical, step-by-step diagnostic process.

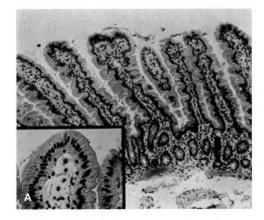 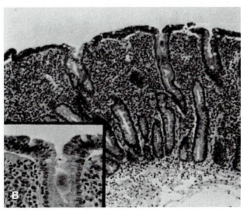

Figure 6.9–3. Jejunal biopsies. **A:** Normal. The villi are long and slender, covered by tall columnar epithelium (inset). **B:** Celiac disease. No villi are recognizable, and there is apparent lengthening of the crypts of Lieberkühn. The lamina propria is infiltrated with plasma cells and lymphocytes. The surface epithelium is flattened and infiltrated with lymphocytes, but the crypt epithelium is normal (inset).

SPECIFIC DISORDERS CAUSING INTESTINAL MALABSORPTION

Maldigestion (Intraluminal Defects)

Pancreatic Insufficiency: The most common cause of pancreatic insufficiency is chronic relapsing pancreatitis. However, in 10% of patients, pancreatic insufficiency appears insidiously without clinically recognizable pancreatitis. This form has been called "silent pancreatitis" or "idiopathic pancreatic atrophy." In occasional older patients, an exaggeration of the aging process causes lipomatous replacement of the pancreas; CT shows an empty gland around a normal pancreatic duct. In still other patients, pancreatic insufficiency is one of the presenting manifestations of carcinoma of the pancreas. In children and young adults, the most common cause of pancreatic insufficiency is cystic fibrosis, so a sweat test should be performed early in the evaluation.

Clinical manifestations: The main clinical manifestations of exocrine pancreatic insufficiency are steatorrhea, abdominal bloating, and weight loss. Since some patients maintain an excellent appetite and a high fat intake, the amount of steatorrhea can be massive: over 80 g of fat excreted per day (normal is less than 6 g). The cachexia and low serum carotene that might be expected with this degree of steatorrhea are not found in most patients with pancreatic insufficiency. The lack of such features helps distinguish these people from patients with more debilitating malabsorptive disorders like celiac disease and Whipple's disease.

Diagnosis: Figure 6.9–1 outlines the ways to determine whether maldigestion is caused by pancreatic insufficiency. Pancreatic calcifications can be seen on plain abdominal x-ray in 40–50% of patients with severe pancreatic steatorrhea. Given that over 90% of pancreatic exocrine function must be lost before steatorrhea appears, it is not surprising that 25% of patients with pancreatic insufficiency are diabetic and another 60% have an abnormal glucose tolerance test, indicating endocrine insufficiency and diabetes. CT or magnetic resonance imaging (MRI) is the best way to delineate pancreas size, shape, neoplasms, and pseudocysts. Sonography is an inexpensive and noninvasive method for following pseudocyst size. Endoscopic retrograde cholangiopancreatography (ERCP) is an invasive but reliable test of pancreatic duct anatomy; the procedure carries a small risk of causing pancreatitis. Percutaneous pancreatic biopsy, guided by CT or sonography, may help explain the nature of a pancreatic mass or duct obstruction. A therapeutic trial with pancreatic enzyme replacement is also useful for diagnosis but does not establish the cause of the pancreatic insufficiency. Adequate pancreatic enzyme replacement reduces but rarely eliminates steatorrhea.

Management: Management of pancreatic exocrine insufficiency requires adequate replacement of the deficient digestive enzymes. Several potent pancreatic enzyme preparations are available. They are best given at least three to six times per day, especially just before meals. Taking an antacid or an H_2 receptor blocker to lessen acid secretion just before taking the pancreatic enzyme may lessen its destruction as it passes through the acid environment of the stomach.

Bile Salt Deficiency (Ileal Insufficiency): Extensive ileal inflammation (particularly Crohn's disease), surgical resection, or bypass of the ileum interrupts the enterohepatic circulation of bile salts and interferes with vitamin B_{12} absorption. With small resections (less than 60 cm), the liver is able to replace most of the bile acids lost, steatorrhea is mild (less than 10 g/day), and diarrhea is caused primarily by bile salts stimulating the colon to secrete fluid. This secretory diarrhea can be controlled with cholestyramine, a resin that binds bile salts.

With larger ileal resections (60–100 cm), the liver cannot synthesize enough bile salts to compensate for those lost into the colon. In patients with a diminished bile salt pool, the bile salt concentration in the upper part of the intestine exceeds the critical micellar concentration only at breakfast. Fat absorption after later meals is greatly impaired. Increased fatty acids passing into the colon also stimulate colonic fluid secretion. Limiting the patient's fat intake controls the diarrhea but can lead to caloric deficiency and weight loss. Patients may be helped if their diet is supplemented by water-soluble medium-chain triglycerides (fatty acid chain length C8–C10), which do not require bile acids for solubilization.

Massive resection of the small bowel, usually necessitated by infarction, presents a major therapeutic challenge. Patients have survived with as little as 6–18 inches of jejunum beyond the ligament of Treitz, especially if the ileocecal sphincter and right colon can be preserved. Some patients whose caloric needs are not met by oral diet alone are helped by long-term parenteral hyperalimentation or a small bowel transplantation.

Bacterial Overgrowth Syndromes: The second major cause of bile salt deficiency is deconjugation of bile acids by colonic bacteria that have overgrown the small bowel. The normal small intestine is sparsely populated with bacteria, in part because the stomach's acidity is lethal to many bacteria, but more important because the motility of the fasting intestine keeps it swept clean. A number of intestinal abnormalities promote stasis of small bowel contents, for example, blind loops, one large or multiple small diverticula, strictures, enteroenteric anastomosis or fistula, gastrocolic fistula, radiation enteritis, and generalized atony of the upper part of the small bowel, as in scleroderma or diabetic visceral neuropathy. All these conditions allow massive proliferation of bacteria to levels exceeding 1 million organisms per milliliter of contents. The bacteria are those of the colonic flora, including large numbers of obligate anaerobes plus facultative anaerobes such as *Escherichia coli* and *Streptococcus faecalis,* all of which are readily capable of deconjugating bile acid and causing steatorrhea. In addition to steatorrhea from bile salt deficiency, the bacterial overgrowth syndromes are characterized by vitamin B_{12} malabsorption because the bacteria consume the vitamin B_{12} before it can reach the absorptive site in the ileum.

Patients with bacterial overgrowth have positive bile salt breath tests. Their D-xylose excretion is low because D-xylose is metabolized by the abnormal intestinal flora and because of spotty nonspecific epithelial damage. Fasting breath hydrogen levels are high because the bacteria metabolize unabsorbed dietary carbohydrates.

Bacterial overgrowth is managed by eliminating the cause of stasis, if possible, or, if not, by giving antibiotics to alter the bacterial flora. Response to treatment depends on the extent, location, and severity of the abnormality as well as the types of bacteria present, their sensitivity to antibiotics, and the extent of the bile salt deconjugation. The most useful antibiotics are metronidazole, tetracycline, and ampicillin.

Malabsorption (Mucosal Defects)

Celiac Disease: Celiac disease (gluten-induced enteropathy) is a chronic, probably hereditary illness in which immunologically mediated inflammation of the proximal small intestine causes malabsorption in both children and adults. More than 90% of patients have HLA haplotypes DR3 and DQW2. The mucosa cannot absorb the products of normal digestion because of damage by the digestion products of gluten, a protein contained in grains (especially wheat and rye) but not corn or rice. Patients who avoid eating foods derived from these grains (a gluten-free diet) enjoy a complete remission, including improvement in the jejunal lesion. Reintroducing gluten causes a relapse and a worsening of the jejunal mucosa.

The characteristic mucosal lesion of celiac disease (see Figure 6.9–3 and "Diagnosis of Mucosal Disease" above) is caused by intraepithelial T-lymphocyte–mediated damage to the epithelial cells that absorb gluten peptides. IgA antibodies to the polypeptide gliadin seem to play a role in the immune process, and most patients have circulating IgA antigliadin antibodies. Accelerated loss of cells from the villus crests leads to compensatory crypt hyperplasia. Although no specific defect in gluten hydrolysis has been identified, an interaction has been suggested between gluten peptides and specific HLA class IID antigen recognition sites (HLA-DR3 and DQW2) on absorbing epithelial cells. This interaction might render the cells subject to immune attack, which in turn might present more gliadin to the cells and increase the intraepithelial lymphocytes' immune response. It has been suggested that the immune interaction is mediated by a previous viral infection with human adenovirus type 12.

Celiac disease has been recognized chiefly in temperate climates. The highest prevalence is in Ireland. At one time, the incidence in County Galway, where almost 80% of the population has HLA types DR3 and DQW2 (in contrast to 20% in the United States), was 1 in 500 live births. The incidence is decreasing, presumably because of more breast feeding and later introduction of gluten-containing foods into the diet. Autosomal dominant inheritance with incomplete penetration has been suggested. Relatives of patients have a 10% incidence of celiac disease. Female patients outnumber males in most reports. Almost all patients are white, but the disease occasionally affects black people.

Some disease associations may help in the search for the susceptibility genes for celiac disease. At least 50% of patients have diabetes mellitus or a close relative with diabetes. Patients with dermatitis herpetiformis, a blistering skin condition, have IgA antigliadin antibodies in their skin and circulation. Although these patients do not have clinical malabsorption, intestinal biopsy shows a high incidence of a celiac-like lesion that heals when gluten is removed from the diet. Since patients with typical celiac disease do not have an increased incidence of dermatitis herpetiformis, the IgA-mediated gluten-induced bowel lesion in dermatitis herpetiformis may be caused by a defect at a different step in gluten handling from that of the celiac lesion. The two disorders also have differences in HLA haplotype patterns.

Clinical manifestations: Fifty percent of patients with celiac disease develop their first symptoms and signs during childhood, as early as 8–12 months of age. The other 50% appear to have their onset between the 20's and 50's; it is not known whether these patients have had the gut lesion since childhood.

The major clinical features in children are diarrhea, weight loss, failure to thrive, muscle wasting, potbelly, and anemia. Although the disease may remit spontaneously around age 5, affected children have occasional diarrhea, an abnormal jejunal mucosa, malabsorption, and some delay in growth and body development. Some patients remain in apparent remission, but others have a return of symptoms in their late 20's or 30's.

Patients with adult-onset celiac disease present with light-colored bulky stools, abdominal bloating, weight loss, weakness, easy fatigability, and perhaps vitamin and mineral deficiencies (see "Clinical Manifestations of Malabsorption" above). These patients have the same jejunal biopsy lesion and excellent response to a gluten-free diet as those with childhood onset. However, before these patients develop specific deficiencies, at a time when their only symptoms are nonspecific bloating, flatulence, and chronic fatigue, at least 25% of them are mistakenly thought to have functional bowel disease. About 50% of adult-onset patients are diagnosed as a result of evaluation for chronic diarrhea and weight loss. Another 25% are diagnosed only when they develop more pronounced effects of malabsorption and specific deficiencies such as iron deficiency, megaloblastic anemia, bleeding tendencies, peripheral edema, or osteoporosis. Most patients with celiac disease also have milk intolerance because lactase levels are decreased in the damaged jejunal epithelium.

As for long-term prognosis, about 10% of patients with celiac disease suffer potentially fatal complications, usually starting during their 60's. Older patients reportedly have an increased incidence of T-cell lymphomas and adenocarcinomas of the small intestine. Adhering to a gluten-free diet may lessen the risk of lymphoma. Unexplained intestinal ulceration and perforation can also be life-threatening.

Diagnosis: Most patients with celiac disease have steatorrhea, low serum carotene levels, low D-xylose absorption, and an abnormal small bowel x-ray (see Figure 6.9–2 and "Diagnosis of Mucosal Disease" above). The diagnosis is verified by a flattened mucosa on small bowel biopsy (see Figure 6.9–3) and by later clinical and histologic improvement with a gluten-free diet. Serum IgG antigliadin antibodies are about 90% specific and 80% sensitive for celiac disease and can be used as a screening test. Another screening test can be IgA class antiendomysial antibodies, resulting from increased gut permeability to dietary antigens.

Perhaps 5% of patients with malabsorption and a flattened intestinal mucosa do not respond (or stop responding) to a gluten-free diet. Possible explanations for this unresponsiveness include (1) lack of strict adherence to the gluten-free diet; (2) rarely, sensitivity to other dietary antigens, such as eggs; (3) a concurrent disorder such as tropical sprue, which responds to antibiotics, folic acid, and vitamin B_{12}; or (4) complication by multiple small bowel ulcerations, small bowel adenocarcinoma, or lymphoma. Some patients with seemingly unresponsive celiac disease require adrenocorticosteroids or other anti-inflammatory or immunosuppressive drugs to suppress the small bowel inflammation.

Management: Adults and children with celiac disease improve quickly on a diet free of wheat, rye, oats, and barley gluten. Improvement is clinical, biochemical, and histologic. Symptoms usually decrease within the first week, and most patients are in remission within 2 months. Patients gain weight promptly, an average of over 20 pounds in the first 2 months. Absorption of all food substances improves quickly, and secondary deficiencies usually correct themselves without specific replacement. The surface epithelium of the jejunum recovers very quickly, reaching its normal height in 7–10 days. Later, the villous pattern improves, and, if patients continue to follow their diet, after 1 year or more the mucosa looks almost normal. Minor dietary indiscretions may be tolerated without producing symptoms, but if patients continue to eat gluten, mucosal damage and malabsorption reappear. Adrenocorticosteroids improve the surface epithelium despite continued gluten ingestion, but the remission obtained is usually incomplete.

AIDS Enteropathy: Many patients with HIV infection or AIDS have absorptive defects resulting from mucosal disease of the upper small bowel. The usual causes are parasitic, bacterial, or viral infestations or infections, but in some patients, "enteropathy" may be a direct effect of HIV. Small bowel x-rays in patients with *M avium-intracellulare* infection can reveal large folds suggesting Whipple's disease. Stool smears or immunologic studies

can help identify *M avium-intracellulare, Giardia lamblia, Cryptosporidium* sp, and *Microsporidium* sp. In at least 25% of patients, small bowel biopsies uncover infectious pathogens or lead to a designation of "AIDS enteropathy." Of patients who are not helped by specific antibiotics, one-third have their secretory diarrhea controlled by octreotide acetate (somatostatin).

Tumors of the gastrointestinal tract, particularly Kaposi's sarcoma and lymphomas, are also especially common in HIV-positive populations.

Lymphatic Obstruction Causing Mucosal Transit Defects

Whipple's Disease: Whipple's disease, a long unexplained and once usually fatal multisystem illness, is now known to be caused by systemic infection with the recently recognized bacterium *Tropheryma whippelii*. The mucosal changes caused by this unusual infection can be readily diagnosed by small bowel mucosal biopsy and are found in more than 95% of patients. Even before the pathogen was identified, the infection was known to be curable with chronic antibiotics that penetrate the blood-brain barrier.

Clinical manifestations: Whipple's disease most often affects white men, whose average age at diagnosis is 43. The organism is commonly found in soil, and the prevalence of disease is especially high among farmers and others who work with soil. About 60% of patients have migratory arthritis or arthralgias affecting large joints, usually without deformity. The arthritis, which may be part of a generalized polyserositis, precedes the onset of diarrhea and steatorrhea. Other prodromal manifestations can include pleuritis, low-grade fever, abdominal swelling, uveitis, ascites, and central nervous system disorders.

The effects of malabsorption often dominate the picture when untreated disease enters a progressive phase. Weight loss, emaciation, and asthenia can be severe. Fifty percent of patients have lymphadenopathy, either local or generalized; 30% have chronic cough, and 25% have fever. Uveitis, ocular palsies, dementia, and other central nervous system manifestations are occasionally either the presenting symptoms or the major symptoms of relapse after antibiotic therapy. Fifty percent of patients have skin pigmentation, usually sparing the buccal membranes. The combination of this pigmentation with chronic illness, weakness, hypotension, and diarrhea may lead to an erroneous diagnosis of Addison's disease (adrenal insufficiency).

Small bowel x-rays often show marked coarsening of the mucosal folds, especially in the jejunum. These findings resemble those of *M avium-intracellulare* in patients with AIDS.

Diagnosis: Whipple's disease is most readily and conclusively diagnosed by intestinal biopsy, even though the characteristic periodic acid-Schiff (PAS)-positive macrophages are found in many tissues, including lymph nodes, brain, and heart. The lamina propria is infiltrated with these PAS-positive granule-laden macrophages. Malabsorption results in part from the macrophages blocking the lamina propria and the lymphatic channels.

The material in the PAS-positive granules is derived from both ingested "bacillary bodies" and *T whippelii*, both of which gradually disappear after successful antibiotic treatment. Eventually, an immunologic test for the organism is expected.

Management: Because central nervous system relapse is resistant to antibiotic therapy, Whipple's disease should be treated aggressively with 2 weeks of high-dose intramuscular penicillin and streptomycin, followed by maintenance therapy with a broad-spectrum antibiotic (eg, trimethoprim-sulfamethoxazole) that crosses the blood-brain barrier.

Carbohydrate Malabsorption: Incompletely absorbed carbohydrates such as lactose (from low intestinal lactase levels), sucrose (from low sucrase-isomaltase levels), fructose (limited absorptive capacity), and sorbitol (nonabsorbable) act as solutes, creating an osmotic gradient-induced diarrhea that is discussed in Chapters 6.7 and 6.8. These poorly absorbed carbohydrates are fermented by colonic bacteria and cause bloating, flatulence, and abdominal cramping. (Hydrogen and CO_2 produced from the fermentation of unabsorbed carbohydrates can be measured in the breath, as tests for carbohydrate malabsorption.) Such annoying though not serious symptoms can be avoided if the patient or clinician recognizes the cause and the patient consumes less of the offending sugar.

Fructose, now the major sweetener in soft drinks, is not well absorbed in large amounts. Excess fructose should be considered in patients with diarrhea, bloating, and flatulence who consume apple juice, grapes, honey, or soft drinks. Similarly, sorbitol, the poorly absorbed carbohydrate used in dietetic chewing gum and mints, may cause bloating or a laxative effect.

Lactase Deficiency and Milk Intolerance: Some otherwise healthy adults experience gastrointestinal symptoms after drinking milk, although they drank milk without difficulty as children. About 1–4 hours after consuming 1 or 2 glassfuls on an empty stomach, these patients have abdominal bloating, cramps, and even diarrhea. However, they may be able to tolerate small amounts of milk, as used in cooking or with cereal or coffee, or if they take the lactose-containing product with a meal.

Milk intolerance is caused by abnormally low levels of lactase, the brush-border enzyme that normally hydrolyzes lactose into its absorbable subunits, glucose and galactose. Genetically determined post–RNA-translational lactase deficiency is found in 2–8% of adults of Scandinavian or Western European extraction, but in 70–100% in adult Native Americans, American blacks, African Bantus, Japanese, Thais, Filipinos, and Ashkenazic Jews. Most of these lactose-intolerant people recognize the problem and drink little or no milk, although they can consume milk in a fermented form, such as cheese or yogurt, without symptoms. Well-meaning providers of milk as part of food relief programs can cause symptoms in the people they are trying to help.

In addition to genetically determined postweaning lactase deficiency, any patient with a disease that produces diffuse mucosal damage, such as celiac disease or tropical sprue may acquire clinically significant lactase deficiency that is reversible if the mucosal lesion heals. Finally, rare infants are born with congenital lactase deficiency.

Lactase deficiency is treated by decreasing intake of milk and ice cream to amounts that do not cause symptoms, by using fermented dairy products, and by adding a source of lactase to hydrolyze the lactose in milk before it is drunk. Yogurt, lactose-hydrolyzed milk, and lactase pills are commercially available.

SUMMARY

▶ Malabsorption of nutrients should be suspected in patients with unexplained weight loss and diarrhea, steatorrhea, and secondary vitamin and mineral deficiencies.

▶ The site of the alteration in either intraluminal digestion or mucosal absorption can be determined by a stepwise series of diagnostic tests. A specific cause can usually be established.

▶ A specific diagnosis often permits specific therapy, such as a gluten-free diet for celiac disease, antibiotics for Whipple's disease, pancreatic extract for pancreatic exocrine insufficiency, and lactose-restricted diet or lactose-hydrolyzed milk for otherwise healthy people who are lactose-intolerant.

SUGGESTED READING

Brasitus TA, Sitrin MD: Intestinal malabsorption syndromes. Annu Rev Med 1990;41:339.

Corrao G et al: Serological screening of coeliac disease: Choosing the optimal procedure according to various prevalence values. Gut 1994;35:771.

Relman DA et al: Identification of the uncultured bacillus of Whipple's disease. N Engl J Med 1992;327:293.

Scrimshaw NS, Murray EB: The acceptability of milk and milk products in populations with a high prevalence of lactose intolerance. Am J Clin Nutr 1988;48(Suppl 4):1079.

Trier JS: Celiac sprue. N Engl J Med 1991;325:1709.

6.10

Inflammatory Bowel Disease

Theodore M. Bayless, MD, and Mary L. Harris, MD

The term "inflammatory bowel disease" encompasses ulcerative colitis and Crohn's disease, two disorders that cause chronic inflammation of the intestinal tract (Table 6.10–1). Although the etiology is unknown, strong genetic influences are suggested by the appearance of both diseases in families and unusually often in Jews. These illnesses usually appear early in life: One-sixth of patients present before age 15, often with severe forms of disease. Genetic influences are more prominent in younger-onset patients than patients who present after age 40. These chronic illnesses, which require expensive medications and often entail hospitalization and surgery, can take a heavy social and economic toll on the average patient, who is 27 years old at the time of diagnosis.

Ulcerative colitis can have three patterns of mucosal inflammation: (1) proctitis and proctosigmoiditis (or distal colitis), (2) left-sided ulcerative colitis, and (3) extensive pancolitis. Patients with inflammation and friability of the rectal mucosa present with rectal bleeding, often mistakenly attributed to hemorrhoids. With more inflammation, the area becomes very sensitive to distention by stool or gas; the patient feels an urgency to defecate and may have 20 or more small-volume bowel movements per day. As more proximal portions of the colon become inflamed, fluid and electrolyte absorption drops, and electrolytes, protein, and blood flow into the colon, causing diarrhea and systemic symptoms.

Crohn's disease can also have several patterns of involvement: jejunoileitis, ileitis, ileocolitis, and colitis. Each subtype of Crohn's disease has its own clinical presentation and typical course. Patients with inflammation of the jejunum and ileum present with cramping abdominal pain after meals and eventually diarrhea. These patients—many of whom are teenagers or young adults—may have prominent extraintestinal manifestations, including arthritis, fever, skin lesions, and delayed growth. Ileitis causes discomfort 1–2 hours after meals; patients lose weight because they voluntarily eat less to avoid discomfort. The inflammation in the ileum can extend transmurally into adjacent structures as tracks or fistulas or can cause perforation or abscesses adjacent to the bowel. This

form of Crohn's disease is known as "fistulizing" or "perforating." It has the worst prognosis of all the forms, often requiring surgical resection every 3 or 4 years. Other patients with ileitis develop intestinal obstruction 8–10 years after the onset of disease because muscle hypertrophy and fibrosis narrow the bowel lumen. This form is known as *stricturing* or *stenosing*. Crohn's disease in the colon causes diarrhea and may be difficult to distinguish from ulcerative colitis.

ETIOLOGY

Several factors influence the expression of both Crohn's disease and ulcerative colitis. Genetic factors are the most obvious yet identified. About 10–15% of patients with Crohn's disease have a family history of Crohn's; another 5–7% have a family history of ulcerative colitis. Among patients with ulcerative colitis, 15% have a family history of ulcerative colitis and 2–3% have a family history of Crohn's. Identical twins have 85% concordance for Crohn's; fraternal twins have the same concordance as patients with a family history. Identical twins with ulcerative colitis have 36% concordance; concordance in fraternal twins is similar to nontwin sibling risk. The fact that children of two Ashkenazic Jews with inflammatory bowel disease have greater than 35% risk of developing it suggests involvement by only a limited number of genes.

The immune system clearly takes part in the response to the initial insult. It has been proposed that instead of responding normally to an offending antigen by activating suppressor T cells, the patient with inflammatory bowel disease mounts an exaggerated helper (T4) lymphocyte response, which then is not physiologically down-regulated. The activated T4 lymphocytes in turn release lymphokines, which activate and recruit monocytes, macrophages, polymorphonuclear leukocytes, and mast cells. These cells amplify the inflammatory response. Evidence that a T4 lymphocyte response is necessary for active Crohn's disease is based in part on anecdotal reports that a few unfortunate patients with Crohn's disease im-

Table 6.10–1. Differential diagnosis of colitis.

	Ulcerative Colitis	Crohn's Disease	Ischemic Colitis
Onset	Gradual or abrupt	Gradual	Abrupt
Symptoms	Rectal bleeding and diarrhea	Diarrhea with little or no bleeding	Sudden pain; rectal bleeding
Perianal inflammation	Occasionally	Common; at times, the presenting symptom	None
Proctoscopic findings	Diffuse inflammation with friability	Normal; or focal, discrete ulcers; or diffuse inflammation	Usually normal
Distribution on x-ray	Starts distally, can extend proximally to involve left half or entire colon	Right side most often involved; often discontinuous and asymmetric	Segmental; splenic flexure often involved
Ileal involvement	Normal or dilated	Sometimes normal, often narrowed	Occasionally involved
Pathologic findings	Diffuse involvement of mucosa	Involvement of mucosa, muscularis, and serosa with deep fissures	Mucosa or transmural
Fistula	None	Common	None

proved clinically as their T4 count fell because of HIV infection. T-cell lymphopheresis has also produced remissions in some patients whose illness did not respond to medication. Antigen-antibody reactions in the joints, skin, and eyes are probably responsible for the arthritis, erythema nodosum, iritis, and other extraintestinal manifestations seen in patients with Crohn's disease or ulcerative colitis.

No specific agent of inflammatory bowel disease has been identified, although attention was focused for a time on *Mycobacterium paratuberculosis,* and more recently (but with even less evidence) on the measles virus. Except for one practice that serves large numbers of possibly interrelated Ashkenazi Jews, there have been few reports of apparent spouse-spouse transmission. Thus, inflammatory bowel disease does not seem to spread like an infection.

CROHN'S DISEASE

The term "Crohn's disease" has replaced older terms including "regional enteritis," "regional" or "terminal ileitis," and "granulomatous colitis." Although the terminal ileum and right colon are the most commonly involved sites, a similar pathologic and clinical disorder can affect any part of the gastrointestinal tract from the mouth to the perianal area. Only one-third of patients with Crohn's disease have granulomatous inflammation. The broad term Crohn's disease does not commit to any one etiology, site, or pathologic response.

Pathology

In one-third of patients, the gross pathologic changes of Crohn's disease are limited to the terminal part of the ileum. About 40% of patients have ileocolitis, which is involvement of the distal ileum and proximal colon. About 5% have ileojejunitis, which is either continuous involvement throughout the small bowel or, more commonly, several sharply demarcated "skip" areas of involved tissue separated by normal bowel; the terminal ileum is often

spared. As much as one-third of young patients with Crohn's disease have subtle microscopic and macroscopic ulceration of the gastric antrum and the duodenum, but the lesions are not often symptomatic.

Up to 20% of patients have involvement limited to the colon. The colonic lesions are often segmental and sometimes spare the rectum; this helps to distinguish them from ulcerative colitis, which always involves the rectum and is continuous rather than segmental. Crohn's disease is also more likely than ulcerative colitis to cause fistulas, benign fibrous strictures, and perianal disease. Despite these differences, in about 10% of patients with chronic inflammatory bowel disease confined to the colon both macroscopically and microscopically, the diagnosis must be classed as "indeterminate." This becomes important when the clinician is considering surgery. Ulcerative colitis can be cured by total colectomy: Disease does not recur in an ileoanal pouch. However, patients with Crohn's disease can have troublesome recurrences in the ileum.

Most patients with Crohn's have focal mucosal inflammation seen microscopically and aphthous ulcers visible macroscopically, both scattered through extensive portions of otherwise normal bowel. The widespread microscopic disease may account in part for the high rate of recurrence (50% at 5–10 years) after surgical resection of all gross disease. With time, the inflammation extends through most layers of the bowel. In contrast, ulcerative colitis usually remains within the mucosa; in only a few patients does fulminant colitis go on to perforate. Noncaseating granulomas (hard tubercles) are found in 30–50% of resected bowel sections from patients with Crohn's disease. These are usually considered diagnostic, since granulomas are unusual in ulcerative colitis.

The pathologic findings in Crohn's correlate with the three distinct courses that the disease can follow. The inflammatory type, which affects 30% of patients, remains localized to the mucosa and submucosa, causing diarrhea plus pain from acute partial obstruction. "Fistulizing" or "perforating" disease affects 20% of patients who have ileitis; aggressive transmural inflammation leads to intra-abdominal fistulas from the diseased bowel wall to another bowel loop or to a nearby organ like the urinary bladder, and some patients suffer free bowel perforation early in the disease.

The third course that Crohn's can follow is stenosing or stricturing disease. About 50% of patients with ileitis follow this route. Early in the course of Crohn's in the small bowel, patients seem to develop muscle hypertrophy, followed by collagen deposition. After about 7–8 years of ileal disease, patients develop a fixed, scarred obstruction that causes painful cramping and requires surgical resection. Most patients go to surgery 8–10 years after the onset of disease or after a previous resection for obstruction. This obstructive process seems to be controlled by inflammatory cytokines that are not inhibited by corticosteroids, anti-inflammatory salicylates, or immunomodulator drugs. In the bowel's effort to decompress the obstructed segment, fistulas can develop through fissures in the thickened bowel wall in the proximal part of a stenotic area, causing secondary fistulas or even perforation.

Theories of Pathogenesis

No unified hypothesis explains the pathogenesis of Crohn's disease and its characteristic inflammatory pattern, which starts as focal inflammatory collections and aphthous ulcers in the mucosa and then becomes transmural. It is not known whether patients with fistulizing disease have a distinct type of Crohn's or whether their cytokine response is simply unable to confine the inflammatory process to the bowel wall. But it is known that after an ileocolonic resection, disease recurs at the neoterminal ileum only when it has contact with the luminal stream and colonic contents—and perhaps the bacteria therein. Conversely, inflammation decreases when the fecal stream is diverted or the bowel is rested with an elemental diet or total parenteral nutrition. It is possible that an infectious agent or antigen from the lumen, perhaps in concert with the intestinal bacterial flora, sets up an inflammatory response in a genetically predisposed host who cannot down-regulate it like a normal person. Also as yet unexplained are the segmental distribution of the inflammatory process, its predilection for the terminal part of the ileum and the right colon, the tendency to recur years after remitting or being resected, and the frequency of perianal disease.

Clinical Manifestations

Crohn's disease usually begins in the teens and 20's. More than 90% of patients have symptoms before age 40. Patients most often present with abdominal cramps, diarrhea, delayed growth (in prepubescent patients), weight loss, fever, anemia, a right lower quadrant abdominal mass (if a complication has developed in the ileal area), or perianal fistulas. Typically, patients with ileitis or ileocolitis have an insidious onset and a long course before they receive a specific diagnosis. The average duration of symptoms before diagnosis and start of therapy used to be

$2^1/_2$ years, but the lag is shortening with better imaging techniques such as sonography and computed tomography (CT), and with a higher index of suspicion for Crohn's disease.

The clinical picture of Crohn's disease depends on which areas of bowel are involved. Patients with ileal involvement may notice a gradual decrease in their sense of well-being, and vague, cramping abdominal pain, often coming 1–2 hours after meals. This discomfort, caused by partial obstruction of the bowel lumen by the inflammatory response, may be localized to the periumbilical area, or, more commonly, to the right lower quadrant. Because of anorexia, nausea, or the fear of abdominal cramps, patients eat less and invariably lose weight. Most patients with small bowel Crohn's disease have an increase in the number of bowel movements, though rarely to more than 5 per day, and their stools become soft and unformed. About 80% of patients with ileal disease have diarrhea.

The intestinal nature of the disease can remain obscure. Patients may have a completely normal physical examination of the right lower quadrant. For months, the only objective evidence of disease may be unexplained low-grade fever, polyarthralgia, iron deficiency anemia, hypoalbuminemia, hemoccult-positive stools, or an elevated erythrocyte sedimentation rate. In a follow-up study of patients originally evaluated for fever of unknown origin, Crohn's disease was the second most common final diagnosis (Chapter 8.2). Children and teenagers who present with fever and arthralgia may be given a misdiagnosis of rheumatic fever or juvenile rheumatoid arthritis. Prepubescent patients may have a slowing of growth 1–2 years before weight gain slows or gastrointestinal symptoms begin. This is because inflammatory mediators impair bone growth and mineralization before the intestinal lesions are extensive enough to cause cramping or diarrhea.

Crohn's disease of the colon is marked by diarrhea, cramps, and occult bleeding. Not all patients have rectal bleeding; by contrast, in ulcerative colitis, bloody diarrhea is part of every flare-up. Gross hemorrhage is rare and represents ulceration over a deep arteriole. Colonic disease may be segmental or diffuse and may involve the rectum. Crohn's proctitis can be difficult to distinguish from ulcerative colitis. In fact, about 5% of patients with apparent distal ulcerative colitis that is unresponsive to the usual anti-inflammatory therapy are later found to have Crohn's proctitis.

Complications

The major complication in the 50% of patients with the stenosing type of Crohn's disease is obstruction. The 20% of patients with fistulizing or perforating Crohn's are most likely to develop fistulas, abscesses, and free perforation. These complications usually require surgery. With perianal disease, fistulas can develop between the rectum and vagina or as painful perianal abscesses. Fulminant colitis, occasionally with toxic megacolon (see "Complications" under "Ulcerative Colitis" below), can complicate the course of Crohn's disease of the colon, especially in young people.

Extensive ileal involvement or lengthy resections impair ileal absorption of bile salts and deplete the bile salt pool, leading to steatorrhea; patients improve on a low-fat diet. After shorter resections (up to 50–60 cm), patients develop watery diarrhea secondary to the laxative effects of the wasted bile salts; the diarrhea may improve with cholestyramine (a bile salt-binding resin) plus antidiarrheal drugs. Patients with Crohn's can develop malabsorption from bacterial overgrowth and interference with the flow of intestinal contents. Patients also have an unusually high frequency of vitamin B_{12} and D deficiencies, gallstones, and oxalate kidney stones caused by hyperoxaluria.

Extraintestinal manifestations appear during active disease, especially in the colon. These features include oral aphthous ulcers, migratory nondeforming arthritis, iritis and episcleritis, and erythema nodosum. Ankylosing spondylitis and sclerosing cholangitis are less common and do not correlate with the degree of activity of the inflammatory bowel disease.

A potential late complication is colon cancer. The risk is as great as that for patients with extensive ulcerative colitis that began in childhood. Some type of colonoscopic surveillance for dysplasia and early colon cancer is essential for patients with extensive colonic Crohn's, especially if the illness started in childhood (see "Complications" under "Ulcerative Colitis" below).

Diagnosis

Crohn's disease is diagnosed by a combination of clinical, radiographic, endoscopic, and pathologic findings. The physician gains confidence in the diagnosis by following the patient's course. Laboratory evidence of inflammation, such as an elevated erythrocyte sedimentation rate or hypoalbuminemia, can support a diagnosis of Crohn's disease, but its absence does not exclude the illness.

The availability of excellent imaging techniques such as barium contrast x-rays and CT should make it unusual for Crohn's to be diagnosed unexpectedly at exploratory laparotomy. A double-contrast barium enema x-ray can show the right colon and the terminal part of the ileum, the areas most often involved in Crohn's. The examiner looks for aphthous ulcers (seen as small filling defects with an opaque center), loss of mucosal detail, cobblestone filling defects, segmental areas of involvement, fistulas, and an asymmetric appearance. The ileal lumen may be narrowed by spasm or scarring, producing the classic "string" sign.

Flexible sigmoidoscopy or colonoscopy with colorectal biopsies can reveal focal inflammation and sometimes granulomas, even when the patient has no gross findings. However, the preparation for colonoscopy or for barium enema x-rays can be risky for acutely ill patients with fulminant colitis. For these patients, flexible sigmoidoscopy and a small bowel series with colon follow-through may

give the clinician enough information to make diagnostic and therapeutic decisions. Small bowel x-rays reveal the proximal extent of disease, skip areas, and stenosis and dilatation indicating partial obstruction. Abdominal CT is the preferred technique for suspected intra-abdominal abscesses.

Other diseases that have the same distribution as Crohn's disease are ileal or ileocecal tuberculosis, yersiniosis, lymphoma, carcinoid tumors, amyloidosis, actinomycosis, histoplasmosis (usually in immunocompromised hosts), carcinoma of the cecum, and amebic involvement of the cecum. Tuberculosis bears special mention. About 50% of patients with intestinal tuberculosis have evidence of pulmonary tuberculosis. The cecum is usually fibrotic and narrowed, and a few patients have typical calcified abdominal nodes. Culture and histologic studies should be done on colonoscopic biopsy specimens and material from fistulas to rule out tuberculosis and actinomycosis. When a positive tuberculin skin test and other clinical features make tuberculosis a possibility, the physician may want to start the patient on antituberculous drugs, especially if corticosteroid or immunomodulator drugs are being considered as treatment for presumed Crohn's disease. Before therapy can begin, a few patients need a laparotomy to distinguish Crohn's disease from tuberculosis or lymphoma.

Management

The aims of treatment should be to suppress active inflammatory disease medically and try to conserve the small bowel. Surgery should be reserved for managing complications (fistulas and abscesses) and for giving a fresh start to patients with obstruction.

Adrenocorticosteroids (eg, prednisone 40–60 mg/day) in combination with other anti-inflammatory drugs (eg, sulfasalazine (see "Management" under "Ulcerative Colitis" below) or delayed-release mesalamine) improve symptoms in over 75% of patients who are treated during the first 4–5 years of uncomplicated disease or during a postresection recurrence. Patients with predominantly ileal involvement are the most responsive. An antibiotic-like metronidazole or tetracycline is added if the involved bowel has deep fissures, fistulas, or evidence of obstruction. The reasons to combine drugs are to reduce corticosteroid side effects and take advantage of the drugs' multiple anti-inflammatory actions.

Symptoms such as fever, anorexia, crampy pain, and abdominal tenderness should abate within the first few days or weeks of treatment. If symptoms do not respond promptly, the physician must suspect obstruction, abscess, or an error in diagnosis. As soon as the patient begins to improve, the corticosteroids are tapered over 2–3 months to a maintenance dose of 20 or 30 mg every other day. Not all authors recommend alternate-day prednisone as maintenance therapy in Crohn's disease, but prepubescent adolescents with ileitis have been shown to grow at a normal rate if their disease activity is controlled with a combination of sulfasalazine and alternate-day prednisone. If prednisone cannot be tapered to alternate days or if the inflammation covers several segments of bowel, immunomodulator therapy (usually azathioprine or 6-mercaptopurine) helps 70% of patients with refractory but uncomplicated disease.

For patients with small bowel Crohn's disease, elemental diets (composed of simple sugars and amino acids that do not require digestion) can give temporary relief while medical therapy is being started. "Bowel rest" with total parenteral nutrition (Chapter 4.10) helps correct many of the nutritional deficits in patients with chronically active Crohn's disease, and suppresses uncomplicated disease in 75% of patients. However, this improvement must be sustained by additional medical therapy such as an immunomodulator; without it, most patients relapse when they resume enteral feeding. Late in the disease, medical treatment may give patients with partial obstruction a several-month reprieve from surgery, but they eventually require resection.

About 40–60% of patients with ileal Crohn's disease need surgery during the first 10 years of symptoms, most often at 8–10 years. Patients require surgery earlier if they develop intra-abdominal abscesses or the rare free perforation. Unfortunately, 50–60% of patients who undergo surgery develop recurrent disease within 10 years. Aggressive transmural disease (abscesses or free perforation) tends to recur soonest. Most abscesses require percutaneous or operative drainage. Physicians usually delay definitive resection of the involved bowel and fistulous tracts until they have controlled the inflammatory reaction and corrected malnutrition; total parenteral nutrition can be helpful. If bowel is resected when the disease is active, the early recurrence rate (within 3–4 years) approaches 50% and complications like sepsis and poor healing can be difficult to manage.

Prognosis

Patients with Crohn's disease today have better chances for long-term survival and an acceptable quality of life. The outlook has been improved by new drug and nutritional therapies, better surgical techniques, better postoperative care, and recognition of the cancer risk. In particular, stricturoplasties are used to prevent the *short bowel syndrome,* a severe malabsorption syndrome resulting from repeated long resections; patients may require long-term home parenteral alimentation or even a small bowel transplantation. Mortality from Crohn's is now not much greater than in the general population, but is generally related to complications—perforation and the short bowel syndrome. Suicide remains a problem, especially among young people with extensive disease, ostomies, or need for long-term hyperalimentation. Although primary psychiatric illness is no more common in patients with inflammatory bowel disease than in the general population, patients are prone to reactive depression and a potential to abuse pain medications; these problems must be sought and treated.

Most patients who are managed with currently standard medical and surgical approaches report a good quality of life, but most patients with severely compromised small intestine function are discontented. Patient support groups and educational materials, such as those supplied by the Crohn's Colitis Foundation of America, help improve overall patient management and satisfaction.

ULCERATIVE COLITIS

Ulcerative colitis invariably involves the mucosa of the rectum, but can also extend to involve the left colon or the entire colon, at which point it is called *pancolitis.* The typical but by no means pathognomonic lesion is the crypt abscess, in which the epithelium of the crypt breaks down and the lumen fills with purulent exudate. The lamina propria is densely infiltrated with polymorphonuclear leukocytes. As crypts are destroyed, the normal mucosal architecture is lost and scarring eventually shortens and narrows the colon.

Theories of Pathogenesis

As with Crohn's disease, the cause of ulcerative colitis is unknown, although genetic and psychosomatic factors may play a role. Different theories for the epithelial destruction in ulcerative colitis have implicated arachidonic acid metabolism, bacterial or immunologic interactions, and, least likely, ischemia followed by generation of free radicals.

Clinical Manifestations

Ulcerative colitis can appear at any age, but it is most likely to begin in early adulthood. The disease may be slightly more common in women than men, but proctitis seems to be increasing in men. About 15% of all patients have a family history of inflammatory bowel disease, and, as with Crohn's disease, the incidence is higher in Jews. Nonsmokers and recent quitters are at statistically increased risk for ulcerative colitis, and, remarkably, nicotine patches have helped some patients with unresponsive ulcerative colitis.

Fifty percent of patients have only proctitis or proctosigmoiditis. Rectal bleeding, with or without diarrhea, is often the first symptom that brings a patient to the doctor. Most patients have small, frequent bowel movements containing pus, blood, and mucus mixed with a little feces. The rectum's threshold for stimulation by fecal contents is lowered, and the patient feels urgency, tenesmus, and cramping. A common complaint is lower abdominal pain that is relieved by defecation. As more of the colon becomes involved in the 50% of patients with left-sided colitis or with pancolitis, the major clinical feature is diarrhea.

Ulcerative colitis is intermittently symptomatic in 70% of patients, continuously active in 15–20%, and rapidly progressive (fulminant) in about 5%. Acute fulminant disease may be the first manifestation of ulcerative colitis or may appear in the course of established disease. Patients with fulminant disease have an almost constant rectal discharge, and rectal bleeding that may be serious enough to require transfusion. They also have fever, hypovolemia, tachycardia, and hypoproteinemia. Potentially lethal complications are toxic megacolon and colonic perforation.

Complications

The complications of ulcerative colitis can be divided into (1) local complications related to colonic disease and (2) systemic and other extracolonic manifestations. Rectal bleeding leads to anemia, which often requires transfusion. In occasional patients, massive or persistent hemorrhage can be controlled only by colectomy.

During acute exacerbations of colitis, patients may have marked dilatation of the colon, with abdominal distention and tenderness. In this situation, known as acute toxic dilatation or toxic megacolon, the colon loses all tone, becomes massively dilated, and may perforate if not treated promptly. In patients with severe active colitis, toxic megacolon can be induced iatrogenically by anticholinergic drugs, opiates, or preparation for barium enema or colonoscopy.

Severe ulcerative colitis can lead to the formation of pseudopolyps, which reflect extensive destruction of the colonic mucosa. They are not premalignant.

As with Crohn's disease, the extracolonic complications of ulcerative colitis generally appear when the colitis is active. About 5% of patients have skin lesions: pustules, erythema multiforme, erythema nodosum, or pyoderma gangrenosum. Arthritis can affect large or small joints, but is especially likely to involve the knees and ankles. Patients with ulcerative colitis also have an unusually high incidence of ankylosing spondylitis; the spine changes may precede colonic disease. Eye complications such as iritis, conjunctivitis, and uveitis usually coincide with colon, skin, or joint activity; they affect 5% of patients with extensive ulcerative colitis or Crohn's colitis.

The most important hepatobiliary complication of ulcerative colitis is sclerosing cholangitis. This usually appears in men after 10–15 years of very mild—even subclinical—pancolitis, and in some patients eventually necessitates liver transplantation. Mild diffuse fatty change is common, but usually without clinical effect. Patients have developed sclerosing cholangitis and bile duct cancer even after total colectomy has eliminated the ulcerative colitis.

Colon cancer not only has an increased incidence in patients with ulcerative colitis, but appears earlier (average age 40) than in the general population (average age 60). Risk factors are (1) involvement of the entire colon; (2) long duration, even if disease is inactive; and (3) onset in childhood. The cancer risk in patients with pancolitis begins 8 years into the course; by the time patients have had pancolitis for 15 years, the cancer incidence may be as high as 10%. Regular follow-up, with rectal and colonoscopic biopsies examined for dysplastic changes, can help identify patients who may develop colon cancer. However, randomly taken colonoscopic biopsies from normal-looking areas may not adequately detect dysplasia, so three to four biopsies should be taken from every 10 cm segment of colon. For patients with pancolitis, surveillance colonoscopy and biopsies should probably be repeated every 1–2 years. In some young patients, the best option may be prophylactic colectomy.

Diagnosis

Ulcerative colitis is a diagnosis of exclusion. Before seriously considering this condition, the physician must rule out the infectious causes of colitis, which include shigella, *Campylobacter,* invasive *Escherichia coli,* salmonella, gonococci, amebae, and antibiotic-associated colitis. In a patient who might have a sexually transmitted disease, the physician should consider proctitis caused by syphilis, gonorrhea, chlamydia, or herpes. Ischemia is in the differential diagnosis of rectal bleeding and of colitis in the elderly (Table 6.10–1), but the most distal rectum, receiving its blood supply from a nonmesenteric source, is usually spared.

No single finding is pathognomonic for idiopathic ulcerative colitis, but the prime test is flexible sigmoidoscopy with mucosal biopsy. In mildly active ulcerative colitis, the rectal mucosa is hyperemic, edematous, granular, and, most characteristically, friable, as manifested by small mucosal bleeding points appearing when the mucosa is rubbed with a cotton swab or the flexible sigmoidoscope. In more severe disease, the mucosa shows a purulent exudate, spontaneous bleeding, and small ulcerations. Because the endoscopic findings are nonspecific, the exudate must be examined microscopically for leukocytes, bacteria, and amebae, and the exudate and stools must be cultured.

Rectal biopsy is useful for supporting a diagnosis of ulcerative colitis and helping to rule out such causes of inflammation as cytomegalovirus and amebiasis. Crohn's disease should be suspected if the rectum is spared or if the biopsy shows focal areas of inflammation (in contrast to the uniform inflammation of ulcerative colitis) or giant cell granulomas. Of note, the hypertonic enemas and irritant laxative suppositories used by some clinics as preparative procedures can cause an acute proctitis that an astute pathologist will recognize.

In acutely ill patients, the extent of disease can be determined by checking a plain abdominal x-ray for a gaseous outline of the transverse colon. More stable patients who can tolerate laxative and enema cleansing of the colon should undergo colonoscopy or an air-contrast barium enema to determine how much of the colon is involved grossly.

Management

The primary goal of treating ulcerative colitis is to decrease acute and chronic inflammation so that the patient can have a complete clinical and endoscopic remission.

The mainstays of medical therapy are anti-inflammatory drugs, especially adrenocorticosteroids and compounds containing 5-aminosalicylic acid (most often sulfasalazine or mesalamine). Various forms of these medications are used both orally and topically (as suppositories and enemas) to reduce rectal and distal colonic inflammation. The 15% of patients whose distal colitis resists the usual therapy may need mesalamine enemas to maintain their remission. Oral prednisone and large doses of sulfasalazine or mesalamine are given for mild-to-moderate left-sided colitis and pancolitis. The 70% of patients who go into remission are kept on sulfasalazine or mesalamine in an effort to stay symptom-free.

About 15–20% of patients with left-sided colitis or pancolitis have a chronic, relatively unresponsive form of the disease. They cannot achieve remission with the usual anti-inflammatory medications, and prednisone side effects often become intolerable. Since colectomy cures this intractable disease, some physicians recommend colectomy for patients who have had to take prednisone daily for months or years.

Perhaps a more acceptable approach for some patients and physicians is to use an immunomodulator, most often azathioprine or 6-mercaptopurine, in an effort to suppress the inflammation at the more basic level of the lymphocyte and its lymphokines. This treatment brings remission to 70% of patients with previously chronic unremitting ulcerative colitis. This is the same success rate that these drugs achieve in chronic unresponsive Crohn's disease. Although there is no evidence that immunomodulator therapy further increases the risk of colon cancer in patients with extensive ulcerative colitis, we tend to urge colectomy, which is curative, for patients with unresponsive colitis of over 8–10 years' duration, rather than starting immunomodulator therapy.

Fulminant ulcerative colitis is a medical-surgical emergency that requires intensive care in the hospital. Initial treatment is directed at correcting the large fluid and electrolyte losses caused by severe diarrhea. Hydrocortisone is given parenterally in an effort to control inflammation. About two-thirds of patients with severe, aggressive colitis who are not responding to bowel rest and intravenous corticosteroids have responded within 1–2 weeks to intravenous cyclosporine, a fungal metabolite with profound inhibitory effects on T lymphocytes. These highly selected patients benefit from brief, tapering treatment with this relatively fast-acting drug, but then require long-term immunomodulator therapy. Unfortunately, after 2 years, two-thirds of these patients still need colectomy. Thus, cyclosporine may delay surgery but cannot obviate it.

Patients with fulminant colitis can suffer a perforation of the colon almost without warning. In patients with ulcerative colitis, mortality rate after perforation is 20%; in contrast, mortality rate with emergency colectomy is below 2%. Toxic megacolon—dilatation of the colon with clinical deterioration—can be a harbinger of impending intestinal perforation. Toxic megacolon can be precipitated by narcotics, anticholinergic medications, and opiate-derived antidiarrheal agents such as loperamide and diphenoxylate with atropine. Megacolon can also be triggered by preparation for or performance of colonoscopy or barium enema. Patients with fulminant colitis must be carefully evaluated by both physicians and surgeons several times a day for signs and symptoms of impending perforation: fever, worsening pain, and continued need for blood transfusions. If patients with severe fulminant colitis do not improve within 48 hours, they should undergo total colectomy with ileostomy.

Surgery cures ulcerative colitis. Elective colectomy has a mortality rate below 1%. The indications for colectomy are (1) unresponsiveness to medical therapy, leaving the patient unable to live a full and active life; (2) growth failure in children; (3) life-threatening complications such as bleeding, toxic megacolon, impending perforation, or chronic malnutrition; (4) severe extracolonic complications such as unresponsive pyoderma gangrenosum, persistent incapacitating arthritis, or progressive eye disease; (5) colonic strictures, which may represent malignancy; and (6) dysplasia or carcinoma.

The procedure should almost always be total colectomy with ileostomy or one of the two internal ileal pouch alternatives. The standard ileostomy, known as the Brooke ileostomy, is a silver dollar-sized ring of ileal mucosa that protrudes from the right lower quadrant of the abdomen. The patient attaches to the mucosa a double-faced adhesive ring and to the ring an emptiable opaque sack that collects the 750–1000 mL of material that the ileum produces each day. Although this is the most reliable surgical technique, it requires the greatest aesthetic adjustment. The burden of self-care for an ileostomy has been lessened by well-fitted appliances and disposable ostomy bags. Many patients also find that ostomy societies can help them adjust to the inconvenience and psychological problems of an ileostomy.

One ileostomy alternative, the Kock pouch (continent) ileostomy, is an internal reservoir made from reshaped ileum. A nickel-sized nipple valve of ileum opens onto the lower abdominal wall, and the patient catheterizes the valve to remove fecal contents. The main disadvantage of the Kock pouch is that for 25–30% of patients, the valve becomes incontinent within 2–5 years and requires surgical repair.

The most popular ileostomy alternative for patients with ulcerative colitis—and for patients with familial adenomatous polyposis, a universally premalignant hereditary condition—is the ileal pouch-anal anastomosis. This operation involves rectal mucosal stripping of all the colitis or polyposis tissue, ileal pull-through, formation of an ileal pouch (usually in a "J" shape), and then ileal-anal anastomosis. After closure of a temporary protective ileostomy, patients can defecate thorough their anus. After 1 year, the average patient has five bowel movements per day. Incontinence is unusual except in patients over age

50, patients with a preexisting anal sphincter defect, and patients with coexisting irritable bowel syndrome. In patients with irritable bowel, the ileal pouch is spastic and causes frequent small and often uncomfortable movements. Despite other complications, including pouchitis in 5% of patients, the ileoanal pouch is an acceptable and successful alternative to a standard ileostomy.

Prognosis

Since the advent of anti-inflammatory drugs, nutritional support, surveillance for dysplasia, and early colectomy for fulminant colitis, survival of patients with ulcerative colitis is similar to that of the general population. Although 90% of patients who have had one attack of ulcerative colitis would, if left untreated, have at least one relapse within 5 years, 70% of patients can be kept in remission by sulfasalazine, mesalamine, or an immunomodulator, usually azathioprine or 6-mercaptopurine. The severity and extent of involvement in the first attack influence both short- and long-term prognosis: The more severe and extensive the disease, the more likely that the patient will eventually need colectomy. Patients with distal colitis are not at increased risk for cancer, nor is colectomy ever needed for intractable disease. About 30% of patients with left-sided colitis or pancolitis eventually undergo colectomy. Because of improved medical control and surgical cure, most patients with ulcerative colitis report a very acceptable quality of life.

SUMMARY

► Crohn's disease and ulcerative colitis are chronic inflammatory bowel diseases that cause abdominal pain, diarrhea, and extra-intestinal manifestations. Both diseases most often appear during adolescence or early adulthood.

► Although the etiology is unknown, the immune system fails to "down-regulate" the inflammatory process. Fortunately, the inflammation is usually amenable to adrenocorticosteroids and 5-aminosalicylate-containing compounds; unresponsive inflammation can usually be suppressed indefinitely with an immunomodulator.

► Colectomy cures ulcerative colitis. Alternatives to ileostomy have made colon removal more acceptable to patients.

► Surgery is used for a "fresh start" in Crohn's disease to remove an obstruction or transmurally extensive process, but more than 50% of patients suffer recurrences after bowel resection.

► Risk of dysplasia (a premalignant condition) and colon cancer is increased in patients with extensive ulcerative colitis or Crohn's disease of long duration, especially if the illness began in childhood. These patients should be followed with colonoscopic biopsies.

SUGGESTED READING

Bayless TM (editor): *Current Management of Inflammatory Bowel Disease.* BC Decker, 1989.

Bayless TM, Harris ML: Prognosis in inflammatory bowel disease. In: Kirsner JB, Shorter RG (editors). *Inflammatory Bowel Disease,* 4th ed. Williams & Wilkins, 1995.

Bayless TM et al: Crohn's disease: Concordance for site and clinical type in affected family members. Potential hereditary influences. Gastroenterology, in press.

Ekbom A et al: The epidemiology of inflammatory bowel disease: A large, population-based study in Sweden. Gastroenterology 1991;100:350.

Podolsky DK: Inflammatory bowel disease. N Engl J Med 1991;325:928, 1008.

Section 7

Liver Disease

John D. Stobo, MD, Section Editor

7.1

Approach to the Patient With Liver Disease

H. Franklin Herlong, MD

Clinical manifestations of liver disease include jaundice, ascites, esophageal variceal hemorrhage, and the mental status changes of hepatic encephalopathy. But serious liver disease may produce only nonspecific constitutional symptoms such as anorexia, fatigue, malaise, weight loss, nausea, or fever. A thin, weak, wasted patient who comes into the emergency room may appear to have cancer or AIDS, when the real problem is liver disease. Nutritional deficits—caused by the anorexia that can accompany liver disease or by patients' drinking alcohol rather than eating nutritious food—can produce more symptoms than does the liver disease itself.

Jaundice, the most specific symptom of liver disease, is caused by impaired clearance of bilirubin in a patient who has a disorder of the bile ducts or liver cells. The differential diagnosis of jaundice is the prototype for evaluating a patient with suspected liver disease (Chapter 7.2). The most common causes of jaundice are viral hepatitis, drug-induced liver disease, and alcoholic liver disease (Chapter 7.3). Although viral hepatitis and drug-induced hepatitis often present acutely, sometimes they begin with nonspecific symptoms or are diagnosed by asymptomatic laboratory abnormalities.

Many liver diseases evolve subtly over months or years or can be detected only through laboratory abnormalities. These disorders include (1) inherited diseases such as α_1-antitrypsin deficiency, hemochromatosis, and Wilson's disease; (2) autoimmune liver diseases such as autoimmune hepatitis, primary biliary cirrhosis, and sclerosing cholangitis, which are most often recognized by elevated aminotransferase or alkaline phosphatase levels, or even by signs of portal hypertension; and (3) the hepatic effects of systemic diseases, such as granulomatous hepatitis, Budd-Chiari syndrome secondary to polycythemia or estrogen-induced hypercoagulability, and hepatic abscess from amebiasis (Chapter 7.4).

Most chronic liver diseases cause scarring in the liver and eventually cirrhosis. The most common manifestations of cirrhosis are often related not to impaired hepatic synthetic function but to alteration in hepatic blood flow, resulting in portal hypertension (Chapter 7.5). The manifestations of portal hypertension, all disabling and some life-threatening, include ascites, esophageal variceal hemorrhage, hepatic encephalopathy, and the hepatorenal syndrome.

EVALUATION OF PATIENTS WITH POSSIBLE LIVER DISEASE

The first step in evaluation is a careful history (Table 7.1–1) . For example, ascites in an intravenous drug user is usually caused by chronic viral hepatitis, whereas ascites in a woman taking oral contraceptives is usually caused by Budd-Chiari syndrome. The problem with some of the common presenting symptoms of liver disease—anorexia, malaise, fatigue, and nausea—is that they are also seen with so many nonhepatic disorders. A more specific clue to liver disease may be some degree of abdominal discomfort, usually caused by distention of the liver capsule; patients tend to describe this as a vague "aching" or "heaviness" in the right upper quadrant. Many patients also complain of abdominal bloating and dyspepsia. A patient who reports the sudden onset of severe right upper quadrant pain radiating to the infrascapular region may have acute obstruction of the cystic duct or common bile duct.

Cholestatic disorders such as primary biliary cirrhosis and sclerosing cholangitis often cause pruritus. It is worst on the soles of the feet and palms of the hands and around pressure areas such as belt or bra lines. The itching is most severe at night and during the summer. Fever is common in patients with acute cholangitis and alcoholic hepatitis, but may not affect those with viral hepatitis. Arthralgias,

Table 7.1–1. Historical clues to liver disease.

Finding	Possible Diagnosis
Family history	Wilson's disease α_1-antitrypsin deficiency Hemochromatosis

Current medications
  Chlorpromazine
  Isoniazid
  Estrogen
	
	Cholestasis
	Hepatitis
	Budd-Chiari syndrome, gallstones

Travel history	Viral hepatitis (especially Africa, Asia) Amebic liver abscess (especially India, Mexico) Echinococcal disease (especially exposure to sheep, goats, dogs in South America, Middle East)
Sexual contacts	Viral hepatitis Syphilitic hepatitis Atypical mycobacterial infection
Alcohol abuse	Alcoholic liver disease
Intravenous drug use	Viral hepatitis Pyogenic abscess

Job history
  Health care worker
  Exposure to environmental toxins
    Beryllium
    Vinyl chloride
	
	Viral hepatitis
	
	Berylliosis
	Angiosarcoma

Exposure to blood or blood products	Viral hepatitis

Pain
  Colic
  Dull ache
  Constant epigastric or back pain
	
	Gallstones
	Viral hepatitis
	Pancreatic carcinoma

Pruritus	Chronic biliary tract obstruction from pancreatic carcinoma Primary biliary cirrhosis
Fever	Cholangitis Alcoholic hepatitis
Chalky (acholic) stools	Biliary tract obstruction from bile duct stricture, pancreatic carcinoma Drug-induced cholestasis

Table 7.1–2. Physical examination of the patient with possible liver disease.

Finding	Possible Diagnosis
Head	
Kayser-Fleischer ring	Wilson's disease
Lacrimal gland enlargement, parotid gland enlargement	Alcoholic cirrhosis
Xanthelasma	Primary biliary cirrhosis, bile duct stricture
Hands	
Clubbing	Cirrhosis
Dupuytren's contracture	Alcoholic cirrhosis
Palmar erythema	Alcoholic cirrhosis
Spider angiomas	Alcoholic cirrhosis
Muehrcke's lines (transverse white-banded nail beds)	Hypoalbuminemia
Azure nail beds	Wilson's disease
Extremities	
Pigmentation	
Permanent "tan"	Cholestasis
Bronze	Hemochromatosis
Excoriations	Pruritus with cholestatic hepatitis
Urticaria	Hepatitis B
Abdomen	
Splenomegaly	Cirrhosis with portal hypertension
Dilated abdominal veins	Cirrhosis with portal hypertension, Budd-Chiari syndrome
Ascites	Cirrhosis with portal hypertension
Hepatic rub	Tumor
General	
Gynecomastia	Alcoholic cirrhosis
Testicular atrophy	Alcoholic cirrhosis
Neurologic	
Asterixis	Hepatic encephalopathy
Hyperreflexia	Hepatic encephalopathy

and rashes such as urticaria, suggest autoimmune liver disease or hepatitis B.

On physical exam, the physician looks for signs of chronic disease, such as weight loss and temporal wasting (Table 7.1–2). Common skin signs of chronic liver disease include jaundice, palmar erythema, and spider angiomas (most often on the face and upper chest). A patient with an altered level of consciousness or a diminished intellect may have hepatic encephalopathy or Wilson's disease. A patient with dilated abdominal veins, with blood flowing away from the umbilicus, has portal-systemic collateral circulation from portal hypertension. A patient who has a protruding abdomen with shifting dullness and a fluid wave has ascites, which may be caused by cirrhosis, cancer, or tuberculous peritonitis. A hard, nodular liver is felt in patients with cirrhosis or liver tumor, whereas a soft, enlarged liver with a smooth, tender edge suggests con-

gestion or fatty infiltration. A hepatic bruit is heard in patients with acute alcoholic hepatitis or hepatocellular carcinoma. A palpably enlarged, nontender gallbladder may indicate pancreatic carcinoma, whereas Murphy's sign (tenderness of the gallbladder, elicited by palpation of the right upper quadrant during deep inspiration) suggests cholelithiasis.

LABORATORY ASSESSMENT

Biochemical and radiologic tests are valuable in detecting liver disease, evaluating the nature and extent of dysfunction, following disease progression, and assessing the effects of therapy. The spectrum of hepatic functions is so broad that no one test is usually sufficient. Proper use of the biochemical tests of hepatic function requires knowledge of the specificity and sensitivity of each test. It is also important to recognize that hepatic dysfunction may be highly selective. For example, reduced ability to synthesize urea is a manifestation of very severe hepatic dysfunction, but bile salts may be cleared abnormally in patients with minimal hepatic injury. All patients with definite or suspected liver disease should have the following determinations:

- Serum bilirubin levels: total and direct-reacting fractions (Chapter 7.2)

- Serum aminotransferase levels: aspartate aminotransferase (AST) and alanine aminotransferase (ALT)

- Serum alkaline phosphatase level; if elevated, 5'-nucleotidase or γ-glutamyl transpeptidase

- Prothrombin time

- Total serum protein with albumin and globulin fractions

Aminotransferase Levels

The aminotransferases are a group of intracellular enzymes found in large quantities in hepatocytes, and released into the blood when these cells are injured. The two principal aminotransferases are aspartate aminotransferase (AST; formerly called SGOT) and alanine aminotransferase (ALT; formerly called SGPT). The highest serum concentrations of the AST and ALT—over 1000 IU/L—are seen in ischemic liver disease, viral hepatitis, and toxic hepatitis caused, for example, by acetaminophen overdose. In patients with obstructive jaundice, the aminotransferases are rarely greater than 10 times normal. Elevation of the aminotransferases for longer than 6 months defines chronic hepatitis. When the aminotransferases have been elevated, a sudden, precipitous drop in a patient who is deteriorating clinically may indicate severe hepatic necrosis with impending liver failure.

The pattern of aminotransferase elevation may also help determine the cause of liver disease. Patients with alcoholic hepatitis have a ratio of AST to ALT greater than 2:1 (normal is 1:1), because the AST is only modestly elevated (less than 300 IU/L) whereas the ALT may be normal. Although ALT is made only in the liver, high concentrations of AST are also made in heart and skeletal muscle. Thus, a high AST does not always signal liver disease: An isolated AST elevation can be seen in alcoholic liver disease but is also characteristic of rhabdomyolysis or acute myocardial infarction.

Serum Alkaline Phosphatase

The serum alkaline phosphatase represents a group of isoenzymes made by liver, bone, intestine, and placenta. In a healthy person, serum levels represent equal contributions from bone and liver. The normal serum level varies with age and sex. During periods of rapid bone growth, normal teenagers have an elevated serum alkaline phosphatase. Serum levels can also exceed the normal range in otherwise healthy elderly people who do not have liver disease. The alkaline phosphatase can be markedly elevated in bone diseases such as Paget's disease, primary hyperparathyroidism, and osteomalacia, as well as in hyperthyroidism.

The alkaline phosphatase is elevated in liver diseases that involve obstruction of the bile ducts, infiltration of the liver (eg, metastatic cancer, granulomatous diseases), or drug-induced cholestasis (eg, phenothiazine). Although the alkaline phosphatase tends to be higher in intrahepatic cholestasis than extrahepatic obstruction, there is considerable overlap. The malignant cells in Hodgkin's disease or renal cell carcinoma can release alkaline phosphatase that raises the patient's serum level even without hepatic involvement. A serum alkaline phosphatase isoenzyme associated with bronchogenic carcinoma has also been described. Isoenzyme analysis can distinguish between bone and liver sources of alkaline phosphatase, but the test is too complex and expensive to use routinely. Instead, patients can be tested with serum 5'-nucleotidase or γ-glutamyl transpeptidase.

Serum 5'-Nucleotidase and γ-Glutamyl Transpeptidase

5'-nucleotidase catalyzes the hydrolysis of nucleotides. This enzyme is found predominantly in the bile canalicular and sinusoidal membranes of the liver; unlike alkaline phosphatase, 5'-nucleotidase is not found in bone. However, both the 5'-nucleotidase and alkaline phosphatase are elevated in the same liver diseases. Thus, measuring the 5'-nucleotidase is most useful in determining whether an elevated serum alkaline phosphatase originates in liver or bone.

γ-glutamyl transpeptidase (GGTP), an enzyme found in kidney, liver, and pancreas, catalyzes the transfer of the γ-glutamyl group of peptides. GGTP elevation is a sensitive indicator of hepatobiliary disease and is elevated in the same liver diseases as the serum alkaline phosphatase and 5'-nucleotidase. The assay for GGTP is more readily available than that for 5'-nucleotidase and can be used to determine whether an elevated serum alkaline phosphatase level is of hepatic origin. A lack of specificity limits use of the GGTP. Drugs (eg, phenytoin, phenobarbital) that induce microsomal enzymes can elevate the GGTP level in patients who do not have liver disease. Moderate alcohol consumption increases the GGTP when all other liver function tests are normal.

Prothrombin Time

The prothrombin time is a measure of the clotting factors II, VII, and X—some of the coagulation proteins synthesized by the liver. Malabsorption of vitamin K can prolong the prothrombin time in patients who do not have liver disease. Prolongation that persists after parenteral administration of vitamin K usually indicates hepatic synthetic failure. A prothrombin time prolonged to more than twice normal is an ominous prognostic sign in acute liver diseases, primarily viral or drug-induced hepatitis.

Serum Proteins

The liver produces the majority of serum proteins, including albumin, fibrinogen, and the alpha and beta globulins. Gamma globulins are produced by plasma cells.

The protein that the liver produces in greatest quantity is albumin. The normal serum albumin level of 3.5–5.0 g/dL is maintained by hepatic synthesis of about 150–200 mg/kg/day. The half-life of serum albumin is 14–20 days. Although the serum albumin is low in most patients with chronic liver disease, it may be normal in patients with severe acute hepatitis.

Many chronic liver disorders have associated abnormalities in serum immunoglobulins. Elevation of the IgG fraction is characteristic of autoimmune liver disease; elevated IgA, of alcoholic liver disease; and elevated IgM, of primary biliary cirrhosis. Many patients with cirrhosis have a polyclonal gammopathy. A low α_1-globulin fraction is characteristic of α_1-antitrypsin deficiency, which may cause chronic liver disease.

IMAGING PROCEDURES AND ENDOSCOPY

Ultrasonography is useful in evaluating patients with hepatomegaly or an unexplained elevation in serum alkaline phosphatase. Ultrasonography may detect dilatation of the bile ducts or focal lesions within the liver; a decrease in the liver's echogenicity suggests fatty infiltration. Ultrasonographic guidance facilitates needle aspiration of hepatic abscesses and cysts, and is useful in directing a liver biopsy toward focal defects. If the physician suspects ascites but cannot confirm it by physical exam, ultrasonography can reliably detect even small amounts. Ultrasonography is also the procedure of choice for detecting gallstones.

Doppler flow studies can assess the patency of the portal and hepatic veins and the hepatic artery. Computed tomography (CT) is useful in diagnosing focal masses within the liver and determining the cause of biliary tract dilatation. Vascular patency can be assessed by CT after injection of contrast material. CT is particularly useful in diagnosing hemangiomas of the liver. Magnetic resonance imaging (MRI) is helpful in identifying focal hepatic lesions and evaluating the hepatic vessels. Technetium-99m (Tc^{99m}) iminodiacetic acid (HIDA) and related compounds are isotopes taken up by liver cells and excreted into the bile. They are useful in determining patency of the cystic duct and common bile duct. Other radioisotope liver scans, such as Tc^{99m} sulfacolloid, are of limited usefulness.

Esophagogastroduodenoscopy provides the earliest evidence of the presence and extent of varices in the esophagus and stomach. Endoscopic retrograde cannulation of the ampulla of Vater with cholangiopancreatography (ERCP) is useful in evaluating the common bile duct, particularly in patients with suspected sclerosing cholangitis. The biliary tract can also be visualized with percutaneous transhepatic cholangiography (Chapter 7.2). The doctor can easily puncture bile ducts dilated by obstruction and then inject cholangiographic dye to outline the biliary system. Percutaneous catheters can be used to relieve biliary tract obstruction. Laparoscopy allows direct visualization of the liver surface and may be useful to guide biopsy of focal lesions.

NEEDLE BIOPSY OF THE LIVER

Needle biopsy is a relatively simple but important procedure in diagnosing liver disease. Liver biopsy is particularly useful in the differential diagnosis of hepatomegaly and hepatocellular disease and in diagnosing hepatic neoplasms, evaluating prolonged fevers, and assessing the effect of therapy in chronic liver diseases. The procedure is contraindicated in patients with a severe coagulopathy or with infected fluid in the right pleural space. When performed by experienced physicians, needle biopsy is safe. Serious problems—bleeding, pneumothorax, and inadvertent puncture of the gallbladder—complicate fewer than 1 in 1000 biopsies.

SUMMARY

▶ Although patients with liver disease can present with specific manifestations like right upper quadrant pain, jaundice, hepatomegaly, ascites, or hepatic encephalopathy, most present with nonspecific constitutional symptoms such as malaise, fatigue, or weight loss.

▶ The most important laboratory tests in diagnosing the cause of liver disease are the aminotransferases and the alkaline phosphatase. The prothrombin time and albumin are most helpful in determining severity.

▶ Imaging procedures are most useful in detecting biliary tract dilatation and assessing focal lesions within the liver. Liver biopsy is most useful in diagnosing and assessing the effectiveness of therapy for chronic hepatitis and for determining the histology of mass lesions in the liver.

SUGGESTED READING

Hulcrantz R et al: Liver investigation in 149 asymptomatic patients with moderately elevated activities of serum aminotransferases. Scand J Gastroenterol 1986;21:109.

Ireland A et al: Raised γ-glutamyltransferase activity and the need for liver biopsy. BMJ 1991;302:388.

Kaplan MM: Alkaline phosphatase. Gastroenterology 1972;62:452.

Jaundice

H. Franklin Herlong, MD

Jaundice, the most common and most specific sign of liver disease, is caused by accumulation of bilirubin in tissues. When the total serum bilirubin level exceeds 3 mg/dL, staining of tissues becomes visible, especially in the skin, mucous membranes, and sclerae. Bilirubin is found in plasma and tissues in both unconjugated (indirect) and conjugated (direct) forms (see "Metabolism of Bilirubin" below). Conjugated bilirubin is easier to detect because it preferentially stains tissues with high elastin content, such as the sclerae and mucous membranes. Jaundice is more apparent in sunlight than artificial light and is less apparent in edematous areas because of the low protein content of the edema fluid. Before causing visible discoloration of the skin or sclerae, bilirubin may appear in the urine, giving it a "tea" color. Testing the urine for bilirubin is perhaps the most sensitive way of detecting early jaundice. It is important to distinguish jaundice from similar skin discoloration caused by other substances such as carotene and quinacrine. Although these substances cause yellowish skin, they do not affect the sclerae.

METABOLISM OF BILIRUBIN

A normal person produces about 300 mg of bilirubin each day (Figure 7.2–1). About 80% is derived from the breakdown of senescent red blood cells in the reticuloendothelial system. The remaining 20% comes from catabolism of other heme compounds such as cytochrome enzymes, catalases, peroxidases, and abortive pre-erythrocyte precursors in the bone marrow. In the phagocytic cells of the reticuloendothelial systems of the spleen, bone marrow, and liver, bilirubin is produced from the breakdown of hemoglobin. The enzyme heme oxygenase cleaves the porphyrin ring of heme to yield biliverdin, a reaction that requires molecular oxygen and releases carbon monoxide. Biliverdin reductase converts biliverdin to bilirubin, a water-insoluble unconjugated compound that binds quickly and tightly to albumin. The unconjugated bilirubin-albumin complex is not filtered at the glomerulus.

At the liver cell membrane, bilirubin is separated from its albumin carrier and taken up by liver cells. Once inside the cell, transfer of bilirubin from the plasma membrane to the endoplasmic reticulum is facilitated by cytoplasmic proteins. At the endoplasmic reticulum, bilirubin is conjugated with uridine diphosphate (UDP) glucuronic acid to form a water-soluble compound. This reaction is catalyzed by the enzyme bilirubin UDP glucuronyl transferase. Conjugated bilirubin is then actively secreted across the canalicular membrane of the hepatocyte into the bile. This active transport of conjugated bilirubin is the rate-limiting step in the excretory pathway of bilirubin. With injury to the hepatocyte or obstruction to bile flow at the level of canaliculus or beyond, conjugated bilirubin is regurgitated into the plasma. Regurgitated conjugated bilirubin is also bound to albumin, but less tightly than unconjugated bilirubin. About 1% of the bilirubin glucuronide-albumin complex is excreted by glomerular filtration.

After secretion into the biliary tree, conjugated bilirubin traverses the intestinal tract to the distal portion of the small intestine and colon, where conjugated bilirubin is catabolized by bacteria to colorless urobilinogens that are later oxidized to colored urobilins. These urobilins give stool its characteristic brown color. Severe reduction in bile flow, caused by obstruction or hepatocellular disease, leaves stool uncolored and chalky-looking (acholic stool). Urobilinogen is efficiently reabsorbed by an enterohepatic circulation, with the majority re-excreted into the bile. Normally, about 1% of urobilinogen escapes reuptake by the liver and can be detected in the urine. A high urinary urobilinogen level is found in patients who have an increased pigment load. No urobilinogen in the urine suggests interruption of the enterohepatic circulation of bile pigments and is found in common bile duct obstruction.

The laboratory reports conjugated bilirubin as "direct" bilirubin because of its binding to diazotized sulfonic acid in the Vandenberg reaction. The unconjugated ("indirect") bilirubin fraction is calculated by subtracting the direct fraction from the total bilirubin.

A useful classification system for jaundice is based on

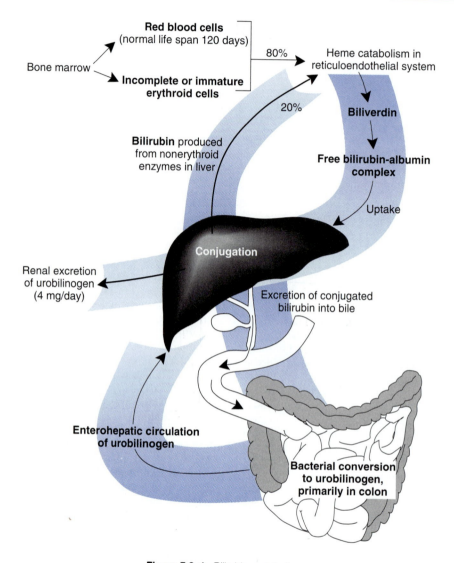

Figure 7.2–1. Bilirubin metabolism.

whether conjugated or unconjugated bilirubin predominates in the blood. Measuring the two bilirubin fractions is the first step in an orderly differential diagnosis of jaundice.

PREDOMINANTLY UNCONJUGATED (INDIRECT) HYPERBILIRUBINEMIA

Unconjugated (indirect) hyperbilirubinemia suggests either an increase in the pigment load presented to the liver or a defect in the uptake or conjugation of bilirubin (Table 7.2–1). Patients with unconjugated hyperbilirubinemia do not have bilirubinuria because unconjugated bilirubin bound to albumin is not excreted into the urine. The normal liver has a considerable reserve capacity to

excrete bilirubin, and a marked increase in pigment production is required to produce hyperbilirubinemia. Even when bilirubin production is increased, such as from hemolysis, as long as hepatic bilirubin clearance is normal, the plasma bilirubin concentration rarely exceeds 4 mg/dL. Higher bilirubin levels imply superimposed hepatocyte dysfunction. Most patients with severe hemolysis have some degree of anemia, but those with a low-grade compensated hemolysis may have an elevated reticulocyte count without anemia. A low serum haptoglobin level and a high urine hemosiderin level are further evidence of hemolysis. Resorption of hemoglobin from areas of tissue trauma, infarction, or burns may elevate the unconjugated bilirubin.

Defective uptake and conjugation of bilirubin may be hereditary or acquired. Medications such as rifampin can

Table 7.2–1. Evaluation of patients with unconjugated (indirect) hyperbilirubinemia.

Causes of High Bilirubin	Clinical and Laboratory Features
Overproduction	
Hemolysis	High reticulocyte count, anemia, positive Coombs' test, low haptoglobin, high urine hemosiderin
Extravasation of blood	Evidence of trauma, postoperative state, pulmonary embolus
Abnormal erythropoiesis	Abnormal Schilling test (pernicious anemia), sideroblastic anemia
Decreased uptake with conjugation	
Gilbert's syndrome	Increased bilirubin with fasting; family history
Glucuronyl transferase deficiency	
Crigler-Najjar syndrome type I (no glucuronyl transferase)	Kernicterus, early death
Crigler-Najjar syndrome type II (low glucuronyl transferase)	Drop in bilirubin level with phenobarbital therapy
Escape through collateral vessels	
Portacaval shunt	Shunt surgery for variceal hemorrhage
Cirrhosis	Hypersplenism, portal hypertension

interfere with uptake and conjugation. In some newborn and premature infants, immaturity of both the glucuronyl transferase system and the cytoplasmic protein receptors leads to unconjugated hyperbilirubinemia. This "physiologic" jaundice reaches its peak within 2–5 days after delivery and usually disappears within 2 weeks. In patients with surgical or endogenous portal-systemic shunts, bilirubin can pass directly from the spleen into the systemic circulation, causing a mild unconjugated jaundice.

Gilbert's Syndrome

Idiopathic unconjugated hyperbilirubinemia (Gilbert's syndrome) is a benign disorder transmitted as an autosomal dominant trait. It is found in 3–7% of adults worldwide, more often in men than women. A high unconjugated bilirubin is found in 15% of the parents of patients with this disorder, and in 25% of siblings. The serum bilirubin level is usually less than 6 mg/dL. The hyperbilirubinemia is often first noted on routine physical examination or blood screening. The bilirubin level fluctuates and may be increased by fasting, intercurrent infection, or strenuous exercise. Jaundice is intermittent but most pronounced during the second and third decades. The liver is otherwise histologically and biochemically normal. The hyperbilirubinemia in Gilbert's syndrome is multifactorial. Hepatic glucuronyl transferase activity is reduced, and alterations in membrane fluidity impair the uptake of bilirubin by liver cells. Some patients have a mild compensated hemolysis. This condition is benign, and the physician should reassure patients that they do not have serious liver disease. They have a normal life expectancy and require no treatment.

Crigler-Najjar Syndrome

The Crigler-Najjar syndrome is a rare form of severe unconjugated hyperbilirubinemia caused by an absence of glucuronyl transferase. The prototype, type I, has autosomal recessive inheritance. Patients are born with severe hyperbilirubinemia (20–31 mg/dL), kernicterus, and colorless bile. Severe jaundice usually begins 3–4 days after birth, with kernicterus (bilirubin encephalopathy) usually developing within 18 months and death shortly thereafter.

Patients with type II Crigler-Najjar syndrome have low levels of glucuronyl transferase, serum bilirubin levels of 9–17 mg/dL, and some bile color. These patients do not acquire kernicterus. Their serum bilirubin responds to phenobarbital, which may be able to induce some production of glucuronyl transferase.

PREDOMINANTLY CONJUGATED (DIRECT) HYPERBILIRUBINEMIA

Elevation in the conjugated (direct) bilirubin level is evidence of a defect in the excretory pathway of bilirubin (Figure 7.2–2). The defect may be caused by a primary inability of liver cells to secrete bile (hepatocellular jaundice) or mechanical obstruction preventing bile from flowing from the canaliculus down to the common bile duct (obstructive jaundice). The physician evaluating a patient with conjugated hyperbilirubinemia should ask: (1) Does the patient have a disease of hepatocyte function or a disorder of the bile ducts? (2) If the jaundice is caused by biliary tract dysfunction, is the problem mechanical obstruction (formerly called "surgical jaundice") of the large bile ducts, or is it intrahepatic bile stasis?

Liver function tests other than the bilirubin are useful in the differential diagnosis of conjugated hyperbilirubinemia (Table 7.2–2). Elevated aminotransferase levels suggest hepatocellular disease, whereas predominant elevation in the alkaline phosphatase suggests biliary tract injury. Individual laboratory tests alone are rarely sufficient to allow an accurate diagnosis. Instead, the physician should form a clinical impression from the history, physical examination, and screening tests (Chapter 7.1).

If extrahepatic biliary tract obstruction appears likely, the bile ducts must be visualized. Ultrasonography and computed tomography (CT) are simple, noninvasive ways

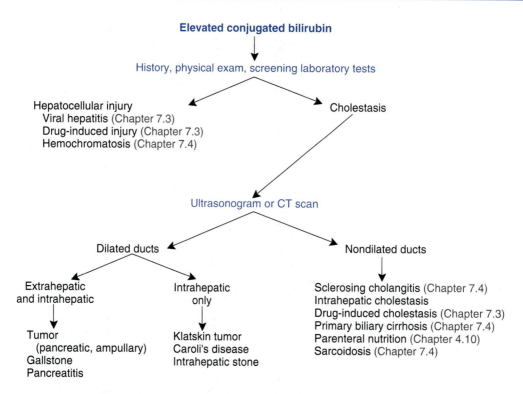

Figure 7.2–2. Evaluation of patients with conjugated hyperbilirubinemia.

of detecting dilated biliary radicles. Both techniques are equally effective, but ultrasonography is more available and less expensive. Dilated intra- and extrahepatic ducts suggest obstruction of the distal common bile duct by tumor (ampullary or pancreatic carcinoma), pancreatic disease, gallstones, or a distal duct stricture. If the common bile duct is normal but the intrahepatic ducts are dilated, the cause may be cholangiocarcinoma at the duct bifurcation (Klatskin tumor), an intrahepatic gallstone, or Caroli's disease, which causes cystic dilatation of the intrahepatic bile ducts. Extrahepatic biliary obstruction without dilated ducts is characteristic of sclerosing cholangitis.

Direct visualization of the biliary tree is often needed to pinpoint the site of obstruction. Percutaneous transhepatic cholangiography is most useful when intrahepatic ducts are dilated. During the procedure, Silastic stents can be placed to drain the obstructed bile ducts. Endoscopic retrograde cholangiopancreatography (ERCP) is most useful when extrahepatic obstruction is suspected but no dilated ducts are seen on an ultrasonogram or CT scan. During ERCP, the doctor may perform a sphincterotomy to retrieve common duct stones or dilate distal duct strictures. Definitive treatment for many patients with extrahepatic biliary tract obstruction requires surgery.

When visualization of the extrahepatic biliary tree excludes mechanical obstruction, the clinician must deter-

Table 7.2–2. Laboratory studies in patients with jaundice.

| Disorder Causing Jaundice | Liver Function Tests | | | | | Urine |
| | Bilirubin | | | | | |
	Indirect	Direct	Alk Phos	AST	ALT	Bilirubin
Hemolytic anemia	↑	N	N	N	N	0
Gilbert's syndrome	↑	N	N	N	N	0
Viral hepatitis	↑	↑↑	N–↑	↑↑	↑↑↑	+
Alcoholic hepatitis	↑	↑↑	N–↑	↑	N–↑	+
				(ratio of AST:ALT = 2:1)		
Drug-induced cholestasis	↑	↑↑	↑	N–↑	N–↑	+
Common bile duct obstruction	↑	↑↑	↑↑	N–↑	N–↑	+
Primary biliary cirrhosis	↑	↑↑	↑↑↑	↑	↑	+

Alk phos, alkaline phosphatase; AST, aspartate aminotransferase; ALT, alanine aminotransferase; N, normal.

mine whether jaundice is caused by hepatocellular disease or a disorder of the intrahepatic bile ducts. Viral hepatitis and toxic liver injury impair excretion of conjugated bilirubin into the canalicular bile. Metabolic disturbances such as ischemia, drug toxicity (eg, from phenothiazines), and sepsis can impair liver cell excretory function. Cholestasis (failure of bile flow) may develop from septal or interlobular bile duct injury in primary biliary cirrhosis, or from compression by granulomatous hepatitis or tumor. Occasionally, a pregnant woman develops intrahepatic cholestasis, especially during the third trimester. The jaundice of pregnancy is caused by increased sensitivity to estrogens during pregnancy. Jaundice can also be caused by estrogen-containing oral contraceptives. A careful history of complications of pregnancy should be taken in any woman who develops jaundice while using an oral contraceptive.

Rare intrahepatic causes of defective excretion of conjugated bilirubin include Dubin-Johnson syndrome, Rotor's syndrome, and benign recurrent cholestasis. Dubin-Johnson syndrome is inherited as an autosomal recessive trait. Patients have normal uptake and conjugation of bilirubin, but impaired secretion of conjugated bilirubin into the bile. Conjugated bilirubin regurgitates into the plasma and can be detected in the urine. The liver looks black because conversion of retained metanephrine glucuronide leaves accumulations of melanin pigment. Like Gilbert's syndrome, Dubin-Johnson syndrome is benign and requires no treatment. Rotor's syndrome is like Dubin-Johnson syndrome, except that the liver does not look black. Patients with benign recurrent cholestasis have recurrent bouts of intrahepatic cholestasis. During attacks, patients may itch, but they have no other evidence of hepatic dysfunction. Between attacks, the liver is completely normal.

COMPLICATIONS OF CHOLESTASIS

Symptoms of impaired bile excretion can develop regardless of the site of obstruction. Symptoms tend to be more severe with prolonged cholestasis. The most common symptom of chronic cholestasis is pruritus, caused by retention of bile salts and other pruritogens normally excreted in the bile. The pruritus of cholestasis is often treated with drugs like cholestyramine that bind bile salts in the intestinal tract and prevent their enterohepatic circulation. Impaired secretion of bile salts impairs micelle formation, causing fat malabsorption with secondary fat-soluble vitamin deficiency states, including night blindness (vitamin A), osteomalacia (vitamin D), and coagulopathy (vitamin K). Prompt correction of the prothrombin time after patients are given parenteral vitamin K implies cholestasis rather than hepatocellular synthetic dysfunction. Patients with chronic cholestasis have high cholesterol levels; when levels exceed 1000 mg/dL, patients develop xanthomas and xanthelasma (see Color Plates).

In patients with cholestasis, hepatic cells undergo anatomic changes that worsen the longer bile flow is obstructed. If obstruction continues for several weeks, necrotic cells in the periportal region are replaced by fibrous bands that may slowly progress to first a biliary and later a macronodular cirrhosis.

SUMMARY

▶ Jaundice results from accumulation of predominantly unconjugated (indirect) or conjugated (direct) bilirubin in blood and tissues.

▶ Conjugated hyperbilirubinemia is caused by hepatocyte disorders that stop bile secretion (hepatocellular jaundice) or by obstruction to bile flow within the bile ducts (obstructive jaundice).

▶ Complications of prolonged cholestasis include pruritus, malabsorption of fat-soluble vitamins, hypercholesterolemia, and biliary cirrhosis.

SUGGESTED READING

Camma C et al: A performance evaluation of the expert system "Jaundice" in comparison with that of three hepatologists. J Hepatol 1991;13:279.

Frank BB: Clinical evaluation of jaundice: A guideline of the Patient Care Committee of the American Gastroenterological Association. JAMA 1989;262:3031.

Schmid R: Bilirubin metabolism: State of the art. Gastroenterology 1978;74:1307.

Watson KJR, Gollan JL: Gilbert's syndrome. Baillieres Clin Gastroenterol 1989;3:337.

7.3

Acute Hepatitis

Mack C. Mitchell, MD

About 90% of patients with liver disease present with acute illness, with jaundice, symptoms of acute hepatocellular injury, or both. The most common cause of acute hepatocellular injury is viral hepatitis; second is exposure to drugs—including alcohol—or toxins. (Rare patients with chronic liver disease, such as chronic hepatitis, Wilson's disease, or alcoholic liver disease, present with features suggesting acute hepatitis.) Although both viral and drug-induced hepatitis generally begin acutely, they can progress to chronic liver disease and cirrhosis (Chapter 7.4). This chapter deals with the full spectrum of each of these diseases, including factors that predispose to the development of chronic liver disease, and the management of both the acute and chronic forms.

Patients with acute inflammation and destruction of hepatic parenchyma (hepatitis) can present to a physician with symptoms and signs ranging from fatigue and anorexia to coma. The challenges to the physician are to determine the duration of hepatitis, uncover the etiology, and plan management. Evaluation of patients with suspected hepatitis requires attention to historical features such as intravenous drug use, exposure to blood or blood products, foreign travel, exposure to people who may have hepatitis, and exposure to drugs or toxins. Since many of the signs and symptoms of hepatitis are not specific to the etiology, the history is crucial in suggesting the cause, which can be confirmed by serology.

VIRAL HEPATITIS

Viruses can cause hepatocellular necrosis either directly by cytopathic effect or indirectly by an immune-mediated attack on the virus-infected hepatocyte. The severity of viral hepatitis is variable. Most disease is asymptomatic or produces only mild symptoms. Less than one-third of patients develop jaundice during the initial phase. At the other extreme, about 1% of patients have a fulminant illness, with profound hepatocellular dysfunction leading to jaundice, coagulopathy, and encephalopathy; this form of hepatitis is usually fatal. In addition to producing acute hepatitis, several of the hepatitis viruses can cause chronic infections with potential for fibrosis and cirrhosis.

Five viruses with primary hepatic manifestations have been identified and characterized by molecular techniques. These agents are called hepatitis A, B, C, D (delta), and E (Table 7.3–1). Although each virus causes similar initial clinical features, the natural histories differ. Other viruses producing systemic infection that can include hepatitis are the herpes viruses, such as cytomegalovirus, Epstein-Barr, and herpes simplex, as well as flaviviruses, which cause dengue and yellow fever.

Clinical Manifestations

Most patients with viral hepatitis present with malaise, fatigue, anorexia, nausea, vague abdominal discomfort, weakness, and dark (tea-colored) urine. The abdominal discomfort, caused by distention of the liver capsule, is usually in the right upper quadrant and may be worsened by eating, bending, or even sleeping on the right side. An occasional patient has severe pain that radiates to the infra- or suprascapular area. Some patients describe bloating and heartburn with the pain. Fewer than one-third of patients have jaundice, which usually appears only after the initial symptoms. Depending on the virus, patients may have a low-grade fever and extrahepatic manifestations. Fever (38–39° C) is common with hepatitis A and E, but less so with hepatitis B, C, and D. Up to 50% of patients with acute hepatitis B have arthralgias and urticaria, suggesting an immune complex pathogenesis. About 10–15% of patients with acute viral hepatitis complain of pruritus and have an elevated direct bilirubin and alkaline phosphatase, indicating cholestasis.

Patients with acute hepatitis have relatively few physical findings. None are specific. Patients with a serum bilirubin higher than 3.0 mg/dL may have scleral icterus. Some patients with viral hepatitis have lymphadenopathy, but this is more likely to be seen in patients with acute mononucleosis, who may also have pharyngitis. Right upper quadrant tenderness and mild hepatomegaly are common findings, but splenomegaly is rare. Ascites and edema suggest either chronic or fulminant hepatitis.

Table 7.3–1. Features of viral hepatitis.

Virus	% of Hepatitis in United States	Incubation Period	Mechanism of Hepatocellular Damage	Incidence of Chronic Hepatitis	Major Mode of Transmission
A	25%	15–40 days	Cytopathic	None	Fecal-oral
B	40–50%	30–180 days	Immune-mediated	Low (5–10%)	Parenteral or mucous membranes
C	25%	30–180 days	Cytopathic or possibly immune-mediated	High (50–70%)	Parenteral or mucous membranes
D	<10%	?	Cytopathic	High (50–70%)	Parenteral
E	<1%	15–40 days	Cytopathic	None	Fecal-oral

The laboratory hallmark of all forms of acute hepatitis is elevated aminotransferases. The alkaline phosphatase is usually normal or minimally elevated, but may be higher in patients with the cholestatic variant of viral hepatitis. All these biochemical tests simply reflect hepatocellular necrosis. The etiology of the hepatic damage must be determined through the history and serologic tests for specific pathogens.

Fulminant Hepatitis

Fulminant hepatitis is defined by the onset of altered mental status, asterixis, or other signs of hepatic encephalopathy within 2 weeks of the first signs or symptoms of acute liver disease. Patients are jaundiced and may develop abdominal distention from accumulation of ascites. Biochemical findings usually include marked elevation in aminotransferases, bilirubin (above 10 mg/dL), and ammonia, along with coagulopathy (prolonged prothrombin time and low platelet count). Thrombocytopenia has been attributed to a cytokine-mediated effect. The prognosis is poor. Mortality rate with medical therapy alone exceeds 80% and approaches 100% in patients over age 45 and patients with other serious medical problems.

Hepatitis A

Hepatitis A accounts for about 25% of cases of clinical hepatitis in the United States. The hepatitis A virus (HAV), a ribonucleic acid (RNA) enterovirus, was the first hepatitis virus to be grown successfully in tissue culture. Hepatitis A has predominantly fecal-oral transmission. The disease occurs sporadically or in epidemics when inadequate sewage disposal and poor hygiene allow fecal contamination of water supplies. HAV may be transmitted by raw or partially cooked shellfish harvested from sewage-contaminated waters. In the United States, outbreaks occur most often in children's day care centers, mental institutions, and military installations. Male homosexuals have a high incidence of hepatitis A. Transmission of HAV by blood transfusion or other parenteral means is extremely rare.

The usual incubation period for hepatitis A is 15–40 days (Figure 7.3–1). HAV is detected in the feces late in the incubation period and early in the acute disease. HAV appears transiently in the blood during the late incubation period. Antibody to HAV (anti-HAV) develops near the onset of the acute illness; when it appears, fecal shedding

of HAV declines. The initial anti-HAV is IgM antibody, which disappears after several months. An IgG anti-HAV appears later and persists, usually for life. IgM anti-HAV indicates acute or very recent infection and is diagnostic of acute hepatitis A, whereas IgG anti-HAV signifies previous infection and immunity to reinfection.

Hepatitis A is usually a mild, self-limited illness. Most patients have nonspecific "flu-like" symptoms of malaise, fatigue, and anorexia. A minority of patients develop jaundice. Mortality from hepatitis A is very low, although fulminant hepatitis A has been reported. There is no chronic carrier state for hepatitis A and no evidence that it causes chronic active hepatitis or cirrhosis.

Hepatitis B

Hepatitis B is the most common cause of acute viral hepatitis in American adults. About 300,000 cases per year are reported to the Centers for Disease Control and Pre-

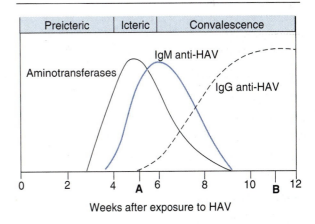

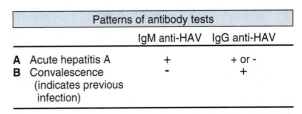

Figure 7.3–1. Usual pattern of serologic changes in hepatitis A.

vention. The hepatitis B virus (HBV), formerly termed the Dane particle, is a DNA virus of the hepadnavirus family. This family includes viruses similar to HBV that cause liver disease in woodchucks, ground squirrels, and Peking ducks. These natural animal models have facilitated the study of HBV and related liver disease.

The hepatitis B virus has a thick lipoprotein outer envelope that expresses the hepatitis B surface antigen (HBsAg, the Australia antigen) and an electron-dense inner core. Unlike many other human viruses, HBV has an endogenous DNA polymerase. The virus replicates by forming HBV RNA, followed by reverse transcription back to DNA, an unusual mechanism for a DNA virus. The process of reverse transcription is thought to have produced a number of mutant viruses, including a pre-core mutant that may cause more severe disease.

Clinical Course: The incubation period for hepatitis B varies from 30–180 days (Figure 7.3–2). The higher the dose of inoculum, the shorter the incubation. Early in the course, the virus replicates actively and HBV DNA accompanies HBsAg in the serum. Deposition of immune complexes and complement accounts for prodromal symptoms such as arthritis and urticaria; in a few patients, immune complexes cause glomerulonephritis. After the prodrome, patients typically develop malaise, fatigue, myalgias, anorexia, and nausea. Patients may also have low-grade fever, right upper quadrant abdominal pain, and dysgeusia. Physical exam reveals mild, tender hepatomegaly in addition to jaundice. Some patients have posterior cervical lymphadenopathy. During the acute phase, rare patients have transient spider angiomas.

Laboratory findings are aminotransferase elevations (above 300 IU/L) and a mild rise in alkaline phosphatase. The leukocyte count is usually normal, with a relative lymphocytosis. Prolongation of the prothrombin time (more than 5 seconds beyond control values) suggests severe hepatitis that may become fulminant.

Serologic Markers: Three circulating particles are known to express HBsAg: the intact virus, a small spherical particle, and a tubular particle. The spherical and tubular particles are immunogenic but not infectious. HBsAg has been found in blood, saliva, semen, urine, feces, and bile. Antibodies to HBsAg are a marker of previous infection or vaccination. They indicate recovery from infection and immunity to reinfection.

Hepatitis B core antigen (HBcAg), a component of the inner core of the hepatitis B virus, is seen in the nuclei of infected hepatocytes. HBcAg is found only in the liver and does not circulate. The hepatitis B e antigen (HBeAg) is not part of the intact virion, but a peptide derived from cleavage of the nascent core protein during viral replication. HBeAg appears transiently in the serum during acute infection, indicates active viral replication, and correlates with circulating intact virus and infectivity. The e antigen persists in most patients who develop chronic hepatitis.

Hepatitis B DNA can also be found in the serum of patients with acute or chronic hepatitis B. Hybridization assays and polymerase chain reaction have both been used

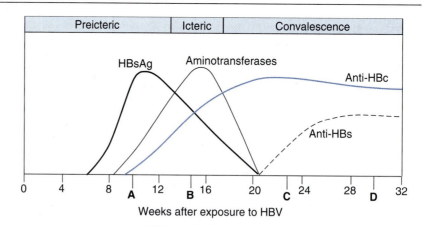

Figure 7.3–2. Usual pattern of serologic changes in hepatitis B.

Usual patterns of hepatitis B antigens and antibodies		
HBsAg	Anti-HBc	Anti-HBs
A Very early +	+ or - (IgM)	-
B Acute +	+ (IgM)	-
C Convalescence +	+ or - (IgM)	+
D Recovery -	+ or - (IgG)	+

to detect small amounts of virus in patients with hepatitis B. HBV DNA is a better marker of infectivity and chronic infection than the e antigen.

Transmission: Although HBV is often transmitted parenterally by blood transfusions or contaminated needles, most patients with acute hepatitis B have no history of apparent parenteral exposure. The incubation period for HBV may be longer after nonparenteral exposure. The major route of transmission for most sporadic cases is considered to be intimate contact, including heterosexual and homosexual sex. Long-term sexual partners of patients with or chronic carriers of hepatitis B have a 20–25% risk of developing HBV infection. Many partners seroconvert without developing symptoms. An infected mother also has a significant risk of transmitting hepatitis B to her newborn baby. In endemic regions, such as the Far East and sub-Saharan Africa, this appears to be the major route of transmission. Infected neonates have a high incidence of chronic hepatitis B infection, which may persist for life. Older children and other household contacts of patients with hepatitis B are at considerably less risk of becoming infected.

Outcomes: Because the hepatitis B virus is not directly cytopathic, the outcome of infection depends largely on the host's immunologic response (Figure 7.3–3). When previously healthy young persons develop acute symptomatic hepatitis B, the prognosis is excellent. Survival of fulminant hepatitis depends on age and is best in patients younger than 20. Chronic HBV infection, defined as persistence of HBsAg for longer than 6 months, develops in 5–10% of patients. Factors influencing the development of a chronic carrier state are (1) clinical expression of the acute disease (anicteric hepatitis is more likely to become chronic), (2) age at time of infection (90% of infected neonates become carriers), (3) gender (the male:female ratio is 5:1), and (4) immune status (immunocompromised hosts are more likely to become carriers). The clinical manifestations of chronic hepatitis B resemble those of

autoimmune hepatitis; the diseases are differentiated by serology (Chapter 7.4).

HBsAg disappears from only 1% of chronic carriers per year. Patients who are chronically HBsAg-positive and have normal aminotransferases are designated "asymptomatic chronic carriers." Chronic carriers are potentially infectious and should be advised to take precautions to reduce their risk of infecting others with HBV. It is not known why, 10–40 years after infection, asymptomatic carriers may develop a more active chronic hepatitis.

Patients who remain HBsAg-positive for longer than 6 months, with elevated aminotransferases, have some form of chronic hepatitis. They need a liver biopsy to determine the severity of their disease. In the past, on the basis of the histologic appearance, chronic viral hepatitis was classified as chronic persistent hepatitis, chronic lobular hepatitis, or chronic active hepatitis. Because the histologic features may change over time, the current trend is to classify the degree of inflammation as mild, moderate, or severe, and to describe the degree of fibrosis.

Chronic hepatitis is a serious liver disease that often progresses to cirrhosis, portal hypertension, and, in occasional patients, death. Many patients have anorexia, malaise, and fatigue, and some already have cirrhosis and signs of portal hypertension when they present. However, chronic active hepatitis can also be discovered incidentally in asymptomatic patients. Liver biopsy shows portal areas markedly infiltrated by mononuclear cells, often with fibro-inflammatory bridging: Fibrous septa isolate groups of liver cells, and the limiting plate is eroded.

An important consequence of chronic hepatitis B infection can be primary hepatocellular carcinoma. Worldwide, hepatocellular carcinoma is the second most common cause of cancer deaths. Although many patients with chronic hepatitis B and primary hepatocellular carcinoma have cirrhosis, this tumor can develop in patients who do not have cirrhosis. The key step in the progression from chronic HBV infection to hepatocellular carcinoma is integration of hepatitis B DNA into the genome of the host's

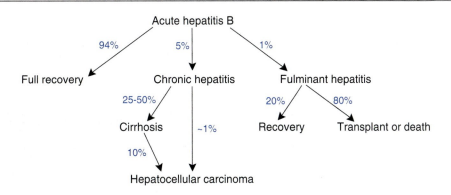

Figure 7.3–3. Outcomes of hepatitis B.

liver cells. This integration alters the cells' gene expression, leading to transformation into clones of cells that become neoplastic.

Hepatitis C

Hepatitis C (HCV), a flavivirus, was the most common cause of post-transfusion hepatitis until 1990, when serologic testing for the virus became commercially available and blood began to be screened.

Serologic Markers: Both enzyme-linked immunosorbent assays (ELISA or EIA) and recombinant immunoblot assays (RIBA) have been developed for serologic detection of hepatitis C infection. These assays test for antibodies to any of four primary antigens. Antibody is usually detectable within 2 months of exposure, but in some patients it is not detected for 6 months. The antibodies assayed do not neutralize virus and do not protect against infection after passive transfer.

The ELISA test for hepatitis C has some false-positive and false-negative results. False-positives occur in some patients who have autoimmune hepatitis with hyperglobulinemia and in occasional asymptomatic volunteer blood donors; the explanation may be a nonspecific reaction to one of the recombinant proteins used in the assay. False-negative results are most frequent in the early stages of infection, before patients have developed an antibody response.

Hepatitis C RNA in serum can be measured by polymerase chain reaction (PCR) or by signal amplification through the branched DNA hybridization assay. The latter is more quantitative but less sensitive than PCR.

Transmission: Until 1990, hepatitis C was most often transmitted by transfusion. Once blood screening tests came into use, the two most common modes of transmission became contaminated needles shared by intravenous drug users and accidental exposure of health care workers. One-third of cases are sporadic, with no known risk factor for infection. The epidemiology of HCV is similar to that of HBV. HCV may be transmitted sexually, but less often than HBV because the virus titer is lower.

Outcomes: Most acute hepatitis C is anicteric, and much is asymptomatic. No specific clinical features permit definitive diagnosis. Because antibody to hepatitis C cannot be detected until 1–6 months after infection, the diagnosis is usually based on risk factors and absence of other viral markers. As with other types of viral hepatitis, the increase in aminotransferases is much greater than the slight elevation in alkaline phosphatase. One characteristic though unexplained feature of hepatitis C is fluctuation of the aminotransferase levels.

In Western countries, hepatitis C rarely causes fulminant hepatitis, but as much as 70% of patients with post-transfusion hepatitis C develop chronic hepatitis. Hepatitis C persists indefinitely in a high percentage of patients, regardless of the source of infection (see Table 7.3–1). The tendency to persist may relate to the poor immune response during infection; that is, patients have humoral responses, but they do not clear the virus.

Aplastic anemia, hemolytic anemia, and agranulocytosis are found in rare patients with hepatitis C. All three are more common in men than women and are more prevalent after acute hepatitis C than hepatitis A or B. Chronic hepatitis C has been associated with a number of immune-mediated illnesses, particularly type II mixed cryoglobulinemia. The liver disease is often quiescent, and some patients' cryoglobulinemia improves if their hepatitis C is treated with interferon-α. Other immune phenomena associated with hepatitis C include Mooren's corneal ulcers, membranous glomerulonephritis, and possibly autoimmune thyroiditis.

After many years, chronic hepatitis C leads to fibrosis and cirrhosis in as much as 30–50% of patients. These patients also seem to have a high incidence of hepatocellular carcinoma. Chronic hepatitis C is especially prevalent in patients with hepatocellular carcinoma in Japan, Spain, and Italy: 70% of these people have viral markers. The prevalence in the United States is only 25%.

Delta Hepatitis (Type D)

The delta agent (HDV) is a defective hepatotropic RNA virus that is pathogenic only in the presence of HBV, which provides it with envelope protein and allows it to replicate. Since the delta agent is inextricably linked to its helper virus, its transmission is similar to that of HBV.

The outcome of delta infection depends on whether the host is infected simultaneously with both hepatitis B and D, or whether the delta agent superinfects a chronic hepatitis B carrier. Coinfection by the delta agent and hepatitis B produces a biphasic acute hepatitis that is often very severe, with fulminant hepatitis in about 30% of patients. In some patients, acute infection with delta causes transient suppression of HBV replication and a brief disappearance of HBsAg from serum; this can temporarily obscure the diagnosis. Because the delta agent cannot live without the hepatitis B virus, delta infection always ends with the clearance of hepatitis B. When chronic hepatitis B carriers become superinfected with the delta agent, most have a relapse of clinical hepatitis and some die.

Delta infection is detected by anti-HDV, which does not clear the infection. The most reliable proof of active delta infection is detection of the delta antigen, either in the liver by immunostaining techniques, or in the serum.

Hepatitis E

Hepatitis E is a cause of both sporadic and epidemic hepatitis in India, Pakistan, Nepal, Southeast Asia, the Middle East, and Mexico. The virus contains single-stranded RNA. Hepatitis E can infect some nonhuman primates as well as humans. Transmission is primarily enteric, through contaminated water. The epidemiology of hepatitis E resembles that of hepatitis A. Hepatitis E has not been reported to cause chronic infection, but a high incidence of fulminant hepatitis has been observed in pregnant women during epidemics. There are no commercial tests for hepatitis E.

Management of Viral Hepatitis

Most patients with acute viral hepatitis recover, given time, rest, and adequate diet. Patients should be hospitalized if they have evidence of significantly impaired coagulation (prothrombin time longer than 16 seconds), encephalopathy, ascites, or dehydration from nausea and vomiting. People without these criteria can be managed as outpatients.

Bed rest is a time-honored recommendation in viral hepatitis. This seems a practical recommendation, since many patients are weak. However, studies of previously healthy military personnel with hepatitis showed that moderate or even forced exercise did not hinder ultimate recovery. On the other hand, the outcome for previously healthy young patients may not apply to an older and more heterogeneous civilian population. A reasonable approach is to encourage rest during symptomatic hepatitis, with gradually increasing activity as the symptoms subside.

A high-calorie, high-protein diet (1 g protein/kg of body weight) seems to shorten symptomatic viral hepatitis. The physician might suggest that patients eat most of their calories in the morning, when they tend to be least nauseated. A mild antiemetic such as diphenhydramine may help to control nausea. If patients develop signs of encephalopathy, their protein intake should be restricted. Specific vitamin deficiencies must be corrected but patients do not need routine vitamin supplements. Patients with severe cholestasis should be given parenteral vitamin K.

Specific Therapy: No specific therapy has been found to improve acute viral hepatitis. Corticosteroids are not indicated, regardless of the cause or severity of the hepatitis. Corticosteroids actually worsen the prognosis of fulminant hepatitis.

Altered mental status in patients with fulminant hepatitis may be caused by hepatic encephalopathy, which affects all patients with fulminant disease, or by cerebral edema, which affects more than 50% of patients. The cerebral edema responds to mannitol but not to corticosteroids. Some physicians recommend that patients who are being considered for a liver transplantation have aggressive monitoring of intracranial pressure with epidural transducers to prevent permanent brain damage. A common complication of fulminant hepatitis is gastrointestinal bleeding from erosive gastritis; this can usually be prevented by prophylactic histamine H_2 blockers. Hypoprothrombinemia and thrombocytopenia do not require prophylactic therapy and should be treated with blood products only during active gastrointestinal bleeding. Pressors are used to manage hypotension and prevent renal failure. There is preliminary evidence that prophylactic antibiotics may prevent endotoxemia, which affects almost 90% of patients with fulminant hepatic failure. The definitive therapy for fulminant viral hepatitis is liver transplantation, which is successful in more than 60% of patients. A graft transplanted for fulminant hepatitis is less likely to get infected than a graft for chronic hepatitis.

Antiviral agents hold promise for treating the severest forms of chronic hepatitis. Interferon has been shown to suppress replication of both hepatitis B and C in about 50% of patients treated, and those who respond have reduced hepatic inflammation.

Prevention and Prophylaxis: Hepatitis A is best prevented by general hygiene measures for avoiding contact with contaminated water and foods. But prevention of spread is made difficult by the shedding of virus during the prodrome and by the many anicteric patients. Immune serum globulin given to contacts of patients with hepatitis A protects against development of overt hepatitis, but not against subclinical infection. A formalin-inactivated vaccine is recommended for travelers to countries where hepatitis A is endemic; primary immunization should be given more than 2 weeks before travel and a booster 6–12 months after the first dose.

Hepatitis B is best prevented by active vaccination with one of several recombinant vaccines. All the vaccines currently in use contain recombinant HBsAg, and some contain pre-S region peptides. The vaccines produce neutralizing antibody in 95% of healthy subjects who receive the complete series of three intramuscular injections. Patients who are immunosuppressed by HIV infection, chronic renal failure, or chronic liver disease have lower rates of seroconversion. In the past, vaccination was recommended for high-risk groups such as health care workers (now mandated by the Occupational Safety and Health Administration), patients on hemodialysis, parenteral drug users, homosexuals, and heterosexual contacts of known hepatitis B carriers. But because targeting high-risk groups failed to lower the incidence of hepatitis B, the Centers for Disease Control and Prevention now recommends universal childhood vaccination.

After accidental percutaneous or permucosal exposure to hepatitis B, people should be given prophylaxis with hepatitis B hyperimmune globulin (HBIG), together with HBV vaccination. Prophylaxis should be given as soon as possible after exposure (within 14 days for sexual contacts). The efficacy is about 75%. Because of the risk of neonatal transmission, all pregnant women should be screened for HBsAg. Babies of hepatitis B-positive mothers should be given both active and passive (HBIG) vaccination within 12 hours after birth.

LIVER INJURY CAUSED BY DRUGS AND OTHER CHEMICALS

Liver damage from drugs and chemical exposure has become the second most common cause of acute hepatitis and an increasingly common cause of chronic liver disease (Table 7.3–2). Drug reactions affecting the liver can

Table 7.3–2. Drug-induced liver injury.

Type of Injury	Examples of Responsible Drugs
Hepatocellular injury	
Acute necrosis	Acetaminophen, carbon tetrachloride
Acute hepatitis	Isoniazid, aspirin, phenytoin
Chronic hepatitis	Isoniazid, α-methyldopa, nitrofurantoin
Steatosis, steatohepatitis	Tetracycline, valproate, corticosteroids, nucleoside analogs, ethanol, amiodarone, perhexiline maleate
Cholestasis	
Inflammatory	Chlorpromazine, erythromycin, amoxicillin-clavulanate
Noninflammatory	Oral contraceptives, rifampicin
Granulomatous inflammation	Many drugs
Vascular injury	
Peliosis hepatitis	Anabolic steroids, oral contraceptives
Hepatic vein thrombosis	Oral contraceptives
Veno-occlusive disease	Antineoplastic agents, particularly when used in high doses before bone marrow transplant
Tumors	
Hepatic adenoma	Oral contraceptives
Hepatocellular carcinoma	Anabolic steroids
Angiosarcoma	Vinyl chloride

Modified and reproduced, with permission, from Mitchell MC: Drug-induced liver damage. In: *Current Therapy in Gastroenterology and Liver Disease,* 4th ed. Bayless TM (editor). CV Mosby, 1994.

have any manifestation from asymptomatic elevation of aminotransferases to fulminant hepatic necrosis.

The mechanisms of drug-induced hepatocellular damage can be divided into two broad categories: direct hepatocellular toxicity and idiosyncratic hepatotoxicity. Direct hepatotoxins characteristically cause reactions that are reproducible and dose-dependent, affect most exposed persons, and appear within several days of exposure. By contrast, idiosyncratic hepatotoxins are unpredictable and poorly reproducible. They affect only a minority of exposed persons, may or may not be dose-dependent, and usually require several weeks of exposure before manifestations appear. True hypersensitivity (allergic) features—fever, lymphadenopathy, arthralgias or arthritis, rash, and eosinophilia—accompany some idiosyncratic reactions but are not required for a diagnosis of idiosyncratic hepatotoxicity.

With both direct and idiosyncratic hepatotoxins, either the parent drug or one of its metabolites may do the damage. Of the many metabolic reactions that the liver performs, the pathway most often responsible for producing hepatotoxic metabolites is oxidation. Oxidation can produce chemically reactive electrophilic metabolites or free radical species of drugs that cause either alkylation or peroxidation of vital macromolecules. Important cellular de-

fenses against this potential damage include glutathione S-transferases, glutathione peroxidase, epoxide hydrolase, and glucuronosyltransferase. Genetic defects in any of these detoxification or activation pathways might render a person susceptible to drug-induced injury.

Diagnosis and Management

Since no definitive test exists, the physician must use the history and exclusion of other causes to implicate drugs in producing hepatotoxicity. Treatment for most hepatic drug reactions is limited to stopping the drug; most patients improve markedly within 2–3 weeks. Specific therapy is available for a few drugs (see below). In general, corticosteroids are not useful in treating drug-induced liver damage.

Rechallenge does not invariably produce a quick recurrence of abnormalities, because some drug hepatotoxicity comes from metabolites that take time to accumulate. Furthermore, rechallenge may be hazardous, causing an exaggerated reaction and even death in hypersensitive patients.

Following are examples of drugs illustrating the major categories of drug-induced hepatotoxicity.

Dose-Related Toxic Injury: Acetaminophen: Excessive doses (more than 10 g) of acetaminophen cause dose-related hepatic necrosis. The liver converts about 90% of acetaminophen to nontoxic glucuronides and sulfates; the remaining 10% is oxidized by cytochrome P-450 to a potentially toxic intermediate. At low doses, this intermediate is detoxified uneventfully by further conjugation with glutathione. But large doses quickly deplete hepatic glutathione stores, and the remaining toxic intermediates bind covalently to cellular macromolecules, leading to cell injury and death.

Most acetaminophen hepatotoxicity results from suicide attempts or accidental swallowing of large doses by children. Alcoholics risk liver damage at relatively low acetaminophen doses because long-term heavy alcohol ingestion both induces cytochrome P-450, which increases formation of toxic metabolites, and decreases hepatic detoxification of acetaminophen. An important contributor to accidental acetaminophen hepatotoxicity is inclusion of acetaminophen in many over-the-counter products that people assume to be safe in unlimited doses.

After acetaminophen overdose, *N*-acetylcysteine can prevent hepatic necrosis by increasing glutathione synthesis. To work best, treatment must be started within 12 hours after an overdose. The drug is ineffective if started more than 24 hours afterward.

Hypersensitivity Hepatitis: Phenytoin: Phenytoin can cause severe and even fatal hepatic necrosis, with symptoms beginning 1–8 weeks after patients start the drug. Many affected patients have fever, exfoliative dermatitis, lymphadenopathy, eosinophilia, and leukocytosis. These clinical features and a finding of granulomas on liver biopsy suggest a hypersensitivity reaction. Patients with the full hypersensitivity syndrome have a poor prognosis. Phenytoin can also cause mild elevation of the aminotransferases, with minimal hepatic inflammation; this reaction does not appear to result from hypersensitivity. There is evidence that toxic intermediates play a role in both types of injury.

Drug-Induced Cholestasis: Chlorpromazine: Clinically apparent cholestatic hepatitis affects 1–2% of patients taking the phenothiazine tranquilizer, chlorpromazine. Chlorpromazine metabolites are thought to cause toxic damage to the bile secretory mechanism. Overt hepatitis characteristically appears during the second to fourth week after patients start the drug. The first phase is a prodrome similar to that in viral hepatitis, with fever, chills, malaise, and anorexia; patients may also have pruritus, arthralgias, and lymphadenopathy. Several days after the onset of constitutional symptoms, patients develop jaundice. Both liver function tests and liver biopsy reveal cholestatic hepatitis. In most patients, the liver function abnormalities resolve gradually over 4–8 weeks after the drug is stopped. In rare patients, the cholestatic reaction has been reported to progress, even to frank biliary cirrhosis.

Hepatic Effects of Oral Contraceptives: Several important side effects of oral contraceptives involve the liver. These effects are caused by the pills' conjugated estrogens, not their progestins. Pills with a lower estrogen content cause fewer hepatic side effects. In susceptible women, jaundice and pruritus begin within the first six cycles of pills and may appear during the first month. (These women are likely to develop a similar syndrome during pregnancy.) Serum bilirubin rarely exceeds 5 mg/dL. Serum alkaline phosphatase and aminotransferases are slightly elevated. Liver biopsy typically shows cholestasis without inflammation. The cholestasis and jaundice usually subside within 1 month after patients stop the pill.

A rare complication of oral contraceptives is formation of hepatic adenoma. This is a benign tumor found almost exclusively in women taking oral contraceptives. In 50% of patients, the adenoma is an asymptomatic mass discovered on routine exam; in the remainder, it is associated with right upper quadrant pain. Patients may have few if any biochemical abnormalities. Occasionally, the adenoma ruptures and causes an intra-abdominal hemorrhage. Some liver cell adenomas regress when patients stop birth control pills.

Other important considerations in the differential diagnosis of intrahepatic masses are hemangioma, a common, benign tumor; hepatocellular carcinoma, for which risk increases slightly with contraceptive use; and focal nodular hyperplasia, which is found much more often in women than men but has not been clearly linked to contraceptives. Hepatic vein thrombosis (Budd-Chiari syndrome) has also been associated with contraceptives.

ISCHEMIC HEPATITIS

Ischemic injury to the liver is an occasional cause of acute hepatitis. Most patients have underlying heart disease, particularly right-sided congestive heart failure leading to passive congestion, which renders the liver more susceptible to ischemic injury. At acute risk are patients with cardiogenic or hypovolemic shock. Most investigators believe that the ischemic injury results from a period of ischemia followed by reperfusion leading to formation of reactive oxygen metabolites that cause oxidant stress to the hepatocytes.

Clinically, ischemic hepatitis is characterized by right upper quadrant pain and tenderness, hepatomegaly, and nausea. Jaundice is uncommon. Many patients have striking aspartate aminotransferase (AST) and alanine aminotransferase (ALT) elevations similar to those often seen after acetaminophen poisoning. The aminotransferases rise abruptly 12–24 hours after the ischemic insult and decline gradually over the next 5–10 days. The AST generally falls faster than the ALT; this can be a clue to the etiology. Most patients recover completely.

ALCOHOLIC LIVER DISEASE

Alcohol is the most common cause of drug-induced liver injury. Unlike most drugs that damage the liver, alcohol toxicity develops not with short-term use but after years of regular heavy drinking. Controversy continues over whether toxicity is dose-related or whether there is a threshold above which toxicity is more likely to develop. The risk of liver damage is known to be higher in men who drink more than 60–80 g (four to six 6 drinks) per day. It is surprising that the prevalence of serious alcohol-related liver damage is low, even in alcoholics. Only 15–20% of alcoholics develop cirrhosis, precursor lesions, or alcoholic hepatitis.

Women are more susceptible than men to the hepatotoxicity of alcohol. Women are at higher risk for liver damage if they drink more than 40–60 g (three to four drinks) per day. There are a number of potential explanations for women's higher risk. The pharmacokinetics of ethanol are different in women and men. Women metabolize less alcohol in the gastric mucosa, allowing for greater absorption and exposure of the liver to ethanol. Furthermore, differences in body composition make women's blood alcohol levels higher. Ethanol distributes preferentially into total body water, which for women is a lower percentage of body weight. The combination of these pharmacokinetic differences accounts for women's greater risk of liver damage.

Ethanol can exacerbate underlying liver disease. There is some evidence that heavy drinkers run an unusually high risk of chronic hepatitis C progressing to cirrhosis. In addition, heterozygotes for α_1-antitrypsin deficiency seem more likely to develop cirrhosis after drinking relatively modest amounts of alcohol.

The mechanism or, more likely, mechanisms of alcoholic liver damage remain unproven. The low incidence of liver injury among heavy drinkers, the long exposure required to produce damage, the lack of a clear dose-response relationship, and clinical features such as fever and leukocytosis suggest that ethanol is not a direct hepatotoxin. Nevertheless, the cause of the disease clearly is ethanol, not other factors like associated nutritional deficiencies.

Female sex and genetic susceptibility contribute significantly to the risk of liver damage in heavy drinkers. Nutritional deficiencies are common in patients with advanced alcoholic liver disease, but malnutrition is more likely a consequence of liver injury than a cause. Specific nutritional deficiencies, particularly of antioxidants, may contribute to risk of injury, but definitive proof is lacking. The type of alcoholic beverage consumed is not important, but the drinking pattern may be: Heavy daily drinking is riskier than sporadic binge drinking.

Spectrum of Alcoholic Liver Disease

Alcoholic liver disease has three broad categories: fatty infiltration of the liver, alcoholic hepatitis, and cirrhosis—the end result of collagen deposition and hepatic regeneration. Cirrhosis is termed "active" if the liver still has evidence of inflammation and "inactive" for fibrosis and regeneration without inflammation (Chapter 7.4).

More than one-third of heavy drinkers have fatty infiltration of the liver. This rarely leads to specific symptoms, but patients occasionally have right upper quadrant discomfort, nausea, and vomiting. Hepatomegaly is caused by the accumulation of triglycerides in hepatocytes. The enlargement may cause pain from stretching of Glisson's capsule. Few patients have jaundice, and it is usually minimal. The aminotransferases may be normal or mildly elevated, with the AST higher than the ALT, a relationship not usually seen in viral or other drug-induced hepatitis. γ-Glutamyl transpeptidase (GGT) is often elevated, but alkaline phosphatase, albumin, and prothrombin time remain normal. On ultrasonography, the liver has increased echogenicity, and on computed tomography, the attenuation of the liver is decreased by the presence of fat.

Alcoholic hepatitis is both a clinical syndrome and a pattern of pathologic changes in the liver. The clinical syndrome is characterized by jaundice, malaise, anorexia, nausea and vomiting, and right upper quadrant pain. Many patients with alcoholic hepatitis have fever unrelated to infection. The sickest patients have ascites, edema, and hepatic encephalopathy. Hepatomegaly is common, but splenomegaly is found only in patients with associated portal hypertension.

Abnormalities in aminotransferases and other liver enzymes are similar to those in patients with fatty liver. In addition, the bilirubin is high and the albumin is low. A prothrombin time prolonged by more than 4 seconds beyond control (ie, prolonged beyond 16 seconds) is a poor prognostic sign, as is marked hyperbilirubinemia. Many patients have mild leukocytosis (15,000–20,000 white blood cells/μL) and many have a mild multifactorial anemia. Other laboratory abnormalities have been described: low serum zinc, high ferritin, low transferrin, low retinol binding protein, and low prealbumin. Most of these features are believed to result from elevated levels of cytokines, particularly tumor necrosis factor-α and interleukins 1 and 6.

The natural history of alcoholic hepatitis is much different from that of simple fatty infiltration of the liver. Patients with fatty liver have a good prognosis. With abstinence, almost all recover completely. In contrast, alcoholic hepatitis often progresses to cirrhosis, particularly in persons who continue to drink. Even with abstinence, 20–25% of patients develop cirrhosis. The prognosis is worse for patients with hepatic encephalopathy unrelated to bleeding or infection and for those with ascites and clinical signs of malnutrition. The short-term mortality of these patients with severe alcoholic hepatitis is over 50%.

Role of Liver Biopsy: Liver biopsy is useful to confirm a diagnosis of alcoholic liver disease, assess its severity, and predict prognosis. The risks of liver biopsy are minimal for patients who clot normally, unless they have ascites. Occasionally, liver biopsy shows more advanced disease than that suspected clinically; this news may help motivate patients to abstain from drinking. Some studies suggest that biopsy detects nonalcoholic liver disease in 15–20% of alcoholics. In patients who have positive serologies for hepatitis C, biopsy can distinguish between viral hepatitis and alcohol as the major cause of liver disease.

Management of Alcoholic Hepatitis and Fatty Liver

Abstinence from alcohol is the cornerstone of managing all forms of alcoholic liver injury. Abstinence improves the rate and completeness of recovery and reduces complications such as gastrointestinal bleeding and infections. The physician should devote considerable effort to treating the underlying alcoholism (Chapter 14.4). To ensure complete abstinence while preventing serious withdrawal complications, the physician should have most patients with serious liver disease begin treatment in the hospital.

Restoring adequate nutrition is critical to recovery from alcoholic hepatitis. Patients with serious alcoholic liver disease have poor nutritional reserve, and many worsen unless they are given nutritional supplements early in treatment. The anorexia and nausea that accompany alcoholic hepatitis have spurred research into the value of both enteral and parenteral nutritional supplements. Although supplements do not reduce mortality, they improve the rate of recovery from both mild and severe alcoholic hepatitis. Patients should be offered a high-protein (1.0–1.5 g/kg), high-calorie diet. Enteral feeding is preferred, but some people benefit from parenteral supplements. Patients should also be given multivitamins, thiamine, and vitamin E.

Many specific treatments have been evaluated. Propylthiouracil, colchicine, and insulin-glucagon infusions have all been reported to improve recovery from alcoholic hepatitis, but have not become part of standard treatment.

Patients with just fatty liver or with mild-to-moderate alcoholic hepatitis require only abstinence and nutritional support.

Severity of alcoholic hepatitis is best predicted by:

$$\text{Severity} = [\text{prothrombin time} \times 4.6] + \text{total bilirubin}$$

Prothrombin time is measured in seconds, and bilirubin in mg/dL. Patients with a severity above 90 have only a 50% chance of surviving 30 days. These findings underscore the importance of laboratory tests in dictating management decisions in alcoholic hepatitis.

Short-term mortality in patients with severe alcoholic hepatitis has been reduced significantly by prednisolone 32 mg per day for 1 month. Thus, patients with severe disease should be treated with corticosteroids unless they have specific contraindications such as active infection, a positive PPD (purified protein derivative) test for tuberculosis, HIV infection, hepatitis B infection, or gastrointestinal bleeding.

Some patients with alcoholic hepatitis have active cirrhosis and portal hypertension. The evaluation and management of cirrhosis and the complications of portal hypertension are discussed in Chapters 7.4 and 7.5.

SUMMARY

▶ The five viruses that cause hepatitis cannot be distinguished by clinical features but are readily differentiated by serologic testing.

▶ Hepatitis C causes chronic infection in 70% of those infected, and hepatitis B becomes chronic in 5–10% of those infected as adults. Both types of chronic hepatitis can progress to cirrhosis, and 10% of patients with cirrhosis develop hepatocellular carcinoma.

▶ Vaccination against hepatitis B prevents the infection and its complications.

▶ Drugs can damage the liver either as direct hepatotoxins that reproducibly cause dose-related injury or as idiosyncratic toxins that affect only susceptible hosts who have a metabolic abnormality or allergic reaction.

▶ Although alcohol is a major cause of liver damage, only 15–20% of heavy drinkers—more women than men—develop serious disease (alcoholic hepatitis, cirrhosis). Alcoholic hepatitis should be managed with abstinence, improved nutrition, supportive care, and, for severe disease, prednisolone.

SUGGESTED READING

Hoofnagle JH, Di Bisceglie AM: Serologic diagnosis of acute and chronic viral hepatitis. Semin Liver Dis 1991;11:73.

Margolis HS, Alter MJ, Hadler SC: Hepatitis B: Evolving epidemiology and implications for control. Semin Liver Dis 1991;11:84.

Mitchell MC: Pathogenesis of alcoholic liver disease. In: *Liver and Biliary Diseases.* Kaplowitz N (editor). Williams & Wilkins, 1992.

Seeff LB: Hepatitis C. Semin Liver Dis 1995;15:1.

Zeldis JB: Molecular biology of viral hepatitis and liver cancer. In: *Liver and Biliary Diseases.* Kaplowitz N (editor). Williams & Wilkins, 1992.

Chronic Liver Disease

H. Franklin Herlong, MD, and Anna Mae Diehl, MD

In contrast to liver diseases that generally present as an acute illness (Chapter 7.3), this chapter concerns liver diseases that more often manifest subtly, evolving over months or years, or that manifest only with laboratory abnormalities. These disorders are (1) inherited diseases of the liver, primarily α_1-antitrypsin deficiency, hemochromatosis, and Wilson's disease (Table 7.4–1); (2) autoimmune diseases of the liver, which are autoimmune hepatitis, primary biliary cirrhosis, and sclerosing cholangitis (Table 7.4–2); and (3) hepatic effects of systemic disease, such as granulomatous hepatitis (Table 7.4–3), Budd-Chiari syndrome secondary to estrogen-induced hypercoagulability, hepatic schistosomiasis, and nonalcoholic steatohepatitis.

LIVER BIOPSY

Liver biopsy permits the staging of the extent and severity of hepatic injury and scarring. The liver's histologic appearance gives some insight into the speed with which liver damage is likely to progress. *Chronic persistent hepatitis* describes a stage of chronic liver injury in which inflammatory infiltration is limited largely to portal triads. If the disease remains at this stage, the patient is unlikely to develop overt liver disease soon; clinical manifestations like jaundice or ascites may appear only if the secondary fibrotic response compromises small vessels and bile ducts in multiple portal triads.

In contrast, *chronic active hepatitis* describes a stage of chronic liver injury in which the inflammatory cells spill out of the portal triads and into adjacent parenchyma. Hepatocytes rimming the portal triad (the "limiting plate" of hepatocytes) are the first to be attacked. Some of these cells are killed (piecemeal necrosis); others are isolated from their normal vascular and stromal contacts by encroaching fibrous tissue. Chronic active hepatitis is likely to lead to progressive—and, eventually, clinically overt—liver damage. As waves of necrosis and secondary fibrosis extend out from multiple portal areas into the liver lobule, they form "bridges" of necrosis and fibrosis that link portal areas. Over time, the fibrotic bridges carve the liver lobule into nodules of parenchyma.

Cirrhosis is a descriptive term for the distortion of normal hepatic architecture that results from progressive hepatocyte necrosis (chronic "hepatitis"), compensatory liver cell proliferation, and associated fibrosis. Cirrhosis is the final stage that chronic liver diseases can reach when the complications of portal hypertension develop. But it is more useful to speak specifically of each disease than to use the generic term "cirrhosis."

Chronic "persistent" and chronic "active" hepatitis are different stages of the same process. In some patients whose index biopsy reveals chronic persistent hepatitis, the process becomes more aggressive; later biopsies may show chronic active hepatitis and eventually cirrhosis. Conversely, treatment can reverse the changes of chronic active hepatitis, so that later biopsies reveal only chronic persistent hepatitis. The intensity of histologic necrosis, inflammation, and fibrosis indicates how soon cirrhosis may develop. Hence, biopsy is the most sensitive and specific test for both detecting chronic liver damage and estimating the rate of disease progression. But because biopsy is invasive, it should be considered only when histologic confirmation is needed to guide management.

Having identified potentially progressive liver disease, the physician should focus on finding the cause of the liver disease in order to interrupt the pathogenetic process and on controlling the clinical complications of liver failure and portal hypertension.

INHERITED LIVER DISEASES

α_1-Antitrypsin Deficiency

The glycoprotein α_1-antitrypsin, the major inhibitor of circulating proteases (Pi), accounts for most circulating α_1-globulin. Hepatic synthesis of α_1-antitrypsin is controlled by multiple alleles. The most common normal allele is designated "M," and the normal phenotype is

Table 7.4–1. Inherited liver diseases.

	Biochemical Features	Associated Disorders	Treatment
α_1-antitrypsin deficiency	↓ α_1-globulin PiZZ phenotype	Lower-lobe emphysema	Liver transplantation
Hemochromatosis	↑ transferrin saturation ↑ ferritin	Arthritis, congestive heart failure, arrhythmias, diabetes, impotence, gray skin	Phlebotomy, deferoxamine, liver transplantation
Wilson's disease	↓ serum ceruloplasmin ↑ urine copper ↓ serum total copper ↑ free copper ↑ hepatic copper	Kayser-Fleischer ring, movement disorders, personality changes, hemolysis, renal tubular defects, premature osteoarthritis	Penicillamine, zinc, liver transplantation

"PiMM." Although uncommon, the abnormal haplotype most often producing liver disease is PiZZ; patients with PiZZ have less than 20% of normal serum α_1-antitrypsin activity. The liver disease presumably results from an inability to transfer the abnormal α_1-antitrypsin from its site of synthesis in the liver to the serum. α_1-Antitrypsin deficiency does not produce specific symptoms of liver disease, but 10–15% of adults with the PiZZ phenotype eventually develop cirrhosis. In some patients, pulmonary involvement leads to emphysema.

The diagnostic criteria for α_1-antitrypsin deficiency are (1) no α_1-globulin peak on serum protein electrophoresis, (2) a low serum α_1-antitrypsin level, and (3) an abnormal Pi phenotype. Liver biopsy is not essential to the diagnosis, but it is helpful in establishing the severity of liver disease. The typical histologic changes in α_1-antitrypsin deficiency are multiple periodic acid-Schiff (PAS)-positive diastase-resistant round bodies in the cytoplasm of hepatocytes. The degree of fibrosis is variable. It is not known whether heterozygotes for PiZ (eg, PiMZ) are at increased risk for significant liver disease. Patients with

PiZZ and cirrhosis are at increased risk for developing hepatocellular carcinoma.

There is no effective therapy for the liver disease caused by α_1-antitrypsin deficiency. Liver transplantation should be considered for patients who have severe liver disease and enough pulmonary function for the operation.

Hemochromatosis

Hemochromatosis is a disease of iron overload. In primary hemochromatosis, total body iron stores are increased from the normal 4 g, up to 50 g. Inherited as an autosomal recessive trait, primary hemochromatosis is the most common genetic liver disease, occurring in about 1 in 500 persons worldwide. Although the hemochromatosis gene has been localized to the region of the sixth chromosome near the HLA complex, the gene product responsible for the clinical manifestations has not been identified. However, it is likely that the defect results in abnormal regulation of intestinal iron absorption.

In most patients with hemochromatosis, the clinical manifestations appear only after age 40 years. Symptoms

Table 7.4–2. Autoimmune liver diseases.

	Biochemical Features	Serologic Tests	Associated Disorders	Treatment
Primary biliary cirrhosis	↑↑ alkaline phosphatase ↑ IgM ↑ AST and ALT ↑ bilirubin	Antimitochondrial antibody	Thyroiditis, renal tubular acidosis, rheumatoid arthritis, CREST syndrome	Ursodeoxycholic acid, liver transplantation
Sclerosing cholangitis	↑↑ alkaline phosphatase ↑ bilirubin ↑ AST and ALT	Antineutrophilic nuclear antibody	Ulcerative colitis, Crohn's disease, bacterial cholangitis, 5-FUDR treatment	Ursodeoxycholic acid, balloon dilatation, liver transplantation
Autoimmune hepatitis				
Subtype 1	↑↑ AST and ALT ↑ alkaline phosphatase ↑ globulins	Antinuclear antibody, anti–smooth muscle antibody	Amenorrhea, acne, immune thrombocytopenic purpura, Coombs-positive anemia, thyroiditis	Corticosteroids, azathioprine
Subtype 2		Liver-kidney microsomal antibody		
Subtype 3		Soluble liver antigen antibody		

AST, aspartate aminotransferase; ALT, alanine aminotransferase; FUDR, 5-fluorouracil.

Table 7.4–3. Granulomatous liver diseases.

Condition	Tests
Sarcoidosis	Biopsy showing noncaseating granulomas in ≥2 organs; ↑ angiotensin converting enzyme level
Infections	
Tuberculosis	PPD, liver biopsy with stain and cultures
Brucellosis	Culture, antibody titers
Syphilis	Fluorescent treponemal antibody-absorption test (FTA-ABS)
Histoplasmosis	Chest x-ray, antibody titers
Epstein-Barr	Monospot, Epstein-Barr antibodies
Cytomegalovirus	IgM anticytomegalovirus
Schistosomiasis	Rectal biopsy
Drugs: allopurinol, phenylbutazone, quinidine	History
Berylliosis	Industrial exposure; chest x-ray, urine beryllium level
Primary biliary cirrhosis	Mitochondrial antibody
Crohn's disease	Endoscopy, barium enema, colonic biopsy

PPD, purified protein derivative.

develop earlier in men than in women, probably because menstrual loss of iron delays the onset in women. Even though hemochromatosis is common, the diagnosis is often not made until patients have developed clinical sequelae. Extrahepatic manifestations produce the earliest signs and symptoms: Hemochromatosis should be suspected in patients who present with unexplained arthritis, particularly pseudogout. Many patients have endocrine disorders such as impotence. Seventy-five percent of all patients with hemochromatosis have diabetes, sometimes with retinopathy, nephropathy, and neuropathy.

Symptomatic heart and liver disease are late manifestations of hemochromatosis. The liver disease produces nonspecific symptoms, most often fatigue and malaise. The liver becomes enlarged only late in the disease. By the time they are diagnosed, many patients already have cirrhosis, often with signs of portal hypertension—splenomegaly, esophageal varices, and ascites. About 25–40% of patients with hemochromatosis develop hepatocellular carcinoma.

Iron deposition in the heart can cause congestive heart failure or, more commonly, supraventricular and ventricular tachyarrhythmias. The congestive heart failure of hemochromatosis often resists the usual therapies for congestive heart failure. Atrioventricular node involvement can lead to heart block.

"Bronzing" of the skin is considered a sign of he-mochromatosis, but is rare. More commonly, the skin is slate gray because of melanin deposition in the basal layers of a thin epidermis.

Hemochromatosis is confirmed by an elevated fasting serum iron saturation of the serum transferrin (>62% for men, >55% for premenopausal women), an elevated serum ferritin, and a high tissue iron level on liver biopsy. The combination of a high transferrin saturation and an elevated serum ferritin is 94% sensitive and 86% specific for hemochromatosis. Considerable iron may be deposited in the liver before the aminotransferases rise. The hepatic iron index is particularly useful in differentiating hemochromatosis from secondary iron overload caused by chronic alcoholism. This index is calculated by dividing the hepatic iron concentration (μg/g of liver tissue) by the patient's age. The index, however, cannot accurately differentiate hemochromatosis from other forms of secondary iron deposition such as chronic hemolytic disorders and multiple transfusions.

Hemochromatosis is managed by repeated phlebotomies to remove excess tissue iron. Patients should have weekly venisections of 500 mL until their serum ferritin falls to 50 μg/dL. Removing iron is most useful when started early in the disease, because removal may do little to reverse late complications such as testicular fibrosis, portal hypertension, and heart disease. Occasionally, patients with hemochromatosis develop chronic refractory anemias. In these patients, venisection is usually not possible; instead, the treatment is chelation with deferoxamine.

Relatives of patients with hemochromatosis should be screened to detect disease before symptoms begin, when therapy is most useful. If a patient's siblings have the patient's HLA haplotype, they are almost sure to be homozygous for primary hemochromatosis. Rarely, spontaneous chromosomal breaks and recombinations result in inheritance of a similar HLA haplotype without inheritance of the tightly linked abnormal iron gene.

Wilson's Disease

Wilson's disease results from an inability to excrete copper from liver cells into the bile, leading to copper accumulations in the liver, central nervous system, cornea, and kidneys. The cause is a genetic defect involving an ATPase that regulates copper transport. Inherited as an autosomal recessive trait, Wilson's disease is the rarest inherited disorder of the liver, affecting about 1 in 300,000 persons worldwide.

Signs and symptoms of Wilson's disease commonly appear by adolescence. Patients may have hepatic or neurologic symptoms, separately or in combination. The hepatic symptoms are nonspecific, most often malaise and fatigue. Jaundice is rare. A few patients present with fulminant hepatic failure, which tends to be complicated by hemolysis. The neurologic symptoms, resulting from copper deposition in the basal ganglia, include rigidity, choreoathetoid movements, and ataxia. Copper deposition in the kidneys causes aminoaciduria, uric aciduria, and phosphaturia. Eye involvement is of particular diagnostic importance: The Kayser-Fleischer ring is a circle of greenish-brown pigment in the periphery of the cornea, caused by copper deposition. Rare patients have only hepatic biochemical abnormalities. Biochemical manifestations are a low serum ceruloplasmin level, a high hepatic copper, and a high urinary copper excretion.

Excess copper is chelated with penicillamine. Many patients require lifetime therapy. Patients with fulminant hepatic failure from Wilson's disease and those with end-stage cirrhosis should be considered for liver transplantation.

AUTOIMMUNE LIVER DISEASE

Primary Biliary Cirrhosis

Primary biliary cirrhosis is a disease of unknown cause that accounts for about 10% of chronic liver disease in women but rarely affects men. The disorder is characterized by progressive—presumably autoimmune—destruction of the smallest bile ducts in the liver. Many patients have biochemical disease for a long time before symptoms appear, but most eventually develop symptoms caused by cholestasis and portal hypertension. The most common symptom is pruritus; it is most severe in the evening and during the summer, and worst on the palms of the hands and soles of the feet. Many patients have fat malabsorption, which can lead to diarrhea. Many also have secondary malabsorption of fat-soluble vitamins. Dramatic hypercholesterolemia is common, with serum cholesterol levels often over 500 mg/dL. It is surprising that patients do not have accelerated atherosclerosis.

The diagnosis requires a combination of clinical, biochemical, serologic, and histologic data. The biochemical profile typically reflects chronic cholestasis. Virtually all patients have high serum alkaline phosphatase, although the extent of elevation does not correlate with the severity of disease. The aminotransferases are modestly elevated, but are not helpful in following the disease course. The blood of more than 95% of patients contains antimitochondrial antibody anti-M_2, directed toward the pyruvate dehydrogenase complex on the inner membrane of the mitochondrion. This antibody is specific to primary biliary cirrhosis.

The severity of primary biliary cirrhosis can be graded by its appearance on liver biopsy. In the earliest stage (grade 1), intense chronic inflammation, often with granulomas, is seen around septal and interlobular bile ducts. As the disease progresses, fibrosis becomes more severe and eventually the bile ducts disappear. Grade 4 is a true histologic cirrhosis with few or no bile ducts.

Management is directed at controlling the symptoms of chronic cholestasis and trying to retard disease progression. Cholestyramine, an ionic resin, binds potential pruritogens in the gut and alleviates most patients' pruri-

tus. Antihistamines are of little value. Malabsorption of fat-soluble vitamins responds to parenteral supplementation.

Medical therapy for primary biliary cirrhosis remains controversial. Although the disease presumably has an immunologic basis, immunosuppressive drug treatment has been disappointing. Ursodeoxycholic acid improves liver function tests and alleviates pruritus in some patients, but whether it slows disease progression is less clear. Primary biliary cirrhosis is the second most common indication for liver transplantation in adults and accounts for about 25% of all liver transplantations performed. Transplantation should be considered for patients with severe jaundice and for those in whom complications of hepatic insufficiency and portal hypertension become refractory to medical therapy.

Sclerosing Cholangitis

Like primary biliary cirrhosis, primary sclerosing cholangitis seems to be an autoimmune phenomenon, but it destroys the larger intrahepatic and extrahepatic bile ducts. Unlike primary biliary cirrhosis, sclerosing cholangitis primarily affects men, and 70% of patients also have inflammatory bowel disease, most often ulcerative colitis. Sclerosing cholangitis is the most common cause of progressive liver disease in patients with ulcerative colitis, affecting about 5%.

Genetic factors play a role in sclerosing cholangitis. About 60% of patients have the HLA-B8 haplotype. In genetically predisposed persons, the bile duct injury seems to be triggered by some exogenous factor, perhaps a virus or bacterium. Unlike primary biliary cirrhosis, sclerosing cholangitis is not associated with a specific antibody like the antimitochondrial antibody anti-M_2. Some patients have high titers of antineutrophilic antibody, but its pathogenetic role has not been identified.

Secondary sclerosing cholangitis is caused by damage to the bile ducts from infection, ischemia, or toxic injury. The arterial blood supply of the common bile duct may be damaged during biliary tract surgery. Ischemic injuries can also be caused by radiation therapy or chemotherapy with intra-arterial 5-fluorouracil deoxyribonucleoside (5-FUDR) infusion. Patients with AIDS develop a biliary tract disease with some of the clinical features of sclerosing cholangitis, caused by opportunistic infection with *Cryptosporidium* or cytomegalovirus. Occasionally, the biliary tract is involved in systemic fibrosing disorders such as retroperitoneal fibrosis, Peyronie's disease, and mediastinal fibrosis.

The preferred test for sclerosing cholangitis is endoscopic retrograde cholangiography. The typical finding is alternating areas of dilatation and stricture in both the intrahepatic and extrahepatic bile ducts. Rare patients have isolated intra- or extrahepatic involvement. Liver biopsy is usually not needed to diagnose sclerosing cholangitis, but may be helpful in following patients' response to therapy.

As with primary biliary cirrhosis, treatment is directed toward controlling the complications of cholestasis and preventing disease progression. Pruritus and malabsorption are treated the same way in both diseases. Patients with sclerosing cholangitis have frequent episodes of bacterial cholangitis, which usually respond to intravenous antibiotics; most patients receive prophylactic oral antibiotics to reduce the number of episodes. If a single dominant stricture causes biliary obstruction, balloon dilatation of the stricture may improve bile flow. About 10% of patients with sclerosing cholangitis develop cholangiocarcinoma. It is suggested by worsening jaundice, weight loss, and abdominal pain, but is very difficult to diagnose early enough to resect.

Most patients with sclerosing cholangitis are given ursodeoxycholic acid. As with primary biliary cirrhosis, many patients have biochemical improvement, but no proven slowing of disease progression. Liver transplantation should be considered for patients who develop ascites, severe jaundice, complications of portal hypertension, or progressive liver failure.

Autoimmune Hepatitis

Accounting for about 10% of chronic liver disease, autoimmune hepatitis is characterized by progressive injury to hepatocytes, caused by abnormalities in immunoregulation. About 75% of patients are women, and most patients are younger than 30 years. The onset of autoimmune hepatitis is usually insidious, although occasional patients present with symptoms of acute hepatitis, mainly jaundice, fatigue, malaise, and arthralgias. The disease is arbitrarily designated "chronic" if it lasts for more than 6 months. However, the physician should consider this diagnosis before waiting 6 months, since prompt corticosteroid therapy can significantly reduce morbidity and mortality.

Autoimmune hepatitis is most often diagnosed when asymptomatic persons are found to have elevated liver enzyme levels or when patients are evaluated for extrahepatic symptoms such as amenorrhea, fatigue, arthralgias, or hemolytic anemia. The physician must exclude toxic, metabolic, and viral conditions for which specific tests are available *and* must identify typical biochemical and serologic features: elevated serum globulin levels, high titers of certain autoantibodies, plasma cell infiltrate on liver biopsy, and a favorable response to corticosteroid therapy. Subgroups of autoimmune hepatitis are identified by autoantibody patterns. The major features of subtype I (classic) are polyclonal hyperglobulinemia and antinuclear and anti-smooth muscle antibodies. Patients with subtype II have no antinuclear or anti-smooth muscle antibodies, but they do have anti-liver-kidney microsomal antibodies (anti-LKM-1). Patients with subtype III also lack antinuclear and anti-smooth muscle antibodies, but have antisoluble liver antigen antibodies.

Moderate doses of corticosteroids promptly relieve the symptoms of autoimmune hepatitis and lower aminotransferase levels. Azathioprine can be used to reduce the needed dose of corticosteroid, particularly in elderly patients who are at high risk for steroid side effects. After 6 months of therapy, the immunosuppressive regimen is slowly tapered. Many patients relapse after stopping treatment, but in most, starting prednisone again (with or without azathioprine) brings the disease back under control.

HEPATIC EFFECTS OF SYSTEMIC DISEASE

Granulomatous Liver Disease

Granulomatous inflammation is found in 5–10% of liver biopsy specimens. In about 25% of these cases, histologic characteristics, culture, and special stains fail to reveal a specific cause. But most hepatic granulomas are part of a generalized multiorgan condition. Sarcoidosis and tuberculosis account for about 50% of cases of multiorgan involvement; many of the rest are caused by drug reactions or infections, some ubiquitous (eg, cytomegalovirus, syphilis), others with geographic concentrations (eg, schistosomiasis, histoplasmosis).

Some patients with granulomatous liver inflammation develop a prolonged febrile illness. In many of these patients, no infectious cause is ever found; the disorder is labeled "idiopathic granulomatous hepatitis." Typically, these patients have modestly elevated aminotransferases, and many have a significantly elevated alkaline phosphatase. Only rare patients develop jaundice. After infectious causes have been ruled out, many of these patients are treated with corticosteroids, which ameliorate both symptoms and biochemical abnormalities.

Budd-Chiari Syndrome

The Budd-Chiari syndrome is a rare disorder caused by occlusion of hepatic veins. In most patients, it develops acutely; some die within days. Other patients develop symptoms and signs like abdominal pain, massive ascites, and tender hepatomegaly over weeks. Eventually, patients may bleed from esophageal varices caused by portal hypertension. Predisposing factors include polycythemia vera, estrogens, pregnancy, hepatocellular carcinoma, and hypercoagulable states secondary to disorders such as paroxysmal nocturnal hemoglobinuria. Symptoms can also be caused by veno-occlusive disease, a concentric narrowing of the terminal hepatic veins and sinusoids, most often affecting allogeneic bone marrow transplant recipients who have undergone radiotherapy and chemotherapy. Worldwide, the most common cause of Budd-Chiari syndrome is membranous occlusion of the suprahepatic vena cava. But in the United States, the most common cause is thrombosis of the hepatic veins, with or without vena cava involvement.

It is surprising that laboratory tests of liver function in Budd-Chiari syndrome show only mild abnormalities. The diagnosis is confirmed by venography showing occluded hepatic veins; sometimes the veins have partially reopened. The caudate lobe of the liver drains directly into the vena cava, and so is infrequently involved in the Budd-Chiari syndrome. As a result, the caudate lobe often hypertrophies and can compress the intrahepatic segment of the vena cava.

Thrombolytic therapy is rarely successful in the treatment of patients with Budd-Chiari syndrome. Most patients need surgery. Peritoneovenous shunts may palliate ascites, but they do nothing to improve the underlying disease. Surgical removal of the venous obstruction is limited to patients with membranous caval webs. Hepatic vein and venal caval thromboses cannot be excised. Patients who have not developed cirrhosis from chronic congestion can be given some form of portosystemic shunt. If the abdominal vena caval pressure is acceptable, a mesocaval shunt converts the portal vein from an inflow to an outflow tract. If the vena cava is occluded or the pressure is too high, a mesoatrial shunt is constructed. Liver transplantation should be considered for patients with advanced liver disease and those who present with the rare fulminant form of Budd-Chiari syndrome.

Hepatic Schistosomiasis

Hepatic schistosomiasis is the most common cause of portal hypertension in the world. The major clinical manifestation of hepatic schistosomiasis is bleeding esophageal varices. This presinusoidal form of portal hypertension rarely causes jaundice, ascites, or hepatic encephalopathy.

Liver disease develops when the ova of *Schistosoma mansoni*, released by mature schistosomes in the mesenteric veins, lodge in the liver's terminal portal veins. The ova elicit a granulomatous response that causes fibrosis and resistance to portal blood flow. Hepatocytes suffer little or no injury, so serum aminotransferase levels are often normal or only minimally elevated. Active schistosomal infection is diagnosed by finding organisms on rectal biopsy. Hepatic involvement is confirmed by finding ova in the portal areas of a liver biopsy. Active *Schistosoma mansoni* infection is treated with praziquantel.

Nonalcoholic Steatohepatitis

In patients who drink little or no alcohol, nonalcoholic steatosis (fatty degeneration) produces a histologic lesion identical with that caused by alcohol. Nonalcoholic steatohepatitis was first recognized in obese women and associated with obesity, diabetes, and hyperlipidemia. Now steatosis is known to be a common condition that can affect persons with normal weight and blood glucose. Intravenous hyperalimentation, jejunoileal bypass, and certain drugs (eg, glucocorticoids, amiodarone, methotrexate) can cause steatosis of the liver.

Most patients with steatosis are asymptomatic, although some complain of fatigue and malaise and some have tender hepatomegaly. The diagnosis is often made incidentally when mild aminotransferase elevations are discovered during a routine examination or when a patient is being evaluated for another disorder such as coronary artery disease or hypertension. The aminotransferases are usually less than twice normal; few patients have the typi-

cal ratio of aspartate aminotransferase (AST) to alanine aminotransferase (ALT) seen in alcoholic liver disease (AST:ALT > 2:1). The most reliable way to diagnose nonalcoholic steatohepatitis is with a liver biopsy that reveals steatosis with mild inflammation. Ultrasonography usually shows a hyperechogenic pattern characteristic of fatty liver, but cannot reliably distinguish steatohepatitis from other liver disorders. A lower CT number on computed tomography also suggests fatty liver.

The natural history of nonalcoholic steatosis is most often indolent, with gradual development of fibrosis. No specific therapy has been established, but recommended empiric management is for patients to lose weight and control their carbohydrate and lipid disorders.

LIVER TRANSPLANTATION

Liver transplantation offers the most effective treatment for patients with advanced liver disease. It is the only way to improve the long-term survival of patients with clinically decompensated cirrhosis. Not all patients with advanced liver disease are candidates for transplantation. Given the risks of perioperative morbidity and mortality, the procedure's expense, and the scarcity of donor organs, patients are carefully screened to exclude concurrent conditions (eg, malignancy, HIV infection, advanced disease in other vital organs, intractable substance abuse) before being offered transplantation as an option. More than 85% of transplant recipients are alive 5 years postoperatively. Most postoperative deaths are from infection and occur within the first 6 months. Most of the patients who survive the perioperative period regain full liver function. Late liver-related deaths are rare.

SUMMARY

▶ Unlike acute liver disease, chronic liver disease often presents with asymptomatic biochemical abnormalities or complications of portal hypertension.

▶ The most important inherited liver diseases are α_1-antitrypsin deficiency, hemochromatosis, and Wilson's disease. Symptoms of these diseases may not develop until adulthood.

▶ Autoimmune chronic liver diseases can involve the hepatocytes (autoimmune hepatitis) or the bile ducts (primary biliary cirrhosis, sclerosing cholangitis).

▶ The liver may be involved in systemic diseases such as granulomatous hepatitis, steatohepatitis, and hypercoagulable states that lead to the Budd-Chiari syndrome.

▶ Liver transplantation is the most effective treatment for patients with advanced liver disease who have no more medical options.

SUGGESTED READING

Conn HO, Atterbury CE: Cirrhosis. In: *Diseases of the Liver,* 7th ed. Schiff L, Schiff E (editors). JB Lippincott, 1993.

Maddrey WC, Combes B: Therapeutic concepts for the management of idiopathic autoimmune chronic hepatitis. Semin Liver Dis 1991;11:248.

Mitchell MC et al: Budd-Chiari syndrome: Etiology, diagnosis and management. Medicine (Baltimore) 1982;61:199.

Powell EE et al: The natural history of nonalcoholic steatohepatitis: A follow-up study of forty-two patients for up to 21 years. Hepatology 1990;11:74.

Stremmel W et al: Wilson's disease: Clinical presentation, treatment, and survival. Ann Intern Med 1991:115:720.

Complications of Portal Hypertension

H. Franklin Herlong, MD

Patients with portal hypertension can develop four major problems: ascites (accumulation of fluid in the abdomen), bacterial peritonitis (infection of peritoneal fluid), the hepatorenal syndrome (functional renal insufficiency caused by cirrhosis), and hepatic encephalopathy (alteration in brain function caused by toxins that the liver normally clears).

PATHOPHYSIOLOGY OF PORTAL HYPERTENSION

The portal vein is formed by the splenic vein and the superior mesenteric vein, which drains the intestinal capillaries (Figure 7.5–1).

Blood in the portal vein normally has a slightly higher pressure (pressure = 5–10 mm Hg) and a higher oxygen content than blood in the systemic veins. Because the portal vein has no valves, the pressure in the portal system normally depends on resistance to blood flow through the liver. When the portal vein reaches the liver, it divides into many small branches that deliver the blood to the extensive sinusoidal system. The hepatic artery usually arises from the celiac axis and enters the liver adjacent to the portal vein. The arterial blood supply also perfuses the hepatic sinusoids. After percolating through the sinusoids, blood is re-collected and discharged into the inferior vena cava via the hepatic veins.

Portal hypertension is a portal pressure that exceeds the inferior vena cava pressure by at least 5 mm Hg. The increase in pressure results either from an increase in blood flow in the portal venous system or from anatomic or functional obstruction to blood flow at any point from the portal system's origin in the splanchnic bed to its exit into the systemic circulation via the hepatic veins (Table 7.5–1). Blood flow may be obstructed by compression or thrombosis of the extrahepatic portal vein, inflammatory obliteration of intrahepatic portal and hepatic vein radicles, or distortion of intrahepatic architecture by collapse, infiltration, or regenerating nodules. Rarely, the major hepatic veins are blocked (Budd-Chiari syndrome), often in conjunction with obstruction in the inferior vena cava. Increased blood flow in the portal system may cause portal hypertension in patients with massive splenomegaly or arteriovenous fistulas or may contribute to portal hypertension in patients with other chronic liver diseases such as cirrhosis.

The causes of obstructive portal hypertension are grouped into two categories according to the site where blood flow is blocked: (1) before the hepatic sinusoids (prehepatic and presinusoidal) or (2) in and beyond them (sinusoidal, postsinusoidal, and posthepatic). Since portal pressure cannot be measured directly, measuring the wedged hepatic venous pressure gives an estimate of the portal venous pressure and helps determine what type of portal hypertension the patient has. The wedged hepatic venous pressure is measured by wedging an end-hole catheter, usually introduced percutaneously through a femoral vein into a peripheral hepatic venule. The catheter creates stasis that extends to the point of anastomotic collateral runoff into the hepatic sinusoids. An elevation in wedged hepatic venous pressure suggests increased resistance to collateral flow in the sinusoidal bed.

Presinusoidal portal hypertension is characterized by an elevated portal venous pressure and a normal wedged hepatic venous pressure, since the sinusoidal pressure is not elevated. Among the important causes of presinusoidal portal hypertension are portal vein thrombosis, schistosomiasis, and arteriovenous fistulas in the splanchnic bed. In patients with massive splenomegaly, increased blood flow in the portal venous system contributes to presinusoidal hypertension. Sinusoidal or postsinusoidal obstruction to portal flow is characterized by an elevated portal pressure and elevated wedged hepatic venous pressure and is found most often in patients with cirrhosis.

CONSEQUENCES OF PORTAL HYPERTENSION

The physiologic consequences of portal hypertension are related both to a decreased blood supply to the liver via the portal vein and to toxins bypassing the liver by shunting through collateral veins and going directly into the systemic circulation. The decrease in the portal com-

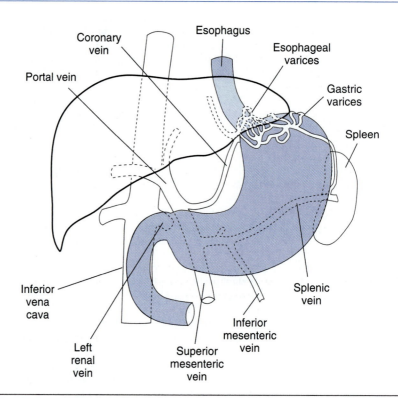

Figure 7.5–1. The portal system.

ponent of hepatic blood flow causes a compensatory increase in the hepatic arterial component, which maintains total liver blood flow at or near normal. The liver thereby becomes more dependent on arterial blood. The physiologic consequences of portal hypertension lead to the direct clinical consequences: bleeding gastroesophageal

Table 7.5–1. Classification of portal hypertension.

Increased resistance to blood flow in the portal venous system
  Prehepatic
    Portal vein thrombosis
    Compression by tumor
  Intrahepatic presinusoidal
    Schistosomiasis
    Sarcoidosis (rare)
    Myeloproliferative disorders (rare)
  Intrahepatic sinusoidal and postsinusoidal
    Alcoholic cirrhosis
    Posthepatitis cirrhosis
    Hemochromatosis
    Biliary cirrhosis
    Hepatolenticular degeneration (Wilson's disease)
    α_1-antitrypsin deficiency
    Veno-occlusive disease
  Posthepatic
    Hepatic venous obstruction (Budd-Chiari syndrome)
    Constrictive pericarditis
    Congestive heart failure

Increased flow in the portal venous system
  Massive splenomegaly
  Arteriovenous fistulas

varices, splenic congestion with hypersplenism, ascites, the hepatorenal syndrome, and hepatic encephalopathy.

Collateral blood vessels linking the portal and systemic veins commonly develop between the coronary vein of the portal system and the azygos veins of the caval system in the submucosa of the lower esophagus and upper part of the stomach (see Figure 7.5–1). These thin-walled vessels (gastroesophageal varices) are poorly supported by the underlying connective tissue and are a common site of major hemorrhage in patients with portal hypertension. One-third of patients with cirrhosis die from variceal hemorrhage (Chapter 6.5). Although gastroesophageal varices most often result from an elevation in portal pressure, an occasional patient has varices from superior vena cava or azygos vein obstruction ("downhill" varices).

Abdominal collateral vessels are prominent in some patients with portal hypertension, and are arranged radially from the umbilicus like the spokes of a wheel (caput medusae). These collateral vessels can be large and cause a vascular bruit (Cruveilhier-Baumgarten syndrome). Abdominal wall vessels may also dilate because of obstruction of either the superior or inferior vena cava, unrelated to portal hypertension. Observing the direction of blood flow in the collateral vessels is important for diagnosis. When portal hypertension causes dilated abdominal collateral vessels, the blood flows away from the umbilicus. In superior vena cava obstruction, the blood in the collateral vessels flows downward from the chest; in inferior vena cava obstruction, the blood flows upward.

Splenomegaly, caused by increased pressure in the splenic vein, is common in patients with an elevated portal venous pressure, but spleen size often does not correlate with the severity of portal hypertension. Hypersplenism causes thrombocytopenia, leukopenia, and anemia; here again, spleen size does not correlate with the severity of pancytopenia.

Ascites

Ascites (fluid in the peritoneal cavity) may be an isolated clinical finding or part of generalized fluid retention with edema. The most common disorders causing ascites are cirrhosis, tumors, and heart failure (Table 7.5–2). Less common causes are tuberculous peritonitis, the nephrotic syndrome, and pancreatitis. Small amounts of ascitic fluid (less than 1 L) may be difficult to detect, especially in obese patients. Both a high index of suspicion and careful physical examination are needed for diagnosis. The physical signs of ascites are bulging of the flanks and shifting dullness to percussion in the abdomen when the patient turns to one side. These signs are unreliable and may not appear until a considerable amount of fluid has accumulated. Ultrasonography of the abdomen is indicated to detect ascites in equivocal cases and to determine the best site for paracentesis in patients who have small amounts of ascites.

The ascitic fluid should be examined by a diagnostic paracentesis when ascites is first detected and in patients with known ascites who develop fever or a marked increase in ascitic fluid volume. Analysis should include determination of the protein and glucose content, amylase levels, blood cell counts and differential count, bacterial culture, fungal and acid-fast bacillus (AFB) cultures, pH, and cytologic exam. One factor helping to determine the cause of ascites is the ratio of serum albumin to ascitic fluid albumin. A ratio of at least 1.1 suggests portal hypertension. A gradient below 1.1 suggests nonhepatic disorders such as tuberculous peritonitis, peritoneal malignancy, and pancreatic ascites.

Bloody ascitic fluid, containing more than 50,000 red blood cells/μL, suggests a neoplasm or pancreatic ascites. Chylous ascites is a milky fluid containing chylomicrons; the cause is lymphatic obstruction, most commonly from tuberculosis, a mediastinal tumor, or trauma to the thoracic duct. An acidic fluid (pH below 7.35) suggests tumor or infection.

In patients with chronic liver disease and cirrhosis but no other complicating factors, ascites means an intraperi-

Table 7.5–2. Causes of ascites.

Cirrhosis
Neoplasms
Congestive heart failure
Hypothyroidism
Tuberculosis
Bacterial peritonitis
Nephrotic syndrome
Pancreatitis

toneal expansion of the extracellular fluid compartment. Important factors in the pathogenesis of ascites in a patient with cirrhosis include elevation of the portal venous pressure, a drop in serum colloid osmotic pressure caused by a decreased serum albumin level, and renal retention of both salt and water. In a patient with portal hypertension, the low serum albumin level reflects both impaired protein synthesis by the liver and dilution caused by a marked expansion of plasma volume. The combination of obstruction to blood flow through the liver and a low serum albumin level drives fluid out of the intrahepatic sinusoids and splanchnic bed, and into the peritoneal cavity. When cell loss, fibrosis, and regenerative nodules raise intrahepatic sinusoidal pressure, more fluid moves into hepatic lymphatic vessels and then into the intraperitoneal space. When fluid is produced faster than the visceral peritoneal lymphatic vessels can reabsorb it, ascites develops. Since ascitic fluid most often comes from hepatic sinusoids, rarely is elevated portal pressure alone—as in portal vein thrombosis—sufficient to cause ascites.

Characteristic abnormalities of salt and water metabolism contributing to ascites in chronic liver disease include increased sodium reabsorption in the proximal renal tubules (secondary to altered renal blood flow), decreased free water clearance, and hyperaldosteronism. Most patients with liver disease and ascites have increased reabsorption of sodium in the proximal renal tubules. The cause may be a humoral agent. Free water clearance is markedly reduced because of inappropriate release and decreased degradation of antidiuretic hormone. In almost all patients with chronic liver disease and ascites, impaired metabolism of aldosterone leads to hyperaldosteronism and thus to increased distal reabsorption of sodium. These complex derangements in portal pressure, plasma colloid osmotic pressure, hepatic lymph production, and salt and walter balance lead to an expansion of total extracellular volume and to ascites.

Edema accompanies ascites in many patients with liver disease, particularly those with severe hypoalbuminemia. About 5% of patients with ascites have a pleural effusion, usually in the right thorax. The effusion is caused in part by ascites from the peritoneal cavity escaping into the chest through anatomic defects in the diaphragm. Some patients develop these pleural effusions even when their ascites is not clinically detectable.

The appearance or worsening of ascites in a patient with known cirrhosis may signify a deterioration in the liver disease. Other complications of cirrhosis that may cause ascites include hepatocellular carcinoma, tuberculous peritonitis, and spontaneous bacterial peritonitis; ascites, with or without abdominal pain, may be the first presentation of any of these conditions. Fever with ascites should alert the clinician to the possibility of tuberculous or bacterial peritonitis. Pancreatic ascites, produced by direct leakage of pancreatic fluid from a disruption of the pancreatic duct, may cause ascites in a patient with chronic alcoholism and is suggested by an elevated amylase level in the abdominal fluid.

Spontaneous Bacterial Peritonitis: Spontaneous bacterial peritonitis develops in about 5% of patients with chronic liver disease, particularly alcoholic cirrhosis. Bacteria can infect ascites in many ways, for example, empyema of the gallbladder, rupture of a colonic diverticulum, or perforation of a peptic ulcer. But most often, no entry site from the gut to the peritoneal cavity is found, and the bacterial infection is labeled "spontaneous." The infection is usually with a single organism, most often an aerobic gram-negative bacillus; anaerobic organisms are rarely to blame. Spontaneous bacterial peritonitis may be caused by septicemia, with gut bacteria entering the portal vein, bypassing the liver, and disseminating through the systemic circulation; or else gut bacteria may move across the edematous gut wall into the ascites. In the occasional patient in whom a nonenteric bacterium is found, the ascites most likely became infected through septicemia. If fluid cultures grow several organisms, especially anaerobes, the physician should suspect direct seeding from the large bowel (eg, diverticulitis). Although spontaneous bacterial peritonitis is characterized by rapidly accumulating ascites, fever, and abdominal pain, the disorder may appear with little or no fever and none of the usual signs of peritoneal inflammation.

The ascitic fluid in spontaneous bacterial peritonitis is characteristically cloudy because of a high leukocyte count (over 300 cells/μL) with predominantly polymorphonuclear cells. The pH is below 7.35. Organisms are seen on Gram's stain in about 25% of patients. Therapy for presumptive bacterial peritonitis should not await fluid culture results. Patients should be started immediately on empiric antibiotics directed toward gram-positive organisms (streptococci and staphylococci) and gram-negative bacilli. Patients with cirrhosis who are given an aminoglycoside should be monitored carefully because they are predisposed to nephrotoxicity.

Management of Ascites in Patients With Liver Disease: The physician should begin by searching for causes of ascites, especially occult gastrointestinal hemorrhage (the mechanism being loss of albumin and decrease in renal blood flow), increased dietary sodium intake, and medications that increase renal sodium retention (Table 7.5–3). After complicating extrahepatic conditions have been excluded or treated, therapy may be directed toward clearing the ascites. The goal is to use the simplest regimen that will induce a diuresis of about 900 mL (1–1$^1/_2$ lb) per day. Patients who have both ascites and peripheral edema can tolerate greater fluid losses. One of the most important factors contributing to ascites is renal retention of sodium. Measuring renal sodium excretion can help the physician plan dietary sodium and diuretic recommendations (Table 7.5–4). In general, patients need fluid restriction only if they develop hyponatremia.

In most patients, ascites can be successfully treated with a combination of salt restriction and diuretics. Refractory ascites is defined as no diuresis (urinary sodium excretion of at most 10 mEq/24 hr) despite maximum di-

Table 7.5–3. Management of ascites in patients with liver disease.

Find cause of ascites
Establish diagnosis of liver disease
Rule out tuberculosis, bacterial peritonitis, and neoplasm

Treat underlying liver disease
If 24-hr urine sodium (mEq) is:

>50	Restrict dietary sodium to 2 g/day
25–50	Give spironolactone
10–25	Restrict dietary sodium to 1 g/day; give furosemide or bumetanide
<10	Give maximal diuretic dose; consider therapeutic paracenteses or peritoneojugular shunt

uretic doses and salt restriction. The patient's tendency to form ascites is so severe that diuretic therapy sufficient to mobilize the ascites leads to volume depletion and prerenal azotemia. Alternative therapies for refractory ascites include therapeutic paracenteses and peritoneovenous shunts.

Repeated therapeutic paracenteses have been used in patients who have severe ascites with markedly impaired urinary sodium excretion. Paracenteses of up to 4 L/24 hr cause no more complications than do potent diuretic regimens. The peritoneojugular (LeVeen) shunt is a long subcutaneous tube that redirects ascites away from the peritoneal cavity to the jugular vein or right atrium. The device is equipped with a one-way pressure-operated valve. When the ascites raises intra-abdominal pressure more than 3 cm over venous pressure, the valve opens and ascitic fluid flows from the peritoneal cavity into the systemic circulation. The peritoneojugular shunt can reduce ascites dramatically, but complications of the implant procedure can be life-threatening. They include clotting of the tube with blood or debris, as well as infection and disseminated intravascular coagulation. If the systemic reinfusion of ascites exceeds the kidney's ability to excrete the fluid, patients can develop hypervolemia that leads to congestive heart failure or bleeding from esophageal varices.

Progressive Renal Failure in Liver Disease (Hepatorenal Syndrome)

Patients with liver disease may develop transient renal insufficiency after a gastrointestinal hemorrhage, overly vigorous diuresis, or intercurrent infection. But some patients with severe liver disease develop progressive, usually fatal renal failure for which no cause is found. This form of renal failure is called the hepatorenal syndrome (Chapters 5.2 and 5.4).

The pathogenesis of the hepatorenal syndrome is unknown. The kidneys are histologically normal and have been used successfully as donor organs for transplant. The volume and distribution of renal blood flow are abnormal; a marked decrease in renal cortical perfusion suggests intrarenal vasoconstriction. Secondary reduction in glomerular filtration leads to marked retention of sodium and free water, as well as to hyponatremia, oliguria, and azotemia.

Table 7.5–4. Complications of diuretic therapy for ascites in patients with liver disease.

Complication	Comments	Treatment
Hyponatremia	Nearly always caused by water retention; total body sodium is normal or high	Record intake and output Avoid IV and oral overhydration Restrict fluids to ≤500 mL/day
Hypokalemia	Often caused by loop diuretics	Give spironolactone to minimize K+ losses If needed, give K+ supplement
Hypochloremic alkalosis	Often caused by diuretic therapy	Give KCl to replace chloride
Azotemia	Progressive rise of creatinine and blood urea nitrogen, with oliguria	Stop all diuretics Monitor venous pressure Avoid overexpanding the intravascular space

Urinary and plasma electrolyte measurements can help differentiate the hepatorenal syndrome from acute tubular necrosis. Patients with the hepatorenal syndrome have a normal urine osmolarity, but their urine contains very little sodium (less than 5 mEq/L) and the ratio of urinary to plasma creatinine is over 30. In contrast, patients with acute tubular necrosis have significant urinary sodium excretion (more than 30 mEq/L), and the ratio of urinary to plasma creatinine is about 1.

Treatment of the hepatorenal syndrome is unsatisfactory; few patients survive. In some patients, renal function improves if the liver disease abates. Treatment must focus on correcting reversible factors and maintaining salt and water balance. Plasma expansion with albumin or blood is indicated if the central venous pressure is less than 6 cm H_2O. Patients should not take prostaglandin synthetase inhibitors such as nonsteroidal anti-inflammatory agents, because these drugs impair synthesis of renal vasodilators and can trigger or worsen renal failure in patients with cirrhosis. In general, vasoactive drugs are not useful.

Hepatic Encephalopathy

Hepatic encephalopathy is a complex neuropsychiatric disorder developing when toxins escape into the systemic circulation because of impaired hepatic clearance in acute or chronic liver disease. The condition is characterized by disturbances in consciousness, personality, behavior, and neuromuscular function. The individual components of the syndrome are nonspecific. Early manifestations include reversal of sleep patterns from night to day, hypersomnia, irritability, neglect of personal appearance, and forgetfulness. In later stages, patients may develop delirium and deep coma. Neurologic signs include hyperreflexia, generalized rigidity, and myoclonus. Many patients have asterixis, which is a nonrhythmic flapping tremor of the wrist and metacarpophalangeal joints, best demonstrated with the arms outstretched and the hands dorsiflexed. Asterixis is not specific to hepatic encephalopathy, but may be found in uremia, chronic heart failure, and chronic lung disease. Few patients with hepatic encephalopathy have seizures.

The most frequently incriminated pathogenetic factor in hepatic encephalopathy is abnormal ammonia metabolism. Ammonia is normally produced in the gut by bacterial ureolysis and is transported through the portal vein to the liver, where it is converted to urea. Evidence that ammonia is a principal toxin in hepatic encephalopathy includes (1) an elevated arterial or cerebrospinal fluid ammonia level in most patients, (2) induction of hepatic encephalopathy in susceptible patients by administration of ammonium salts, (3) relief of encephalopathy when treatment reduces the blood ammonia level, and (4) encephalopathy in children in whom inherited deficiencies of the enzymes of the Krebs-Henseleit cycle lead to hyperammonemia.

Evidence against ammonia as the only toxin includes (1) no close correlation between blood ammonia levels and clinical degree of encephalopathy and (2) encephalopathy in some patients who have a normal blood ammonia level. Other compounds that may act as toxins in producing hepatic encephalopathy include endogenous benzodiazepine-like substances (GABA-ergic neurotransmission), mercaptans derived from methionine metabolism, and biogenic amines (eg, γ-aminobutyric acid) that affect neurochemical transmission in the brain. Most likely, hepatic encephalopathy is caused by several toxins acting in combination.

Other abnormalities commonly seen in hepatic encephalopathy include an elevated cerebrospinal fluid glutamine level and plasma amino acid abnormalities (high levels of methionine, phenylalanine, and tyrosine, and low levels of the branched-chain amino acids valine, leucine, and isoleucine). The electroencephalogram shows nonspecific slow-wave activity (delta waves less than 4 Hz), predominantly over the frontal regions. Many patients have triphasic waves, but they are not pathognomonic for hepatic encephalopathy.

Factors important in the pathogenesis of hepatic encephalopathy are hepatocellular dysfunction and shunting of blood so that it bypasses the liver cells and goes directly into the systemic circulation. Most patients have both factors. Portal blood may bypass the liver cells through extrahepatic or intrahepatic shunts. The neurologic syndrome is believed to develop when one or more toxic intestinal products normally metabolized by the liver is introduced into the systemic circulation.

Hepatic encephalopathy may arise without an apparent cause during acute or chronic liver disease or may have an obvious trigger. Important exogenous triggers include increased dietary protein, certain drugs (particularly sedatives and analgesics), infection, gastrointestinal hemorrhage, azotemia, and overzealous use of diuretics, leading to hypovolemia and hypokalemia. Gastrointestinal hemorrhage can precipitate hepatic encephalopathy not only because hypovolemia decreases liver perfusion but because blood in the gut is a rich source of ammonia.

Management: The objectives of managing hepatic encephalopathy are (1) lowering the levels of ammonia and other toxic substances by reducing or excluding dietary protein and (2) cleansing nitrogenous materials from the gut (Table 7.5–5). Patients may get additional benefit from nonabsorbable antibiotics that reduce colonic bacteria. The physician must provide general support of confused or comatose patients and must search aggressively for factors such as gastrointestinal hemorrhage, dietary indiscretion, and drugs that may have triggered or worsened the syndrome. Alternative explanations for coma and depressed mentation in patients with liver disease must not be overlooked. The physician should exclude subdural hematoma, hypoglycemia, meningitis, and sedative overdose before starting specific therapy for hepatic encephalopathy.

Mental status may improve if toxins are eliminated from the gut by enemas. Protein should be excluded from the diet until the encephalopathy has been controlled. Protein is gradually restarted in 10 g increments every 3–5 days. Volume depletion and electrolyte disturbances should be corrected. Sedatives and analgesics can precipitate encephalopathy in patients with advanced liver disease.

Lactulose is the most important drug in management of hepatic encephalopathy. This synthetic disaccharide is degraded by intestinal bacteria, acidifying the contents of the lower gut, trapping ammonia before it can enter the blood. Lactulose also produces an osmotic, fermentative diarrhea that increases elimination of toxins. The drug can be given orally or by retention enema. Lactulose regularly reduces blood ammonia levels and lessens the frequency of episodes of hepatic encephalopathy in patients with chronic liver disease. Instead of lactulose, patients can be given the nonabsorbable antibiotic neomycin. Neomycin produces bacteriostasis with inhibition of urea-splitting and deaminating bacteria. The dangers of long-term

Table 7.5–5. Management of hepatic encephalopathy.

Search for precipitating factors
  Excess nitrogen load
  Electrolyte abnormalities
  Drugs (eg, tranquilizers, sedatives)
  Infection
Management
  For minimal encephalopathy
    Reduce dietary protein to 20–40 g/day
    Give lactulose
  For moderate to severe encephalopathy
    Remove all protein from diet
    Induce vigorous catharsis with enemas
    Give 1000–1500 calories/day as oral or IV carbohydrate
    Give lactulose
  When patients improve
    Restart dietary protein in 10-g increments every 3–5 days
    Continue lactulose until patient can tolerate 50 g protein/day; then consider stopping drug

neomycin treatment include ototoxicity, malabsorption, and renal tubular toxicity. In some patients, the combination of lactulose and neomycin is more effective than either used alone.

Some patients' encephalopathy is reversed by flumazenil, a benzodiazepine antagonist, which presumably blocks the central nervous system effects of an endogenous benzodiazepine-like substance.

SUMMARY

▶ Portal hypertension results from altered hepatic blood flow, caused most often by cirrhosis, portal vein thrombosis, infiltrative diseases of the liver, or hepatic vein occlusion.

▶ Since portal hypertension is often caused by disorders for which there is no specific treatment, therapy is directed toward controlling its consequences, primarily ascites, bacterial peritonitis, hepatic encephalopathy, and variceal hemorrhage.

▶ Management of ascites and hepatic encephalopathy requires a search for precipitating factors. Specific treatment for ascites is salt restriction and diuretics; for encephalopathy, lactulose.

SUGGESTED READING

Akriviadis EA, Runyon BA: Utility of an algorithm in differentiating spontaneous from secondary bacterial peritonitis. Gastroenterology 1990;98:127.

Conn HO: Complications of portal hypertension. Curr Hepatol 1993;13:223.

Epstein M: The hepatorenal syndrome: Newer perspectives. N Engl J Med 1992;327:1810.

Gonwa TA et al: Pathogenesis and outcome of hepatorenal syndrome in patients undergoing orthotopic liver transplant. Transplantation 1989;47:395.

Runyon BA: Care of patients with ascites. N Engl J Med 1994;330:337.

Section 8

Infectious Disease

David B. Hellmann, MD, Section Editor

8.1

Approach to the Patient With an Infectious Disease

John G. Bartlett, MD, and Patricia Charache, MD

Infectious diseases are pathologic processes caused by microbes or microbial products. These diverse conditions, among the most common encountered in both office and hospital practice, have several salient features.

- Infectious diseases are caused by pathogens that are classified as bacteria, mycobacteria, bacteria-like organisms, viruses, fungi, or parasites.

- Because infectious diseases can involve any organ system, they make a great impact on other medical disciplines.

- Many infectious diseases and most serious infections can be treated by antimicrobial drugs or prevented by good public health measures.

- New pathogens and new infectious diseases are continually being identified (Table 8.1–1). The development of new vaccines and antimicrobial drugs is not keeping pace with the new microbes.

- Patterns of infectious disease transmission are described as epidemics (clusters of cases confined in space and time), endemics (cases confined in space over prolonged periods), or sporadic (isolated) cases. The mechanism of transmission is also characteristic of some microbes and epidemiologic patterns. Infections may spread from person to person (contagious), from animal to person (zoonosis), from insect to animal or person (vector-borne), or from an environmental source such as water or food (water-borne or food-borne).

Control and treatment of infectious diseases have radically changed medical practice since 1900, when tuberculosis, rheumatic fever, typhoid fever, and similar devastating infections were the most common causes of hospitalization and death. The tremendous improvements brought by public health advances, vaccines, and antibiotics are widely viewed as medicine's greatest achievements.

The largest single lethal epidemic in the history of medicine was the 14th century's bubonic plague, which killed 25 million people. Ranking second was the influenza epidemic of 1918–1919, which killed 20 million. With industrialization, tuberculosis became epidemic in the United States and was the most common cause of death around 1900. Much of the control of tuberculosis can be credited to learning the pathogen's mechanism of transmission and intervening with public health policies to prevent person-to-person spread.

The potential value of vaccines to control infectious diseases was first reported in 1798 by Edward Jenner, who wrote about the use of cowpox vaccine to prevent smallpox. His idea eventually evolved into a planned program for global eradication of smallpox. The program worked: The last case of smallpox was recorded in 1976. Smallpox is the only disease that has been eliminated from the earth. The World Health Organization has identified poliomyelitis as the next candidate for global eradication through a vaccine program. Diseases that vaccine programs have almost eliminated from the developed world are poliomyelitis, measles, rubella, mumps, pertussis, tetanus, and diphtheria (Table 8.1–2). Most recently, vaccines have been introduced for *Haemophilus influenzae* type B, hepatitis A, hepatitis B, *Streptococcus pneumoniae*, varicella zoster, and typhoid fever.

The first antimicrobial drugs were the sulfonamides, introduced in the mid-1930's. Next came penicillin in the 1940's. The discovery of antimicrobial drugs has been described as the greatest life-saving technologic development in the history of medicine, and these drugs have been credited with extending the average American's life expectancy by at least 10 years.

Table 8.1–1. Microbial pathogens identified since 1975.

Disease	Pathogen (Year Discovered)
Acute hemorrhagic fever	Ebola virus (1976)
Cryptosporidiosis	*Cryptosporidium* (1976)
Genital warts (carcinoma), cervical cancer, laryngeal papillomatosis	Human papillomavirus 16 and 18 (1976)
(Delta) hepatitis	Delta agent (1977)
Legionnaires' disease	*Legionella pneumophila* (1977)
Antibiotic-associated colitis	*Clostridium difficile* (1978)
Toxic shock syndrome	*Staphylococcus aureus* (1978)
Adult T-cell leukemia, tropical spastic paraparesis	HTLV-I (1980)
Lyme disease	*Borrelia burgdorferi* (1982)
Hemorrhagic colitis, hemolytic-uremic syndrome	*Escherichia coli* 0157:H7 (1982)
Korean hemorrhagic fever, hemorrhagic fever with renal failure syndrome	Hantavirus (1982)
Erythema infectiosum, aplastic crisis, acute arthritis, hydrops fetalis	Parvovirus B19 (1983)
Peptic ulcer disease, gastric cancer	*Helicobacter pylori* (1983)
AIDS	HIV (1983)
Chlamydia pneumonia	*Chlamydia pneumoniae* (1986)
Roseola infantum	Herpes 6 virus (1986)
Ehrlichiosis	*Ehrlichiosis canis* (1986)
Non-A, non-B hepatitis	Hepatitis C virus (1989)
Cat-scratch disease, bacillary angiomatosis, trench fever	*Bartonella* (formerly *Rochalimaea*) *henselae* or *quintana* (1990)
Whipple's disease	*Tropheryma whippelii* (1992)
Hantavirus pulmonary syndrome (HPS)	Sin nombre virus (1993)
Kaposi's sarcoma	Kaposi's sarcoma herpes virus (1995)

Table 8.1–2. Impact of vaccines on selected infections in the United States.

Disease	Number of Cases		% Reduction
	Maximum (Year)	1994	
Diphtheria	206,939 (1921)	1	99.9%
Measles	894,134 (1941)	876	99.9%
Mumps	152,209 (1968)	1212	99.2%
Pertussis	265,269 (1934)	3198	98.8%
Polio (paralytic)	21,269 (1952)	1	99.9%
Rubella	57,686 (1969)	211	99.7%
Congenital rubella	20,000 (1964)	6	99.9%
Tetanus	1,560 (1923)	34	97.8%

paradoxically, immune complexes, cytokine release, and the inflammatory reaction all are expressed as disease.

Depending on the pathogen's virulence, a different number of microbes is needed to cause infection. As few as 10 *Shigella* organisms produce diarrheal disease, whereas over 100,000 *Salmonella* organisms are required to produce disease. Smaller numbers of organisms are eliminated by normal host defenses.

Host defense mechanisms are an elaborate system of properties that protect normal people from infection. Humans are sterile in utero, but after birth spend an entire lifetime defending against the hostile world of microbes. The mucocutaneous barrier (skin and skin structures, and cells lining the pulmonary, gastrointestinal, and genitourinary tracts) is a simple shield, polymorphonuclear cells are nonspecific scavengers of multiple microbes, cell-mediated immunity is a complex array of cell-cytokine interactions designed to defend the host, and humoral antibody provides an antigen-specific response that helps eradicate the microbe.

CLASSIFICATION OF PATHOGENS

Pathogens are classified as bacteria, mycobacteria, bacteria-like organisms (eg, mycoplasma, rickettsiae, chlamydiae), viruses, fungi, or parasites. These microbes vary in size, growth requirements, methods of detection, and susceptibility to antimicrobial drugs (Table 8.1–3). In general, bacteria can be seen microscopically with magnification × 1000. They have a rigid peptidoglycan-containing cell wall, they are prokaryotic, they contain both RNA and DNA, most grow on cell-free media, and most can be treated with antimicrobial drugs. In contrast, most viruses can be seen only by electron microscopy. They have no cell wall, they contain only RNA or only DNA, they require tissue culture (cell-incorporated media) for growth, and relatively few are treatable with antimicrobial drugs.

Fungi are widely distributed in nature, are eukaryotic, and are more complex and usually larger than bacteria. Most have a rigid cell wall containing chitin and polysaccharides, and most can be grown on cell-free media. Parasites are categorized as helminths (worms), ectoparasites (lice, scabies, mites, ticks, and maggots), and protozoa. Protozoa tend to have complex life cycles and

PATHOPHYSIOLOGY

Infectious diseases are governed by the equation:

Disease severity =

$$\frac{\text{(virulence of microbe)} \times \text{(number of microbes)}}{\text{host defense mechanisms}}$$

A microbe's *virulence* is its ability to cause disease. Virulence factors include the organism's ability to adhere to and penetrate normal protective barrier surfaces, invade cells, spread through tissue planes, evade normal host defenses, and wall itself off within protective polysaccharide capsules that resist phagocytosis. Some microbes produce toxins that impair host molecular functions directly or destroy host cells through enzymes. Another virulence factor is the way in which the organism activates host defenses;

Table 8.1–3. Diagnostic properties of microbial pathogens.

Microbe	Diameter*	Visualization	Growth Outside Host Cell	Laboratory Media	Normal Flora	Usual Method of Disease Detection	Susceptibility to Antibiotics
Bacteria and bacteria-like organisms							
Aerobic and anaerobic	0.5–1 μm	Gram's stain	Yes	Agar, broth	Yes	Culture	Virtually all
Spirochetes	0.2 μm	Darkfield exam, immunofluorescence	Yes	Experimental animals	Yes	Serology, darkfield exam	All (penicillin, tetracycline, etc.)
Rickettsiae	0.5 μm	Giemsa stain, immunoperoxidase	No	Tissue culture, embryonated eggs	No	Serology, special stains	All (tetracycline, chloramphenicol, etc.)
Chlamydiae	0.3 μm	Immunofluorescence, electron microscopy	No	Tissue culture, embryonated eggs	No	Culture, serology	All (tetracycline, erythromycin)
Mycoplasma	0.3 μm	Electron microscopy, acridine orange	Yes	Hypertonic media	Yes (not *M pneumoniae*)	Serology, culture	All (tetracycline, erythromycin)
Mycobacteria	0.5–1 μm	Acid-fast stain	Yes	Solid media, radiometric broth	Yes (not *M tuberculosis*)	Culture	Most
Viruses	0.02–0.3 μm	Immunofluorescence (some), electron microscopy, in situ hybridization	No	Tissue culture	Yes (latent herpesviruses; enteroviruses, adenovirus)	Culture, serology, probes	Few
Fungi	1–20 μm	KOH mount, calcafluor white	Yes	Agar	Yes (especially *Candida* sp)	Culture, serology	Most (amphotericin)
Parasites	10–≥50 μm	Acid-fast and Giemsa stains, fluorescent microscopy	Variable	Rarely done	Yes	Visualization, immuno-diagnostics	Most

*The resolving power of the naked eye is 100 μm. The resolving power of light microscopy is 0.2 μm.

specific patterns of geographic distribution. Few protozoa require cultivation because nearly all can be identified with light microscopy. Most can be treated with antiparasitic drugs.

TYPES OF INFECTIONS

Community-Acquired Versus Nosocomial Infections

Community-acquired infections account for an estimated 600 million physician visits per year in the United States. The most common infections seen in office practice are respiratory tract infections—the common cold, influenza, bronchitis, and pharyngitis. These conditions are usually caused by viruses and are self-limited and not treatable with antimicrobial drugs. The most common treatable infections seen in office practice are bacterial infections: streptococcal pharyngitis, otitis media, sinusitis, urinary tract infections, sexually transmitted diseases, and lower respiratory tract infections. The major pathogens in these infections are *Streptococcus pyogenes* (group A streptococci), *H influenzae, S pneumoniae, Escherichia coli, Neisseria gonorrhoeae,* and *Chlamydia trachomatis.*

Each year, about 2.5 million Americans are hospitalized for infectious diseases. These hospitalizations ac-

count for 10% of the 281 million patient days spent in acute care facilities. The infections that most often necessitate hospital admission are urinary tract infections (pyelonephritis), lower respiratory tract infections, and infectious complications of HIV. The current estimate is that, not counting HIV-related infections, about 90% of all community-acquired infections requiring hospitalization of adults are caused by bacteria, and 6% by viruses.

Nosocomial infections are infections acquired within a hospital and are not established or incubating at the time of admission. About 5% of all hospitalized patients develop a nosocomial infection. Fifty percent of these infections could be prevented if medical personnel followed infection control guidelines established by the Centers for Disease Control and Prevention—primarily, washing their hands before touching each patient. The most common nosocomial infections involve the urinary tract, surgical wounds, and lower respiratory tract. Hospital-acquired pneumonia accounts for only about 12% of nosocomial infections, but is most often lethal. Nosocomial infections kill nearly 1% of all hospitalized patients and contribute to the deaths of an additional 3%.

The ecology and microbiology of nosocomial infections differ markedly from those of community-acquired infections. Bacteria are responsible for 90% of nosocomial infections, and fungi (especially *Candida albicans*) for most of the rest. The major hospital pathogens are *Staphylococ-*

cus aureus, enterococci, gram-negative bacilli (especially *Pseudomonas aeruginosa,* which is rarely acquired in the community), and *Candida* sp. These organisms are endemic to many hospitals and easily colonize patients who have been rendered susceptible by antibiotic treatment, debilitating conditions, and medical procedures, especially invasive procedures that breach mucocutaneous barriers. Infections caused by these organisms are often difficult to treat, partly because most patients have serious associated conditions and partly because the organisms can be resistant to commonly used antibiotics.

Infections in Developing Versus Developed Countries

Infectious diseases differ substantially between the developed and the developing world. In the Third World countries of Asia, Africa, and Latin America, the most prevalent pathogens reflect crowding, poor sanitation, and limited health care resources. Diseases that have historically plagued the developing world include tuberculosis, pneumonia, and diarrheal diseases; so have such infections as malaria, schistosomiasis, amebiasis, hookworm, ascariasis, filariasis, dengue, measles, whooping cough, cholera, typhoid fever, and trichuriasis, which no longer cause major problems in any developed country (Table 8.1–4). Recent rates of tuberculosis and AIDS, problematic throughout the world, have escalated, with the greatest severity in developing countries.

Infections in Immunocompromised Versus Immunocompetent Hosts

As already mentioned (see "Pathophysiology" above), severity of infection depends on microbial virulence multiplied by inoculum size, then divided by host defenses.

Table 8.1–4. Prevalence and mortality of infectious diseases in Africa, Asia, and Latin America, 1977–1978.

Disease	Infections	Deaths
Diarrhea	4,000,000,000	7,500,000
Respiratory tract infections	?	4,500,000
Tuberculosis	1,700,000,000	3,000,000
Malaria	800,000,000	1,200,000
Measles	85,000,000	900,000
Schistosomiasis	200,000,000	750,000
Whooping cough	70,000,000	350,000
Neonatal tetanus	150,000	125,000
Chagas' disease	12,000,000	60,000
Diphtheria	40,000,000	55,000
Hookworm	800,000,000	55,000
Onchocerciasis	30,000,000	35,000
Amebiasis	400,000,000	30,000
Meningitis	150,000	30,000
Typhoid fever	1,000,000	25,000
Ascariasis	900,000,000	20,000
Poliomyelitis	80,000,000	15,000
African trypanosomiasis	1,000,000	5,000
Dengue	3,500,000	100

Modified and reproduced, with permission, from Warren KS: Tropical medicine or tropical health: The Heath Clark lectures, 1988. Rev Infect Dis 1990;12:142.

Many microbes cause disease in any host if the inoculum is sufficient. There are other microbes against which the healthy host is generally protected because the organism lacks the virulence to overcome normal defenses. But the immunocompromised host may be vulnerable (Table 8.1–5). For example, histoplasmosis can affect any person who is immunologically naive and receives a sufficient inoculum, but *Pneumocystis carinii* causes disease in adults only if they have severely defective cell-mediated immunity.

Increasing numbers of people are immunosuppressed because of population aging, growing rates of cancer chemotherapy and organ transplantations, and the epidemic of HIV infection. Patients in all these categories share compromised cell-mediated immunity, which renders them susceptible to low-virulence "opportunistic" pathogens. At the same time, these patients are no more vulnerable than healthy hosts to virulent microbes like rhinovirus, influenza virus, and organisms (eg, the Norwalk agent) causing diarrheal disease. The type of vulnerability is defined by the immune defect. Thus, the patient with hypogammaglobulinemia is susceptible to encapsulated bacteria that can be cleared only by antibody and phagocytosis, but this person is not at particular risk for candidiasis, *P carinii,* or other pathogens that are eradicated by cell-mediated immunity. These observations provide the rationale for vaccines, prophylactic antimicrobial drugs, and algorithms for evaluating suspected infection according to type of host defense defect.

Endogenous Versus Exogenous Infections

Exogenous infections are caused by microbes from external sources—the environment, animals, and other people. Exogenous pathogens produce most infections, including such classic diseases as tuberculosis, cholera, typhoid fever, influenza, and the common cold. But an increasing number of infections involve endogenous pathogens. Most mucocutaneous surfaces harbor bacteria. Saliva contains about 1 billion bacteria/mL. The stomach contents harbor few swallowed organisms because gastric acidity creates a formidable barrier. Rapid transit keeps bacterial counts low in the small intestine. But the colon contains 1 trillion bacteria/g of stool. Large concentrations of bacteria are also found in the female genital tract and urethra, although the fallopian tubes, uterus, and proximal urethra and bladder are normally sterile. Current estimates are that normal people harbor about 10,000,000,000,000,000 (10^{15}, or 10 quadrillion) microbes from at least 400 species of bacteria and fungi.

Endogenous infections can develop when a mucosal barrier is breached or when flora innocuous to one anatomic site is transported to an "unprotected" site. Examples are aspiration pneumonia (from aspiration of oral or gastric flora), intra-abdominal infections (from migration of intestinal bacteria), urinary tract infections (urethral flora), wound infections (skin flora), and infections of the female genital tract (genital tract flora).

Table 8.1–5. Pathogens associated with immunodeficiency states.

Conditions	Usual Cause	Pathogens
Neutropenia (<500/mL)	Cancer chemotherapy, adverse drug reaction, leukemia	Bacteria: aerobic gram-negative bacteria (coliforms and pseudomonads) Fungi: *Aspergillus*
Impaired cell-mediated immunity	Organ transplant, HIV infection, lymphoma (especially Hodgkin's disease), corticosteroid therapy	Bacteria: intracellular species, eg, *Listeria, Salmonella,* mycobacteria (*Mycobacterium tuberculosis, M avium*), *Legionella, Nocardia* Viruses: cytomegalovirus, *H simplex,* varicella zoster Parasites: *Pneumocystis carinii, Toxoplasma, Strongyloides stercoralis, Cryptosporidium* Fungi: *Candida, Phycomyces (Mucor), Cryptococcus*
Hypogammaglobulinemia or dysgammaglobulinemia	Multiple myeloma, congenital or acquired deficiency, chronic lymphocytic leukemia	Bacteria: encapsulated species, eg, *Streptococcus pneumoniae, Haemophilus influenzae* type B Parasites: *Giardia* Viruses: enteroviruses
Complement deficiencies C2, C3 C5 C6–8 Alternative pathway	Congenital	Bacteria: *S pneumoniae, H influenzae* *S pneumoniae, S aureus,* Enterobacteriaceae *Neisseria meningitidis* *S pneumoniae, H influenzae, Salmonella*
Hyposplenism	Splenectomy, hemolytic anemia	*S pneumoniae, H influenzae, Capnocytophaga canimorsus*

MICROBIOLOGIC DIAGNOSIS

The unifying factor in infectious disease diagnosis is detection of the pathogen or its toxin by microscopy, culture, antigen detection, molecular probes, or specific antibody response.

Bacteria are classified by their morphology and appearance on Gram's stain as bacilli (rods) or cocci (spheres), which are gram-positive or gram-negative. Most bacteria grow on cell-free media, either broth or agar, to which the microbiological laboratory may have added growth-promoting or growth-inhibiting components based on the specimen source, the pathogens sought, and the normal flora expected.

Interpretation of culture results always depends on the clinical data. For example, the number of organisms cultured means more or less, depending on the setting. Nearly all bacterial infections have relatively large numbers of organisms at the infected site—usually more than 100,000/mL of body fluid or g of tissue. But even small numbers of bacteria from normally sterile sites must be taken seriously if they correlate with clinical findings. Some organisms are virtually always pathogenic or are never normal flora: *Mycobacterium tuberculosis, Legionella* sp, *Shigella,* influenza A virus, pathogenic fungi (*Blastomyces, Histoplasma,* and *Coccidioides*), *Mycoplasma pneumoniae, Chlamydia pneumoniae,* and *Corynebacterium diphtheriae.* Not of concern are small numbers of organisms such as coagulase-negative staphylococci, diphtheroids, and *Bacillus* sp, which are common skin organisms that often contaminate cultures and are not meaningful.

The time required for testing varies. Stain results can be available within 15–20 minutes, bacterial cultures generally require 24–48 hours, fungal cultures usually take 48–72 hours, and mycobacterial cultures may take 2–3 weeks. These differences reflect replication times for growth on artificial media, ranging from 20 minutes for most bacteria to 24 hours for mycobacteria.

Stains and Antigen Detection

The stains available for identifying organisms in body fluids or tissues include Gram's stain for bacteria, KOH mounts for fungi, Giemsa and trichrome stains for parasites, and acid-fast stains for mycobacteria, *Nocardia,* and *Cryptosporidium.* There are also stains for specific antigens, for example, fluorescein-conjugated stain to detect *Legionella, C pneumoniae,* pertussis, parapertussis, *Actinomyces israelii,* respiratory syncytial virus, herpes simplex virus, influenza A, and *P carinii.*

Alternative antigen detection methods are latex particle agglutination, counterimmunoelectrophoresis, and the enzyme-linked immunosorbent assay (ELISA). Among the organisms that can be identified with these techniques are *S pneumoniae, H influenzae* type B, group B streptococci, group A streptococci, *N gonorrhoeae, N meningitidis, Cryptococcus,* adenovirus, rotavirus, and *C pneumoniae.* Molecular probes, with or without DNA amplification by polymerase chain reaction (Chapter 10.2), allow detection of organisms that are not normal flora, such as *Chlamydia, N gonorrhoeae, Histoplasma,* HIV, human T-cell leukemia virus (HTLV-I), hepatitis C virus, parvovirus B19, papillomaviruses, *Legionella, Bartonella* (formerly *Rochalimaea*) *henselae* (cause of cat-scratch disease), and *Ehrlichia canis.* These methods also permit detection of toxin-producing bacterial strains, such as toxin-producing *E coli* (Chapter 6.7) and staphylococci that produce toxic shock syndrome toxin (TSST-1), as well as detection of antibiotic resistance genes.

Measuring the patient's immune response by indirect

fluorescence, particle agglutination, or ELISA can be a sensitive way of diagnosing infection caused by pathogens not generally prevalent in the community. An IgM antibody response without IgG, or a rising IgG titer, signals recent exposure. The key advantages of this approach are the availability of sensitive tests and the ability to make a diagnosis when the pathogen cannot be recovered. The primary disadvantages rest in the fact that the immune response appears late in the course of most diseases and that it may not be available when needed. Furthermore, a finding of IgG indicates exposure to the pathogen but cannot distinguish a recent immune response from one long ago.

PRINCIPLES OF MANAGEMENT AND VACCINATION

The foundation of therapy for most established infections is antimicrobial drugs. These drugs, designed to kill microbes or at least inhibit their growth, are classified by the target organisms as antibacterial, antiviral, antiparasitic, and antifungal agents. Antimicrobial treatment should be as specific as possible. Once the putative pathogen has been cultured, treatment for most bacterial infections is determined by in vitro tests of organism sensitivity to antibacterial drugs or by predicted patterns of susceptibility; viruses, parasites, fungi, and some bacterial infections are treated empirically. The physician tries to determine the infection site and the microbes likely to be involved and, when possible, does stains, antigen detection tests, and cultures to identify the pathogen. Often, however, initial therapy must be chosen empirically to cover microbes likely to be causing the observed pattern of disease; then, as the search narrows, the physician adjusts the therapy while avoiding unnecessary toxicity and cost. If the infection is thought not to require antimicrobial treatment, the patient may be given supportive care and followed up. An important part of management for any focal collection or abscess is drainage, often by surgery. Another therapeutic option is bolstering host defenses, but this is not well established for most infectious diseases.

Vaccines are effective in preventing infections by microbes containing a stable antigen that has limited variants and against which type-specific antibodies are protective. Diseases amenable to vaccines include measles, mumps,

and chickenpox. A microbe that is not amenable to vaccines is rhinovirus (the main cause of the common cold), because it has more than 100 antigenic types. Thus, repeated upper respiratory tract infections involving different viruses from this group are the rule rather than the exception. As for influenza, the antigenic variants are not stable: Antigenic shifts and drifts explain the need for annual vaccination. Last year's vaccine may be only partially protective because this year's epidemic strain may be slightly different. This year's vaccine is preferred.

Physicians dealing with infections have certain obligations to society. Contagious conditions like tuberculosis, typhoid fever, syphilis, gonorrhea, and poliovirus must be reported to health departments to enable public health officials to intervene when appropriate. Another concern is the need to curb the unbridled enthusiasm for antibiotics by both physicians and the public. Abuse of these drugs promotes microbial resistance and now threatens much of the progress celebrated in this chapter.

SUMMARY

▶ Infectious diseases afflict everyone; they are the most common reasons for physician consultation and the most common causes of death in the developing world.

▶ The greatest accomplishments in the history of medicine have been the antimicrobial drug treatment of infectious diseases and their prevention with vaccines and public health measures.

▶ The types of microbes that can infect an individual depend on the person's age, defenses (immunocompetent versus immunosuppressed), geography (developed versus developing country), and site of acquisition (community-acquired versus hospital-acquired).

▶ Infectious diseases are governed by the equation:

$$\text{Disease severity} = \frac{(\text{virulence of microbe}) \times (\text{number of microbes})}{\text{host defense mechanisms}}$$

▶ Management of infectious diseases involves differential diagnosis, appropriate use of the laboratory to detect the pathogen, and careful decisions about when to treat with antimicrobial drugs and which drugs to give.

SUGGESTED READING

Cohen ML: Epidemiology of drug resistance: Implications for a post-antimicrobial era. Science 1992;257:1050.

Ellner JJ et al: Tuberculosis symposium: Emerging problems and promise. J Infect Dis 1993;168:537.

Murphy FA: New, emerging, and reemerging infectious diseases. Adv Virus Res 1994;43:1.

Pinner RW et al: Trends in infectious diseases mortality in the United States. JAMA 1996;275:189.

Tompkins LS: The use of molecular methods in infectious diseases. N Engl J Med 1992;327:1290.

Warren KS: Tropical medicine or tropical health: The Heath Clark lectures, 1988. Rev Infect Dis 1990;12:142.

Fever of Unknown Origin

Patrick A. Murphy, MD, PhD

Many diseases cause fever, but in only a few patients is protracted fever the only or chief presenting complaint. Fever of unknown origin (FUO) is defined as a fever that has persisted for at least 3 weeks, whose maximum is at least 38.3°C (101°F) on at least two occasions, and whose cause is not apparent after routine history and physical examination. Because FUO usually indicates serious disease, which if not diagnosed and treated is likely to be fatal, it merits the physician's intensive investigation and continuing concern.

CAUSES

About 85% of FUOs are caused by disorders that fall into three categories (Table 8.2–1). About 40% of cases are caused by infection, 30% by tumors, and 15% by rheumatic diseases. Tropical infectious diseases are not common in the United States, but are important considerations in people who have lived or visited abroad.

A patient's age and sex do not rule in or out any of the causes of FUO, but they do bias the probabilities. Most fevers in children or young adults have an infectious cause; if these patients have a tumor, it is likely to be a leukemia or lymphoma. Most old people with FUO turn out to have an adenocarcinoma with or without superinfection. Rheumatic diseases depend much more on age and sex. Takayasu's disease is "young female arteritis," whereas giant cell arteritis is almost unheard of before age 50 and is common in the 80's. Systemic lupus erythematosus tends to occur in those between ages 20 and 50 and is much more common in women than men.

Localized Infections

The infections that cause fever of unknown origin can be divided into two types: localized and generalized. In the first type, the patient has localized pus somewhere, but in a site where it gives rise to few symptoms or signs. If the patient is conscious and mentally normal, the only places where pus can hide without causing symptoms are the abdomen, chest, and spine. Computed tomography

(CT) ensures that the source of this kind of fever is soon discovered, although it may not be possible to diagnose the infection on the first CT scan.

Most abscesses arise from a contained perforation of some part of the gut, because of a process such as colon cancer, diverticulitis, Crohn's disease, or peptic ulcer. Patients who have had a recent operation may have a leaking anastomosis or a peritoneal abscess in the subphrenic or pelvic area. Gallstones can lead to empyema of the gallbladder, ascending cholangitis, pancreatitis, and liver abscess. Urinary stones can cause pyonephrosis or a perinephric abscess.

Some intra-abdominal abscesses arise from hematogenous spread of bacteria from elsewhere. Staphylococcal psoas abscess, with or without vertebral osteomyelitis, is seen in drug abusers and occasionally in people who do not use drugs. Hematogenous abscesses can also develop in the spleen, liver, and kidneys.

Most osteomyelitis produces obvious symptoms of local disease, and the nature of the problem is apparent. However, vertebral osteomyelitis can be caused by a number of organisms that invade the bloodstream, including staphylococci, brucellae, gram-negative rods, and tubercle bacilli. The patient's only symptom may be vague backache.

In patients who are obtunded, psychotic, or demented, abscesses can be found in places where they would ordinarily produce severe symptoms. Purulent sinusitis, prostatic abscess, septic arthritis of the knee, and ischiorectal abscesses may be found in demented persons who are unaware of them. The best way of detecting these abscesses is with repeated complete physical exams. This is particularly important with decubitus ulcers, which can be extensive under skin that looks minimally abnormal.

Generalized Infections

More difficult to diagnose are infections in which the organisms are disseminated throughout the body. The main diseases in this category are endocarditis and miliary tuberculosis. Each of these diseases accounts for 5–10%

Table 8.2–1. Causes of fever of unknown origin.

Percentage of Patients	Causes
40	Infections (local or generalized)
30	Tumors (with or without infection)
15	Rheumatic diseases
~5	Factitious fever
10	Miscellaneous: inflammatory bowel disease, allergic reactions (eg, to drugs), granulomatous reactions (eg, sarcoid), rarities (eg, familial Mediterranean fever)

of all cases of FUO. To these, the modern era has added HIV infection and its complicating superinfections.

Untreated bacterial endocarditis can continue undetected for up to 18 months. For most of this time, patients may have few or no cardiac symptoms. However, something abnormal can generally be heard on auscultation of the heart. Most patients have an obvious cardiac murmur indicating valve disease. Some have only a systolic murmur whose significance is not at first apparent, such as the early, short systolic murmur of bicuspid aortic valve. If several observers checking the patient over a long time do not hear a murmur, endocarditis is unlikely. The only form of endocarditis that might not cause a murmur is right-sided endocarditis in drug addicts, but this, too, is unusual.

Most patients with endocarditis have a positive blood culture, usually for a streptococcus. The hallmark of endocarditis is continuous bacteremia, with every blood culture positive. If the patient has not recently received an antibiotic, three blood cultures will establish the diagnosis with 99% probability; doing more is not routinely worthwhile.

Culture-negative bacterial endocarditis is rare. Even if the patient has been given one or several doses of an antibiotic, the blood culture is still positive over 90% of the time, and that percentage can be raised by waiting for a few days and repeating the cultures or by using resin bottles. A few nutritionally fastidious organisms, such as certain streptococci, grow very slowly or require enriched media, but a good laboratory can eventually grow them.

Some bacteria, such as *Coxiella burnetii* and *Chlamydia psittaci,* can cause endocarditis but cannot grow on any artificial medium. Moreover, although fungi can grow on many media, it is curiously difficult to get a positive blood culture in those few patients who have fungal endocarditis. The usual clue to these diagnoses is large vegetations on a heart valve on echocardiogram. Emboli are common, and removal of the embolus may allow a pathologic diagnosis.

Even today, disseminated (miliary) tuberculosis is commonly diagnosed at autopsy. Chest x-ray is part of the routine investigation of anyone who is sick and febrile; therefore, pulmonary tuberculosis is easy to diagnose. But miliary tuberculosis can be very subtle. Many patients are elderly and already ill with diabetes, alcoholism, or cancer, and the onset of accelerated deterioration may be missed. Most young patients have underlying HIV infec-

tion. The tubercles are microscopic, and they barely disturb organ function until very late in the disease course. Bone marrow involvement may cause pancytopenia, and granulomas in the liver may raise the alkaline phosphatase. These laboratory findings, along with fever, a high erythrocyte sedimentation rate, and progressive weight loss, may be patients' only abnormalities until they develop tuberculous meningitis, by which time it may be too late.

The site from which tuberculosis disseminates is usually a caseous node in the abdomen or mediastinum and may be visible on CT scan. The purified protein derivative skin test may not help in diagnosis: About 20% of patients with disseminated tuberculosis have negative test results, and many patients sick from other causes have positive results because of longstanding, inactive tuberculosis. The diagnosis can often be made by biopsy of liver or bone marrow. But biopsy should be done only if there is laboratory evidence of organ abnormality: For example, if the alkaline phosphatase is normal, it is unlikely that liver biopsy will show caseating granulomas. Occasionally, the tubercle bacillus can be cultured from urine, cerebrospinal fluid, a biopsy, or even blood. Some patients must still be diagnosed by a trial of antituberculous therapy.

HIV infection and its complications are discussed in Chapter 8.10. The serologic tests are both sensitive and specific and diagnose 99% of HIV-infected patients. The acute HIV seroconversion syndrome can be diagnosed by demonstrating viral p24 antigen or nucleic acid in the blood, and most patients undergo seroconversion within 1 or 2 months. The real diagnostic problem is in older patients who have no obvious risk factors and in whom HIV may not be suspected. The explanation may be a forgotten blood transfusion or a secretly bisexual husband.

Many generalized infections can be acquired only in particular parts of the world (Table 8.2–2; Chapter 8.15). People who have never left the United States can acquire malaria only under exceptional circumstances. But for people who have just returned from a trip to Ghana, it is hardly worth considering any other diagnosis. If the patient has a travel history, the physician should remember not only infections like visceral leishmaniasis, which is usually chronic, but those like typhoid and typhus, which are generally over in less than 3 weeks but sometimes cause prolonged illness. Once an infection is considered in the differential diagnosis, the physician can generally rule it in or out by a laboratory test, so the crucial step is to think of it.

Table 8.2–2. Common prolonged tropical infections causing fever of unknown origin.

Malaria (most common)
Leishmaniasis
Amebic liver abscess
Trypanosomiasis
Typhoid, other forms of salmonellosis
Brucellosis
Louse-borne relapsing fever

Table 8.2–3. Infections acquired in certain regions of the United States, causing fever of unknown origin.

Infection	Region
Coccidioidomycosis	Southwest
Tick-borne relapsing fever	Rocky Mountain states
Histoplasmosis	Ohio River Valley
Plague	Arizona, New Mexico

The physician should also ask patients about travel within the United States (Table 8.2–3). Coccidioidomycosis is acquired only in the southwestern United States, but exposure may be brief and the disease may manifest long after the patient has returned home. Most fungal diseases have a long latency and can be activated by immunosuppression. A kidney transplant recipient who develops manifestations of histoplasmosis may have acquired the infection while growing up in the Ohio Valley.

Certain infections can be acquired in particular occupations and avocations. In the United States, brucellosis is seen essentially only in people who raise or slaughter pigs. Tularemia affects those who butcher wild rabbits or hares. Listeriosis can affect those who drink unpasteurized milk. Cat-scratch disease is caused by a scratch, usually from a kitten.

Lastly, there are generalized infections that can be acquired anywhere. In addition to HIV, the most common viruses are cytomegalic inclusion disease and Epstein-Barr virus infection, especially affecting patients over 40. Both viruses usually produce at least mild and occasionally severe hepatitis. Hepatitis B or C may also present as a chronic illness with fever and hepatitis. In people with immune defects, viruses that ordinarily produce acute infection can cause prolonged illness. Rotaviruses, enteroviruses, and parvovirus B19 can cause chronic infection in people who have defective synthesis of antibodies.

Most untreated septicemic bacterial diseases end quickly, because the patient either dies or becomes immune. However, even apart from endocarditis, a few septicemic bacterial diseases occasionally persist long enough to qualify as causes of FUO. *Streptobacillus moniliformis, Yersinia enterocolitica,* gonococci, and meningococci all can cause subacute sepsis. Rickettsial infections cause prolonged fever only rarely, and they usually produce a diagnostic rash.

As the duration of fever stretches into months, it becomes less and less likely that a septicemic bacterial illness is responsible. The equilibrium between bacterium and patient is too unstable to persist for long periods. However, a bacterium may persist by establishing some local focus of infection, such as endocarditis, spondylitis, or a splenic abscess.

Fungal infection is always chronic, and cryptococcosis is not geographically confined. Most normal hosts have pulmonary or central nervous system symptoms and signs, but the disease can cause chronic fever. The parasitic disease toxoplasmosis is also cosmopolitan and can cause

FUO. Both of these infections are more common in immunosuppressed persons, and they are common causes of FUO in persons with AIDS.

Tumors

Most tumors cause fever because of related infection. Tumors ulcerate, perforate, or obstruct some drainage pathway, and become infected with normal flora. Most such tumors are adenocarcinomas and are seen most often in older patients. Adenocarcinomas that are not infected are seldom a source of fever, unless they outgrow their blood supply and undergo necrosis. Sometimes the tumor acts as an antigen, and an antitumor response causes the fever; this is well known to occur with hypernephroma.

About two-thirds of all noninfected tumors that cause FUO are lymphomas. They tend to involve the mediastinal or abdominal nodes, since lymphomas with palpable nodes are easy to diagnose. Patients with leukemia, preleukemia, and myelodysplastic syndromes can also present with prolonged fever; few patients have a completely normal blood smear, but the abnormalities may be subtle and diagnosis often requires bone marrow examination. FUO can also be caused by atrial myxoma, a rare benign tumor.

Leukemia and lymphoma cause fever by the tumor cells' producing endogenous pyrogens such as interleukin-1 and tumor necrosis factor. Since these lymphokines are produced mainly by macrophages, fever is an unusual manifestation of purely lymphocytic tumors such as myeloma and chronic lymphocytic leukemia.

The easy availability of CT and magnetic resonance imaging (MRI) has revolutionized the diagnosis of FUO caused by tumors. With few exceptions, if a carcinoma or a lymphoma is not visible on the chest or abdominal CT scan, it does not exist.

Rheumatic Diseases

Decades ago, few physicians had experience with rheumatic diseases, although these diseases caused fully 20% of cases of FUO. The situation has changed because of the widespread availability of serologic tests. The rheumatic diseases that still present as FUO are those for which no serologic test is available and a clinical diagnosis is required (Table 8.2–4)—most commonly giant cell arteritis (Chapter 3.5) and Still's disease. Patients with these diseases often present with high fever and severe weight loss, with few other physical signs and no specific laboratory abnormalities.

Table 8.2–4. The chief rheumatic diseases causing fever of unknown origin.

Disease	Age Group Affected
Giant cell arteritis	Common in people >60
Still's disease	Children and young adults
Periarteritis nodosa	Middle-aged men
Wegener's granulomatosis	Middle age
Lymphomatoid granulomatosis	Middle-aged men
Takayasu's disease	Young women

Miscellaneous Causes

Inflammatory bowel disease that presents as FUO is virtually always Crohn's disease (Chapter 6.10). Most patients have some abdominal pain or diarrhea, but it may be mild and patients may have had it for so long that they do not mention it unless asked. Crohn's disease is generally visible on abdominal CT scan.

Allergic reactions to drugs account for 3% of all cases of FUO. Usually, the responsible medication is a new one, but patients can develop allergic reactions to drugs that they have taken for years. The internist should make sure to know about drugs prescribed by specialists such as dentists, gynecologists, and ophthalmologists and should ask patients about over-the-counter medications that they take for complaints like headaches, constipation, and sinusitis. In general, drug fever responds to withdrawal of the drug; rechallenge is rarely indicated.

Allergic reactions to inhaled substances can also cause fever. Most allergies relate to particular occupations, such as Monday morning fever in cotton mills and metal fume fever in the nickel industry. Such fevers are seldom mysterious, but the patient's occupation and hobbies should be considered for possible relevance.

Most of the remaining miscellaneous causes of FUO are granulomatous conditions with or without small vessel vasculitis. Presumably, these conditions reflect an immune response to some unknown antigen. Sarcoidosis and granulomatous hepatitis are not final diagnoses, but histologic patterns. The differential diagnosis of noncaseating granulomas of the liver or bone marrow is very broad and strikingly similar to that of FUO. The differential diagnosis includes many infections (eg, tuberculosis, fungi), tumors, collagen vascular diseases, and drugs. Thus, the physician who finds granulomatous pathology on biopsy has not really made any progress toward reaching a diagnosis. If the granulomatous reaction is causing severe symptoms and no agent is evident after an exhaustive search, it may be necessary to suppress the granulomas with corticosteroids. But the physician should remain aware that the agent is unknown and may become apparent later. Patients with what looked like sarcoid have been treated with corticosteroids, and after initial improvement have died with disseminated tuberculosis or histoplasmosis.

FUO has other causes, but most are usually easy to diagnose, such as thyrotoxicosis, adrenal insufficiency, pheochromocytoma, and alcoholic hepatitis. However, Whipple's disease is difficult to diagnose because the symptoms are so variable. Another obscure cause of fever can be slow dissection of the aorta. Multiple pulmonary emboli, thrombophlebitis, and deep-seated hematomas rarely present as fever with no other signs.

Familial Mediterranean fever is easy to diagnose because the clinical pattern is unique: recurrent attacks of serous inflammation with abdominal or chest pain, plus fever, a high neutrophil count, and a high erythrocyte sedimentation rate. Between attacks, the patient is perfectly well. Inquiry shows similar symptoms in an ancestor from a Mediterranean country.

Factitious fever and other psychiatric conditions account for about 5% of hospitalized patients with FUO and for a much greater proportion of outpatients. Most patients who feign illness do it in one of two ways: Either they bring extensive records of temperatures measured at home, or they inject themselves with something, such as urine, saliva, or even feces, which makes them febrile. Those in the first group are easier to diagnose: If patients have no abnormal physical signs, have not lost weight, are not anemic, have a normal erythrocyte sedimentation rate, and have never had a fever documented by a medical professional, they are unlikely to have a real illness. The main clue to patients in the second group is striking variation in symptoms from day to day and even from hour to hour. Another clue can be inconstant or unlikely bacteriologic data. For example, persons with factitious illness often have blood cultures positive for multiple organisms, blood cultures positive for mouth flora, or changing bacteriology from day to day.

In addition to the few patients who actively feign illness, there are many more patients who have some objective evidence of disease, but in whom the psychological distress is out of all proportion to the physical illness. Most psychologically distressed patients do not satisfy the criterion of 38.3°C (101°F) or higher on two separate occasions.

EVALUATION OF A PATIENT WITH FEVER OF UNKNOWN ORIGIN

The essential first step is to take a detailed history and perform a complete physical exam that pays special attention to possibilities suggested by the history. Every patient should be given routine laboratory tests—urinalysis, complete blood count, erythrocyte sedimentation rate, blood chemistry panels, and a chest x-ray. If all of these are normal, go no farther. The patient has either recovered or perhaps has never really been ill.

Generally, at least one of the tests is abnormal, but it does not point to any particular diagnosis. At this point, the physician must order specific tests, and the history is supremely important in this decision. Every test cannot be carried out, so that each test should be performed for a reason rather than blindly. Every patient should have several blood cultures and CT scans of the chest and abdomen. If both types of test results are negative, the patient probably does not have endocarditis, abscess, or tumor.

Sonograms, gallium or indium scans, bone scans, and MRI scans usually add little to the information provided by CT. The physician may have to repeat the CT scan later (eg, to detect a slowly developing liver or perinephric abscess), but if it is persistently negative, the more likely diagnoses are generalized infections, rheumatic diseases, and miscellaneous causes.

It is important to be critical about positive serologic tests. A positive test for Lyme disease, leptospirosis, or even typhoid is not necessarily relevant to the FUO. Symptomless members of the general public are seropositive for Lyme disease or leptospirosis, and anyone who has ever received typhoid vaccine is likely to have high titers of anti-H agglutinin.

Often, exhaustive investigation fails to lead to a diagnosis, and the physician considers treating blindly. This is best postponed or avoided. But the patient who is febrile and anemic and has lost 50 lb should be started on a powerful nonsteroidal anti-inflammatory agent such as indomethacin. If the patient does not improve within 2 weeks, the physician needs to weigh the relative attractions of corticosteroids and antituberculous therapy. It is preferable not to give both simultaneously, because if the patient's fever abates, it is hard to decide why.

Even if the patient with FUO responds to blind treatment, the diagnosis is still unknown, may be serious, and may surface later. The physician should continue to see the patient at intervals and investigate any new symptoms.

A few patients with FUO never get a definite diagnosis. If the fever has continued for more than 1 year, "no diagnosis" becomes the most common diagnosis. The outlook is relatively good: In most of these patients, the fever eventually subsides spontaneously.

SUMMARY

▶ Fever of unknown origin is defined as a fever that lasts longer than 3 weeks, that reaches at least 38.3°C (101°F) on at least two occasions separated by at least 24 hours, and whose cause is not apparent after routine examination.

▶ Most cases of FUO are caused by serious disease: about 40% by infections, 30% by tumors, and 15% by collagen vascular diseases. The remaining cases have many diagnoses, some of which are also serious.

▶ Factitious fever, a patient's actively faking illness for some secondary gain, accounts for about 5% of cases of FUO and usually implies a major psychiatric problem.

▶ In some patients, no cause for FUO is found despite exhaustive investigation. If fever continues for more than 1 year, it is likely that no cause will be found. The prognosis is good: Most of these patients recover spontaneously.

SUGGESTED READING

Guyton AC: Body temperature, temperature regulation, and fever. In: *Textbook of Medical Physiology,* 8th ed. WB Saunders, 1991.

Knockaert DC et al: Fever of unknown origin in the 1980s: An update of the diagnostic spectrum. Arch Intern Med 1992;152:51.

Larson EB, Featherstone HJ, Petersdorf RG: Fever of undetermined origin: Diagnosis and follow-up of 105 cases, 1970–1980. Medicine 1982;61:269.

Petersdorf RG: Fever of unknown origin: An old friend revisited (editorial). Arch Intern Med 1992;152:21.

Petersdorf RG, Beeson PB: Fever of unexplained origin: Report on 100 cases. Medicine 1961;40:1.

Central Nervous System Infections

Diane E. Griffin, MD, PhD

Central nervous system (CNS) infection should be suspected in any patient who presents acutely with fever, headache, and stiff neck (meningismus). CNS infection should be considered also in any patient who has an unexplained change in mental status, even without meningismus or fever. Although CNS infections are relatively rare, their potential severity demands swift and knowledgeable evaluation. Infection can be localized to the meninges (meningitis), spread diffusely in the brain parenchyma (encephalitis) or spinal cord (myelitis), or cause focal lesions (abscess). Disease can range from acute but benign forms of viral meningitis, to quickly fatal bacterial meningitis, to slowly progressive mental deterioration from fungal, mycobacterial, or persistent viral infection. Prompt treatment is effective against many of the more severe pathogens, and outcome is often determined by the speed and appropriateness of the therapy.

EVALUATION

Clinical Assessment

Initial assessment requires a careful history, with attention to the tempo of the disease, potential exposures to infectious agents, and host factors that may increase susceptibility to certain infections. The physical examination is directed at localizing the site of the neurologic disease and finding evidence of systemic infection. Evaluation is supplemented by examination of the cerebrospinal fluid (CSF), and, when indicated, imaging studies.

The history and physical exam should include evaluation for cranial trauma, level of consciousness, cranial nerve palsies, focal deficits, meningismus, and increased intracranial pressure. If the patient has papilledema, lumbar puncture may be contraindicated. A history of recent open trauma or surgery suggests infection with staphylococcal and gram-negative organisms from the environment and skin. The physician should search for other foci of infection and for physical signs suggesting a specific microbe. Cutaneous petechiae and purpura strongly suggest meningococcal infection, although Rocky Mountain

spotted fever, typhus, and enterovirus infections can also produce a spotty rash. Meningitis in a patient with middle ear or sinus infection, CSF rhinorrhea, or pneumonia suggests the pneumococcus, whereas mumps virus would be the likely cause of encephalitis in an individual with parotitis.

Evidence of CNS infection may be attributed to or masked by other processes. Physicians may ascribe fever to a recognized infection elsewhere or may blame altered CNS function on alcoholism, head trauma, stroke, brain tumor, subarachnoid hemorrhage, or senility. Physicians evaluating a patient with altered CNS function must rule out treatable CNS infection, particularly bacterial meningitis. The usual method is lumbar puncture and CSF exam (Table 8.3–1). Physicians may need to start treatment before lumbar puncture if they suspect that the patient has an overwhelming bacterial infection or if the lumbar puncture will be delayed for any reason (see below).

Cerebrospinal Fluid Examination: Lumbar puncture is riskiest when patients have evidence of increased intracranial pressure caused by a mass lesion within the cranial vault. When CSF is removed, the intracranial pressure dynamics change and the brain may shift downward through the tentorial notch or foramen magnum. This is particularly likely to happen in patients with a large, asymmetric supratentorial or posterior fossa mass. Herniation is seldom seen with diffuse increases in intracranial volume, as occurs with generalized infection or meningitis. The physician suspects a mass if the history or physical findings suggest a focal lesion or funduscopic exam shows increased intracranial pressure; then the patient should have an imaging scan such as computed tomography (CT) before the lumbar puncture. Otherwise, the lumbar puncture should not be delayed, since the information gained from examining CSF is crucial for both differential diagnosis and prompt treatment.

Normal CSF is crystal clear. It contains at most five mononuclear cells/μL and at most 45 mg/dL protein, has a glucose concentration greater than 50% of the blood glucose, and has a pressure below 180 mm H_2O. CNS infec-

Table 8.3–1. Typical cerebrospinal fluid (CSF) findings in central nervous system infections.

CSF Finding	Most Common Infections
Cells (normal ≤4 cells/μL)	
10–100	Viral, early bacterial, spirochetal, fungal meningitis; encephalitis; abscesses
>1000	Bacterial meningitis
>50% polymorphonuclear	Bacterial, early viral, amebic meningitis
>50% mononuclear	Viral, spirochetal, fungal, mycobacterial meningitis
Protein (normal <45 mg/dL)	
45–100 mg/dL	Viral meningitis or encephalitis; bacterial meningitis
>200 mg/dL	Abscesses; bacterial, fungal, and mycobacterial meningitis
Glucose (normal >50% of blood level)	
Low	Bacterial, mycobacterial, or fungal meningitis
Normal	Viral meningitis or encephalitis; abscesses

Table 8.3–2. Causes of CSF pleocytosis with negative cultures.

Category	Examples
Infections	
Difficult to culture	Lyme disease, leptospirosis, syphilis, fungi, mycoplasma, viruses
Infected "neighboring" structures	Brain abscess, epidural abscess
Rheumatic diseases	Systemic lupus erythematosus, Behçet's syndrome, central nervous system angiitis
Neoplasms	Carcinomatous meningitis
Drug reactions	Meningitis from nonsteroidal anti-inflammatory drugs
Miscellaneous	Sarcoidosis, Mollaret's meningitis, Vogt-Koyanagi (Harada) syndrome

tion usually increases the number of cells (pleocytosis), increases the protein, or decreases the glucose (see Table 8.3–1). In patients suspected of having infection, the cells should be counted and a differential count carried out. Lymphocytes usually predominate in mycobacterial, fungal, rickettsial, and viral infections, whereas polymorphonuclear leukocytes predominate in bacterial and amebic infections. The CSF protein content increases with most infections: The rise may be slight with viral infections and is usually greater with bacterial, fungal, or tuberculous infections. A high protein content may be the only CSF abnormality in a patient with a brain abscess. The CSF glucose is usually low in untreated bacterial meningitis and often low in fungal and tuberculous meningitis. The CSF glucose may also be depressed in some viral encephalitides, CNS sarcoidosis, CNS tumors, and subarachnoid hemorrhage. The CSF glucose probably drops because of altered glucose transport between blood and CSF.

It is often possible to identify the pathogen in the CSF. Mycobacteria, amebae, bacteria, and fungi may be seen by direct microscopy with a wet mount or with acid-fast, Gram's, or India ink stain. Microbial antigens also may be detected immunologically by latex agglutination, radioimmunoassay, or enzyme immunoassay. Microbial nucleic acid may be detected by polymerase chain reaction. CSF should be cultured for fungi, mycobacteria, bacteria, and viruses, because cultures may be positive when other tests are negative and may provide important information such as species and antibiotic sensitivity. Since CNS infection is often a complication of systemic disease, the differential diagnosis should guide the choice of other relevant sites to culture (eg, blood, stool, throat, sputum, and urine).

The term "aseptic meningitis" describes a sterile CSF with pleocytosis. Aseptic meningitis has many causes, in-

cluding infections that are difficult to culture (eg, viruses, spirochetes) or "hidden" (eg, brain abscess) (Table 8.3–2). Noninfectious causes of aseptic meningitis include rheumatic diseases, sarcoidosis, drugs, and neoplasms.

Imaging Studies

Few patients need plain films of the skull or spine, but these may help identify trauma or vertebral disease predisposing to infection. CT scan with contrast may or may not confirm meningeal infection, but it is useful in diagnosing epidural, subdural, and parenchymal brain abscesses. Magnetic resonance imaging (MRI) is more sensitive for revealing such parenchymal infections as progressive multifocal leukoencephalopathy, herpes simplex virus encephalitis, the white matter lesions of HIV-associated dementia, bacterial cerebritis before the capsule develops, and spinal cord lesions. Myelography and MRI are highly sensitive in diagnosing spinal epidural abscess.

TYPES OF CENTRAL NERVOUS SYSTEM INFECTIONS

Meningitis

The organisms that cause meningitis most often reach the CNS through the bloodstream. Meningitis commonly presents with headache and fever. Inflammation of the meninges causes reflex paraspinous muscle spasm that is reflected by an opisthotonic posture (head bent backward and body bowed forward), nuchal rigidity, inability to straighten a raised leg (Kernig's sign), and flexion of the leg when the head is flexed (Brudzinski's sign). Chronic meningeal inflammation can lead to cranial nerve palsies.

Viral Meningitis: A number of viruses can cause viral meningitis, a disease that most often attacks children and young adults (Figure 8.3–1). The most common causes are enteroviruses (echovirus, coxsackievirus, and polio), mumps virus, HIV, herpes simplex virus type 2, and the arthropod-borne viruses (in the United States: eastern equine, western equine, St. Louis, and California encephalitis viruses). The most likely cause varies with the

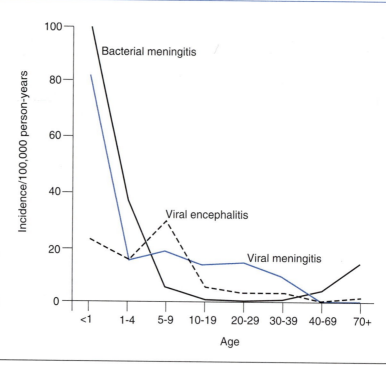

Figure 8.3–1. Major types of central nervous system infections: incidence/100,000 person-years, according to age. (Modified and reproduced, with permission, from Nicolosi A et al: Epidemiology of central nervous system infections in Olmsted County, Minnesota, 1950–1981. J Infect Dis 1986;154:399. Copyright 1986, University of Chicago. All rights reserved.)

season. Mumps, a common cause of encephalitis before widespread immunization was begun, took its greatest toll in the springtime. In temperate climates, enteroviruses (which cause over 50% of all cases of viral meningitis) and arthropod-borne viruses are most common in the summer and fall, often causing community-wide outbreaks.

Typical symptoms are headache, photophobia, stiff neck, and fever, sometimes following a prodrome a few days long. The disease is usually brief: Most patients improve in 1–3 days. No treatment is needed. CSF cell counts are usually 20–1000/µL (see Table 8.3–1). Early in the illness, polymorphonuclear leukocytes may predominate, but mononuclear cells soon take over. The etiology is determined by isolating the virus from the CSF or showing a significant rise in virus-specific antibodies in the serum or CSF during the illness. Enteroviruses are most often isolated from the pharynx, stool, or urine. All methods for specific diagnosis take time. Before assuming an untreatable viral cause, the physician must rule out CNS infections like herpes encephalitis, which require specific therapy and have a poor prognosis if untreated. Repeat CSF exams to document the shift from polymorphonuclear to mononuclear leukocytes often help differentiate viral from bacterial meningitis.

Meningitis Caused by Spirochetes: Three spirochetal diseases—syphilis, Lyme disease, and leptospirosis—can cause meningitis or meningoencephalitis that resembles viral infection. Syphilis is a sexually transmitted disease that characteristically begins with a painless genital ulcer (Chapter 8.9). Several weeks later, patients can develop meningitis along with other signs (eg, fever, rash, lym-

phadenopathy) of secondary syphilis. Lyme disease, transmitted by ticks, characteristically begins with an annular skin lesion that may be followed by meningitis and encephalitis (Chapter 8.16); many patients develop cranial nerve palsies, especially of the facial nerves. Leptospirosis, transmitted by contact with infected animal urine, causes fever, headache, conjunctivitis, impaired renal function, jaundice, cough, and meningitis (Chapter 8.16). The disease may be mild and self-limited or quickly fatal.

For all of these spirochetal diseases, CSF findings are similar to those in viral meningitis (see Table 8.3–1) and the diagnosis is usually made by testing serum or CSF for antibody. Left untreated, late meningovascular syphilis impairs the pupillary light reflex, and tertiary Lyme disease causes headache, intellectual impairment, and focal neurologic deficits.

Bacterial Meningitis: Many types of bacteria can cause meningitis. But in patients who have no direct site of entry, a few organisms predominate: *Haemophilus influenzae, Neisseria meningitidis,* and *Streptococcus pneumoniae.* These are all encapsulated bacteria that usually enter the CNS through the bloodstream. Age is an important host determinant of bacterial meningitis (Table 8.3–3). Infants, possibly because of their immature immune status, are uniquely susceptible to CNS infection with *Listeria,* enteric gram-negative bacilli, and group B streptococci. As maternal antibody wanes and de novo production of antibody to bacterial polysaccharides lags, babies become susceptible to other bacterial pathogens, such as *H influenzae* and *N meningitidis.* Older people, especially those with liver disease, also become more

Table 8.3–3. Most common organisms causing CNS infection.

Risk Category	Infectious Agents
Normal (age 20–60)	Enteroviruses, *Neisseria meningitidis*, *Streptococcus pneumoniae*, herpes simplex virus
Normal (age >60)	*S pneumoniae*, gram-negative bacilli, *Listeria*
Splenectomy	*S pneumoniae*
AIDS	*Cryptococcus*, *Toxoplasma*, JC virus (progressive multifocal leukoencephalopathy), cytomegalovirus
Trauma	Gram-negative bacilli, staphylococci

susceptible to enteric gram-negative organisms; these pathogens account for 25% of all CNS infections in persons over 65.

Factors that increase susceptibility by facilitating entry of bacteria into the CNS are altered barriers to infection and impaired clearance of organisms from the blood. *S pneumoniae* is a common cause of bacterial meningitis in persons who have a history of head trauma causing CSF rhinorrhea and in persons who do not have a functional spleen. *N meningitidis* may affect young adults who are deficient in one of the complement components (detected by the CH_{50} assay) needed to work with antibody to lyse and clear this organism. *Staphylococcus aureus* and the gram-negative enteric rods often infect the CNS after cranial trauma or neurosurgery. *Staphylococcus epidermidis* is especially likely to cause CNS infection in patients with implanted shunts or reservoirs. *Listeria* meningitis occurs most often in neonates, the elderly, and individuals with compromised cellular immunity. The physical exam of all patients with suspected meningitis should include a careful search for a focus of infection that may have given rise to bacterial meningitis by direct extension or by production of a bacteremia.

Most adults with acute bacterial meningitis present with signs of meningeal irritation. Those without such signs are likely to be elderly and to have gram-negative meningitis. Bacterial meningitis can be fulminant, progressing quickly from apparent good health through headache, fever, and meningismus to coma and death. The immediate differentiation of bacterial meningitis from other varieties of CNS infection depends on physical findings and CSF exam. Bacterial meningitis is strongly suggested by a high cell count (>100/μL) with more than 50% polymorphonuclear leukocytes and by a low glucose (see Table 8.3–1). Bacteria seen on a Gram's stain of centrifuged CSF permit tentative identification of the pathogen. Immunologic tests can quickly detect bacterial antigen in CSF. The bacterial etiology is confirmed by culturing the organism from CSF or blood.

Differentiating bacterial meningitis from other types of meningitis becomes more difficult after patients have received partially effective antibiotics for even 1 or 2 days. Gram's stain of the CSF is less likely to be positive, and the organism may not grow on culture. But the CSF usu-

ally continues to suggest a bacterial process, since several days of therapy are required to reverse the characteristic polymorphonuclear pleocytosis, high protein, and low glucose.

Tuberculous Meningitis: Tuberculous meningitis is caused by hematogenous spread of miliary tuberculosis (Chapter 8.14) or by reactivation and rupture of a previously latent CNS tubercle. The disease progresses over several days to several weeks, with steadily increasing symptoms. The predominant clinical features are headache, nuchal rigidity, lethargy, and progressive deterioration of mental function. The chronic, fibrosing nature of the meningitis can lead to cranial nerve palsies and obstructive hydrocephalus (manifested by headache, nausea and vomiting, mental deterioration, or spastic paraparesis), or produce localized infarction secondary to vasculitis. Patients with miliary CNS disease may have demonstrable tuberculosis involving other organs, but negative purified protein derivative (PPD) skin tests. Many patients with reactivated CNS tuberculosis do not have demonstrable infection in other organs, but most have positive skin tests and many have a history of exposure to tuberculosis.

Examined early in tuberculous meningitis, the CSF may look similar to that in viral meningitis: mononuclear pleocytosis, elevated protein, and normal glucose (see Table 8.3–1). Later in the course, the glucose is usually low. Most patients must be started on treatment without a definitive diagnosis, since the organisms are rarely seen on acid-fast stains of the CSF and therapy cannot be delayed for the 6 weeks needed to obtain culture results.

Fungal Meningitis: The fungi that most often cause meningitis are *Cryptococcus*, *Coccidioides*, *Histoplasma*, and *Blastomyces*. Of these, cryptococcal meningitis is most common. It is a subacute disease, primarily seen in the elderly and in persons immunosuppressed by either underlying disease (eg, AIDS) or chemotherapy. Initial CNS symptoms may be mild and nonspecific, but they gradually progress to clumsiness, somnolence, and blurred vision. Chronic cryptococcal meningitis should be considered in the differential diagnosis of delirium or dementia in the elderly. Recurrent headache and mental impairment can evolve slowly over many months and have a waxing and waning course. Few patients have fever or nuchal rigidity. Dementia may develop secondary to direct infection of the brain parenchyma or to hydrocephalus.

Meningitis caused by *Coccidioides immitis* usually appears within 6 months after the primary pulmonary infection and involves predominantly the basilar meninges. The most common symptom is headache, but patients may have fever, confusion, seizures, stiff neck, diplopia, ataxia, and focal neurologic deficits. The disease should be suspected in a patient who has a compatible clinical picture and a history of travel or residence in the American southwest, where the organism is endemic. Meningitis can also be caused by *Histoplasma capsulatum*, a fungus endemic to the southeastern United States. Disseminated histoplasmosis can cause hepatosplenomegaly, fever, lymphadenopathy, weight loss, and an ulcerated or indurated lesion in the nasopharynx. Disseminated blastomycosis can also present as chronic meningitis.

CSF findings in fungal meningitis are usually similar to those of tuberculous meningitis (see Table 8.3–1), but some patients with cryptococcal meningitis (particularly patients with AIDS) have an entirely normal CSF. Cryptococcal capsular antigen is usually detectable in the CSF by immunologic methods, but culture remains the most sensitive test. Other fungal infections are most often diagnosed by serology, although cultures of CSF are occasionally positive.

Parenchymal Infection

The brain parenchyma can become infected through local spread of organisms from a contiguous source of infection (usually resulting in a single lesion) or through hematogenous spread (often resulting in multiple lesions). Disease within the brain parenchyma can cause seizures, altered consciousness, acute changes in personality or behavior, and focal neurologic deficits. Patients may have no signs of meningeal irritation.

Viral Encephalomyelitis: Viral infection of the brain parenchyma can be focal or diffuse. Viruses can infect neurons, leading directly to seizures, paralysis, or changes in mental status. The severity of viral encephalitis is related to the etiology and the patient's age. Cytomegalovirus and Epstein-Barr, western equine, Venezuelan equine, St. Louis, and California encephalitis viruses all cause relatively mild disease that is rarely fatal. Although the long-term outlook is poor, the acute meningoencephalitis associated with HIV seroconversion is self-limited. Mortality is greater and sequelae more severe, when acute encephalitis is caused by infection with herpes simplex virus type 1, varicella zoster, eastern equine encephalitis, Japanese encephalitis, or rabies virus.

With severe disease, patients' mental status typically deteriorates over several days from lethargy to confusion, stupor, and then coma. The hypothalamus may be involved, causing severe hyper- or hypothermia and diabetes insipidus. Common signs of herpes simplex virus type 1 encephalitis are focal seizures, bizarre behavior, hallucinations, and aphasia suggesting the typical temporal lobe localization. Rabies may begin with local paresthesias at the site of the bite and progress to agitation and muscle spasms or ascending paralysis. Acute contralateral hemiparesis may follow herpes zoster ophthalmicus related to a localized cerebral angiitis. Certain of the "slow virus infections" (eg, Creutzfeldt-Jakob disease, subacute sclerosing panencephalitis, progressive multifocal leukoencephalopathy) begin insidiously, progress slowly, and do not cause fever. A history of travel or insect bites may be important since the arthropod-borne viruses are geographically restricted and appear only during the seasons of their vectors.

Myelitis can occur with or without encephalitis. Transverse myelitis produces lower limb weakness, a sensory level, and loss of bowel and bladder control. An intraparenchymal lesion is suggested by sacral sparing or dissociated sensory loss, whereas local pain suggests an extramedullary lesion more likely caused by a bacterial abscess. Anterior spinal artery occlusion may be secondary to infectious vasculitis (caused by tuberculosis, syphilis, schistosomiasis). Classic poliomyelitis, with primary infection of anterior horn cells, presents with flaccid paralysis and muscle pain.

Other Causes of Encephalomyelitis: Rickettsiae, spirochetes, and some bacteria can cause an encephalomyelitis similar to that produced by viruses. Rocky Mountain spotted fever is transmitted by ticks, with the highest incidence in the spring and early summer when ticks are most abundant (Chapter 8.16). The severe headache characteristic of this disease may precede the rash, and neurologic deterioration may be rapid. The most common spirochetal diseases causing encephalitis are Lyme disease and syphilis. The most common bacterial cause is *Listeria*. Whipple's disease may begin insidiously, with dementia, myoclonus, and ataxia but not significant malabsorption. In addition to these CNS infections, the autoimmune disease acute disseminated or postinfectious encephalomyelitis can complicate viral exanthems (particularly measles) and respiratory infections. This acute demyelinating disease causes new-onset fever and neurologic signs, particularly seizures, altered mental status, and focal deficits.

Localized Intracranial Bacterial Infection: The common localized intracranial bacterial infections are brain abscess, subdural empyema, epidural abscess, and septic thrombophlebitis of the major venous sinuses. Abscesses originating from hematogenous spread or a contiguous source of infection (eg, the ear, paranasal sinuses) begin as localized cerebritis with softening, necrosis, inflammation, and edema. As the process continues, fibroblasts proliferate at the periphery to encapsulate the infected area. Symptoms can be caused by local destruction of tissue, but most often result from pressure from the expanding lesion and surrounding edema. Clinical signs can develop rapidly, or slowly over several weeks. Brain abscess most often presents with increasingly severe headache, followed by nausea and vomiting. Temperature may be normal, particularly in older people and patients with temporal lobe abscesses. Increased intracranial pressure can cause papilledema and third and sixth cranial nerve palsies. The bacteria that form a brain abscess reflect the infected focus of origin. Anaerobes are common, but many patients have more than one bacterial strain; streptococci, enterobacteria, and staphylococci are frequent aerobic pathogens.

Epidural abscesses typically spread laterally and are often thin, since the dura is relatively adherent to the skull. However, subdural abscesses may be large, space-occupying lesions. Infections in both of these parameningeal sites usually result from direct invasion of microorganisms, but occasionally blood-borne organisms localize in a closed sterile area that was previously traumatized.

The signs of suppurative intracranial thrombophlebitis depend on the veins involved. Cortical vein thrombosis can cause impaired consciousness, focal neurologic deficits, seizures, and increased intracranial pressure. Cavernous sinus thrombosis usually follows facial infection and quickly causes proptosis, ophthalmoplegia, and retinal hemorrhage. As with brain abscesses, the organisms reflect those at the original site of infection.

Important techniques to detect and differentiate these localized infections include neurologic exam, CT scanning (for brain abscesses and subdural empyema), MRI, and arteriography (for subdural empyema and thrombophlebitis). Skull films may show mastoiditis or sinusitis. Lumbar puncture is of limited value and may be dangerous. CSF pressure is often elevated, and protein or cells may be increased, but these findings are not diagnostic. Bacteria are found in the CSF only if the infection has extended to the meninges.

Infection in the Immunocompromised Host

The host is an important determinant of susceptibility to certain CNS infections. Patients who have trouble clearing organisms from the blood because of asplenia or humoral immune defects tend to have more frequent and fulminant infections with common bacterial pathogens (eg, *S pneumoniae, N meningitidis,*). In patients with defective humoral immunity, enteroviral infections can present as subacute disease involving liver, skin, and CNS. Patients with defective cellular immunity are susceptible to new infection with unusual pathogens and to reactivated infection with organisms (eg, tuberculosis, fungi) previously contained by the immune response. Opportunistic infections of the CNS are second only to pulmonary infections in causing morbidity and mortality in chronically immunosuppressed patients.

Symptoms are as variable as the pathogens, but many patients present with nonspecific complaints of recurrent headache and memory loss evolving over many days to weeks. Patients may have focal deficits. Many of the diseases are difficult to diagnose. The CSF may be normal or only slightly abnormal. Serology often does not help, because of the underlying immunodeficiency. *Cryptococcus, Candida,* and *Listeria* cause meningitis and may be cultured from the CSF, but brain biopsy or aspiration is required to diagnose *Toxoplasma* or progressive multifocal leukoencephalopathy (PML) definitively.

MANAGEMENT

Treatment of CNS infections is guided by a determination of the most likely pathogen and a knowledge of drugs' bactericidal activity and their ability to penetrate into the CNS. If lumbar puncture is delayed for any rea-

son, treatment may need to be started before the CSF is examined and cultured. Drugs (eg, chloramphenicol, rifampin, metronidazole) that penetrate cells usually achieve excellent levels in the CNS at doses routinely used for systemic infection. The usefulness of drugs (eg, penicillin) that penetrate the CNS less well is determined by the ability to give large doses without causing toxicity. In general, drug doses must be chosen to achieve high plasma concentrations.

Few drugs are currently available for viral diseases of the CNS. Acyclovir is effective for herpes simplex virus and varicella zoster virus. Ganciclovir is effective for cytomegalovirus. Many other acute viral infections (eg, enterovirus, mumps) in the normal host resolve without specific treatment. The subarachnoid space is relatively deficient in host defenses, since it contains low protein (antibody, complement) levels and few phagocytes. Therefore, drugs or drug combinations should be bactericidal. Many of the most common causes of bacterial meningitis are effectively treated with penicillin, ampicillin, or a third-generation cephalosporin (eg, ceftriaxone) that penetrates the CNS well. Persons who have close contact with patients with meningococcal meningitis should receive rifampin prophylaxis. Brain abscesses that are not yet well encapsulated can often be treated with antibiotics alone; encapsulated abscesses should be drained by aspiration and may need to be excised. The standard treatment for fungal meningitis remains amphotericin, sometimes supplemented with flucytosine. Fluconazole penetrates the CNS well and can be used as primary or suppressive therapy for some fungal infections. Encephalitis and bacterial meningitis require 14–21 days of therapy. Abscesses and fungal meningitis generally require treatment for 6 weeks.

SUMMARY

▶ Central nervous system infections require prompt evaluation to localize the site of infection and identify the most likely pathogen.

▶ Headache, fever, and stiff neck are the most common presenting symptoms of acute meningitis.

▶ Chronic meningitis should be in the differential diagnosis of any patient who has unexplained mental status changes, even without fever or meningismus.

▶ Examining the CSF for cells, protein, glucose, and organisms is often the most informative laboratory test. Imaging studies are essential to evaluate infection in the parenchyma or a parameningeal site.

▶ Treatment may need to be started before lumbar puncture if the patient is suspected of having an overwhelming bacterial infection or if the lumbar puncture will be delayed for any reason.

SUGGESTED READING

Berlin LE et al: Aseptic meningitis in infants <2 years of age: Diagnosis and etiology. J Infect Dis 1993;168:888.

Durand ML et al: Acute bacterial meningitis in adults: A review of 493 episodes. N Engl J Med 1993;328:21.

Koskiniemi M et al: Epidemiology of encephalitis in children: A 20-year survey. Ann Neurol 1991;29:492.

Seydoux C, Francioli P: Bacterial brain abscesses: Factors influencing mortality and sequelae. Clin Infect Dis 1992;15:394.

Upper Respiratory Tract Infections

John J. Mann, MD, and Katharine S. Harrison, MD

Patients with upper respiratory tract infection can present with coryza, pharyngitis, sinusitis, otitis media, or bronchitis. Most upper respiratory illnesses are caused by viruses, have no specific therapy, and resolve spontaneously. However, some upper respiratory illnesses are caused or complicated by bacterial infections that can produce serious problems if not treated appropriately with antibiotics. Rheumatic fever following untreated streptococcal pharyngitis, and meningitis following middle ear infection, are but two examples of how a minor upper respiratory illness can have major (yet often preventable) consequences. The primary challenge that physicians face with upper respiratory infections is knowing when to limit care to supportive measures and when to suspect or treat important bacterial infections.

THE COMMON COLD

The common cold can be caused by many viruses, including rhinovirus, coronavirus, adenovirus, parainfluenza, respiratory syncytial, and influenza viruses. The most common symptoms of a cold are a runny nose, sneezing, and a dry cough, with or without mild sore throat. Colds can also present with headache, myalgia, and fever as well as coryza. The nasal discharge is clear and the cough is nonproductive. The tympanic membrane may be retracted but should not be inflamed.

Until recently, upper airway colds were believed to affect only the nose and pharynx. Sinus involvement was considered to be caused by bacterial superinfection following the viral infection. Now it is known that the viral infection itself routinely involves the sinuses and can cause sinusitis.

Patients with a cold may be helped by decongestants, antipyretics, and cough suppressants, especially those containing codeine. Antibiotics have no use in routine management of the common cold. They are always ineffective, often expensive, and, in rare patients, the cause of serious side effects (eg, anaphylaxis, rashes, Stevens-Johnson reaction). Antibiotics may be prescribed for complications such as otitis media or sinusitis (see "Sinusitis" below), and for patients with special risk factors such as serious underlying conditions, respiratory allergy, chronic lung disease, or immune suppression.

PHARYNGITIS

Pharyngitis is primarily caused by a viral or bacterial infection. Bacterial pharyngitis is usually more serious and is treated with antibiotics. Acute epiglottitis is a life-threatening condition, which requires early recognition and, possibly, surgical intervention. In addition, pharyngitis may be a manifestation of an acute infection such as mononucleosis or AIDS.

Viral Pharyngitis

Probably more than 80% of cases of pharyngitis are caused by the same viruses that cause the common cold, such as the rhinoviruses and coronaviruses (Table 8.4–1). Typically, the normal adult infected with one of these viruses develops a mild-to-moderate sore throat, often in conjunction with coryza or nasal congestion. The patient appears uncomfortable, sounds hoarse, and may have a modest fever, an erythematous pharynx, and minimal cervical lymphadenopathy. Such a patient does not require antibiotics. Supportive care is sufficient.

Bacterial Pharyngitis

Determining whether a patient with a sore throat has an important infection such as streptococcal pharyngitis or epiglottitis depends on the clinical presentation and the host. A central dilemma arises in recognizing the patient who has streptococcal pharyngitis. Antibiotic treatment for such a patient not only alleviates the symptoms, but also prevents the poststreptococcal complications of acute glomerulonephritis and rheumatic fever. About 15% of cases of pharyngitis are caused by group A β-hemolytic streptococci (*Streptococcus pyogenes*), and a few cases are caused by group C. Classically, patients with strep throat have pharyngeal exudates, enlarged and tender anterior

Table 8.4–1. Microbial causes of acute pharyngitis.

	Organism	Clinical Features
Viruses	Rhinovirus	Common cold
	Coronavirus	Common cold
	Adenovirus	Conjunctivitis
	Influenza	Ill-appearing patient, influenza, high fever
	Parainfluenza	Common cold, cough
	Coxsackievirus	Herpangina, pleurodynia
	Epstein-Barr virus ⎫ Cytomegalovirus ⎭	Adolescent or young adult, posterior cervical lymphadenopathy
	Herpes simplex types I and II	Gingivitis, stomatitis
	HIV	Primary HIV infection, mononucleosis-like syndrome
Bacteria	*Streptococcus pyogenes*	Fever, exudates
	Mixed anaerobes	Pain, fetid breath
	Neisseria gonorrhoeae	Oral-genital contact
	Neisseria meningitidis	Systemic infection
	Corynebacterium diphtheriae	Membranous pharyngitis
	Yersinia enterocolitica	Abdominal pain, colitis
	Treponema pallidum	Secondary syphilis
Other pathogens	*Mycoplasma pneumoniae*	Pneumonia
	Chlamydia pneumoniae, strain TWAR	Young adult, hoarseness, bronchitis

cervical lymph nodes, fever above 38.3°C (101°F), and leukocytosis. However, the clinical presentation is often indistinguishable from that of benign viral pharyngitis.

Less common bacterial causes of pharyngitis include *M pneumoniae* and the TWAR strain of *C pneumoniae*. The TWAR strain most often affects teenagers and young adults and can produce hoarseness, a sign usually attributed to viral laryngitis. Rarely, sore throat is caused by other bacterial pathogens such as *Corynebacterium diphtheriae, Yersinia enterocolitica, Neisseria meningitidis, Neisseria gonorrhoeae,* and *Treponema pallidum. N gonorrhoeae* and *T pallidum* infections are complications of oral-genital sex. Anaerobic infection can cause a number of syndromes, including pharyngitis (Vincent's angina), stomatitis (trench mouth), peritonsillar abscess (quinsy), and sublingual and submandibular space abscess (Ludwig's angina). Ludwig's angina causes severe pain, putrid breath, acute necrosis, and pseudomembrane formation.

Despite the diagnostic difficulties, several observations argue against the routine use of throat cultures and other tests. First, cultures can be misleading because some adults are asymptomatic carriers and some cultures are falsely negative. Second, rheumatic fever usually follows an obviously symptomatic streptococcal pharyngitis. Third, rheumatic fever today is rare and does not justify the expense of routine cultures in adults. Fourth, even if patients sustain one attack of rheumatic fever, long-term antibiotic prophylaxis can usually prevent them from developing rheumatic heart disease.

Thus, it is reasonable not to do routine throat cultures but to prescribe antibiotics for patients who have a severe sore throat, a history of contact with a person who had a streptococcal infection, a personal or family history of rheumatic fever or glomerulonephritis, or a history of frequent sinusitis or bronchitis after pharyngitis. Antibiotics should also be given to all patients with splenectomy, hy-

pogammaglobulinemia, or other immune suppression. For a few patients who may not need antibiotics, withholding this treatment causes psychological stress, which then provokes multiple phone calls or office visits. A brief course of antibiotic therapy may prevent great frustration for both patient and physician.

To prevent rheumatic fever, an effective oral antibiotic must be given for 10 days, although the pharyngeal symptoms abate before 10 days. Erythromycin, amoxicillin, or penicillin is effective. Erythromycin has the advantage of covering other causes of pharyngitis (eg, *Mycoplasma pneumoniae, Chlamydia pneumoniae*); its disadvantage is that it more often causes gastrointestinal upset. Patients with doubtful compliance can be given a long-acting parenteral penicillin such as benzathine penicillin.

Complicated Pharyngeal Infections

Acute epiglottitis is a life-threatening infection in which early recognition is key to successful management. Epiglottitis usually affects young children, but more than 10% of patients are adults. The most common pathogen is *Haemophilus influenzae* type b; other pathogens include staphylococci, *Streptococcus pneumoniae,* and group A streptococci. The onset is acute, and airway obstruction can cause abrupt respiratory failure. Symptoms include severe sore throat, chills, painful dysphagia, excessive secretions with drooling, a noncroupy cough, and pain on speaking, but without true hoarseness. Most patients are febrile, appear acutely ill, and prefer sitting to lying down. The anterior neck is tender, sometimes with visible swelling and erythema. If pharyngitis is present, it is mild and the uvula may be swollen. Stridor indicates impending airway obstruction. Visualizing the epiglottis may be difficult and may precipitate airway obstruction, so it should be attempted only by a trained physician in an acute care facility. When visualized, the epiglottis is markedly swollen and usually cherry red, but sometimes pale. The vocal cords and other infra-epiglottic structures are normal. Lateral soft tissue x-rays of the neck may show a hemispherical mass at the base of the tongue and narrowing of the upper airway.

The key to effective treatment of acute epiglottitis is early recognition and prevention of airway obstruction. At the first sign of airway compromise such as stridor, endotracheal intubation should be performed in an operating room. After the examiner obtains blood and a swab from the epiglottis for cultures, the patient may be started on intravenous ceftriaxone. Patients should improve within 36–48 hours. The artificial airway can be removed when patients are afebrile and alert and when direct visualization shows that the epiglottitis is resolving.

Other complicated respiratory infections are peritonsillar abscess, lateral or retropharyngeal space abscesses, and infections involving the submandibular, sublingual, and submaxillary spaces (Ludwig's angina). Prompt recognition of these syndromes is important because of the risk of airway obstruction or of the infection spreading to the mediastinum, deep cervical structures, jugular veins, or central nervous system. Patients should be given empiric antibiotic treatment with intravenous clindamycin or cefoxitin, with an aminoglycoside added in immunocompromised hosts.

Some patients suffer relapse after treatment of a seemingly typical streptococcal sore throat. Therapeutic choices for these patients include short-term retreatment with the same or a different antibiotic, a longer antibiotic course (4–8 weeks), or a penicillinase-resistant antibiotic such as clindamycin. Tonsillectomy is rarely indicated, but it is the only option acceptable to some patients.

Occasionally, pharyngitis is a manifestation of an important viral or fungal infection. Infectious mononucleosis caused by the Epstein-Barr virus often manifests in teenagers or young adults as a severe sore throat, fever, and lymphadenopathy that is most often posterior cervical. This pharyngitis must be distinguished from group A streptococci, because giving penicillin or related drugs to patients with mononucleosis is not only ineffective but also much more likely to cause a drug rash. Acute HIV infection can also present with pharyngitis. Patients on corticosteroids or with T-cell defects including AIDS are at risk for *Candida* pharyngitis, often easily recognized by the "flecks of cottage cheese" distributed diffusely over the buccal mucosa, tongue, and posterior pharynx. Especially in patients with AIDS, oral candidiasis can progress to esophagitis.

Patients with pharyngitis often present with ulceration of the mucous membranes. Included in the differential diagnosis are aphthous ulcers, herpes simplex, anaerobic stomatitis, syphilis, herpangina (caused by coxsackieviruses and distinguished by small vesicles in the pharynx), and fungal infection, especially histoplasmosis. Inflammatory noninfectious causes include Behçet's syndrome, erythema multiforme, pemphigus, pemphigoid, Wegener's granulomatosis, systemic lupus erythematosus, and Still's disease.

Extrarespiratory causes of sore throat include reflux esophagitis, angina pectoris, dissecting aortic aneurysm, vitamin deficiency, lymphoma, leukemia, and thyroiditis, which can be recognized by a tender thyroid gland.

COMPLICATIONS OF STREPTOCOCCAL PHARYNGITIS

The sequelae of streptococcal pharyngitis include suppurative complications from local extension of the infection, and nonsuppurative complications—scarlet fever, acute rheumatic fever, and acute glomerulonephritis. Infection around the tonsils may lead to peritonsillar abscess or quinsy or abscess of lymph tissue in the posterior pharyngeal wall. Secondary infection of the ears or sinuses can extend locally to cause central nervous system complications such as brain abscess, meningitis, and venous thrombosis of the intracranial sinuses. Septicemia and pneumonia complicating *S pyogenes* pharyngitis are exceedingly rare, except in debilitated patients.

Scarlet Fever

Scarlet fever, which usually affects children, develops from an infection with streptococci harboring a bacteriophage that codes for an erythrogenic toxin. On the second day, a rash develops on the upper torso and spreads to the remainder of the trunk, sparing the face, palms, and soles. The skin shows multiple tiny erythematous papules that blanch on pressure. The face is flushed and circumoral pallor is classic. The tongue is covered with a yellowish-white layer that coats the red papillae as "white strawberries." This turns to a beefy "red strawberry" tongue as the coating disappears. Scarlet fever usually follows pharyngitis, but it can follow streptococcal infections at other sites. The rash must be differentiated from viral exanthems, drug reactions, and the rash of toxic shock syndrome, which is usually caused by *Staphylococcus aureus*.

Severe group A streptococcal infections producing a toxic shock-like syndrome and scarlatinal toxin have recently been reported from several areas of the United States. The clinical picture is shock, renal impairment, adult respiratory distress syndrome, necrotizing fasciitis, and bullous skin lesions. Blood cultures are usually positive for group A β-hemolytic streptococci of different M and T types. The toxin A elaborated by these bacteria is the same scarlatinal toxin that produces scarlet fever. This toxic shock syndrome complicates group A streptococcal soft tissue infections more often than it complicates pharyngitis. Mortality rate is 30–50%. Treatment should be aggressive, including antibiotics, débridement, and intensive care support.

Rheumatic Fever

Although the incidence of acute rheumatic fever has declined precipitously in the antibiotic era, there have been recent reports of outbreaks in the United States, mostly limited to children and military recruits. Acute rheumatic fever appears about 3 weeks after streptococcal pharyngitis; this long latent period allows the physician to prevent rheumatic fever by treating the infection. Rheumatic fever is caused by an autoimmune process in which persons with certain HLA class II antigens make antibody to the M protein of specific strains of group A β-hemolytic streptococci. These antibodies cross-react with cardiac tissue antigens.

Acute rheumatic fever targets the heart, joints, central nervous system, and skin, but its only long-term morbidity derives from its cardiac effects. There is no test for the disease. Diagnosis depends on the Jones criteria (Table 8.4–2). In brief, patients present with either arthritis or carditis, the latter producing new-onset mitral regurgitation. Very rare patients present with chorea. The other major criteria—erythema marginatum and subcutaneous nodules—always appear in conjunction with the arthritis or carditis. The acute illness can be severe, with mitral regurgitation and heart failure, but most patients have a low-grade illness and look deceptively well.

Acute rheumatic fever is treated by eradicating the streptococcal infection, giving high-dose aspirin for arthritis and giving prednisone for valvulitis.

Patients who have had one episode of rheumatic fever are at risk for recurrences after bouts of streptococcal pharyngitis. Preventing recurrences is extremely important in preventing rheumatic heart disease, which develops as chronic mitral valve disease in about 50% of patients who have acute rheumatic fever. For this reason, all young people who have had rheumatic fever should receive daily penicillin prophylaxis until their early 20's; patients af-

Table 8.4–2. Jones criteria (revised) for guidance in the diagnosis of acute rheumatic fever.

Major criteria
Carditis
Polyarthritis
Chorea
Erythema marginatum
Subcutaneous nodules

Minor criteria
Clinical
  Arthralgia
  Fever
Laboratory
  Elevated acute phase reactants: erythrocyte sedimentation
    rate, C-reactive protein
  Prolonged PR interval

Evidence of preceding group A streptococcal infection
Positive throat culture or rapid streptococcal antigen test
Elevated or rising streptococcal antibody titer

Acute rheumatic fever is likely if the patient has:
• 2 major criteria + evidence of streptococcal infection
• 1 major criterion + 2 minor criteria + evidence of
  streptococcal infection

Modified and reproduced, with permission, from: Guidelines for the diagnosis of rheumatic fever: Jones criteria, 1992 update. JAMA 1992;268:2069. © 1992, American Medical Association.

fected in their late teens should receive prophylaxis for at least 5 years. Some experts recommend long-term daily prophylaxis for patients at high risk for streptococcal exposure, such as parents of young children, elementary school teachers, and prison inmates. Some recommend lifetime prophylaxis for patients who have had carditis.

Patients with rheumatic valve damage risk developing endocarditis from any bacteremia, so they need additional antibiotic prophylaxis against endocarditis when they are having some surgical and dental procedures (Chapter 9.6). Patients with a history of acute rheumatic fever but no evidence of valve damage do not need endocarditis prophylaxis.

Acute Glomerulonephritis

Acute glomerulonephritis develops after infection with certain strains of group A or C streptococci. The mechanism of renal injury is unknown. One hypothesis is that it is immune-mediated, with injury caused by deposition of preformed complexes of streptococcal antigen and antibody. On a microscopic level, the kidneys of patients with poststreptococcal nephritis have increased glomerular cellularity because of endothelial and mesangial cell proliferation. Complement C3 and properdin are also found, thus supporting a role for the alternate complement pathway.

Poststreptococcal nephritis can develop in patients of any age and can be severe in adults. On average, it appears 10 days after pharyngitis and 3 weeks or longer after pyoderma. In most patients, the nephritis resolves spontaneously within weeks, but in a few people it progresses to chronic and sometimes permanent renal disease. Unlike rheumatic fever, nephritis rarely recurs, but streptococcal infections can exacerbate chronic glomerulonephritis.

Although penicillin prevents rheumatic fever, it is less effective in preventing glomerulonephritis. Patients should be treated to prevent spread to others, and a strong case can be made for prophylaxis of asymptomatic close contacts. After recovering from the glomerulonephritis, patients do not need long-term penicillin, probably because the type-specific antibody generated by the infection is protective.

TRACHEOBRONCHITIS

Patients with tracheobronchitis characteristically have an incessant cough. Symptoms of tracheobronchitis may begin with fever or headache, with or without sore throat and coryza. Dyspnea is not a feature. There are no signs of consolidation. Most tracheobronchitis is caused by viruses, and patients recover spontaneously. Bacterial superinfection can occur, especially in patients with chronic lung diseases such as chronic obstructive pulmonary disease, asthma, and cystic fibrosis. In adults, the most common cause of tracheobronchitis without sore throat or coryza is influenza virus. Coxsackie- and echoviruses also cause illness in adults; rhinovirus, parainfluenza, and respiratory syncytial virus are seen more frequently in children. *M pneumoniae* is an occasional, treatable cause of bronchitis. *Moraxella catarrhalis* most commonly causes tracheitis in patients with chronic pulmonary disease. In college students, *M pneumoniae* and *C pneumoniae* strain TWAR cause about 5% of tracheitis and 20% of pneumonia.

In most healthy adults, bronchitis is self-limited. For patients with chronic pulmonary disease, whose airways may be colonized with pneumococci, streptococci, or *H influenzae*, a viral infection of the trachea causing lysis of the protective epithelial cells may then lead to a severe bacterial bronchopneumonia. For this reason, it is wise to treat these patients with an antibiotic such as amoxicillin-clavulanate, trimethoprim-sulfamethoxazole, or erythromycin. These drugs also cover *Moraxella*, and erythromycin covers *Mycoplasma* as well as *Chlamydia*.

Other challenging patients present with a spasmodic cough, usually following a viral infection. The cough is distinctive—brassy, forceful, recurrent, nonproductive, and precipitated by deep breathing, rapid speech, or the supine position. Only time relieves the symptoms. Patients should be warned that the cough will persist for 3–6 weeks. Treatment should include reassurance, humidity, and cough suppressants. Antibiotics, antihistamines, decongestants, and systemic corticosteroids are of no value.

INFLUENZA

The influenza viruses are the most important agents causing acute respiratory disease. Because influenza is a well-studied epidemic viral disease, because of its prevalence and importance, and because it is a representative localized viral respiratory infection with prominent systemic manifestations, influenza is used here to illustrate some general epidemiologic, clinical, and immunologic features of viral disease. Although the fatality rate is usually low, influenza affects enormous numbers of people. During the influenza epidemic in the winter of 1962–1963, the United States had an estimated 80 million cases, and 70,000 deaths occurred from influenza and pneumonia. Pandemics (worldwide epidemics) of influenza have been recorded at the rate of about four per century since 1610. The most severe pandemic occurred in 1917–1918, when an estimated 10 million people died.

The only important source of influenza virus is infected people. The virus is readily found in respiratory secretions during the first few days of illness, but is rarely detectable for longer than the first week. Persistent carriers have not been found. There is evidence that inapparent or mild infections are more common than clinical disease; thus, the viruses may persist in a population by causing sporadic mild illnesses resembling the common cold.

The viral types influenza A and B appear during the winter in the northern hemisphere. The viruses are named according to their hemagglutinin or neuraminidase glycoproteins (H and N) on the viral coat. "Antigenic shift" is a change of peptide antigens, caused by genetic RNA reassortment. Antigenic shifts may herald the beginning of a pandemic. Minor changes in the coat proteins, known as "antigenic drift," occur every few years, and the new virus is immunologically favored over the old.

Major influenza epidemics are caused only by type A strains. No part of the world escapes for long. Widespread type A influenza recurs every 2–4 years. Nearly all epidemics in the northern hemisphere reach their peak in January and February. Type B influenza usually causes less severe epidemics, often localized to schools, military camps, and other closed populations. Type B epidemics occur in 4- to 6-year cycles. Influenza type C rarely causes epidemic disease.

Epidemics in any one locality tend to last for only 6–8 weeks. The short, explosive nature of the epidemics may be explained by the short incubation period (2–3 days), ease of transmission, widespread seeding of the virus before the outbreak, and high attack rates—50–75% when subclinical infections are included.

Clinical Presentation

The manifestations of influenza range from those of a mild upper respiratory illness to a severe pneumonia with involvement of many lobes. There is little to distinguish isolated cases of influenza from disease caused by other common upper respiratory tract pathogens, but it is easy to spot a characteristic pattern in groups of patients. The knowledge that influenza is prevalent is the most important clue to the diagnosis.

The incubation period is usually 2–3 days. Typically, patients have the sudden onset of prostration, myalgia, headache, and retro-orbital pain. Fever of 39.5–40°C (103–104°F) may begin within a few hours. Bradycardia is common, but the most severely ill usually have tachycardia. Typical are a flushed face and hot, dry skin. Rarely, heliotrope (reddish-purple) cyanosis suggests influenza pneumonia, a pneumonia caused entirely by replication of influenza virus in the lung.

Systemic symptoms predominate during the first 24–48 hours of illness. As they subside, respiratory symptoms become prominent. Pharyngitis alone is unusual, but it is often combined with coryza, conjunctivitis, nasopharyngitis, tracheobronchitis, and bronchitis. All patients have mucosal hyperemia, which occasionally progresses to hemorrhagic necrosis of the tracheobronchial mucosa. Scattered rhonchi or moist rales in the lungs are found in as many as one-third of patients with uncomplicated infections, but few patients have radiographic evidence of lung involvement. A dry, hacking cough and retrosternal burning are often the most distressing parts of the illness.

Leukopenia and lymphopenia are often seen early in influenza, but mild leukocytosis is more common. Brisk leukocytosis (>15,000 white blood cells/μL) suggests a secondary bacterial infection. Secondary bacterial pulmonary infections are most frequent during the late stages of the illness and are heralded by the sudden return of high fever and prostration or by the appearance of dyspnea and cyanosis.

Gastrointestinal manifestations are rare in patients with influenza. Neurologic involvement, including meningoencephalitis, is not unusual during outbreaks. Guillain-Barré syndrome, transverse myelitis, and encephalitis have been reported in a few patients, associated with but not necessarily as a result of influenza infection. Similarly, cardiac complications such as myocarditis are thought to be nonspecific complications of influenza infection in the elderly. Reye's syndrome, a hepatic and central nervous system disorder, occurs primarily in children aged 2–16 years who have been given aspirin during a viral illness. Primary influenza pneumonia affects elderly persons, patients with chronic pulmonary or cardiovascular diseases, and pregnant women.

Patients with influenza can develop secondary bacterial infection of the ears, sinuses, bronchi, or lungs. Bacterial pneumonia with *S pneumoniae, S aureus*, or *H influenzae* is the most serious complication and the cause of most deaths during epidemics. Even without bacterial complications, influenza is particularly severe in the elderly, patients with lung disease, and the immunocompromised. Many patients contract the infection from ill health care workers. For this reason, all of these patient groups and all health care workers should be given influenza vaccine.

Management

Most patients with influenza need only supportive therapy, since the illness is usually self-limited, although severe. Amantadine, a dopaminergic agonist, has been shown to reduce symptoms in about 50% of patients with influenza A. Because of its neurologic effect, however, it can produce seizures in older patients. Amantadine or rimantadine can also be used prophylactically in epidemics, until patients make antibodies in response to influenza vaccine. Affected children should not be given aspirin, to avoid risking Reye's syndrome. In patients ill enough to seek a physician's care and in patients with chronic underlying disease, antibiotics are also given to prevent secondary bacterial superinfection. Secondary bacterial infection must be treated aggressively with broad-spectrum antibiotics, maintenance of oxygenation, and, if necessary, intubation and advanced respiratory support.

SINUSITIS

Sinusitis develops when anatomic or physiologic obstruction prevents free drainage through the narrow ostia. This obstruction causes stasis of secretions, impaired ciliary activity, and infection, presumably by bacteria. The ostia can be obstructed by viral upper respiratory infection, allergy, allergic polyps, nasal septal deviation, or dental infection. The obstruction is aggravated by smoking, pollution, swimming, and flying.

Patients with acute sinusitis have localized pain, which typically starts in the late morning, is worse in the late afternoon, and is intensified by drinking alcohol or leaning forward. A purulent nasal discharge, rarely found in the common cold or pharyngitis, is typical of sinusitis. Patients may have a decreased sense of smell and a sensation of swelling of the skin overlying the frontal or maxillary sinuses. On examination, patients have tenderness to palpitation over the frontal and maxillary sinuses and poor transillumination. When sinusitis becomes more chronic, it often means an underlying allergic state. This is suggested by a compatible history, pale turbinates, swollen nasal mucosa, or nasal polyps.

Normally, sinuses are sterile. Nasopharyngeal cultures do not correlate well with sinus cultures and should not be used. In acute sinusitis, the most common pathogens are *S pneumoniae*, anaerobic bacteria, *H influenzae*, and a variety of streptococci. In chronic sinusitis, the primary pathogens are anaerobes.

Uncomplicated mild acute sinusitis may not require any treatment. In patients with more severe or persistent symptoms, treatment should be directed toward controlling the infection and restoring drainage. The infection can be easily controlled by any one of several antibiotics—erythromycin, penicillin, amoxicillin, or trimethoprim-sulfamethoxazole. It is much more difficult to restore normal sinus drainage. Useful approaches are hydration, avoiding smoking, inhaling steam, and treating any underlying allergic state with an antihistamine, nasal cortisone spray, or, if needed, occasional systemic corticosteroids. Some patients with unresponsive acute sinusitis require surgery to allow immediate drainage. The role of surgery in patients with chronic sinusitis is less well defined, and surgery in these patients may be overused. A better understanding of the pathophysiology of chronic sinusitis and the development of less invasive endoscopic surgery have led to a more rational surgical approach in chronic sinusitis.

A few patients with sinusitis develop complications requiring urgent, aggressive treatment. Serious complications of sinusitis include, in increasing order of severity, orbital edema, orbital cellulitis, orbital abscess, cavernous sinus thrombosis, meningitis, brain abscess, subdural abscess or empyema, and extradural abscess. Complications are indicated by generalized headaches, high fever, shaking chills, leukocytosis greater than $15,000/\mu L$, swelling of soft tissues of the face, blurred vision, diplopia, and persistent retro-ocular pain. If the infection progresses, patients can develop ptosis, exophthalmos, and diplopia. If the infection spreads to the central nervous system, patients have signs of increased intracranial pressure, meningitis, and deterioration of mental status.

Other challenging patients have hyperplastic sinusitis, characterized by marked tissue swelling caused by the combination of allergy and infection. Symptoms range from mild congestion to severe pain and nasal obstruction. Aggravating factors include extrinsic allergies, intrinsic allergies, nasal polyps, smoking, flying, drugs, and conditions that cause drying of the mucous membranes. Management should be individualized, and patients must be given careful instructions to start treatment promptly on their own. Initial treatment includes an antibiotic (erythromycin or amoxicillin), antihistamine, and nasal cortisone spray. Patients who do not respond to treatment develop fatigue, persistent cough, broadening of the nose, a typical "potato-in-the-nose" voice, and tender sinuses with poor transillumination. The throat is unremarkable and the chest is clear. Blood count may show eosinophilia, which can be a very useful marker for diagnosis and treatment. At this point, the antihistamine and nasal cortisone should be stopped, the same antibiotic continued, and a short course of prednisone started. Most patients respond dramatically within 36–48 hours. Most need to resume nasal cortisone spray on day 10 of treatment and continue it for weeks to months, depending on their underlying disease. Some patients require this routine two to four times a year. An otolaryngologist should be consulted for the rare patient who might benefit from polyp removal or surgical drainage.

When a patient presents with what appears to be progressive invasive sinusitis that is not responding to therapy, the physician should consider noninfectious entities such as tumors, vasculitis (particularly Wegener's granulomatosis), midline granuloma, and sarcoidosis. It is also worth considering less common infections such as tuberculosis, mucormycosis (particularly in patients with diabetes mellitus), progressive granulomatous aspergillosis of the sinuses, and other fungal infections.

OTITIS MEDIA

Otitis media is an inflammation of the middle ear caused by fluid accumulation in the middle ear. It is the most common cause of office visits by children up to age 5 years, but it is much less common in adults.

The pathogenesis of middle ear infection revolves around obstruction of the eustachian tubes, which both equalize pressure in and drain the middle ear. The mucosae of the middle ear are ciliated, mucus-secreting, respiratory-type epithelia. If drainage is obstructed, secretions from the epithelia can build up and become infected, most often by *S pneumoniae* or *H influenzae*. Although *H influenzae* otitis media is usually nontypeable, type B has been identified in some patients, and 25% of these patients present in a septic state with evidence of bacteremia or meningitis. *M catarrhalis* has also been recognized as an important pathogen. Viruses commonly cause otitis

media in children, but not in adults. *M pneumoniae*, which can cause hemorrhagic bullous myringitis, has only rarely been isolated from patients with middle ear infection. *Chlamydia trachomatis* does not cause otitis in adults.

The signs and symptoms of acute otitis media include ear pain, drainage, hearing loss, vertigo, nystagmus, and tinnitus. Erythema of the tympanic membrane suggests otitis media and is diagnostic if the patient also has middle ear fluid. This fluid can persist for up to 2–4 weeks after treatment of the ear infection, and produce short-term hearing loss.

Microbiologic studies of otitis media so consistently show the same types of organisms that fluid need not be cultured unless the patient is septic, immunocompromised, or not responding to initial antibiotics. Amoxicillin, ampicillin, or erythromycin is the drug of choice. Also acceptable are trimethoprim-sulfamethoxazole and amoxicillin-clavulanate. Chronic or recurrent otitis media in a previously unaffected adult should prompt the physician to evaluate the patient for an underlying disorder such as acquired hypogammaglobulinemia, Wegener's granulomatosis, and obstruction of the nasopharynx by mass or tumor.

SUMMARY

► Most upper respiratory tract infections are viral and self-limited and do not require treatment.

► Pharyngitis caused by group A β-hemolytic streptococci requires antibiotic treatment in an attempt to prevent rheumatic fever and glomerulonephritis.

► The influenza viruses are the most important agents causing acute respiratory disease. In epidemics, most deaths occur among elderly patients and patients with underlying respiratory diseases.

► Antibiotic therapy for acute sinusitis is directed against the most common pathogens—*Streptococcus pneumoniae*, other streptococci, anaerobic bacteria, and *Haemophilus influenzae*.

► Anaerobic bacteria are the almost universal cause of chronic sinusitis. Treatment requires prolonged antibiotics and restoration of drainage.

SUGGESTED READING

Dajani A et al: Treatment of acute streptococcal pharyngitis and prevention of rheumatic fever: A statement for health professionals. *Pediatrics* 1995;96:758.

Guidelines for the diagnosis of rheumatic fever: Jones criteria, 1992 update. JAMA 1992;268:2069.

Gwaltney JM Jr et al: Computed tomographic study of the common cold. N Engl J Med 1994;330:25.

Huovinen P et al: Pharyngitis in adults: The presence and coexistence of viruses and bacterial organisms. Ann Intern Med 1989;110:612.

Stevens DL et al: Severe group A streptococcal infections associated with a toxic shock-like syndrome and scarlet fever toxin A. N Engl J Med 1989;321:1.

8.5

Lower Respiratory Tract Infections

John G. Bartlett, MD

Patients with pneumonia typically present with cough, fever, and sputum production. Pneumonia is the most common serious acute infectious disease in both industrialized and underdeveloped countries. At the turn of the century, only cardiovascular disease killed more Americans than did pneumonia. According to William Osler in 1901, "The most widespread and fatal of all acute diseases, pneumonia is now the 'Captain of the Men of Death.'" Since that time, mortality from pneumonia has fallen nearly 10-fold, but it has not dropped substantially since 1950. The annual rate remains 20–30 deaths per 100,000 population. Pneumonia is still the most common lethal infectious disease in the United States. *Pneumocystis carinii* pneumonia is the most common identifiable cause of death in patients with HIV infection, and pulmonary tuberculosis rivals HIV as the world's greatest public health problem.

Despite these shifts in epidemiology and in population at risk, most patients with lower respiratory tract infections are previously healthy individuals who respond well to standard antibiotics. Only about 25% of patients with pneumonia require hospitalization, and most patients recover without sequelae. An exception is hospital-acquired pneumonia, which has a high mortality rate and is the most common cause of death from nosocomial infection.

Though a major cause of morbidity and mortality, pneumonia can usually be treated with antimicrobial drugs. The challenges to the physician are early recognition, appropriate tests to identify the infecting microbe, and pathogen-specific antibiotic treatment.

PRESENTATION AND EVALUATION

Classically, patients with lower respiratory tract infections present with a combination of cough, fever, and sputum production. Other common features are chills, chest pain aggravated by inspiration (pleurisy), and dyspnea. Any patient with this presentation should be evaluated for pneumonia. The usual tests are a chest x-ray, complete blood count, and lab studies to determine the pathogen.

The chest x-ray is critical for detecting an inflammatory process in the pulmonary parenchyma, as shown by a pulmonary infiltrate. An infiltrate is almost essential to the diagnosis of pneumonia. Most patients with typical complaints but a negative x-ray have only viral bronchitis, or sinusitis with a postnasal discharge. An infiltrate combined with typical symptoms usually means pneumonia, although this picture can be produced by noninfectious conditions such as pulmonary infarction, pulmonary edema, adult respiratory distress syndrome, and neoplasms (Chapter 2.9). Only rare patients with a clear chest x-ray have pneumonia, but four commonly quoted explanations are given for false-negatives. (1) Very early in the course of pneumonia (especially the first 24 hours of pneumococcal pneumonia), the infiltrate may not yet have developed. (2) It is often claimed that severe dehydration prevents a pulmonary infiltrate, but neither animal experiments nor logic supports the probability that dehydration could be so severe as to blunt or eliminate an inflammatory reaction in the lung or elsewhere. (3) Theoretically, severe neutropenia could account for a false-negative chest x-ray, but this possibility does not have strong clinical support. (4) At least initially, about 20–30% of patients with *P carinii* pneumonia have a negative chest x-ray; here the evidence is solid, based on detection of the microbe and response to appropriate antibiotics.

The chest x-ray can also reveal the extent of involvement (one or several lobes), the type of process (interstitial versus alveolar pattern as a clue to etiology), cavitation (which suggests specific pathogens), adenopathy (which also influences the differential diagnosis), and underlying diseases such as cancer, tuberculosis, and chronic lung disease. In general, febrile patients with a pulmonary infiltrate have conditions that can be treated with antibiotics; the same symptoms without an infiltrate usually mean less serious disease that is less likely to respond to antibiotics.

A complete blood count is usually obtained. Anemia can be an important indicator of chronic disease. The peripheral leukocyte count in patients with pneumonia is usually 10,000–18,000/μL. Severe leukopenia suggests viral infection, severe pneumococcal pneumonia, or pneumonia secondary to a primary cause of neutropenia such as pancytopenia, cancer chemotherapy, or AIDS (neutropenia can be caused by HIV itself, or by zidovudine or ganciclovir treatment). In patients with a secondary pneumonia, the usual pathogens are gram-negative bacteria or, in persons with AIDS, opportunistic infections. Severe leukocytosis suggests bacterial infection but does not point to specific bacteria. Thus, a hematocrit of 35% in an 18-year-old male college student with a pulmonary infiltrate suggests that the pneumonia is complicating a chronic disease. Similarly, a peripheral leukocyte count of 40,000/mm³ in this patient suggests something other than the usual types of pneumonia in a college student.

Identifying the Infecting Microbe

A major goal in the management of pneumonia is identifying the etiologic agent. In general, treatment is much simpler when the pathogen is known (see also Table 2.2–3. The alternative is to treat patients empirically, based on probabilities; this approach is potentially risky and not intellectually satisfying, but usually successful and required until culture results become available. Recovering the pathogen is confounded by two problems. First, the usual specimens are contaminated by the normal flora of the upper airways. Second, many of the common pulmonary pathogens cannot be detected with the routine cultures offered by most microbiology laboratories. Table 8.5–1 summarizes likely and less likely pulmonary pathogens and distinguishes two types of organisms: those that can be detected by routine sputum studies and those that require alternative tests. Table 8.5–2 summarizes the major causes of pulmonary infections according to the host's age.

All patients with acute pneumonia should have blood cultures and cultures of any pleural fluid. Since these specimens are not contaminated by normal flora, recovery of likely pulmonary pathogens is virtually diagnostic of the causative agent. The time-honored specimen in most patients with pneumonia is expectorated sputum for Gram's stain and culture. Unfortunately, sputum is inevitably contaminated by the bacteria residing in the

upper airways. Overgrowth of contaminating bacteria may mask the growth of fastidious pathogens, especially *Streptococcus pneumoniae* and *Haemophilus influenzae*. Contaminating bacteria may also cause confusion, since some contaminants, such as *Staphylococcus aureus* and gram-negative bacilli, can also be pathogens.

Four procedures notably improve the diagnostic accuracy of expectorated sputum beyond simple clinical correlations. (1) Encourage the patient to cough deeply so as to provide a good specimen from the lower airways (specimen must be obtained before antibiotics are started). (2) Screen sputum in the laboratory under low power magnification, and restrict cultures to specimens that show many polymorphonuclear cells and few contaminating epithelial cells. (3) Correlate Gram's stain with culture results. (4) Perform the quellung test, a quick way to identify pneu-

Table 8.5–1. Causes of community-acquired pneumonia in adults.

Bacteria recovered from expectorated sputum

Common	Uncommon
Streptococcus pneumoniae Haemophilus influenzae	Moraxella catarrhalis Staphylococcus aureus Group A beta-hemolytic streptococci Neisseria meningitidis Gram-negative bacilli

Microorganisms not recovered from expectorated sputum with conventional cultures ("atypical pneumonia")

	Common	Uncommon
Bacteria	Legionella sp Anaerobic bacteria Chlamydia pneumoniae Mycoplasma pneumoniae	Nocardia Actinomyces Mycobacterium sp Chlamydia psittaci
Viruses	Influenza	Respiratory syncytial virus Parainfluenza Herpesvirus exanthems Adenoviruses
Rickettsia		Coxiella burnetii
Parasites	Pneumocystis carinii	

Table 8.5–2. Causes of community-acquired pneumonia by host age (from most to least common).

	6 Weeks–18 Years	18–40 Years	40–65 Years*	>65 Years*
Most common	Haemophilus influenzae Mycoplasma Viruses† Chlamydia pneumoniae Streptococcus pneumoniae	Mycoplasma C pneumoniae S pneumoniae Pneumocystis carinii (AIDS)	S pneumoniae Anaerobes H influenzae	S pneumoniae Anaerobes H influenzae Gram-negative bacilli Viruses†
Less common	Staphylococcus aureus	Haemophilus influenzae	Viruses Mycoplasma Legionella C pneumoniae S aureus	Legionella C pneumoniae S aureus

*Major causes of nosocomial pneumonia are gram-negative bacilli (*Klebsiella* sp, *Pseudomonas aeruginosa*, *Enterobacter*, and *Escherichia coli*), *Staphylococcus aureus*, and anaerobes.
†Major viral pathogens are respiratory syncytial virus, parainfluenza, and adenovirus; the only common viral pathogen in middle-aged adults is influenza.

mococci based on capsular swelling after application of omniserum antibody to capsular polysaccharide.

Alternative specimens from the lower airways include induced sputum, bronchoscopic specimens, transthoracic aspirates, transtracheal aspirates, and open lung biopsy (Chapter 2.2). These studies are generally reserved for special circumstances, especially pneumonia in the compromised host, chronic pneumonia, and enigmatic pulmonary diseases. Such procedures are justified by an inability to obtain an adequate expectorated specimen, the need for an uncontaminated specimen, or the need for tissue. Bronchoscopic aspirates or bronchoalveolar lavage specimens are also subject to contamination with saliva; the quality of these specimens can be improved with quantitative cultures or specimens obtained with telescoping cannulas designed to reduce salivary contamination.

Regardless of the specimen source, some organisms are virtually always considered pathogens because they rarely if ever contaminate the upper airways. These organisms include *Mycobacterium tuberculosis, Mycoplasma pneumoniae, Chlamydia pneumoniae, Legionella* sp, some viruses (respiratory syncytial virus, influenza, parainfluenza), and pathogenic fungi *(Histoplasma capsulatum, Blastomyces dermatitidis, Coccidioides immitis)*. Regardless of the specimen source, other organisms mean little because they lack the pathogenic potential to cause pneumonitis. Organisms in this category include *Staphylococcus epidermidis,* enterococci, most alpha-hemolytic streptococci, and *Candida* sp.

ETIOLOGIC AGENTS OF PNEUMONIA

Streptococcus pneumoniae

In the pre-penicillin era, *S pneumoniae* was the dominant organism in community-acquired pneumonia. In studies from that time, the pneumococcus could be recovered from expectorated sputum or transthoracic aspirates in about 80% of all patients hospitalized with pneumonia and in 96% of those with lobar consolidation on chest x-ray (Figure 8.5–1). The apparent steep drop in recovery of the pneumococcus since that time is explained either by less efficient microbiologic studies or by a true change in the causes of pneumonia. Most recent reports show a yield of 10–40% among adults who are hospitalized for community-acquired pneumonia. Despite the real decrease in frequency, *S pneumoniae* remains the most often-identified pathogen in patients who develop pneumonia severe enough to require hospitalization. It continues to account for a high mortality rate in patients over age 70 and patients with AIDS, alcoholism, cancer, and other disorders of host defenses.

The classic clinical presentation is an upper respiratory tract infection followed by a shaking chill and then fever, dyspnea, and blood-tinged sputum ("rusty sputum"). Before penicillin, the natural history of the disease included fever, dyspnea, and tachypnea for 10–14 days, followed by a recovery that was as dramatic as the onset. Nevertheless, during recovery the x-ray showed little improvement in lobar consolidation. This observation indicates that

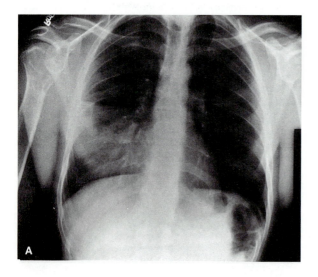

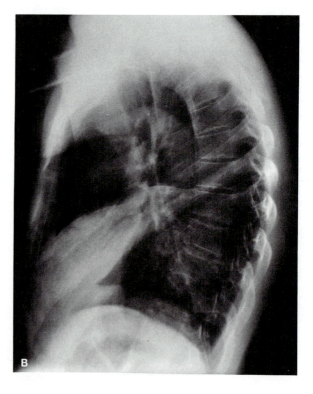

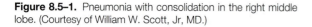

Figure 8.5–1. Pneumonia with consolidation in the right middle lobe. (Courtesy of William W. Scott, Jr, MD.)

there is far more to pneumococcal pneumonia than pulmonary inflammation.

S pneumoniae is relatively difficult to recover from expectorated sputum. The pneumococcus resembles other alpha-hemolytic streptococci on culture media, and any recent antibiotic exposure is likely to preclude recovery. The yield with sputum culture is only about 50% in patients with bacteremic pneumococcal pneumonia.

Penicillin-resistant strains are becoming a major management problem, especially since these strains are often resistant to other drugs as well. Even with penicillin-sensitive strains, the mortality for pneumococcal pneumonia with bacteremia is 20–45%. Complications of pneumococcal pneumonia include empyema, endocarditis, pericarditis, meningitis, and septic arthritis. Poor prognostic indicators besides bacteremia are multiple lobe involvement, advanced age, serious associated conditions (especially lung cancer, AIDS, and alcoholism), and certain alterations in host defenses (asplenia, complement deficiency, agammaglobulinemia, and neutropenia).

Haemophilus influenzae

According to bacteriologic studies of expectorated sputum, *H influenzae* accounts for about 10–15% of cases of community-acquired pneumonia in adults. Some experts believe that this infection is especially prevalent in patients with chronic obstructive lung disease. The infection's clinical features are not distinctive. Like the pneumococcus, *H influenzae* is difficult to recover from expectorated sputum because it is fastidious and easily overgrown by normal oral flora. About 15–30% of strains produce beta-lactamase and are thus resistant to ampicillin; erythromycin, too, is often ineffective. Preferred drugs are most oral cephalosporins, quinolones, and beta-lactam-betalactamase inhibitors.

Staphylococcus aureus

S aureus causes pneumonia in three settings: in young children, as a superinfection in patients with influenza, and as hospital-acquired pneumonia. Children frequently have bullous disease and empyema. Most adults have pneumonia without lobar consolidation; occasional patients develop acute or chronic pulmonary abscesses. *S aureus* is easily recovered from expectorated secretions and should be readily recognized on a direct Gram's stain as large gram-positive cocci arranged in clusters. Nearly all strains are resistant to penicillin, and about 20–40% of nosocomial strains are also resistant to methicillin. Nafcillin, oxacillin, or cefazolin is preferred for methicillin-sensitive strains. Vancomycin is preferred for methicillin-resistant strains.

Gram-Negative Bacteria

These organisms are the major cause of nosocomial pneumonia, especially pneumonia acquired in intensive care units. The predominant organisms are *Pseudomonas aeruginosa*, *Klebsiella* sp, and *Enterobacter* sp, but there are many others. In the pre-antibiotic era, *Klebsiella* re-

portedly caused a serious form of pneumonia in alcoholics and other compromised hosts. Characteristic features included upper lobe involvement, early cavitation, and sputum that resembled currant jelly. This form of *Klebsiella* pulmonary infection was never common and now is very rare.

Gram-negative bacilli are easily recovered from pulmonary secretions including expectorated sputum, tracheostomy or endotracheal tube aspirates, and bronchoscopy specimens. The major problem with these organisms is their frequency as contaminants, especially in patients who have recently received antibiotics. The physician should remember that gram-negative organisms rarely cause community-acquired pneumonia, but they are common, often devastating, pathogens in hospital-acquired pneumonia. An important early clue is large numbers of typical organisms on direct Gram's stains of respiratory secretions.

Anaerobic Bacteria

Anaerobic bacteria are organisms that constitute the dominant normal flora of the upper airways and are especially prominent in the gingival crevices. Anaerobes are the major pathogens in pulmonary infections caused by aspiration and its sequela, lung abscess. Many patients have a condition that predisposes to aspiration: altered consciousness, neurologic deficits, or dysphagia. Many have gingivitis or periodontitis. The typical patient is an alcoholic who aspirates gingival crevice material while in a stupor; because of the patient's suppressed consciousness, this material is not cleared by the cough reflex. First, the patient develops pneumonia, usually involving a segment of the lung that is dependent in the recumbent position—a superior segment of a lower lobe or a posterior segment of an upper lobe. Later, the patient develops tissue necrosis with abscess formation or a bronchopleural fistula leading to an empyema, or both.

Anaerobic bacterial infection of the lung tends to be a more subtle process than other bacterial infections of the lower airways. Many patients present with symptoms of several weeks' or even months' duration, usually with other evidence of chronic disease, such as weight loss and anemia. Clues to anaerobic infection include (1) a host who is prone to aspiration, has infection in a dependent lung segment, and may have periodontal disease; (2) putrid discharge from sputum, breath, or empyema fluid, presumably reflecting the short-chain volatile fatty acids and amines produced by these organisms (this finding is considered diagnostic of anaerobic infection); (3) tissue necrosis with abscess formation, or a bronchopleural fistula with empyema (few of the agents that cause pneumonia produce cavitation, but anaerobic bacteria are the most likely); (4) chronic symptoms, which are common with this infection but uncommon with most bacterial lung infections other than mycobacteria.

The microbiologic diagnosis of anaerobic conditions is extremely difficult to confirm because specimens must be devoid of normal flora for meaningful culture. Appropriate specimens include transthoracic aspirates, pleural fluid, and transtracheal aspirates. Furthermore, many laboratories have great difficulty in recovering and identifying oxygen-sensitive bacteria. The result is that most patients are recognized by the clinical features and treated empirically with penicillin, clindamycin, or penicillin plus metronidazole.

Viruses

Viruses often cause upper respiratory tract infections and bronchitis, but they cause pneumonia in only a few settings. (1) Influenza virus occasionally causes primary influenza pneumonia or, more frequently, sets the stage for secondary bacterial infection. (2) Viruses—most often influenza, parainfluenza, and respiratory syncytial virus—are the primary pulmonary pathogens in young children. (3) In immunocompromised hosts, especially recipients of bone marrow or organ transplants, cytomegalovirus is a common cause of pneumonia.

Few clinical laboratories can perform viral cultures to detect common viral agents of pneumonia. But a fluorescent antibody stain is available to identify respiratory syncytial virus, which is the most important viral agent in children, and methods are well established to find cytomegalovirus in all types of organ transplant recipients through cultures, fluorescent antibody stains, and antigen detection on respiratory secretions usually obtained by bronchoscopy.

"Atypical Organisms"

"Atypical organisms" are pneumonia-causing microbes—especially *Mycoplasma pneumoniae, Legionella sp, and Chlamydia pneumoniae*—that cannot be detected with conventional stain and culture of expectorated sputum (see Table 8.5–1). The term "atypical pneumonia" is traced to Relman, who in 1938 described a form of pneumonia that was less serious than pneumococcal pneumonia and for which no likely pathogen could be found with the usual cultures of expectorated sputum. Later studies showed the cause of this disease to be an agent that Eaton described in the 1950's as a transferrable pathogen that would pass through a 0.45 μm filter. The "Eaton agent" was first assumed to be a virus, but later shown to be *M pneumoniae.* This agent is now recognized as the most common cause of lower respiratory tract infections in young adults such as college students, but the organism is uncommon in older patients and rarely causes severe disease. *M pneumoniae* is also unusual in that in many patients it causes extrapulmonary manifestations including bullous myringitis, hemolytic anemia, hepatitis, pancreatitis, pericarditis, myocarditis, erythema multiforme, and neurologic syndromes such as aseptic meningitis, meningoencephalitis, and neuropathies. The organism can be recovered from throat washes, but few laboratories can cultivate mycoplasma. The usual way to establish the diagnosis is with serology, but results are not available until long after all treatment decisions have been made. Thus, *M pneumoniae* is treated empirically, based on the clinical features of "atypical pneumonia" in young adults. The two drugs with established merit are tetracyclines and erythromycins.

The second form of "atypical pneumonia" is usually caused by *Legionella pneumophila,* or, less often, *Legionella micdadei* or *Legionella bozemanii.* These organisms account for 2–5% of all community-acquired pneumonia, and they may also be responsible for outbreaks or epidemics of pneumonia. Several epidemics have been traced to contaminated water supplies, with exposure through air conditioning systems and hospital showers. Patients receiving corticosteroids are unusually susceptible. Mortality from *Legionella* infections is high, especially in compromised hosts and nosocomial cases. The typical presentation is high fever and relatively mild pulmonary symptoms. In general, the diagnosis is established with direct fluorescent antibody staining of sputum, sputum culture, or antigen assays of urine. All these tests show good specificity, but they lack sensitivity; thus, negative tests do not exclude the diagnosis. Erythromycin is the only antibiotic with established merit for this intracellular pathogen, although many drugs show good activity in vitro.

Chlamydia pneumoniae is the newest of the "atypicals." This organism was originally described as causing a mild, self-limited pneumonia similar to mycoplasma pneumonia in young, otherwise healthy adults. But *C pneumoniae* occasionally causes pneumonitis in older people and may be responsible for up to 5–10% of nosocomial pneumonias. The clinical presentation of *C pneumoniae* is unique only in that (1) this infection is less likely than mycoplasma pneumonia to cause extrapulmonary manifestations; (2) compromised hosts do not appear uniquely susceptible; and (3) many patients have pharyngitis and a persistent cough. The diagnosis is best established with fluorescent antibody stains of sputum, polymerase chain reaction tests, or serology, but most patients are just treated empirically with erythromycin or a tetracycline.

"Opportunists"

This term is applied to organisms that have little pathogenic propensity except in patients with diminished defenses. Patients at risk for opportunistic infections include those receiving chronic corticosteroids or cancer chemotherapy; those with lymphoma, Hodgkin's disease, or AIDS; and organ transplant recipients. The specific defect in defenses dictates the usual type of infection (Table 8.5–3). Patients with neutropenia are especially prone to gram-negative bacillary pneumonia and aspergillosis, whereas patients with complement deficiencies, agammaglobulinemia, or asplenia are especially prone to infections with encapsulated organisms such as *S pneumoniae, H influenzae,* and *Neisseria meningitidis.* With compromised cell-mediated immunity, the range of pathogens is extensive, including *Mycobacterium tuberculosis, Nocardia,* cytomegalovirus, *P carinii, Aspergillus,* and *Cryptococcus.* Diagnostic methods depend on the clinical setting, x-ray changes, and associated disease.

Table 8.5–3. Microbial correlations with pulmonary infections in immunocompromised patients.

Clinical Observation	Common (and Less Common) Pathogens
Type of immune defect (and examples)	
Humoral (agammaglobulinemia)	*Streptococcus pneumoniae, Haemophilus influenzae (Neisseria meningitidis, Pseudomonas aeruginosa)*
Complement (congenital defects)	*S pneumoniae, H influenzae (N meningitidis)*
Asplenia (sickle cell disease, traumatic or surgical asplenia)	*S pneumoniae, H influenzae (N meningitidis)*
Neutropenia (aplastic anemia, cancer chemotherapy, AIDS)	Gram-negative bacilli, *Aspergillus*
Cell-mediated immunity (AIDS, corticosteroids, organ transplant, cancer chemotherapy, lymphoma)	*Pneumocystis carinii, Nocardia, Aspergillus, Phycomyces, Cryptococcus, Legionella, Mycobacterium tuberculosis, Mycobacterium avium-intracellulare;* herpesviruses, eg, cytomegalovirus, herpes simplex
Changes on chest x-ray	
Diffuse interstitial infiltrates	*P carinii,* cytomegalovirus *(Cryptococcus, Aspergillus)*
Localized infiltrate	Bacteria, *Nocardia,* mycobacteria, *Cryptococcus, Aspergillus, Phycomyces*
Nodules or cavitation	*Nocardia,* mycobacteria, anaerobes, gram-negative bacilli, *Aspergillus, Cryptococcus*
Tempo of disease	
Rapid	Bacteria, cytomegalovirus
Subacute	Cytomegalovirus, *Cryptococcus, Aspergillus, Phycomyces*

PATHOGEN BY HOST SETTING

Although a great many organisms can cause pneumonia, only a few are likely to affect a particular type of host. The following descriptions of representative hosts account for the majority of cases of pneumonia in adults.

Pneumonia in a Previously Healthy College Student

A typical pneumonia patient is a previously healthy 18-year-old student who has had cough, fever, and shortness of breath for 2–3 days. Despite these symptoms, most patients remain ambulatory (ie, have "walking pneumonia"). Often, other students in the dormitory or on campus have similar symptoms. If the chest x-ray is normal, the most likely cause is a viral infection; the patient needs no further tests, just symptomatic treatment and prevention of person-to-person spread. If the patient has a pulmonary infiltrate, the most likely treatable causes are *M pneumoniae, C pneumoniae,* and *S pneumoniae.* The evaluation is usually limited to bacteriologic studies of expectorated sputum. If pneumococci are found, the patient is given penicillin; if the sputum is negative, the patient gets erythromycin or tetracycline. Both erythromycin and tetracycline are active against all three of the major possible pathogens. Few patients require hospitalization, and most patients recover with no sequelae.

Community-Acquired Pneumonia Requiring Hospitalization of an Older Adult

A typical patient is a previously healthy 50-year-old who develops an upper respiratory tract infection followed by cough, fever, and sputum production. In about 50% of patients, expectorated sputum reveals a likely bacterial pathogen. The microbiologist's interpretation of the

Gram's stain is 90% accurate in predicting the organism that will later be recovered in culture. Most patients in whom *S pneumoniae* is cultured have a positive quellung test on initial exam. Thus, Gram's stain and culture are useful in guiding therapeutic decisions in about 50% of patients. In the other 50%, Gram's stain is interpreted as "mixed flora," "sparse bacteria," "normal flora," or another nonspecific designation. An additional 10–20% of patients have sparse polymorphonuclear cells, indicating either failure to procure a specimen from the lower airways or excessive contamination from the upper airways.

When bacteria are recovered in community-acquired pneumonia, the major pathogen is *S pneumoniae. H influenzae* accounts for 5–15% of cases, and rare cases are caused by *S aureus,* gram-negative bacilli, or *Moraxella catarrhalis. Legionella* is occasionally responsible, but diagnosis requires special tests (see "Atypical Organisms" above). When tests do not show the usual bacterial pathogens, other possibilities include *C pneumoniae,* anaerobic bacteria, and influenza. Rare causes are *M pneumoniae, Chlamydia psittaci,* and Q fever (Chapter 8.16).

Most clinical laboratories are prepared to test sputum for conventional aerobic bacteria, legionella, mycobacteria, and fungi. But even when research laboratories perform tests for all recognized agents, a substantial number of cases remain enigmatic. As confusing as the diagnosis may be, management is simple. Patients with specific pathogens are treated with the appropriate antimicrobial drug, and those with enigmatic infections are usually managed with a combination of drugs such as erythromycin and cefuroxime. The rationale for this combination is it is active against virtually all treatable bacteria and "atypical organisms" that cause common forms of community-acquired pneumonia.

Nosocomial Pneumonia

Nosocomial pneumonia is a distinctive category because the microbiologic menu is unique and the mortality rate is high. A typical patient is a 65-year-old man in the intensive care unit with a tracheostomy, who develops fever, purulent secretions, and a pulmonary infiltrate. Respiratory secretions are likely to yield gram-negative bacilli, *S aureus,* or both. Anaerobic bacteria might be implicated, since the patient is so prone to aspiration. Many patients have combinations of these organisms. The most serious condition is gram-negative bacillary pneumonia, which, despite appropriate antibiotics, may progress to bacteremia or the adult respiratory distress syndrome (Chapter 2.7).

The suggested mechanism is colonization of the oropharynx by organisms from the host's colonic flora and then aspiration of these organisms in oral or gastric secretions. The patient's propensity to have the upper airways colonized by gram-negative bacteria correlates directly with the severity of the underlying disease. Thus, pharyngeal colonization with gram-negative bacilli affects 3–10% of patients on the psychiatry ward, 15–30% on the general medical ward, and 50–70% in intensive care units. These colonization rates are independent of antibiotic exposure. *P aeruginosa* is the most likely pathogen in intensive care units and carries the worst prognosis.

Most management decisions are straightforward, because unlike *S pneumoniae* and *H influenzae,* the likely nosocomial pathogens—gram-negative bacilli and *S aureus*—are easy to recover from respiratory secretions. Stains and cultures showing large numbers of gram-negative bacteria should prompt aggressive treatment, for example, with an aminoglycoside and a third-generation cephalosporin or antipseudomonad penicillin (ticarcillin, mezlocillin, or piperacillin). If *S aureus* is seen on Gram's stain, vancomycin should be added pending sensitivity tests.

Pulmonary Infection in the Compromised Host

The typical patient is a 30-year-old man with HIV infection and a CD4 cell count of 50/μL, presenting with dry cough, fever, and progressive dyspnea over several days or weeks. If the chest x-ray shows bilateral interstitial infiltrates, the great probability is *P carinii* pneumonia, a diagnosis that is usually established with induced sputum or bronchoalveolar lavage. The physician encountering this patient is most likely to be misled if the patient was not previously known to have HIV infection—especially if he has no declared risk—or if the x-ray is atypical or normal. If the patient's symptoms, disease stage, x-ray findings, or sputum analysis do not fit the classic presentation of *P carinii,* the physician should consider any of the pathogens that are likely to cause pneumonia in patients with defective cell-mediated immunity: *Mycobacterium tuberculosis, S pneumoniae, H influenzae, Cryptococcus, Nocardia, Aspergillus, Mycobacterium avium-intracellulare,* and cytomegalovirus.

Another typical compromised host is an adult who received a bone marrow transplant 50 days ago and now has fever, cough, and bilateral infiltrates on chest x-ray. Extensive tests generally show one of two possibilities: cytomegalovirus or idiopathic pneumonitis. If the infiltrate is pleural-based and shows a cavity, the strongest possibility is aspergillosis. Likely pathogens can be predicted quite accurately by the clinical findings and specific host defect. Nevertheless, pneumonia in the compromised host remains a difficult diagnostic problem. Many patients are given empiric treatment, but their antibiotic regimen may need to be altered repeatedly if they do not respond. The wide range of treatable pathogens justifies aggressive attempts to pinpoint the cause.

SUMMARY

▶ Pneumonia is "captain of the men of death," "the old man's friend," and the most common fatal infectious disease in the United States.

▶ A major goal in the management of pneumonia is identifying the pathogen. This may be difficult because of problems inherent in interpreting stains and cultures of expectorated sputum.

▶ The cause of pneumonia can often be predicted according to the host's age and circumstances.

▶ Empiric treatment usually succeeds in treating the young adult with "walking pneumonia," the older adult with pneumonia severe enough to require hospitalization, and the hospitalized patient with nosocomial pneumonia. Only immunocompromised hosts regularly require invasive diagnostic studies.

SUGGESTED READING

Austrian R: Pneumococcal pneumonia: Diagnostic, epidemiologic, therapeutic and prophylactic considerations. Chest 1986; 90:738.

Bartlett JG: Anaerobic bacterial infections of the lung. Chest 1987;91:901.

Bartlett JG, Mundy L: Community-acquired pneumonia. N Engl J Med 1995;333:1618.

Hofmann J et al: The prevalence of drug-resistant *Streptococcus pneumoniae* in Atlanta. N Engl J Med 1995;333:481.

Niederman MS et al: Guidelines for the initial management of adults with community-acquired pneumonia: Diagnosis, assessment of severity, and initial antibiotic therapy. Am Rev Respir Dis 1993;148:1418.

8.6

Endocarditis

John J. Mann, MD, and Katharine S. Harrison, MD

Infective endocarditis, one of the most important infections in adults, is caused by microorganisms attaching to the endocardium and damaging the tissue. Many patients with endocarditis present with nonlocalizing symptoms of infection such as fever, plus signs of endocardial damage that range in severity from a subtle murmur to acute aortic regurgitation with pulmonary edema. Other patients present with stroke, arthritis, or other symptoms that at first glance seem unrelated to endocarditis.

People usually develop endocarditis because they have an abnormal heart valve that resists bacterial seeding less effectively than does normal endocardium and they have developed a bacteremia. Thus, the patient predisposed to endocarditis may be an elderly man with a prosthetic aortic valve, a middle-aged woman with mitral valve prolapse, or a young person whose intravenous drug use has caused repeated episodes of bacteremia. Depending on the virulence of the infecting organism, the patient's symptoms evolve subacutely over weeks to months or develop acutely and progress quickly to heart failure as valve tissue is rapidly destroyed.

The diagnosis and treatment of endocarditis can be as straightforward as recognizing the implication of fever with a new murmur, obtaining blood cultures, and giving antibiotics. Often, the diagnosis is obscure and the management complicated. Whether the challenge is identifying fastidious or unusual organisms, managing the tenuous and quickly changing hemodynamics of a patient with acute valvular regurgitation, or timing surgery for a patient in whom endocarditis has caused a stroke, managing endocarditis successfully can call on all of a physician's skills. These skills, plus antibiotics and heart surgery, explain why, for most patients, the prognosis of infective endocarditis has been transformed from certain death to recovery and cure.

PATHOGENESIS

Endocarditis develops through the hematogenous spread of organisms to endocardial tissue. Previously damaged endocardium or repetitive bacteremia increases the risk.

That everyone experiences frequent transient bacteremia (eg, from brushing teeth) but few develop endocarditis, testifies to how well the endocardium normally resists the deposition of microorganisms. Damage to the endocardium—from rheumatic fever, calcific degeneration, congenital malformation, or previous endocarditis—leads to deposition of thrombin and platelets and makes the valve surface much more hospitable to infection by circulating organisms. Turbulent blood flow, as seen with a ventricular septal defect, also predisposes to formation of thrombi and adherence of bacteria in the endocardium or on heart valves.

Endocarditis develops much more often on the left side of the heart (mitral or aortic valve) than on the right (tricuspid or pulmonic valve), reflecting how much more often the left-sided valves are damaged or abnormal. Right-sided endocarditis develops primarily in intravenous drug users and patients with congenital heart disease or a catheter dwelling (and perhaps damaging the endocardium) in the right side of the heart. Even the usually resistant normal endocardium can be overwhelmed by protracted or frequent bacteremia such as that caused by intravenous drug use or an infected intravascular catheter.

The ability of bacteria to cause endocarditis depends on their ability to adhere to endocardial structures. The usual gram-negative aerobic bacilli and most anaerobic bacteria lack this ability, and thus rarely cause native valve endocarditis. But because aerobic gram-negative bacteria can more easily infect implanted foreign material, these organisms more often cause prosthetic valve endocarditis.

The inflammatory and immune responses to the chronically infected endocardium explain many of the clinical manifestations discussed in the following text. The recruitment of polymorphonuclear cells to the nidus of infection leads to the release of cytokines that secondarily cause fever, myalgia, and weight loss. Progression of the infection damages valves, leading to murmur and hemodynamic abnormalities. Hematogenous spread of the bacteria, either as microscopic organisms or as macroscopic vegetations, can cause septic arthritis, meningitis, osteomyelitis, splenic abscess, stroke, or Osler's nodes (see "Presentation" below).

A chronic infection like endocarditis elicits not only an inflammatory response, but also an immunologic reaction, characterized by the production of antibodies to bacterial cell wall fragments. Wherever these circulating immune complexes deposit, they activate complement and damage tissue. This process can cause hypocomplementemia, glomerulonephritis (with proteinuria, hematuria, and renal insufficiency), petechiae, and purpura.

MICROBIOLOGY

Almost any microorganism except a virus can cause endocarditis, but certain organisms are predisposed to infecting native or prosthetic heart valves in different populations at risk (Table 8.6–1). Knowing the most likely cause of a patient's endocarditis is important because often antibiotics must be started before the organism is identified.

The most common microbes isolated from native valve endocarditis are streptococci, with viridans streptococci accounting for about 35% of cases, enterococci about 10%, and other streptococcal species about 15%. The usual portal of entry for streptococci is the mouth; therefore, recent dental procedures, poor dental hygiene, gin-

givitis, tonsillectomy, and viral upper respiratory tract infections make streptococcal bacteremia and endocarditis more likely. Some streptococci come from other sources. Occasional patients with *Streptococcus pneumoniae* pneumonia, bacteremia, and meningitis develop pneumococcal endocarditis of the aortic valve. Enterococcal endocarditis accounts for 10% of cases. *Streptococcus bovis* deserves special mention because about 20% of patients with *S bovis* endocarditis or bacteremia have a significant gastrointestinal neoplasm such as polyps or carcinoma. *Staphylococcus aureus* causes about 30% of endocarditis cases. The usual sources of staphylococci are furuncles, cardiac surgery, infected wounds, intravenous drug injections through contaminated skin, and occasionally osteomyelitis.

Gram-negative aerobic bacilli, once a rare cause of native valve endocarditis, have recently achieved an incidence of up to 7% in some series of native valve endocarditis. Most of these gram-negative bacilli belong to a group of fastidious nonenteric organisms called "HACEK," an acronym for **H**aemophilus species, **A**ctinobacillus actinomycetemcomitans, **C**ardiobacterium hominis, **E**ikenella corrodens, and **K**ingella species. These organisms tend to produce symptoms of a chronic illness, including weight loss, anemia, and fatigue. Routine blood cultures are often negative. Endocarditis from enteric gram-negative bacilli is unusual unless the patient uses intravenous drugs; *Pseudomonas aeruginosa, Salmonella* sp, and *Serratia* are the most common isolates.

Anaerobic nonstreptococcal endocarditis remains uncommon, but is an increasing cause of endocarditis. Most infections are with the *Bacteroides* sp found in the oral cavity and intestinal tract. Patients at risk for fungal endocarditis are intravenous drug users, patients with prosthetic valves, and hospitalized patients with central venous lines who have received prolonged courses of intravenous antibiotics.

Unusual causes of endocarditis include *Listeria monocytogenes*, usually found in an immunocompromised host, and *Legionella* on prosthetic valves. *Erysipelothrix, Coxiella burnetii* (the agent of Q fever), *Chlamydia psittaci* and *C trachomatis*, and *Brucella* are usually found in patients who have been exposed to animals. *Bartonella quintana* is a newly recognized agent of endocarditis.

The risk of prosthetic valve endocarditis is higher during the first 6–12 months after surgery (3–4% risk). Early prosthetic valve endocarditis (<2 months after surgery) is most often caused by coagulase-negative staphylococci such as *Staphylococcus epidermidis*, followed by viridans streptococci and *S aureus*. Other causes are aerobic gram-negative bacilli, diphtheroids, and fungi, particularly *Candida* sp and *Aspergillus*. In contrast, late prosthetic valve endocarditis (>2 months postoperatively) is most often caused by *S aureus, S epidermidis,* and streptococci.

The intravenous drug user who presents with symptoms of endocarditis is most likely infected with *S aureus*. The infection represents hematogenous spread of staphylococci from the skin, nose, and throat. As mentioned, the

Table 8.6–1. Bacteriology of infective endocarditis according to host.

Percentage of Infections	Most Common Pathogens
All Patients	
60	Streptococci, especially *S viridans*, group D enterococci, *S pneumoniae, S bovis*
30	Staphylococci, especially *S aureus*
<5	Anaerobes, especially *Bacteroides*
<5	Gram-negative bacteria
Intravenous Drug Users	
60	*S aureus*
20	*S viridans*, other streptococci
10	Gram-negative bacteria, especially enteric bacilli, *Salmonella, Serratia, Pseudomonas aeruginosa*
8	Enterococci
Prosthetic Heart Valve Recipients	
Early endocarditis (<2 mo after surgery)	
30	*Staphylococcus epidermidis*
20	*S aureus*
20	Aerobic gram-negative bacteria
10	Diphtheroids
10	Fungi (especially *Candida, Aspergillus*)
Late endocarditis (>2 mo after surgery)	
35	*S aureus, S epidermidis*
25	Streptococci
10	Enterococci
10	Gram-negative bacteria
5	Fungi
5	Diphtheroids

Note: Immunosuppressed patients are not at special risk for endocarditis. They are susceptible to the same organisms as immunocompetent persons.

intravenous drug user is also at risk for fungal endocarditis, particularly *Candida parapsilosis,* and gram-negative infection, particularly *Pseudomonas.*

CLINICAL FEATURES

The protean manifestations of endocarditis range from subtle abnormalities of the skin or nails to dramatic lesions of the heart or brain (Table 8.6–2). Because the manifestations can change over time, the physician must examine patients repeatedly to detect the full range of clinical features.

Endocarditis is classified as subacute or acute, depending on the severity of constitutional symptoms and valve damage, the pace of evolution, and the likelihood and severity of emboli. The virulence of the infecting organism chiefly determines whether the disease is subacute or acute. Subacute endocarditis is most often caused by *Streptococcus viridans:* The onset is insidious, the constitutional symptoms modest, and the endocardial damage often minor. In contrast, *S aureus* typically produces acute disease, with an abrupt onset of high fever, prominent leukocytosis, and rapid, severe destruction of valve tissue. Congestive heart failure often complicates acute endocarditis.

Presentation

Fever: The onset of subacute endocarditis is often vague and insidious, marked by anorexia, easy fatigability, weight loss, malaise, and low-grade fever. The fever is especially important because it is the most common manifestation of endocarditis and often the earliest sign that convinces both patient and doctor that the patient is ill. Little about the fever is characteristic, although generally it is intermittent, irregular, and mild (38.3–39°C) (101–102.2°F), and not associated with shaking chills. Afebrile periods are rarely prolonged. Temperature may be normal in patients who have severe congestive heart failure or uremia and in patients receiving antibiotics or corticosteroids.

Heart Murmur and Other Cardiac Presentations: Another cardinal manifestation of endocarditis is murmur, heard in 85% of patients. Murmurs from endocarditis are not always loud. Many patients have only an apical systolic murmur. But an unimpressive murmur can camouflage severe valve damage. For example, when aortic regurgitation develops quickly because the infection has ruptured the aortic leaflets, the left end-diastolic pressure rises and tends to equalize with the aortic pressure; this prevents the development of classic signs of severe regurgitation, which depend on a wide pulse pressure. The severity of this valve lesion is best assessed by echocardiography.

Many patients with right-sided endocarditis have no murmur, but the majority of patients with left-sided endocarditis have some murmur. Every patient with a murmur and unexplained fever for more than 1 week should be suspected of having endocarditis.

Skin Manifestations: A number of skin findings provide important clues to endocarditis (see Table 8.6–2). Janeway lesions are red macules and papules—usually nontender—on the palms and soles; these lesions, caused by septic emboli, are nearly pathognomonic for endocarditis. Osler's nodes are raised red lesions in the pads of fingers and toes; these tender lesions, representing immune complex deposition, are seen in other diseases in addition to endocarditis. Osler's nodes appear in more than 25% of patients with subacute endocarditis and are rare in patients with acute disease.

Nontender splinter hemorrhages in the nail beds are not specific for endocarditis. Petechiae are most often seen in the oral mucosa (especially on the palate), in the retina and conjunctiva, over the upper chest, and on the distal extremities. Retinal hemorrhages (Roth's spots) also strongly suggest endocarditis. Since Osler's nodes, splinter hemorrhages, and petechiae all result from the deposition of circulating immune complexes, the lesions may continue to appear for several days after antibiotics are started. Anemia and clubbing of the fingers also suggest endocarditis, but often appear too late to help with early diagnosis.

Abdominal Manifestations: Splenomegaly is found in nearly 50% of patients with subacute infective endocarditis, but in fewer than 25% of those with acute disease. The sudden appearance of splenomegaly with left upper quadrant pain and a friction rub in the region of the spleen sug-

Table 8.6–2. Manifestations of infective endocarditis.

System Affected	Manifestations
General	Anorexia, weakness, malaise, fever, weight loss
Cardiac	Murmur, congestive heart failure
Cutaneous	Osler's nodes, Janeway lesions, splinter hemorrhages, pallor, icterus, pustular rash, petechiae, purpura
Gastrointestinal	Splenomegaly, abdominal pain, left upper quadrant pain from splenic infarct, mesenteric vascular occlusion, abnormal liver function tests
Central nervous system	Emboli, mycotic aneurysms, brain abscess, meningitis, stroke, paresis, diffuse encephalitis, coma, subarachnoid hemorrhage
Ocular	Roth's spots
Musculoskeletal	Myalgia, arthralgia, arthritis, back pain, clubbing, osteomyelitis
Renal	Hematuria, proteinuria, renal insufficiency
Pulmonary	Multiple abscesses in right-sided endocarditis
Hematologic	Leukocytosis, anemia, elevated erythrocyte sedimentation rate, hypocomplementemia, hyperglobulinemia, positive tests for rheumatoid factor and antinuclear antibody

gests splenic infarction. The spleen is the most frequently recognized site of infarction, but renal infarcts are almost as common. Splenic abscess, caused by septic emboli, should be considered when a patient treated with appropriate antibiotics for longer than 1 week remains febrile (see "Persistent or Recurrent Fever" below).

Neurologic Manifestations: At least one-third of patients with endocarditis have neurologic complications. A sudden neurologic event may dominate the clinical picture, masking the underlying heart infection. Stroke, particularly in a young person, should suggest bacterial endocarditis.

The most common neurologic complications appearing at any time during endocarditis are cerebral embolism (usually to the middle cerebral arterial system) and aseptic meningitis. The most common complications tending to appear early in the course are mycotic aneurysm, brain abscess, and purulent meningitis. A mycotic aneurysm usually remains clinically silent until it ruptures; then the patient presents with sudden, severe headache and rapid deterioration of level of consciousness.

Nephritis and Uremia: Many patients with endocarditis develop focal embolic glomerulitis; a repeated search for hematuria and intermittent albuminuria is important in establishing the diagnosis. Especially in patients with staphylococcal or culture-negative endocarditis, the outstanding feature of the endocarditis may be a diffuse proliferative glomerulonephritis, probably caused by circulating antigen-antibody complexes, and occasionally producing renal failure. In these patients, endocarditis can easily be mistaken for systemic lupus erythematosus.

Emboli and Vascular Accidents: Since almost all patients with infective endocarditis have friable, easily dislodged valve vegetations, it is not surprising that many patients suffer embolic phenomena. These can be the first manifestation of endocarditis and can be fatal. Emboli can involve any organ, but are most common in spleen, kidney, heart, and brain, and, with right-sided endocarditis, lung. Suppurative pulmonary emboli are particularly common in narcotic addicts with staphylococcal infections of the tricuspid valve.

Lung Involvement: Patients with right-sided endocarditis can have such prominent pulmonary involvement that they are first thought to have pneumonia. Pulmonary involvement in right-sided endocarditis typically presents with multiple pulmonary abscesses, pneumonia, or pleural effusion. In contrast, lung involvement in what appears to be left-sided endocarditis should make the clinician search for an alternate diagnosis or a complication such as congestive heart failure.

Laboratory Features

Most patients with endocarditis have a normocytic, normochromic anemia and an elevated erythrocyte sedimentation rate. Tracking these two abnormalities is useful in monitoring the results of therapy. In subacute endocarditis, the white blood cell count is often normal or minimally elevated. Leukocytosis with a left shift implies acute endocarditis or a complication. The rapid development of anemia indicates acute infection. Hyperglobulinemia and significant titers of rheumatoid factor are seen in about 50% of patients with subacute endocarditis. Microscopic hematuria is common; a few patients develop full-blown glomerulonephritis, with red blood cell casts, proteinuria, and low serum complement.

DIAGNOSIS

With proper technique, positive venous blood cultures can be obtained in almost all patients with infective endocarditis. The frequency of positive cultures is equally great with right- or left-sided endocarditis. Bacteremia is characteristically continuous. The usual pathogens can be readily isolated within a few days, but for some organisms, such as the members of the HACEK group, isolation may require 3–4 weeks. With newer culture systems that detect carbon dioxide produced by metabolizing bacteria, more than 90% of cultures that will become positive do so within a 7-day incubation. Prior antibiotic therapy may delay growth or necessitate that cultures be repeated after the antibiotics have been stopped. A patient who has a recurrent febrile illness, with a short remission induced by antibiotic treatment and with persistently negative blood cultures, must be suspected of having infective endocarditis, particularly if the person has had valvular or congenital heart disease.

Diagnosis of acute endocarditis rarely requires more than three cultures, whereas subacute disease may require four to six. If this number fails to yield a diagnosis, processing methods should be modified; further cultures using the failed techniques are not warranted. A separate venipuncture should be used for each culture. The time of day at which blood is drawn is of little importance. Arterial blood cultures are of no special value, but bone marrow cultures may be useful when unusual organisms are suspected or when venous cultures remain sterile. Resin designed to remove antibiotics may be used for patients on antibiotics, although its value is not established. The resin bottle may also be helpful when hemophilus or meningococcus is suspected.

Echocardiography can identify vegetations in many patients with endocarditis, but is indicated only when the diagnosis is not otherwise confirmed, when a complication such as an abscess is suspected, or when the clinician wants to assess the severity of valve damage. A large vegetation means a higher risk of complications such as the acute development of congestive heart failure, major embolization, and death. Patients with large vegetations need careful monitoring, and many require urgent cardiac surgery.

Transthoracic echocardiography is simpler and less expensive than transesophageal echocardiography, but less sensitive in detecting vegetations and particularly in detecting abscesses. Transesophageal echocardiography is the method of choice when infective endocarditis is suspected in a patient who has a prosthetic heart valve. Transesophageal echocardiography can detect 85% of vegetations and almost 50% of complications in native valve endocarditis, and nearly 90% of vegetations and 30% of complications in prosthetic valve endocarditis. But even with these sophisticated imaging techniques, a negative result does not completely exclude endocarditis.

MANAGEMENT

Starting antibiotic therapy is a major step because it forever alters the clinical picture. The physician should start antibiotics only when the clinical features are so characteristic that no new facts could alter the diagnosis or when the findings suggest acute, destructive endocarditis.

Initial empiric therapy and therapy of culture-negative endocarditis is based on analysis of the clinical features and the patient's risk factors (Table 8.6–3). For subacute native valve endocarditis, the recommended drugs are oxacillin, penicillin, and gentamicin. For acute endocarditis or prosthetic valve endocarditis, empiric treatment should include at least vancomycin and gentamicin.

Antibiotic treatment of endocarditis is predicated on the fact that the infecting organisms must be killed by the antibiotic alone, without help from neutrophils. Therefore, treatment requires a bactericidal rather than a bacteriostatic drug regimen. Endocarditis is always fatal if untreated, and extremely dangerous if undertreated. In vitro experiments and animal models of endocarditis have shown synergism between cell wall-active antibiotics like penicillin and aminoglycosides like gentamicin; this synergism is essential for the complete killing of resistant streptococci as well as enterococci.

Careful in vitro sensitivity testing of recovered organisms is crucial. Tube dilution sensitivity studies should include determinations of minimum inhibitory concentration (MIC) and minimum bactericidal concentration (MBC). After the antibiotic regimen has been started, the ability of the patient's serum to inhibit or kill the infecting

Table 8.6–3. Treatment of infective endocarditis.

Treatment based on organism
Streptococcus: Penicillin ± gentamicin
Enterococcus: Ampicillin + gentamicin
Staphylococcus aureus: Oxacillin (or vancomycin) ± gentamicin
S epidermidis: Vancomycin ± gentamicin

Empiric treatment based on clinical setting
Native valve endocarditis
  Subacute: Penicillin + gentamicin
  Acute: Penicillin + oxacillin (or vancomycin) + gentamicin
Prosthetic valve endocarditis: Vancomycin + gentamicin ± rifampin
Intravenous drug user: Vancomycin + gentamicin

organism can also be determined. It is traditional to recommend a serum MBC of at least 1:8 to ensure cure. Peak serum bactericidal titers of at least 1:64 and trough serum bactericidal titers of at least 1:32 predict bacteriologic cure in most patients. However, the serum bactericidal test can be a poor predictor of bactericidal failure and clinical outcome.

Streptococci that are killed by ≤0.1 µg/mL of penicillin are classified as penicillin-sensitive. These are the most common causes of native valve endocarditis, and include *S viridans* and *S bovis*. Cephalothin or vancomycin can be used in penicillin-allergic patients, although these patients should be given cephalosporins cautiously. For enterococci and streptococci that are resistant to greater than 0.1 µg/mL of penicillin, ampicillin or penicillin is given synergistically with an aminoglycoside.

Staphylococcus aureus is a destructive organism that causes acute endocarditis with significant morbidity. The course is often complicated by endocardial abscesses, valve destruction, and suppurative emboli. If the *S aureus* is sensitive, it is treated with a semisynthetic penicillin such as nafcillin or oxacillin. There is some controversy as to gentamicin's role: In vitro and in animal models, gentamicin enhances killing of the staphylococci, but clinically, the addition of gentamicin to a semisynthetic penicillin increases renal toxicity without improving the cure rate. This combination does have a role to play in initial treatment and in treatment of critically ill patients, treatment of tolerant organisms, and short-course therapy for patients who have trouble following a medication regimen.

The term "methicillin-resistant *Staphylococcus aureus*" applies to organisms that resist all penicillins, β-lactamases, and cephalosporins. Treating these organisms as well as most coagulase-negative staphylococci requires vancomycin. Prosthetic valve endocarditis is often caused by methicillin-resistant or coagulase-negative staphylococci. Initial treatment should be vancomycin and gentamicin; many experts favor also giving rifampin.

Culture-negative endocarditis is rare except in a setting of previous antibiotic therapy, improper culture media, cultures discarded too soon (before 3 weeks), or an incorrect diagnosis. Because the prognosis is worse in patients with negative cultures, these people should be treated vigorously with a semisynthetic penicillin and an aminoglycoside, to cover the possible pathogens. If patients do not respond within 2 weeks, the physician should consider another diagnosis.

Duration of antibiotic therapy is not a well-settled issue. Of patients with uncomplicated disease caused by a penicillin-sensitive organism, 99% are cured by a 2-week regimen. If the endocarditis has lasted for longer than 3 months or if the patient has a prosthetic valve or suppurative complications, a course of 4–6 week or longer is suggested. *S aureus* endocarditis in intravenous drug users has been cured with a 2-week short course of nafcillin and tobramycin. For intravenous drug users with right-sided endocarditis, a proposed, potentially effective treatment is oral ciprofloxacin plus rifampin for 28 days.

Monitoring and Management of Complications

The major goal in treating endocarditis is to sterilize the vegetation. Management should be based on observing the patient's temperature response and searching for a new or changing murmur, congestive heart failure, and emboli to skin, joints, or brain. The fever should improve within the first week of treatment, but patients can remain febrile for 2–3 weeks. Blood cultures should become sterile within 2–5 days of starting treatment. It may take as long as several weeks for patients to notice improvement in their appetite, strength, and general well-being. Blood counts, erythrocyte sedimentation rate, and urinalysis should be followed up until they return to normal. The electrocardiogram and echocardiogram should be repeated only if the patient develops a complication such as heart block or cardiac abscess.

Common Management Problems

Persistent or Recurrent Fever: If fever persists or recurs during the treatment of proven endocarditis, the clinician should search for different causes in patients with sensitive organisms and patients with resistant organisms. During treatment of resistant organisms such as staphylococci, persistent fever usually results from failure to sterilize the valve infection, from a local abscess, or from septic emboli to the kidneys, spleen, joints, or brain. If the answer is not apparent after repeated physical exams, the patient should undergo computed tomography (CT) of the abdomen and head, bone scans, and a repeat echocardiogram.

Recurrent fever in patients with endocarditis caused by sensitive organisms is usually explained by treatment complications or development of an unrelated condition. Complications of treatment include drug fever, thrombophlebitis, sterile abscesses at injection sites, and bland emboli, usually to the spleen or kidneys. Unrelated conditions that can affect chronically ill patients with endocarditis are pneumonia, pulmonary emboli, and urinary tract infections.

Persistent fever in a patient who is otherwise doing well does not require a change in antibiotic treatment. If drug fever is suspected, all nonessential drugs should be stopped. If an equally effective alternate antibiotic regimen is available, it should be used. If no effective alternate exists, the patient and physician may tolerate the fever or treat it symptomatically with antipyretics, including corticosteroids if absolutely necessary.

Role of Surgery: In the pre-antibiotic era, patients with endocarditis were most likely to die from the bacterial infection. Nowadays, the most common cause of death is congestive heart failure. Heart failure is caused by acute endocarditis, virulent microorganisms, and aortic insufficiency, or, less commonly, mitral insufficiency.

Heart failure caused by valve destruction from infective endocarditis is the strongest and most urgent indication for cardiac surgery. Rupture of the sinus of Valsalva from extension of aortic valve endocarditis also causes acute heart failure and requires emergency surgery. Other strong indications for surgery are an unstable prosthetic valve, fungal endocarditis, and bacteria that are responding poorly to all antibiotic regimens.

Relative indications for cardiac surgery in native and prosthetic valve endocarditis are relapse of the infection, evidence of intracardiac extension of the infection (eg, rupture of the chordae tendineae or papillary muscle), heart block, abscess, recurrent emboli, large (>1 cm) vegetations, and renal failure.

In general, extracardiac manifestations of infective endocarditis are managed by simply controlling the valve infection. But occasionally, extracardiac complications require more specific treatment. With pathogens like *S aureus*, emboli can lead to frank pyogenic abscesses that require surgical drainage. Splenectomy is rarely required to treat splenic abscess. Strokes from emboli are treated conservatively; anticoagulation is given only to patients with prosthetic valves. Occasionally, a cerebral abscess needs surgical drainage. Management of mycotic aneurysm is controversial; most experts reserve surgery for large or symptomatic aneurysms.

Renal failure in endocarditis is caused by immune glomerulonephritis. Usually, controlling the valve infection improves kidney function. But some patients progress to permanent renal failure, which can be treated only by dialysis.

Prophylaxis

Because infective endocarditis is potentially fatal, giving antibiotics to prevent infection is thought—although not proven—to be worthwhile. Only about 15% of cases of endocarditis can be clearly attributed to prior medical, surgical, or dental procedures, but because these procedures are common, prophylaxis might prevent a large number of cases of endocarditis. There has been much debate about which underlying cardiac lesions and which procedures deserve prophylaxis. The decision to give antibiotic prophylaxis must be based on the nature of the cardiac lesion and the risk and type of bacteremia associated with a given procedure. For procedures above the diaphragm, prophylaxis is directed against *S viridans*; for procedures below the diaphragm, treatment is directed against enterococci.

All patients with a history of endocarditis or with a prosthetic valve need antibiotic prophylaxis. When the procedure carries a moderate risk of bacteremia, prophylaxis should also be given to patients who have congenital malformations or acquired valve lesions and to patients who have mitral valve prolapse with valvular regurgitation as manifested by a murmur. Patients with mitral valve prolapse alone (without a murmur) present a frequent and difficult problem. Some experts recommend prophylaxis for all such patients; other experts recommend none. The authors recommend prophylaxis for all patients with mitral valve prolapse unless echocardiogram has shown their valve leaflets to be normal. The reader is advised to consult the current recommendations of the American Heart Association.

SUMMARY

▶ Endocarditis develops through the hematogenous spread of organisms to endocardial tissue. The chief risk factors are previous endocardial damage (from rheumatic fever, calcific degeneration, congenital abnormalities, or previous endocarditis) and abnormal bacteremia (eg, from intravenous drug use, infected intravascular catheters).

▶ Early recognition of the infection is important to prevent cardiac and extracardiac complications. Blood cultures must be obtained before antibiotic treatment is started in any patient with fever and risk for endocarditis.

▶ The most common causes of endocarditis are streptococci and staphylococci; gram-negative endocarditis is rare except in intravenous drug users and prosthetic valve recipients.

▶ Heart failure from endocarditis requires urgent surgery.

▶ Preventing endocarditis is the responsibility of all physicians and dentists, who should be familiar with the official American Heart Association recommendations.

SUGGESTED READING

Dajani AS et al: Prevention of bacterial endocarditis: Recommendations by the American Heart Association. JAMA 1990; 264:2919.

Daniel WG et al: Improvement in the diagnosis of abscesses associated with endocarditis by transesophageal echocardiography. N Engl J Med 1991;324:795.

Drancourt M et L: *Bartonella (Rochalimaea) quintana* endocarditis in three homeless men. N Engl J Med 1995; 332:419.

Karp RB: Role of surgery in infective endocarditis. Cardiovasc Clin 1987;17:141.

Wilson WR et al: Antibiotic treatment of adults with infective endocarditis due to streptococci, enterococci, staphylococci, and HACEK microorganisms. JAMA 1995;274:1706.

Intra-Abdominal Infections

John G. Bartlett, MD

Intra-abdominal sepsis is any infection within the abdominal cavity but outside the lumen of the gastrointestinal tract. Such an infection can involve the serosal surfaces, peritoneum, or parenchymal organs such as the liver, gallbladder, spleen, or pancreas.

The following principles describe most types of intra-abdominal sepsis:

- The infection almost always involves the flora of the gastrointestinal tract—bacteria that have been displaced from their normal location.

- Nearly all intra-abdominal sepsis follows two stages: first inflammation, then abscess formation.

- The most common causes of intra-abdominal sepsis are appendicitis, diverticulitis, and infections following abdominal surgery. Appendicitis, diverticulitis, and cholecystitis are caused by obstruction that leads to infection in the distal segment.

- Nearly all patients with intra-abdominal sepsis present with abdominal pain and tenderness, fever, and leukocytosis. Many patients also have nausea, vomiting, and diarrhea.

- Common complications are disruption of the vascular supply with gangrene, perforation of the distal segment, bacteremia, and extension of the infection by fistula formation.

- Most patients are treated with empirically chosen antibiotics and surgery.

PATHOGENESIS

Most infections of the abdominal cavity involve bacteria that normally colonize the gastrointestinal tract. The usual mechanism for infections involving serosal surfaces is a break in the mucosal barrier, mainly caused by a perforated peptic ulcer, diverticulitis, appendicitis, inflammatory bowel disease, penetrating abdominal trauma, colon cancer, or intestinal surgery. Peritonitis results when the infection extends to the peritoneum by direct spread through the bowel mucosa, by perforation, or by bacteremia.

Inoculum

The types and concentrations of bacteria in the inoculum depend on which part of the gastrointestinal tract is involved (Table 8.7–1; Figure 8.7–1). The stomach usually harbors a sparse flora of penicillin-sensitive, gram-positive bacteria originating in saliva. Stomach acid kills most bacteria; patients with gastric achlorhydria from aging or from use of antacids or H_2 blocking drugs are likely to have much higher bacterial concentrations. The small bowel also has few bacteria, but here the major limiting factor is peristalsis, which simply propels bacteria distally along with the intestinal contents. Thus, perforation of the stomach or small bowel under otherwise physiologic conditions results in contamination with relatively few bacteria, usually about 100–100,000 bacteria/mL of gastric or small bowel contents. The predominant bacteria are those that dominate in saliva and survive gastric acid, especially streptococci, lactobacilli, some anaerobes (but not *Bacteroides fragilis*), and occasional coliforms (see below) and *Candida*.

The colon harbors the body's largest microbial population: Bacterial concentrations approach 1 billion/g of intestinal contents, with over 99% anaerobes. This concentration approaches the geometric limit within which bacteria can occupy space. The dry weight of stool is almost entirely bacteria. A person's colon harbors an estimated 400 species; many species are found in virtually all humans, others in only some people. Every person has a distinctive combination of species that remains a lifelong bacterial "signature."

Infections such as diverticulitis, appendicitis, and infections following colonic surgery—all of which involve colonic bacteria—reflect this polymicrobial flora. Most infections are mixed, with the dominant aerobe being *Escherichia coli* and the dominant anaerobe, *B fragilis*. Both organisms are normal constituents of the colonic flora,

Table 8.7–1. Types of intra-abdominal sepsis.

Type of Infection	Predisposing Factors	Usual Pathogens
Monomicrobial		
Cholecystitis	Cholelithiasis	*Escherichia coli*, other coliforms, streptococci
Spontaneous bacterial peritonitis	Ascites	*E coli*, other coliforms
Infected pancreatic pseudocyst	Pancreatitis	Same as above
Polymicrobial		
Peritonitis or intra-abdominal abscess	Perforated ulcer Colonic perforation	Streptococci; less often, coliforms *E coli, Bacteroides fragilis*, streptococci, coliforms, others
Diverticulitis	Diverticula	*E coli, B fragilis*, streptococci, coliforms, others
Appendicitis	Appendiceal fecalith	Same as above
Liver abscess	Biliary tract disease	Same as above

and both possess virulence factors that contribute to intra-abdominal sepsis. *E coli,* and possibly other coliforms, appear to play an especially important role in causing peritonitis, whereas *B fragilis* seems to play a critical role in abscess formation (see "Defenses" below).

The term *coliform* applies to members of the Enterobacteriaceae family, which includes the fermenting enteric gram-negative bacilli, for example, *E coli, Klebsiella, Proteus,* and *Enterobacter.* All of these organisms seem to have similar pathogenic potential in intra-abdominal sepsis. *E coli* is the most common pathogen simply because it is the dominant coliform in the intestinal tract. Likewise, *B fragilis* is the most common anaerobic gram-negative bacillus in intra-abdominal sepsis, but other species of *Bacteroides* are often found as well. All the *Bacteroides* seem to have similar virulence properties, including a polysaccharide capsule and the potential to produce short-chain volatile acids.

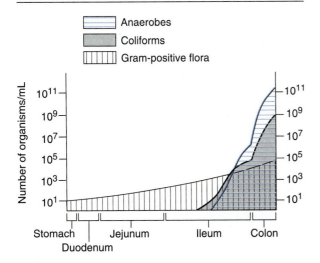

Figure 8.7–1. Normal bacterial flora in different parts of the gastrointestinal tract.

Defenses

The peritoneal cavity is the largest preformed extravascular space in the body, with a surface area almost as large as the total cutaneous surface. The cavity usually contains less than 100 mL of peritoneal fluid; normal fluid is clear and has fewer than 150 cells/mL—about 50% macrophages and 40% lymphocytes. The only part of the peritoneal surface that can clear bacteria independent of an inflammatory reaction is the inferior surface of the diaphragm, which contains lymphatic channels that drain from the peritoneal cavity to the anterior mediastinal lymphatics and then to the systemic circulation. Diaphragmatic clearance is the first line of defense when bacteria enter the peritoneal cavity. The negative pressure of diaphragmatic movement facilitates clearance by drawing bacteria toward the diaphragm. Lymphatic clearance can eliminate bacteria quickly but can be overwhelmed, leading to bacteremia.

The second line of defense is the inflammatory response, which generally begins within minutes of a bacterial challenge. The first phase is an influx of polymorphonuclear leukocytes. Bacteria then activate the alternative complement pathway: Opsonic and chemotactic factors C3 and C5a are released and opsonized bacteria are phagocytized. The surviving bacteria form a phlegmon—an inflammatory mass with neutrophils and edema fluid. The phlegmon can progress to an abscess by developing a collagen outer wall (see "Intra-abdominal Abscesses" below). An abscess has the advantage of localizing the microbial insult but the disadvantage of protecting the microbes from host defenses.

CLINICAL MANIFESTATIONS AND DIAGNOSIS

Intra-abdominal sepsis has two phases: peritonitis followed by abscess. In the acute stage, patients may have free perforation of the intestine, leading to generalized peritonitis with free-flowing exudate. Alternatively, and more often, the infection is successfully restricted to its site of origin with a phlegmon. Either form of infection may be accompanied by bacteremia. Depending on the inoculum size, mortality can be high. In survivors, the peritonitis resolves, followed days to years later by the second phase of intra-abdominal sepsis: abscess formation.

Peritonitis

Patients with generalized peritonitis develop a classic "acute surgical abdomen" with a rapid, acute inflammatory reaction that may produce a net flow of 300–500 mL of fluid per hour into the peritoneal cavity. An example is acute perforation of a peptic ulcer, which suddenly releases onto the peritoneal surface an inoculum containing both acid, which causes a florid chemical peritonitis, and gastric bacteria, which cause bacterial peritonitis.

Patients with generalized peritonitis present with severe pain that usually begins suddenly and may be diffuse or localized. Physical exam shows generalized tenderness, rebound tenderness, and involuntary muscular guarding indicating inflammation of the parietal peritoneum. Most patients also have fever, leukocytosis, nausea, vomiting, ileus, abdominal distention with hyperresonance, and diminished or no bowel sounds. The flux of fluid into the abdomen leads to dehydration with hypotension and oliguria.

In localized peritonitis, the inflammatory response is restricted, usually to a disease site such as a ruptured appendix or diverticulum. Helping to limit the infection are the inflammatory reaction and the mobility of the mesentery, which adheres to sites of perforation. Localized peritonitis presents much more indolently and subtly than generalized peritonitis. The first symptom is often a vague pain reflecting irritation of the visceral peritoneum; early signs are minimal. The infection site may become more obvious later when the parietal peritoneum of the anterior abdominal wall becomes involved and causes localized tenderness. Many patients also have fever and leukocytosis.

Intra-Abdominal Abscess

An abscess is a loculated collection that usually contains viable bacteria, polymorphonuclear cells, and necrotic debris (pus) entrapped within a collagen wall or capsule. A phlegmon is an inflammatory mass that precedes an abscess and contains all the same elements except the collagen wall. This distinction has important treatment implications: Most phlegmons respond to antibiotics, but abscesses require drainage. Antibiotics penetrate abscesses but usually cannot eliminate bacteria, either because the drugs are less active in anaerobic or acidic conditions or because the bacteria are not in a growth phase.

Intra-abdominal abscesses develop in three patterns:

1. An abscess can follow immediately in the wake of generalized peritonitis.
2. The course can be biphasic: acute peritonitis, followed by an abscess within days, months, or even years.

3. The course can be insidious, with no obvious initial insult and only the late sequela of an abscess.

Abscesses can develop anywhere in the abdominal cavity. Many are at the organism's portal of entry. For example, a peri-appendiceal or diverticular abscess is the late sequela of a phlegmon at the original site. But with free perforation or a leak that is not successfully localized to the portal of entry, abscesses may be distributed throughout the abdomen. Most often they develop either in the subphrenic area, reflecting the negative pressure created by diaphragmatic movement, or in the lower quadrants or pelvis, reflecting gravitational flow.

Most patients with an intra-abdominal abscess have fever and abdominal pain and tenderness. Specific findings depend on the location and size of the abscess. Some patients who present with minimal pain pose the enigma of "fever of unknown origin" (Chapter 8.2); this is most common with intraloop, intramesenteric, and subphrenic abscesses, which produce little or no pain and generally no palpable mass. Pelvic abscesses may be palpated on rectal or vaginal examination, but patients' symptoms are often so vague that the appropriate examination is not done. About one-third of intra-abdominal abscesses follow intestinal surgery; this poses a special diagnostic problem because it is difficult to interpret clinical signs in the postoperative state.

Laboratory clues to an intra-abdominal abscess are leukocytosis and a chest x-ray showing an otherwise unexplained pleural effusion or elevated diaphragm, a plain film of the abdomen showing ileus or gas outside the intestinal tract, and positive blood cultures for coliforms or *Bacteroides* sp. The usual preferred method for detecting intra-abdominal abscesses is computed tomography (CT), which defines abdominal anatomy with a sensitivity and specificity of 95%. Ultrasonography is less reliable but has two advantages: It can be done at the bedside, and it does not expose patients to radiation. Ultrasonography may be the preferred way of detecting pelvic abscesses. Other imaging options are indium-labeled neutrophil scans and magnetic resonance imaging.

MANAGEMENT

The physician managing a patient with intra-abdominal sepsis should provide supportive care, give antibiotics to cover for both aerobes and anaerobes, and determine the role and timing of surgery or percutaneous drainage.

Choice of antibiotics is simpler if the bacteriology has been determined, but this is often unrealistic because of limited access to the infected site and, even when useful specimens are obtained, the delay in laboratory reporting. Most intra-abdominal sepsis is treated empirically, based on pathogens predicted by published bacteriologic and clinical studies. Although most infected sites have multiple aerobic and anaerobic bacteria, there is no evidence that antibiotics should be directed against every bacterium. The important pathogens to treat are coliforms, primarily *E coli,* and anaerobic bacteria, primarily *B fragilis.* The usual empiric approach is to treat the coliforms with one drug such as a third-generation cephalosporin or an aminoglycoside and to treat the anaerobes with a second drug such as metronidazole, cefoxitin, or clindamycin.

Most patients with intra-abdominal sepsis require surgery or a drainage procedure to correct the underlying defect and to drain focal collections. Intra-abdominal abscesses tend to respond poorly to antibiotics; in fact, in the pre-penicillin era, drainage alone was usually satisfactory. The major question at present concerns the best method for drainage. Traditional drainage has been surgical, but percutaneous drainage under ultrasound or CT guidance is equally effective in most patients.

COMMON FORMS OF INTRA-ABDOMINAL SEPSIS

Appendicitis

Appendicitis is acute inflammation of the appendix, most often affecting persons 5–30 years old. Appendicitis is common and curable and is one of the most important conditions in the differential diagnosis of the acute abdomen. The cause is usually not known, but some patients have obstruction from fecaliths or stones, and rare patients have a tumor or parasitic infection. Most patients present with fever, leukocytosis, and abdominal pain that is at first referred to the epigastric or periumbilical area and later localizes to the right lower quadrant. Other common symptoms are anorexia and nausea with or without vomiting. Physical exam usually shows tenderness to palpation, most often confined to McBurney's point in the right lower quadrant. Late complications are perforation leading to generalized or localized peritonitis, as well as abscess formation and gangrene. The usual treatment is removal of the appendix, and antibiotics directed against the colonic flora. Overall mortality rate is 0.2–2%, and it is highest in patients older than 60 years and patients whose appendix perforates.

Diverticulitis

Focal inflammation of the wall of a diverticulum is generally caused by inspissated stool and is most common in patients over 40. The major symptoms are fever and pain, usually in the left lower quadrant, since the sigmoid and descending colon are the predominant sites of diverticula. The pain may be intermittent at first, but it generally becomes constant and resembles that of acute appendicitis. This is why acute diverticulitis is sometimes called "left-sided appendicitis." Physical exam generally reveals fever and localized tenderness, both direct and rebound. Abdominal x-rays may show collections of air and fluid in the left lower quadrant or free air under the diaphragm (in-

dicating perforation). Major complications are perforation, intestinal obstruction, fistula, and abscesses. Scans are especially useful in showing inflammation and abscesses. Most patients with uncomplicated diverticulitis can be treated with antibiotics and a diet of clear liquids. Many patients with complications require surgery.

Cholecystitis

Acute cholecystitis results from obstruction and chronic inflammation of the cystic duct. Only about 50% of patients have bacteria in the bile, and bacterial infection is thought to be a secondary rather than a primary process. Critical to the pathogenesis is obstruction, usually caused by a stone, although 2–5% of patients present with abdominal pain in the right subcostal region, often accompanied by fever, anorexia, nausea, and vomiting. Physical exam shows tenderness to palpation in the right subcostal region with Murphy's sign—subhepatic tenderness that increases as the patient takes a deep breath during palpation. To establish the diagnosis, ultrasonography is the simplest and best method for detecting stones in the gallbladder, and radionuclide scans are the best way to verify a clinical impression of acute cholecystitis. Complications include perforation leading to bile peritonitis, abscesses (usually pericholecystic), empyema (pus-filled gallbladder), and a fistula that may communicate with the duodenum.

The usual treatment is removal of the gallbladder. This should be reserved for patients with an established diagnosis and adequate preoperative preparation. Antibiotics are given to prevent bacteremia and suppurative complications. The most common bacteria isolated from bile are *E coli,* other coliforms, and *Enterococcus* sp; anaerobic bacteria are infrequently implicated, except with ascending cholangitis. The usual surgical procedure is cholecystectomy, sometimes done acutely and sometimes delayed until after a "cooling-off period" of a few weeks.

Liver Abscess

Liver abscess is generally caused by *Entamoeba histolytica* (amebic liver abscess) or colonic coliforms and anaerobes (pyogenic liver abscess). People usually develop amebic abscesses after travel to or residence in an endemic area. The source of infection is enteric (the gut), although few patients have concurrent amebic colitis. Most patients with pyogenic abscesses have associated biliary tract infection or infection in organs drained by the portal vein, such as appendicitis or diverticulitis. Both types of liver abscesses manifest with fever, abdominal pain, and anorexia. The liver may be enlarged and show focal tenderness. Laboratory tests show leukocytosis and abnormal liver function tests, especially an elevated alkaline phosphatase and low serum albumin. The diagnosis is readily confirmed by CT with contrast. Amebic liver abscesses respond well to antibiotic treatment, usually metronidazole. Pyogenic abscesses are treated with antibiotics and surgical or percutaneous drainage.

SUMMARY

▶ Intra-abdominal sepsis is a biphasic disease: acute peritonitis followed by abscess formation.

▶ Peritonitis can manifest classically with an acute surgical abdomen or can be localized and subtle, as with appendicitis or diverticulitis. Both presentations can lead to intra-abdominal abscesses.

▶ An inoculum of stomach contents has relatively few bacteria, most of which are sensitive to penicillin. An inoculum of colon contents usually has a polymicrobial flora of aerobes and anaerobes; the most common isolates are *E coli* and *B fragilis*.

▶ Management of intra-abdominal sepsis should include supportive care, empiric antibiotics to cover for *E coli* and *B fragilis,* and, usually, surgery or percutaneous drainage.

SUGGESTED READING

Altemeier WA et al: Intra-abdominal abscesses. Am J Surg 1973; 125:70.

Bartlett JG et al: A review: Lessons from an animal model of intra-abdominal sepsis. Arch Surg 1978;113:853.

Dellinger EP et al: Quality standard for antimicrobial prophylaxis in surgical procedures. Clin Infect Dis 1994;18:422.

Gerzof SG et al: Percutaneous catheter drainage of abdominal abscesses: A five-year experience. N Engl J Med 1981;305:653.

Solomkin JS et al: Antibiotic trials in intra-abdominal infections: A critical evaluation of study design and outcome reporting. Ann Surg 1984;200:29.

Solomkin JS et al: Results of a multicenter trial comparing imipenem/cilastatin to tobramycin/clindamycin for intra-abdominal infections. Ann Surg 1990;212:581.

Urinary Tract Infections

Janet E. Horn, MD

Urinary tract infections (UTIs) are the most common of all bacterial infections, usually affecting otherwise healthy people of any age. Most people can be easily treated as outpatients. Left untreated, UTIs can have devastating consequences, including protracted illness and even death. Although UTIs are generally considered simple to diagnose and treat, they can manifest with subtle clinical and laboratory findings and can be complicated.

DEFINITIONS

Urinary tract infection is a general term; many more specific terms are used to denote the anatomic site of infection. Most commonly, the site is indicated as a lower or upper tract infection. Lower tract infections involve (1) the urethra (urethritis in either men or women, or acute urethral syndrome in women), (2) the superficial mucosa of the bladder (cystitis), or (3) the prostate or epididymis in men (prostatitis or epididymitis). Upper tract infections involve the renal parenchyma and may be called *pyelonephritis.* Other types of upper tract infections are perinephric abscesses and intrarenal abscesses. Upper tract infections are more serious and more difficult to eradicate than lower tract infections.

Another way to categorize UTIs is as uncomplicated or complicated. Although imprecisely defined, an uncomplicated UTI is cystitis in a patient who has no congenital or acquired structural abnormality or neurologic dysfunction. All other UTIs, including any UTI in a pregnant woman, are considered complicated. Examples are UTIs related to a long-term indwelling urinary catheter, a neurogenic bladder, or a fistula between the urinary tract and the gastrointestinal tract.

Another frequently used term is *asymptomatic bacteriuria*, that is, 100,000 or more colony-forming units/mL (CFU/mL) of bacteria in the urine of a patient who has no symptoms.

PATHOPHYSIOLOGY

Urine is normally sterile. Bacteria infect the normally sterile urinary tract either by traveling from the bloodstream to the kidneys (hematogenous spread) or by infecting the urethra and traveling upward toward the bladder and kidneys (ascending infection). More than 95% of UTIs are caused by ascending infection. Women develop ascending infections when bacteria normally found in fecal flora colonize the vaginal vestibule, enter the urethra, and spread to the bladder.

Four major factors influence the development of a UTI: anatomy of the genitourinary tract, host defense mechanisms, the presence and virulence of bacteria, and behaviors that increase the risk of UTI, such as failure to empty the bladder completely.

During the first year of life, bacteria in the urine (bacteriuria) and pyelonephritis are more common in boys than girls, because boys are more likely to have congenital anomalies of the genitourinary tract (Table 8.8–1). From age 1 year until about 50, UTI is for the most part a disease of females; the male's longer urethra protects against bacteria ascending into the bladder. Men over age 50 have an increasing incidence of bacteriuria, because they have more of a tendency to develop urinary obstruction from prostatic hypertrophy.

Other anatomic factors can increase the risk of acquiring a UTI. These are reflux of the normal valve-like mechanism of the ureterovesical junction; obstruction of the genitourinary tract by stones or gynecologic abnormalities such as fibroid tumors; and instrumentation of the urinary tract.

The following are host defense factors against UTIs:

1. Normal periurethral flora, which inhibits growth and adhesion of pathogens
2. Prostatic antibacterial factor, which naturally suppresses bacterial activity

Table 8.8–1. Risk factors for urinary tract infection.

Both sexes
Congenital and other anatomic abnormalities
Stones
Ureterovesical reflux
Inadequate emptying of bladder, prolonged intervals between
   emptyings
Urinary tract instrumentation

Women
Sexual intercourse
Use of diaphragm with spermicide
Obstruction by gynecologic abnormalities (eg, fibroid tumors)
Pregnancy
"Nonsecretor" Lewis blood group
P_1 blood group phenotype

Men
Lack of circumcision
Active anal intercourse
Obstruction by prostatic hypertrophy
Female sexual partner with vaginal colonization by fecal flora

3. Urinary and vaginal acidity, which inhibits bacterial growth
4. Urinary and perineal immunoglobulins, which in some people prevent bacteria from adhering to the urinary tract
5. Normal bladder emptying mechanism, which may prevent bacteria from multiplying
6. Mucopolysaccharide lining of the bladder, which can prevent bacterial adherence

Interruption of any of the above defense mechanisms can lead to a UTI.

Studies have shown that some women with recurrent UTIs have a genetic predisposition. Women who have the "nonsecretor" Lewis blood group are prone to recurrent UTIs because some of their urogenital epithelial cells tend to adhere to specific strains of bacteria. For unknown reasons, women with the P_1 blood group phenotype are also prone to recurrent UTIs.

Certain behaviors also increase the risk for UTI. Normal micturition usually eliminates organisms, and bacterial growth is inhibited by a low urinary pH, high or low urine osmolarity, high urea concentration, and high organic acid content. A significant residual urine volume promotes infection. In women who have an anatomically normal urinary tract and normal micturition patterns, a major predisposing risk factor for UTI is vaginal intercourse. Use of a diaphragm with spermicide also increases women's risk of bacteriuria by altering both the vaginal pH and the natural flora. Men practicing active anal intercourse are at risk of acquiring a UTI through exposure to fecal flora.

MICROBIOLOGY

As might be expected, most UTIs are caused by bacteria of the family Enterobacteriaceae, especially *Escherichia coli* but also *Klebsiella, Enterobacter, Serratia,*

Proteus, and *Providencia* sp (Table 8.8–2). *E coli* accounts for almost 80% of all UTIs. Group D streptococci (enterococci) and *Pseudomonas* sp account for 5–10% of uncomplicated UTIs. In young women, *Staphylococcus saprophyticus* is a significant pathogen. Over 95% of UTIs are caused by a single bacterial species. When mixed species grow from a urine culture in an uncomplicated UTI, the culture is probably contaminated. However, mixed species can cause complicated UTIs, such as those in patients with an indwelling catheter.

All the bacteria just mentioned can cause a simple urethritis or cystitis, or can ascend to the kidneys and cause pyelonephritis. In contrast, the sexually transmitted bacteria (eg, *Neisseria gonorrhoeae, Chlamydia trachomatis, Ureaplasma urealyticum*) infect only the urethra in women and men, and the epididymis and prostate in men. These organisms never cause upper urinary tract infection.

Other organisms can cause urinary tract infections, but only in unusual circumstances. Fungal cystitis, for instance, is found mainly in patients who are immunocompromised, have received long-term antibiotics, or have indwelling catheters. Renal tuberculosis, which occurs as part of a disseminated mycobacterial infection, can cause a descending infection that manifests as sterile pyuria (see "Microscopic Examination" below). Viruses such as adenovirus can cause hemorrhagic cystitis. But these organisms are the exception rather than the rule in causing UTIs.

Laboratory Diagnosis

Microscopic Examination: Laboratory diagnosis of UTI is based on finding bacteriuria and pyuria (leukocytes in the urine). The first test should be the simple and cost-effective microscopic examination of uncentrifuged and centrifuged urine. Uncentrifuged urine showing one or more bacterium per oil immersion field suggests 100,000 CFU of bacteria per mL of urine. When several oil immersion fields must be searched to find one bacterium, the counts usually range from 10,000 to 100,000 bacteria per mL of urine. Gram's stain of uncentrifuged urine is helpful in determining bacteriuria. In a patient with symptoms, centrifuged urine containing 10 or more white blood cells

Table 8.8–2. Major etiologic agents of genitourinary infections.

Cystitis and pyelonephritis
Enterobacteriaceae (especially *Escherichia coli* in women)
Group D enterococci
Staphylococcus saprophyticus (in women)

Urethritis
Chlamydia trachomatis
Neisseria gonorrhoeae
Ureaplasma urealyticum
Herpes simplex virus
Mycoplasma hominis

Less common infections
Pseudomonas aeruginosa
Other resistant gram-negative organisms
Fungi

per high-power field has a sensitivity of almost 95% in diagnosing UTI. Microscopic examination of centrifuged urine showing more than 20 bacteria under high, dry power correlates with 100,000 bacteria per mL of urine.

Several factors can falsely reduce the numbers of white blood cells or bacteria seen microscopically in the urine: an improperly collected specimen (see "Urine Culture" below), a very dilute specimen, and previous antibiotic treatment.

Urine Culture: Although the urine culture is the "gold standard" for diagnosing UTI, not every patient needs it. Nonetheless, physicians should know how to obtain and interpret a urine culture.

The urine for culture must be collected with extreme care. A clean-catch urine specimen is obtained from a woman after she has carefully washed her external genitalia with four sterile soapy gauze pads and another four gauze pads containing warm water. The patient is instructed to use each pad to wash the external genitalia from front to back. By following these instructions, she should prevent contamination from the urethra, vagina, and perineum.

A man prepares for a clean-catch urine specimen by retracting the foreskin of the penis, if uncircumcised, and washing the glans with one soaped gauze and one plain gauze.

After washing, patients are asked to void a little urine into the toilet, and then void the remainder into a sterile cup. This is a "midstream collection." In patients who are obese or acutely ill, and thus unable to provide a clean-catch midstream urine collection, a specimen may have to be obtained by an "in-and-out" urethral catheterization.

Older criteria for interpreting urine cultures defined UTI as bacteriuria of more than 100,000 CFU/mL. However, the criteria have changed. In a symptomatic woman with pyuria, a UTI is defined as growth of 10,000–100,000 CFU/mL of a single or predominant organism. In a symptomatic man with pyuria, a UTI is growth of at least 1000 CFU/mL of a single or predominant organism. Occasionally, urine cultures reveal two or more species of bacteria, but no predominant organism. This usually means a contaminated specimen, and the culture should be repeated.

Several factors can affect the culturing of pathogens from urine. As mentioned above, improper collection of a urine sample undermines the accuracy of the culture results. Delays in processing urine specimens can decrease the accuracy of a culture. Storing urine at room temperature for longer than 1 hour, or in a refrigerator for longer than 48 hours, significantly increases bacterial counts. Lastly, unusual or fastidious microorganisms require special transport media or culture techniques; a negative culture in a patient with pyuria may mean fastidious organisms such as mycobacteria, or sexually transmitted organisms—*C trachomatis* or *N gonorrhoeae*.

Rapid Diagnostic Tests: Many tests enable detection of pyuria and bacteriuria faster than urine culture. The most reliable quick way to detect pyuria is the chemical measurement of leukocyte esterase by urine dipstick. This test has a sensitivity of 75–96% in detecting pyuria indicative of infection. Since the dipstick test is slightly less sensitive than microscopic examination for leukocytes, it may be used as an alternative when urine microscopy is not available, or as a first diagnostic step. A finding of nitrates on the dipstick usually indicates bacteria, but this test is less well studied than that for pyuria.

DIAGNOSIS AND MANAGEMENT

Urinary Tract Infections in Women

Acute Uncomplicated Cystitis: The most common presenting symptoms of cystitis are burning on urination (dysuria), frequent urination, urgency, hesitancy on beginning the flow, and blood in the urine (hematuria). In a sexually active woman, however, dysuria may be the presenting symptom not only of cystitis, but also of acute urethritis caused by a sexually transmitted organism (Chapter 8.9) or of vaginitis caused by *Trichomonas* or *Candida*. These three diagnoses can usually be differentiated by a careful history, physical examination, and urinalysis (Table 8.8–3). A urine culture can confirm the UTI.

Acute cystitis usually presents with an abrupt onset of multiple symptoms including frequency, urgency, dysuria, and low back or suprapubic pain. The physical exam is unremarkable or reveals only suprapubic tenderness. Urinalysis usually shows pyuria. Urine culture shows 100 to over 100,000 CFU/mL.

Table 8.8–3. Differentiating cystitis from urethritis and vaginitis.

	Cystitis	Urethritis	Vaginitis
Urinary symptoms	Abrupt onset of frequency, urgency, dysuria, low back or suprapubic pain	Gradual onset of dysuria	Gradual onset of dysuria
Vaginal discharge	No	Yes	Yes
Pelvic exam	Suprapubic tenderness	Cervicitis, cervical discharge	Vaginitis
Pyuria	Yes	Sometimes	No
Positive urine culture	Yes	No	No

Adapted from information appearing in *The New England Journal of Medicine.* Stamm WE, Hooton TM: Management of urinary tract infections in adults. N Engl J Med 1993;329:1328.

Most women with acute urethritis (acute urethral syndrome) give a history of a new sexual partner, vaginal discharge or bleeding, and the gradual onset of very mild urinary symptoms, usually dysuria alone. Pelvic exam usually reveals cervicitis, cervical discharge, or herpetic lesions in the vulvovaginal area. Urinalysis may or may not show pyuria. Urine culture usually shows at most 100 CFU/mL.

Vaginitis usually causes the same symptoms as urethritis. Pelvic exam reveals vaginitis, and urinalysis does not show pyuria.

Recommended therapy for uncomplicated cystitis is a 3–7-day course of an antimicrobial drug. A single dose may also be given, but the cure rate is lower and recurrences more likely. Since cystitis in women is usually caused by *E coli, Klebsiella,* or *Proteus,* an antibiotic effective against such Enterobacteriaceae may be started in patients who present typically and have pyuria on microscopy or leukocyte esterase testing, but without a urine culture. The most effective antibiotics are trimethoprim-sulfamethoxazole, tetracyclines, first-generation cephalosporins, and fluoroquinolones. Amoxicillin may also be tried, but about one-third of bacterial strains causing cystitis are resistant. After completing antibiotic therapy for cystitis, only patients who have persistent or recurrent symptoms need follow-up.

Recurrent Cystitis: About 20% of women who have had cystitis will have recurrent infections. Although recurrences can be caused by a persistent focus of infection, such as a partially treated pyelonephritis, most recurrences are exogenous reinfections resulting from the same predisposing factors that caused the first episode, such as genetic susceptibility, incomplete emptying of the bladder, and use of diaphragms and spermicides (see "Pathophysiology" above). Few patients have anatomic or functional abnormalities of the urinary tract; thus, few need extensive radiographic or invasive evaluation.

Women with recurrent cystitis (≥3 episodes within 6 months) should have at least one episode documented by urine culture. Then they may be started on a low dose of an antibiotic, usually trimethoprim, trimethoprim-sulfamethoxazole, norfloxacin, or cephalexin, in the form of continuous prophylaxis, postcoital prophylaxis, or patient-initiated therapy whenever symptoms begin. Decisions about further evaluation (cystoscopy, intravenous pyelogram, and others) depend on a number of factors, such as whether the patient continues to have UTIs while on prophylaxis or has had multiple episodes of pyelonephritis.

Urinary Tract Infections in Men

Men younger than 50 years rarely have UTIs. Until recently, any UTI in a man younger than 50 was thought to mean an underlying urologic abnormality meriting extensive investigation of the genitourinary tract. Now young men, like women, are known to have risk factors for UTIs: noncircumcision, active anal intercourse, and a sexual partner with vaginal colonization of uropathogens. It is recommended that young men with UTIs be evaluated simply with urinalysis and urine culture, followed by 7 days of antimicrobial therapy. All children and all men with no risk factors should be further evaluated for anatomic abnormalities. Evaluation is not usually indicated for patients with an enlarged prostate or a history of active anal intercourse.

UTIs in men can mimic acute urethritis secondary to sexually transmitted organisms and should be evaluated as such (Chapter 8.9). Men over age 50 who present with urinary symptoms must also be evaluated for prostatitis by rectal exam and urinalysis and may require a longer course of antibiotics.

Acute Pyelonephritis

Patients with acute pyelonephritis may present with all the symptoms of cystitis plus flank pain and a fever, and they may be acutely ill with nausea, vomiting, and unstable vital signs. *E coli* causes more than 80% of episodes of pyelonephritis. The presumptive diagnosis is established by microscopic examination of unspun urine, which almost always shows pyuria and usually shows bacteria. Urine cultures should always be obtained, as should two sets of blood cultures in patients who appear acutely ill with tachycardia and high fever, and require hospitalization.

If patients have only a mild systemic illness, without nausea and vomiting, they should be started on empiric oral therapy as outpatients while awaiting culture results. Moderately to severely ill patients, patients with nausea and vomiting who cannot tolerate oral antibiotics, and pregnant women should be hospitalized. Hospitalization should also be considered for patients with complicated underlying conditions such as diabetes and immunosuppression. Hospitalized patients should be begun on parenteral antibiotics; treatment should be continued for 2 weeks, although it may be switched to oral antibiotics once the patient's signs and symptoms have improved. Most patients begin to feel better within 48–72 hours of starting appropriate antibiotics. For patients who do not improve, the physician should use imaging techniques to seek possible obstruction, urologic abnormalities, and perinephric and intrarenal abscesses.

Complicated Urinary Tract Infections

Complicated UTIs are generally infections in patients with anatomically or functionally abnormal genitourinary tracts. Examples of complicated UTIs are those in pregnant women (pregnancy interferes with urinary tract function) and those in men or women with known abnormal urinary tract anatomy, neurogenic bladders, or indwelling catheters. All patients in these categories should have a microscopic urinalysis and urine culture performed whenever they develop a UTI.

Catheter-Associated Urinary Tract Infections: The most common source of gram-negative bacteriuria in hospitalized patients is indwelling catheters. Because bacteria adhere to the catheter surface and may promote the growth of biofilms that protect bacteria from antibiotics, routine therapy often fails. If a patient with a UTI has had the catheter in place for longer than 2 weeks, the physician should consider replacing it. UTIs can be prevented by sterile insertion and care of the catheter, prompt removal, and use of a closed collecting system.

Almost all patients with chronic indwelling catheters develop bacteriuria, often from colonization. The bacteriuria should be treated only if it causes symptoms or if the patient becomes toxic.

SUMMARY

▶ Urinary tract infections (UTIs) are the most common of all bacterial infections. They may be categorized by the site of infection: lower (cystitis) or upper (pyelo-nephritis). Most UTIs are caused by Enterobacteri-aceae: *Escherichia coli, Klebsiella,* or *Proteus.*

▶ The most common risk factors for UTI are sexual intercourse (for women), prostatic hypertrophy (for men), diabetes, instrumentation, chronic catheterization, and anatomic abnormalities.

▶ Pyuria is sensitive and specific in diagnosing urinary tract infection. Urine culture is not needed routinely, but should be obtained in men with infections and in women with complicated cystitis, pyelonephritis, or recurrent infections.

▶ Urethritis and vaginitis can mimic cystitis, but are distinguished by genital examination and urinalysis.

▶ Patients with pyelonephritis who do not improve after 48–72 hours of antibiotics should be evaluated for obstruction, urologic abnormalities, and perinephric and intrarenal abscesses.

SUGGESTED READING

Andriole VT (editor): Urinary tract infections. Infect Dis Clin North Am 1987;1:713.

Rubin RH: Infections of the urinary tract. In: *Scientific American Medicine.* Rubinstein E, Federman DD (editors). Scientific American, January 1992.

Stamm WE, Hooton TM: Management of urinary tract infections in adults. N Engl J Med 1993;329:1328.

Ward TT, Jones SR: Genitourinary tract infections. In: *A Practical Approach to Infectious Diseases,* 3rd ed. Reese RE, Betts RF (editors). Little, Brown, 1991.

Sexually Transmitted Diseases

Thomas C. Quinn, MD

Any physician who demands justification for learning about sexually transmitted diseases need consider only the epidemic numbers of people affected, the extraordinary diversity of presentations, and the enormous benefit of treatment. Each year, 250 million people worldwide acquire a sexually transmitted disease. Each year in the United States, 1 of 20 people contracts a new sexually transmitted disease, an incidence approaching that of a developing country. Twenty-five percent of Americans contract a sexually transmitted disease at some point in their lives. Any sexually active person—regardless of age, race, sexual preference, or marital status—is potentially at risk.

Sexually transmitted diseases have many causes (Table 8.9–1). Since the 1970s, the field of sexually transmitted diseases has evolved from emphasizing the traditional (and still prevalent) venereal diseases, gonorrhea and syphilis, to focusing on the increasingly common syndromes caused by *Chlamydia trachomatis,* herpes simplex virus, hepatitis B virus, human papillomavirus, and HIV. At least 56 million Americans—more than one in five—are believed to be infected with a sexually transmitted virus other than HIV. In addition to bacteria and viruses, sexually transmitted diseases can be caused by protozoa and ectoparasites.

Osler's claim that "he who knows syphilis knows medicine" acknowledges the diverse ways that patients with syphilis can present. The penile chancre of syphilis, the urethritis of gonorrhea, the anorexia and jaundice of hepatitis B, and the genital ulcers of herpes simplex illustrate the diversity of the early presentations of those with sexually transmitted diseases. However, the infection often goes undetected at first, becoming evident years or decades later when the patient develops chronic sequelae (Table 8.9–2). Illustrating the range and importance of late presentations are infertility from gonorrhea or *C trachomatis,* aortic regurgitation from syphilis, cervical cancer from human papillomavirus, cirrhosis from hepatitis B, and AIDS from HIV.

The total benefit of treating and preventing sexually transmitted diseases is greater than the sum of the parts. Early treatment can both prevent late complications like infertility and keep sexually transmitted diseases from interacting and potentiating each other. For example, people who have a genital ulcer from syphilis increase their risk of contracting HIV, if exposed. In fact, a person with any sexually transmitted disease increases the risk of acquiring HIV. Thus, one of the possible best ways to prevent HIV is to diagnose other sexually transmitted diseases and treat them effectively.

SCREENING AND PREVENTING SEXUALLY TRANSMITTED DISEASES

With all types of sexually transmitted disease, many patients do not know that they are infected, either because they are asymptomatic or because they have such mild symptoms that they do not seek medical care. These persons are at risk for complications and for spreading the infection to others. Therefore, every primary care provider should screen patients for unrecognized sexually transmitted diseases.

A complete sexual history should include both questions about sexual function and questions about the patient's sexual preference, numbers of sexual partners, recent changes in sexual partners, and prior sexually transmitted diseases. Physicians may at first be uncomfortable asking such questions, but few patients mind answering them. In fact, patients whose primary care provider includes a complete sexual history as part of their initial evaluation feel that their physician is better prepared to care for them than are physicians who have not taken such a history.

Sexually transmitted diseases can affect every part of the physical examination. However, as described below in the discussions of individual infections, the most common abnormalities are found in the skin (eg, genital warts, palmar macules of secondary syphilis), pharynx (eg, thrush

Acknowledgment: This chapter is adapted from a chapter by Drs. Quinn and Bradley Bender in the 22nd edition of *The Principles and Practice of Medicine.*

Table 8.9–1. Sexually transmitted infections.

Pathogen	Disease	Complications	Diagnostic Assay	Treatment
Bacteria				
Neisseria gonorrhoeae	Urethritis, cervicitis, proctitis, pharyngitis, conjunctivitis	Pelvic inflammatory disease, urethral strictures, septic arthritis, endocarditis, epididymitis, prostatitis, infertility, ectopic pregnancy, prematurity, blindness	Gram's stain; culture on selective media; DNA amplification	Quinolones or cephalosporins plus therapy for chlamydia
Treponema pallidum	Syphilis	Tabes dorsalis, Charcot joints, meningovascular syphilis, dementia, aortitis, gummas, congenital syphilis	1°: darkfield microscopy and serology (RPR/VDRL/FTA) 2°: serology 3°: serology, lumbar puncture	1°, 2°, latent: IM benzathine penicillin G 3°: IV aqueous penicillin G
Chlamydia trachomatis	Urethritis, cervicitis, proctitis, lymphogranuloma venereum	Pelvic inflammatory disease, epididymitis, infertility, ectopic pregnancy, prematurity, neonatal pneumonia	Tissue culture; antigen detection; direct fluorescent antibody; DNA amplification	Azithromycin, doxycycline, or erythromycin
Ureaplasma urealyticum	Urethritis	Prostatitis	Isolation in culture	Azithromycin, doxycycline, or erythromycin
Mycoplasma hominis	Urethritis	Pelvic inflammatory disease	Isolation in culture	Azithromycin, doxycycline, or erythromycin
Haemophilus ducreyi	Chancroid	Spontaneous rupture of fluctuant nodes	Selective media; Gram's stain	Azithromycin, or ceftriaxone, or erythromycin
Mobiluncus species, anaerobes	Bacterial vaginosis	Postpartum endometritis	Three of the following criteria: 1. homogeneous white vaginal discharge 2. clue cells on microscopic exam 3. pH of vaginal fluid >4.5 4. fishy amine odor after KOH added (whiff test)	Metronidazole (oral or gel); clindamycin cream
Fungi				
Candida albicans	Vaginitis		KOH wet prep	Azole antifungals (cream, tablet, or suppository)
Viruses				
Herpes simplex virus	Genital herpes, proctitis, pharyngitis	Recurrent attacks, disseminated disease, meningitis, neonatal herpes, autonomic dysfunction	Tissue culture; antigen detection	Acyclovir or famciclovir
Hepatitis A, B, C viruses	Hepatitis	Hepatitis, cirrhosis, hepatoma, vasculitis	Serology	Interferon? (see Chapter 7.3)
Cytomegalovirus	Infectious mononucleosis syndrome	Congenital birth defects, prematurity, pneumonia (in immunocompromised patients), inflammatory colitis	Tissue culture; serology	Ganciclovir or foscarnet
Human papillomavirus	Condyloma acuminatum	Cervical and anorectal carcinoma caused by human papillomavirus 16 or 18	Warts visible on clinical exam; DNA amplification	Cryotherapy, podofilox, podophyllin, trichloroacetic acid
Poxvirus	Molluscum contagiosum		Cytoplasmic inclusions on microscopy	Removal of caseous center
HIV	AIDS	Kaposi's sarcoma, *Pneumocystis carinii* pneumonia and other opportunistic infections	Serology; culture; DNA amplification	Antiretroviral drugs (see Chapter 8.10)
Protozoa				
Trichomonas vaginalis	Vaginitis		Saline wet prep	Metronidazole
Ectoparasites				
Sarcoptes scabiei var *hominis*	Scabies	Norwegian scabies in immuno-suppressed patients	Clinical	Lindane; permethrin
Phthirus pubis	Pubic lice		Clinical	Lindane; permethrin

RPR, rapid plasma reagin; VDRL, Venereal Disease Research Laboratory; FTA, fluorescent antibody-absorption test.
Modified and reproduced from: Centers for Disease Control and Prevention: 1993 sexually transmitted diseases treatment guidelines. Morb Mort Wkly Rep 1993:42:RR-14.

Table 8.9–2. Major sexually transmitted disease syndromes, sequelae, and pathogens.

Syndrome	Pathogen
Primary syndromes	
Urethritis	Neisseria gonorrhoeae, Chlamydia trachomatis, Ureaplasma urealyticum, Trichomonas vaginalis
Cervicitis	N gonorrhoeae, C trachomatis, herpes simplex virus, T vaginalis
Vaginitis or vaginosis	T vaginalis, Candida albicans, Mobiluncus sp, anaerobes, Gardnerella vaginalis
Genital ulcers	Treponema pallidum, herpes simplex virus, Haemophilus ducreyi (chancroid)
Genital warts	Human papillomavirus, T pallidum (secondary syphilis)
Ectoparasite infestation	Sarcoptes scabiei, Phthirius (pediculosis) pubis, Molluscum contagiosum
Proctitis	C trachomatis, N gonorrhoeae, herpes simplex virus, T pallidum
Proctocolitis	Shigella, Salmonella, Campylobacter, Entamoeba histolytica
Enteritis	Giardia lamblia
Primary, secondary, tertiary syphilis, including latent, cardiovascular, and neurosyphilis	T pallidum
Sequelae	
Pelvic inflammatory disease and sequelae (infertility and ectopic pregnancy)	C trachomatis, N gonorrhoeae, Mycoplasma hominis, anaerobes
Fitz-Hugh–Curtis syndrome	N gonorrhoeae, C trachomatis
Acute or chronic arthritis	N gonorrhoeae, C trachomatis, hepatitis B virus, enteric infections
Acute or chronic hepatitis	Hepatitis A, B, C viruses; cytomegalovirus, Epstein-Barr virus, T pallidum
Adverse outcomes of pregnancy	C trachomatis, N gonorrhoeae, T pallidum, cytomegalovirus, primary herpes simplex virus, HIV, bacterial vaginosis
Fetal and neonatal infections	C trachomatis, N gonorrhoeae, cytomegalovirus, herpes simplex virus, T pallidum, HIV
Epididymitis	N gonorrhoeae, C trachomatis
Genital tract neoplasia	Human papillomavirus 16, 18
AIDS	HIV

of HIV, erythema of gonococcal pharyngitis), genitals (eg, ulcers of herpes simplex or primary syphilis), rectum (eg, proctitis of gonorrhea), and lymph nodes (eg, inguinal adenopathy with chancroid).

Laboratory screening for HIV and syphilis is justified in asymptomatic patients with no physical findings if the patients are at high risk. At risk are men and women who have had two or more sex partners in the past year, those with anonymous partners, those who engage in anal intercourse, and those having sexual contact with other high-risk persons (homosexuals, intravenous drug users, prostitutes). Suspicious physical findings should also prompt testing. All pregnant women and all sexually active women younger than 25 years should be tested for gonorrhea and chlamydia.

Although the plague-like spread of sexually transmitted diseases might suggest otherwise, all these diseases are preventable. Therefore, physicians should not only screen for these diseases but should teach patients safe-sex practices. Physicians should not assume sexual sophistication. They should show teenagers, men, and women how to use condoms and should emphasize the proven value of latex condoms in preventing sexual transmission of infection. Doctors should explain that all barrier contraceptives, primarily condoms, diaphragms, and spermicides, reduce their risk of contracting a sexually transmitted disease. In contrast, birth control pills may actually increase the risk for gonorrhea or chlamydia, and some types of intrauterine devices increase the risk of pelvic inflammatory disease occurring in women who acquire a sexually transmitted disease.

GONORRHEA

Although the incidence has declined steadily since 1977, in 1993 more than 400,000 cases of gonorrhea were reported in the United States, making gonorrhea the most common reportable disease. The pathogen is *Neisseria gonorrhoeae,* a gram-negative diplococcus typically found within polymorphonuclear leukocytes in the discharge from body sites such as the urethra and cervix. The organism is capable of infecting or colonizing a wide range of columnar and transitional epithelial mucous membranes. These include the urethra of men and women, genital glands such as Tyson's or Cowper's in men and Bartholin's in women, uterine cervical canal and fallopian tubes, epididymis, anal canal, distal rectum, conjunctiva, and pharynx. Many infections of the endocervix, anal canal, and pharynx are asymptomatic.

Except in neonates and some young children, gonorrhea is transmitted sexually, via vaginal or anal intercourse, fellatio, or cunnilingus. *N gonorrhoeae* infection is more common and more severe in women than in men. Likewise, the complications of gonorrhea in women (pelvic inflammatory disease, perihepatitis [Fitz-Hugh–Curtis syndrome], infertility, and premature delivery) are more common and more serious than the rare epididymitis or urethral stricture that can develop in men.

Localized Infections

Men: Urethritis is the most common manifestation of gonorrhea in men. The usual incubation period is 2–5 days after sexual contact, but can be as long as 2–3 weeks.

The penile discharge begins thin and mucoid, but becomes grossly purulent. Many men complain of meatal irritation, dysuria, and frequent urination. If patients ignore their symptoms or if the infection is only partially treated, it can persist, producing few or no symptoms, and can spread to cause epididymitis, prostatitis, and, rarely, disseminated gonococcal infection.

Homosexual men who engage in receptive anal intercourse are susceptible to anorectal gonococcal infections. In 20–50% of infected men, the disease is asymptomatic. Those who have symptoms may complain only of pruritus, discomfort, tenesmus, and mucopurulent discharge. Gonococcal pharyngitis is most common in persons who perform fellatio, but can also be acquired by anilingus or cunnilingus. Symptomatic patients present nonspecifically, with a sore throat, pharyngeal erythema or exudate, and cervical adenopathy. But because most pharyngeal infections are asymptomatic, the physician must routinely do urethral, rectal, and throat cultures in high-risk persons such as homosexual men.

Women: Gonorrhea in women is manifested by urethritis with frequent urination and dysuria, and by cervicitis with a purulent cervical-vaginal discharge, dyspareunia, abnormal menstrual flow, and pelvic pain or discomfort. Up to 50% of women with cervical gonorrhea have anorectal involvement, which is usually asymptomatic. Anorectal gonorrhea is often the result of rectal-vaginal contamination and does not necessarily imply that the patient has participated in anal intercourse. However, women who engage in anal intercourse or fellatio are as susceptible to gonococcal proctitis or pharyngitis, respectively, as homosexual men who engage in these practices. Anorectal gonorrhea causes anal itching, painful defecation, mucopurulent discharge, and constipation; signs include erythema and edema of the anal crypts, anal discharge, and, rarely, rectal bleeding from ulcerative proctitis.

One of the most serious complications of cervical gonorrhea is pelvic inflammatory disease, which develops in 10–20% of infected women (see "Pelvic Inflammatory Disease" below). In prepubescent girls, the vaginal mucosa is susceptible to gonococcal invasion, leading to vulvovaginitis. Gonorrhea in prepubertal patients more than 1 year old is prima facie evidence of sexual molestation.

Disseminated Gonococcal Infection

Blood-borne dissemination of *N gonorrhoeae* is rare, probably occurring in less than 1% of all gonococcal infections. Actual rates depend on the infecting strain and host defenses. Strains that are prone to disseminate tend to be nutritionally deficient auxotypes. Compared with other strains, these are less likely to cause local symptoms; they are most resistant to the bactericidal action of normal human sera and complement, more difficult to culture, and more susceptible to antibiotics.

Disseminated infection causes fever, polyarthralgias, and a rash. The rash usually consists of less than 20 petechial, papular, hemorrhagic, or necrotic lesions on the distal extremities. Scrapings from lesions occasionally show intracellular gram-negative diplococci representing *N gonorrhoeae*. Two-thirds of patients develop tenosynovitis of the wrists, ankles, and knees, without frank arthritis. However, one-third develop a monoarthritis, and *N gonorrhoeae* is the most common cause of infectious arthritis in young adults (Chapter 3.11). Recurrent bouts of disseminated gonococcal infection have been described in patients who have defects in the terminal components of the complement cascade.

Diagnosis and Management

Despite new tests designed to detect *N gonorrhoeae* in specimens from mucous membranes, the best methods remain a Gram's stain smear and cultures that are directly inoculated onto selective media, such as Thayer-Martin, Martin-Lewis, and NYC. A Gram's stain smear of urethral exudate shows intracellular gram-negative diplococci in more than 90% of symptomatic men with gonococcal urethritis. A Gram's stain smear of cervical exudate is positive in about 40–60% of infected women. The Gram's stain is positive in only 30–50% of patients with rectal gonorrhea. Gram's stains of pharyngeal exudate are not useful because they can be confused with *Neisseria* sp normal to the pharynx. Although a negative Gram's stain does not rule out gonorrhea, a positive stain for intracellular gram-negative diplococci taken from the urethra, cervix, or rectum strongly supports gonococcal infection. Of patients with disseminated gonococcal infection, 20% have positive blood cultures; 50% of patients with swollen joints have positive synovial fluid cultures.

Regardless of the result of the Gram's stain, all patients with suspected gonorrhea should have cultures of specimens obtained from multiple sites. The sensitivity (true positive) of a single culture swab is 90–98% in symptomatic men with urethritis and 80–90% in women with cervicitis. Rectal and pharyngeal cultures are slightly less sensitive, and patients may need repeated cultures.

Because of the increasing prevalence of gonococcal strains resistant to penicillin, the currently recommended drugs are second- and third-generation cephalosporins such as ceftriaxone or cefixime, or quinolones such as ciprofloxacin or ofloxacin. Unfortunately, resistance to quinolones has been reported in some patients. Thus, all isolates should be tested for antibiotic susceptibility. Patients with complications such as epididymitis, disseminated gonococcal infection, or pelvic inflammatory disease should be hospitalized and treated with an intravenous cephalosporin. Coinfection with *C trachomatis* is so common that it should be presumed and treated empirically with doxycycline or azithromycin.

SYPHILIS

After penicillin was introduced in the late 1940s, the number of cases of primary and secondary syphilis in the United States plummeted. In the 1970s and early 1980s, syphilis was most common among sexually active homosexual men. From 1985 to 1990, the rate of infection rose dramatically to its highest level in 40 years, largely among minority group heterosexuals in large metropolitan areas. Some of the outbreaks were linked to the exchange of sex for drugs, particularly crack cocaine. Interest in syphilis has also been renewed by the recognition of how syphilis and HIV can interact. Having HIV predisposes a person to developing more severe forms of syphilis, whereas having a genital ulcer from syphilis increases the risk of acquiring HIV. Thus, controlling syphilis may help to reduce transmission of HIV.

Acquired Syphilis

Treponema pallidum, the spirochete that causes syphilis, is transmitted by intimate sexual contact with penetration of the mucous membranes and seemingly unbroken skin through minute abrasions. The disease passes through a number of stages (Table 8.9–3).

Primary Stage: After sexual contact with an infected partner, the organism penetrates the skin, replicates at the site of primary inoculation, and spreads systemically. The typical chancre appears 21 days after exposure (range 10–90 days) as a painless papule that evolves into a painless ulcer 2–20 mm in diameter, with an indurated edge. The lesion usually appears on the penis, labia, or cervix, but can be at any site of inoculation. Genital lesions may be accompanied by firm, nontender inguinal adenopathy. The chancre heals within 2–6 weeks, leaving no scar. The primary stage may go unrecognized.

Secondary Stage: In 25% of patients, the primary stage overlaps with the secondary stage, which begins 6 weeks to 6 months after exposure and lasts for 1–3 months. The characteristic finding at this stage is a maculopapular rash with symmetric red lesions. The rash can involve any part of the body, but lesions on the palms (Figure 8.9–1) and soles strongly suggest secondary syphilis. The secondary stage is systemic; many patients complain of weight loss, fever, and malaise. Some patients have a generalized nontender lymphadenopathy, and some have a patchy alopecia at the same time as the rash. Condyloma lata—flat, wart-like lesions—may be found in intertriginous areas and

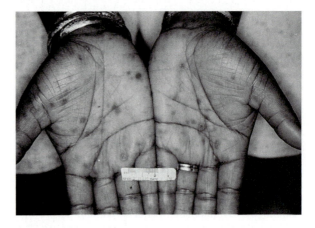

Figure 8.9–1. Palmar rash of secondary syphilis. Lesions do not respect crease lines. (Courtesy of Jonathan M. Zenilman, MD, and Anne M. Rompalo, MD.)

around the anal canal. These must be differentiated from condyloma acuminata, which are fleshy genital warts (see "Human Papillomavirus" below). Mucous patches, found in about one-third of patients, are superficial gray erosions of the mucous membranes. All skin lesions are infectious, particularly condyloma lata and mucous patches.

About 15–30% of patients with secondary-stage syphilis have abnormal cerebrospinal fluid with increased protein or cells; however, clinical meningitis is rare. Hepatitis, immune complex nephropathy, arthritis, periostitis, uveitis, and proctitis are seen, although not often. One of these conditions may be a patient's only manifestation of secondary syphilis.

Latent Stage: After the secondary stage, patients enter a clinically silent (latent) stage, which is divided into early (<1 year) and late (>1 year) latent syphilis. Patients can have relapses of secondary syphilis during this time. Most relapses occur during the first year and are typically milder than during the secondary stage.

Table 8.9–3. Syphilis in untreated patients.

Stage	Typical Findings	Average Onset After Exposure	Course	Serology (% Reactive)	
				VDRL	FTA-ABS
Primary	Chancre	21 days (range 10–90)	2–12 wk	72	91
Secondary	Rash, condyloma lata, mucous patches, fever, lymphadenopathy, patchy alopecia	6 wk–6 mo	1–3 mo	100	100
Early latent	Relapses of secondary syphilis	<1 yr	≤1 yr	73	97
Late latent	None	>1 yr	Lifelong unless tertiary syphilis appears	73	97
Tertiary	Neurosyphilis, cardiovascular syphilis, gummas	1 yr until death	Until death	77	99

VDRL, Venereal Disease Research Laboratory test; FTA-ABS, fluorescent treponemal antibody-absorption test.

Tertiary Stage: Before antibiotics, about 30% of patients developed tertiary syphilis. The wide availability of penicillin has made this stage rare today. The three forms of tertiary disease are cardiovascular syphilis, neurosyphilis, and benign gummas.

Cardiovascular syphilis is rare, but most likely to be seen in men and blacks. Endarteritis obliterans destroys the elastic tissues; this causes aneurysmal dilatation of the ascending aorta, leading to heart failure and coronary ostial obstruction. Aortitis may affect up to 30–50% of patients with untreated syphilis.

Neurosyphilis affects 4–6% of untreated patients. Some patients have asymptomatic neurosyphilis, whose only manifestations are a reactive blood serology and abnormal cerebrospinal fluid. Meningovascular syphilis is the acute onset of delirium, seizures, headache, and focal neurologic deficits. Tabes dorsalis causes signs of posterior spinal column involvement, with ataxia, areflexia, sensory deficits, "lightning pains" in the extremities, impotence, and urine retention or incontinence. The sensory deficits can lead to trophic joint changes (Charcot joints). General paresis presents as dementia, with the insidious onset of personality changes, irritability, insomnia, poor judgment, and declining mental capacity. The Argyll-Robertson pupil seen in both general paresis and tabes dorsalis is a small, irregular pupil that can accommodate but fails to react to light.

Gummas are late syphilitic lesions that, microscopically, are nonspecific granulomas. Essentially any organ can be involved, but most often affected are the skin, bones, cartilage, liver, oral cavity, and upper respiratory tract.

Syphilis in Pregnant Women: Women who acquire syphilis while pregnant or who become pregnant during the first year of the disease have an 80–90% chance of transmitting the infection to the fetus. The risk is lower but still exists during late latent syphilis. All pregnant women should be given serologic screening for syphilis. Treatment before the 19th week prevents congenital infection. Later treatment can prevent further disease progression.

Congenital Syphilis

Congenital syphilis results from transplacental spread of *T pallidum* from mother to fetus. Transmission is rare before the fourth month of gestation, and early abortion is not seen. Untreated maternal infection may lead to prematurity, stillbirth, neonatal death, and early or late congenital syphilis. Treating the mother during the first 4 months of pregnancy virtually eliminates the risk of congenital syphilis.

Early congenital syphilis begins during the first 2 years of life and may be manifested by nasal discharge (snuffles) followed by mucocutaneous lesions; unlike adults, rash in babies may be vesicular or even bullous. Many babies develop pseudoparalysis from painful osteochondritis. Also common are hepatosplenomegaly, lymphadenopathy, anemia, thrombocytopenia, and leukocytosis.

Late congenital syphilis is defined as features that appear after 2 years of age. This stage is analogous to tertiary syphilis in adults, except that cardiovascular disease is rare. Periostitis and osteochondritis lead to frontal bossing, anterior bowing of the tibia (saber shin), and deafness from cochlear degeneration. Characteristic dental abnormalities are Hutchinson's teeth (widely space, tapered incisors with a central notch) and mulberry molars (6-year molars with multiple small cusps). Interstitial keratitis presents with photophobia, pain, tearing, and blurred vision. Hutchinson's triad is interstitial keratitis, neural deafness, and the typical dentition. Up to one-third of infected children have asymptomatic neurosyphilis; the symptomatic forms, such as general paresis, tabes dorsalis, and localized gummas, usually appear during adolescence.

Diagnosis and Management

Syphilis cannot be cultured. Diagnosis is usually based on two types of serologic tests. (1) Patients are screened by the Venereal Disease Research Laboratory (VDRL) or rapid plasma reagin (RPR) test; both tests measure antibodies to reaginic, nontreponemal antigen. (2) The diagnosis is confirmed by the fluorescent treponemal antibody-absorption test (FTA), which detects antibody to *T pallidum.* The tests have different sensitivities for each stage of syphilis (see Table 8.9–3). The VDRL or RPR can be false-positive in patients with autoimmune disease, especially systemic lupus erythematosus (SLE), as well as patients with chronic viral infections, drug addicts, and the elderly. Most patients with false-positive results have a low titer (<1:8) and a negative FTA. False-positive FTAs are rare and are seen chiefly in patients with SLE. False-positive FTAs can be identified by a beaded immunofluorescence pattern. Once patients have a positive FTA, they may remain positive for life.

Darkfield examination to visualize spirochetes can be done on a chancre or the lesions of secondary or congenital syphilis. The serous fluid from the lesion is placed on a slide, covered, and examined under a microscope outfitted with a darkfield condenser. Spirochetes seen in the fluid are pathognomonic for syphilis. The test cannot be done on oral or rectal lesions because the large number of normal commensal spirochetes might cause a false-positive.

Penicillin is the treatment of choice for all stages of syphilis. Patients who have had syphilis for less than 1 year need only one large intramuscular dose of benzathine penicillin G. Those who have had syphilis for over 1 year but do not have neurosyphilis should receive the same large dose once a week for 3 consecutive weeks. Patients who are allergic to penicillin should be given oral tetracycline in an intensive 15-day regimen for early infections and 30 days for late infections.

Neurosyphilis is harder to treat because benzathine penicillin does not reliably provide treponemicidal levels of penicillin in the cerebrospinal fluid. Therefore, it is recommended that patients be admitted to the hospital and treated with intravenous aqueous crystalline penicillin G for 10 days. An infectious disease specialist should be consulted for patients who have penicillin allergy and neurosyphilis.

After treatment for syphilis, many patients develop shaking chills, fever, myalgias, headache, tachycardia, and exacerbation of local inflammatory reactions at involved sites (Jarisch-Herxheimer reaction). This reaction affects 50% of patients with primary syphilis, 75% with secondary syphilis, and 30% with neurosyphilis. The pathogenesis is not known, but the reaction is treated with antihistamines.

Follow-up of patients with syphilis is especially important. VDRL titers are recommended at 1, 3, 6, and 12 months. The titer should revert to negative or should decrease by fourfold dilutions and remain low. If this does not happen, the patient should be retreated. Penicillin-resistant treponemes have not been described.

CHLAMYDIA TRACHOMATIS

Chlamydia trachomatis, a gram-negative, obligate intracellular bacterium, is the most common sexually transmitted bacterium in developed countries. The incidence in the United States is 4 million infections per year, 10 times the rate of gonorrhea. The clinical manifestations of chlamydia are similar to those of gonorrhea, but usually milder, and asymptomatic infections are much more common. The two organisms also have similar epidemiologic patterns, with the highest prevalence in poor teenagers; many people harbor both infections at once.

Chlamydial Infections in Men

C trachomatis is found in up to 35–50% of patients with nongonococcal urethritis. This condition usually affects young, sexually active men. After a 1- to 3-week incubation, many patients develop a mucopurulent discharge, dysuria, and pruritus. Although the discharge is less purulent in gonococcal urethritis, the two syndromes can be difficult to differentiate on clinical grounds. Postgonococcal urethritis, a persistent urethral discharge in men who have been treated successfully for gonorrhea, most often results from concomitant chlamydial infection. The usual antibiotics given to treat gonorrhea are inactive against chlamydia.

Complications of chlamydial urethritis are epididymitis and Reiter's syndrome. About one-third of epididymitis cases in young, sexually active men are caused by gonococcal infection; most of the rest are caused by *C trachomatis.* Reiter's syndrome (Chapter 3.7) is characterized by urethritis, conjunctivitis, arthritis, and a rash. About 40–70% of men with acute Reiter's syndrome have *C trachomatis* isolated from the urethra, but it is not known whether chlamydia causes Reiter's syndrome or is merely associated with the urethritis.

Homosexual men can develop an inflammatory proctitis from chlamydial infection. Like gonococcal proctitis, most chlamydial proctitis is asymptomatic or mild, with major complaints being anorectal discharge, constipation, tenesmus, and pruritus; many patients have a red rectal mucosa and mucopurulent discharge. However, infection with the LGV serovars of *C trachomatis* (see "Lymphogranuloma Venereum" below) may induce a more severe ulcerative proctitis, which clinically and histopathologically resembles granulomatous colitis or Crohn's disease.

Chlamydial Infections in Women

The most common manifestation of *C trachomatis* infection in women is cervicitis. The cervicitis may be mild or asymptomatic. Patients may complain of a vaginal discharge. The cervix is red and friable, with a mucopurulent discharge from the os. As with urethritis in men, many women have concurrent infections with *C trachomatis* and *N gonorrhoeae.* After treatment for gonorrhea, persistent symptoms of mucopurulent endocervicitis are the female counterpart of postgonococcal urethritis in men.

The most important complication of chlamydial infection in women is acute salpingitis. *C trachomatis* is a leading cause of acute salpingitis. This complication is clinically milder than when it results from gonococcal or anaerobic bacterial infection, but the risk of infertility may be higher. In addition, *C trachomatis* is probably the most common cause of the acute urethral syndrome, characterized by dysuria and pyuria, with urine cultures showing bacterial counts less than 100,000/mL. Babies born to women with cervical *C trachomatis* can acquire the infection and develop conjunctivitis or pneumonia.

Lymphogranuloma Venereum

The *C trachomatis* serovars L1, L2, and L3 cause lymphogranuloma venereum, which is a systemic sexually transmitted infection. After a 1- to 3-week incubation, a small painless papule appears at the site of inoculation, healing spontaneously within a few days. But several weeks later, patients, especially men, develop a prominent inguinal lymphadenopathy. In two-thirds of patients, the adenopathy is unilateral, and in one-third, bilateral. In 20% of patients, enlargement of nodes above and below the inguinal ligament causes the "groove sign." Over the next month, the nodes enlarge and become fluctuant (filled with pus); they are often called *buboes.* If treatment is delayed, the overlying skin becomes inflamed and draining fistulas may appear. Many patients have systemic symptoms of fever, myalgias, and malaise. Neglected patients may develop late complications such as anorectal strictures or rectovaginal fistulas.

Diagnosis and Management

Chlamydial infections are difficult to diagnose for several reasons. First, they are usually mild or asymptomatic. Second, many patients have coincident infections with gonorrhea, which may lead the physician to overlook the possibility of chlamydial coinfection. Third, *C trachomatis* is an obligate intracellular parasite that must be cultivated in tissue culture facilities that are not available to all physicians. Diagnosis has been made easier as new techniques have become available using antibodies to identify *C trachomatis* antigens, or polymerase chain reactions (PCR) (Chapter 10.2) to identify *C trachomatis* DNA.

The key to diagnosis remains clinical suspicion. Men with urethritis and a Gram's stain showing polymorphonuclear leukocytes without intracellular diplococci should be treated empirically for nongonococcal urethritis, with doxycycline or azithromycin. Women with cervicitis or salpingitis and negative Gram's stain and culture for *N gonorrhoeae* should be presumed to have *C trachomatis* infection. Cultures should be done to confirm the pathogen, but treatment should not await the results.

Doxycycline or azithromycin is recommended for treating chlamydial infections. Doxycycline is given orally for 7 days; azithromycin is more expensive but is given in one oral dose. Patients do not need to be retested for *C trachomatis* after completing treatment with either drug, unless symptoms persist or reinfection is suspected. Pregnant women should not take doxycycline; they should be treated with azithromycin or erythromycin. As with other sexually transmitted infections, treatment of sex partners helps to prevent reinfection of the patient.

HERPES SIMPLEX VIRUS

Herpes simplex virus (herpesvirus hominis) is a DNA-containing virus and a member of the herpesvirus group, which also includes varicella zoster, cytomegalovirus, and Epstein-Barr virus. There are two types of herpesviruses: type I (HSV-I), which causes 90% of oral labial herpes (fever blisters and pharyngitis), and type II (HSV-II), which causes 90% of genital herpetic ulcers in the United States. About 500,000 Americans develop new genital herpes each year, and 30% of adult Americans have evidence of previous HSV-II infection. The most distinguishing and clinically significant feature of herpes simplex is its ability to establish a latent infection within sensory nerve ganglia of the spinal cord. Reactivation of the latent infection causes recurrences of viral lesions in the area of the original infection.

Genital Herpes

Initial Episode: Genital herpes is transmitted through direct contact with an infected individual. The person transmitting the infection need not have symptoms or ulcers: About 1–2% of infected persons shed virus when they are symptom-free and have no lesions. Asymptomatic shedding is now believed to account for most herpes transmission. After an incubation period of 2–7 days, the newly infected person develops systemic symptoms such as fever, malaise, headaches, and myalgias, all of which ease over the next week. The local lesions begin as multiple painful vesicles, ulcerate after 3–4 days, then crust and re-epithelialize over the next week (see Color Plates). In severe cases, new vesicles also form during this time. Typically, herpes simplex can be isolated from the lesions until they have re-epithelialized. The lesions are most commonly seen on the gland and shaft of the penis in men, and the labia, vagina, and cervix in women. Most patients with

newly acquired genital herpes simplex infection have tender, nonfluctuant inguinal lymphadenopathy. People who participate in receptive anal intercourse can develop herpes proctitis, which causes fever, severe anorectal pain, constipation, difficulty starting to urinate, sacral dermatome paresthesias, tenesmus, and perianal ulcers.

Reactivation: The causes of herpes simplex reactivation are unknown, but psychological stress and menstruation are risk factors. Recurrent infections are generally milder than primary infections. About 50% of patients have a prodrome of numbness or a burning or tingling sensation in the area where new vesicles will form, but fewer than 10% have systemic symptoms. After the prodrome has lasted a few hours to several days, patients develop 4–6 small, painful, pruritic vesicles. These ulcerate and form either multiple small ulcers or 1–2 large ones. Recurrent lesions last about 10 days. Recurrences are much more common in patients whose primary genital herpes infection is with HSV-II than in those with HSV-I.

Complications

The most important complication of genital herpes is transmission of the infection from mother to baby during delivery. The baby acquires the virus by direct contact with herpetic lesions while passing through the cervix and vagina. Untreated neonatal herpes is often fatal or causes significant neurologic sequelae. Cesarean section delivery largely eliminates this risk and has become mandatory for women who come to term with active lesions or are known to be shedding virus.

Other complications of genital herpes are more common in women than men and occur mostly with primary infections. About 20–30% of patients develop aseptic meningitis. Some have autonomic nervous system disorders (urinary retention, impotence, decreased rectal sphincter tone), sacral paresthesias, and myelitis. If patients touch a lesion and then touch their eye or another mucous membrane, they can spread the infection, giving themselves typical herpetic ulcers or herpes keratitis. Local herpetic lesions can develop in small breaks in the skin. When the terminal phalanx is involved, the condition is called *herpetic whitlow*. In immunosuppressed patients, herpes simplex infection can disseminate and involve many organ systems; the mortality is high.

Diagnosis and Management

The diagnosis of genital herpes is suggested by the clinical presentation and confirmed by smear or culture. Either a Tzanck smear of a labial lesion or a Papanicolaou (Pap) smear of a cervical lesion can show the multinucleated giant cells that are diagnostic. Patients with primary herpes simplex infections have at least a fourfold increase in complement-fixing serum antibodies; in recurrent infections, serology is often nonspecific and nondiagnostic.

Acyclovir has been the drug of choice for treatment of herpes. A newer antiherpes drug, famciclovir, appears from limited trials to be equally effective. Oral acyclovir for primary herpes simplex lesions decreases viral shedding, formation of new lesions, and pruritus. However, a 10-day course of acyclovir given for symptomatic herpes cannot reduce the number or severity of recurrences. Patients with complications severe enough to require hospitalization should be given intravenous acyclovir.

The only patients who should be treated for recurrences of genital herpes are those who typically have severe symptoms and who are able to begin therapy during the prodrome or within 2 days of the onset of lesions. Acyclovir may shorten the clinical course by about 1 day. For persons who have six or more recurrences per year, daily treatment with acyclovir reduces the frequency of attacks by 75% or more. After patients stop acyclovir, their attacks may come as often as they did before treatment. The suppressive regimen is contraindicated in pregnant women.

Counseling is especially important in the management of herpes. Many patients feel extremely guilty about the disease and, despite the proliferation of public information about herpes, continue to be ill-informed. The physician should emphasize to patients the high infectivity of active lesions and the low transmission rate during remissions, as well as the marked variability of the course within patients and its relation to stress. Because genital herpes increases the risk for carcinoma of the cervix, women should be advised to get yearly Pap tests.

PELVIC INFLAMMATORY DISEASE

Pelvic inflammatory disease is the syndrome caused by ascending spread of microorganisms from the vagina and cervix to the endometrium, fallopian tubes, and contiguous structures. Pelvic inflammatory disease is one of the most serious complications of sexually transmitted diseases in women and is probably the most common serious infection in women of child-bearing age. This disease is the major preventable cause of female infertility and ectopic pregnancy in the United States and worldwide. Other complications of pelvic inflammatory disease are abscesses of the salpinx or ovary, rupture of the abscess, and, rarely, death. Chronic complications, although less severe, are more common. The risk of infertility is about 20% after one episode of pelvic inflammatory disease, 35% after two, and 75% after three or more. Chronic abdominal pain with dyspareunia can be particularly distressing. Women who have had pelvic inflammatory disease have a seven- to tenfold higher-than-normal rate of ectopic pregnancies.

Acute pelvic inflammatory disease is almost exclusively an infection of sexually active women. About 75% of patients with pelvic inflammatory disease are under 25 years old, and 75% are nulliparous. Reasons for young women's susceptibility include more sexual partners, high frequency of anovulatory cycles (probably because of hormonal influences), lower prevalence of immunity to sexually transmitted pathogens, and possibly a delay in getting medical care. Other risk factors include a history of gonorrhea or salpingitis and use of an intrauterine contraceptive device.

The etiology of pelvic inflammatory disease is complex and polymicrobial. Two major groups of organisms are thought to be responsible. An exogenous sexually transmitted pathogen (*N gonorrhoeae, C trachomatis,* or *Mycoplasma*) starts the process, followed by overgrowth of endogenous microorganisms, which are primarily facultative or strictly anaerobic.

Pelvic inflammatory disease is often classified as being of gonococcal or nongonococcal origin; gonococcal disease is defined by the recovery of *N gonorrhoeae* from cervical culture. In addition to the cervix, many physicians use culdocentesis to sample the peritoneum. The peritoneum shows one of three patterns of infection: *N gonorrhoeae* alone, *N gonorrhoeae* with mixed aerobic and anaerobic bacteria, or mixed aerobic and anaerobic bacteria without the gonococcus. The aerobic organisms include gram-negative bacilli, streptococci, staphylococci, and *Haemophilus* sp. The anaerobic organisms include *Bacteroides fragilis,* other *Bacteroides* sp, *Clostridium* sp, peptococci, and peptostreptococci. *Mycoplasma hominis* has been isolated, but its role in pelvic inflammatory disease remains uncertain.

All the above-mentioned aerobes and anaerobes are also found in nongonococcal pelvic inflammatory disease, along with *C trachomatis. C trachomatis,* either alone or in conjunction with mixed aerobes and anaerobes, is responsible for more cases than is gonorrhea. The role of other organisms, such as those seen in bacterial vaginosis, is controversial.

Gonococcal pelvic inflammatory disease begins with cervical infection. Susceptible women have intracanalicular spread of the organism to the uterine cavity and fallopian tubes, provoking an inflammatory response that leads to either endometritis or salpingitis. Other organisms are thought to invade secondarily. When *C trachomatis* is isolated, it has probably followed the same path as the gonococcus. Because chlamydia produces a less intense inflammatory response and milder clinical manifestations, it is sometimes called "silent pelvic inflammatory disease." However, chlamydia can induce scarring in the fallopian tube, which, over several months, may lead to anaerobic abscesses. When peritoneal exudate from a salpingitis spreads to the right upper quadrant, the patient may develop perihepatitis.

Diagnosis and Management

Pelvic inflammatory disease has a different presentation in different women. Patients with acute disease typically report abdominal pain or discomfort for up to 2 weeks. The symptoms of gonococcal pelvic inflammatory disease may begin soon after menses; those of nongonococcal disease can appear at any time during the cycle. Patients report varying degrees of dysuria, vaginal discharge, abnormal vaginal bleeding, dyspareunia, pain on defecation, nausea, vomiting, fever, and chills. Women with perihepatitis may also complain of right upper quadrant pain, radiating to the right shoulder. Lower abdominal tenderness may be mild to severe; many patients have rebound tenderness. In most women with either gonococcal or chlamydial disease, vaginal speculum examination reveals a mucopurulent cervicitis. On rectovaginal exam, patients may have tenderness on cervical motion and on palpation of the adnexal area. The differential diagnosis should include acute appendicitis, ectopic pregnancy, endometriosis, ovarian cyst or tumor, and urinary tract disease. Sonography, laparoscopy, and culdocentesis are often used to confirm pelvic inflammatory disease and rule out other conditions.

Empiric treatment should be started in women who have, at the least, tenderness in the lower abdomen and adnexa as well as on cervical motion, all with no established cause. Women with severe signs should have a more elaborate evaluation because incorrect diagnosis and management may cause unnecessary morbidity. Treatment should include empiric broad-spectrum coverage for likely pathogens, including *N gonorrhoeae, C trachomatis,* gram-negative facultative bacteria, anaerobes, and streptococci. No single regimen has been established. One possible regimen is a second- or third-generation cephalosporin such as cefoxitin or cefotetan, plus doxycycline; another is a combination of clindamycin and gentamicin.

CHANCROID

Chancroid is a disease of one or more genital ulcers caused by *Haemophilus ducreyi,* a facultative anaerobic gram-negative coccobacillus. Chancroid is endemic in tropical and subtropical countries, and in recent years has become more common in the United States, particularly in cities. After an incubation period of 2–14 days (median 7 days), a small, painful papule appears at the site of inoculation and ulcerates in 1–2 days. Lack of circumcision is an established risk factor in men. Women have more numerous ulcers, which cluster around the cervix and are generally less painful than men's lesions. Many men and women have unilateral, tender, fluctuant inguinal lymphadenopathy. The differential diagnosis includes herpes, primary syphilis, granuloma inguinale, and lymphogranuloma venereum.

The diagnosis of chancroid is made by culturing the edge of the ulcer or a lymph node aspirate on supplemented chocolate agar. Treatment is with azithromycin, ceftriaxone, or erythromycin. The susceptibility of *H ducreyi* to these drugs varies widely and influences drug choice. Fluctuant nodes should be aspirated as needed, to minimize the risk of spontaneous rupture.

HUMAN PAPILLOMAVIRUS

Office visits for anogenital warts (condyloma acuminata) have increased more than ninefold since the 1960s. Anogenital warts are caused by human papillomaviruses, which are double-stranded DNA viruses transmitted through sexual intercourse. After an incubation period of 1–2 months, the disease appears as pink or brown cauliflower-like lesions on the glans penis, vulva, urethra, cervix, perineum, or anorectal region. The lesions may be mildly pruritic, but mainly are cosmetically unappealing. These warts must be differentiated from the highly infectious condyloma lata of secondary syphilis. Most flat genital warts are condyloma lata; condyloma acuminata are raised. The distinction can also be made by darkfield microscopy for spirochetes.

Treatment of papillomavirus is primarily for cosmetic purposes, and, depending on the site, consists of topical podophyllin, cryosurgery, electrocauterization, or surgery. Because cervical warts (particularly those caused by human papillomavirus 16 or 18) increase the risk for cervical neoplasms, affected women should get routine Pap smears.

ECTOPARASITES

Ectoparasites are parasites that live on the integument of their hosts. The two most common ectoparasites are *Phthirus pubis* (pubic or crab louse), which causes pediculosis pubis, and *Sarcoptes scabiei* var *hominis* (scab mite), which causes scabies. These infections are transmitted by prolonged personal contact, including sexual intercourse.

The primary symptom of pediculosis is itching, primarily in the genital area, although any hairy part of the body can be involved. A close look at affected areas shows nits (eggs) attached to the hair shaft 0.5–1 inch from its base. The yellow-gray pinhead-sized lice can be seen on the skin. Many patients have reddish papules caused by local irritation. The diagnosis can be made clinically or by examining hair combings under the low-power microscope.

Like pediculosis, scabies causes pruritus, which is typically worst at night. The lesions are pathognomonic—wavy, thready, usually symmetric burrows 1–10 mm long, made by the female mite. The most common sites are the interdigital web spaces of the hand, the flexor aspect of the wrist and elbow, the belt line, the penis and scrotum in men, and around the nipples in women. Immunodeficient patients can be infested with thousands of mites, a condition called Norwegian scabies.

The epidemiology of ectoparasite conditions differs from that of most sexually transmitted diseases, with a higher prevalence in heterosexuals than homosexuals. Simply sleeping with an infected person all night is more hazardous than a brief sexual contact. Topical lindane is the treatment of choice for both pediculosis and scabies. A single application is usually effective for scabies; many patients with pediculosis need a second application 1 week later. Overuse may cause neurotoxicity (seizures), especially in children. All members of a household should be treated at the same time, and on the day of treatment all their bed linens and clothing should be laundered. The pruritus of scabies may continue for several weeks after treatment because of persistent antigens in the skin.

GRANULOMA INGUINALE

Granuloma inguinale (donovanosis) is a sexually transmitted disease caused by *Calymmatobacterium granulomatis,* an encapsulated, short, gram-negative bacillus. Like chancroid, this disease is much more common in tropical and subtropical countries. The incubation period is 2–4 weeks. The infection begins as a painless, indurated papule, but after 1–4 weeks it becomes a beefy, granulomatous ulcer with raised borders. Few patients have lymphadenopathy, but the surrounding induration can extend into the inguinal region, causing a pseudobubo. The lesion resembles squamous cell carcinoma, which may also complicate longstanding cases. Thus, biopsy is essential when the diagnosis is uncertain.

Diagnosis of granuloma inguinale is made by Wright's or Giemsa stain of a scraping of the ulcer bed or biopsied tissue. Blue-black bipolar-staining bacilli (Donovan bodies) in the cytoplasm of large mononuclear cells is pathognomonic. Contrary to the disease's name, the lesions do not contain granulomas.

Treatment is with tetracycline, which should be continued until the lesions have healed completely.

MOLLUSCUM CONTAGIOSUM

Molluscum contagiosum is a benign epidermal neoplasm caused by a poxvirus. This DNA virus is difficult to grow in tissue culture, and the disease has a long incubation period of up to 6 months. The lesion begins as a flesh-colored 2- to 5-mm papule, which then becomes umbilicated; a cheesy material can be expressed from the center. Many patients have multiple lesions. Diagnosis is made by the lesion's appearance and can be confirmed by biopsy or by examining the expressed caseous material, which should show molluscum bodies—basophilic cytoplasmic inclusions filled with the virion.

The physician treats the lesions by nicking the center with a scalpel or needle, then pressing on the lesion to force out the caseous center. Many lesions resolve without any treatment. Resistant lesions can be treated by podophyllin 20% compound or by cryotherapy with liquid nitrogen.

GENITAL ULCERS

The cause of genital ulcers differs in different parts of the world. In the United States and other industrialized countries, 40–65% of patients with ulcers have genital herpes, 15–20% have syphilis, 1–2% have chancroid, and the rest have nonvenereal lesions. Trauma, either direct or secondary to excoriation, is the most common cause of nonvenereal genital ulcers.

Despite the characteristic picture in some patients (Table 8.9–4), the clinical diagnosis should always be confirmed by the laboratory. Some patients have two or more simultaneous pathogens. Since most test results are not immediately available, empiric therapy with benzathine penicillin is recommended for patients with lesions typical of syphilis (1–2 painless ulcers that begin as papules and then develop firm, indurated bases), and ceftriaxone for patients with suspected chancroid (typically, painful ulcers with undermined edges and necrotic bases).

Genital ulcer diseases have become an increasing focus of research and public health concern because, even more than other sexually transmitted diseases, they appear to facilitate transmission of HIV. HIV has a complex interrelationship (epidemiologic synergy) with some sexually transmitted diseases. Risk of HIV transmission increases about three- to fivefold in patients with genital ulcer diseases, as well as in some patients with nonulcerative diseases such as chlamydia, gonorrhea, and trichomoniasis. In turn, HIV infection may prolong or augment the infectivity of several of these diseases by altering their clinical presentation, natural history, or response to standard tests and therapy. Sexually transmitted diseases may facilitate HIV transmission directly by disrupting epithelial barriers in the genital tract. Genital ulcer diseases break the mu-

Table 8.9–4. Clues in the differential diagnosis of genital ulcer caused by an infectious disease.

	Herpes	Syphilis	Chancroid	Lymphogranuloma Venereum	Granuloma Inguinale
History	Recurrences	Homosexual and bisexual men	Overseas contact	Overseas contact, or homosexual or bisexual men	Overseas contact
Systemic symptoms	In primary herpes	In secondary syphilis	No	Gastrointestinal symptoms in some patients	No
Number of ulcers	Many	1–2	1–3	1	1
Vesicles	Some patients	Few patients	Few patients	Few patients	Few patients
Pain	Most patients	Few patients	Most patients	Some patients	Few patients
Induration	Few patients	Most patients	Few patients	Few patients	Most patients
Adenopathy	Tender	Firm, nontender	Tender, may suppurate	Tender; groove sign	Pseudobubo

Table 8.9–5. Diagnosis and management of vaginitis.

Cause	Symptoms	Discharge			Diagnosis	Therapy
		Odor	Color	Consistency		
Candida sp	Pruritus, irritation	None	White	Thick, curd-like, scant	Fungal elements on 10% KOH preparation	Intravaginal miconazole or clotrimazole
Trichomonas vaginalis	Profuse discharge, pruritus	Foul	Yellow, green	Frothy, profuse	Motile trichomonads on wet mount	Metronidazole
Bacterial vaginosis	Vaginal odor, thin discharge	Fishy odor on 10% KOH preparation	Clear, white	Thin, homogeneous	Clue cells on wet mount, vaginal pH >4.5	Metronidazole

cosal lining of the genital tract, thereby possibly increasing both susceptibility to HIV and infectiousness of HIV. HIV has been isolated directly from genital ulcers in both men and women. Thus, HIV should be considered in any patient who has any other sexually transmitted disease, and vice versa.

VAGINAL DISCHARGE

Many women with symptomatic sexually acquired infections present with abnormal vaginal discharges, which can also manifest as abnormal vaginal odor and dysuria (Table 8.9–5). Abnormal vaginal discharge may result from vaginal infections, cervical infections, local reactions to chemical irritants, and retained foreign bodies (eg, tampons, condoms). Gonorrhea and chlamydia rarely cause vaginal discharge.

A crucial first diagnostic step is differentiating vaginal from cervical discharges, during the speculum exam. Cervicovaginal secretions pooled on the posterior blade of the speculum are the wrong specimens to use in evaluating vaginal discharge. Vaginal discharge specimens should be collected from the lateral vaginal walls. The three main causes of infectious vaginitis—*Candida, Trichomonas,* and bacterial vaginosis—are distinguished chiefly by the gross characteristics of the discharge and by microscopic examination (see Table 8.9–5). Women with clinically diagnosed cervicitis should be treated for chlamydia or gonorrhea if the local prevalence is high.

EPIDIDYMITIS

The epididymis, a thin tubular structure adjacent to the posterior surface of the testis, stores sperm until ejaculation. Patients with epididymitis present with either a sudden or a gradual onset of local pain. The scrotum on the involved side is usually red and swollen. Gentle palpation generally reveals that the swelling is limited to the cord.

Most epididymitis in sexually active men younger than 35 years is caused by a sexually transmitted disease, either gonorrhea or chlamydia. Most patients also have a sponta-

neous or expressible urethral discharge. Treatment is guided by Gram's stain of the discharge. Patients with gram-negative intracellular diplococci should be treated for gonorrhea, followed by 10 days of oral doxycycline. Patients who do not have diplococci should be treated for *C trachomatis.*

Most epididymitis in men older than 35 years is caused by a uropathogen. The age difference in etiology seems to be explained by both a lower incidence of sexually transmitted diseases in older men and a higher incidence of acquired genitourinary tract abnormalities such as prostatic hypertrophy and stones. Many older patients have other symptoms of a urinary tract infection; many have concurrent prostatitis. Treatment is guided by the results of midstream urine culture.

Tuberculosis was once a common cause of epididymitis worldwide, and still is in many places, although not in the United States. Most patients have concurrent involvement of the kidney, prostate, or seminal vesicles.

Two important diseases that can be confused with epididymitis are torsion of the testicle and testicular carcinoma. Torsion of the testicle is most common in adolescents. Patients have pain and swelling that involves the testis more than the epididymis. The testes may be high in the scrotum. Few patients have pyuria or a urethral discharge. Surgical exploration is often indicated.

The incidence of testicular carcinoma peaks during the 20s, the same age as the peak for epididymitis. Even though most tumors are painless, pain does not rule out carcinoma. When the diagnosis is difficult or patients do not respond promptly to antimicrobial drugs, urologic consultation is warranted.

SUMMARY

▶ Twenty-five percent of Americans contract a sexually transmitted disease at some point in their life. Any sexually active person, regardless of age, race, sexual preference, or marital status, is potentially at risk.

▶ Sexually transmitted diseases can be prevented by teaching patients to use safe-sex practices.

▶ Early diagnosis and treatment, particularly for bacterial sexually transmitted diseases, can prevent most late complications. Treatment of viral sexually transmitted diseases is usually palliative rather than curative.

▶ Late complications of sexually transmitted diseases can include pelvic inflammatory disease, infertility, cervical and anorectal cancer, and AIDS.

▶ Sexually transmitted diseases can interact; for example, having a genital ulcer from syphilis increases the likelihood of a person's acquiring HIV, if exposed.

SUGGESTED READING

Benedetti J, Corey L, Ashley R: Recurrence rates in genital herpes after symptomatic first-episode infection. Ann Intern Med 1994;121:847.

Hillier SL et al: Association between bacterial vaginosis and preterm delivery of a low-birth-weight infant. N Engl J Med 1995;333:1737.

Quinn TC, Zenilman J, Rompalo A: Sexually transmitted diseases: Advances in diagnosis and treatment. Adv Intern Med 1994;39:149.

Recommendations for the prevention and management of *Chlamydia trachomatis* infections, 1993. Morb Mort Wkly Rep 1993;42(RR-12):1.

Rolfs RT: Treatment of syphilis, 1993. Clin Infect Dis 1995;20 (Suppl 1):S23.

Schmid GP, Fontanarosa PB: Evolving strategies for management of the nongonococcal urethritis syndrome. JAMA 1995; 274:577.

Sexually transmitted diseases treatment guidelines, 1993. Morb Mort Wkly Rep 1993;42(RR-14):1.

Wald A et al: Virologic characteristics of subclinical and symptomatic genital herpes infections. N Engl J Med 1995;333:770.

Wasserheit JN: Epidemiological synergy: Interrelationships between human immunodeficiency virus infection and other sexually transmitted diseases. Sex Transm Dis 1992;19:61.

8.10

HIV Infection and AIDS

Richard E. Chaisson, MD, and Thomas C. Quinn, MD

The human immunodeficiency virus (HIV) is a retrovirus that infects and ultimately depletes the CD4+ (helper/inducer) population of T lymphocytes. As levels of these cells fall, patients develop the acquired immunodeficiency syndrome (AIDS), an as yet incurable state of profound cellular immunodeficiency that puts them at high risk for opportunistic infections and malignancies. AIDS is defined as either a specific opportunistic disease or a CD4+ count of less than 200/μL (or CD4+ cells accounting for <14% of lymphocytes) in a person who has HIV. HIV is transmitted by three main routes: through any form of sexual intercourse, through percutaneous inoculation of blood or other infected materials (injected drugs, blood or blood product transfusion, needlestick), and through exposure (from mother to child) to infected blood and tissues in utero or during birth, or from infected breast milk.

In 1996, an estimated 1 million persons in the United States were infected with HIV, and an estimated 18 million persons were infected worldwide. Because many of these people are young and advanced HIV infection appears to be uniformly fatal, in the United States AIDS has become the leading cause of death in men 25–44 years old and the third leading cause of death in women 25–44.

Although the incubation period varies greatly, the median time from HIV exposure to the development of AIDS-related opportunistic disease is about 11 years. Many patients with HIV infection present for medical care after undergoing a voluntary serologic test for HIV. Patients who do not know that they are infected most often present with *Pneumocystis carinii* pneumonia, oral candidiasis, bacterial pneumonia, cytopenia (particularly thrombocytopenia), or Kaposi's sarcoma.

Caring for patients with HIV infection can be enormously challenging. Not only must these patients deal with complex and quickly changing medical and therapeutic issues and the probability of early death, but they confront myriad social problems. Because AIDS first appeared in socially ostracized populations, for many people the disease carries considerable social stigma. Moreover, some patients have behaviors or conditions (eg, injected drug use) that may put them at odds with their physician's recommendations. Caregivers who are willing to help patients with these many concerns can find the work as gratifying as it is challenging.

NATURAL HISTORY

During acute HIV infection, the virus appears to replicate freely in the peripheral blood, from which it probably seeds the central nervous system and lymphatic tissue (Figure 8.10–1). Viremia peaks about 2–3 weeks after infection, reaching very high levels.

Many newly infected people have no clinical manifestations of primary HIV infection. However, 50–70% of patients develop an acute retroviral syndrome, usually starting 2–4 weeks after HIV exposure, but sometimes delayed as long as 6 weeks. Patients present with a febrile illness of abrupt onset, which resembles acute mononucleosis and lasts 1–2 weeks. Symptoms may include myalgias, lymphadenopathy, pharyngitis, rash, diarrhea, nausea and vomiting, hepatosplenomegaly, thrush, and mucocutaneous ulcerations of the mouth, esophagus, and genitals. The erythematous maculopapular rash seen in 70% of patients with the acute retroviral syndrome is generally symmetric, with 5–10 mm lesions on the face, trunk, palms, and soles. Many patients have neurologic involvement—meningoencephalitis, peripheral neuropathy, facial palsy, Guillain-Barré syndrome, brachial neuritis, radiculopathy, cognitive impairment, or psychosis.

The first immune response to HIV infection is cytotoxic T lymphocytes, which appear at about 2–3 weeks. The T cells bring a three-to-five log decrease in HIV concentrations in peripheral blood, much better than any antiviral drug can achieve. The development of cellular immunity and the abrupt decline in virus titer suggest that at first the host immune system at least partially suppresses HIV infection. About 6–12 weeks after infection, the patient begins producing IgG, IgA, and IgM antibodies against HIV antigens in serum or plasma. These antibodies, which con-

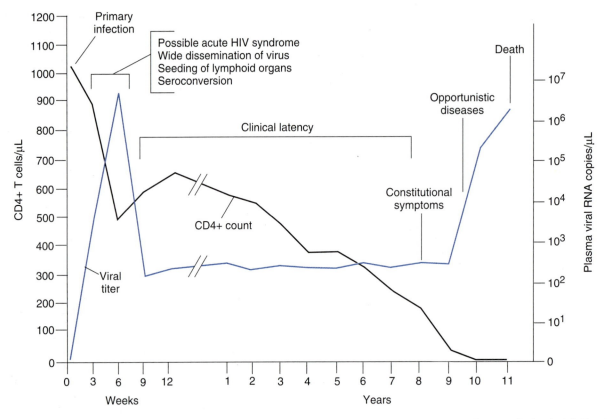

Figure 8.10–1. Hypothetical natural history of untreated HIV infection. (Modified, with permission, from Pantaleo G, Graziosi C, Fauci AS: New concepts in the immunopathogenesis of human immunodeficiency virus infection. N Engl J Med 1993;328:327.)

tinue to circulate for the rest of the patient's life, are the basis of tests for HIV (see "Diagnosis" below).

When the acute retroviral syndrome resolves, most people become asymptomatic for the next few years. During this period, peripheral blood mononuclear cells carry relatively little virus; rather, lymphoid tissue is the major reservoir. Some patients develop a syndrome of persistent generalized lymphadenopathy, defined as enlarged lymph nodes in two noncontiguous extrainguinal sites. The lymph nodes of patients with this syndrome show extremely high concentrations of HIV as extracellular virus trapped in the follicular dendritic cell network, and as intracellular virus in CD4+ cells, predominantly in a latent form.

Although most patients remain symptom-free for the first few years after infection, their immune deterioration progresses, manifested by gradual attrition of circulating CD4+ T lymphocytes, skin test anergy, and autoimmune phenomena such as immune-mediated thrombocytopenia. The best measure of immunologic depression is the CD4+ cell count. During the first few years, the CD4+ count falls by an average of only 30 cells/μL/yr, although with considerable individual variation. But after 5–8 years of infection, the rate of depletion increases to 50–100

cells/mm³/yr. This accelerated decline predicts AIDS developing within 18–24 months. Levels of viral RNA can be measured in plasma. An elevated viral load (more than 30,000–50,000 RNA copies/μL) in plasma predicts increased risk for illness developing within 2–3 years. Measurement of viral load is also useful in gauging response after treatment is started.

Early in HIV disease, when CD4+ counts are still over 500/μL, the only clinical manifestation may be an unusual susceptibility to virulent pathogens (eg, *Streptococcus pneumoniae*) that cause disease in normal hosts. As CD4+ counts fall below 500/μL, patients tend to develop pneumococcal or other bacterial pneumonia, reactivation of varicella zoster virus (shingles), and tuberculosis.

At 7–8 years after infection with HIV, most patients with CD4+ counts over 200–300/μL are still asymptomatic. But their immune system is persistently activated, as shown by increased cytokine expression and increased levels of gamma globulin, neopterin, acid-labile interferon, β_2-microglobulin, and interleukin-2 receptors. This is when patients may begin to develop unexplained constitutional symptoms—weight loss, fever, and night sweats. Other clinical features are generally limited to autoimmune phenomena such as thrombocytopenia and to an increasing range of infections. In addition to pneumococcal pneumonia, pulmonary tuberculosis, and shingles, these might include fungal skin infections and oral, vaginal, and esophageal candidiasis. Noninfectious diseases that may be seen during this stage include cervical intraepithelial neoplasia, cervical carcinoma, Kaposi's sarcoma, and B-cell lymphoma. It is possible that these illnesses have an infectious etiology; for example, cervical intraepithelial neoplasia may be caused by a human papillomavirus.

When the CD4+ count falls lower than 200/μL, the risk rises greatly for progressive malignancies and for opportunistic infections such as *P carinii* pneumonia, disseminated or chronic herpes simplex virus infection, central nervous system toxoplasmosis, cryptococcosis, disseminated histoplasmosis and coccidioidomycosis, chronic cryptosporidiosis, microsporidiosis, disseminated tuberculosis, and nontuberculous mycobacterial infections. Most opportunistic infections in persons with advanced HIV disease are reactivations of old infections that the cellular immune system had held in check. When these patients acquire a new virulent pathogen, such as *Mycobacterium tuberculosis,* it may progress unusually quickly.

Patients with CD4+ counts under 50/μL can develop disseminated cytomegalovirus, particularly chorioretinitis, and disseminated *Mycobacterium avium* complex. Progressive diarrheal wasting syndromes, painful peripheral neuropathy, and HIV-associated dementia may become more severe. With current therapies, these patients have a median survival of 12–18 months.

In addition to injuring and killing CD4+ lymphocytes, HIV impairs other aspects of immunity, further increasing risk for opportunistic disease. Early in HIV infection, B lymphocytes proliferate spontaneously and synthesize large amounts of immunoglobulins, causing a polyclonal gammopathy. Paradoxically, the B-lymphocyte response to new antigens is markedly impaired, and patients have a high incidence of bacterial infections that would normally be controlled by humoral immune responses. HIV directly infects monocytes and macrophages, but, unlike CD4+ lymphocytes, does not kill them. Infected macrophages carry HIV to tissues and organs, including the brain, where the virus may cause direct and indirect damage. HIV interferes with cytokine production, further hampering cellular immune responses. For example, HIV-infected persons produce too little gamma interferon, which activates macrophages to kill intracellular pathogens, and too little interleukin-2, which is responsible for T-cell proliferation.

DIAGNOSIS

Since exposed persons take several weeks to develop antibody to HIV, diagnosis of the acute retroviral syndrome requires direct measurement of viral constituents, such as the viral p24 antigen, viral culture, or amplification of viral nucleic acids by polymerase chain reaction. Beyond the first 6–12 weeks after infection, persons with

suspected HIV infection should be screened with an enzyme-linked immunosorbent assay (ELISA), which detects antibodies to HIV core proteins and surface glycoproteins. Although ELISA is highly sensitive and specific, it does generate false-positive results, especially in persons with autoimmune disease. A positive ELISA must be confirmed with a more specific test. The usual test is the Western blot, in which HIV antigens are separated by electrophoresis and specific antibodies in sera can bind to viral antigens and be visualized.

HIV serology is recommended in the evaluation of people with suspected HIV-related illnesses, those with sexually transmitted diseases, those with a history of high-risk behavior (use of injected drugs, sexual contact with an infected person or a person at risk), those who received blood product transfusions between 1977 and 1985, those contemplating pregnancy, and those undergoing medical procedures that HIV might complicate (eg, organ transplantation). Routine screening for HIV has been proposed for hospital or community settings where the prevalence of HIV infection exceeds 1%. Consent and confidentiality laws vary widely in the United States, but in general the physician contemplating HIV serology must obtain the patient's written consent and inform the patient of the test's potential risks and benefits. Persons who are positive for HIV antibodies by both ELISA and a confirming test should be informed that they are infected with HIV and should understand the natural history of the infection, the need for ongoing medical care, and the risks and means of transmitting the virus to others.

ORGAN SYSTEM COMPLICATIONS

HIV itself produces few clinical syndromes. The virus does most of its damage by causing autoimmune phenomena and by inducing immunodeficiency that opens the way to opportunistic infections and malignancies (Table 8.10–1).

Respiratory Disease

P carinii pneumonia was once the most common opportunistic infection and the leading cause of death in patients with AIDS. Now that the infection can be prevented with chemoprophylaxis, many other respiratory pathogens have emerged in HIV-infected persons. Pneumococci and other common bacteria are frequent causes of community-acquired pneumonia. Patients' risk of bacterial pneumonia is increased by smoking tobacco or other drugs. In the later stages of HIV disease, bacterial pneumonias caused by *Pseudomonas aeruginosa* and other gram-negative bacilli become more prevalent. Tuberculosis (Chapter 8.14) tends to occur as reactivation of latent tuberculous infection when CD4+ cell counts are 200–500/μL, although patients can contract primary tuberculosis at virtually any CD4+ count. Epidemics of both drug-susceptible and drug-resistant tuberculosis have occurred in HIV-infected persons exposed to tuberculosis while institutional-

Table 8.10–1. Major organ system complications of HIV disease by CD4+ cell count.

Conditions	CD4+ ≥300/μL	CD4+ <200/μL
Lymphadenopathy	Persistent generalized lymphadenopathy (syphilis, lymphoma, Kaposi's sarcoma, tuberculosis)	Persistent generalized lymphadenopathy, tuberculosis, Kaposi's sarcoma, *Mycobacterium avium* complex
Eye (fundi)		
Exudate and hemorrhage		Cytomegalovirus retinitis, toxoplasmic chorioretinitis
Cotton wool spots	HIV retinopathy	HIV retinopathy
Mouth		
White patches	Thrush, oral hairy leukoplakia	Thrush, oral hairy leukoplakia
Ulcers	Herpes simplex virus, aphthous ulcers	Herpes simplex virus, aphthous ulcers (cytomegalovirus)
Red-purple nodular lesions	Kaposi's sarcoma	Kaposi's sarcoma
Dysphagia	Candidiasis	Candidiasis (herpes simplex virus, cytomegalovirus, aphthous ulcers)
Abdomen		
Diarrhea	*Salmonella, Clostridium difficile, Campylobacter, Shigella*	*Cryptosporidium*, bacteria, *Microsporidia, M avium* complex, cytomegalovirus, AIDS enteropathy, small bowel overgrowth (histoplasmosis, *Isospora*, blue-green algae, *C difficile*)
Hepatomegaly	Hepatitis (usually B or C)	Hepatitis, cytomegalovirus, *M avium* complex, lymphoma, HIV, fatty liver secondary to malnutrition
Splenomegaly	Tuberculosis, lymphoma	Lymphoma, *M avium* complex, histoplasmosis, HIV
Skin		
Purple-black nodular lesions	Kaposi's sarcoma (bacillary angiomatosis, nodular prurigo)	Kaposi's sarcoma (bacillary angiomatosis, nodular prurigo)
Vesicles	Herpes simplex, herpes zoster	Herpes simplex, herpes zoster (cytomegalovirus)
Maculopapular lesions	Drug reaction, syphilis	Drug reaction, syphilis
Plaques, scaling lesions	Seborrhea (psoriasis, eczema)	Seborrhea (psoriasis, eczema)
Umbilicated papules	Molluscum contagiosum	Molluscum contagiosum (cryptococcosis)
Petechiae, purpura	Immune thrombocytopenic purpura	Immune thrombocytopenic purpura
Nodules		Cryptococcosis, histoplasmosis
Lungs		
Pneumonia	*Streptococcus pneumoniae, Haemophilus influenzae*, tuberculosis	*Pneumocystis carinii* pneumonia (tuberculosis, Kaposi's sarcoma, cytomegalovirus, cryptococcosis, bacterial infection, lymphoid interstitial pneumonia)
Cavitary nodules	Tuberculosis (*Staphylococcus aureus* in IV drug users)	Tuberculosis (cryptococcosis, *Nocardia*, Kaposi's sarcoma, lymphoma, *M avium* complex, *M kansasii*, atypical *P carinii* pneumonia, *Rhodococcus, Pseudomonas*)
Neurologic disorders		
Aseptic meningitis	Viral, neurosyphilis	Cryptococcal meningitis, *Listeria* meningitis
Chronic meningitis	Tuberculosis, fungal meningitis	Cryptococcosis or tuberculosis
Dementia	Trauma, tumor, depression, hypothyroidism	HIV-associated dementia
Constitutional features		
Fever of unknown origin, weight loss, etc.	Lymphoma, tuberculosis	*M avium* complex, cytomegalovirus, histoplasmosis, HIV, cryptococcosis, *P carinii* pneumonia, lymphoma

*Less common complications are shown in parentheses.
Modified and reproduced, with permission, from Bartlett J: *Medical Management of HIV Infection*. Physicians & Scientists Publishing Company, 1994.

ized. *P carinii* is unusual in patients with CD4+ cell counts higher than 200/μL, but it is increasingly prevalent at lower levels.

The evaluation of the HIV-infected patient with respiratory symptoms begins with a history detailing duration and severity of symptoms, exposure to individuals with respiratory infections, smoking history, and use of chemoprophylaxis. The physical exam should focus on signs of consolidation. Laboratory findings are generally nonspecific, but patients with high white blood cell counts are more likely to have a bacterial infection than *P carinii* pneumonia. Chest x-rays are an important tool in the workup of pulmonary disease, although patients with *P carinii* may have normal chest films. Focal consolidation strongly suggests bacterial pneumonia or tuberculosis. Diffuse infiltrates are the most common presentation of *P carinii*, but may also be seen with tuberculosis, bacterial pneumonia, interstitial pneumonitis, and opportunistic lung cancers. Cavitary lesions are sometimes found in patients with mycobacterial disease, but may also be seen in those with bacterial pneumonias, fungal pneumonias, and lymphomas. Many patients with HIV-related tuberculosis have intrathoracic adenopathy and pleural effusions, although these findings are nonspecific. Patients who have respiratory symptoms but normal chest x-rays should have pulmonary disease confirmed by more sensitive means such as pulmonary function tests, exercise oximetry, gallium scanning, or computed tomography.

If patients are expectorating sputum spontaneously, it should be stained and cultured for bacteria and mycobacteria. Patients with possible *P carinii* pneumonia who do not expectorate sputum should undergo sputum induction with hypertonic saline. Specimens of induced sputum should be stained for *P carinii* by standard (Giemsa) or immunofluorescence assays and stained and cultured for bacteria and mycobacteria. Routine cytologic exam and viral and fungal cultures have a very low yield, but sputum induction has a sensitivity of 75–90% for *P carinii.*

Patients with a negative sputum induction should be evaluated with a more sensitive test, such as bronchoscopy with bronchoalveolar lavage. This is crucial, since patients who have signs and symptoms of *P carinii* pneumonia but a negative sputum induction have a 50% probability that bronchoscopy will make the diagnosis. Patients whose sputum or lavage fluid is purulent may be treated with antimicrobial drugs for presumed bacterial pneumonia and reevaluated if symptoms persist. If the workup is unrevealing, the physician should consider giving presumptive therapy for tuberculosis while mycobacterial cultures are pending.

First-line treatment for *P carinii* pneumonia is trimethoprim with either sulfamethoxazole or dapsone. Second-line choices are intravenous pentamidine, oral atovaquone, or oral clindamycin and primaquine. Patients with moderate to severe *P carinii* pneumonia (PAO$_2$-PaO$_2$ gradient >35 torr) should also receive adjuvant corticosteroids.

Central Nervous System Disease

Central nervous system complications tend to occur late in HIV disease and can present subtly or severely. The most common opportunistic complications involving the brain and meninges are cryptococcal meningitis, cerebral toxoplasmosis, central nervous system lymphoma, cytomegalovirus encephalitis, and progressive multifocal leukoencephalopathy. Less common infections are *Listeria monocytogenes,* tuberculosis, and histoplasmosis. HIV itself can cause a subcortical dementia, manifesting with impaired memory and cognition, apathy, and psychomotor retardation. In addition to intracranial disease, HIV can involve the spinal cord (vacuolar myelopathy), and the central nervous system can be involved by cytomegalovirus, herpes simplex virus, or lymphomas.

Physical exam should focus on mental status (Chapters 14.1 and 14.2), cranial and peripheral nerves, and cerebellar function. Neurologic exam should focus on assessment for cognitive defects like mental slowing and problems with concentration and memory. Motor function should be evaluated for imbalance, incoordination, and difficulty with complex motor tasks. Many patients have problems with rapid, alternating movements, as well as hyperreflexia and ataxia. Neuropsychological testing should seek slowed verbal responses and difficulty with complex sequencing, problem solving, performance under time

pressure, and visual-motor integration such as path finding. Neuroradiographic studies may show cerebral atrophy with or without abnormal white matter.

Psychological evaluation is also important. At some time during HIV infection—most often the advanced stages—20–30% of patients develop major depression, which may be unrelated to any personal or family history of depression (Chapter 14.3). Symptoms include a sudden drop in mood, energy, and self-attitude, with morning insomnia, anorexia, decreased libido, low energy, flat affect, feelings of guilt, and a self-denigrating attitude. Most patients respond well to antidepressant drugs.

Delirium is also common (Chapter 14.2). It is distinguished from dementia by acute onset, a "waxing and waning" mental state, disrupted sleep, speech that is often incoherent, and reduced awareness. Delirious patients should be thoroughly evaluated for infectious or metabolic causes, with a cranial imaging study and a lumbar puncture with the cerebrospinal fluid evaluated for cell count, chemistries, cryptococcal antigen, and cultures. If a specific cause for the delirium cannot be found, most patients respond to low-dose neuroleptic drugs.

Gastrointestinal Disease

Oral lesions are a prominent feature of HIV infection and AIDS. Oral thrush (candidiasis) is a marker of advanced immunosuppression. The most common form of thrush is pseudomembranous candidiasis, which presents as a removable white plaque on any oral mucosal surface. Plaques may be as small as 1–2 mm or may be large and widespread. When they are wiped off, they leave a red or even bleeding mucosal surface. An erythematous form of thrush is smooth red patches on the hard or soft palate, buccal mucosa, or dorsal surface of the tongue. Occasionally, *Candida* causes hyperkeratoses, which are white lesions that cannot be wiped off but that regress with prolonged antifungal therapy. This form of candidal leukoplakia appears on the buccal mucosa, tongue, and hard palate and may be confused with hairy leukoplakia.

Hairy leukoplakia produces a white thickening of the oral mucosa, often with vertical folds or corrugations (see Color Plates). The lesions may measure only a few millimeters or may involve the entire dorsal surface of the tongue. Biopsy reveals epithelial hyperplasia with a thickened parakeratin layer showing surface irregularities, projections (hairs), vacuolated prickle cells, and very little inflammation. The differential diagnosis includes *Candida* leukoplakia, smokers' leukoplakia, epithelial dysplasia, oral cancer, and a white sponge nevus in the plaque form of lichen planus. Almost all patients with hairy leukoplakia are HIV-positive, and about 75% have HIV viremia.

Oral lesions caused by herpes simplex virus are a common feature of HIV infection. The condition usually presents as recurrent crops of small, painful, ulcerating vesicles on the palate or gingiva. Oral ulcers may also be caused by cytomegalovirus.

Neoplastic oral lesions include Kaposi's sarcoma, lymphoma, and squamous cell carcinoma. Kaposi's sarcoma may appear as red or purple macules, papules, or nodules within the oral cavity. The lesions are often symptomless, but traumatic ulceration with inflammation and infection can cause pain.

Esophageal disease in the HIV-infected patient can cause dysphagia (difficulty swallowing), odynophagia (painful swallowing), retrosternal pain, fever, and inanition. A patient who has oropharyngeal candidiasis and symptoms of esophageal disease very likely has *Candida* esophagitis and should be treated presumptively with an oral azole antifungal drug. Patients who do not have thrush or whose symptoms fail to resolve with antifungal therapy should be evaluated by endoscopy. Other esophageal diseases in HIV include cytomegalovirus esophagitis, herpes esophagitis, aphthous ulcers, lymphoma, and conventional esophageal diseases.

Upper gastrointestinal disease may be caused by infections or malignancies of the stomach or small bowel. Common complications in patients with advanced HIV disease include infection with cytomegalovirus, *M avium* complex, *Cryptosporidium,* or *Microsporida,* as well as Kaposi's sarcoma and lymphoma. Patients with diarrhea and upper gastrointestinal tract symptoms (eg, epigastric cramping, nausea, and large-volume watery stool) should have stool examined for *Cryptosporidium, Microsporida,* ova and parasites, and *Clostridium difficile* toxin and cultured for conventional bacterial pathogens.

Lower gastrointestinal tract infections are suggested by cramping abdominal pain, small-volume diarrheal stools, tenesmus, hematochezia, and rectal pain. Community-acquired causes are *Shigella, Campylobacter, Salmonella,* and other gram-negative bacilli, all of which may be unusually severe in persons with HIV disease. *C difficile* toxin-induced pseudomembranous colitis can develop in patients who have recently received antimicrobial drugs. Cytomegalovirus colitis causes severe abdominal pain, often without diarrhea. Lower gastrointestinal tract infections are diagnosed by stool cultures, *C difficile* toxin assay, and ova and parasite exam, or, if these tests are negative, by colonoscopy.

Nutritional assessment is important, since wasting is a common feature of late-stage disease. Contributing factors are increased metabolic requirements, malabsorption, and patients not eating enough because of depression, anorexia, and oral and esophageal lesions. Patients who have lost weight may benefit from consultation with a nutritionist as well as nutritional supplements and an appetite stimulant such as megestrol acetate. The value of vitamin supplements, low-dose corticosteroids, indomethacin, and other drugs is unclear.

Hematologic Manifestations

Hematologic abnormalities, found at all stages of HIV disease, involve the bone marrow, cellular elements of the peripheral blood, and coagulation pathways. Contributing are HIV's direct suppressive effect plus ineffective hematopoiesis, infections infiltrating the bone marrow, nutritional deficiencies, peripheral consumption of platelets secondary to splenomegaly or immune dysregulation, and drug effects.

Anemia is the most common blood abnormality in HIV-infected persons. About 65–85% of patients with overt AIDS have anemia, most often the anemia of chronic disease, with low reticulocyte counts and low erythropoietin levels. Patients have adequate iron stores in the reticuloendothelial system, but cannot use this stored iron. The result is ineffective erythropoiesis and a normocytic, normochromic anemia. Ineffective erythropoiesis may also result from HIV infection of erythroid precursors or from inappropriate release of tumor necrosis factor, which inhibits red blood cell production in vitro. Iron deficiency, with a microcytic, hypochromic anemia, may be caused by chronic blood loss from Kaposi's sarcoma or lymphomatous involvement of the gastrointestinal tract. Thrombocytopenia with resultant occult bleeding occasionally leads to iron deficiency anemia. Infiltrative disease of the bone marrow by *M avium* complex is a common cause of isolated anemia, usually without concomitant suppression of other cell lines. In contrast, lymphoma can cause profound anemia with depression of other cell lines.

The HIV-infected patient's most common platelet abnormality is thrombocytopenia. Many patients produce platelet-associated antibodies, which cause the platelets to be destroyed by the reticuloendothelial system. Circulating immune complexes can precipitate on platelets' surface, also causing the platelets to be cleared by the reticuloendothelial system. As patients become sicker, more circulating immune complexes and hypergammaglobulinemia seem to block the spleen's ability to remove these antibody-coated platelets from the circulation. Thus, the platelet count may rise. Most patients with HIV-related idiopathic thrombocytopenic purpura have only minor submucosal bleeding, characterized by petechiae, ecchymoses, and occasional epistaxis.

Many HIV-infected persons have drug-induced anemia, thrombocytopenia, and neutropenia. Medications to treat infections such as *P carinii* pneumonia, toxoplasmosis, and cytomegalovirus retinitis or colitis often cause neutropenia. Similarly, zidovudine (see "Inhibition of Viral Replication" below) can cause macrocytic anemia and neutropenia. Myelosuppression caused by many of these drugs can be reversed by stopping the drug or lowering the dose. Alternatively, patients can be given an additional drug such as colony-stimulating factor (CSF), which stimulates production of macrophages (GM-CSF) or granulocytes (G-CSF). Human recombinant erythropoietin may also be given to HIV-infected patients who have anemia secondary to antiretroviral therapy.

Ocular Disease

HIV involves the eyes in four main ways: (1) a noninfectious microangiopathy, most often in the retina (HIV retinopathy); (2) opportunistic eye infections such as cytomegalovirus; (3) ocular adnexal involvement by the neoplasms seen in AIDS; and (4) neuro-ophthalmic lesions. Cytomegalovirus retinitis is the most common opportunistic eye infection in patients with HIV and a major cause of impaired vision. Asymptomatic patients should be instructed about signs and symptoms of cytomegalovirus retinitis to watch for. Patients should seek immediate evaluation if they develop floaters (semitransparent bodies perceived to be floating in the field of vision), blurred vision, sudden loss of vision, unilateral vision change, or subtle field defects. The chance for early diagnosis is greatest when eye exams are a routine part of primary care visits and patients monitor their own visual symptoms. All patients with CD4+ counts lower than 50/mm^3 need routine ophthalmologic visits (eg, every 3 months) with a careful history of visual disturbance and an eye exam with funduscopy.

Cotton wool spots, the most common feature of HIV retinopathy, have been reported in 25–90% of patients with AIDS. Cotton wool spots are microinfarcts in the nerve fiber layer of the retina. The cause is ischemia that disrupts axonal transport, causing axons in the nerve fiber to swell and produce the characteristic opaque white patches.

Skin Lesions

Skin disease complicates HIV infection in up to 90% of patients. The most common neoplasm in HIV-infected persons is the once-rare Kaposi's sarcoma, which usually presents first in the skin. Many patients' early skin tumors are palpable, firm nodules, 0.5–2 cm in diameter, although some early lesions look like small ecchymoses. In more advanced disease, the tumors become confluent and cover large areas of skin. In light-skinned individuals, the lesions are typically violaceous; in dark-skinned individuals, they are brown or black (see Color Plates). Kaposi's sarcoma often involves the viscera, most frequently the gastrointestinal tract and lungs. Routine exams of the skin and mouth are key to early diagnosis. Suspected lesions should be confirmed histologically.

The pathogenesis of Kaposi's sarcoma in HIV-infected people is thought to be related to infection with a herpesvirus (HHV-8). A sexually transmitted agent is suggested by the nearly exclusive confinement of this neoplasm to male homosexuals and by a decline in the incidence of Kaposi's in male homosexuals during a period when they were engaging in safer sex.

Another skin manifestation of HIV infection is bacillary angiomatosis. This disease is an uncommon subacute or chronic bacterial infection caused by *Bartonella quintana* or *B henselae* (formerly *Rochalimaea quintana* and *R henselae*). The agent is extremely difficult to culture, so the diagnosis is usually established by identifying the pathogen histopathologically in affected tissue. The skin lesions present as friable vascular papules, subcutaneous nodules, or cellulitic plaques. Lesions can appear anywhere on the skin and on mucosal surfaces, especially the respiratory tract and conjunctiva. Indicators of chronic infection are fever, night sweats, anemia, and a high ery-

throcyte sedimentation rate. Many patients have visceral disease, with or without skin lesions; the major forms are liver and spleen involvement (bacillary peliosis), osteolytic bone lesions, lymphadenopathy, and bacteremia. Ultrasonography may show echogenic lesions in the liver, and computed tomography shows a heterogenous liver parenchyma. The physician should consider bacillary angiomatosis in any HIV-infected person who has vascular lesions of the skin, viscera, or bone. A biopsy of infected tissue should confirm the diagnosis; the organism can be identified by Warthin-Starry stain.

Many HIV-infected patients also develop staphylococcal skin infections—folliculitis, impetigo, ecthyma, abscesses, and cellulitis. Herpes simplex and varicella zoster virus infections often appear during both the asymptomatic and advanced stages of AIDS. Shingles in a person younger than age 65 should raise suspicion of HIV infection.

Patients with HIV disease can also have hypersensitivity reactions to medications. About 20% of persons treated with trimethoprim-sulfamethoxazole for *P carinii* pneumonia develop a widespread maculopapular rash. The rash may resolve with continued treatment, but it often persists and progresses, forcing the drug to be stopped. Even insect bite reactions can be extremely florid, presenting as nonfollicular papules or cellulitic plaques with marked pruritus.

Cardiac, Endocrine, and Renal Complications

Pulmonary, gastrointestinal, hematologic, and neurologic dysfunction remain the principal manifestations of HIV infection. But as antiretroviral therapy and prophylaxis of opportunistic infections have allowed patients to live longer, more organ systems have become involved.

Among the cardiac manifestations is myocarditis, which may be idiopathic or caused by cytomegalovirus, coxsackie B virus, or HIV itself. Congestive cardiomyopathy has been described in patients with AIDS; the pathologic hallmark is biventricular dilatation. Dilated cardiomyopathy can be caused not only by infection but by nutritional deficiency, cardiotoxins, drugs, and immunologic mechanisms. Many autopsies of patients with AIDS show nonbacterial thrombotic (marantic) endocarditis, in which sterile thrombi can develop on any valve and then embolize; lesions are often found in chronically ill persons, particularly those with malignancy.

HIV-infected persons carry unusually high burdens of *Staphylococcus aureus* in their skin, nose, and pharynx. HIV-positive intravenous drug users may have a high incidence of staphylococcal endocarditis.

A final major cardiac manifestation of AIDS is pericardial effusion. Most such effusions are sterile and of uncertain clinical significance. Symptomatic pericardial effusion and tamponade are often infectious, caused by *M tuberculosis, M avium* complex, or *Cryptococcus.*

The most common site of endocrine involvement in HIV-infected patients is the adrenal gland; the most common adrenal infection is cytomegalovirus adrenalitis, characterized by intranuclear cytoplasmic inclusions. Many HIV-positive people have lipid depletion (typical of chronic disease in general), adrenal infection with *Cryptococcus* or mycobacteria, and adrenal infiltration with Kaposi's sarcoma. People with advanced HIV disease may have clinical adrenal insufficiency. Measuring adrenal function in patients with AIDS is complicated by drugs (eg, ketoconazole, rifampin) that affect steroidogenesis and steroid metabolism. HIV can also affect the gonads, thyroid, and pancreas.

Renal function in HIV-infected patients may be disturbed by systemic infection, sepsis, dehydration, ischemia, or exposure to nephrotoxic drugs. An HIV-specific nephropathy is characterized by focal and segmental glomerulosclerosis, with intraglomerular deposition of IgM and C3.

HIV Complications in Women

With the increasing spread of HIV among women, HIV-associated gynecologic conditions have become an important concern. As their immunosuppression increases, women may manifest opportunistic infections of the reproductive tract, most commonly *Candida* vaginitis. In addition, gynecologic conditions such as cervicitis, salpingitis, genital ulcers, genital warts, and cervical dysplastic epithelial changes may be more frequent and severe—and less responsive to treatment—among HIV-infected than noninfected women. The risk of HIV-infected patients for human papillomavirus-associated epithelial malignancy rises as their immunosuppression worsens. Anal dysplasia and squamous cell carcinoma have higher-than-normal rates in HIV-infected women and in homosexual men. These lesions can be readily detected by Papanicolaou (Pap) smear of the cervical or anal epithelium. The morphology of these lesions extends from relatively benign koilocytic atypia, which signifies human papillomavirus infection, to the more poorly differentiated epithelium of high-grade dysplastic lesions. Squamous intraepithelial lesions and invasive cervical carcinoma also appear to be more common among HIV-infected women.

All HIV-infected women should have a complete gynecologic exam, including vaginal and rectal exams and Pap smear, at least twice during the year after diagnosis and then yearly if the first Pap smear is normal. Patients with a

Table 8.10–2. Laboratory tests for patients with HIV infection.

Test	Recommended Frequency
Complete blood count	Baseline, then every 3–6 months
CD4+ count	Baseline, then every 3–6 months
Plasma HIV	Baseline, then every 6–12 months
Blood chemistries	Baseline, then as needed
Serologic test for syphilis	Baseline, then yearly
Hepatitis B serology	Baseline
PPD (Mantoux method)	Baseline; if negative, yearly
Toxoplasma IgG serology	Baseline
Varicella zoster antibody	Baseline (optional)
Measles antibody	Baseline (for patients born after 1957)

PPD, purified protein derivative.

Table 8.10–3. AIDS Surveillance Case Definition for adolescents and adults.*

	CD4+ cells/μL (% of Normal Lymphocytes)		
Clinical Categories	1 ≥500 (≥29%)	2 200–499 (14–28%)	3 ≤199 (≤13%)
A No symptoms *or* acute HIV infection *or* persistent generalized lymphadenopathy	A1	A2	A3
B Symptoms other than A or C (see Table 8.10–4)	B1	B2	B3
C AIDS indicator condition (see Table 8.10–5)	C1	C2	C3

*Shaded categories are considered to be AIDS.
Modified from: 1993 revised classification system for HIV infection and expanded surveillance case definition for AIDS among adolescents and adults. Morb Mort Wkly Rep 1992;41(RR-17).

history of human papillomavirus infection or with squamous intraepithelial lesions on Pap smear should be examined every 6 months. Colposcopy (examination of the vagina and cervix by a magnifying lens) may provide detailed follow-up of women with HIV-related problems of the cervix.

MANAGEMENT

Evaluation and Staging

All patients with confirmed HIV infection should have an evaluation to determine the stage of their HIV disease and assess their need for specific therapies. The physician should get a detailed history of past illnesses, symptoms, and medications. Some laboratory tests should be done as a baseline, and some repeated later (Table 8.10–2). The CD4+ lymphocyte count is important for determining prognosis and for guiding therapy. All patients should have a tuberculin skin test, and those with 5 mm or more induration should receive isoniazid chemoprophylaxis. Patients should have a baseline hepatitis B serology, and those at risk for acquiring the disease (particularly homosexuals and injection drug users) should be given recombinant hepatitis B vaccine. *Toxoplasma* serology identifies patients at risk for developing toxoplasmic encephalitis; they may be candidates for chemoprophylaxis. Patients who do not have a history of chickenpox but are exposed to children with chickenpox may benefit from a varicella zoster antibody test, and, if the test result is negative, from varicella zoster immune globulin. A measles antibody test can be done in unvaccinated patients born after 1957. All patients should be given polyvalent pneumococcal polysaccharide vaccine every 6 years.

HIV-infected persons are classified according to their clinical features and CD4+ cell counts (Tables 8.10–3 through 8.10–5). Clinically, patients are classified into three groups: (1) those who are asymptomatic; (2) those

Table 8.10–4. Examples of "B" conditions.*

Bacillary angiomatosis
Thrush or vulvovaginal candidiasis that is persistent, frequent, or poorly responsive to therapy
Cervical dysplasia, moderate or severe
Cervical carcinoma in situ
Constitutional symptoms such as fever (≥38.5°C [101.3°F]) or diarrhea for >1 month
Oral hairy leukoplakia
Herpes zoster involving 2 episodes or >1 dermatome
Immune thrombocytopenic purpura
Listeriosis
Pelvic inflammatory disease, especially if complicated by a tubo-ovarian abscess
Peripheral neuropathy

*1993 AIDS Surveillance Case Definition (see Table 8.10–3). These are symptomatic conditions (not included in Category A or C) that are (1) attributed to HIV infection or indicative of a defect in cell-mediated immunity, or (2) considered to have a clinical course or management that is complicated by HIV infection.
Modified from: 1993 revised classification system for HIV infection and expanded surveillance case definition for AIDS among adolescents and adults. Morb Mort Wkly Rep 1992;41(RR-17).

Table 8.10–5. "C" conditions defining AIDS.*

Candidiasis of bronchi, trachea, or lungs
Candidiasis, esophageal
Cervical cancer, invasive
Coccidioidomycosis, disseminated or extrapulmonary
Cryptococcosis, extrapulmonary
Cryptosporidiosis, chronic intestinal (>1 month)
Cytomegalovirus disease (other than liver, spleen, or lymph nodes)
Cytomegalovirus retinitis with loss of vision
Encephalopathy, HIV-related
Herpes simplex: chronic ulcer(s) (>1 month), or bronchitis, pneumonitis, or esophagitis
Histoplasmosis, disseminated or extrapulmonary
Isosporiasis, chronic intestinal (>1 month)
Kaposi's sarcoma
Lymphoma, Burkitt's
Lymphoma, immunoblastic
Lymphoma, primary, of brain
Mycobacterium avium complex or *M kansasii,* disseminated or extrapulmonary
Mycobacterium tuberculosis, any site (pulmonary or extrapulmonary)
Mycobacterium, other species or unidentified species, disseminated or extrapulmonary
Pneumocystis carinii pneumonia
Pneumonia, recurrent bacterial
Progressive multifocal leukoencephalopathy
Salmonella septicemia, recurrent
Toxoplasmosis of brain
Wasting syndrome caused by HIV

*1993 AIDS Surveillance Case Definition (see Table 8.10–3). Modified from: 1993 revised classification system for HIV infection and expanded surveillance case definition for AIDS among adolescents and adults. Morb Mort Wkly Rep 1992;41(RR-17).

who have non-life-threatening infections and other manifestations of HIV infection, such as shingles, oral thrush, and seborrheic dermatitis; and (3) those who have serious opportunistic infections and malignancies. The CD4+ count categories are 500/μL or higher, 200–499/μL, and less than 200/mm³.

How often HIV-infected persons need CD4+ cell counts depends on the stage of their disease. Those with CD4+ counts of 500/μL or more should be tested every 6 months. When the CD4+ approaches a level at which a clinical decision is made (eg, antiretroviral therapy to be started when the CD4+ count is <500/μL), the test should be repeated every 3 months. Patients with lower CD4+ counts should have tests every 3–6 months, depending on the therapeutic implications.

Plasma HIV RNA levels should be measured initially and then once or twice a year, depending on the patient's clinical course and therapy. (Patients with high CD4+ counts and a low viral load need less frequent testing.) Viral RNA elevations of 0.6 log or greater may indicate the beginning of treatment failure.

Inhibition of Viral Replication

Drugs of several classes are approved for controlling HIV replication. The most effective approach may be combination therapy with two to three drugs that act at different stages in the viral life cycle or that thwart different mechanisms of viral resistance. Currently available agents include inhibitors of HIV reverse transcriptase (mostly nucleoside analogs) and inhibitors of HIV protease.

Zidovudine (formerly called AZT) is a thymidine analog that prolongs life and reduces risk for opportunistic disease in patients with advanced HIV infection. Zidovudine is more effective when given in combination with other nucleoside analogs, protease inhibitors, or both. Zi-

dovudine's main side effects are nausea, headache, anemia, and granulocytopenia. The drug generally produces increases in platelet counts, especially in patients with HIV-related immune thrombocytopenia; the mechanism of this effect may be inhibition of HIV replication in megakaryocytes.

Didanosine (ddI) is an inosine nucleoside that is metabolized to dideoxyadenosine. Didanosine is more effective than zidovudine at preventing progression in patients with HIV disease, although some studies suggest that it should be given with zidovudine. Didanosine can cause peripheral neuropathy, and it causes severe or fatal pancreatitis in about 2% of patients.

Zalcitabine (ddC) is a cytosine nucleoside. Although inferior to zidovudine as initial therapy in advanced HIV disease, zalcitabine is effective when combined with zidovudine. Zalcitabine and zidovudine given together produce significantly higher increases in CD4+ cell counts than either drug alone. Like didanosine, zalcitabine can cause peripheral neuropathy and severe or fatal pancreatitis.

Lamivudine (3TC) is a cytosine analog that enhances the efficacy of zidovudine. Lamivudine induces the emergence of an HIV-mutant with a reverse transcriptase codon mutation that increases susceptibility to zidovudine. Over time, patients given both agents are less likely

Table 8.10–6. Recommended therapies for patients with HIV infection.

Patient Group	Therapies	Comments
All patients	Isoniazid if PPD-positive or exposed to infectious tuberculosis Pneumococcal vaccine	Consider antiretroviral therapy for high plasma HIV RNA load
CD4+ 200–500	Didanosine + zidovudine, or Zidovudine + lamivudine ± protease inhibitor	Therapy prolongs survival; optimal regimen unknown
CD4+ <200	Trimethoprim-sulfamethoxazole or dapsone or aerosol pentamidine 2 nucleoside analogs + protease inhibitor	*Pneumocystis* prophylaxis
CD4+ <100 and *Toxoplasma*-positive by IgG	Trimethoprim-sulfamethoxazole or dapsone-pyrimethamine	*Toxoplasma* prophylaxis
CD4+ <75	Clarithromycin or azithromycin or rifabutin	*M avium* complex prophylaxis
CD4+ <50 and CMV-positive by PCR	Oral ganciclovir	CMV prophylaxis

PPD, purified protein derivative; CMV, cytomegalovirus; PCR, polymerase chain reaction.

to develop zidovudine-resistant infection, and susceptibility to zidovudine can be restored in patients with resistant virus. Lamivudine appears to be well-tolerated when given with zidovudine. The efficacy of lamivudine given in combination with other nucleoside drugs such as didanosine and stavudine is not yet known.

Stavudine (d4T), like zidovudine, is a thymidine analog. Stavudine is approved for patients who do not tolerate or respond to other antiretroviral drugs. Its efficacy relative to other approved drugs has not been well described. Common side effects of stavudine are peripheral neuropathy and hematologic toxicity.

The available protease inhibitor drugs include saquinavir, ritonavir, and indinavir. These agents competitively inhibit HIV viral protease, an enzyme essential for assembly of infectious virions. These drugs are considerably more potent than nucleoside analogs. However, unless protease inhibitors are given in combination with other agents, resistance to the inhibitors begins within several weeks after patients start therapy. These drugs are highly protein-bound, and are metabolized by P450 cytochromes—features that raise important concerns about bioavailability and drug-drug interactions. The long-term safety and tolerability of the protease inhibitors have not been determined.

Prophylaxis

Prophylaxis of specific HIV-related opportunistic infections reduces both morbidity and mortality. Prophylactic therapy should be based on the patient's stage of disease and the pathogen's prevalence and virulence (see Table 8.10–6). Tuberculosis prophylaxis should be given to any HIV-infected patient who has a positive tuberculin skin test, a history of a positive test, or close contact with a person who has tuberculosis. Similarly, all patients with HIV should receive pneumococcal polysaccharide vaccine during the initial workup, as the disease is common and can occur at any CD4+ cell level. Prophylaxis against *P carinii* pneumonia is recommended for patients who have had one bout and for all patients with a CD4+ count under

$200/mm^3$, because they are at high risk. Patients with quickly falling CD4+ counts or with severe constitutional symptoms may also benefit from *P carinii* prophylaxis.

Trimethoprim-sulfamethoxazole is extremely effective in preventing *P carinii* and has the added benefit of reducing the incidence of serious bacterial infections and toxoplasmosis. Alternatives for *P carinii* prophylaxis are aerosolized pentamidine and oral dapsone, although neither drug protects against other pathogens. Rifabutin, clarithromycin, and azithromycin all reduce the risk of disseminated *M avium* complex infection by 50–70% and should be given to all HIV-infected persons with CD4+ counts of less than $75/\mu L$. Oral ganciclovir has been shown to reduce the incidence of cytomegalovirus infections in HIV-infected patients with CD4+ counts of less than $50/\mu L$. The most appropriate use of oral ganciclovir may be for selected patients with CD4+ counts below $50 \mu L$ *and* blood shown to be positive for cytomegalovirus by polymerase chain reaction.

PREVENTION OF HIV TRANSMISSION

HIV transmission through blood and blood products, donated tissue and organs, and accidental infection of health care workers is prevented mainly by routine HIV screening of donated blood and by universal precautions. The basis of these precautions is that *all* patients' blood and other potentially infectious body fluids should be considered infectious, and caregivers should use gloves, goggles, and other barriers to prevent direct contact.

Sexual transmission of HIV is largely preventable by "safe sex" practices that reduce or eliminate risk. The standard recommendations for avoiding sexual transmission are a monogamous relationship with someone who has been HIV antibody-negative for at least 6 months, avoiding sexual intercourse with a person known to be HIV-seropositive, and using latex condoms with nonoxynol-9 for insertive vaginal or anal sex. How closely people follow these guidelines often depends on the risk they perceive in their partner and the benefit they perceive in using the intervention. Safe sex works only if both partners commit to it. Other sexually transmitted diseases such as genital ulcers and cervical infections must be controlled, since they increase HIV transmission (Chapter 8.9).

Factors shown to reduce HIV risk among intravenous drug users are the cleaning of needles, bleach distribution, avoiding sharing needles, needle exchange programs, skilled counselors, and enrollment in a drug treatment program.

One of the successes of HIV prevention has been the screening of blood donors for HIV antibody begun in 1985. The risk of receiving infected blood is now 1:153,000; the main risk is from donors who have recently become infected and are still antibody-negative. The process for heat treatment of factor VIII, instituted in 1984, has virtually eliminated new infections in persons with hemophilia.

Despite the thousands of health care workers exposed to needlestick injuries or blood from HIV-infected or high-risk patients, only a few people have likely been infected while providing health care. The risk of contracting HIV from a single needlestick injury is less than 0.4%, compared with a 20% risk of contracting hepatitis B. The risk from mucous membrane contact or inoculation of broken skin with HIV-infected blood or other body fluids is too low to be measured, even though at least 1000 exposures of this type have been studied. Nevertheless, a small risk multiplied many times is a very real risk, and rigorous attention must be paid to protecting health care workers. There is some evidence suggesting that postexposure prophylaxis with antiretroviral agents reduces the risk of acquiring HIV infection after a needlestick injury, although a number of treatment failures have been reported.

Zidovudine can reduce the risk of a mother transmitting HIV to her infant. When zidovudine is given to HIV-infected women during the second and third trimesters of pregnancy and to their babies for the first 6 weeks of life, transmission is reduced from 25% to 8%. Pregnant women with a higher than 0.1% probability of HIV infection should be offered HIV screening with counseling and follow-up.

SUMMARY

▶ HIV infection causes progressive immunodeficiency, with risk of opportunistic complications increasing with increasing length of infection.

▶ In the United States, AIDS has become the leading cause of death in men 25–44 years old and the third leading cause of death in women 25–44.

▶ Levels of CD4+ lymphocytes and plasma HIV RNA help stage the patient, predict which infections the patient is liable to develop, and determine the timing and nature of treatments.

▶ Prophylaxis against opportunistic diseases significantly reduces morbidity and mortality in advanced HIV disease. Antiretroviral therapy may prolong survival in advanced HIV disease and delay progression of symptomless early disease.

▶ HIV transmission is prevented by routine HIV screening of donated blood, universal precautions, and safe sex practices.

SUGGESTED READING

Chaisson RE, Volberding PA: Clinical manifestations of HIV infection. In: *Principles and Practice of Infectious Diseases,* 4th ed. Mandell GL, Bennett JE, Dolin R (editors). Churchill Livingstone, 1995.

Fauci AS: Multifactorial nature of human immunodeficiency virus disease: Implications for therapy. Science 1993;262:1011.

Ho DD et al: Rapid turnover of plasma virions and CD4 lymphocytes in HIV-1 infection. Nature 1995;373:123.

Mellors JW et al: Quantitation of HIV-1 RNA in plasma predicts outcome after seroconversion. Ann Intern Med 1995;122:573.

Moore RD, Chaisson RE: Natural history of opportunistic disease in an HIV-infected urban clinical cohort. Ann Intern Med 1996;124:633.

Pantaleo G, Graziosi C, Fauci AS: New concepts in the immunopathogenesis of human immunodeficiency virus infection. N Engl J Med 1993;328:327.

Sande MA, Volberding PA (editors): *The Medical Management of AIDS,* 4th ed. WB Saunders, 1995.

Volberding PA et al: A comparison of immediate with deferred zidovudine therapy for asymptomatic HIV-infected adults with CD4 cell counts of 500 or more per cubic millimeter. N Engl J Med 1995;333:401.

Systemic Viral Infections

John F. Modlin, MD

Most acute viral infections cause transient central nervous system, respiratory, or gastrointestinal symptoms, with only minor constitutional effects. But a few viruses produce more specific systemic illnesses. HIV, hepatitis B and C, and other viral infections that can cause chronic disease are covered elsewhere in the book. This chapter focuses on selected viral infections that usually cause acute systemic illness.

INFECTIOUS MONONUCLEOSIS

Infectious mononucleosis is an acute illness of sore throat, fever, adenopathy, and lymphocytosis, usually caused by the Epstein-Barr virus. A few cases are produced by human cytomegalovirus or the coccidian parasite *Toxoplasma gondii.* Primary infections with HIV-1 may also resemble infectious mononucleosis. Epstein-Barr virus and cytomegalovirus are both members of the human herpesvirus family. Epstein-Barr virus preferentially infects B lymphocytes; cytomegalovirus is found principally in neutrophils. Activated T lymphocytes, although not directly infected, play a prominent role in causing illness.

Epstein-Barr virus and cytomegalovirus infect people at all ages, but infectious mononucleosis mainly affects teenagers and young adults from middle and upper socioeconomic strata who escaped Epstein-Barr virus infection earlier in life. College students develop mononucleosis at an annual rate of 0.5–12%. Infectious mononucleosis is known popularly as "the kissing disease" because it is usually transmitted by intimate oral contact with an asymptomatic person who is shedding the virus. Both cytomegalovirus and Epstein-Barr virus mononucleosis can also be transmitted by transfusion of fresh blood or by transplanted organs, so the illness first develops in some patients after coronary artery bypass surgery (postperfusion syndrome) or organ transplantation.

Clinical Features

After an incubation period of 30–50 days (shorter for transfusion-acquired disease), people infected with Epstein-Barr virus have an abrupt onset of fever, malaise, and pharyngitis. Many patients also complain of chills, headache, photophobia, anorexia, dysphagia, myalgia, or a distaste for cigarettes. Physical examination often reveals periorbital edema, enlarged tonsils with erythema and exudate, palatine petechiae, cervical adenopathy, and splenomegaly. Less common findings are jaundice and hepatomegaly. A maculopapular rash develops in about 10% of patients, especially those who have been given ampicillin; ampicillin causes a generalized rash in about 90% of patients who receive it during acute infectious mononucleosis. A blood count drawn during the acute illness shows a peripheral blood white blood cell count of 12,000–50,000/mm^3, with most of the increase in lymphocytes. At least 8–10% of all white blood cells are atypical lymphocytes (reactive T lymphocytes with an enlarged nucleus, increased cytoplasm content with basophilia, and prominent nucleoli; Figure 8.11–1). More than 80% of patients have mildly elevated serum transaminases.

Epstein-Barr virus and cytomegalovirus infections produce nearly identical clinical and laboratory features. The difference is that cytomegalovirus mononucleosis does not cause an exudative pharyngitis or extensive lymphadenopathy. Primary HIV infection (Chapter 8.10) causes a mononucleosis-like illness lasting 2–4 weeks and consisting of fever, adenitis, sore throat, rash, and myalgias; the HIV serologic assay is often negative at this early stage. Unlike patients with Epstein-Barr virus mononucleosis, those with primary HIV do not have exudative pharyngitis, and less than 50% have atypical lymphocytes.

Diagnosis

In practice, the diagnosis of Epstein-Barr virus mononucleosis rests on finding serum heterophile antibodies (immunoglobulins that bind to nonhuman red blood cell antigens). The classic heterophile reaction is mediated by a patient's IgM antibody, which agglutinates sheep red blood cells after adsorption of the test serum with guinea pig red blood cells. Many clinical laboratories now use "slide" or "spot" tests with horse or ox red blood cells, which are more sensitive and specific than tests based on sheep cells. Heterophile antibodies can be found in 75%

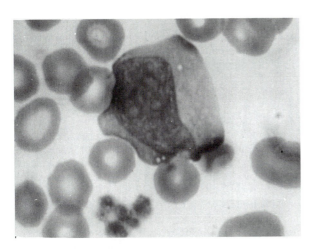

Figure 8.11–1. Atypical lymphocyte in infectious mononucleosis: enlarged T cell with an indented and lobulated nucleus, vacuolated cytoplasm, and indentation of the lymphocyte membrane by adjacent red cells ("Dutch skirting"). (Courtesy of Stuart E. Selonick, MD.)

of patients with Epstein-Barr virus mononucleosis by the seventh day of illness, and in 95–97% by the 21st day. The antibodies may persist for up to 1 year afterward. In atypical or complicated cases, it may be desirable to test the patient's serum for antibodies directed against a number of Epstein-Barr virus-specific antigens (early antigen, viral capsid antigen, and viral nuclear antigen), which are increasingly available at commercial laboratories. Cytomegalovirus mononucleosis is heterophile-negative; the diagnosis requires recovery of cytomegalovirus from the blood, urine, or oropharynx, or a rise in the cytomegalovirus-specific antibody titer.

Complications

The symptoms of Epstein-Barr virus infectious mononucleosis abate slowly. Fifty percent of patients are free of symptoms by 2 weeks, 80% by 3 weeks, and 97% by 4 weeks. Complications include hemolytic anemia, immune thrombocytopenia, neutropenia, upper airway obstruction, pneumonia, myopericarditis, splenic rupture, severe hepatitis, and bacterial superinfection. The central nervous system becomes involved in less than 1% of patients; Epstein-Barr virus mononucleosis can cause encephalitis, aseptic meningitis, transverse myelitis, hearing loss, cranial nerve palsies, and peripheral neuropathy, especially Guillain-Barré syndrome.

Rare patients have recurrent fever, malaise, pharyngitis, cervical adenopathy, or neuropsychiatric symptoms for months or years after acute Epstein-Barr virus mononucleosis. However, a defined relation between Epstein-Barr virus infection and chronic fatigue syndrome remains elusive. Patients with a rare X-linked deficiency syndrome develop acquired agammaglobulinemia (Chapter 9.5) or lymphomas after Epstein-Barr virus mononucleosis. Ex-

cept in these patients, mononucleosis-related deaths are very rare and are usually secondary to central nervous system disease, splenic rupture, or upper airway obstruction from severe tonsillitis.

Management

To minimize the risk of splenic rupture, acutely ill patients should be advised to avoid strenuous exercise and contact sports. Corticosteroids are sometimes useful in managing airway obstruction or thrombocytopenia, but should generally be avoided otherwise, since they do not alter the natural history of the illness. Acyclovir, which has moderate activity against Epstein-Barr virus in vitro, reduces oropharyngeal shedding but has little effect on the clinical course and does not prevent latent infection.

MEASLES

Measles (rubeola) is caused by a member of the *Morbillivirus* genus of the family Paramyxoviridae. The virus is one of the most infectious agents known. Primary infection confers lifelong immunity to disease. Before measles vaccines were deployed in the 1960s, virtually all children became infected. Since then, the widespread use of measles vaccine in developed countries has greatly reduced the incidence of measles. However, those who are not vaccinated and escape childhood exposure to measles remain susceptible as adults. In addition, some teenagers and young adults remain susceptible because of primary vaccine failure or become susceptible again because of waning immunity after childhood vaccination. As a result, in recent years more than 40% of reported measles cases in the United States have been in persons over age 15. Many adults acquire the disease during outbreaks at colleges and other institutions.

Clinical Features

Measles virus is transmitted through the respiratory tract. After an incubation period of 9–11 days, patients develop fever and symptoms of upper respiratory tract infection, usually cough, coryza, and conjunctivitis. Within 2–3 days, most patients develop Koplik's spots—blue-white punctate lesions on the buccal mucosa. On the third or fourth day, a red maculopapular rash begins on the face and quickly extends to the trunk and extremities while becoming confluent on the face and neck. In uncomplicated infections, the fever and respiratory symptoms begin to abate quickly after 4–5 days, and the rash fades, sometimes with desquamation.

Complications

Measles is usually mild in children, but it can be severe in infants and adults. Many patients develop respiratory complications such as otitis media, croup, bronchitis, bronchiectasis, and pneumonia. Central nervous system complications are unusual, but serious. Postinfectious encephalitis, which affects 1 in 1000 children with measles, generally appears abruptly during convalescence from the primary illness. Recurrence of fever, diminished consciousness, and generalized seizures are typical of measles encephalitis. The mortality rate is as high as 20%, and about one-third of survivors are left with significant neurologic impairment.

Subacute sclerosing panencephalitis (SSPE) is an extremely rare (5–10 in 1,000,000 measles cases), progressive, degenerative late disease of the central nervous system. Measles virus has been isolated from brain tissue in some patients; all have a high titer of measles antibody in the cerebrospinal fluid. Central nervous system symptoms begin a mean of 7 years after measles. Most patients with SSPE have had measles before age 2.

Diagnosis

Measles is most often a clinical diagnosis. When the physician seeks laboratory confirmation, the easiest and most reliable means is determining acute and convalescent measles hemagglutination inhibition antibody titers. Antibody is usually detectable when the rash appears and peaks in 3–4 weeks. A fourfold rise is diagnostic. Virus can be isolated from throat washings during the prodrome and the first 1–2 days of the rash. The Centers for Disease Control and Prevention now recommends that all suspected cases of measles in the United States be confirmed in the laboratory.

Immunization

Immune serum globulin prevents or modifies measles when given at any time during the incubation period. Immune serum globulin is recommended for all susceptible measles contacts, especially infants 4–12 months old. Live attenuated measles vaccine confers long-term immunity in 95% or more of recipients. Persons with waning vaccine-induced immunity who become exposed to the virus may develop asymptomatic or mild disease. Measles vaccine is recommended for all immunocompetent persons older than 12 months; a second dose is now recommended for children aged 6 or older, teenagers, and young adults born after 1957.

RUBELLA

Rubella infects children, teenagers, and young adults. The illness is generally mild and rarely causes serious complications. The primary clinical and public health importance of rubella is pregnant women transmitting the infection to the fetus and causing chronic infection and congenital abnormalities. Once a universal disease in the United States, rubella has had a dramatic drop in incidence since the live attenuated rubella vaccine was introduced in 1969. Still, serologic surveys in several American cities show that 15–25% of persons over age 15 remain susceptible, a percentage that has not fallen substantially since the vaccine was introduced. In isolated, remote populations, susceptibility may be higher.

Clinical Features

Rubella virus is highly communicable, with respiratory transmission. Infected persons may shed rubella virus in the upper respiratory tract starting 1 week before the onset of acute illness and continuing for as long as 2 weeks afterward. About 50% of rubella infections are asymptomatic. Symptomatic infections have an incubation period of 14–18 days; then patients develop rash, fever, and mild upper respiratory tract symptoms all at once. The rash is typically salmon-pink, macular, and pruritic; it begins on the face and neck, spreads to the trunk and proximal extremities, and fades within 1–3 days. If patients have any fever, it is generally low grade. Posterior cervical and occipital adenopathy is a hallmark of rubella and may be the only symptom. Node enlargement begins as early as 7 days before the rash and peaks with onset of the rash. The occasional patient who has generalized adenopathy and splenomegaly may be given a mistaken diagnosis of infectious mononucleosis. Pharyngitis and conjunctivitis are common.

Complications

Many patients have only mild illness. Virtually everyone recovers within 3–4 days. The major complication is acute polyarthropathy, usually affecting the proximal interphalangeal joints, metacarpophalangeal joints, wrists, elbows, or knees. Some patients develop tenosynovitis or carpal tunnel syndrome. Joint symptoms usually begin during convalescence and persist for days to several weeks. The pathogenesis of the arthritis may involve immune complexes; rubella virus has been isolated from the joint fluid of patients who have developed acute arthritis after receiving live attenuated rubella virus vaccine. Rare complications of rubella are thrombocytopenic purpura, pancytopenia, orchitis, and postinfectious meningoencephalitis.

Diagnosis

The diagnosis of rubella is usually confirmed by a rise in specific humoral antibody titer. Serum antibody appears within 1–3 days of the onset of the rash and peaks 2–6 weeks later. The hemagglutination inhibition test remains the gold standard for diagnosing acute rubella. Titers lower than 1:8 are considered negative, and seroconversion to positive—a fourfold rise in titer—indicates recent rubella. Many immune persons have a negative rubella hemagglutination inhibition titer because the test is less sensitive than newer serologic methods like enzyme immunoassay (ELISA) and latex agglutination. None of the newer methods is sufficiently standardized to make a specific diagnosis of acute rubella, but they are widely used for serologic screening, for example, of pregnant women and hospital employees.

IgM antibody appears first, peaks in 2–6 weeks, and declines to undetectable levels within 6 months. IgM antibody thus indicates recent rubella infection. Rubella-specific IgM serology is especially useful in diagnosing congenital rubella syndrome in newborns. Both acquired and congenital rubella can also be diagnosed by recovering rubella virus in cell culture, but the isolation procedure is long, laborious, and not widely available.

Rubella During Pregnancy

The risk of fetal rubella infection and the risk of the infection causing congenital anomalies are both highest when the mother becomes infected during the first month of pregnancy; thereafter, both risks decline. Congenital anomalies, most often cataracts, deafness, and congenital heart disease, are detected early in life in 60% of babies born to mothers who had rubella during the first month of pregnancy. Estimates for the second month are 25–40%, and for the third month 10–30%.

Immunization

The RA 27/3 virus is the rubella vaccine strain distributed in the United States. It produces seroconversion in 95% of susceptible seronegative persons and boosts the antibody titer in previously seropositive persons with low antibody titers. RA 27/3 vaccine causes fever in 4% of seronegative recipients and rash in 10%. The vaccine's most important adverse effects are arthralgia and arthritis, which occur about as often as with natural rubella. The risk is highest among women, 15–25% of whom develop arthralgia and arthritis. The risk in men is 5–10%, and in boys and girls, 2–10%. Joint symptoms generally appear 7–21 days after vaccination, most often in the fingers, hands, wrists, and knees. Most joint pains resolve within 1 week, but they have been known to recur and persist for up to 8 years.

Rubella vaccine virus is shed in very low titers in the nasopharynx of vaccinated persons. However, studies in schools, institutions, and families have shown that susceptible contacts remain seronegative, so it is safe to immunize contacts of pregnant women. Although rubella vaccine is contraindicated for pregnant women, studies show that the vaccine virus has virtually no teratogenic potential.

Reinfection

Many persons who are immune to rubella because of either natural disease or vaccination become reinfected through exposure to natural disease or a booster dose of live virus vaccine. Reinfection is almost always asymptomatic. It produces an anamnestic humoral IgG antibody response with little or no rubella-specific IgM. Reinfection probably poses little risk to fetuses.

VARICELLA

Varicella (chickenpox) is a common acute illness characterized by fever and a vesicular rash; it principally affects children (see Color Plates). Varicella is the manifestation of primary infection with varicella zoster virus, a member of the human herpesvirus family. Reactivation of latent varicella zoster infection later in life is the cause of herpes zoster (shingles), a painful vesicular eruption that is usually limited to the dermatome innervated by a single sensory nerve (see "Herpes Zoster" below). The clinical course of both varicella and zoster worsens with older age and with cell-mediated immunodeficiency.

Seroprevalence surveys show that 50% of children in most urban areas of the United States acquire antibody to varicella zoster virus by age 6 years, and more than 95% have antibody by age 13. In the tropics and some isolated areas, over 20% of adults remain susceptible. Infection confers lifelong immunity to varicella, although many persons get subclinical reinfections. About 4% persons develop herpes zoster sometime later in life.

Varicella zoster virus is highly contagious, easily spreading from person to person among those susceptible within households and institutions such as day care centers, schools, and hospital wards. Respiratory transmission is assumed; airborne spread is well documented in hospitals. The virus can be transmitted by persons who are shedding virus (starting 1–2 days before the varicella rash appears) and persons with active herpes zoster. Persons with either varicella or zoster become less infectious as their skin lesions dry and crust.

Clinical Features

In as many as 10–20% of patients, varicella zoster is asymptomatic or mild enough to escape notice. Clinical disease follows an incubation period that normally lasts 11–21 days, but may be 30 days or less in persons who have been given varicella zoster immune globulin. In normal children, the illness begins with a low-grade fever, followed within 12–48 hours by a generalized, itchy rash. Several crops of lesions may develop over 1–5 days, usually on the trunk and sparing the limbs. Lesions begin as papules, but quickly evolve into 1–4-mm vesicles with thin red bases. Histologically, the lesions are confined to the epidermis, with some inflammatory cells extending down into the dermis. The vesicles evolve into small pustules, with polymorphonuclear cells infiltrating the vesicular fluid. Lesions crust over within 2–5 days after they appear, then quickly heal without scarring.

Often appearing at the same time as the rash is an exanthem of shallow ulcers of the oral mucous membranes. In most patients, varicella causes only mild discomfort and little limitation of activity. Secondary cases within the same household may be more severe than the index case.

Immunocompromised persons, especially patients receiving chemotherapy and recipients of organ transplants, develop high fever and a more extensive rash during varicella. Individual lesions are larger, extend deeper into the dermis, and resolve more slowly. At least 30% of immunocompromised children with varicella develop visceral involvement: hepatitis, pneumonia, encephalitis, or myocarditis. Varicella pneumonia is life-threatening, killing as many as 5–10% of immunocompromised patients who are not given varicella zoster immune globulin (VZIG) prophylaxis or treated with acyclovir.

Varicella in otherwise healthy adults may also be more

severe than in normal children, with a prodrome of fever, chills, and myalgia. Adults also have a higher rate of complications and death. A study of varicella in military personnel found that 16% had x-ray evidence of pneumonia, even though only 2–4% had symptoms suggesting lower respiratory tract involvement. Pregnancy increases the risk of varicella complications.

Complications

The most common complication of varicella in healthy children is secondary bacterial infection of the skin, most often cellulitis, impetigo, or erysipelas, caused by staphylococci or streptococci. Acute cerebellar ataxia can develop 1–3 weeks after the rash; most patients recover completely in days to weeks. About 30% of patients with acute cerebellar ataxia have a low-grade cerebrospinal fluid pleocytosis. Less common central nervous system complications are Reye's syndrome, postinfectious encephalitis, aseptic meningitis, Guillain-Barré syndrome, and transverse myelitis. Arthritis, nephritis, nephrotic syndrome, and orchitis may accompany or follow acute varicella. Hematologic complications are thrombocytopenia and epistaxis. Hemorrhagic varicella is a dreaded form of the disease, causing purpura fulminans and diffuse intravascular coagulation.

Varicella During Pregnancy

Varicella infecting a woman during the first trimester of pregnancy can cause an unusual but well-documented syndrome of congenital malformations in the fetus. Affected infants can have circumferential limb lesions, limb atrophy, eye defects, and cerebral atrophy. When the mother develops varicella during the perinatal period, the newborn risks a severe, even fatal infection.

Diagnosis

The diagnosis of varicella is usually based on a history of exposure to varicella or herpes zoster and a finding of the typical vesicular rash. Clinicians can diagnose the infection simply and quickly by scraping cells from the base of one or more lesions and applying Giemsa stain to reveal multinucleated cells and intranuclear inclusions (Tzanck prep). Varicella zoster virus may be recovered from vesicular fluid in cell culture. Acute infection can be proved serologically by at least a fourfold rise in specific varicella zoster virus antibody titer; the "gold standard" of serologic tests is the fluorescent antimembrane antibody method.

Management

Varicella in normal children requires no therapy beyond relieving the pruritus that often accompanies the rash. Children should not be given aspirin, because of its role in the development of Reye's syndrome. Adults with varicella are generally observed without treatment unless they develop signs of visceral disease. Immunocompromised patients of any age with varicella should be treated with specific antiviral therapy: Intravenous acyclovir hastens recovery and reduces the risk and severity of visceral complications.

Immunization

Varicella can be prevented by either passive or active immunization. Human varicella zoster immune globulin (VZIG) prevents or modifies infection in susceptible immunocompromised patients who receive it within 3 days after being exposed to the virus. VZIG has no effect when given late in the incubation period or after symptoms begin. VZIG recipients may remain seronegative, develop subclinical varicella zoster virus infection with seroconversion, or develop mild varicella. Active immunization with live attenuated varicella zoster virus vaccine prevents clinical varicella in about 80% of children with acute leukemia, and modifies illness in the minority who develop symptoms after exposure.

HERPES ZOSTER (SHINGLES)

Herpes zoster is an acute, painful vesicular rash resulting from reactivation of latent varicella zoster virus in a sensory nerve ganglion and infection of the dermatome innervated by the involved cranial or spinal nerve. About 10% of persons experience zoster during their lifetime; the rate of disease increases substantially with advancing age. Immunosuppressed patients and infants of mothers who had chickenpox during pregnancy are also at higher risk for zoster. Most persons have only a single episode, but about 4% of zoster cases are recurrences.

Pathogenesis

Zoster appears unilaterally in the distribution of the involved dermatome. The thoracic and lumbar nerves are commonly involved, although any sensory nerve can be affected, including the trigeminal nerve. Intense neuralgic pain may precede the rash by 1–3 days. The rash begins as clustered maculopapular lesions; these quickly coalesce and develop vesicles. Immunocompetent persons stop forming new lesions within 3–5 days, but healing may take 2–3 weeks. Postherpetic neuralgia, a troublesome complication that is most common among elderly patients, can persist for weeks to months after the rash resolves. Immunocompromised patients may continue to form new lesions within the involved dermatome for 10–14 days and may also develop extradermatomal skin lesions, disseminated cutaneous zoster (which resembles chickenpox), or involvement of the lungs, liver, or central nervous system.

Diagnosis and Management

Although zoster is readily confirmed by isolating varicella zoster virus from skin lesions or showing a boost in viral antibody, the diagnosis is usually based on the history and physical examination. Two licensed antiviral agents, acyclovir and famciclovir, are active against the virus in vitro, but are only marginally active when given orally; thus, uncomplicated zoster in normal hosts is usually managed without these expensive drugs. There is evidence that famciclovir shortens postherpetic neuralgia, so this drug may be indicated for patients at high risk, such as the elderly. Immunocompromised patients may require hospital admission and intravenous acyclovir. Corticosteroids have no role in the management of zoster. Zoster in otherwise healthy persons is not an indication to search for underlying occult disease.

SUMMARY

▶ Infectious mononucleosis, usually caused by Epstein-Barr virus, is characterized by sore throat, cervical adenopathy, splenomegaly, and atypical lymphocytosis. Management includes proscribing strenuous exercise (to minimize risk of splenic rupture), not prescribing ampicillin (because of a high incidence of rash), and recognizing uncommon complications such as severe thrombocytopenia.

▶ Measles is often a severe disease in adults. Adults born after 1957 who have not had measles or received measles vaccine should be immunized.

▶ Rubella infection in a pregnant woman can cause congenital abnormalities in her child. Another important complication of rubella in adults is a polyarthropathy that usually remits after several weeks. Pregnant women should be screened serologically for evidence of immunity.

▶ Varicella zoster virus causes chickenpox and, often after a dormant period, zoster. Important complications of zoster include dissemination (in the immunosuppressed host), eye disease, and postherpetic neuralgia.

SUGGESTED READING

Evans AS, Niederman JC, McCollum RW: Seroepidemiologic studies of infectious mononucleosis with EB virus. N Engl J Med 1968;279:1121.

Gardner P et al: Adult immunizations. Ann Intern Med 1996; 124:35.

Rubella and congenital rubella syndrome: United States, 1985–1988. Morb Mort Wkly Rep 1989;38:173.

Weller TH: Varicella and herpes zoster: Changing concepts of the natural history, control, and importance of a not-so-benign virus. N Engl J Med 1983;309:1362, 1434.

8.12

Infections of Skin, Soft Tissue, and Bone

John G. Bartlett, MD

Most patients with skin and soft tissue infections present with a lesion that is painful, red, swollen, and warm. Skin and soft tissue infections are classified as primary or secondary and as superficial or deep. Primary superficial infections include impetigo, erysipelas, cellulitis, lymphangitis, and folliculitis; the major pathogens are group A streptococci and *Staphylococcus aureus.* Secondary superficial infections result from a skin break such as a decubitus ulcer, diabetic foot ulcer, bite, burn, intravenous line, or surgical wound; a wider range of pathogens may cause these infections. Superficial infections are common and easily recognized, but management is often confounded by misunderstanding of the bacterial diagnosis and confusion over how to exclude fasciitis and myositis.

Deep soft tissue infections affect subcutaneous tissues, spreading along a fascial plane or even within the muscle it encloses. These infections are often devastating. They typically involve three types of organisms: group A streptococci, *Clostridium perfringens* or other species of clostridia, and mixed flora with aerobic and anaerobic bacteria.

Osteomyelitis (bone inflammation caused by a microbial infection) can result from hematogenous spread from any focal source of infection, but can also result from direct extension of a superficial infection.

INFECTIONS OF SKIN AND SOFT TISSUE

Pathophysiology

The skin consists of an outer layer, the epidermis, which is attached to an inner layer, the dermis (Figure 8.12–1). The epidermis lacks a vascular supply and is relatively isolated from systemic host defenses. The dermis contains lymphatic and vascular structures that provide access to immune defense mechanisms, but these structures may also facilitate the circumferential spread of lymphangitis or cellulitis. Below the dermis is the subcutaneous tissue, which contains the skin appendages, for example, sweat glands, hair follicles, sebaceous glands, and apocrine glands. Because these appendages traverse the superficial layers, they promote spread of superficial infections to the deeper layers. Most soft tissue infections are superficial, meaning that they are restricted to the dermis, subcutaneous tissue, and skin appendages. The deep fascia envelops the muscles and forms the barrier that prevents superficial infections from spreading to the muscle compartments.

Bacterial cultures of the skin show a permanent resident flora and a transient flora; total bacterial concentrations vary from 100–1,000,000/cm^2, depending on the anatomic site. The lowest counts are on exposed, cool, dry surfaces such as the extremities and face. Large concentrations are found in warm, moist areas like the anterior nares, axillae, perineum, and toe webs. The resident flora is a stable bacterial population, the major components being *Staphylococcus epidermidis, Propionibacterium acnes,* and diphtheroids. Gram-negative bacilli are found in warm, moist areas. *S aureus* is usually transient, rather than part of the resident flora. Anaerobic streptococci are not part of the normal flora.

Electron microscopy shows that bacteria inhabit the superficial two or three desquamating layers of the epidermis; deeper structures are protected by the anatomic barrier of intact dermis. Most infections result from bacteria entering directly through a breach in the cutaneous barrier, as with trauma, but pathogenic microbes can also be spread to these sites from deeper structures, for example, through the bloodstream.

It is difficult to produce soft tissue infections by placing bacteria on intact skin. Factors contributing to infection include the microbe's virulence, the inoculum size, reduced vascular supply, occlusive dressings on the skin, a foreign body, compromised host defenses, and edema disrupting lymphatic or venous drainage.

Clinical Presentation

Most infections of the skin and soft tissue are easily found by discovery of local symptoms and obvious signs of local inflammation. Most patients complain of pain at the site of the lesion. The hallmarks of inflammation are tenderness, redness, swelling, and warmth. The lesion

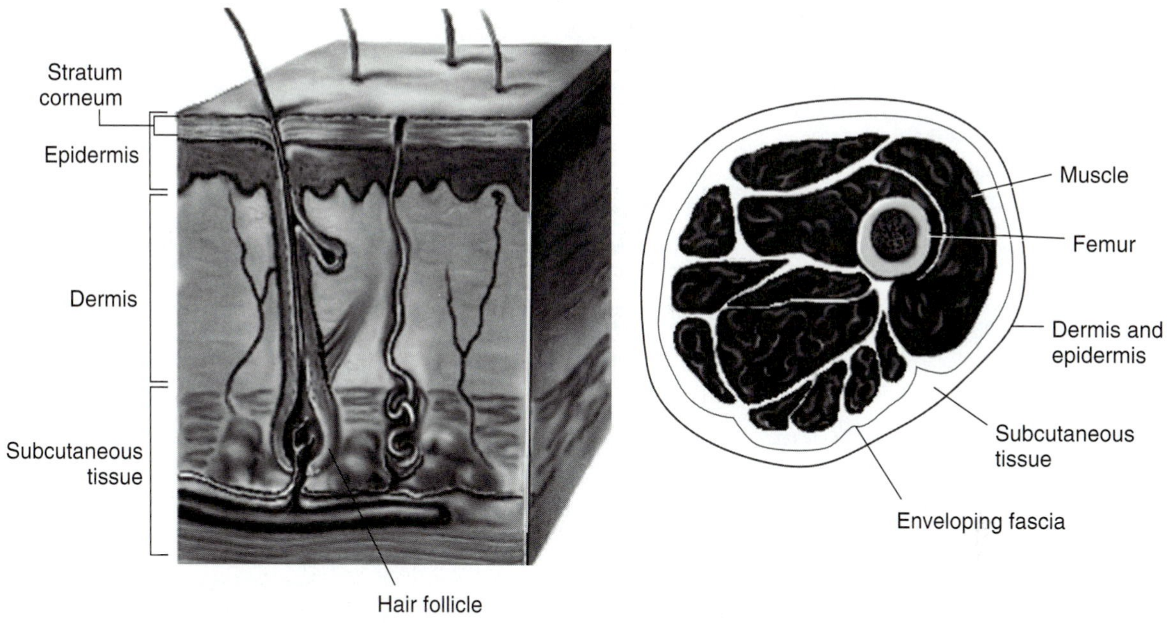

Figure 8.12–1. Cross section of skin and soft tissue, showing the planes of involvement in infections.

may drain serous or purulent fluid, which serves as an important source of material for Gram's stain and culture. Systemic signs of infection—fever, malaise, and leukocytosis—depend on the type and severity of the process.

In the differential diagnosis, the physician must distinguish dermal infections from primary dermatologic conditions and must differentiate primary infection of the skin or soft tissue from systemic infection with skin involvement. Dermatologic conditions are generally confined to the skin, often involve noncontiguous areas, and are less likely to be accompanied by systemic signs. Most patients who have a systemic infection with cutaneous involvement have disease in multiple organ systems plus constitutional signs such as fever and leukocytosis. Most primary infections of the skin and soft tissue are confined to a focal area and may or may not be accompanied by constitutional signs.

Microbial Diagnosis

Most skin and soft tissue infections are caused by bacteria. Cultures must distinguish pathogens from contaminants, as determined by the method used to obtain specimens, the organisms recovered, the number of organisms recovered, and correlation with direct Gram's stain. Virtually all bacterial infections of the skin and other anatomic sites involve more than 100,000 bacteria/mL of secretion or gram of tissue from biopsy. Most laboratories do not perform quantitative bacteriology, but they do report semiquantitative culture results as light, moderate, or heavy growth.

The major organisms that can cause infection at low concentrations are group A streptococci, possibly because they do much of their damage through their microbial products or toxins traversing the tissue. About the only time that *S epidermidis, P acnes,* and diphtheroids cause soft tissue infections is when a patient has an intravenous line. Cultures of open ulcers virtually always yield bacteria, but because they are part of the normal surface flora, they are not necessarily pathogenic. It is important to prepare the culture site with antiseptics; aspirates or biopsy specimens taken without surface contamination are more likely to identify true pathogens.

Superficial Soft Tissue Infections

Primary Superficial Infections:

Impetigo: This superficial infection of the skin is usually caused by group A β-hemolytic streptococci, although many patients also have *S aureus* (Table 8.12–1). Impetigo is a communicable infection, with spread from person to person often facilitated by crowding and poor hygiene. Most patients are children. The infection is restricted to the epidermis and does not produce a systemic response of fever or leukocytosis. The usual treatment is an oral cephalosporin or a penicillinase-resistant penicillin.

Erysipelas: This is a superficial infection with prominent involvement of lymphatics. The usual cause is group A β-hemolytic streptococci, but again occasional cases are caused by *S aureus* or other streptococci, such as group B, C, or G. The lesion is bright red and indurated, with a highly characteristic elevated, sharply demarcated border. Patients have fever and leukocytosis. The putative agent is

Table 8.12–1. Primary superficial soft tissue infections.

Disorder	Organism	Usual Host or Site	Clinical Features
Impetigo	*Streptococcus pyogenes* (also *Staphylococcus aureus;* group B, C, or G streptococci)	Children; exposed areas of the body; sometimes epidemic	Painless vesicles with red halos, progressing to painless pustules and crusted lesions
Bullous impetigo	*S aureus*	Newborn and young children	Vesicles, progressing to flaccid bullae
Erysipelas	*S pyogenes* (also group B, C, or G streptococci; *S aureus*)	Young children, older adults; predisposition in areas of lymphatic obstruction or edema	Painful, red, edematous, indurated, raised lesions with sharply demarcated margins; often, fever and leukocytosis
Lymphangitis	*S pyogenes* (also *S aureus*)	Extremity	Red streak with regional adenopathy
Cellulitis	*S pyogenes, S aureus,* others	Sometimes areas of prior trauma or ulceration	Painful, tender redness with no elevation or sharp demarcation; variable systemic signs
Folliculitis	*S aureus* (also *Pseudomonas aeruginosa, Candida albicans*)	Any area with hair follicles; areas exposed in swimming pool or whirlpool (*P aeruginosa*)	Small red papules with central pustule; no systemic signs
Furunculosis, furuncle	*S aureus*	Areas of friction, sweat, and hair follicles: neck, face, axillae, buttocks	Firm red nodule, progressing to fluctuant, painful mass with spontaneous drainage; sometimes fever and leukocytosis
Carbuncle	*S aureus*	Patients with diabetes mellitus; most often posterior neck, back, thigh	Multiple abscesses, connecting in subcutaneous tissue and draining along hair follicles
Paronychia	*S aureus, S pyogenes, P aeruginosa, Candida*	Frequent hand immersion; nail fold	Periungual redness and swelling, with separation of nail fold from nail plate

often difficult to recover. The usual treatment is intravenous penicillin or clindamycin.

Lymphangitis: Acute lymphangitis produces straight red streaks that extend from the site of infection or portal of entry to regional lymph nodes that are enlarged and tender. Most acute lymphangitis is caused by group A β-hemolytic streptococci and is treated with penicillin or erythromycin. Other forms include rat-bite fever, caused by either *Spirillum minus* or *Streptobacillus moniliformis,* and filariasis, caused by *Wuchereria bancrofti* and usually contracted during travel to Africa, South America, or southeast Asia. Chronic lymphangitis, developing over weeks, is a much more subtle process caused by *Sporothrix schenckii, Mycobacterium marinum, Mycobacterium kansasii,* filariasis, or *Nocardia.*

Cellulitis: This is a common form of a spreading infection involving the dermis and subcutaneous tissue. Cellulitis sometimes follows local trauma or superficial ulceration that breaks the cutaneous barrier. There may be no clear portal of entry, especially in patients with alcoholism, obesity, or edema. Typical findings are tenderness, redness, warmth, and edema. In advanced cellulitis, the skin lesion is not sharply demarcated and systemic symptoms are variable. Multiple organisms have been implicated, but the most common are *S aureus* and group A streptococci. It is often very difficult to recover the responsible microbe, even with deep aspiration of the skin or biopsies of the lesion. The usual treatment is a cephalosporin, a penicillinase-resistant penicillin (nafcillin or oxacillin), or clindamycin.

Abscesses: Subcutaneous abscesses are purulent collections within a closed space. *S aureus* is implicated in 25–50% of patients and is the major pathogen in abscesses above the waist. When *S aureus* is found, it is usually the sole organism and is readily apparent on Gram's stain and culture. Anaerobic bacteria are the dominant organisms in subcutaneous abscesses below the waist, such as infected sebaceous cysts and pilonidal cysts. In infections involving anaerobes, the pus is often putrid and the Gram's stain shows mixed flora. Whatever the microbial pattern, patients present with pain, swelling, tenderness, and redness at the infected site, sometimes with spontaneous drainage. Mature lesions are fluctuant (pus-filled), well-encapsulated, and amenable to surgical incision and drainage. Severe infections are usually treated with a cephalosporin, nafcillin, oxacillin, or clindamycin.

Most subcutaneous abscesses are hair follicle infections: folliculitis, furunculosis, and carbuncles. These infections develop at sites subject to sweating and friction, such as the face, neck, axillae, and buttocks. Folliculitis, an infection restricted to hair follicles, manifests as multiple red papules. Furunculosis is a more extensive infection, with red, firm, painful nodules that become fluctuant and may drain. A carbuncle is a confluent infection characterized by extensive penetration into the subcutaneous tissue, with a large abscess that presents as a tender mass, sometimes with multiple draining sites. Contributing to the development of hair follicle infections are obesity, neutropenia, poor hygiene, seborrhea, corticosteroid therapy, occlusive dressings, trauma, and diabetes mellitus. These lesions require surgical drainage and intravenous antibiotics such as nafcillin, oxacillin, or a cephalosporin.

Exposure may also be important. Epidemics have been reported, for example, folliculitis spread through swimming pools or whirlpools. These infections characteristically involve *Pseudomonas aeruginosa.* The usual treatment is warm compresses and hygienic soap.

Infections Secondary to Preexisting Cutaneous Lesions: These infections are complications of a previous insult, generally an obvious breach in the mucocutaneous barrier, as from trauma or surgery (Table 8.12–2).

Infected ulcers: Decubitus ulcers, diabetic foot ulcers, and ischemic ulcers are susceptible to invasion by bacteria, usually flora of the skin or colon. Characteristic clinical features can be pain and tenderness (which are blunted in patients with neurotrophic ulcers), purulent drainage, and a systemic response of fever and leukocytosis. A common complication of chronically infected ulcers, especially those close to bone, is osteomyelitis. Occasional patients develop bacteremia.

Contributing to the pathogenesis of infected ulcers is loss of the cutaneous integrity that acts as a mechanical barrier to infection. Other factors are vascular insufficiency and accompanying neuropathy. Many diabetic patients have such severe neuropathy that they are unaware of their infection until it is well advanced.

A minority of patients are infected with a single microbe, which is usually *S aureus* or a group A streptococcus. Most patients have a polymicrobial infection

dominated by coliforms, streptococci, and anaerobes. Single-microbe infections can be easily distinguished from polymicrobial infections by Gram's stain of purulent exudate. Culture results must be interpreted cautiously: Because open lesions always harbor resident flora, the physician must differentiate pathogens from contaminants or colonizing bacteria, using as criteria the microbe's virulence, the relative concentrations of bacteria, and the infection's clinical features. Group A streptococci tend to cause spreading infections that often reach regional lymph nodes and do not tend to form abscesses. Although *S aureus,* too, can cause cellulitis, this organism is more likely to cause focal infection. Many mixed aerobic-anaerobic abscesses have a putrid discharge and a chronic course. The most important management issues are the need for débridement, decisions about adequacy of vascular supply and the role of vascular surgery with large-vessel disease, avoidance of pressure, and the role of antibiotics. In general, antibiotics are recommended for patients with systemic signs of infection (fever, leukocytosis), extensive cellulitis, regional adenopathy, or complications such as osteomyelitis. Commonly given are cefoxitin, ciprofloxacin plus metronidazole, or regimens used in intra-abdominal sepsis (Chapter 8.7).

Bites: Infected bites can be similar to other soft tissue infections resulting from trauma. The pathogens come from either the oral flora of the biter species or from the patient's adjacent skin flora that has entered the breach in the cutaneous barrier. With human bites, the major pathogens are *Eikenella corrodens* and anaerobic bacteria, especially *Prevotella melaninogenica,* fusobacteria, and

Table 8.12–2. Infections secondary to preexisting cutaneous lesions.

Lesion or Setting	Major Pathogens
Bites by humans, dogs, cats	Oral anaerobes, *Staphylococcus aureus, Pasteurella multocida*
Burns	*Pseudomonas aeruginosa* and other gram-negative bacilli, *Streptococcus pyogenes* and other streptococci, *S aureus, Candida, Aspergillus*
Decubitus ulcers	Usually polymicrobial: coliforms, *P aeruginosa,* anaerobes (*Bacteroides fragilis,* clostridia), streptococci, *S aureus*
Diabetic foot ulcers	Usually polymicrobial: coliforms, *P aeruginosa,* anaerobes, streptococci, *S aureus*
Vascular gangrene	*S aureus,* coliforms, anaerobes, streptococci
Sebaceous cysts	Anaerobic bacteria
Pilonidal cysts	Anaerobic bacteria
Dermatologic conditions with secondary infection: eczema, dermatophytes, acne, vesicular or bullous lesions	*S pyogenes, S aureus* (lesions in perineum, groin, buttocks: colonic flora with coliforms and anaerobes)
Intertrigo	*S aureus,* coliforms, *Candida*
Cutaneous surgical wounds Clean surgery Clean-contaminated or dirty surgery Colon Pelvic Biliary tract Gastroduodenal Trauma	*S aureus, S pyogenes* Usually polymicrobial: anaerobes, coliforms, streptococci Usually polymicrobial: anaerobes, coliforms, streptococci Coliforms, clostridia, streptococci Coliforms, streptococci *S aureus, S pyogenes,* clostridia
Intravenous infusion sites	*S aureus,* coliforms, *P aeruginosa, Staphylococcus epidermidis, Candida*

anaerobic or microaerophilic streptococci. A variant of this lesion is the "clenched fist injury," an infection that the patient develops over the knuckles after punching an opponent's teeth. Effective treatment is amoxicillin-clavulanate or clindamycin. With dog and cat bites, the most common pathogen is *Pasteurella multocida,* a small gram-negative coccobacillus found in the mouths of virtually all cats, most dogs, and many rodents. The usual lesion is red, with edema, central ulceration, and a seropurulent discharge. The patient may have spreading cellulitis, lymphangitis, lymphadenopathy, abscess formation, or osteomyelitis. The drug of choice is penicillin.

Another consequence of animal bites can be cat-scratch disease (Chapter 8.16), caused by *Bartonella henselae* or *Bartonella quintana* (formerly *Rochalimaea henselae* and *Rochalimaea quintana*). As suggested by the name, this infection is most often caused by a cat scratch or bite or simply by exposure to cats. The first lesion is a red papule, followed 10–14 days later by tender regional adenopathy, which usually regresses spontaneously within 6 weeks. Cat-scratch disease is usually not treated with antibiotics.

Rat-bite fever is an acute febrile illness caused by *Streptobacillus moniliformis* or *Spirillum minus* after the bite of a rat, mouse, or other rodent (Chapter 8.16). *S moniliformis* is a pleomorphic gram-negative bacillus that may be recovered from blood, abscesses, or joint fluid. After a 5–10-day incubation, this organism causes a systemic illness with relapsing fever and a generalized morbilliform (measles-like) or petechial rash. *S minus* is a spirochete that may be detected by darkfield examination of exudate from the infected site. This organism, too, causes relapsing fever with a generalized rash, but the incubation period is 7–21 days and the bite site usually shows suppuration, ulceration, lymphangitis, and local adenopathy. Both forms of rat-bite fever are treated with penicillin.

Burns: Sepsis is the major cause of death in patients with thermal injury. Cutaneous burn wound infections may be superficial, but they may be deep and severe, with "burn wound sepsis." Full-thickness burns (burns that involve all layers of the skin) are complicated by vascular occlusion that persists for 2–3 weeks before circulation is restored. The result is coagulation necrosis with large accumulations of nonviable tissue, the "burn eschar" that provides a highly susceptible culture medium for microbial invasion. Surface bacteria are destroyed with the original injury, but the wound becomes colonized within 48 hours.

Burn wound isolates represent both the patient's endogenous flora and the hospital flora. Major pathogens during the first 2 days are gram-positive bacteria, especially group A streptococci, less often *S aureus.* By the third day, gram-negative bacteria appear, and the major pathogens of late infections are *P aeruginosa, Providencia stuartii, Enterobacter cloacae, Serratia marcescens,* and *Klebsiella* sp. These organisms proliferate in the eschar and are likely to invade the underlying subcutaneous tissue before the eschar separates with autografting by granulation tissue. Less common pathogens are fungi (*Candida* sp, *Aspergillus, Mucor,* and *Geotrichum*) and herpes simplex virus. Efforts to reduce infections include the use of topical antibiotics.

The signs of burn wound sepsis tend to appear late, and there may be minimal findings at the burn site. Patients most often present with altered mental status, tachycardia, tachypnea, fever or hypothermia, thrombocytopenia, leukocytosis or leukopenia, and hypotension. Evaluation should include blood cultures and cultures of the burn site, preferably from a biopsy with quantitative or semiquantitative cultures. The results of these cultures are used to select antibiotics.

Infections associated with intravenous lines: Metal and plastic devices placed percutaneously provide access to the vascular circulation, but these lines are also prone to infections because of the break in the cutaneous barrier, direct access to the vascular circulation, and the presence of a foreign body, which always promotes infection. Risk of infection increases with prolonged use, placement by cutdown rather than percutaneous puncture, and use of plastic catheters instead of needles. Lines (eg, Hickman catheter) inserted by tunneling through subcutaneous tissue require meticulous placement and care, since they are usually left in place for prolonged periods.

Patients on intravenous therapy develop three major types of infections. The major pathogens for all three types are the patient's skin flora, primarily *S aureus* and *S epidermidis.* Less common pathogens are *P aeruginosa,* other gram-negative bacteria, and *Candida* species.

The most common complication of intravenous therapy is occult infection at the infusion site. Patients have positive blood cultures but no local evidence of infection. The diagnosis is supported by recovery of the same organism from the blood as from the intravenous cannula and by inability to find any other likely portal of entry. The standard way to evaluate the catheter as a source of infection is to remove it, sever its distal segment, and roll the segment on microbiology media; 15 colonies of bacteria are the criterion for an infected line.

The second most common intravenous line infection is local. The skin is red and tender, often with purulent drainage at the needle insertion site. But the same picture can also indicate mechanical or chemical irritation without infection, and many of the drugs infused are common causes of "chemical phlebitis."

The least common infection, suppurative thrombophlebitis, often presents with similar findings at the needle insertion site, but there is suppuration within the vessel lumen or wall and purulent exudate may be expressed. Many patients have a palpable cord and persistent or refractory bacteremia. The main difference between suppurative thrombophlebitis and the uncomplicated focal infection previously described is that suppurative thrombophlebitis is characterized by abscesses within the vessel wall. This complication is rare but important to recognize because it necessitates excision of the vein.

Surgical wounds: The risk of surgical wound infection depends primarily on whether the surgery is clean, clean–contaminated, contaminated, or dirty. Clean surgery is defined as an operation involving sterile body sites that have no inflammation. Clean–contaminated surgery is an operation in which the surgeon enters the respiratory tract or gastrointestinal tract but does not spill a significant amount of its contents. Contaminated surgery is an operation in which sites have inflammation but no pus or in which significant amounts of material spill from the respiratory or gastrointestinal tract. Dirty surgery involves pus or a perforated viscus.

As expected, the risk of wound infection increases as surgery becomes more contaminated. The rate is less than 1% with clean surgery and 15–20% with contaminated surgery. Other factors that influence the frequency of wound infection include obesity, surgical technique, duration of surgery, method used to prepare the incision site (shaved sites have higher rates of infection), and use of prophylactic antibiotics. In general, prophylactic antibiotics are not recommended for clean surgery, since the incidence of infection is so low and the risk of drug side effects outweighs the potential benefits. In contrast, many patients who are to undergo contaminated surgery are given prophylactic antibiotics directed against the flora at the site.

Wound infections are easily recognized by the local signs of inflammation—redness, induration, and tenderness, often with purulent discharge. Patients may also have fever and leukocytosis. The etiologic diagnosis is readily established by Gram's stain and culture of exudate from the wound. Most infections from clean surgery are caused by *S aureus*. Most infections from contaminated surgery reflect the flora at the site, usually a mixture of aerobic and anaerobic bacteria. *S aureus* usually originates from the patient's skin, but this and other bacteria can be spread by "horizontal transmission," that is, transmission by health care workers as they move from patient to patient without wearing gloves or adequately washing their hands. Most wound infections can be successfully treated by suture removal and local débridement; most patients with severe infections are also given systemic antibiotics.

Deep and Devastating Primary Soft Tissue Infections

Beneath the subcutaneous tissue lies the fascia. The fascia envelops muscle, creating a formidable barrier to penetration. "Deep and devastating" soft tissue infections are deep because they involve the fascial plane, the contents of the fascia (compartment infections or myonecrosis), or both, and devastating because they cause substantial morbidity and mortality. These infections are not common, but they are important to recognize because of their potential severity and because they are diagnosed and treated differently from superficial soft tissue infections.

Deep and devastating infections are classified by the pathogen, the involved tissue plane, characteristics of the clinical presentation, or a combination of these factors. The simplest classification distinguishes two sites, fascia and muscle compartment, and how they are affected by three types of bacteria—clostridia, streptococci (classically group A, but other groups as well), and mixed aerobes and anaerobes (Table 8.12–3).

Diagnosis: Five major clinical features suggest deep and devastating soft tissue infections:

1. Severe pain that is usually spontaneous, that is, severe even without manipulation.
2. Bullous lesions. When infection occludes deep vessels that traverse the fascia or muscle compartment, cutaneous necrosis can lead to bullae. But bullous lesions can also be found in patients with erysipelas, some forms of cellulitis, some disseminated infections (eg, meningococcemia, purpura fulminans, erythema gangrenosum, toxic shock syndrome, disseminated intravascular coagulation), some toxins (eg, brown recluse spider bites), and some primary dermatologic conditions, such as pyoderma gangrenosum.
3. Gas in the soft tissue. Gas can often be detected by palpation (crepitation), x-ray, or scanning. The gases, volatile acids produced by anaerobic bacteria, probably account for the characteristic putrid odor of these infections.
4. Systemic toxicity, manifested by, for example, fever, leukocytosis, delirium, and renal failure.
5. Rapid spread, generally along the fascial plane. The borders of the infection can advance as much as 1–2 cm/hour.

The clinician who suspects a deep and devastating soft tissue infection based on the patient's presentation must quickly confirm and localize it, usually with computed tomography (CT) or magnetic resonance imaging (MRI).

Types:

Fasciitis: Necrotizing fasciitis is a deep infection that spreads along the fascial cleft between the subcutaneous tissue and the deep fascia. A portal of entry may be provided by a break in the skin, as from a drug injection,

Table 8.12–3. Deep and devastating soft tissue infections: Anatomic patterns of pathogens.

Bacteria	Anatomic Pattern	
	Fasciitis	Muscle Compartment Infection
Clostridia	Crepitant cellulitis	Gas gangrene
Streptococci	Streptococcal gangrene	Streptococcal myonecrosis
Mixed aerobic and anaerobic bacteria	Necrotizing fasciitis	Necrotizing synergistic cellulitis

decubitus ulcer, diabetic foot ulcer, enterostomy, or perirectal abscess. Some patients have no apparent predisposing lesion. More than 50% of patients with necrotizing fasciitis have diabetes mellitus.

The more common form of necrotizing fasciitis is caused by mixtures of coliforms, streptococci, and anaerobes. The less common form is caused by streptococci, especially group A; toxins produced by these streptococci can cause toxic shock syndrome, a life-threatening condition with shock and multiple organ failure. The two types of pathogens can be easily distinguished by the putrid discharge and gas formation that are characteristic of anaerobic infections, and by Gram's stain of exudate. The diagnosis is suspected in patients who have serious soft tissue infections, generally with regional swelling, severe local pain, and rapid spread. The diagnosis is established by a CT or MRI scan that shows an exudate extending along the fascial plane or by surgery that reveals exudate extending along the fascial plane and permitting passage of a probe.

Compartment infections: These are infections within muscle. There are four microbial patterns: clostridial infections, streptococcal infections, mixed infections involving aerobes and anaerobes, and muscle abscesses, usually caused by *S aureus.*

Clostridial myonecrosis (gas gangrene) is a devastating infection that usually follows trauma or surgery and is characterized by myonecrosis and profound systemic toxicity. The most common clinical settings are a traumatic injury or penetrating wound; surgery, especially of the intestines or biliary tract; uterine gas gangrene, usually following septic abortion; soft tissue infections associated with vascular insufficiency; intestinal gas gangrene, usually found in patients with leukemia, neutropenia, or colon cancer; and, most rarely, spontaneous gas gangrene.

The first symptom is sudden, severe pain at the site of injury. The skin is first pale, then turns magenta or bronze, often with necrosis and hemorrhagic bullae. The tempo of disease varies, but in many patients it progresses over hours or days to hemolytic anemia, hypotension, and renal failure. Systemic toxicity is ascribed to exotoxins produced by clostridia. The most serious is alpha toxin, a phospholipase that destroys cell membranes, alters capillary permeability, and causes severe hemolysis.

The clostridium most often implicated in gas gangrene is *C perfringens.* This organism is found in nearly all soil samples and is usually part of the normal colonic flora. Although an estimated 30–80% of serious traumatic wounds are contaminated with *C perfringens* spores, the frequency of gas gangrene is very low. Local factors that seem to increase the risk are poor vascular supply, foreign bodies, and concurrent infections. Patients are managed with amputation and penicillin.

Streptococcal myonecrosis resembles gas gangrene except that the tempo of the disease is less fulminant, local pain is not prominent in the early stages, soft tissue gas is uncommon, and Gram's stain of exudate shows polymorphonuclear cells and gram-positive cocci in chains. Like patients with clostridial myonecrosis, those with streptococcal myonecrosis may develop shock and multiple organ failure, but the cause is the toxins produced by group A streptococci.

The most common muscle infection is caused by a combination of aerobic and anaerobic bacteria and is sometimes called *synergistic necrotizing cellulitis.* This condition is similar to necrotizing fasciitis involving a mixed flora, but the infection has extended beneath the fascia to involve muscle. Most patients have diabetes, many are obese, and many have had renal failure. The usual sites of involvement are the perirectal area and legs. Common clinical features are bullous skin lesions, severe pain, and gas in the soft tissue. The diagnosis is established by the characteristic clinical features, CT or MRI showing myonecrosis with or without fasciitis, analysis of aspirates from the lesion, or surgical exploration. Aspirates typically show "dishwater pus," a thin, grayish fluid with an extremely putrid odor; Gram's stains and culture show a combination of coliforms, streptococci, and anaerobes. Treatment is surgical débridement combined with antibiotics directed against the fecal flora.

Pyomyositis is not really a devastating soft tissue infection but is important to recognize. This focal purulent collection within muscle is almost always caused by *S aureus.* The infection is uncommon in industrialized countries, but common in the tropics, where it is called "tropical pyomyositis" (Chapter 13.12). Most patients present with the insidious onset of pain, swelling, and tenderness, usually involving a single muscle group of a leg or the trunk, for example, a psoas abscess. CT scan with contrast or MRI scan readily demonstrates the lesion, and needle aspirate of the purulent collection usually shows *S aureus* on Gram's stain and culture. Treatment is drainage combined with antibiotics directed against *S aureus,* such as nafcillin, oxacillin, a cephalosporin, or vancomycin.

OSTEOMYELITIS

Infections of bone are classified in three major groups: osteomyelitis caused by hematogenous spread of infection, osteomyelitis secondary to a contiguous focus of infection, and osteomyelitis associated with vascular insufficiency (Table 8.12–4).

Types

Hematogenous Spread: Hematogenous osteomyelitis accounts for about 20% of all bone infections. It is classically described as a disease of children, in whom it usually involves the metaphysis of long bones, especially the femur or tibia. The relatively high incidence during growth seems to reflect particular susceptibility of the vascular network of the metaphysis. At least one-third of patients have a history of blunt trauma to the involved area. The infection starts in the metaphysial sinusoidal

Table 8.12–4. Types of osteomyelitis.

	Hematogenous	Secondary to Contiguous Infection	Complication of Vascular Insufficiency
% of all cases	20%	50%	30%
Age	1–16 yr and >50 yr	>40 yr	>50 yr
Bones involved	Long bones in children, vertebrae in adults	Hip, femur, tibia	Feet
Predisposing causes	Trauma, bacteremia	Surgery, soft tissue infection	Diabetes mellitus, vascular insufficiency
Major bacteria	*Staphylococcus aureus,* gram-negative bacilli	Often polymicrobial: *S aureus,* gram-negative bacilli	Usually polymicrobial: gram-negative bacilli, anaerobes, streptococci, *S aureus*
Presentation First episode Recurrence	Fever, local pain, swelling, tenderness, limited movement Sinus drainage ± pain	Fever, local pain, swelling, tenderness, limited movement Sinus drainage ± pain	Ulceration, drainage ± pain

veins. It is contained by the epiphyseal growth plate and tends to spread laterally, perforating the cortex and lifting the loose periosteum.

Hematogenous osteomyelitis involving long bones is rare in adults, and adults' long bone infections present differently from those in children. Because adults' growth cartilage has been resorbed, the subarticular space is more vulnerable; because the periosteum is firmly attached, subperiosteal abscesses are less likely to form.

In adults, especially those over age 50, the most common form of hematogenous osteomyelitis affects the vertebrae. The first site of infection is the richly vascularized bone adjacent to the cartilage. Eventually, involvement extends to adjacent bone plates and the intervening intervertebral disks of the thoracolumbar, lumbar, or lumbosacral spine. The infection may extend longitudinally to involve other vertebrae, anteriorly to cause a paraspinal abscess, or posteriorly to form an epidural abscess. Epidural abscess is considered a serious complication because it can lead to meningitis or to cord compression with paraplegia. In only about 50% of patients with vertebral osteomyelitis can a likely primary source for hematogenous dissemination be found. The most common sources are the genitourinary tract, skin, and respiratory tract.

S aureus is implicated in 50–70% of cases of hematogenous osteomyelitis. Enterobacteriaceae account for 20–30% of cases and are more common in adults than in children. Other organisms also may be involved. *P aeruginosa* is unusual, except in drug addicts or after penetrating trauma of the foot.

The classic presentation of acute hematogenous osteomyelitis is a precipitous onset of pain, swelling, chills, and fever. The usual symptoms of vertebral osteomyelitis are fever, back pain, and stiffness. Many patients have a less acute form, with vague symptoms for 1–2 months before they seek medical help. These patients have few constitutional complaints; the dominant symptom is local pain.

Many patients with recurrent or chronic osteomyelitis report the recurrence merely as increased drainage and pain at the same site as before. One well-described variant of chronic osteomyelitis, seen primarily in young adults, is Brodie's abscess, a subacute pyogenic osteomyelitis affecting the metaphysis of long bones and usually caused by *S aureus.* The major symptom is local pain without fever.

Contiguous Spread: Osteomyelitis secondary to a contiguous focus of infection accounts for about 50% of all cases. Most patients are over 40 years old. The most common precipitating factor is surgery, especially open reduction of fractures involving the hip, femoral shaft, or tibial shaft. The next most common source is a soft tissue infection involving the fingers or toes. Less common associated conditions include craniotomy, disk surgery, infected teeth, and radiation therapy for malignant tumors, especially of the mandible. Contiguous-spread infections usually become apparent within 1 month of the precipitating event, although many patients have chronic or recurrent infections that may be seen years or even decades later. The most common pathogen is *S aureus,* followed by Enterobacteriaceae, *P aeruginosa,* and streptococci. Many of these infections, especially those not caused by *S aureus,* involve multiple bacteria. Most infections developing from decubitus ulcers and diabetic foot ulcers involve a polymicrobial flora, including both coliforms and anaerobes.

Vascular Insufficiency: Osteomyelitis associated with vascular insufficiency accounts for about one-third of all cases. Most patients have diabetes or severe atherosclerosis and most are over 50 years old. The major site of infection is the toes or small bones of the feet. Patients present with draining ulcers, with or without pain. These infections usually involve multiple bacteria, including Enterobacteriaceae, *S aureus,* anaerobes, and streptococci.

Diagnosis and Management

The most important tests for osteomyelitis are x-rays or radionuclide studies to prove bone involvement, and cultures to identify the pathogen. The first radiographic changes, lytic lesions, become visible only 10–14 days into the course. New bone forms slowly, so it is not detected on x-ray for at least 1 month. Technetium and gallium scans are positive as early as 3 days after symptoms appear, but they do not differentiate cellulitis from osteomyelitis. One of the most reliable signs of osteomyelitis associated with ulcers is bone felt during a probing of the wound.

Conclusive bacteriologic studies require isolating the pathogen from either the bone lesion or blood cultures. Blood cultures are positive in about half of patients with acute untreated hematogenous osteomyelitis. Direct bone aspiration yields positive cultures in about 60% of patients, and surgical biopsy in about 90%. Cultures from draining sinus tracts correlate poorly with cultures obtained directly from bone, especially when organisms other than *S aureus* are recovered. Thus, the preferred test is bone biopsy or deep aspiration; cultures of wound drainage must be interpreted with caution.

Most patients with acute osteomyelitis respond to systemic antibiotics given for 4–6 weeks. Chronic osteomyelitis is much more challenging to treat because of the frequent number of relapses. The keys to management are surgical removal of sequestra and any associated foreign bodies (such as prosthetic devices), and prolonged antibiotics directed against implicated bacteria.

SUMMARY

▶ Superficial infections of the skin and soft tissue classically involve two types of microbes: group A streptococci and *Staphylococcus aureus.* Major superficial infections, which are differentiated by their clinical features, are impetigo, erysipelas, lymphangitis, furunculosis, and cellulitis.

▶ Bacteria involved in classic deep soft tissue infections are clostridia, group A streptococci, and mixed aerobes and anaerobes. Deep soft tissue infections affect fascia (fasciitis) and muscle (myositis).

▶ Superficial infections are treated primarily with antibiotics. Deep infections are treated primarily with surgery.

▶ Osteomyelitis results from hematogenous or contiguous spread of infection, or from vascular insufficiency.

SUGGESTED READING

Bisno AL, Stevens DL: Streptococcal infections of skin and soft tissues. N Engl J Med 1996;334:240.

MacLennan JD: The histotoxic clostridial infections of man. Bacteriol Rev 1962;26:177.

Smith JW, Piercy EA: Infectious arthritis. Clin Infect Dis 1995; 20:225.

Stone HH, Martin JD Jr: Synergistic necrotizing cellulitis. Ann Surg 1972;175:702.

Swartz MN: Section on Skin and Soft Tissue Infections. In: *Principles and Practice of Infectious Diseases,* 4th ed. Mandell GL, Bennett JE, Dolin R (editors). Churchill Livingstone, 1995.

Waldvogel FA, Vasey H: Osteomyelitis: The past decade. N Engl J Med 1980;303:360.

8.13

Fungal Infections

John G. Bartlett, MD

Fungal infections are sometimes referred to as "mycoses" or "mycotic infections." Fungal infections show an enormous range of presentations, from minor vaginal candidiasis or athlete's foot to life-threatening aspergillosis in a patient with a bone marrow transplant. The variability in presentations results from the differing virulence of fungi and the host's immune status (see below). Although some fungi are important pathogens for normal persons, most serious fungal infections affect immunocompromised hosts. In fact, fungal infections are among the leading causes of serious complications in persons with AIDS, organ transplant recipients, and patients receiving cancer chemotherapy. Improving the outcome for these patients requires early recognition, diagnosis, and treatment of the mycotic infection. Better yet is prevention: This is now becoming standard practice in selected patient groups.

The diagnosis and treatment of fungal infections are especially challenging. Unlike bacterial infections, most serious fungal infections develop insidiously, and most require specialized laboratory techniques to establish the diagnosis. Also unlike bacterial infections, for which there are usually several safe, effective treatments, therapy for serious fungal infections commonly comes down to one or two choices.

CLASSIFICATION

Most fungi are widely distributed in nature, primarily in soil and organic debris. The most convenient way to classify fungi is as pathogenic or opportunistic (Table 8.13–1). Pathogenic fungi can infect the healthy host. They include *Histoplasma capsulatum, Coccidioides immitis,* and *Blastomyces dermatitidis.* In general, opportunistic fungal infections are found only in the compromised host and primarily in the host with specific immune defects such as neutropenia or defective cell-mediated immunity. A third category of fungi, not discussed in this chapter, is the dermatophytic fungi that cause infections confined to the skin, hair, and nails.

Fungi differ from bacteria in being eukaryotic and in reproducing sexually or asexually. Many fungi are biphasic, having one form in nature and another at body temperature in the infected person.

Pathogenic Fungi

All three pathogenic fungi first infect the respiratory tract through inhalation. The response to this challenge is variable and is at least somewhat influenced by host immune defenses. Most normal persons remain asymptomatic, but some develop a flu-like illness, and occasional patients develop severe pulmonary disease or disseminated infection. Severe disease, especially disseminated disease, is most common in persons who have compromised cell-mediated immunity or another condition that impairs host defenses.

Opportunistic Fungi

The healthy host rarely becomes infected through contact with opportunistic fungi, simply because normal host defenses are sufficient, regardless of the inoculum size. Specific risk factors dictate the pathogenic potential of individual fungi: Neutropenia predisposes to infections with *Aspergillus* and *Candida,* while defective cell-mediated immunity predisposes to infections with *Candida, Aspergillus, Phycomycetes,* and *Cryptococcus.* Examples of conditions impairing cell-mediated immunity are corticosteroid therapy, AIDS, cancer, chemotherapy, and lymphomas. Antibiotics predispose to *Candida* infections, especially thrush and *Candida* vaginitis.

PATHOPHYSIOLOGY

Fungal infections may be classified as localized or disseminated. Localized infections are restricted to the site of entry, usually the lung, where they cause acute or chronic pulmonary disease. Disseminated infections involve distant sites, which usually reflect widespread hematogenous spread. Disseminated infections may in-

Table 8.13–1. Comparison of pathogenic and opportunistic fungal infections.

	Pathogenic Fungi	Opportunistic Fungi
Examples	Histoplasmosis Blastomycosis Coccidioidomycosis	Candidiasis Phycomycosis Aspergillosis Cryptococcosis
Geographic distribution	Endemic areas	Ubiquitous
Host	Usually healthy; disease may be more severe in compromised host	Usually compromised with neutropenia or defective cell-mediated immunity
Diagnosis	Recovery of fungi or demonstration with stains of exudate or tissue	Many are common contaminants; proof of pathogenic role may require histologic evidence of invasion

volve one or many organs, and the site of entry may be a dominant, trivial, or completely inapparent part of the presentation.

A fascinating and poorly understood component of fungal infections is the propensity of certain fungi to spread to specific anatomic sites (Table 8.13–2). The analogy with tuberculosis is useful. *Mycobacterium tuberculosis* may cause disease in the healthy host, most often in the lungs, the site of entry. Clinically advanced pulmonary disease and disseminated disease are more common and more severe in persons with certain defects in host defenses, primarily conditions (see "Opportunistic Fungi" above) that cause defective cell-mediated immunity. When the infection disseminates, specific organs seem to be particularly susceptible—to tuberculosis as well as fungi (see Table 8.13–2).

DIAGNOSIS

Fungal infections can be identified by culture, stains, or serologic tests. There are two general diagnostic rules. First, recovery of pathogenic fungi from any specimen generally indicates disease, but recovery of opportunistic fungi from specimens contaminated by normal flora is always suspect. Second, each fungus has its own diagnostic idiosyncrasies (see "Pathogenic Mycoses" below); some fungi are usually diagnosed by cultures, and others by stains or serologic tests.

PATHOGENIC MYCOSES

Histoplasmosis

Histoplasma capsulatum is a biphasic fungus: The environmental form is mycelia and the tissue form is yeast. The organism is distributed throughout the world, but the most prevalent areas are river valleys of the temperate and tropical zones. In the United States, the endemic areas are the middle west, primarily the Mississippi, Tennessee, and Ohio river valleys, and the river valley areas of the east, especially the St. Lawrence River basin. At least 80% of residents of the Mississippi and Ohio river valleys have positive skin tests to histoplasmin, indicating prior infection. The organism can easily be recovered from the soil, especially when it contains bird or bat guano. Epidemics have occurred in closed areas such as caves, silos, and attics, where there may be a common source of exposure. Wind and digging at construction sites may also cause exposures, sometimes far from the source. Epidemics can involve large areas; the largest histoplasmosis epidemic ever reported was in Indianapolis in 1980–1981, with an estimated 10,000 cases.

Pathophysiology: The mechanism of fungal infection is inhalation of microconidia from the mycelia form in soil or from aerosolized feces of birds or bats. After inhalation, the organism changes to the yeast form and is phagocytized by macrophages. Infected macrophages spread to lymph nodes and other parts of the reticuloendothelial system. The host responds with antigen-specific cellular immunity that contains the infection with granuloma formation, fibrosis, and, eventually, calcification. Lack of this cell-mediated immune response allows uncontrolled infection, with wide dissemination to liver, spleen, lymph nodes, and bone marrow. Infection in the healthy host may be detected by a positive skin test, indicating prior infection; by a chest x-ray showing a nodule or calcification of the lung parenchyma, perhaps with hilar adenopathy; or by splenic calcification, indicating previous dissemination.

Clinical Forms: The major clinical forms of histoplasmosis are primary pulmonary histoplasmosis, chronic pulmonary histoplasmosis, and disseminated infection. In more than 90% of patients, the initial infection is either asymptomatic or simply regarded as an influenza-like condition that does not require medical attention. When patients with the acute form have symptoms, the most common are cough, fever, myalgias, and pleurisy. The severity of symptoms tends to correlate directly with inoculum size. Previous exposure to the antigen confers partial protection. In many patients, chest x-ray shows localized or diffuse infiltrates; unlike bacterial pneumonias, histoplasmosis often causes hilar or mediastinal lymphadenopathy. Less common symptoms include erythema nodosum, erythema multiforme, and arthralgias, all most

Table 8.13–2. Epidemiologic and clinical features of fungal infections.

Fungus	Epidemiology		Clinical Features		
	Distribution	Acquisition	Forms	Sites of Dissemination	Host
Histoplasmosis (*Histoplasma capsulatum*)	Along river basins; bat and bird habitats	Inhaled	Primary pulmonary, chronic pulmonary, localized (eye, mediastinitis), disseminated	Liver, spleen, marrow, mucous membranes, lymph nodes	Healthy people; progressive disease in patients with defective CMI (especially AIDS)
Coccidioidomycosis (*Coccidioides immitis*)	Southwest US	Inhaled	Primary pulmonary, chronic pulmonary, disseminated	Skin, joints, bone, meninges	Healthy people; progressive disease in dark-skinned races and patients with defective CMI
Blastomycosis (*Blastomyces dermatitidis*)	South and north central US	Inhaled	Primary pulmonary, chronic pulmonary, disseminated	Skin, bones, joints, genitourinary tract	Healthy people
Cryptococcosis (*Cryptococcus neoformans*)	Worldwide bird habitats	Inhaled	Primary pulmonary, chronic pulmonary, disseminated	Meninges, skin, prostate	Patients with AIDS or otherwise defective CMI; patients with diabetes
Candidiasis (*Candida albicans* and other sp)	Normal flora of skin, gut, genital tract	Endogenous	Mucocutaneous, localized (peritonitis, urinary tract infection, endocarditis), fungemia (line sepsis), disseminated	Liver, spleen, kidney, eye	Patients with defective CMI; patients receiving antibiotics; patients with neutropenia
Aspergillosis (*Aspergillus fumigatus* and other sp)	Worldwide	Inhaled or cutaneous	Primary pulmonary, bronchoallergic, fungus ball, invasive, localized (infusion sites, burns, sinuses), disseminated	Skin, central nervous system, liver	Patients with neutropenia or defective CMI
Phycomycosis (*Absidia, Rhizopus, Mucor*)	Worldwide	Inhaled or cutaneous	Rhinocerebral, pulmonary	—	Patients with defective CMI or diabetic ketoacidosis

CMI, cell-mediated immunity.

likely to be seen in previously healthy young women. These symptoms generally resolve without treatment.

The most common sequel is chronic pulmonary histoplasmosis, with persistent cough, fever, and malaise. This complication is seen most often in men with chronic obstructive airway disease, and its clinical features and x-ray changes may resemble tuberculosis. In most patients, symptoms resolve spontaneously over 2–4 months, leaving residual pulmonary fibrosis. About 20% of patients have progression to chronic cavitary disease with thick-walled cavities, fibrosis, and respiratory failure.

Disseminated histoplasmosis means extrapulmonary histoplasmosis. Immunocompetent hosts may have no symptoms of disseminated infection, or they may have indolent constitutional symptoms (fever, malaise, weight loss) combined with laboratory or physical findings indicating the favored sites of involvement: hepatosplenomegaly, lymphadenopathy, oral ulcers resembling carcinoma, bone marrow suppression (with anemia, leukopenia, and thrombocytopenia), or adrenal insufficiency. In the previously healthy host, biopsies of affected organs show well-formed granulomas.

Common forms of disseminated histoplasmosis in

adults are dissemination at the time of the original pulmonary infection and reactivation of silent foci as a result of depressed cell-mediated immunity, as seen with AIDS, organ transplantation, or corticosteroid treatment. Reactivated disease progresses faster and biopsies show large numbers of typical intracellular yeast forms with minimal granuloma formation. Again, common presentations are fever of unknown origin, marrow failure, oral ulcers, and other sites of dissemination, including gastrointestinal tract involvement with enteritis or ileocecitis, adrenal gland involvement with adrenal insufficiency, or central nervous system involvement with cerebritis, meningitis, or meningoencephalitis.

Two special late complications of histoplasmosis are chronic mediastinitis and chorioretinitis. Chronic mediastinitis may be granulomatous or fibrotic. The clinical presentation and location of both types of mediastinal lesions are essentially identical, suggesting that they are different stages of the same process. Many patients are asymptomatic, with chest x-rays showing a widened superior mediastinum, with or without calcifications. When present, symptoms usually reflect compression of adjacent structures, such as the superior vena cava, esophagus, or tracheobronchial tree. Chorioretinitis is ascribed to a hypersensitivity response to *H capsulatum*. The diagnosis is generally based on fundoscopic examination, and treatment is corticosteroids, laser photocoagulation, or both.

Diagnosis and Management: Histoplasmosis can be diagnosed by cultures from pulmonary secretions or from sites of disseminated disease, by tissue stains showing characteristic yeast forms, or by radioimmunoassay detecting antigen in urine or blood. Sputum cultures infrequently yield *H capsulatum* in patients with self-limited pulmonary disease, but are positive in 50–70% of patients with chronic cavitary histoplasmosis and in 50–90% of sites of disseminated disease. Histopathologic studies reveal typical ovoid yeast forms measuring $2–3 \times 3–4$ μm, usually within macrophages. The preferred stain is periodic acid-Schiff (PAS), methenamine silver, or Giemsa. The organism stains poorly with hematoxylin-eosin and often goes undetected if this is the only stain used.

Use of the histoplasmin skin test is limited by the high percentage of positive results in persons from endemic areas. Another strike against skin tests is that they make any later serologic test for histoplasmosis uninterpretable. Serologic tests include complement fixation methods with mycelia or yeast from antigens that typically show a titer of 1:32 or higher, or, preferably, paired sera showing a fourfold rise over 3 weeks. The immunodiffusion test detects antibodies to *Histoplasma* antigens with M and H bands and is considered significant when both bands are shown. These serologic tests are relatively insensitive in acute pulmonary histoplasmosis and in disseminated infection in the compromised host.

Treatment is usually restricted to patients with progressive pulmonary disease, chronic cavitary disease, and symptomatic disseminated disease. The drug most often used is amphotericin B or itraconazole.

Coccidioidomycosis

Coccidioides immitis is a diphasic fungus with mycelial forms in nature, and, in tissue, large spherules 10–50 μm in diameter, containing endospores. The organism is found in semi-arid climates, primarily the southwestern United States and parts of South and Central America. The endemic area in the United States includes New Mexico, Arizona, Texas, and California. Because the largest endemic area in the United States is the southern portion of the San Joaquin Valley, this disease is sometimes called "valley fever."

Coccidioidomycosis begins with inhalation of arthrospores. As with histoplasmosis, the course of the infection is determined largely by inoculum size and host resistance. The acute infection is commonly arrested by development of immunity at 2–3 weeks and may remain dormant for years. Reactivation is unusual except in patients with compromised cell-mediated immunity.

Clinical forms are similar to those described for histoplasmosis: primary pulmonary coccidioidomycosis, chronic progressive pulmonary disease, and disseminated coccidioidomycosis. Most infections cause no symptoms or cause a mild flu-like illness. Common symptoms are cough, fever, and pleurisy, all beginning 5–21 days after exposure. Occasional patients with the acute pulmonary infection develop erythema nodosum, erythema multiforme, and arthralgias; this syndrome is most common in young white women. Chest x-rays of the acute pulmonary form show focal infiltrates, especially single or multiple nodules that are sometimes associated with hilar adenopathy or pleural effusion. These lesions usually resolve without treatment, but there may be a residual nodule that resembles carcinoma. Another sequel is cavitary or cystic disease that is often asymptomatic but may cause hemoptysis, pleurisy, or rupture into the pleural space, leading to a pyopneumothorax.

Disseminated disease is most common in men, especially blacks, Filipinos, and persons with compromised cell-mediated immunity. The initial infection may disseminate or a latent focus of infection may reactivate. The most common sites of disseminated disease are the skin and subcutaneous tissue, bones, joints, and meninges. Disseminated disease should be suspected in patients who have dark skin or defective cell-mediated immunity, and who present with unexplained meningitis, arthritis, or skin nodules.

Coccidioidomycosis is diagnosed with culture of *Coccidioides immitis* from pulmonary secretions or sites of dissemination, although the yield is relatively low. Alternatively and equally specific is demonstration of the large and highly characteristic spherules in exudate, with KOH wet mount or biopsies using hematoxylin-eosin, PAS, or methenamine silver. Gram's stain does not show spherules. Skin tests are generally useful for epidemiologic studies; skin test conversion may be shown with the initial acute infection, and skin test reversion from positive to negative supports the probability of disseminated disease. Serologic tests are not altered by the coccidioidin skin test, and the serologic titer tends to correlate directly with the severity of disease. A complement fixation test generally becomes positive around the third week of illness, and titers that persist at 1:32 or higher suggest disseminated disease. A positive complement fixation from cerebrospinal fluid is considered diagnostic of coccidioidomycosis meningitis.

Treatment is rarely advocated for patients with primary pulmonary coccidioidomycosis, since it generally resolves spontaneously. Some authorities recommend treating patients who are at high risk for disseminated disease. Most patients with progressive pulmonary coccidioidomycosis are treated, as are virtually all patients with disseminated disease. The most used drugs are amphotericin B, ketoconazole, and itraconazole.

Blastomycosis

Blastomyces dermatitidis is a dimorphic fungus with mycelia that produce conidia in nature, and large encapsulated yeasts measuring 8–15 μm in infected tissue. The endemic area in the United States is the southeastern, south central, and midwestern states, and regions adjacent to the Great Lakes. The fungus is presumed to reside in soil, but cultures of soil samples in endemic areas infrequently yield the organism.

Blastomycosis is acquired by inhalation of conidia spores, leading to primary infection in the lung. Most patients are asymptomatic or have only a flu-like illness that does not merit medical attention. The incubation period after a point source exposure is about 40 days. Patients with pulmonary infections may present much as do patients with bacterial pneumonias; chronic pulmonary infections often cause chronic symptoms suggesting tuberculosis. Typical symptoms are chronic cough, pleurisy, hemoptysis, weight loss, and low-grade fever. Chest x-ray usually shows an infiltrate or nodular densities, most often in the lower lobes. Complications include chronic pulmonary infections with cavities, pleural involvement, pulmonary fibrosis, and hematogenous spread. Disseminated disease most often involves the skin and subcutaneous tissue, prostate gland, bones, and joints. Unlike histoplasmosis and coccidioidomycosis, disseminated blastomycosis is not usually associated with compromised host defenses.

The diagnosis of blastomycosis is generally made by KOH stains of sputum or exudate from infected sites, by recovering the organism in culture, or by demonstrating typical morphologic forms in biopsy specimens. The organism characteristically appears as a large yeast 8–15 μm long, often with a single budding daughter cell attached with a broad base. The preferred stains are PAS and methenamine silver. There is no useful skin, serologic, or antigen detection test.

In the past, treatment was advocated for virtually everyone with blastomycosis. More recently, this recommendation has been restricted to patients with progressive pulmonary disease, severe pulmonary disease, and disseminated disease. The typical drugs used are amphotericin B and ketoconazole.

OPPORTUNISTIC MYCOSES

Cryptococcosis

Cryptococcus neoformans is a spherical or ovoid yeast 4–7 μm in diameter, enveloped by a thick, gelatinous polysaccharide capsule that sometimes has budding cells with a narrow attachment. The organism occurs widely in nature and is found in exceptionally high concentrations in pigeon feces. Nevertheless, for most patients with cryptococcal infection, the source is unknown.

The infection is usually acquired by inhalation, resulting in a pneumonitis that may cause cough, fever, and sputum production, or it may be clinically silent. Chest x-rays may show one or more nodules, infiltrates, a miliary pattern (many small nodules), cavitary pulmonary disease, hilar adenopathy, and pleural effusion. Often, pulmonary nodules or small cavities are found in asymptomatic patients, who may then mistakenly be evaluated for bronchogenic neoplasm or tuberculosis.

C neoformans has two distinctive properties. First, it represents something of a bridge in the classification of fungi as opportunists or pathogens, since it often causes pulmonary disease and occasionally causes disseminated disease in an otherwise healthy host. The second unique feature is that cryptococcus has an extraordinary tropism for the meninges. *C neoformans* is the most common causes of meningitis in patients with AIDS and is second only to *Listeria* in causing meningitis in patients with other defects in cell-mediated immunity. Less common sites for disseminated disease are the skin, mucous membranes, bone, and prostate.

Pulmonary cryptococcosis may be diagnosed by cultures of sputum or bronchial washings prepared with selective media such as Sabouraud's medium, or by India ink preparations of respiratory secretions. The yield from these specimens is poor, and chronic pulmonary cryptococcosis is often not established until the patient undergoes thoracotomy for a suspected neoplasm. The organism is second only to *Candida* sp as a cause of fungemia and positive fungal urine cultures, since both fungi grow in the media used to process these specimens. Some patients with pulmonary disease and most patients with disseminated disease have cryptococcal antigen detected with the latex agglutination test.

All patients who have cryptococcal antigen recovered from any site should undergo lumbar puncture to search for cryptococcal meningitis. Patients with cryptococcal meningitis may present with typical findings of headache, stiff neck, and fever, or they may have no meningeal symptoms. Typical cerebrospinal fluid findings are increased protein, lymphocytosis, and a positive cryptococcal antigen assay. The assay for this antigen in cerebrospinal fluid is possibly the best assay available for detection of a microbe in body fluid.

If normal patients have disease only in the chest and if their cerebrospinal fluid is normal, their disease is probably self-limited and they do not need treatment. If patients are immunocompromised or have progressive pulmonary disease or disseminated disease (including meningitis), they should be treated. The usual treatment is fluconazole, amphotericin B, or amphotericin B plus flucytosine. Patients with AIDS require lifelong treatment to prevent relapse.

Candidiasis

There are many species of *Candida,* and the species found most frequently in the normal flora and at infected sites is *Candida albicans.* In normal flora, *C albicans* organisms appear as egg-shaped yeasts that may be budding; in infected tissues or exudates, they appear as pseudohyphae (chains of elongated yeast). *Candida* is the most common fungus recovered in clinical specimens, reflecting that it is in normal flora, easily cultivated on the media used to detect bacteria, and a common cause of mucocutaneous infections. Routine cultures of healthy persons yield these organisms in 20–30% of respiratory tract specimens, 30–50% of vaginal swabs, and 50–70% of stool specimens. In contrast to other fungal infections, candidiasis is usually thought to be endogenous. The organism is also found in soil, food, and hospitals.

The clinical manifestations of candidiasis are highly variable, depending on the host. They may be classified as mucocutaneous infections, fungemia, focal infections of deep organs or foreign bodies (eg, intravenous lines, prosthetic heart valves, prosthetic joints), and disseminated candidiasis.

Mucocutaneous infections are extremely common, affecting otherwise healthy hosts as well as patients with diabetes mellitus, antibiotic exposure, defective cell-mediated immunity, or neutropenia. Mucocutaneous infections are surface infections in which the fungi do not invade beyond the basement membrane. These infections include oral candidiasis (thrush) and *Candida* vaginitis, dermatitis, intertriginous infection, cheilosis, and cystitis. Thrush, characterized by curd-like patches on the mucous membranes, is found in 80–90% of patients with advanced HIV infection. *Candida* vaginitis, also characterized by curd-like patches, is especially common as a complication of diabetes, antibiotic treatment, or HIV infection. Mucocutaneous candidiasis invading beyond the basement membrane manifests as *Candida* esophagitis, enteritis, or colitis. Chronic mucocutaneous candidiasis is a rare disease related to specific defects in T-cell function and characterized by hypoparathyroidism and persistent superficial *Candida* infections of the skin, nails, mucous membranes, and scalp (Chapter 9.5).

Candida sp are the only fungi often isolated from blood cultures. *C albicans* is most frequently recovered, followed by *C tropicalis, C parapsilosis,* and *C krusei.* The physician should suspect disseminated candidiasis or endocarditis when blood cultures are persistently positive. Endocarditis develops most often in patients with a prosthetic heart valve and less often in intravenous drug abusers.

Disseminated candidiasis is generally restricted to compromised hosts, primarily patients with leukemia or lymphomas and patients receiving cancer chemotherapy. (Although many patients with HIV infection have thrush, few have disseminated candidiasis.) Candidiasis often spreads after patients with neutropenia or those taking corticosteroids are given multiple broad-spectrum antibiotics. The most common sites of disseminated disease are the kidneys, eyes, and skin. Funduscopic exam may show typical raised white lesions that resemble colonies of *Candida* growing on blood agar plates and are considered diagnostic of disseminated candidiasis. Many patients with renal involvement have renal abscesses and progressive renal insufficiency. Nevertheless, urine cultures that yield *Candida* sp must be interpreted cautiously, since many patients have colonization of the lower urinary tract but no clear evidence of disseminated or invasive disease.

Focal *Candida* infections of deep structures include peritonitis, urinary tract infection, hepatosplenic infection, meningitis, and infection of practically any organ system. Peritonitis usually develops after perforation of the upper intestine or as a complication of peritoneal dialysis. Hepatosplenic candidiasis is usually seen in patients with leukemia who are in remission and have had prolonged neutropenia secondary to chemotherapy. *Candida* is an unusual isolate in cerebrospinal fluid, but is one of the more common causes of meningitis in the compromised host.

The diagnosis of superficial *Candida* infections, such as thrush and vaginitis, requires little more than seeing typical lesions. Superficial *Candida* infections may be verified by swabs or scrapings of infected sites for KOH wet mount. Gram's stain or recovery from blood cultures may be difficult, even in patients with endocarditis. Endocarditis is suggested by negative blood cultures, large heart valve vegetations, a typical host (a patient with a prosthetic valve or an intravenous drug user), and no response to empiric antibacterial treatment. Deep and disseminated disease may also be difficult to detect, since most *Candida* isolates represent contamination from the mucocutaneous surfaces, where *Candida* is normal flora. Disseminated disease is documented by typical organisms on stain or culture of biopsy specimens, by repeatedly positive blood cultures for *Candida* sp in typical clinical settings, or by *Candida* endophthalmitis.

In most patients, mucocutaneous *Candida* infection is treated effectively by topical drugs such as nystatin or clotrimazole or by oral drugs such as ketoconazole or fluconazole. Line-associated candidemia is usually treated with fluconazole, combined with removal of indwelling vascular devices. Patients with disseminated candidiasis require amphotericin B with or without flucytosine, and patients with *Candida* endocarditis require both antifungal treatment and valve replacement.

Phycomycosis

Fungi belonging to the order Mucorales include the genera *Mucor, Rhizopus, Absidia,* and *Cunninghamella.* These organisms are broad, nonseptate hyphae 10–15 µm long with right-angled branching. They are distributed throughout the world in decaying matter, manure, and soil. These fungi are highly invasive and, like *Aspergillus,* have a marked tendency to invade blood vessels, leading to thrombosis and tissue necrosis. Their effects can be devastating.

The organisms may be acquired by inhalation, ingestion, or contamination of wounds by spores. Two types of hosts are susceptible: diabetic patients with ketoacidosis and patients with defective cell-mediated immunity. In patients with diabetes, the most characteristic form of disease is rhinocerebral mucormycosis complicating ketoacidosis; this form is also found in patients with hematologic malignancies causing neutropenia. The infection spreads through contiguous structures, with minimal respect for anatomic boundaries. When the orbit becomes involved, the infection can cause ophthalmoplegia and can invade the nervous system, destroying cranial nerves II, IV, V, and VI. The infection may extend to the carotid artery, cavernous sinuses, meninges, and brain.

The second common form of the disease is pulmonary mucormycosis, which generally afflicts patients with hematologic malignancy or cancer chemotherapy complicated by neutropenia or defective cell-mediated immunity. The clinical presentation and chest x-ray often simulate those of pulmonary embolism and infarction, and the x-ray may show cavitation. Disseminated disease is uncommon.

Diagnosis of mucormycosis is generally based on finding the usual clinical features in a typical host, and finding a typical hyphal form in tissue biopsies or KOH preparations. *Mucor* is one of the few fungi seen well with hematoxylin and eosin stains. The organism is difficult to culture.

Mucormycosis infections are among the most devastating encountered in medicine. The rhinocerebral form requires aggressive surgical debridement, prompt steps to control diabetic ketoacidosis, and high doses of amphotericin B. The pulmonary form requires aggressive use of amphotericin B combined with attempts to correct the deficits in host defenses.

Aspergillosis

Aspergillus sp occur in nature as hyphae with conidia and in tissue as septate hyphae 2–5 μm in diameter with 45° angled branching. The organism is distributed throughout the world, most frequently in decaying vegetation, but also in house dust, air samples, plants, and heroin. The dominant species in clinical disease is *Aspergillus fumigatus*, followed by *A flavus, A niger,* and *A terreus*.

Aspergillus infection usually follows inhalation of airborne spores. Epidemics can occur in hospitals, usually reflecting inadequate air filtration; only immunocompromised hosts are affected. The major host factors predisposing to *Aspergillus* infection are neutropenia and burns. Defective cell-mediated immunity also plays a role.

The clinical features of *Aspergillus* depend on the host. Among the many possible manifestations are aspergilloma (fungus ball), allergic bronchopulmonary aspergillosis, invasive pulmonary aspergillosis, and disseminated disease.

An *aspergilloma* is a tangled mass of hyphae inside a pulmonary cavity produced by another disease, such as sarcoidosis, or within an abscess or thin-wall cyst caused by tuberculosis, lung abscess, or histoplasmosis (for example). Usually, an aspergilloma is merely a curiosity on a chest x-ray or computed tomography scan. But some patients have hemoptysis, and some have progressive disease invading the lungs over months or even years.

Allergic bronchopulmonary aspergillosis affects patients with asthma. This is a hypersensitivity reaction to *Aspergillus* antigens colonizing the bronchial mucosa. Allergic bronchopulmonary aspergillosis is a common form of the PIE syndrome (pulmonary infiltrate with eosinophilia).

Invasive pulmonary aspergillosis is a serious infection found only in compromised hosts, especially patients with leukemia or lymphomas, persons receiving cancer chemotherapy, and organ transplant recipients. Both neutropenia and defective cell-mediated immunity may play a role.

Neutropenia is especially common. The usual clinical presentation is bronchopneumonia or vascular invasion with thrombosis and infarction, sometimes with cavity formation. A pleural cavity in a bone marrow transplant recipient is usually caused by *Aspergillus*.

Another characteristic presentation in compromised hosts is focal cutaneous infection by airborne spores at sites of intravenous infusions. Local infection may be complicated by the organ disseminating to the brain, kidneys, liver, and other organs.

Aspergillus, like *Mucor,* is difficult to culture and is more often seen than grown. A positive culture must be interpreted cautiously, since *Aspergillus* may be an airborne contaminant or may colonize sites without causing disease. Usually, the preferred tests are KOH stains of exudate and impression smears or biopsies with methenamine silver or PAS stains. Serology measuring *Aspergillus* precipitants in serum is usually positive in the allergic bronchopulmonary form and often positive with aspergillomas, but not helpful with invasive or disseminated disease.

Therapy depends on the form of aspergillosis. The bronchoallergic form is generally treated with corticosteroids and tends to respond well. Aspergillomas are generally observed rather than treated; patients may need amphotericin B, surgery, or both, if they have persistent hemoptysis or evidence of progressive invasion. Patients with invasive pulmonary or disseminated disease need to be treated aggressively with amphotericin B; equally important are attempts to reestablish normal defense mechanisms.

SUMMARY

▶ Pathogenic fungi *(Histoplasma capsulatum, Coccidioides immitis,* and *Blastomyces dermatitidis)* are virulent enough to infect healthy hosts. The usual sequence is inhalation of mycelia leading to pneumonitis that may or may not be symptomatic, and possibly to wide hematogenous dissemination. Progressive lung disease and infection at extrapulmonary sites are more common in patients with compromised defenses.

▶ Opportunistic fungi *(Cryptococcus neoformans, Candida* sp, *Aspergillus* sp, and *Phycomycetes)* usually cause disease only when host defenses are compromised, primarily with defective cell-mediated immunity or neutropenia. The range of pathogenic processes and clinical presentations is diverse. As with pathogenic fungi, a common pattern is infection at the site of inoculation, sometimes with progressive disease at that site or dissemination to other organs.

▶ The usual tests for fungi are stains and cultures to detect the organisms.

▶ The typical treatments are amphotericin B or azoles.

SUGGESTED READING

Ampel NM, Wieden MA, Galgiani JN: Coccidioidomycosis: Clinical update. Rev Infect Dis 1989;11:897.

Diamond RD: The growing problem of mycoses in patients infected with the human immunodeficiency virus. Rev Infect Dis 1991;13:480.

Fungal infection in HIV-infected persons. American Thoracic Society. Am J Respir Crit Care Med 1995;152:816.

Horn R et al: Fungemia in a cancer hospital: Changing frequency, earlier onset, and results of therapy. Rev Infect Dis 1985;7:646.

Wheat LJ et al: A large urban outbreak of histoplasmosis: Clinical features. Ann Intern Med 1981;94:331.

Young RC et al: Aspergillosis: The spectrum of the disease in 98 patients. Medicine 1970;49:147.

Mycobacterial Infections

Thomas R. Moench, MD

Mycobacteria are extraordinary pathogens that can cause chronic infection and disease nearly unique among bacteria. *Mycobacterium tuberculosis,* the mycobacterium of greatest virulence and importance, infects one-third of the world's population and causes 8 million new cases of active tuberculosis each year. In addition to causing chronic and severe morbidity, tuberculosis kills 3 million people each year, more than any other infectious disease. After decades of progressively declining incidence in the developed world, tuberculosis rates have begun rising alarmingly because of the AIDS epidemic, immigration from high prevalence areas, deteriorating social conditions, and relaxation of tuberculosis control measures. Equally alarming has been the increase in resistant strains of this virulent pathogen, made possible by interruption of the prolonged therapy required for cure.

Since the manifestations of tuberculosis are diverse, the physician must consider it in the differential diagnosis of a great many patients' presenting complaints. If diagnosed and managed skillfully, tuberculosis can almost always be cured. But if it goes untreated, the mortality is high: Two of three patients with untreated active tuberculosis die within 3 years. Treatment that is inadequate because of either patient nonadherence or physician error can allow outgrowth of resistant organisms, greatly diminishing the potential for cure and posing a serious risk of transmission to others.

Other mycobacteria cause serious pulmonary and extrapulmonary disease in patients with compromised immune defenses. Many of these organisms are difficult to treat because they are resistant to antimicrobial drugs and because patients require prolonged therapy. Chief among these organisms is a group called the *Mycobacterium avium* complex, which has emerged as a common and important pathogen in patients with AIDS.

MYCOBACTERIUM TUBERCULOSIS

Pathophysiology

M tuberculosis infection is acquired by inhaling organisms within aerosol droplets expelled primarily during coughing by persons who have pulmonary or laryngeal tu-

berculosis. Since only very small droplets (<5 μm in diameter) can bypass the nasal turbinates and bronchial mucociliary defenses to reach the alveoli, infection typically occurs only after months of exposure to contaminated air. Occasionally, infectious droplets are so abundant as to cause infection after only a few hours of exposure.

After they are inhaled into the alveoli, mycobacteria replicate locally and then spread throughout the body via the blood and lymphatic systems. During this "primary infection" phase, the patient generally feels well. Immunocompetent persons mount an immune response in which antigen-specific T cells activate macrophages and induce them to engulf and kill the mycobacteria. This cellular immune response effectively contains the infection in 95% of immunocompetent persons. The other 5% develop "progressive primary infection," manifested either as localized disease (progressive pneumonia or tuberculous pleurisy) or as widespread systemic disease (miliary tuberculosis). Even among those whose infection was successfully contained, most continue to harbor viable organisms for decades, and their only evidence of infection may be a positive tuberculin skin test (see below). However, 5% of these individuals develop "reactivation" disease at some time during their lives. Reactivation is most common in the upper lobes, but can occur elsewhere in or outside the lung.

Patients with deficient cellular immunity, such as that induced by HIV infection, are unable to contain mycobacterial replication and spread. Extraordinarily high percentages of these patients suffer progressive primary infection. Likewise, patients with a contained *M tuberculosis* infection who are later infected with HIV are at very high risk for reactivation disease as they become immunosuppressed.

Pulmonary Tuberculosis

Patients with pulmonary tuberculosis typically have both systemic and pulmonary symptoms. Systemic complaints include fever, chills, night sweats, anorexia, weight loss, and fatigue. The cardinal pulmonary symptom, which should always raise suspicion of tuberculosis, is chronic productive cough lasting more than 3 weeks, with or without hemoptysis. This symptom is especially important because patients with cough are far more infectious than those without. Patients may also suffer pleuritic chest pain caused by pleural inflammation. The physician should always inquire about tuberculosis contacts or prior treatment for tuberculosis and should contact local public health authorities who may have information about a patient's tuberculosis history. The index of suspicion for tuberculosis should be especially high in patients who have risk factors for tuberculosis infection or disease, such as HIV infection, alcoholism, immunosuppression, silicosis, poor nutrition, diabetes, renal dialysis, organ transplant, and previous residence in Asia, Africa, or Latin America. Physical findings include rales, signs of consolidation, and pleural effusion.

The key tests for pulmonary tuberculosis are chest x-ray, purified protein derivative (PPD) skin test, acid-fast bacillus (AFB) stain of sputum smears, and sputum mycobacterial culture. A normal chest x-ray quickly rules out active pulmonary tuberculosis, and generally determines that the patient is not an infectious risk. When the lung is involved by tuberculosis, the range of x-ray abnormalities is broad. The most characteristic finding in patients with reactivation pulmonary tuberculosis is a cavitary infiltrate in a posterior-apical segment of an upper lobe or in a superior segment of a lower lobe (Figure 8.14–1). Formation of cavities correlates with a million-fold increase in the density of organisms. Patients with cavitary disease are much more infectious than those without, and their large populations of organisms are more prone to develop resistance when drug therapy has been inadequate or the patients nonadherent.

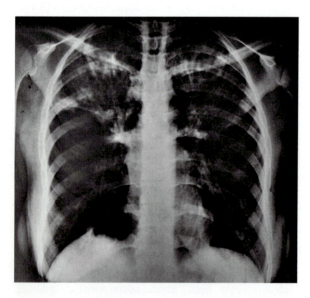

Figure 8.14–1. Reactivation pulmonary tuberculosis. This chest x-ray shows the most characteristic finding: cavitary infiltrates in both upper lobes. (Courtesy of Paul S. Wheeler, MD.)

Not all patients present with these characteristic x-ray findings. Noncavitary infiltrates, nondescript lower lobe infiltrates, diffuse interstitial infiltrates, mass lesions, and many other findings are compatible with pulmonary tuberculosis.

Infection in immunocompetent persons, with or without active disease, can be diagnosed by the PPD skin test. The PPD detects mycobacteria-specific cellular immunity manifested when lymphocytes and macrophages infiltrate and indurate the skin at the site where mycobacterial proteins have been injected. Infection is very likely if induration of 10 mm or more is seen 48–72 hours after intradermal injection with a 5-tuberculin unit (TU) dose of PPD. Induration of 5–10 mm also suggests infection with *M tuberculosis,* especially in HIV-infected patients and contacts of patients with active tuberculosis.

About 80% of immunocompetent individuals with active tuberculosis react to PPD testing with induration of 10 mm or more. Since less than 8% of the general population has such reactions, a positive skin test supports a diagnosis of tuberculosis, but a negative skin test does not rule it out. Almost all immunocompetent patients with tuberculosis and false-negative skin tests show positive responses if retested after several weeks of therapy. This initial unresponsiveness (anergy) is thought to be a temporary immunologic consequence of the patient's generally poor condition. Retesting can be of diagnostic benefit in patients who have been started empirically on antituberculous drugs.

Examination of sputum smears for acid-fast bacilli (AFB) is a rapid way to detect mycobacteria and differentiate them from other bacteria. Because of mycolic acids in their cell walls, all species of mycobacteria (and another important but less common pathogen, *Nocardia*) retain certain lipophilic dyes; other bacteria, lacking mycolic acids, are stripped of dye by an acid wash. AFB smears help in quickly detecting the most infectious patients with tuberculosis. Smear-negative patients can also be infectious, but they pose a risk at least 10-fold lower than patients with AFB visible on smears. Positive smears allow only a presumptive diagnosis of tuberculosis, since other mycobacteria give indistinguishable positive smears. Nor do negative smears rule out active disease; nearly 50% of patients with positive cultures have negative smears.

Definitive diagnosis of pulmonary tuberculosis requires mycobacterial culture of the sputum. Culture is more sensitive than smear, it definitively identifies the organism, and it allows determination of the organism's susceptibility to antituberculous drugs. Culture requires secretions from deep in the lung. If patients are likely to have pulmonary tuberculosis but cannot give adequate specimens by coughing and spitting, they should have sputum induction by aerosol inhalation, or, if that does not work, bronchoscopy.

Differential Diagnosis: Conditions that may mimic pulmonary tuberculosis include pulmonary diseases caused by other mycobacteria, as well as sarcoidosis, nocardiosis, anaerobic aspiration pneumonia, *Pneumocystis carinii* pneumonia, fungal infections, pulmonary infarction, and cancer. Because many patients with AIDS have multiple simultaneous infections, the definitive diagnosis of another pathogen does not exclude coexisting tuberculosis.

Management: The principles of chemotherapy for tuberculosis are governed by several peculiarities of the organism. *M tuberculosis* grows slowly: The doubling time is 20 hours—many times that of most bacteria. Growth is also intermittent, with long periods of complete dormancy. The need for prolonged treatment is explained by the fact that only actively growing organisms are susceptible to antituberculous chemotherapy. Populations of *M tuberculosis* include spontaneous mutants that resist individual antituberculous drugs, at a frequency of one resistant mutant for every 1 million to 100 million organisms. Many patients with cavitary disease have more than a billion organisms. Resistant organisms are likely to develop—and eventually predominate—under the selective pressure of a single antituberculous drug. Thus, there is a need for more than one drug in patients with active disease and large populations of organisms. The only patients who should receive a single drug are those taking preventive treatment for an asymptomatic infection with few organisms (see "Preventive Treatment" below).

Treatment of active disease: The main obstacle to the reliable cure of tuberculosis is the difficulty in ensuring patients' consistent adherence to their necessarily prolonged therapy. Because symptoms generally disappear after several weeks of treatment, many patients stop taking their medicine well before they have completed the regimen. Full adherence to the intended course averages only 75%, and in many inner city populations it is less than 60%.

A second obstacle to successful therapy grows from the first: When patients do not complete therapy, resistant strains are selected. The increasing resistance of *M tuberculosis* to isoniazid and other antituberculous drugs is the consequence of nonadherence, poorly supervised therapy, or inappropriate prescribing. Resistant organisms are fully virulent and communicable and constitute a serious public health threat. Isoniazid resistance has reached a prevalence of 30–50% in countries where antituberculous drugs are commonly available without prescription. In the United States, the prevalence of resistance was relatively low until the mid-1980's and has since been increasing. Moreover, alarming outbreaks involving strains that are resistant to multiple drugs have recently been reported, primarily among HIV-infected persons in prisons, shelters, hospitals, and nursing homes. Currently, areas of the country where tuberculosis is most prevalent have a substantial rate of isoniazid-resistant organisms.

For these reasons, new regimens containing increased numbers of drugs have become standard therapy for tuberculosis (Table 8.14–1), providing greater certainty that the initial regimen will include at least two drugs to which the infecting organism is sensitive. These regimens have the additional advantage of providing reliable cure with shorter therapy (6 months), thus increasing the likelihood of patients' completing their treatment.

In 1994, the American Thoracic Society and the Centers for Disease Control and Prevention recommended a new regimen for initial treatment of tuberculosis: isoniazid, rifampin, pyrazinamide, and a fourth drug, either ethambutol or streptomycin. All patients should have drug susceptibility testing performed on the initial isolate. If the isolate is documented to be susceptible to isoniazid and rifampin, the fourth drug is stopped, and pyrazinamide is stopped after the patient has completed 2 months or more of therapy. Isoniazid and rifampin are continued for a total of 6 months. In localities where the rate of isoniazid resistance is documented to be less than 4%, initial therapy need not include a fourth drug unless the patient has other risk factors for drug resistance, such as immigration from a developing country, previous antituberculous therapy, or

Table 8.14–1. Treatment of *Mycobacterium tuberculosis* infections.

Condition	Usual Treatment	Comments
Active pulmonary tuberculosis	Standard regimen when drug sensitivities are unknown: Isoniazid, rifampin, pyrazinamide, and ethambutol (or streptomycin) for 6 months	Monitor with monthly sputum culture
	Standard regimen after documenting sensitivity to isoniazid and rifampin: As above, but once organism is proven sensitive to isoniazid and rifampin, ethambutol (or streptomycin) is stopped, and pyrazinamide is stopped after 2 months of therapy; continue isoniazid and rifampin for a total of 6 months	Monitor with monthly sputum culture
Miliary tuberculosis	Standard regimen	Begin therapy as soon as diagnosis is suspected
Meningeal tuberculosis	Standard regimen + corticosteroids; continue isoniazid and rifampin for a total of 12 months	Begin therapy as soon as diagnosis is suspected
Other sites of extrapulmonary tuberculosis	Standard regimen	
Asymptomatic infection (positive PPD)	Isoniazid for 6–12 months (12 months if HIV coinfection)	Table 8.14–2 explains which patients to treat

PPD, purified protein derivative.

contact with persons with known or suspected drug-resistant tuberculosis. By these criteria, greater than 90% of patients must be started on the four-drug regimen.

Directly observed therapy (taking each dose of antituberculous medication while being watched by a responsible person such as a health care provider) has long been an effective way to increase adherence to antituberculous treatment regimens. Strong arguments for the wide use of directly observed therapy come from recent documentation that (1) many patients fail to complete prescribed therapy and it is difficult to predict which patients will fail to adhere to their regimen; (2) nonadherence leads to increases in drug-resistant strains; (3) twice- or thrice-weekly dosing is highly effective; and (4) multiple-drug regimens can provide reliable cures in only 6 months. Directly observed therapy should be considered for all patients; it is mandatory for patients whose sputum cultures are still positive after 3 months of treatment.

Preventive treatment: If the PPD skin test is positive but patients are asymptomatic, they can be treated with antituberculous therapy to reduce their chances of developing active disease (Table 8.14–2). This therapy reduces the risk of disease by 70% overall and by more than 90% in patients who follow their treatment regimen carefully. Although often called "prophylaxis," preventive treatment is really treatment of subclinical infection with low-level replication. Single-drug therapy is acceptable for these patients, whose relatively few organisms put them at low risk for selection of resistant strains. The standard regimen is isoniazid for 6–12 months.

Because it can cause hepatitis, isoniazid is not given to everyone who has a positive skin test. Present policy is to give it only to infected persons who have some factor increasing their risk for symptomatic disease: persons who are also infected with HIV, close contacts of patients with newly active tuberculosis, persons whose skin test became positive within the past 2 years, persons with a history of inadequately treated tuberculosis, previously untreated persons whose chest x-ray shows lesions compatible with healed tuberculosis, and patients with other medical conditions that increase the risk of active disease (see Table 8.14–2). Persons younger than 35 have a lower risk of iso-

Table 8.14–2. Indications for prophylactic treatment of patients with asymptomatic *Mycobacterium tuberculosis* infection detected by tuberculin skin test.*

HIV infection
History of inadequately treated tuberculosis
Close contact with a person who has newly acquired tuberculosis
Chest x-ray showing lesions compatible with healed, previously untreated tuberculosis
Conversion of PPD skin test during past 2 yr
Other conditions that increase risk for active tuberculosis: intravenous drug use, end-stage renal disease, poorly controlled diabetes mellitus, silicosis, malnutrition, gastrectomy, immunosuppressive therapy, reticuloendothelial malignancy
Age <35

PPD, purified protein derivative.
*Sequence shows highest to lowest risk for reactivation if not treated.

niazid-induced hepatitis than older persons. In the past, these young people were started on preventive treatment after a positive skin test, even if they did not have other risk factors. Now the issue is controversial, but a good case can be made for treating these patients: With proper monitoring, their risk of isoniazid hepatotoxicity is extremely low, and, because they have a long predicted life span, they derive great benefit from the lowered risk of reactivation disease.

Monitoring: Antituberculous chemotherapy requires close monitoring to ensure adherence, to detect drug toxicity, and, with active disease, to ensure that the patient is responding to treatment. The crucial measure of adequate response is monthly sputum cultures to determine that the patient's sputum is free of organisms. Failure to sterilize the sputum within 3 months strongly suggests nonadherence or drug resistance. Patients in this situation should be given their drugs under direct supervision and the sensitivity tests repeated. If resistance is proved, referral to or consultation with a physician experienced in treating resistant tuberculosis is strongly advised. A patient who makes a delayed but ultimately adequate bacteriologic response should have the treatment period extended. All patients should be seen monthly and asked if they are having any of the common side effects of their drugs, especially symptoms of hepatitis. Patients at greater risk for hepatitis—older people, patients with preexisting liver disease, and heavy drinkers—should have serum transaminase determinations, and their therapy should be interrupted if levels exceed five times normal. A final sputum culture should be obtained at the end of therapy.

Infection control: The most important tool for preventing transmission of tuberculosis is prompt detection and treatment of infectious patients. The physician should be especially vigilant for patients who may be most infectious: those with cavitary or laryngeal disease, those with visible AFB on smears, and those who are coughing. Most infectious patients can be detected if all persons with unexplained signs or symptoms of pulmonary disease are evaluated with AFB smears.

Many patients with tuberculosis can be treated at home. Patients hospitalized with documented or suspected infectious tuberculosis should be isolated in rooms with negative pressure and six nonrecirculated air changes per hour. Masks for patient and staff probably provide some protection. Cough-inducing procedures (sputum induction, aerosol treatments, bronchoscopy) should be performed in isolation rooms or booths. Precautions should be maintained until three sputum smears are negative for AFB, the cough improves, or patients have received 2 weeks of effective treatment, by which time most are noninfectious. Patients with multidrug-resistant tuberculosis may require longer isolation.

Extrapulmonary Tuberculosis

About 15% of patients with active tuberculosis have disease outside the lung, and the rate is increasing because of its greater prevalence in patients infected with HIV.

Extrapulmonary disease poses special diagnostic challenges because the clinical presentation varies with the site of infection, many patients require biopsies for diagnosis, and some patients have only a few organisms, which are difficult to demonstrate by AFB stain or culture. A positive PPD skin test can be a crucial clue to extrapulmonary tuberculosis, since it increases the suspicion of tuberculosis. Patients with extrapulmonary tuberculosis may not have pulmonary disease, but it should always be sought, particularly since sputum AFB smears and mycobacterial cultures are the most straightforward, noninvasive tests. Further tests include biopsies or aspirates of sites suggested by the patient's presentation.

Lymphatic tuberculosis can involve any lymph node group, but typically causes adenitis of the cervical region (scrofula) and only rarely causes generalized adenopathy. The adenopathy is tender and most patients are otherwise well, with no constitutional signs or evidence of tuberculosis elsewhere. Diagnosis usually requires excisional biopsy of a node for histologic examination and culture. The major differential diagnosis is that of adenitis caused by other mycobacteria, but it also includes adenitis from pyogenic bacteria, cat-scratch disease, fungi, and malignancy.

Tuberculous pleurisy develops when a tuberculous pulmonary focus ruptures through the adjacent visceral pleura into the pleural space. Pleurisy may be a manifestation of primary tuberculosis or of reactivation. The presentation may be insidious or acute, the latter the result of a vigorous inflammatory response to the sudden release of mycobacterial antigen into the pleural space. Symptoms include fever and unilateral pleuritic pain. Pleural fluid can usually be detected on physical examination as dullness to percussion, decreased breath sounds, and decreased fremitus. Some patients have a pleural friction rub. The pleural fluid is exudative (Chapter 2.10), with mononuclear inflammatory cells. A positive PPD skin test in a patient with an exudative pleural effusion strongly suggests tuberculous pleurisy. The diagnosis is confirmed by percutaneous pleural biopsy for histology and culture. Other diseases that may present a similar picture are parapneumonic effusions caused by other bacterial pneumonias, effusions caused by pulmonary embolism, and malignant effusion. Tuberculosis can involve other serosal surfaces, leading to tuberculous pericarditis or peritonitis.

Genitourinary tuberculosis can involve the urinary tract at any level. Most patients have minimal symptoms, although some experience dysuria, gross hematuria, or flank pain. The urinary sediment is almost always abnormal, containing red blood cells, white blood cells, or both. The diagnosis can usually be made by urine mycobacterial culture. The physician should suspect renal tuberculosis when a patient has an active urine sediment, suggesting urinary tract infection, but negative cultures for the common bacterial uropathogens (sterile pyuria). The male genital tract may be seeded when organisms from preexisting renal tuberculosis enter the urine. The female genital tract may become involved by reactivation of latent foci in the fallopian tubes.

Skeletal tuberculosis can involve any bone or joint, but most commonly involves the vertebral bodies or the epiphyses of the long bones. Tuberculous spondylitis (Pott's disease) may present with fever, back pain, gibbus spinal deformity (hump), paraspinal abscess, or spinal cord or nerve root impingement. The differential diagnosis includes vertebral osteomyelitis caused by other bacteria, as well as subdural or epidural abscess and vertebral metastases. Peripheral skeletal tuberculosis generally presents as a large-joint monoarticular arthritis with combined involvement of the joint space and osteomyelitis of adjacent bone. An insidious onset and minimal inflammatory findings distinguish skeletal tuberculosis from septic arthritis caused by pyogenic organisms.

Miliary tuberculosis is a rapidly lethal dissemination of either progressive primary or reactivation tuberculosis. Symptoms are usually nonspecific constitutional complaints, including fever, weight loss, weakness, and fatigue. In most patients, the chest x-ray eventually shows diffusely scattered 2–3-mm nodules (the size of millet seeds, hence "miliary" tuberculosis), but this pattern may not be visible at first presentation. The differential diagnosis is that of fever of unknown origin, since the symptoms are nonspecific (Chapter 8.2). Diagnostic clues include the characteristic chest x-ray, meningeal signs (since tuberculous meningitis often accompanies miliary tuberculosis), hepatosplenomegaly, and an elevated alkaline phosphatase. The diagnosis of miliary tuberculosis is confirmed by culture of samples from various locations, especially liver and bone marrow.

Tuberculous meningitis can complicate miliary tuberculosis or develop locally when an adjacent tuberculous focus ruptures into the subarachnoid space (Chapter 8.3). Patients with tuberculous meningitis typically present with a prodrome of fever, malaise, and headache, lasting one to several weeks, followed by more specific symptoms of meningismus, cranial nerve palsies, and progressive obtundation. Examination of the spinal fluid typically reveals a lymphocytic pleocytosis, elevated protein, and low glucose; initial findings may be atypical (predominantly neutrophils, normal glucose), but generally later shift to the typical pattern. The diagnosis is made by lumbar puncture on at least four occasions, each yielding 15 mL of spinal fluid for AFB smear and culture of the centrifuged pellet.

Management: Patients with extrapulmonary tuberculosis generally respond well to the standard regimen for pulmonary tuberculosis (see "Treatment of Active Disease" above). One crucial difference is that the physician who has a clinical suspicion of meningeal or miliary tuberculosis must start to treat immediately, rather than waiting for laboratory confirmation. Without empiric treatment, these forms of extrapulmonary disease are quickly fatal. Once treatment has begun, the physician can gather samples for AFB stains and cultures. The drugs only slightly reduce the yield of cultures on samples obtained during the first week of therapy. Another difference from the standard regimen is the recommendation to extend the therapy for meningitis to 12 months to prevent a disastrous central nervous system relapse. Surgery is sometimes indicated in skeletal tuberculosis, for example, to drain a paraspinal abscess or stabilize the spine. Finally, corticosteroids are of proven benefit for patients with meningitis and probably also help patients with pericarditis.

Tuberculosis and HIV

Much of the resurgence of tuberculosis in the United States since the mid-1980s has been caused by the HIV pandemic. The risk of active tuberculosis in patients infected with both *M tuberculosis* and HIV is 30 times higher than in HIV-negative persons, and the risk in patients with AIDS is 500 times higher. So intertwined are these two infections that the physician must search for *M tuberculosis* in every patient infected with HIV, and for HIV infection in every patient with active tuberculosis. All patients with tuberculosis should be tested for HIV antibodies, all HIV-infected persons should have PPD skin tests, and all HIV-infected patients with pulmonary signs or symptoms should be evaluated with chest x-ray and sputum AFB smear and culture. Such a high index of suspicion is justified by the extraordinary morbidity and mortality of tuberculosis in HIV-infected persons, by the fact that tuberculosis is often the first infectious complication in HIV-infected persons, by the contagiousness of untreated patients, by the availability of effective preventive therapy, and by the excellent chance for complete cure of tuberculosis—nearly unique among the infections of patients with AIDS.

Tuberculosis in HIV-infected persons can present conventionally, but its often atypical presentation can pose diagnostic challenges. In contrast to the 15% incidence of extrapulmonary disease in non-HIV-infected patients with active tuberculosis, 60% of HIV-infected patients with active tuberculosis have extrapulmonary disease, particularly lymphatic, central nervous system, and miliary. They are also far more likely to suffer rapidly progressive disease. Chest x-rays often show changes typical for tuberculosis, but are less likely to show cavitation or upper lobe disease and more likely to show hilar adenopathy, miliary disease, or infiltrates that are easily confused with other HIV-related pulmonary conditions. Finally, false-negative PPD skin tests become progressively more common as immunologic function deteriorates.

The physician should try vigorously to diagnose or exclude tuberculosis in all patients with HIV infection and any signs or symptoms of pulmonary disease, by obtaining chest x-rays, expectorated or induced sputum for AFB smears, and sputum and blood mycobacterial cultures. (Although *M tuberculosis* is rarely isolated from the blood of non-HIV-infected patients with tuberculosis, it is often found in the blood of patients with HIV.) Additional cultures should be obtained from extrapulmonary sites, according to the patient's signs and symptoms.

Individuals who have HIV and a positive PPD but no evidence of active tuberculosis should receive isoniazid prophylaxis for 12 months. This generally well-tolerated treatment substantially reduces these patients' extraordinarily high risk for progression to active disease. Prophylaxis should also be given to all HIV-infected persons of all ages (1) who have PPD skin test induration greater than 5 mm; (2) who have at some time had positive skin tests, even if they are now negative; and (3) who, regardless of skin test results, are at high risk for tuberculosis because they are intravenous drug users, previous residents of high prevalence facilities (eg, prisons, shelters) or geographic areas (developing countries), or close contacts of patients with infectious tuberculosis.

The treatment regimens for HIV-infected individuals with active tuberculosis are the same as those for HIV-negative patients. Patients whose organisms are drug-sensitive and who complete therapy are unlikely to suffer relapse.

OTHER MYCOBACTERIA

Mycobacteria other than the classic human pathogens, *M tuberculosis* and *M leprae,* are widespread throughout the environment. Although less virulent than *M tuberculosis,* they are capable of causing severe disease in patients with compromised cellular immunity or pulmonary mucosal defenses. Humans acquire these mycobacteria from environmental sources rather than from human sources, since the organisms are ubiquitous free-living species in soil and water or are pathogens or commensals of many animal species. The most important syndromes caused by mycobacteria are pneumonia, skin lesions, and systemic dissemination, with clinical and histologic findings very similar to those of tuberculosis.

The most significant mycobacteria affecting humans are listed in Table 8.14–3. A group of several closely related organisms, the *M avium* complex, are of particular importance, since they are the most common nontuberculous mycobacteria to cause disease and are particularly resistant to treatment. They cause adenitis in children; in immunocompetent adults, they cause pulmonary disease much like tuberculosis, nearly always in patients with preexisting chronic pulmonary disease (eg, obstructive lung disease, pneumoconiosis). In many patients with AIDS, *M avium* complex disseminates and causes a syndrome of fever, wasting, and anemia, with or without diarrhea and

Table 8.14–3. Nontuberculous mycobacteria.

Organism	Systems Affected	Route of Entry
M avium complex	Respiratory, disseminated	Inhalation, food, water
M kansasii	Respiratory	Inhalation
M fortuitum	Skin, musculoskeletal	Surgical or traumatic inoculation
M chelonei	Skin, musculoskeletal	Surgical or traumatic inoculation
M marinum	Skin	Traumatic inoculation

abdominal pain. Patients with symptomatic disease can be treated with multidrug regimens.

M kansasii most often causes pneumonia, usually in patients with chronic pulmonary disease; disseminated disease is less common and largely restricted to patients with AIDS. In most patients, the organism is very sensitive to antituberculous drugs and can be cured almost as reliably as tuberculosis. *M fortuitum* and *M chelonei* typically cause disease weeks to months after contaminating surgical or traumatic wounds of the skin, soft tissue, or bone. Treatment is surgical débridement to the extent possible, followed by antimicrobial therapy. *M marinum* most often infects an extremity injured by an object contaminated with sea or aquarium water.

Diagnosing disease caused by these organisms is made difficult by their ubiquity. Although the isolation of *M tuberculosis* proves infection, isolation of other mycobacteria may represent merely harmless colonization or contamination of the specimen by environmental sources. Clinical significance must be proved by evidence of a compatible disease and either by repeated isolation of multiple colonies of the same species of mycobacteria from pulmonary secretions or by isolation of mycobacterium from a normally sterile site such as the pleural fluid. In patients with AIDS, *M avium* complex is usually easily diagnosed by mycobacterial blood culture.

Mycobacterium leprae

Leprosy is a chronic infection of the skin, mucous membranes, nasal structures, and peripheral nerves, caused by *Mycobacterium leprae.* More than 12 million persons worldwide suffer from this disease, and several hundred cases are reported each year in the United States, most of them in immigrants from endemic countries. Like *M tuberculosis,* but unlike other mycobacteria, *M leprae* is not a free-living organism or an infection of other animals. Like tuberculosis, it is thought to be spread by close contact with an infected individual.

Patients' complaints and physical findings are usually dominated by their skin lesions. These very diverse lesions can include macules, plaques with raised borders, nodules, and papules. Erythema and hypopigmentation are common, as is diffuse thickening of the skin of the face and edema of the hands and feet. Many patients also complain of nasal stuffiness, nosebleeds, numbness, and arthralgia. Extracutaneous physical findings include pal-

pable nerve thickening, peripheral neuropathy, neuropathic deformities of the hands and feet, nasal deformities, testicular atrophy, and gynecomastia. The differential diagnosis includes neuropathies as well as rheumatic syndromes such as scleroderma, systemic lupus erythematosus, erythema nodosum, and Wegener's granulomatosis. *M leprae* cannot be cultivated in vitro, so diagnosis depends on the clinical findings supplemented by skin biopsy and histologic stains.

Like tuberculosis, leprosy requires prolonged multipledrug therapy. Also like tuberculosis, therapy is often complicated by nonadherence, thus potentially by resistance to drugs. The currently recommended treatment is dapsone, clofazimine, and rifampin. If patients continue this regimen for 2 years, their infection can be cured, but serious disfigurement may be irreversible.

SUMMARY

▶ The cardinal symptom of pulmonary tuberculosis is chronic productive cough, found in nearly all patients with infectious tuberculosis. Unexplained fever or suspicion of occult malignancy should also prompt evaluation for tuberculosis.

▶ Patients with HIV infection are at extraordinarily high risk for tuberculosis and other mycobacterial diseases, especially disseminated *Mycobacterium avium* complex disease.

▶ Key tests for tuberculosis are the tuberculin skin test, chest x-ray, acid-fast bacillus (AFB) stain of sputum, and sputum mycobacterial culture.

▶ Patients with active tuberculosis should be treated with four drugs until their isolate is shown not to be drug-resistant.

▶ Leprosy, though difficult to diagnose in the United States because of its rarity, can be cured. Other low-virulence, widely distributed mycobacteria can infect patients whose mucosal or immune defenses are compromised, or gain entry by surgical or traumatic inoculation. Although more commonly drug-resistant than *M tuberculosis,* many of these infections can be cured with multiple drugs.

SUGGESTED READING

Barnes PF, Barrows SA: Tuberculosis in the 1990s. Ann Intern Med 1993;119:400.

Bass JB Jr et al: Treatment of tuberculosis and tuberculosis infection in adults and children. American Thoracic Society and The Centers for Disease Control and Prevention. Am J Respir Crit Care Med 1994;149:1359.

Bayer R, Wilkinson D: Directly observed therapy for tuberculosis: History of an idea. Lancet 1995;345:1545.

Division of Tuberculosis Elimination of the Centers for Disease Control, and The American Thoracic Society: Core Curriculum on Tuberculosis, 2nd ed, April 1991. Available from: Division of Tuberculosis Elimination, Centers for Disease Control and Prevention, 1600 Clifton Road (E10), Atlanta, GA 30333. (404) 639–3311.

Wolinsky E: Mycobacterial diseases other than tuberculosis. Clin Infect Dis 1992;15:1.

Geographic Medicine and Travelers' Diseases

R. Bradley Sack, MD, ScD

The term "geographic medicine" has been used to denote illnesses that historically were confined to specific locations, particularly the tropics. A more timely and practical definition is "infectious diseases of the developing world." Before the advent of easy worldwide transportation, these diseases were indeed confined to certain geographic areas limited by mountains or oceans and were slow to spread. These barriers have essentially disappeared, and diseases can be carried to any part of the world within 1 or 2 days. Travelers may come home with illnesses that may not be familiar to medical practitioners in the United States. Since it is now recognized that new infectious diseases are emerging in various parts of the world—for example, Ebola virus infections in Africa—it is vital that physicians at least be aware of these new diseases and the possibility that they may be introduced into the United States. This chapter summarizes the basics of recognizing and treating some of the more common infectious geographic illnesses.

WHEN TO SUSPECT A GEOGRAPHIC ILLNESS

During all routine medical histories, the physician should ask patients whether they have traveled to or lived in the developing world. Geographic diseases are almost always acquired through direct exposure during travel; indirect transmission without travel is usually explained by either a large infecting dose or insect vectors. For example, outbreaks of typhoid fever in the United States have been caused by *Salmonella typhi* carriers, who have come from the developing world; airport cargo handlers can contract malaria if they are bitten by mosquitoes arriving in the cargo.

Several aspects of the travel history are critical to pinpointing the type of illness.

Exact Time of Travel: Geographic diseases have known incubation periods and seasonal characteristics. Malaria, for instance, cannot be manifested clinically until at least 7 days after a mosquito bite, and dengue fever has an incubation period of 5–8 days. Therefore, a febrile illness beginning 1 day after a 3-day stay in Haiti cannot be either malaria or dengue. Furthermore, some illnesses have distinct seasonal transmission; for example, Japanese encephalitis is transmitted only during the summer, and in some countries malaria is not transmitted during the cold months.

Places Visited: It is important to know both the countries and the cities visited. Knowing which countries allows the doctor to suspect the illnesses reported from those countries and the drugs to which the pathogens are known to be most sensitive. Knowing which cities allows the doctor to further narrow infection risks. For example, Peru is known to have malaria only in jungle areas and to have bartonellosis only in the Andes Mountains. Therefore, visitors to Peru's capital city, Lima, are not at risk for either disease. Certain cities are also associated with specific illnesses: Visitors to St. Petersburg, Russia, are known to have a high rate of giardiasis. Jakarta, Indonesia, is known for its high rate of typhoid fever. Some illnesses are acquired primarily in rural areas and jungles. For example, Japanese encephalitis is contracted primarily by mosquitoes in rural areas, and yellow fever by mosquitoes in jungles.

Style of Travel: Persons traveling first class have a lower risk of contracting enteric illnesses than do budget travelers and backpackers. Persons who travel on luxury cruise ships are at little risk, regardless of their itinerary, except for the brief times that they go ashore.

Types of Prevention Used: The doctor can better assess risks by knowing what immunizations patients received before travel and whether they used malaria prophylaxis, prophylactic antibiotics to prevent diarrhea, or repellent and bed nets to prevent mosquito bites.

Known Exposures During Travel: The physician should ask whether travelers were bitten by such disease vectors as mosquitoes, ticks, or larger animals. Travelers who have eaten unusual foods such as raw or undercooked seafood may contract a *Vibrio* enteric infection, whereas eating food from street vendors suggests exposure to *S typhi.*

Medications Taken During Travel: Travelers may have taken with them medicines such as antibiotics for diarrhea, or they may have sought medical treatment on their trip. Since medications may influence the clinical course of the disease, the doctor should find out what, if any, medications were taken and whether any injections or blood transfusions were received. In addition, exposure to blood products may suggest hepatitis B or HIV infection.

SYMPTOMS

The most common complaints of travelers returning from the developing world are diarrhea, respiratory symptoms, fevers, and rashes. These symptoms are generally nonspecific, but a detailed history may give clues to the diagnosis (Table 8.15–1).

Diarrhea

Diarrhea is the most common symptom in returning travelers. The onset is usually abrupt, often preceded by vomiting. Patients have frequent watery stools, nausea, loss of appetite, and, occasionally, low-grade fever. This syndrome of traveler's diarrhea is a secretory diarrhea, typically caused by enterotoxigenic *Escherichia coli* that have colonized the small bowel.

A less common form of traveler's diarrhea, invasive diarrhea or dysentery, is characterized by one or a combination of gross blood, pus, and mucus in the stools, along with abdominal cramping and fever. The typical pathogen is *Shigella,* or less often *Campylobacter.*

Respiratory Symptoms

Most respiratory infections of travelers are caused by viruses (particularly common in China). Pleuritic chest pain and high fever suggest a lower respiratory tract infection, probably bacterial. The common bacterial respiratory pathogens are generally the same worldwide, and unusual organisms would not be anticipated. Chronic respiratory symptoms suggest tuberculosis.

Fever

Malaria and typhoid are the most worrisome causes of fever in returning travelers. The fever of malaria is often periodic and associated with chills and sweating, whereas the fever of typhoid is more sustained. Patients may need to record their temperatures 4–6 times a day for several days after returning home to be able to characterize the fever.

Rashes

Important clues include insect bites, unusual skin exposures, and medications that can elicit an allergic response.

DIAGNOSIS

During the physical examination, the physician should pay careful attention to any skin lesions and to lymphadenopathy (tuberculosis, filariasis), organomegaly (malaria, typhoid, kala-azar), and hepatic tenderness (hepatitis, liver abscess). Patients with suspected onchocercosis need special eye exams.

Possible causes suggested by the history and physical

Table 8.15–1. Major geographic illnesses for which travelers are at risk, and recommendations for prevention.

Illnesses	Recommendations for Prevention	Locations
Enteric diseases: traveler's diarrhea, cholera, typhoid, shigellosis, amebiasis, intestinal parasites	Water and food precautions Immunization: typhoid	All developing countries where water and sanitation are poor and health care is less than adequate
Diseases transmitted enterically: hepatitis A, poliomyelitis	Water and food precautions Immunizations: hepatitis A, polio	
Diphtheria, measles, hepatitis B	Immunizations: diphtheria-tetanus, measles, hepatitis B	
Tuberculosis, HIV	Avoid personal exposure; avoid injections and blood transfusions from local practitioners	

Malaria:
 Chloroquine-sensitive
  Plasmodium falciparum
 Chloroquine-resistant
  Plasmodium falciparum
	Mosquito repellent and bed nets to prevent mosquito bites
	 Chloroquine 1 wk before, weekly during, and
	  4 wk after travel
	 Mefloquine 1 wk before, weekly during, and
	  4 wk after travel
		Mexico, Central America, Middle East
		
		South America, central and southern Africa, Asia

Yellow fever	Yellow fever immunization needed for both prophylaxis and legal entry into some countries	Tropical areas of South America and Africa
Schistosomiasis	Avoiding swimming in unprotected fresh water	Widespread
Filariasis and onchocercosis	Avoiding bites of mosquitoes and blackflies	Widespread tropical areas

See "Suggested Reading" for maps of high-risk locations.

exam dictate the laboratory tests to perform. To assess body homeostasis and inflammation, the physician should order a hematocrit, white blood count and differential (including eosinophil count), blood urea nitrogen (or creatinine), urinalysis, and chest x-ray. Tests of skin or body fluids aid in identifying specific pathogens. The tuberculin skin test is helpful for a person who has lived in a developing country for a long time, particularly one who was skin-test-negative when departing for travel. Cultures of blood and bone marrow are used to diagnose typhoid and other bacteremias. Cultures of cerebrospinal fluid, urine, and other body fluids may also be needed.

Blood smears (thin and thick film) are taken for malaria and microfilaria. Stool is examined for leukocytes, cultured for bacterial enteropathogens, and checked for ova and parasites. Urine is studied for schistosome eggs.

Duodenal aspirates obtained by a "string capsule" may be useful in identifying *Strongyloides* and *S typhi*. In this test, the patient swallows a capsule that contains a coiled string. When the capsule dissolves in the stomach, the string unwinds into the small intestine, becomes coated with intestinal mucus, and is retrieved by being pulled out through the mouth.

Skin biopsies (or superficial skin snips) may be taken for tissue diagnosis of leprosy and onchocercosis. Biopsies may be taken from the rectum for schistosomiasis and amebiasis, from the spleen for kala-azar, and from the pleura for tuberculosis.

Serologic assays that provide immunologic evidence of infection are most helpful in persons who have visited endemic areas, since any antibody titer denotes recent infection. For persons *living* in endemic areas, serologic tests are less useful, since many show evidence of past infection. Serologic tests have been developed for many parasitic infections, such as filariasis, strongyloidiasis, and Chagas' disease, but they available only at research institutions such as the National Institutes of Health (NIH) and the Centers for Disease Control and Prevention (CDC).

Some infections can be practically diagnosed only by serologic tests. Rickettsial and nearly all viral illnesses must be diagnosed serologically, since cultures and other methods for primary identification are not generally available. A serologic assay for antibodies to *Entamoeba histolytica* is useful in diagnosing invasive amebiasis, particularly liver abscess.

Radiographic techniques permit visualization of lesions in the liver (abscess, *Echinococcus* cysts), brain (cysticercosis), and abdomen (*Echinococcus* cysts). Ultrasonography is useful for defining fibrosis of the liver caused by schistosomiasis.

MANAGEMENT

Although management of most geographic illnesses is beyond the scope of this chapter, a few illnesses that demand immediate treatment will be discussed.

Plasmodium falciparum malaria is a life-threatening illness that requires urgent therapy; most of the deaths in the United States result from delayed diagnosis. The physician who suspects malaria should immediately make thick and thin blood smears to identify the characteristic protozoal forms and may need to repeat the smears every few hours to demonstrate the parasite.

As soon as the diagnosis is confirmed, therapy should be started. Mildly and moderately sick patients can take oral treatment; the choice of drug depends on the parasite's sensitivity, determined by the geographic area where it was acquired and the species identified from the blood smear. Severely ill patients require parenteral medication. For patients suspected of having chloroquine-resistant falciparum malaria, the preferred drug is intravenous quinidine, plus oral tetracycline when tolerated, and general supportive therapy. Quinidine must be given with cardiac monitoring. Response to therapy should be followed clinically as well as by checking thin blood smears for the percentage of red cells parasitized.

Rickettsial infections occur worldwide, often with names designating a geographic area, for example, Kenya tick-bite fever. Since there is no rapid diagnostic test for rickettsial infection, treatment must be based on the characteristic history and physical findings, usually fever and a typical macular rash. The rash begins 3–5 days after the fever, starts around the wrists and ankles, and spreads to the rest of the body within 1–2 days. The drug of choice is tetracycline or long-acting doxycycline. A serologic test confirms the diagnosis retrospectively.

For nonspecific diarrhea, travelers should take an antibiotic for moderate to severe symptoms, usually watery diarrhea or, less commonly, bloody stools. A stool culture is optional and used primarily for confirmation. The drug of choice is a fluoroquinolone (norfloxacin or ciprofloxacin) or trimethoprim-sulfamethoxazole. Symptoms predictably resolve within 24–36 hours after starting treatment. The diarrhea is self-limited, but without antibiotics it usually lasts 2–5 days. Patients should also take an oral rehydration solution to prevent dehydration secondary to the loss of large volumes of stool. Patients may resume a normal diet when they feel ready.

Milder diarrhea that does not interfere with normal activity can be treated with an antimotility drug (eg, loperamide [not to be taken by very young children]) or bismuth subsalicylate. The antimotility drug decreases the frequency of diarrheal stools and may be particularly helpful in providing relief during prolonged travel such as a bus ride.

PREVENTION

All travelers are at risk for geographic illnesses when visiting areas where water quality and sanitation are poor and health care is less than adequate (see Table 8.15–1). During a 3-week trip, 30–50% of travelers will develop acute diarrhea. Before leaving home, travelers should obtain pertinent health information, immunizations and malaria prophylaxis as needed, and antibiotics and oral rehydration solution packets to treat acute diarrhea. Specialized medical clinics for international travelers are available in most major metropolitan areas of the United States. Travelers should be informed about possible illnesses in the area to be visited.

Travel to the developing world will be associated with a minimal risk if travelers follow the following guidelines:

1. Because enteric pathogens have fecal-oral transmission in food, water, and ice, eat raw fruits and vegetables only if they can be peeled and drink only water that has been chlorinated, iodinated, boiled, or in a sealed bottle.
2. Use mosquito repellent and bed nets to decrease the risk of malaria in endemic areas.
3. Do not swim in unprotected fresh water in areas where schistosomiasis is endemic.
4. Avoid injections or blood transfusions from local medical practitioners. (Reusable needles and syringes may not be adequately sterilized between injections, and blood may not be screened for hepatitis B surface antigen and HIV antibody.)

Some immunizations, as a primary series or as boosters, should be given to most visitors to the developing world, since the risks exist everywhere; these include vaccines against diphtheria-tetanus, hepatitis A, typhoid, and polio (except in the Western Hemisphere, where polio has been eradicated). Other vaccines should be given to travelers going to areas where specific diseases are prevalent (eg, meningococcal vaccine for sub-Saharan Africa, Japanese encephalitis vaccine for Thailand and parts of Southeast Asia) or to areas considered high risk for exposure (eg, rabies vaccine for places with many stray dogs).

Proof of yellow fever immunization is required to enter many countries, particularly if the traveler has visited a yellow fever area within the past 10 days. Immunization is required primarily to prevent introducing yellow fever into new countries. Therefore, travelers need yellow fever vaccine both to protect themselves from the disease and to gain legal entry into countries on their itinerary.

No country requires cholera immunization, nor does the World Health Organization (WHO) recommend it for travel anywhere in the world. Injectable vaccine does not prevent transmission of cholera and gives minimal protection. Oral vaccines are being developed.

Immunization recommendations and requirements change periodically. The best way to stay current is to consult annual CDC and WHO publications (see Suggested Reading).

Malaria prophylaxis with chloroquine or mefloquine should be given to all persons visiting high-risk areas and during seasons when they might be at risk. Consult recent CDC and WHO publications for updates. Although chloroquine and mefloquine have low incidences of side effects, this possibility should be fully explained to travelers so that they can stop taking the drug, if necessary.

When prevention of traveler's diarrhea is essential, persons traveling for less than 3 weeks may benefit from prophylaxis with daily antibiotics. The drugs of choice are the fluoroquinolones, which reduce the risk of diarrhea by 80–90%. The only significant risk of prophylactic antibiotics is drug reactions, which, although rare, may require discontinuation of the drug.

For treating acute diarrhea, all travelers to the developing world should be given antibiotics and oral hydration solution packets—and detailed instructions on how to use them—to take along on their trip. Bismuth subsalicylate and antimotility drugs may also be recommended (see "Management" above).

SUMMARY

▶ A history of travel to, or residence in, the developing world is essential to suspecting a "geographic" infectious illness. This question should be part of all routine medical histories.

▶ The most common complaints of travelers returning from the developing world are diarrhea, respiratory symptoms, fevers, and rashes.

▶ Malaria and typhoid are the most worrisome causes of fever in returning travelers. *Plasmodium falciparum* malaria is life-threatening and may require urgent treatment.

▶ Most travelers' diseases are preventable. To stay healthy, all visitors to the developing world need special information, immunizations, and medications before their travel.

SUGGESTED READING

Advice for travelers. Med Lett Drugs Ther 1996;38:17.

Drugs for parasitic infections. Med Lett Drugs Ther 1995;37:99.

Health Hints for the Tropics, 11th ed. American Society of Tropical Medicine and Hygiene, Northbrook, IL, 1993.

Health Information for International Travel. US Department of Health and Human Services, Centers for Disease Control and Prevention, Atlanta (a new edition is published every year).

International Travel and Health: Vaccination Requirements and Health Advice. World Health Organization, Geneva (a new edition is published every year).

Sears SD, Sack DA: Medical advice for the international traveler. In: *Principles of Ambulatory Medicine,* 4th ed. Barker LR, Burton JR, Zieve PD (editors). Williams & Wilkins, 1995.

Warren KS, Mahmoud AAF (editors): *Tropical and Geographical Medicine,* 2nd ed. McGraw-Hill, 1990.

Animal-Borne Diseases

Thomas R. Moench, MD

Animal-borne diseases can be extraordinarily lethal (eg, rabies, plague, Rocky Mountain spotted fever) and extraordinarily infectious (eg, Q fever, tularemia). Furthermore, they can mimic noninfectious rheumatologic and neoplastic diseases (eg, Lyme disease, cat-scratch disease). Most animal-borne infections present as fever, usually with skin lesions or lymphadenopathy, and often with neurologic signs, musculoskeletal complaints, pneumonia, and diarrhea (Table 8.16–1). Some patients have no localizing signs; they present with fever of unknown origin. Even urban populations commonly come in contact with animals, so infection by animal-borne pathogens is not exotic, but routine. Physicians must be familiar with these infections and ready to narrow the broad range of diagnostic possibilities by considering a patient's presentation and exposures.

People respond to infectious agents in only a limited number of ways; thus, their symptoms and signs are usually not specific to a single pathogen. The physician must seek other clues. Most pathogens rely on living hosts for amplification, dispersal, and transmission. Although some human pathogens are so specialized that their only reservoir is man, the majority also infect other species. A few pathogens (eg, salmonella) are very widespread among species, but most are more restricted. Thus, determining the animal hosts (Table 8.16–2) and vectors (Table 8.16–3) to which patients have been exposed can suggest the range of pathogens that may be causing their illness. When patients' presentations are considered along with their exposure history, the wide range of possible pathogens may shrink to a manageable number and guide initial empiric therapy. Directed tests can then efficiently yield a diagnosis and permit definitive treatment.

Human pathogens may cause disease in animal hosts, or they may be commensals, living in or on the host without harming it. Organisms are transferred to humans in diverse ways. The most direct is inoculation (by animal bites or scratches). Persons who touch animals can acquire surface organisms or organisms in secretions. Secretions, excrement, hair, feathers, or dander may transmit pathogens indirectly by aerosolization or by con-

taminating food, water, or objects that humans then inhale, swallow, or otherwise contact. Finally, many pathogens are transmitted by ectoparasite vectors, particularly ticks, mosquitoes, flies, lice, fleas, and mites (see Table 8.16–2).

Although patients know when they have been bitten by an animal, they may not recognize tick bites or be aware of exposure to contaminated air, water, or food. Thus, the physician should inquire not only about pets and occupational exposure to animals but also about indirect exposures such as travel, outdoor activities, insect bites, rodent infestation, unpasteurized dairy products, traditional foods, and water source.

There are many more animal-borne diseases that can be listed in this chapter's tables or covered in the text. Representative diseases are discussed below in an effort to increase familiarity with the most common and important of the infections seen in the United States and to illustrate the diversity of transmission mechanisms and some of the major syndromes that these diseases can produce.

LYME DISEASE

Lyme disease, caused by the spirochete *Borrelia burgdorferi,* has quickly increased in incidence and geographic range since the early 1980's and is now more common in the United States than all other vector-borne diseases combined.

The manifestations of Lyme disease are sometimes divided into primary, secondary, and tertiary stages, by analogy to the prototype spirochetal disease, syphilis. Primary manifestations are those localized to the inoculation site shortly after the infecting bite, secondary manifestations are those of early disseminated disease, and tertiary manifestations are the late features of persistent infection.

Although Lyme disease is justly famous for the diversity of its manifestations, in most patients the initial illness (primary stage) is characteristic enough to allow a confident clinical diagnosis. About 1 week (range 2–30 days) after a deer tick bite, most patients develop a non-

Table 8.16–1. Clinical features of animal-borne diseases, in roughly descending order of frequency in the United States.*

Features or Syndrome	Disease
Fever without localizing signs	Malaria, brucellosis, babesiosis, ehrlichiosis, *Bartonella* bacteremia
Rash	Lyme disease, Rocky Mountain spotted fever, leptospirosis, rat-bite fever, erysipeloid, bacillary angiomatosis
Lymphadenopathy	Cat-scratch disease, toxoplasmosis, tularemia, brucellosis, leptospirosis, plague, rat-bite fever, dengue fever
Pneumonia	Tularemia, psittacosis, Q fever, *Rhodococcus equi,* plague, Hantavirus
Rheumatologic disease	Lyme disease, brucellosis, leptospirosis, dengue fever, rat-bite fever
Central nervous system disease	Toxoplasmosis, Lyme disease, arbovirus encephalitis, leptospirosis, brucellosis, lymphocytic choriomeningitis virus, herpesvirus simiae, rabies
Liver disease	Leptospirosis, Q fever, psittacosis
Diarrhea	Campylobacteriosis, salmonellosis, cryptosporidiosis, yersiniosis
Renal disease	Leptospirosis, hemorrhagic fever with renal syndrome

*Almost all patients present with fever.

Table 8.16–2. Pathogens or diseases associated with species.

Species	Bites and Scratches	Ectoparasites	Secretions and Aerosols
Pets			
Dogs	*Staphylococcus aureus, Pasteurella, Capnocytophaga canimorsus* (dysgonic fermenter-2), brucellosis, rabies, tularemia, *Bartonella henselae*	Tularemia, Rocky Mountain spotted fever, Lyme disease, ehrlichiosis	*Leptospira,* salmonellosis, *Campylobacter, Toxocara canis,* echinococcosis
Cats	*Pasteurella, B henselae,* tularemia, plague, rabies	Lyme disease, tularemia, plague, *B henselae*	Toxoplasmosis, salmonellosis, *Campylobacter,* Q fever, *Toxocara cati*
Birds	Erysipeloid		Psittacosis, salmonellosis
Turtles			Salmonellosis
Livestock			
Cows	Rabies		Brucellosis, leptospirosis, cryptosporidiosis, salmonellosis
Sheep and goats			Brucellosis, Q fever, orf, echinococcosis, salmonellosis
Horses	Rabies	Viral encephalitis	*Rhodococcus equi,* brucellosis, glanders, leptospirosis, salmonellosis
Swine			Brucellosis, leptospirosis, cryptosporidiosis, salmonellosis
Fowl		Viral encephalitis	Psittacosis, salmonellosis
Wild animals			
Rabbits		Tularemia, plague	Tularemia, plague
Deer		Lyme disease, tularemia	
Raccoons	Rabies		
Skunks	Rabies		
Foxes	Rabies		
Bats	Rabies		
Mice	Hantavirus	Lyme disease, typhus, plague	Leptospirosis, Hantavirus
Laboratory animals			
Rats	Rat-bite fever		Leptospirosis, Hantavirus, lymphocytic choriomeningitis virus, rat-bite fever
Mice and hamsters	Hantavirus		Leptospirosis, lymphocytic choriomeningitis virus, Hantavirus
Monkeys	Herpesvirus simiae, simian immunodeficiency virus		Hepatitis A, shigellosis, measles, tuberculosis

Table 8.16–3. Diseases transmitted by arthropods.

Arthropod	Disease
Ticks	Lyme disease, Rocky Mountain spotted fever, tularemia, Q fever, ehrlichiosis, relapsing fever, Colorado tick fever, viral encephalitis, babesiosis
Mosquitoes	Malaria, viral encephalitis, dengue fever, yellow fever, filariasis, dirofilariasis
Flies	Tularemia, onchocerciasis, trypanosomiasis, bartonellosis
Lice	Murine typhus, trench fever, epidemic typhus
Fleas	Plague, murine typhus, leishmaniasis
Mites	Rickettsial pox, scrub typhus

pruritic rash called *erythema migrans* (see Color Plates). This erythematous rash expands, but typically the center clears, giving the rash a ring shape; a residual punctum is often found in the center, at the site of the infecting bite. About 50% of patients have mild constitutional symptoms of fever, myalgias, arthralgias, and meningismus.

The physician must recognize the many variations on these early signs and symptoms. Fewer than 50% of patients report a tick bite, since the tick most often transmits the infection while in its inconspicuous poppy-seed–sized nymphal form. Twenty percent of patients do not have erythema migrans at all. Of those who have the rash, it does not always follow expected patterns. It may appear as multiple concentric rings, the center may not clear, or the rash may remain stationary for weeks. The site of the bite occasionally manifests vesiculation, necrosis, ulceration, scaling, or purpura. If patients are bitten on their back, they may not notice the rash.

Early disseminated Lyme disease (secondary stage) presents with more severe constitutional symptoms: high fever, severe headache, meningismus, and musculoskeletal pain. About 50% of patients have multiple annular lesions similar to the initial rash. Some people develop aseptic meningitis, facial (Bell's) palsy, peripheral neuritis, migratory arthritis, or cardiac conduction abnormalities.

The late manifestations of Lyme disease are also diverse and can involve many organ systems. Untreated patients can develop chronic monoarticular or asymmetric oligoarticular arthritis. Chronic neurologic manifestations include fatigue, headache, hearing loss, encephalomyelitis, demyelinating disease, and polyneuropathy. Late cutaneous manifestations include atrophic patches on the distal extremities (acrodermatitis chronica atrophicans); erythematous swellings at the ear lobe, nipple, or areola (*Borrelia* lymphocytoma); and localized scleroderma.

Earliest diagnosis and treatment give the best chance of curing Lyme disease quickly and preventing its later complications; however, this can be difficult. During the early erythema migrans phase, the diagnosis must be based on clinical findings, which may be equivocal. Testing for antibodies to *B burgdorferi* is of limited value during this phase, since only 10–40% of patients are seropositive. Later in the disease, too, serologic tests are occasionally negative because early treatment can suppress the antibody response. In parts of the country where the prevalence of Lyme disease is high, patients with typical erythema migrans present little diagnostic difficulty (Figure 8.16–1). Those who have atypical skin lesions or are from low-prevalence regions can be studied with skin

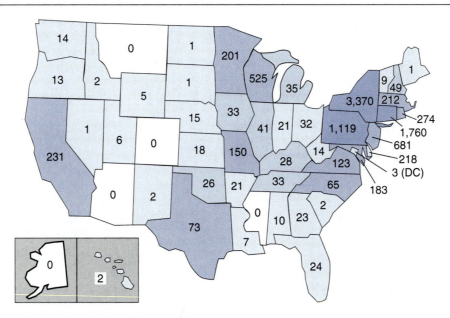

Figure 8.16–1. Distribution of Lyme disease in the United States (preliminary totals for 1992). (Courtesy of the Centers for Disease Control and Prevention.)

biopsy at the periphery of the lesion for histology and silver stain or monoclonal antibody demonstration of *B burgdorferi*.

Diagnosing Lyme disease becomes more difficult during the later stages and when the patient has no history of erythema migrans. Clinical manifestations are highly diverse and nonspecific, and serologic tests, although often helpful to confirm the diagnosis, have limitations in both sensitivity and specificity (false-negatives and false-positives). Moreover, even true positive serologic tests may reflect previous infection that is irrelevant to the patient's presenting complaints. Direct culture is insensitive and not widely available. Improved serologic tests and, preferably, direct spirochetal antigen detection or nucleic acid amplification (polymerase chain reaction) are being developed and are sorely needed. Initial reports of polymerase chain reaction detection of *B burgdorferi* in joint fluid are very promising.

Early Lyme disease is treated with doxycycline or amoxicillin. A prolonged course of 3–4 weeks is advisable to minimize the risk of late complications. Minor neurologic (facial nerve palsy without cerebrospinal fluid pleocytosis) or cardiac (first-degree heart block) involvement can also be treated with an oral antibiotic. More severe neurologic or cardiac disease, or serious or refractory arthritis, should be treated with 2–4 weeks of parenteral ceftriaxone.

Lyme disease can be prevented by avoiding infected habitats, using protective clothing and insect repellents, taking prompt showers and changing clothes after outdoor exposure, and inspecting daily for ticks on skin, scalp, clothing, and pets.

ROCKY MOUNTAIN SPOTTED FEVER

Few pathogens can kill as quickly as *Rickettsia rickettsii*, the agent of Rocky Mountain spotted fever, even in young and previously healthy victims. The organism invades and destroys endothelial cells, producing diffuse vasculitis, increased vascular permeability, edema, hypovolemia, and shock; 20% of untreated patients die. Early diagnosis is essential but difficult.

The illness typically begins with fever, myalgias, and headache, starting about a week after a tick bite. A maculopapular rash appears 3–5 days after the fever, typically beginning on the wrists and ankles; often later it becomes petechial and extends to the palms and soles. The triad of fever, headache, and rash should always spark strong consideration of Rocky Mountain spotted fever. The geographic distribution shows that, despite its name, Rocky Mountain spotted fever is most common in the south central and southeastern United States (Figure 8.16–2).

The diagnosis is hardest in the 10% of patients who do not develop a rash and in patients whose rash appears late. Prominent local symptoms can distract attention from the systemic nature of the illness and its possible rickettsial cause: Prominent gastrointestinal symptoms may suggest gastroenteritis or an acute abdominal emergency, whereas a neurologic presentation may suggest other causes such as meningitis or encephalitis.

Typical manifestations of Rocky Mountain spotted fever are characteristic enough to allow a confident clinical diagnosis. In some patients, the diagnosis can be confirmed quickly by immunohistologic staining of skin biopsy sections for *R rickettsii* antigens. Serologic tests allow only a

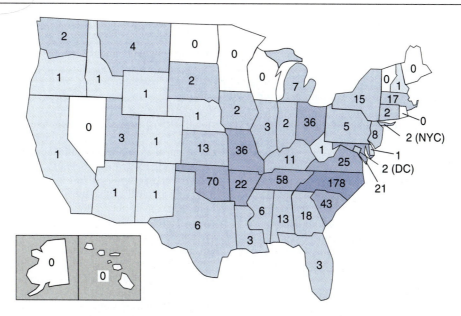

Figure 8.16–2. Distribution of Rocky Mountain spotted fever in the United States (totals for 1990). (Courtesy of the Centers for Disease Control and Prevention.)

retrospective diagnosis. The differential diagnosis of Rocky Mountain spotted fever is broad and includes other rickettsial infections (particularly ehrlichiosis in patients who do not have a rash), drug reaction, measles, rubella, mononucleosis, meningococcemia, disseminated gonococcal infection, and leptospirosis.

Doxycycline is the drug of choice, but chloramphenicol is also highly active and preferred for pregnant women and young children. These drugs have reduced mortality to about 5%, and even less when they are started early. Treatment is usually oral, but should be intravenous in patients who have hypoperfusion from severe disease, or nausea and vomiting. Many seriously ill patients require intensive support, including careful maintenance of intravascular volume.

LEPTOSPIROSIS

Leptospirosis is a systemic infection caused by spirochetes of the genus *Leptospira,* commonly found in many mammalian species and occasionally causing disease in humans. Most important, dogs, ruminants, rodents, and cats may chronically harbor leptospira without evident illness, and excrete the organism in the urine. People can become infected through pets or rodent-infested living areas or by coming in contact with water contaminated with infected urine. Infection is also common in heavily exposed groups such as slaughterhouse workers, farmers, and veterinarians. Most infections are subclinical, but the organism has the potential to cause anything from a mild anicteric illness to a severe icteric multisystem illness that can be fatal.

About 90% of patients with symptomatic disease have anicteric leptospirosis, which presents with headache, fever, myalgias, and often nausea, vomiting, diarrhea, or abdominal pain. Patients improve after 4–7 days, but some then enter a secondary "immune" phase: Their original symptoms recur and often progress to aseptic meningitis and more intense gastrointestinal symptoms. Characteristically, they complain of eye pain and photophobia, and examination shows conjunctival injection and meningeal signs. This immune phase nearly always resolves uneventfully in 1–4 weeks, even without specific therapy.

Patients with icteric leptospirosis are severely ill, generally with many systems involved. Liver disease causes acute jaundice, moderately elevated alkaline phosphatase, and modestly elevated serum transaminases. Renal function is often impaired, occasionally requiring temporary dialysis. Underlying the organ dysfunction is vasculitis caused by spirochetal endothelial damage; this can also lead to capillary leak syndrome, with hypovolemia, thrombocytopenia, and hemorrhage.

The diagnosis of leptospirosis, like that of syphilis, can be confirmed by darkfield exam, silver stain, culture, or serology. Darkfield exam can provide a rapid diagnosis by demonstrating spirochetes, but usually only in cerebrospinal fluid, since urine and blood contain too few organisms. Silver stain can reveal organisms in biopsy material. Culture requires special techniques and media, but heparinized blood can be sent to reference laboratories with reasonably good yield, since the organism is hardy. Serology is rarely diagnostic until 2–4 weeks after onset of disease, thus giving mainly retrospective confirmation.

Even when started late, antimicrobial therapy shortens the course of leptospirosis and improves outcome. Parenteral penicillin G or ampicillin is given to seriously ill patients; oral amoxicillin or doxycycline is appropriate for those less ill. Rodent control and vaccination of farm animals and pets have reduced but not eliminated transmission.

CAT-SCRATCH DISEASE AND RELATED ILLNESSES

Cat-scratch disease is a bacterial infection that characteristically presents as fever and lymphadenopathy after a cat scratch. Several days after the scratch, a papule or pustule arises at the site, followed in 1–7 weeks by tender regional adenopathy lasting 2–4 months. Fifty percent of patients look and feel well except for their adenopathy. Most of the rest have mild fever and flu-like symptoms. A small percentage are much sicker, with highly diverse complications that can include a prolonged and severe febrile illness, granulomatous hepatitis, encephalopathy, aseptic meningitis, radiculitis, neuroretinitis, granulomatous conjunctivitis, atypical pneumonia, and osteolytic bone lesions. Although cat-scratch disease is generally considered an illness of children, at least 20% of patients are adults.

The disease most commonly follows a cat scratch or bite, but can also follow a dog scratch or bite. Some people with intact skin are infected by contact with a cat, probably through mucosal transmission, fleas, or ticks. Fewer than 1% of patients are infected without animal contact, by puncture wounds, as from thorns or splinters.

Most cases of cat-scratch disease are caused by *Bartonella henselae* (formerly *Rochalimaea henselae*), a small, slow-growing, gram-negative bacillus related to *Bartonella quintana* (formerly *Rochalimaea quintana*), the agent of trench fever epidemics during World War I and distantly related to *Brucella* and *Rickettsia* species. A newly available serologic test for *B henselae* will help diagnose individual cases, and doubtless will also bring to light additional manifestations of this already many-faceted disease. About 10% of patients with typical cat-scratch disease are negative for antibodies to *B henselae;* this may reflect infections with other organisms or limited sensitivity of the test.

B henselae also causes three recently recognized and increasingly common syndromes that have substantial clinical differences from cat-scratch disease: bacillary angiomatosis, bacillary peliosis hepatis, and isolated fever and bacteremia. The first two infections predominantly affect immunosuppressed adults, most often patients with AIDS, producing vasoproliferative lesions. Bacillary angiomatosis presents as multiple enlarging cranberry-like skin papules composed of proliferating small blood vessels infiltrated with polymorphonuclear cells and bacteria. The disease may also involve nearly any other organ, and usually produces fever, weight loss, and malaise. The cause can be B henselae or, less commonly, *B quintana.* Bacillary peliosis hepatis is a liver disorder that on histologic study shows blood-filled cystic spaces containing abundant silver-stained bacteria. Bacillary peliosis hepatis can accompany bacillary angiomatosis or occur independently. Patients present with constitutional symptoms, abdominal pain, and hepatomegaly. Lastly, *B henselae* can present as febrile bacteremia without local features. This syndrome is again most common in immunosuppressed patients, in whom it tends to persist, but it also causes a brief, self-limited illness in immunocompetent individuals.

B henselae infection can be diagnosed by culturing the organism from blood or lymph node by the lysis-centrifugation blood culture method, with prolonged incubation and subculture onto chocolate agar plates. A new serologic assay that detects antibody to *B henselae* should prove useful, since few members of the general population are seropositive.

Prolonged courses (4–6 weeks) of either erythromycin or doxycycline can cure *B henselae* infections in both immunocompetent and immunocompromised patients. In contrast, most patients with cat-scratch disease improve spontaneously without specific therapy. Early studies did not show antibiotics helped to shorten cat-scratch disease, but their role is being reexamined in light of the responsiveness of other *B henselae* infections, as well as the present ability to culture the pathogen and choose therapy according to documented sensitivity testing.

TULAREMIA

Francisella tularensis, the cause of tularemia, is a highly infectious, virulent bacterium capable of infecting humans and many other kinds of animals. The infection is most often transmitted by contamination of minor skin breaks or even intact skin, but can also be acquired by arthropod or mammal bites, inhalation of aerosols, or ingestion of contaminated food or water. The most important reservoirs are rabbits, ticks, deer, dogs, and cats.

In 80% of patients, tularemia presents in an ulceroglandular form. Patients develop a papule, pustule, or ulcer at the site of inoculation 3–6 days after exposure to an infected animal or a tick bite. The bacteria replicate at the inoculation site, causing bacteremia and then reticuloendothelial sequestration. Patients then develop tender regional lymphadenopathy, fever, and malaise. Pneumonia or other localized infections can complicate the syndrome, but usually do not, and the prognosis is relatively good.

The other major syndrome is typhoidal tularemia—tu-

laremia without involved nodes or an evident inoculation site. Patients with this form seem to have deficient ability to contain the infection. Many more of these patients develop pneumonia, and the disease is more often fatal. One in four untreated patients dies.

Tularemia is easiest to recognize in patients who present with the ulceroglandular syndrome, but must be considered as well in patients who present with fever without localizing signs and in patients with "atypical pneumonia." Atypical pneumonia is pneumonitis that is detected by physical or radiographic exam but that is causing minimal pulmonary symptoms, only a nonproductive cough, or sputum production without purulence or without evident organisms on Gram or acid-fast stains. Several animal-borne diseases can cause atypical pneumonia—especially tularemia, psittacosis, Q fever, and, rarely, ehrlichiosis, brucellosis, leptospirosis, pasteurellosis, and cat-scratch disease. Nonanimal-borne causes include respiratory viruses, *Mycoplasma pneumoniae, Chlamydia pneumoniae,* and legionellosis (Chapter 8.5).

Tularemia can be cultured from the inoculation ulcer or from blood, sputum, nodes, or a throat swab, but requires a cystine-rich medium for optimal growth. The diagnosis can be made quickly by immunofluorescent staining of ulcer exudate. Serologic tests can provide retrospective confirmation.

Streptomycin is the best established therapy for tularemia and should be given when the diagnosis is sure. Although inferior to streptomycin, the tetracyclines are active against the broad range of expected pathogens; they are especially useful in treating atypical pneumonia when epidemiologic features suggest an animal-borne disease but the diagnosis is not yet established.

BRUCELLOSIS

Brucellosis is caused by a group of closely related gram-negative coccobacilli whose natural hosts are domesticated animals. When these organisms infect humans, they cause a severe and prolonged systemic febrile illness, often exacerbated by focal suppurative complications. The most important reservoir species are swine, cattle, goats, sheep, and dogs. The infection is transmitted by mucous membranes or abraded skin coming in contact with infected blood or meat or by eating contaminated food or inhaling infectious aerosols. Thus, the populations at risk include farmers, slaughterhouse workers, veterinarians, microbiology laboratory workers, travelers to endemic areas (Latin America and the Mediterranean basin), and people ingesting unpasteurized milk or cheese, particularly traditional products imported from endemic areas.

After an incubation period of 1 week to 3 months, nearly all patients develop fever, sweats, chills, and weakness, and many have headache, anorexia, weight loss, myalgias, and arthralgias. *Brucella* organisms localize in the reticuloendothelial system as intracellular parasites within phagocytic cells, often producing lymphadenopathy, splenomegaly, or hepatomegaly. Focal complications can develop in other organs as well, most prominently the skeletal system: More than 50% of patients suffer sacroiliitis, peripheral arthritis, or vertebral osteomyelitis. The central nervous system can also be involved, with meningoencephalitis or myelitis. Other complications are pneumonia, epididymo-orchitis, endocarditis, granulomatous hepatitis, and marrow suppression.

Definitive diagnosis is by culture, usually of blood or bone marrow aspirate. Physicians should alert the laboratory when they suspect brucellosis, so that cultures can be held for prolonged periods, special techniques can be used, and laboratory workers can take precautions to reduce their hazard. Since brucellosis is a prolonged illness, many patients seroconvert during active disease, and serologic tests (agglutination or ELISA) may be clinically useful.

Brucellosis requires prolonged multidrug therapy, with agents active in the intracellular compartment to ensure eradication and prevent relapse. Two regimens have proved to be highly effective. One is streptomycin plus tetracycline taken for 3 weeks, followed by 3 weeks of tetracycline alone. The other, doxycycline plus rifampin for 6 weeks, is less toxic, more convenient, and generally preferred. Patients with focal suppurative complications may be cured only by longer antimicrobial courses and surgical drainage.

SUMMARY

▶ Most pathogens rely on living hosts for amplification and dispersal, and many pathogens can be transmitted from animals to humans.

▶ Animal-borne organisms can be transmitted by direct inoculation via bites, by direct contact with secretions or aerosols, indirectly by ectoparasite vectors, or through contaminated water or food.

▶ Animal-borne infections may present as isolated fever, or fever with rash, lymphadenopathy, pneumonia, diarrhea, or neurologic or rheumatologic disorders.

▶ The range of likely pathogens can be narrowed by considering the patient's animal exposure history and the pathogens compatible with the presenting syndrome.

SUGGESTED READING

Barbour AG, Fish D: The biological and social phenomenon of Lyme disease. Science 1993;260:1610.

Elliot DL et al: Pet-associated illness. N Engl J Med 1985; 313:985.

Goldstein EJC: Bite wounds and infection. Clin Infect Dis 1992; 14:633.

Nocton JJ, Steere AC: Lyme disease. Adv Intern Med 1995; 40:69.

Schwartzman WA: Infections due to *Rochalimaea*: Expanding clinical spectrum. Clin Infect Dis 1992;15:893.

Section 9

Allergy and Immunology

John D. Stobo, MD, Section Editor

Approach to the Patient with Allergy

Philip S. Norman, MD

An allergy is a hypersensitivity state produced when exposure to a substance provokes an immune response that causes harmful reactions when the person is exposed to the substance again. Allergic symptoms can vary from a harmless rash to life-threatening shock. Classic symptoms are itching, swelling (from increased capillary permeability), hypersecretion, and smooth muscle contraction. Symptoms usually begin within minutes after exposure to an allergen (immediate-phase reaction), but typically fade within 30–60 minutes. Sometimes symptoms recur 4–6 hours later in a second wave of inflammation (late-phase reaction), which can last for hours. When a patient is exposed to the allergen continuously, the immediate and late-phase reactions overlap, making them impossible to distinguish. With prolonged exposure, tissue may be damaged or even scarred. Accurate diagnosis of allergy is crucial both to allow correct treatment and because allergic reactions can mimic other diseases.

MECHANISMS OF ALLERGIC REACTION

The substance that elicits an allergic reaction is an *allergen.* An allergen is a form of antigen—a substance that can provoke a specific immune response in the form of antibody or T lymphocytes and can later react with those immune components. Sometimes the allergen is a protein or carbohydrate—a large molecule that by itself can trigger the allergic response. At other times, the allergen is a small molecule that can provoke an allergic response only after it combines with a protein in tissue or serum. The process of a low molecular weight "hapten" combining with a higher molecular weight molecule to make a biologically complete allergen is "haptenation."

When people are exposed to a substance that is allergenic to them, their immune system responds by producing specific IgE antibody (Figure 9.1–1). Antigen-processing cells process the antigen and present it to T cells; the T cells help B cells to differentiate into IgE-secreting plasma cells. The IgE attaches to the surface of mast cells—connective tissue cells of unknown function, found primarily in the respiratory tract, gastrointestinal tract, and skin. When people are later exposed to the same allergen, it binds to and cross-links the IgE antibody on these mast cells. Antigen-induced cross-linking of the IgE molecules causes the mast cells to release histamine, prostaglandins, leukotrienes, and other mediators. These substances increase vascular permeability and cause smooth muscle contraction, leading to allergic symptoms. This rapidly occurring response is the immediate phase of allergic reactions. It is the principal mechanism for anaphylaxis (Chapter 9.4).

When allergic patients are reexposed to an allergen, they can also develop a late-phase reaction 4–6 hours after exposure. In this reaction, the processed allergen is presented to specific Th2 cells. When activated, these cells release interleukins that induce eosinophils and basophils to release mediators capable of causing allergic symptoms. Mediator release by these eosinophils and basophils is facilitated by the mediators released from mast cells during the acute phase reaction.

An allergic reaction is likely when (1) symptoms occur only during or after exposure to a specific environment or substance, or at a certain time of year; (2) the patient has many circulating eosinophils (an elevation in circulating eosinophils is helpful, but a normal eosinophil count does not exclude an allergic reaction); and (3) reactions typically occur in organs rich in mast cells—the respiratory tract, gastrointestinal tract, and skin.

Occasionally, mast cells are activated by stimuli other than those that produce immune reactions. Neural, chemical, and physical stimuli can directly induce mast cells to release mediators, producing symptoms that resemble allergic reactions even though the patient has not been exposed to an allergen. When such a reaction is sudden and catastrophic, as can occur after intravenous injection of hypertonic iodinated contrast media, it is called an *anaphylactoid reaction* (Chapter 9.4). In the respiratory tract, mediators can be released in response to physical stimuli such as cold air and can lead to late-phase reactions. These mediators may be important in rhinitis and asthma.

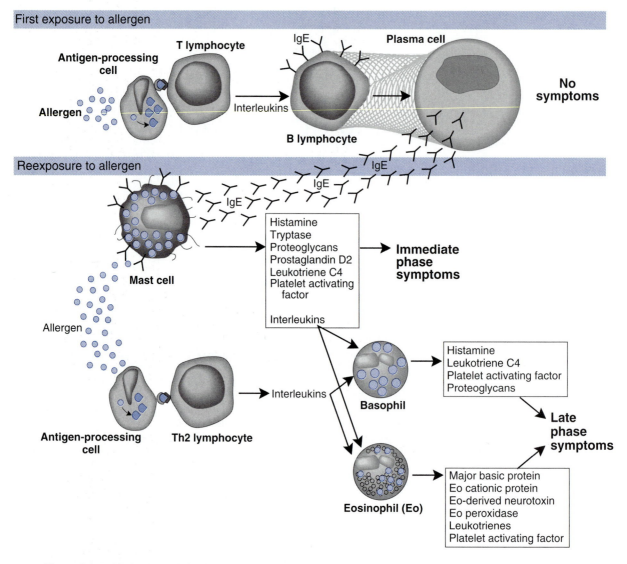

Figure 9.1–1. Mechanisms of allergic reactions: immediate and late phases. See description under "Mechanisms" in text.

CLINICAL MANIFESTATIONS OF ALLERGIC REACTIONS

Respiratory Symptoms

Since the nose is the main filter for inspired air, airborne allergens most often cause nasal symptoms, such as sneezing, hypersecretion of watery mucus, and mucosal swelling that blocks the airway. These symptoms resemble those of a common cold. They can be transient when exposure to the allergen is brief or persistent when exposure continues. Some airborne particles are small enough (less than about 5 mm in diameter) to evade the nasal filter and deposit in the lung. Mild reactions may cause only tracheal itching and cough. More severe reactions produce asthma, manifested by wheezing and respiratory distress

from bronchial smooth muscle spasm, hypersecretion of tenacious mucus, and an airway narrowed by mucosal swelling.

Gastrointestinal Symptoms

Eating allergens in food can first cause burning or itching in the mouth, then nausea, vomiting, or diarrhea that persists until the allergen has transited the gastrointestinal tract. When some of the allergen is absorbed into the circulation, it may activate mast cells in the skin, causing hives. In extreme cases, absorbed allergen causes enough mediator release to produce anaphylaxis, with hypotension, tracheal edema, and cardiorespiratory collapse. In infants, food allergy can lead to eczema, and babies may fail to thrive as long as they continue to eat the offending foods. Almost any food containing protein has the potential to incite antibody production and induce an allergic response. However, most food allergies are caused by a few common foods: milk, egg, wheat, peanut, and soy.

Cutaneous Symptoms

The skin is a good enough barrier to prevent direct absorption of most protein antigens. Rarely, small molecular weight allergens, such as platinum salts, are absorbed directly and cause hives. More often, hives are caused by ingestion of foods or drugs; presumably, enough of the antigen escapes digestion to enter the circulation and trigger mediator-containing cells in the skin.

The venom of bees, yellow jackets, hornets, wasps, and fire ants contains protein allergens that the insects inject directly under the skin. When a sensitized person quickly absorbs the venom systemically, the allergens can cause anaphylaxis. A person who survives this potentially fatal reaction will require prophylactic treatment, such as immunotherapy (Chapter 9.4). More frequently, sensitized people do not get anaphylaxis; instead, they have a late-phase local swelling at the site of the sting, caused by inflammatory cells entering the site and releasing their mediators. This late reaction is life-threatening only when the sting is in the mouth or neck, where extensive swelling may encroach on the airway.

DIAGNOSIS

The physician's principal tool in diagnosing allergies is the history relating allergic exposures to symptoms. This requires a thorough knowledge of potential allergens and the circumstances of their appearance. Table 9.1–1 outlines the most common allergens.

Exposure History

Allergic symptoms tend to be episodic and related to the respiratory tract, skin, or gastrointestinal tract. The physician should ask patients about symptoms in these systems, whether the symptoms are brief (minutes or hours) or more prolonged (days, weeks, or months), and whether any of the symptoms relate to time of year or specific foods or environmental exposures.

Airborne Allergens: Airborne pollens cause allergic rhinitis, often called "hay fever," which is usually seasonal. The specific pollens and the time of their appearance vary from one locale to another. Whatever the location, the offenders are trees, grasses, and weeds that depend on wind-borne pollen (as opposed to insect- or bird-borne pollen) for propagation. Other outdoor allergens include molds and fungi that grow on decaying vegetation and produce airborne spores.

Indoor allergens are less likely to be seasonal and thus may cause perennial allergies. House dust mites, tiny (300-mm) arachnids that live in house dust and subsist on human skin scales, leave a highly allergenic detritus that is a major cause of rhinitis and asthma. Danders (shed epidermal scales) from pets are the other major indoor allergen in homes. The leavings and dead bodies of cockroaches are also highly allergenic. Molds growing on damp walls or in poorly cleaned humidifiers may evolve allergenic spores from mycelia.

Allergens in the Work Place: The physician may suspect occupational exposure to allergens when the patient gets better on weekends or vacations. The allergens may be typical proteins such as wheat flour, which causes "baker's asthma," or chemicals such as toluene diisocyanate, a plasticizer used in paints and plastics. Animal allergens may cause respiratory symptoms in persons engaged in veterinary and animal husbandry. Persons with outdoor occupations may have more severe pollen and mold hay fever than office or factory workers.

Family History

Although it is not completely understood why some people develop an allergic reaction to an antigen and others do not, heredity plays a role. Allergies tend to run in families and recur in individuals. A few allergies are related to specific HLA-D genotypes; other allergies are more complex. Patients should be asked about a past or family history of allergy or of conditions typically allergic, such as childhood eczema, allergic rhinitis, asthma, and hives. Such a history helps build a case for suspicious current symptoms being allergic.

Difficulties in Interpreting the History

Most allergic people have multiple allergies. Overlapping exposures and symptoms in several organs may complicate specific diagnosis by history alone. Furthermore, many patients with respiratory allergies are bothered by atmospheric irritants such as tobacco smoke, automobile exhaust, cooking odors, and perfumes. Patients regard themselves as allergic to these substances, although they cause no immunologic response but simply irritate membranes already disturbed by allergic exposures. Furthermore, many allergic persons respond excessively to cold air, with a worsening of rhinitis or with asthma, particularly during exercise.

Allergic reactions can mimic other conditions. For example, the fever, glomerulonephritis, and lymphadenopathy that are part of a "serum sickness" reaction to a drug can mimic a lymphoma or collagen-vascular disease. Recurrent cough and shortness of breath caused by an allergic reaction to an inhaled allergen can be mistaken for intrinsic pulmonary disease.

Table 9.1–1. Common allergens.

Airborne
  Outdoor: tree, grass, and weed pollens; mold spores
  Indoor: house dust mites, animal danders, cockroaches, mold spores
Foods: wheat, milk, egg, soy, peanuts, other nuts, grains, meats
Drugs: penicillin and analogs, sulfa drugs, insulin
Insect venoms: yellow jacket, honey bee, hornet, wasp, fire ant

Allergy Testing

Although the history is the most important part of evaluating for allergy, it is often inconclusive. Tests for IgE antibodies to suspected allergens can be used to confirm a diagnosis. Skin tests are most expeditious. Allergen is introduced into the cleansed skin of the forearm or back by either pricking through a drop of allergen solution or injecting dilute solution into the skin with a fine needle. If the patient has skin mast cells with IgE for that allergen, a wheal-and-flare reaction develops in 15–30 minutes. Responses are compared with a nonreactive saline control and a histamine solution control.

For patients with skin disease or an aversion to skin testing, an alternative is serologic tests for specific IgE antibodies. In these tests, a solid phase carrier, such as a paper disk, is coated with allergen. The patient's diluted serum is added to the solid phase. After incubation, excess serum is washed away. Nonhuman anti-IgE antibody with either a radioactive marker or an enzyme marker is added. After incubation and washing, the amount of marker antibody attached to the solid phase is measured.

Serologic tests are less sensitive but more specific than skin tests. Both skin and serologic tests are generally satisfactory with airborne and insect sting allergens. Considerable research has gone into identifying the allergenic proteins in these substances and standardizing commercial extracts for diagnostic reliability. Positive responses to skin and serologic tests, when combined with a compatible history, are sufficient for diagnosis and planning management.

With food allergies, the research is less advanced. Diagnostic materials are less reliable and a positive result less meaningful. Specialists sometimes resort to blinded challenges, putting freeze-dried food powders into capsules so that patients will not know whether they have ingested the food or a placebo. For the next several hours, the patients are observed for allergic manifestations.

MANAGEMENT

There are three approaches to managing allergy: (1) eliminate exposure to the allergen; (2) lessen the effects of released allergic mediators; and (3) blunt the IgE-mediated response to the allergen (Table 9.1–2).

Table 9.1–2. Therapeutic approaches in allergic conditions.

Avoidance of the allergen
Drugs that interfere with the effects of released allergic mediators
  Physiologic antagonists
    Sympathomimetics (eg, epinephrine, decongestants)
    Theophyllines
  Mediator antagonists (eg, H$_1$-blocking antihistamines)
  Inhibitors of mediator release (eg, cromolyn)
  Anti-inflammatory drugs (eg, corticosteroids)
Immunotherapy to blunt the IgE-mediated response to the
  allergen

Eliminating Exposure to Allergens

Eliminating indoor respiratory allergens can occasion major changes in lifestyle. Household pets should go to a new home, and the patient's home should then be cleaned of residual hair and dander. Although extermination of cockroaches is effective, house dust mites, being arachnids, resist ordinary insecticides. Patients can significantly decrease mite exposure by removing dust-catching rugs, draperies, and overstuffed furniture; vacuum cleaning regularly; enclosing mattresses and pillows with mite-proof covers; and regularly laundering bedclothes with water heated to more than 60°C (140°F). Some laboratories can assess the mite allergen content of house dust samples to test the effectiveness of these measures. Protective masks and clothing can reduce or eliminate work exposures, but a change in job is even better. Patients cannot completely avoid outdoor pollens and molds, but indoor air conditioning with filtration provides at least a temporary haven from exposure.

It is easy to avoid foods that are eaten occasionally and are readily identifiable, such as fruits, vegetables, and seafood. But some common foodstuffs are so ubiquitous that avoiding them requires patients to study labels on all processed foods and to be wary of unidentified items. Peanuts, the most common cause of fatal food anaphylaxis, are sometimes ground up, processed, and served disguised in cakes, candies, and meat products. Eggs and milk are found in many foods that seem innocuous.

Drug Treatment of Mediators of Allergy

Antihistamines, β-adrenergic bronchodilators, α-adrenergic agents (epinephrine, decongestants), and theophyllines all have physiologic actions that counteract some allergic mediators and reverse specific symptoms of allergic reactions. Antihistamines are specific antagonists at H$_1$ receptors. Cromolyn seems to prevent or interrupt some allergic responses by mechanisms still poorly understood. Corticosteroids are specifically useful for the inflammation with eosinophils and basophils that characterizes late-phase allergic responses; thus, they are of little use for immediate or anaphylactic reactions, but they suppress ongoing late reactions.

Because allergic reactions are usually limited to the site of exposure, local application of anti-allergic medications often puts a therapeutic concentration of drug where it is needed, with but small risk of side effects. Thus, eye drops, nose sprays, skin creams, and inhaled aerosols can localize drug treatment. For best results, inhaled aerosols of drugs for asthma must deposit uniformly in the airways; patients require considerable training to learn to use aerosols correctly. Patients who have frequent asthma attacks should learn to monitor their pulmonary function several times a day. Many patients can recognize the beginnings of an attack and start taking medication before their daily routine is disrupted or they need emergency treatment.

Immunotherapy

The most specific form of treatment is modulating the immune response to allergens. Injecting extracts of allergens (immunotherapy) redirects antibody synthesis from IgE to IgG production. IgG antibodies combine with allergens and prevent union with IgE antibody fixed to effector cells. Such immunotherapy also down-regulates T-cell responses to allergens. Often, the clinician mixes extracts specific for the person's allergies, and gives the mixture as a series of subcutaneous injections every 1–2 weeks. Since patients are at risk for anaphylaxis until IgG antibodies appear, the initial doses must be small and later doses raised slowly. If patients develop minor symptoms of systemic allergy, later doses should be held steady or lowered temporarily until the patient begins to develop resistance. Injections must be given in a setting where well-trained personnel have epinephrine and other materials to treat anaphylaxis.

With these precautions, immunotherapy safely protects most people from severe allergic reactions to insect venoms and respiratory allergens. However, it may not completely relieve symptoms, so that patients subjected to heavy exposure may still need drug treatment. Immunotherapy to food allergens is not recommended because effective techniques have not been developed.

Long-Term Management

Since allergies are almost never "cured," management is a continuing process in which patient, family, and physician are partners. The process often requires eliminating environmental exposures, changing lifestyle, receiving drug treatment, and undergoing immunologic therapy. Managing allergies in children invariably involves parents and siblings. In adults, the spouse or employer often must be involved. Successful management requires continuing education of patients and those who surround them at home and work.

SUMMARY

▶ Allergic responses range from a mild rash to shock, but are most often episodic and related to the respiratory tract, skin, or gastrointestinal tract.

▶ Early manifestations of allergy are caused by IgE-mediated liberation of mediators from mast cells. When inflammation with eosinophils and basophils is invoked, symptoms can recur hours later (late phase).

▶ The diagnosis of an allergic reaction is made by the history, and in some patients can be confirmed by laboratory tests for immunoglobulin that has specificity for the allergen.

▶ The treatment of choice for allergy is avoiding the allergen. Patients who cannot avoid the allergen should receive either immunotherapy or long-term drug therapy.

SUGGESTED READING

Creticos PS et al: Ragweed immunotherapy in adult asthma. N Engl J Med 1996;334:501.

Multiauthored Section V on "Allergic Diseases." In: *Samter's Immunologic Diseases,* 5th ed. Frank MM et al (editors). Little, Brown, 1994.

Ownby DR: Clinical significance of IgE. In: *Allergy: Principles and Practice,* 4th ed. Middleton E Jr et al (editors). CV Mosby, 1993.

Sampson HA: Adverse reactions to foods. In: *Allergy: Principles and Practice,* 4th ed. Middleton E Jr et al (editors). CV Mosby, 1993.

9.2

Urticaria and Angioedema

Martin D. Valentine, MD

Urticaria (hives) appears as discrete raised red lesions of variable size, with sharp, visible borders, usually accompanied by intense pruritus (itching) (Table 9.2–1; see also Color Plates and Chapter 15.5). Angioedema appears as a diffuse, poorly demarcated swelling, often the same color as normal skin, and accompanied by burning rather than itching. Histologically, urticaria involves the superficial layers of the skin (Figure 9.2–1) and angioedema involves the deeper layers. Both conditions result from immunologic reactions or physical stimuli that cause the generation and release of inflammatory mediators, primarily histamine. Both conditions can be cutaneous manifestations of allergy or of systemic disease.

When confronted with a patient who has urticaria or angioedema, the physician must address three concerns: Is the cause a transient or reversible phenomenon and how can I make the patient more comfortable until it resolves? Is it a manifestation of a systemic disease? Is it hereditary angioedema?

DIAGNOSIS

The history is central to addressing the three major concerns about urticaria and angioedema. The physician should ask patients the following questions:

1. How long have you noticed these lesions? Urticaria or angioedema lasting less than 6 weeks is considered acute; 6 weeks or longer, chronic (Table 9.2–2). Acute urticaria or angioedema usually has a definable etiology—an allergic reaction to a drug or food, a reaction to an insect bite, part of an acute viral infection, or a response to a physical stimulus. When the cause is found, patients can be reassured, the inciting agent avoided, and, if necessary, short-term therapy given to make patients more comfortable until the rash resolves spontaneously (see "Management" below).

In contrast, the cause of chronic urticaria or angioedema is elusive and can be precisely determined in only 10% of patients. In the 90% of patients in whom a cause cannot be found, the lesions usually resolve on their own, and the goal is to alleviate the symptoms until they do. In the remaining 10% of patients, the skin lesions are a manifestation of a systemic disorder, most often a chronic occult infection, collagen vascular disease (eg, systemic lupus erythematosus), myeloproliferative disorder, lymphoma, or hyperthyroid Graves' disease. For patients with chronic urticaria or angioedema, the physician must aim the questions in the history at gaining clues to a possible underlying disorder.

2. Do the lesions consistently appear in one place, eg, the soles of your feet or palms of your hands? Urticaria induced by pressure (pressure urticaria) is manifested by painful nodules full of trapped extravascular fluid, on the soles of the feet. Urticaria on the palms can be caused by vibration, such as operating a jackhammer.

3. Does something trigger this reaction—food, medications, exposure to cold or heat, exposure to the sun? Foods such as shellfish can induce immune-mediated urticaria in individuals who have IgE antibodies against protein antigens in the food. Drugs can induce urticaria through both IgE-mediated reactions and reactions that do not involve IgE (Chapter 9.3). Certain drugs, including vancomycin, codeine, morphine, and iodinated radiographic contrast materials, can cause direct release of histamine and other mediators from mast cells.

An increase in body temperature, such as after vigorous exercise, can induce cholinergic urticaria. Exposure to the sun can induce solar urticaria, and exposure to cold can induce a diffuse urticaria or angioedema. Cold urticaria is thought to develop when cold exposure causes cold-reactive IgE antibodies to bind to IgE receptors on the surface of basophils and mast cells. It

Table 9.2–1. Urticaria versus angioedema: Clinical manifestations.

Feature	Urticaria	Angioedema
Erythema	Yes	No
Pruritus	Yes	No
Burning sensation	No	Yes
Lesion margins	Sharp	Diffuse
Histologic location in skin	Superficial	Deep
Histamine release produces lesions	Yes	Yes

Table 9.2–2. Common causes: Acute versus chronic urticaria.

Acute (<6 weeks)
Bacterial and viral infections
Drug and food allergens
Physical stimuli
Idiopathic urticaria

Chronic (≥6 weeks)
Idiopathic urticaria
Chronic infections
Collagen vascular diseases
Myeloproliferative disorders
Lymphoma
Graves' disease

is not known whether cholinergic and solar urticaria operate by a similar mechanism.
4. How long do individual lesions last? Urticaria and angioedema lesions that last not minutes or hours, but a day or longer, are characteristic of systemic vasculitis.
5. Has anyone in your family had angioedema? A "yes" to this question is a clue to hereditary angioedema (see below). Although this disorder can be acquired, it is usually familial with autosomal dominant inheritance.

The history guides the physical examination. For patients with chronic urticaria or angioedema, the physician should concentrate on looking for signs of systemic illness (Table 9.2–3). If the history and physical examination do not reveal the etiology, it is unlikely to be found through laboratory tests.

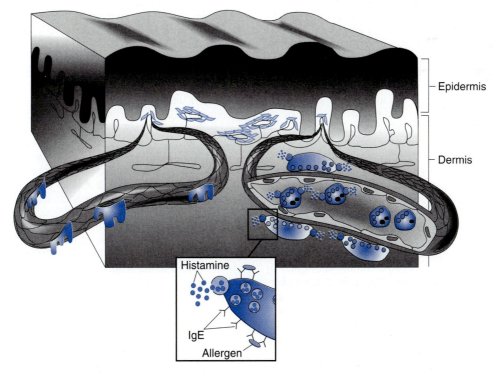

Figure 9.2–1. Urticaria. Histamine and other chemical mediators of increased vascular permeability are released from mast cell and basophil granules when a specific allergen bridges pairs of IgE antibody molecules on cell surface receptors (inset) or when the granules are exposed to physical or chemical liberators of inflammatory mediators. Histamine stimulates nerve endings, causing itch, and produces local swelling by allowing plasma to leak between cell junctions into the extravascular space.

Table 9.2–3. Search for systemic conditions in patients with chronic urticaria or angioedema.

Aspect of Physical Exam	Condition Sought
Inflamed blood vessels in fundi	Vasculitis
Lymphadenopathy, splenomegaly	Myeloproliferative disease, lymphoma
Exophthalmos; warm, dry skin; rapid pulse	Hyperthyroidism
Sinus tenderness	Chronic sinusitis
Right upper quadrant abdominal tenderness	Chronic inflammation of gallbladder

MANAGEMENT

When the physician identifies an inciting agent or associated condition, the next task is to remove or treat it. If no agent or condition can be found, the patient should be treated with the smallest effective dose of histamine antagonists. Particularly effective are H_1 antihistamines such as hydroxyzine. The primary side effect of these drugs is sedation. They are best taken at bedtime, since the sedative effect may wear off overnight, whereas the cutaneous benefit lasts through the next day.

Many patients with cold urticaria respond well to cyproheptadine. The physician can minimize this drug's sedation by starting patients on a very small dose and gradually increasing the dose until it is effective. A dose response can be checked by observing the effect of different doses of the drug when an ice cube is applied to the forearm. Some patients who do not respond well to an H_1 antagonist alone do respond to an H_1 and H_2 antihistamine given together; a few respond to an H_2 drug alone.

Other drugs that may be tried for cold urticaria or chronic idiopathic urticaria are β-receptor agonists and tricyclic antidepressants. In theory, selective β-adrenergic agonists like terbutaline better inhibit histamine release, but in practice, nonselective drugs like epinephrine and ephedrine may be more effective because they stimulate both α- and β-receptors. By stimulating α-receptors, these drugs constrict postcapillary venules. Thus, they seem to reverse the histamine-induced leaks of intravascular fluid to the extravascular space. Among the tricyclic antidepressants, doxepin has been helpful in chronic urticaria; other tricyclics may also be tried. The tricyclics can cause sedation and anticholinergic symptoms like dry mouth. When all else fails, the physician can give corticosteroids, but the potentially long duration of the urticaria or angioedema militates against drugs like steroids that cause long-term side effects.

Patients with chronic urticaria should be advised to prevent facial flushing and increased cutaneous blood flow by avoiding hot peppers and spicy foods, hot baths and showers, and vigorous exercise. Patients should also avoid dry skin, because it intensifies itching; especially in the winter, they can be helped by moisturizers.

HEREDITARY ANGIOEDEMA

A dangerous familial form of angioedema was first described by William Osler, in a kindred that had a history of premature death from airway edema and asphyxiation. Hereditary angioedema was at first called "angioneurotic," wrongly implying a "nervous" etiology. Attacks can be provoked by immunologic events whose mechanisms in activating complement are well understood (eg, drug exposure, infection), as well as by physical agents whose ability to activate complement has not been explained.

Typical patients present in the late teens with a history of angioedema, perhaps involving the larynx or pharynx, initiated by local trauma such as dental treatment. Many patients have suffered episodes of abdominal pain caused by angioedema in the intestinal wall. The pain may have been severe enough to necessitate exploratory surgery, and the failure to reach a diagnosis may have led their physicians to doubt the history. A parent has had recurrent attacks of angioedema, and relatives may have died from asphyxiation caused by airway obstruction. Antihistamines have not helped at all, and epinephrine and corticosteroids but little.

Hereditary angioedema is caused by deficiency of the serum inhibitor of C1 esterase, an enzyme that can activate the first component of complement. Without this inhibitor, the complement cascade is continuously activated, generating components that increase vascular permeability. Between attacks, complement stays activated at a low level. The continuing activation is reflected by a drop in C4, which is a substrate of the uninhibited C1 esterase. A patient with a normal serum C4 level is very unlikely to have hereditary angioedema. But when the C4 is low, the diagnosis can be confirmed by checking the serum level of the C1 inhibitor. In most patients with C1 inhibitor deficiency, the inhibitor is absent both functionally and immunochemically. However, 10–15% of patients have a nonfunctioning variant of the inhibitor. The variant reacts normally on immunochemical assay; it can be detected only by an assay that measures C1 esterase inhibitor function. The physician should suspect the variant when in spite of a normal C1 inhibitor level, a patient with a history compatible with hereditary angioedema history has a consistently low C4. Patients with congenital C4 deficiency have normal C1 esterase inhibitor levels.

In some patients, the deficiency of C1 esterase inhibitor is not inherited but acquired. These patients' inhibitor is consumed by an excess of activated C1 esterase. This can happen in a disease that produces circulating immune complexes. Acquired C1 inhibitor deficiency is seen primarily in patients with B-cell lymphoma, but it can develop with other malignancies.

Treatment for both inherited and acquired C1 inhibitor deficiency is an androgen such as danazol or stanozolol. Such drugs increase hepatic synthesis of the inhibitor and restore C4 levels to normal. The plasminogen inhibitors ε-aminocaproic acid and tranexamic acid have also been of benefit, but are not often used because they can damage the liver. Plasma transfusions may help during acute attacks. Purified C1 inhibitor, which is also effective, is not available in the United States. Epinephrine, antihistamines, and corticosteroids do not help.

SUMMARY

▶ Acute urticaria or angioedema (lasting less than 6 weeks) is self-limited. It is usually caused by infection, allergy, or physical stimuli and is often diagnosed by history alone.

▶ In 90% of patients with chronic urticaria or angioedema (6 weeks or more), the cause is never found, and the lesion resolves spontaneously. The other 10% of patients have an underlying systemic disease such as a chronic infection, collagen vascular disease, myeloproliferative disorder, or Graves' disease.

▶ Idiopathic urticaria should be treated symptomatically.

▶ Hereditary angioedema, caused by a deficiency in C1 esterase inhibitor, can be lethal unless attacks are prevented with danazol or stanozolol.

SUGGESTED READING

Arndt KA, Jick H: Rates of cutaneous reactions to drugs: A report from the Boston Collaborative Drug Surveillance Program. JAMA 1976;235:918.

Casale TB et al: Guide to physical urticarias. J Allergy Clin Immunol 1988;82:758.

Kaplan AP: Urticaria and angioedema. In: *Allergy*. Kaplan AP (editor). Churchill Livingstone, 1985.

Sim TC, Grant JA: Hereditary angioedema: Its diagnostic and management perspectives. Am J Med 1990;88:656.

Stafford CT: Urticaria as a sign of systemic disease. Ann Allergy 1990;64:264.

Drug Allergy

Jacqueline A. Pongracic, MD, and N. Franklin Adkinson, Jr, MD

Reactions to drugs can be life-threatening and require immediate treatment. This is especially true of anaphylactic reactions that cause bronchospasm and hypotension (Chapter 9.4). Furthermore, drug reactions can mimic systemic illness. Patients in whom a drug causes fever, rash, lymphadenopathy, and thrombocytopenia may be misdiagnosed as having a lymphoma or collagen vascular disease.

Our understanding of immune-mediated drug allergy is based largely on studies of penicillin allergy. The ubiquity and strong protein reactivity of penicillins and related beta-lactam antibiotics make them responsible for more allergic reactions than any other commonly used drug class. About 10% of hospitalized patients have a history of allergic reactions to penicillin. This chapter will use as a prototype the penicillins and related antibiotics that have a beta-lactam ring—cephalosporins, carbapenems, and monobactams. The chapter will cover immunologic testing in the diagnosis of drug allergy, risk factor assessment, management, and pseudoallergic drug reactions.

DRUGS AS ALLERGENS

A drug's chemical properties determine its propensity to act as an allergen. Drugs made of large molecules may independently induce immune responses. These drugs (eg, insulin, chymopapain, heterologous antisera) are called "complete antigens" because they are antigenic by themselves. Most drugs, however, are low molecular weight compounds that can become antigenic only after they form an immunogenic conjugate by covalently binding to a higher molecular weight carrier, usually a serum or cell surface protein. Through this process, known as *haptenation,* low molecular weight drugs such as penicillin and sulfonamides (haptens) form multivalent antigens and become potentially allergenic. The immunogenicity of a drug acting as a hapten correlates with its ability to interact with protein carriers.

TESTS FOR DRUG ALLERGY

Of the many immunologic tests that have been studied for drug allergy, the only test with strong predictive value is intradermal skin testing for penicillin IgE antibodies. Unfortunately, the predictive value of negative skin tests is not known for most other haptenic drugs, in large part because the antigenic determinants for most drugs have not been found.

Reliable skin testing has been developed for penicillin because the immunochemistry of its metabolites has been carefully worked out. Under physiologic conditions, the beta-lactam ring of penicillin opens to form a covalent (amide) bond with serum proteins, producing the penicilloyl determinant. This is called the *major antigenic determinant* because more than 95% of penicillin antibodies are directed against this immunogenic conjugate. *Minor antigenic determinants* are generated when serum proteins interact with the sulfide group on penicillin's thiazolidine ring. Although few anti-penicillin antibodies are directed against the minor determinants, they are important because IgE antibody against them causes most anaphylactic reactions.

Skin testing with penicillin alone has an unacceptably high rate of false-negatives. This is because penicillin can evoke a positive skin response only when it conjugates efficiently with host proteins. The test is much more sensitive if it is done with a preformed conjugate of penicillin G and poly-L-lysine, which together form the major determinant analog, penicilloyl-polylysine. Penicilloyl-polylysine skin testing identifies as many as 90% of patients at risk for IgE-mediated allergic reactions.

A mixture of minor determinants (penicilloate, peniloate, and penicillin) has been formulated and shown to be an indispensable companion reagent for skin testing. Unfortunately, the reagent is not yet commercially available in the United States. As an alternative, some authorities have suggested using penicillin G at a concentration of 6000 U/mL to skin test for minor determinant antigens. However, this substitute reagent is not sufficient to evaluate risk in patients who have a history of anaphylaxis; these patients require the three-part minor determinant mixture.

Skin testing starts with a prick or puncture test with each reagent. If both tests are negative, patients should get intradermal tests, which are definitive. Patients are given two intradermal injections of the mixture of minor determinants, or, as an alternative, penicillin G and penicilloyl-polylysine. If patients do not show a wheal-and-flare response within 15 minutes, their chances of having a serious allergic reaction are less than 1%. Diluent and histamine phosphate must also be tested as negative and positive controls.

In different studies, skin tests are positive in only 15–65% of patients with a history of penicillin allergy. The wide range in reported prevalence is probably explained by differences in patient selection criteria and time elapsed since the last reaction, reflecting the half-life of IgE antibodies. Of patients who have a history of penicillin allergy and positive skin tests, only 50–70% have allergic reactions upon later exposure to penicillin. Negative skin tests are much more predictive. To date, there have been no reports of anaphylaxis in persons who had negative penicillin skin tests with both the major and minor determinants. Of patients with a history of penicillin allergy who had negative skin tests, about 2–15% developed transient pruritus and urticaria when later given penicillin. Skin tests are not predictive of non-IgE-mediated penicillin reactions such as drug fever, exfoliative dermatitis, maculopapular rashes, interstitial nephritis, serum sickness, and hemolytic anemia.

Intradermal drug testing based on the principles of penicillin testing may be useful for other drugs known to induce IgE-mediated responses. These include insulin, chymopapain, local anesthetics, muscle relaxants, thiopental, cephalosporins, heterologous antisera, antituberculous drugs, anticonvulsants, quinidine, cisplatin, and penicillamine. Patients are at high risk for an allergic reaction if they have positive tests at concentrations that do not produce irritant responses in nonallergic persons.

In vitro measurements of drug-specific IgE by radioallergosorbent testing (RAST) have been developed for several drugs, but are not widely available. With penicillin, RAST is available only for the major determinant and has inferential value only when positive. With all drugs, RAST is less sensitive than intradermal skin testing, so a negative test result does not rule out drug allergy.

MANAGING ALLERGIC DRUG REACTIONS

Managing a drug reaction consists of three steps: (1) stop the offending drug; (2) treat the drug reaction; and (3) desensitize patients if it is absolutely necessary that they use the drug.

A drug that causes a serious reaction must be stopped immediately. A patient who is taking several drugs should stop the drug or drugs most likely to be allergenic. Some manifestations of a reaction can take time to dissipate after the offending drug is stopped. Drug-induced fever can last as long as 2 weeks. The antinuclear antibody response to hydralazine can persist for months.

With some allergic drug reactions, such as mild urticaria and maculopapular rash late in a course of penicillin therapy, the patient may be continued on the drug, sometimes at a lower dose and with careful observation. This is known as "treating through" the reaction. However, multisystem reactions such as serum sickness rarely resolve unless the drug is stopped; attempting to treat through can further damage critical organs.

Treatment for a drug reaction depends on the manifestations. Antihistamines are useful for pruritus and urticaria, corticosteroids are necessary for severe and systemic reactions like serum sickness and exfoliative dermatitis, and drugs combating hypotension and bronchospasm are required for anaphylaxis.

Ideally, patients should not use any drug to which they are known to be allergic. They should be given a non-cross-reacting drug instead. Most drugs have safe, effective substitutes. For example, with most infectious diseases, penicillin-allergic patients can be given non-beta-lactam antibiotics.

For the rare patient for whom alternative therapy is impossible or ineffective, the physician should consider drug desensitization. Desensitization protocols for penicillin and insulin have been developed and may be used in conditions such as neurosyphilis, refractory bacterial endocarditis, and insulin-dependent diabetes mellitus. Beginning with a very small amount of drug, patients are given gradually increasing amounts as tolerated, up to a full therapeutic dose. Although desensitization carries some risk, it is relatively safe and effective. It requires informed consent and careful monitoring, either in an intensive care unit or on an inpatient unit with staff and facilities that can treat anaphylaxis.

Patients who have had a drug reaction should be clearly told the name of the offending drug and the reaction it caused, and they should be instructed to mention this to every health care worker they see in the future, whether or not they are asked about allergies. If the drug reaction has been life-threatening, patients should be encouraged to wear a medical identification bracelet indicating the offending drug and type of reaction.

ASSESSMENT OF PATIENTS WITH DRUG ALLERGY

The most important part of the assessment of patients with suspected drug allergy is the history. A meticulous history usually reveals the culpable agent. Patients should be asked about all current medicines and the route and frequency of administration, about whether they were exposed to these medicines before the current course of treatment, and about how well they have tolerated these medicines. It can be helpful to ask how much time elapsed from first dose to onset of symptoms. A primary immune response usually takes 10–14 days; with prior sensitization, however, a patient may have an allergic reaction minutes after the first dose.

Many patients are unaware that they have become sensitized to a drug, either because the sensitization produced only a mild reaction or because they were reacting to a cross-reactive molecule in a drug or substance otherwise unrelated to the offending drug.

Risk factors for drug allergy depend on host and treatment considerations. An important host factor is age: Adults have a higher incidence of drug allergy than children. Genetic or metabolic factors may also affect a person's ability to generate a drug-specific immune response. For example, for unknown reasons, only 10% of inpatients receiving penicillin make drug-specific IgE antibody. IgE antibody levels usually fall over time, but they can disappear within 4 weeks or persist indefinitely; a long antibody half-life increases the cumulative risk for future reactions. Dose and duration of treatment are important determinants of type II (cytotoxic) and III (immune complex) reactions. Parenteral administration seems to increase the risk of acute allergic reactions, but this could be explained by higher dose rather than route.

IDIOSYNCRATIC AND PSEUDOALLERGIC DRUG REACTIONS

Many drug reactions look allergic but are not immune-mediated. Some of these reactions are caused by drug idiosyncrasy, attributable to a genetic or metabolic defect. The best-studied idiosyncratic drug reaction is primaquine-induced hemolytic anemia, which occurs in persons deficient in the enzyme glucose-6-phosphate dehydrogenase. Another example is the increased risk for hydralazine-induced lupus in those who are slow acetylators of hydralazine.

Sometimes idiosyncratic drug reactions are called "pseudoallergic" or "anaphylactoid" (Table 9.3–1). In contrast to allergic reactions, these can occur when patients are first exposed to drugs and diagnostic agents. These reactions do not require prior sensitization, nor do

Table 9.3–1. The most common causes of allergic and pseudoallergic drug reactions.

Allergic (immune-mediated)
Antibiotics (penicillin)
Hormones (insulin)
Enzymes (chymopapain)
Pseudoallergic (non–immune-mediated)
Nonsteroidal anti-inflammatory drugs (aspirin)
Radiocontrast media
Opiates

they involve production of antibody or antigen-specific T cells. For example, in susceptible patients, exposure to aspirin and most nonsteroidal anti-inflammatory drugs (NSAIDs) can induce urticaria, angioedema, rhinitis, and asthma. Most patients who get pseudoallergic skin reactions to aspirin and related drugs have underlying urticaria or angioedema. Patients who get respiratory manifestations typically are middle-aged adults with a history of nonallergic rhinitis, sinusitis, nasal polyposis, or steroid-dependent asthma.

The mechanism of pseudoallergic NSAID reactions is not fully understood. Despite their clinical cross-reactivity, these aspirin-like analgesics are structurally unrelated, so an immune response to a common antigenic determinant is improbable. Also arguing against an immune response is the frequency of patients reacting to these drugs on first exposure. Given the NSAIDs' common function as cyclooxygenase inhibitors, a possible mechanism is a shunting of arachidonic acid metabolites from the cyclooxygenase pathway to the lipoxygenase pathway, thereby increasing leukotriene production.

Patients with a history of anaphylactoid reactions to aspirin should avoid not only aspirin but all other NSAIDs. Safe alternatives include acetaminophen and sodium salicylate, neither of which inhibits cyclooxygenase. When long-term aspirin or other NSAIDs are indicated for treatment of chronic diseases, specific sensitivity should first be confirmed. Skin testing is not helpful, since these reactions are not IgE-mediated. The recommended test is double-blinded, placebo-controlled provocative challenge. Challenge-positive patients who need chronic treatment with NSAIDs may be desensitized by being given small and gradually increasing doses under supervision.

Angiotensin converting enzyme (ACE) inhibitors, which are used to treat hypertension and congestive heart failure, can cause pseudoallergic reactions of cough, angioedema, and rhinitis. The most common symptom is chronic cough, rarely producing sputum. Pulmonary function studies are most often normal. The angioedema is usually mild, but can be so severe as to require emergency intubation and tracheostomy. Symptoms resolve gradually after the drug is stopped. The mechanism of ACE inhibitor reactions may be related to reduced degradation of substance P and bradykinin, which are mediators causing bronchospasm and edema. As with aspirin and NSAIDs, structurally different ACE inhibitors like captopril and enalapril can cross-react. If a patient reacts to one of these agents, the drug should be stopped and all ACE inhibitors avoided.

Many patients have anaphylactoid reactions to radiocontrast media, and a few die from hypovolemic shock (Chapters 9.2 and 9.4). Conventional radiocontrast media are iodinated, hypertonic, water-soluble, aromatic salts. A newer agent, metrizamide, is isotonic and produces many fewer reactions, but its cost has limited its use. Most serious radiocontrast media reactions begin 1–3 minutes after intravenous injection. Self-limited pruritus, urticaria, rhinitis, and bronchospasm are most common, but some patients develop life-threatening angioedema, bronchospasm, or hypotension.

The pathogenesis of radiocontrast media reactions is incompletely understood, and there is no way to predict which history-negative individuals are at risk. Since these reactions occur by non-IgE-mediated effects on mast cells, skin testing is useless. Iodide sensitivity is irrelevant. However, a history of rhinitis or asthma increases the risk of radiocontrast media reaction three- or fourfold, perhaps because atopic individuals tend to have more mediators released from their mast cells and basophils.

Patients who have had radiocontrast media reactions are at risk for recurrent reactions. The risk is substantially lower in procedures for which the radiocontrast medium is injected into a nonvascular space, as for a retrograde pyelogram or oral cholecystogram. The incidence and severity of anaphylactoid reactions to radiocontrast media can be reduced by pretreating patients with H_1 antihistamines and corticosteroids. In one study, adding ephedrine to the premedication regimen appeared to reduce the risk further, but ephedrine is not recommended for the elderly or for patients with cardiovascular disease.

SUMMARY

▶ Drug reactions can be life-threatening, and can mimic systemic illnesses such as lymphoma and collagen vascular disease.

▶ An offending drug is best identified by a thorough history. The only reliable skin test is for reactivity to penicillin. A patient with a negative result from a properly performed skin test is unlikely to suffer penicillin anaphylaxis.

▶ Drug reactions are treated by stopping the offending drug, treating the manifestations, and changing to a non-cross-reacting drug. If the offending drug must be continued, the patient should be desensitized.

▶ Patients should be informed about their drug allergy and encouraged to wear a medical identification bracelet.

▶ Pseudoallergic and anaphylactoid drug reactions resemble true drug allergy clinically, but do not involve antibody production or T-cell sensitization; they can occur on first exposure to the drug.

SUGGESTED READING

Anderson JA: Allergic reactions to drugs and biological agents. JAMA 1992;268:2844.

Sullivan TJ: Drug allergy. In: *Allergy: Principles and Practice,* 4th ed. Middleton E Jr et al (editors). CV Mosby, 1993.

VanArsdel PP (editor): Drug allergy. Immunol Allerg Clin North Am 1991;11:461.

Weiss ME, Adkinson NF: Immediate hypersensitivity reactions to penicillin and related antibiotics. Clin Allergy 1988;18:515.

9.4

Anaphylaxis

("without protection")

Bruce S. Bochner, MD, and Lawrence M. Lichtenstein, MD, PhD

In the early 1900's, Portier and Richet observed a paradoxical immunologic effect when they tried to enhance dogs' resistance to sea anemone toxin by injecting them with it. When the dogs were reinjected weeks later with even tiny doses of the toxin, several died minutes later from cardiorespiratory collapse. The investigators later coined the term "anaphylaxis" (meaning "anti"-protection) to describe this acquired response. They determined that such a reaction required prior exposure to the foreign substance (antigen) and a period of weeks to establish the response. It was later found that a number of antigens, including proteins and carbohydrates, could elicit the same response. It was also found that anaphylactic sensitivity could be transferred from one animal to another by injecting or infusing a serum-derived factor, initially referred to as "reagin" and later identified as immunoglobulin E (IgE).

The term anaphylaxis denotes a spectrum of reactions. At one end are relatively mild allergic reactions confined, for example, to the skin and manifesting as pruritus or urticaria (Chapter 9.2). At the other end of the spectrum are severe reactions in the tracheobronchial tree manifesting as laryngospasm or asthma or in the cardiovascular system as hypotension. Patients can present in extreme distress, gasping for air as vasoactive substances cause edema of the airway and constriction of smooth muscles surrounding bronchioles, or in shock as the same mediators cause fluid from the intravascular space to leak into tissues.

All anaphylactic reactions require antigen-induced cross-linking of specific IgE molecules on the surface of mast cells or basophils, causing the cells to release vasoactive mediators. Reactions mimicking anaphylaxis can occur in persons who were not previously sensitized to an antigen. These are called *anaphylactoid reactions*. They involve the release of the same mediators as in anaphylaxis, but by pathways independent of IgE antibodies.

MECHANISMS

The inciting antigen of anaphylaxis can be an exogenous protein or an antigen generated when a foreign low molecular weight substance such as penicillin combines with endogenous serum or tissue proteins through haptenation (Chapters 9.1 and 9.3). If many individuals are exposed to the same antigen by the same route, only a few develop IgE antibodies, and only a few are at risk for anaphylaxis on re-exposure. Some of the variability can be accounted for by individual differences in the half-life of IgE antibodies or the plasma cells that produce them. Antigens that induce an IgE response have no consistent features, although many are enzymes. Why only a minority of people make IgE and become allergic remains unknown; genetic factors are thought to play a role.

After an antigen triggers antibody-producing plasma cells to secrete IgE, the antibody readily binds to receptors for the Fc portion on mast cells and basophils throughout the body (Figure 9.4–1). These cells, armed with antigen-specific IgE, can be stimulated on re-exposure to the antigen. On re-exposure, the antigen cross-links IgE molecules on the cell surface, initiating a series of events that within seconds or minutes leads to the release of numerous chemical mediators, including histamine, many kinds of prostaglandins and leukotrienes, and perhaps cytokines as well. These mediators cause the clinical manifestations of anaphylaxis.

Anaphylactoid reactions are produced by two pathways that do not involve IgE and do not require previous exposure to the inciting agent (see Figure 9.4–1). The first pathway starts with activation of complement, for example, by immune complexes. Activated complement leads to generation of the protein fragments C3a and C5a, which in turn can stimulate mediator release by mast cells and basophils through specific complement receptors, independent of IgE. The second non-IgE pathway is the direct release of mediators from mast cells and basophils, induced by opiates or hyperosmolar solutions, such as radiocontrast media or mannitol, or by morphine and other opiates.

Although anaphylactic and anaphylactoid reactions have different mechanisms and although anaphylactic reactions tend to be more severe, the clinical manifestations of the two reactions and their treatment are often similar.

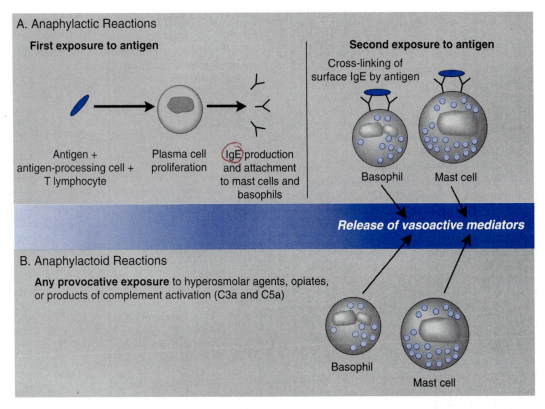

Figure 9.4–1. Anaphylactic and anaphylactoid reactions. **A:** Anaphylactic reactions require an initial exposure to the antigen, leading to IgE synthesis by plasma cells. The IgE then attaches to circulating basophils and tissue mast cells through their high-affinity IgE receptors. Re-exposure to the antigen leads to cross-linking of surface-bound IgE, and to degranulation. **B:** Anaphylactoid reactions do not require prior exposure and do not involve IgE. They are caused by degranulating substances (hypertonic solutions, certain drugs, proteins from complement activation) acting directly on mast cells and basophils.

CLINICAL FEATURES

Most anaphylactic reactions start quickly and evolve over minutes, but rare patients have reactions beginning hours after they are exposed to the antigen. A few patients have biphasic reactions, in which symptoms gradually recur many hours after the first episode; these, too, may be life-threatening. Biphasic reactions may be an example of the late-phase allergic response, an IgE-dependent reaction consisting of delayed edema and tissue infiltration with eosinophils and other leukocytes. Because of the risk of late reactions after anaphylaxis, all patients, regardless of their initial clinical course, should be kept under observation for at least 24 hours in the hospital or at home by their family.

Anaphylaxis most often involves the skin, airways, and cardiovascular system (Table 9.4–1). Most patients have one or more forms of cutaneous involvement, commonly of the mucous membranes of the eyes, nose, and mouth. A very serious development is upper airway obstruction caused by edema of the larynx or epiglottis. The edema can cause respiratory obstruction with stridor, or complete airway obstruction. Bronchoconstriction and edema of the lower airways can cause dyspnea, wheezing, and a sensation of chest tightness. These complications can be difficult to manage, and can lead to hypoxemia and hypercapnia.

The cardiovascular collapse is thought to result primarily from extensive vasodilatation and plasma leakage, major factors in causing the tissue edema mentioned above. The cardiac, neurologic, and gastrointestinal manifestations are caused either by insufficient perfusion or directly by anaphylactic mediators.

Table 9.4–1. Typical manifestations of anaphylactic reactions.

Organ System	Manifestations
Cutaneous	Pruritus, erythema, urticaria, edema
Upper airway	Pruritus, edema*
Lower airway	Dyspnea, wheezing, bronchospasm*
Cardiovascular	Hypotension,* arrhythmias
Neurologic	Dizziness, confusion, syncope, seizures
Gastrointestinal	Nausea, vomiting, crampy abdominal pain, diarrhea

*Often responsible for life-threatening reactions.

Bronchospasm, urticaria, edema, hypotension, and other changes that occur during anaphylaxis can be mimicked by inhaling, injecting, or infusing histamine, but not all the events can be explained by histamine or other known mediators derived from mast cells and basophils. As yet unidentified cells and mediators must also be involved.

ETIOLOGY

Several factors influence the initial site of an anaphylactic reaction, as well as the severity. These factors include the route, rate, and quantity of antigen exposure; the patient's predisposition to produce IgE antibody; and pre-existing conditions (eg, asthma) or treatments (eg, beta-blockers). Since the tissue mast cell and peripheral blood basophil are thought to mediate IgE-dependent anaphylactic reactions, the site where these cells are exposed to allergen is usually the first site of anaphylactic symptoms. For example, an antigen given intravenously is quickly distributed throughout the body, and may elicit a more severe multiorgan reaction than the same agent given orally. In contrast, gastrointestinal symptoms may be prominent during reactions to a food or oral drug allergen, whereas subcutaneous or intramuscular injection of the same allergen may first elicit a local skin response. Nevertheless, both sensitization and systemic reactions can occur by any route, and patients may have life-threatening reactions to tiny quantities of antigen.

The list of agents suspected or proven to cause anaphylactic or anaphylactoid reactions is long and will probably keep growing as new drugs are introduced (Table 9.4–2). Most of the responsible agents are proteins, but low molecular weight substances (eg, drugs acting as haptens, certain polysaccharides) can also cause true IgE-dependent anaphylaxis.

DIAGNOSIS AND DIFFERENTIAL DIAGNOSIS

Anaphylaxis is a clinical diagnosis that can be made only when the history and physical examination verify that any combination of the clinical features (see Table 9.4–1) developed after the patient was exposed to a foreign substance. By itself, no single sign, symptom, or test is diagnostic. Elevated blood levels of mediators such as histamine or tryptase (a neutral protease released only by mast cells) during a reaction are helpful, but they are relatively insensitive and seldom available. Demonstrating IgE to the suspected agent, by skin test or other means, supports but in no way confirms the diagnosis. Demonstrating the absence of IgE may be more helpful. If the physician can reliably document that a patient has negative skin tests to a food or drug suspected of having caused anaphylaxis in the past, the patient can eat or use that substance again without special risk. Finally, challenge tests (exposing patients to the suspected agent to

Table 9.4–2. Agents that can cause anaphylactic and anaphylactoid reactions.

Mechanism	Typical Agents
Anaphylactic reactions	
IgE-mediated reaction against native proteins	Venoms (*Hymenoptera,* fire ant)
	Airborne allergens (pollens, molds, danders)
	Foods (peanut, milk, egg, seafood, grains)
	Enzymes (trypsin, streptokinase, chymopapain)
	Heterologous sera (tetanus antitoxin, anti-lymphocyte globulin)
	Human proteins (insulin, ACTH, vasopressin, serum and seminal proteins)
	Others (protamine, latex)
IgE-mediated reaction against hapten–protein conjugates	Antibiotics (penicillins, cephalosporins, sulfonamides)
	Ethylene oxide
Anaphylactoid reactions	
Complement activation	Human proteins (gamma globulin, other blood products)
	Dialysis (contact of blood with cuprammonium cellulose dialysis membranes)
Direct activation of mediator release from mast cells or basophils	Hypertonic solutions (radiocontrast media, mannitol)
	Drugs (opiates, dextran)

Modified and reproduced, with permission, from Bochner BS, Lichtenstein LM: Current concepts: Anaphylaxis. N Engl J Med 1991;324:1785.

check for anaphylactic sensitivity) are seldom worth the risk, particularly when alternative drugs of different chemical classes are available.

MANAGEMENT

Prevention

Avoidance and prevention are the best strategies for those at risk for anaphylaxis (Table 9.4–3). Sometimes, however, high-risk patients must be treated with suspected materials (eg, radiocontrast media) or allergens (eg, beta-lactam antibiotics when alternative antibiotics are not available or effective). The physician can follow several protocols that reduce the probability and severity of anaphylaxis in these patients: (1) radiocontrast sensitivity—prophylaxis with antihistamines and corticosteroids in an attempt to prevent the release and effect of anaphylactic mediators during radiocontrast reactions; (2) acute desensitization—cautiously giving gradually larger oral or parenteral doses of the suspected agent over several hours to induce temporary but sustained tolerance, so that the patient can receive a full course of treatment; or (3) chronic desensitization (allergy shots, immunotherapy)—giving the agent parenterally in gradually increasing doses on a weekly to monthly schedule over at least several years. Since all three approaches involve exposing sensitive pa-

Table 9.4–3. Anaphylaxis prevention.

General measures
 Identify allergens and persons at risk
 Avoid exposure (the only effective treatment for food allergy)
 Equip high-risk outpatients with injectable epinephrine and
  medical identification bracelet

Specific measures
 Drug prophylaxis, eg, radiographic contrast media (pretreat with
  corticosteroids and antihistamines)
 Acute desensitization, eg, penicillins, insulin, aspirin
 Chronic desensitization, eg, *Hymenoptera* (bee sting) venoms,
  imported fire ant venom

Modified and reproduced, with permission, from Bochner BS, Lichtenstein LM: Current concepts: Anaphylaxis. N Engl J Med 1991;324:1785.

tients to known triggers of anaphylaxis, these measures should be performed in a monitored setting where anaphylactic reactions can be effectively managed.

Management of Anaphylactic Reactions

Despite awareness and efforts at prevention, an estimated 1 in 3000 inpatients has an anaphylactic reaction. The continuing high rate is explained in part by failure to anticipate the reaction. A physician administering any agent that can induce anaphylaxis must obtain a careful history, must be suspicious and cautious, and must recognize the event early to prevent the serious complications that can develop so quickly.

Successful treatment depends on quick clinical assessment, stopping the suspected agent, and close monitoring of vital signs. The goals of acute treatment are protecting the airway and maintaining adequate oxygenation, cardiac output, and tissue perfusion. The physician should have at hand the equipment and drugs needed for cardiopulmonary resuscitation, including endotracheal intubation and tracheotomy.

Epinephrine, intravenous fluids, and oxygen are the mainstays of therapy for anaphylaxis, used alone or in combination, depending on the site and severity of reaction. Rarely, dopamine and other vasopressors are needed for severe reactions. Corticosteroids and antihistamines (especially H_1 receptor antagonists) are not generally useful early in a reaction. They should be given after other agents have stabilized the acute symptoms, usually within 1–2 hours, to relieve pruritus and prevent or attenuate late reactions. Even when anaphylactic reactions are expected and promptly treated, they may respond slowly or incompletely to treatment, and symptoms can recur. Everyone experiencing an anaphylactic reaction should be closely monitored for at least 24 hours.

The goal of long-term management is to identify the inciting agent and either take measures to avoid it or, in cases like anaphylaxis to bee stings, desensitize the patient. If the agent cannot be identified or patients cannot be desensitized, they should be equipped with injectable epinephrine and taught how to treat themselves. Patients must be cautioned that the purpose of self-injected epinephrine is to start therapy during the time that it takes to seek emergency medical help. Patients should still go to the emergency room, because severe anaphylactic reactions may require additional treatment. All patients with life-threatening anaphylaxis should wear a medical identification bracelet.

SUMMARY

▶ Anaphylaxis requires prior sensitization by an antigen. A reaction occurs when re-exposure to the antigen cross-links antigen-specific IgE molecules bound to IgE receptors on the surface of mast cells and basophils, liberating vasoactive substances from the cells.

▶ Anaphylactoid reactions do not require prior sensitization by antigen. These reactions are caused by release of the same vasoactive mediators from basophils and mast cells, by either complement activation or direct interaction with cells, not by mechanisms that involve IgE.

▶ Anaphylactic and anaphylactoid reactions most often involve the skin, airways, and cardiovascular system. Common symptoms are hives, respiratory distress (eg, inspiratory stridor, wheezing), and shock.

▶ Epinephrine, oxygen, and intravenous fluids are the agents of choice in treating anaphylactic and anaphylactoid reactions. Because symptoms can recur long after the initial episode, patients should be observed for 24 hours.

▶ Patients at risk should be identified and helped to avoid the inciting agent.

SUGGESTED READING

Austen KF, Metcalfe DD: Anaphylactic syndrome. In: *Samter's Immunological Diseases,* 5th ed. Frank MM et al (editors), Little, Brown, & Co, 1995.

Bochner BS, Lichtenstein LM: Current concepts: Anaphylaxis. N Engl J Med 1991;324:1785.

Schwartz LB et al: Tryptase levels as an indicator of mast-cell activation in systemic anaphylaxis and mastocytosis. N Engl J Med 1987;316:1622.

Smith PL et al: Physiologic manifestations of human anaphylaxis. J Clin Invest 1980;66:1072.

Valentine MD: Anaphylaxis and stinging insect hypersensitivity. JAMA 1992;268:2830.

Primary Immunodeficiency Diseases

Howard M. Lederman, MD, PhD, and Jerry A. Winkelstein, MD

The primary immunodeficiency diseases used to be viewed as rare disorders, usually characterized by severe infections and seen most often in infants and young children. Recently, however, it has become clear that these diseases are more common than previously thought; that they can present with clinical manifestations other than infections, notably autoimmune disorders; that they are seen nearly as often in adolescents and adults as in infants and children; and that their clinical expression can be mild. Immunodeficiency diseases may present so subtly in adults that only a physician alert to the possibility of immunodeficiency will make the diagnosis. Once diagnosed, many of these diseases can be treated effectively.

Each of the more than 50 primary immunodeficiency diseases is caused by a defect in one or more of the four components of immunity: B cells, T cells, complement, and phagocytic cells (neutrophils and macrophages). Understanding immune system physiology helps the physician understand how defects in each of these components contribute to a particular patient's condition.

Immunodeficiency can also develop secondary to other conditions, among them viral infection (eg, AIDS, measles, Epstein-Barr virus), medical treatment (eg, corticosteroids, chemotherapy), and malignancy (eg, myeloma, chronic lymphocytic leukemia). Physicians must be able to determine whether an adult presenting with an immunodeficiency has it as a primary or secondary disorder.

CLINICAL MANIFESTATIONS

Infectious Manifestations

The hallmark of primary immunodeficiency diseases is susceptibility to infection (Table 9.5–1). Individual infections may be no more severe than those in a normal host; what is striking about these infections is that they are chronic or recurrent. On occasion, infections are unusually severe (eg, sepsis), lead to an unexpected complication (eg, fistula formation), or are caused by an organism of relatively low virulence (eg, *Pneumocystis carinii* pneumonia). It is difficult to assign a precise frequency of recurrent infections that defines increased susceptibility. As a guideline, the physician should suspect immunodeficiency when a patient has more than one pneumonia per decade, chronic sinusitis, chronic bronchitis without a history of smoking or occupational exposure, or onset of ear infections in adulthood. The most common presenting manifestations of immunodeficiency are recurrent sinopulmonary infections, particularly sinusitis, bronchitis, and pneumonia, but some patients present with recurrent systemic infections such as bacteremia and meningitis. Recurrent infections at a single site should prompt investigation of nonimmunologic abnormalities. For example, recurrent pyelonephritis should suggest obstruction to urine outflow, and recurrent meningitis could be caused by a cribriform plate defect.

Not all immunodeficient patients are diagnosed after recurrent infections. In some patients, the first infection may be unusual enough to raise the question of immunodeficiency. For example, someone who presents with *P carinii* pneumonia is likely to be immunodeficient even if it is the person's first recognized opportunistic infection. Similarly, since few immunocompetent persons develop oral thrush, it should suggest immunodeficiency.

The type of pathogen and site of the infection can give valuable insight into the type of immune defect (Table 9.5–2). For example, persons with B-cell defects are unusually susceptible to encapsulated bacteria (eg, pneumococci, streptococci, *Haemophilus influenzae*) and enteroviruses (eg, coxsackieviruses, echoviruses). Those with T-cell deficiencies characteristically have infections with fungi, mycobacteria, pneumocystis, and viruses. Patients with complement deficiencies often present with blood-borne infections like bacteremia and meningitis, caused by encapsulated bacteria (eg, streptococci, gonococci, pneumococci, meningococci). Finally, phagocytic disorders are characterized by infections of the skin and reticuloendothelial system, caused by bacteria (staphylococci) and fungi (*Candida, Aspergillus*).

Table 9.5–1. Characteristics of infections, suggesting immunodeficiency.

Characteristic	Examples
Infection with an organism of low virulence	*Pneumocystis carinii* pneumonia, candidiasis
Chronic or recurrent infections without an obvious explanation	Chronic bronchitis without a history of smoking
Infection of unusual severity	Pneumonia with empyema or bacterial sepsis
Infection that leads to an unexpected complication	Abscess, osteomyelitis

Gastrointestinal Manifestations

Chronic diarrhea, malabsorption, and malnutrition can be manifestations of the primary immunodeficiency diseases. Sometimes the cause is clearly infectious. Chronic giardiasis, rotavirus infection, and cryptosporidiosis are among the infections documented to cause chronic diarrhea in patients with primary immunodeficiency. Bacterial overgrowth of the small bowel is also a major cause of malabsorption, which can lead to chronic diarrhea. This condition is difficult to treat; it recurs in many patients with antibody deficiency disorders. Immunodeficient patients can also suffer gastrointestinal complications from autoimmune and chronic inflammatory diseases, including inflammatory bowel diseases, gluten-sensitive enteropathy, atrophic gastritis with pernicious anemia, villous atrophy, and nodular lymphoid hyperplasia.

Hematologic Manifestations

Patients with primary immunodeficiency diseases can have anemia, thrombocytopenia, or leukopenia. These blood abnormalities may be secondary consequences of infection or manifestations of autoimmunity. The most common of the blood abnormalities are autoimmune hemolytic anemia, idiopathic thrombocytopenic purpura, and pernicious anemia; they are most often seen in patients with B-cell or T-cell disorders such as IgA defi-

Table 9.5–2. Types of infections, reflecting type of immunodeficiency.

Type of Immunodeficiency	Infection
B cell	Pyogenic bacteria (pneumococci, streptococci, *Haemophilus influenzae*), enteroviruses (coxsackieviruses, echoviruses)
T cell	Fungi, mycobacteria (typical and atypical), *Pneumocystis carinii,* viruses, *Listeria monocytogenes*
Complement	Encapsulated bacteria (streptococci, gonococci, pneumococci, meningococci)
Phagocytosis	Skin and reticuloendothelial system infection with bacteria (staphylococci) and fungi (*Candida, Aspergillus*)

ciency, common variable immunodeficiency, and chronic mucocutaneous candidiasis. Patients with some T- or B-cell disorders also have an increased susceptibility to malignancy. Most malignancies are of lymphoreticular origin (lymphomas, thymoma), but some are epithelial (carcinoma).

Autoimmune and Rheumatic Manifestations

Immunodeficient patients can present with clinical features similar to those seen in rheumatic or autoimmune diseases. The basic abnormality that leads to immunodeficiency may also lead to faulty discrimination between self and nonself, and thus to autoimmune disease. Autoimmune and rheumatic diseases are more frequently seen in patients with common variable immunodeficiency, selective IgA deficiency, chronic mucocutaneous candidiasis, and deficiencies of the classic pathway of complement.

In some immunodeficient patients, the manifestations of autoimmune or rheumatic disorders are limited to a single type of cell or tissue, as in autoimmune hemolytic anemia or autoimmune thyroiditis. These illnesses may occur years before patients manifest increased susceptibility to infection. On occasion, the clinical manifestations involve a number of tissues and thus resemble vasculitis, systemic lupus erythematosus, dermatomyositis, or rheumatoid arthritis. For instance, patients with deficiencies of complement may present with systemic lupus erythematosus.

Occasionally, a disorder that appears to be autoimmune is actually caused by an infectious agent. For example, the dermatomyositis seen in some patients with X-linked agammaglobulinemia is not an autoimmune disease but a manifestation of a chronic enterovirus infection.

LABORATORY EVALUATION

Once the possibility of a primary immunodeficiency disease has been raised by clinical findings, laboratory tests are used to document and delineate the immunologic defect. The types of infections and symptoms may help to focus the laboratory workup on specific parts of the immune system (Table 9.5–3).

B-Lymphocyte Function

The first test of B-lymphocyte function is measurement of serum immunoglobulins. Neither serum protein electrophoresis nor immunoelectrophoresis is useful for this purpose, because neither is sensitive enough or able to measure individual immunoglobulin classes precisely. Instead, individual classes (IgG, IgA, IgM) should be measured in order to identify patients with panhypogammaglobulinemia as well as those with deficiencies of a single class, such as selective IgA deficiency. Sometimes the total serum IgG is normal or near normal, but the patient has a deficiency of an IgG subclass. IgG has four subclasses (IgG_{1-4}), and selective deficiencies of each have been described (see "IgG Subclass Deficiencies" below). Thus, when a patient is strongly suspected of hav-

Table 9.5–3. Evaluation of suspected defects in host defense.

Suspected Abnormality	Diagnostic Tests	
	Initial	Additional
B cell	Quantitative immunoglobulins (IgG, IgA, IgM)	Antibody response to immunization Quantitative IgG subclasses Lymphocyte enumeration (B and T)
T cell	CBC with differential Delayed hypersensitivity skin tests	Lymphocyte enumeration (CD3, CD4, CD8) HIV serology Lymphocyte proliferation in response to mitogens, antigens
Complement	Total hemolytic complement (CH_{50})	Quantitation of individual components
Phagocytosis	CBC with differential	Nitroblue tetrazolium (NBT) test White blood cell chemotaxis, phagocytosis, bacterial killing

CBC, complete blood count.

ing a humoral immunodeficiency but the total serum IgG is normal, individual IgG subclasses should be measured.

Another part of evaluating humoral immunity is assessment of antibody function. It is most useful to measure antibody titers generated in response to immunizations with a protein antigen (eg, tetanus toxoid) and a polysaccharide antigen (eg, pneumococcal capsular polysaccharides).

If patients are found to have low immunoglobulin levels or little antibody produced in response to immunization, the evaluation should proceed with enumeration of B lymphocytes in the blood. Further specialized tests, such as in vitro studies of mitogen- or antigen-driven B-cell proliferation, may be helpful in delineating the functional B-cell defect.

T-Lymphocyte Function

Testing for defects in cell-mediated immunity is relatively difficult because of the lack of good screening tests. Delayed hypersensitivity skin testing with a panel of antigens can be used as a screen in older children and adults. A positive test for delayed hypersensitivity generally indicates intact cell-mediated immunity. There are many limitations to these tests, however. Standardized antigens other than tuberculin have not been developed for use by intracutaneous injection (a Mantoux-type procedure), and licensed devices for percutaneous injection of multiple antigens do not deliver consistent amounts of antigen into the skin. A positive test to some antigens does not ensure that the patient has normal cell-mediated immunity to all antigens. For example, patients with chronic mucocutaneous candidiasis have a lacunar defect in which cell-mediated immunity is generally intact, except for the response to *Candida*. Some persons do not react to a specific antigen because they have not had prior exposure. Finally, some viral infections, some cancers, and most chemotherapeutic and immunosuppressive drugs can induce transient depressions of delayed hypersensitivity. For all these reasons, an abnormal (negative) delayed hypersensitivity skin test does not necessarily reflect abnormal T-lymphocyte function.

Other information about T lymphocytes can be obtained by enumerating peripheral blood T lymphocytes using fluorescein-conjugated monoclonal antibodies to cell surface determinants. Total T (CD2 or CD3), "helper" T (CD4), and "suppressor" T (CD8) cells can be measured with monoclonal antibodies. All patients with reduced T-lymphocyte function or reduced CD4 cell number should have a serologic test for HIV infection. Another test of T-cell function is measurement of lymphocyte proliferation in vitro after stimulation with mitogens, antigens, or allogeneic cells. This test is most useful in confirming the validity of negative delayed hypersensitivity skin tests.

Complement System

Most of the genetically determined deficiencies of the classic activating pathway of C3 (C1, C4, and C2), of C3 itself, and of the terminal components (C5, C6, C7, C8, and C9) can be detected with antibody-sensitized sheep erythrocytes in a total serum hemolytic complement (CH_{50}) assay, since this assay depends on the functional integrity of C1 through C9. Further identification of the deficient component rests on both functional and immunochemical tests specific for each component.

Phagocytic Cells

Evaluation of phagocytic cells entails assessing both their number and their function. Disorders such as congenital agranulocytosis and cyclic neutropenia, which are characterized by a deficiency in phagocyte number, can usually be detected with a white blood cell count and differential. Anatomic or functional (eg, as a result of infarctions from sickle cell disease) asplenia can be inferred from Howell-Jolly bodies on a peripheral blood film (see Color Plates).

Assessment of phagocytic cell function depends on a number of functional assays. In vitro assays can test directed cell motility (chemotaxis), ingestion (phagocytosis), and intracellular killing (bactericidal activity). In addition, there are assays that indirectly assess phagocytic killing by measuring the metabolic changes in cells that accompany or are responsible for intracellular killing. The most widely used metabolic assay is the nitroblue tetrazolium (NBT) dye test.

SPECIFIC IMMUNODEFICIENCY DISEASES

Of the more than 50 primary immunodeficiency diseases, most are genetically determined. The others occur sporadically and do not appear to be the direct consequence of a genetic defect. Many of these diseases first appear during adolescence or adulthood. Left untreated, patients with immunodeficiency diseases may have a poor quality of life, but treatment markedly improves many patients' lives. Early diagnosis is important so that patients can start treatment before they suffer irreversible end-organ damage. The rest of the chapter covers the disorders that are most often seen in adults.

Selective IgA Deficiency

Selective IgA deficiency is the most prevalent primary immunodeficiency disease, affecting about 1 in 600 people worldwide. The disease can present in adults. Selective IgA deficiency is defined as a serum IgA level below 5 mg/dL, with normal levels of other immunoglobulin classes, normal serum antibody responses, and normal cell-mediated immunity. This definition may be too restrictive. Patients with IgA levels of 5–10 mg/dL share some clinical manifestations. Furthermore, many patients previously classified as having selective IgA deficiency are now known to have associated immunologic abnormalities, most often deficiency of IgG_2 or IgG_4. Selective IgA deficiency usually occurs sporadically, but it can run in families.

For reasons that are not known, many patients with selective IgA deficiency are normal, whereas others are unusually susceptible to infections. As might be expected by IgA's role as the predominant secretory immunoglobulin, the most common sites of infection are mucosal surfaces; bacterial sepsis and meningitis are rare. As many as 50% of patients with IgA deficiency have chronic otitis, sinusitis, or pneumonia. Those with chronic respiratory infections are most likely to have an associated IgG subclass deficiency. Since those with IgG subclass deficiency and associated deficiencies of antibody production can be treated with gamma globulin, IgG subclasses and antibody responses to immunization should be measured in the workup of all IgA-deficient patients.

The second major mucosal target for infections is the small intestine. *Giardia lamblia* is the most frequently identified pathogen in patients with selective IgA deficiency, although this infection often goes unrecognized because the symptoms are chronic and indolent.

Autoimmune and rheumatic diseases are also associated with selective IgA deficiency. The main diseases are juvenile rheumatoid arthritis (Still's disease), systemic lupus erythematosus, autoimmune thyroiditis, pernicious anemia, inflammatory bowel diseases, and gluten-sensitive enteropathy. No unifying etiology has been established to explain the association of these disorders with selective IgA deficiency.

Immunoglobulin therapy is generally contraindicated in selective IgA deficiency unless the patient has an associated defect in the production of IgG antibodies. Commercial gamma-globulin preparations contain trace amounts of IgA that are sufficient to sensitize the patient to IgA, and, on rare occasions, to induce anaphylaxis. Similar reactions can occur with blood products such as plasma, red blood cells, or platelets. Use of washed red cells may reduce the risk.

Common Variable Immunodeficiency

Common variable immunodeficiency describes a heterogenous group of disorders in patients who have hypogammaglobulinemia, sometimes accompanied by T-cell dysfunction. The etiology of these diseases is unclear. There is no recognizable pattern of inheritance, although common variable immunodeficiency clusters in some families. Most patients do not manifest symptoms until the second or third decade of life; some patients present after age 50. Individuals can also develop hypogammaglobulinemia as a result of lymphoreticular malignancy (eg, chronic lymphocytic leukemia, multiple myeloma). Therefore, all patients with acquired hypogammaglobulinemia should have a carefully examined peripheral blood smear, as well as immunofixation electrophoresis of serum and urine.

The most common manifestations of common variable immunodeficiency are chronic or recurrent infections of the respiratory and gastrointestinal tracts. For example, persons with no history of infections may develop recurrent otitis media or bronchitis. Individual infections may be no more severe than in the general population, but they are chronic or recurrent. The most frequently identified pathogens are *Streptococcus pneumoniae, H influenzae* type b, streptococci, and staphylococci, but nontypeable *H influenzae*, a variety of gram-negative bacilli, and mycoplasma can become important pathogens in patients with chronic lung disease. There is also a surprisingly high incidence of gastrointestinal disease. As many as 30% of patients have chronic diarrhea, most often caused by *G lamblia* or bacterial overgrowth. These infections often continue, although less frequently, after patients start gamma-globulin therapy.

Patients with common variable immunodeficiency have associated autoimmune diseases. Chronic idiopathic diarrhea with malabsorption is common; small bowel biopsies typically show villous blunting, epithelial atrophy, and nodular lymphoid hyperplasia. There is a high incidence of inflammatory bowel disease, gluten-sensitive enteropathy, and collagenous colitis. Important hematologic abnormalities are autoimmune hemolytic anemia, autoimmune thrombocytopenia, leukopenia, pernicious anemia, and persistent splenomegaly. A few patients develop the clinical and pathologic findings of sarcoidosis, although they do not have hypergammaglobulinemia. Rheumatoid arthritis and other collagen vascular diseases are also found more often than expected.

Patients with common variable immunodeficiency, especially older people, also have a high incidence of malignancy. Non-Hodgkin's lymphoma is most common, followed closely by other lymphoreticular neoplasms and carcinoma of the stomach. In patients with multiple myeloma, production of normal serum immunoglobulins is depressed to levels at which patients develop pyogenic infections. In patients with light-chain disease, serum immunoglobulins can be depressed without producing a detectable serum "M" spike (Chapter 12.7). Therefore, when persons over age 50 present with depressed serum immunoglobulins, even without a serum M spike, the physician should consider light-chain myeloma.

Prophylactic gamma globulin and aggressive treatment of infections can greatly improve outcome, especially when treatment is started before patients develop serious end-organ damage. Treatment reduces the occurrence of infections and increases patients' function and longevity. Patients with common variable immunodeficiency should not receive live viral vaccines (measles, mumps, rubella, or oral polio), nor should household contacts be given the live (oral) polio vaccine because of the patient's risk of contracting vaccine-associated poliomyelitis.

X-Linked Agammaglobulinemia

X-linked agammaglobulinemia causes developmental arrest in B-lymphocyte differentiation, and patients usually present in the first year or two of life. Males with X-linked agammaglobulinemia have no mature B-lymphocytes in their blood and lymphoid tissues, no plasma cells, and severe panhypogammaglobulinemia. Cell-mediated immune function is normal.

The most common sites of infection are in the respiratory tract, particularly the paranasal sinuses and the lungs. The spectrum of microorganisms is similar to that seen in patients with common variable immunodeficiency (see above). Bacterial meningitis, sepsis, arthritis, and osteomyelitis occur much less often, but still more than in the normal population. Of note, autoimmune diseases are not a problem.

A particularly severe and somewhat unique problem in patients with X-linked agammaglobulinemia is the propensity to develop disseminated enteroviral infections. Echovirus, coxsackievirus, and adenovirus have caused chronic and often fatal hepatitis, pneumonitis, meningoencephalitis, and gastroenteritis. In some patients, the enterovirus infection also takes the form of a dermatomyositis-like syndrome.

Early recognition and initiation of gamma-globulin therapy are key to preventing chronic pulmonary disease in patients with X-linked agammaglobulinemia. If treatment is delayed, most patients develop chronic obstructive pulmonary disease before age 20. If diagnosed and treated in early childhood, most patients have a relatively normal incidence of infections and survive to adulthood without any sequelae of chronic disease. Unfortunately, however, gamma-globulin therapy may not completely prevent infections because the antibody spectrum reflects the exposure of the donor pool but not the exposure of the patient and perhaps because gamma globulin contains only IgG.

Patients with X-linked agammaglobulinemia follow the same restrictions on live viral vaccines as patients with common variable immunodeficiency (see above).

IgG Subclass Deficiencies

The four subclasses of IgG (IgG$_1$, IgG$_2$, IgG$_3$, IgG$_4$) differ somewhat in their biologic activities. The IgG response to protein antigens occurs predominantly within the IgG$_1$ and IgG$_3$ subclasses. The IgG response to polysaccharide antigens, such as bacterial capsular polysaccharides, occurs predominantly within the IgG$_2$ and IgG$_4$ subclasses. Deficiencies of IgG subclasses usually occur in association with other primary immunodeficiency diseases such as selective IgA deficiency, Wiskott-Aldrich syndrome, and ataxia-telangiectasia. Isolated IgG subclass deficiencies are uncommon. Often, the clue to diagnosis is borderline or low-normal total serum IgG levels in a patient with recurrent sinopulmonary infections. Persons with this disorder may not present until adulthood.

Patients with selective deficiencies of IgG$_2$, or of IgG$_2$ and IgG$_4$, may have recurrent pyogenic infections of the respiratory tract. They may benefit from antibiotic prophylaxis or from therapy with gamma globulin. Only a few patients have been identified with isolated deficiencies of IgG$_3$ or IgG$_4$; their biologic significance is uncertain. Isolated IgG$_1$ deficiency has not been reported.

Complement Deficiencies

The complement system has over 20 components, and genetically determined deficiencies have been described for each. Most are inherited as autosomal recessive traits, although one—properdin deficiency—is X-linked recessive.

The clinical presentation of complement deficiencies depends to some extent on which component is deficient. The third component (C3) is an important opsonin, whereas C5 through C9 assemble into a membrane attack complex and are responsible for bactericidal activity. Deficiencies of C1, C4, C2, and C3 are characterized by susceptibility to encapsulated bacteria, as well as predisposition to rheumatic disorders such as systemic lupus erythematosus. In contrast, patients with deficiencies of C5, C6, C7, C8, or C9 have a selective susceptibility to systemic meningococcal and gonococcal infections, since normal host defense against these organisms depends in large part on serum bactericidal activity. Although complement deficiencies can manifest in children, many patients do not show an increased susceptibility to infection or rheumatic diseases until adulthood.

There is no specific therapy for complement deficiencies, but immunization against *H influenzae, S pneumoniae,* and *Neisseria meningitidis* is probably of some value.

Chronic Granulomatous Disease

Chronic granulomatous disease is a disorder of phagocytic cells in which both polymorphonuclear leukocytes and monocytes have markedly deficient killing of certain intracellular bacteria and fungi. Phagocytic cells are unable to reduce molecular oxygen and make reactive oxygen products such as hydrogen peroxide and superoxide, which are necessary for the intracellular killing of bacteria and fungi. As a result, patients are unduly susceptible to bacteria and fungi that are catalase-positive and have no net production of peroxide. These microorganisms include staphylococci, some gram-negative enteric organisms (eg, *Escherichia coli, Pseudomonas,* salmonella), certain fungi (eg, *Candida, Aspergillus*), and mycobacteria. The infections most often involve the lungs, lymph nodes, soft tissues, and bone, and are characterized histologically by formation of granulomas. Catalase-positive organisms (eg, streptococci), which produce peroxide, supply the missing metabolite to the phagocytic cell and are readily killed.

Chronic granulomatous disease can be caused by any of a variety of genetic defects that affect components of the electron transport system. The disorder has both X-linked recessive and autosomal recessive forms. Patients usually present in infancy or childhood, but there are patients with milder variants in whom the diagnosis is not made until adolescence or later.

Management has traditionally consisted of antibiotics for prophylaxis and avoidance of swimming in nonchlorinated water. Although not generally used in the United States, bacillus Calmette-Guérin (BCG) vaccine should never be used in patients with chronic granulomatous disease because the BCG organism can cause a serious, chronic infection. Recombinant γ-interferon appears beneficial for both prophylaxis and therapy.

Chronic Mucocutaneous Candidiasis

Chronic mucocutaneous candidiasis is an illness of persistent, severe *Candida* infections of mucous membranes, skin, and nails, occurring in patients who do not have another identifiable underlying illness or a defined defect that impairs cell-mediated immunity. Patients may present at any age, although the incidence of underlying malignancy increases with age. The first step in evaluating any patient with suspected chronic mucocutaneous candidiasis must be to rule out other disorders such as AIDS and lymphoreticular malignancy, particularly thymoma. Most patients with primary mucocutaneous candidiasis have a limited defect in immunity, such as the inability to mount a cell-mediated immune response only to *Candida albicans.*

Patients most often develop the *Candida* infections on the oral mucosa, fingernails, perineum, and esophagus. Invasive candidiasis is rare. Although laboratory abnormalities are typically limited to impaired T-lymphocyte responses to *Candida,* patients are susceptible to severe non-*Candida* infections caused by pyogenic bacteria, a variety of fungi, and herpesviruses. Patients with chronic mucocutaneous candidiasis also have a high incidence of endocrinopathies, particularly diabetes mellitus, hypoparathyroidism, adrenal insufficiency, thyroiditis, and gonadal failure. Many patients also have autoimmune hematologic diseases, such as autoimmune hemolytic anemia, idiopathic thrombocytopenic purpura, and autoimmune neutropenia. These disorders may precede the candidiasis, or vice versa, and may present at any age.

Treatment of chronic mucocutaneous candidiasis focuses on both treating the *Candida* infections with a systemic antifungal drug like fluconazole, and giving supportive and hormone replacement therapy for endocrinopathy and autoimmune disease.

SUMMARY

▶ The hallmark of immunodeficiency diseases is infections that are frequent, recurrent, or unusually severe. They can be caused by organisms of low virulence and can lead to complications.

▶ It is now recognized that immunodeficiency can manifest in adulthood, often in subtle ways (eg, more than one episode of pneumonia per decade).

▶ Immunodeficient patients can also present with gastrointestinal, rheumatic, autoimmune, or hematologic abnormalities.

▶ Secondary causes (eg, HIV infection, lymphoreticular malignancy) should be suspected in all adults presenting with immunodeficiency.

▶ Early diagnosis is important so that treatment can be started before patients suffer irreversible end-organ damage.

SUGGESTED READING

Buckley RH: Immunodeficiency diseases. JAMA 1992;268: 2797.

Cunningham-Rundles C: Clinical and immunologic analyses of 103 patients with common variable immunodeficiency. J Clin Immunol 1989;9:22.

Curnutte JT: Chronic granulomatous disease: The solving of a clinical riddle at the molecular level. Clin Immunol Immunopathol 1993;67:S2.

Figueroa JE, Densen P: Infectious diseases associated with complement deficiencies. Clin Microbiol Rev 1991;4:359.

Rosen FS, Cooper MD, Wedgwood RJP: The primary immunodeficiencies. N Engl J Med 1995;333:431.

Strober W, Sneller MC: IgA deficiency. Ann Allergy 1991; 66:363.

Section 10

Medical Genetics

John D. Stobo, MD, Section Editor

10.1

Approach to the Patient with a Hereditary Disorder

Reed Edwin Pyeritz, MD, PhD

Virtually all the disorders that fall under the jurisdiction of internal medicine have genes involved in their etiology and pathogenesis. This notion is different from the popular perception of "genetic diseases" as being limited to uncommon conditions caused by mutations in single genes. The importance of the genome is clear when one considers the fundamental nature of most disease. Pathology arises because of the body's inability to confront a challenge. Whether it is an infectious agent, a toxin, hypoxemia, or the body's own immune system, the challenge overwhelms the body's homeostatic system.

Homeostasis is controlled by genes, which set the bounds on how well a given homeostatic system can cope. This explains why people of different genetic constitutions respond differently to the same challenge. The reason why a patient does not follow all the rules for signs and symptoms, natural history, and response to therapy may be inborn variation in the genome. Against this background, it may seem narrow-minded to think of genetic disease primarily in the limited sphere of hereditary disorders, and before doing so we should comment on the ways that inherited characteristics can modulate the expression of disease.

GENES AND DISEASE

Multifactorial Disorders

Human afflictions can be grouped into four major overlapping categories, all of which involve the genome. One group is diseases caused by two or more genes, combined with environmental factors. These sorts of disorders have often been termed "multifactorial." Among these disorders are insulin-dependent diabetes, inflammatory bowel disease, coronary artery disease, and chronic obstructive pulmonary disease. Variants of certain genes are known to predispose strongly to each of these disorders, but other factors such as diet and smoking also determine whether and when disease appears.

Acquired Mutations

A second group of diseases is caused largely by mutations that were not present at birth but occur in somatic cells during a person's life. The most common and best-studied example is neoplasia. All tumors seem to arise in part from mutations of oncogenes or tumor suppressor genes in somatic cells. Usually, more than one gene locus must be altered—in the case of suppressor genes, both copies (alleles) of a gene. The fact that people can inherit one or more of these gene alterations accounts for much of the familial susceptibility to cancer, but even these people must have additional somatic mutations before they develop tumors. Similarly, disorders of autoimmunity seem to be determined in part by somatic mutations of immune response genes. Growing evidence suggests that many neurodegenerative disorders such as Parkinson's disease are caused by somatic mutations in the mitochondrial genome (see "Mitochondrial Mutations" below).

Chromosomal Disorders

In general, gross distortions of chromosome number or structure cause problems prenatally and during childhood. Occasionally, however, healthy persons carry chromosome translocations (chromosomes that have been rearranged through breakage and reunion) in which no important genetic material appears to have been duplicated or deleted (a balanced rearrangement). Such translocations cause problems only if material is duplicated or lost during meiosis and passed to a child in an unbalanced state. For example, about 5% of cases of Down syndrome occurs when a healthy parent with a balanced rearrangement of chromosome 21 gives a child two copies of the critical alleles.

The most common gross chromosome aberrations seen in adults are not inherited, but arise in somatic cells and contribute to neoplastic transformation. These aberrations disrupt a limited number of genes and behave much as the somatic cell gene mutations mentioned above.

Mendelian Disorders

The final group of disorders comprises the conditions and traits whose inheritance pattern indicates that a single gene is responsible. Transmission of the resulting phenotype, the gene's clinical manifestation, follows the rules established by Gregor Mendel, with some refinements described below. Although thousands of mendelian disorders have been identified, only a few affect large numbers of people. Examples are sickle cell disease, cystic fibrosis, hypercholesterolemia caused by low-density lipoprotein (LDL) receptor defects, hemochromatosis, and adult polycystic kidney disease. Taken together, however, the mendelian disorders account for considerable morbidity and mortality in both children and adults. The rest of this chapter considers how to approach patients who may have such a disorder.

THE FAMILY HISTORY

Of the many aspects of the workup that should alert physicians to genetic factors being particularly relevant to a patient's condition, by far the most important is a thorough family history (Table 10.1–1). It is often useful to draw and label a pedigree diagram of the family to keep in the chart and update as needed. Several texts explain in detail how to construct a pedigree (see Rimoin et al and Pyeritz references in "Suggested Reading").

A good first question to ask is, "Does any condition run in your family?" Even if the patient says "no," the interviewer should ask specifically and in detail about all first-degree relatives—parents, siblings, and children. The interviewer should record their sex, age, ethnic derivation, consanguineous matings, age at death, cause of death, and any important conditions and malformations. Some questions should be focused by the patient's complaints: "Has anyone in your family had a condition similar to yours?" Other questions should be broad: "Has anyone in your family suffered several miscarriages?" A physician who suspects a specific diagnosis, such as Marfan's syndrome, might then continue with questions aimed at learning whether any of the patient's relatives were unusually tall, had pectus excavatum, or died of aortic dissection.

There are two reasons why physicians should ask in the family history about diseases like tuberculosis and cancer. First, not all diseases that "run in families" are caused primarily by mutant genes. People who live together are more likely to share microbes, dietary deficiencies, car-

Table 10.1–1. History and physical examination: Findings suggesting important genetic considerations in diagnosis and management.

Present illness
Unusually early age of onset of a common disorder
Exposure to mutagenic or teratogenic agents
Patient born to a mother ≥35 yr old

Family history
Relatives having had signs and symptoms similar to those of the patient's present illness
Any disorders affecting multiple relatives, especially if of early onset
Parental consanguinity
Ethnicity in which specific disorders are especially common
Reproductive failure: sterility, infertility; multiple miscarriages, stillbirths, or neonatal deaths
Multiple cases of mental retardation, congenital deformity, disturbance of growth or pubertal development, or neuromuscular difficulties

Physical examination
Major congenital malformation
Dysmorphic features
Ambiguous genitalia or abnormal sexual development
Unusually tall or short stature, or abnormal body proportions
Mental retardation or developmental delay

cinogens, and so forth. Second, even infectious and nutritional diseases have genetic determinants that render some people more susceptible, and the family history can provide clues to unsuspected risk factors.

Some of the points in Table 10.1–1 are most relevant to patients of childbearing age or intent. Others are focused on patients of particular ethnic derivations. For example, all patients of African descent should be asked whether they or their relatives have sickle cell disease and whether they know if they are carriers. People of Mediterranean ancestry should be asked about glucose-6-phosphate dehydrogenase (G6PD) deficiency and thalassemia.

Many patients do not know all the details about their relatives. Distance, divorce, and death all conspire against the historian. The family history does not need to be completed during the first conversation. The interviewer can assign the patient or accompanying relatives to seek answers to any pertinent questions.

The family information that the physician gathers may not turn out to help in diagnosing or managing the patient's chief complaint. But it should ease concerns about potential contributing or confounding problems, and it will certainly have focused and solidified the review of systems.

MENDELIAN INHERITANCE

The uncommon disorders caused by mutations at a single gene are those that follow the patterns of classic mendelian inheritance. Specific genes or alleles are often spoken of as being "dominant" or "recessive," but such designations are misleading. These terms describe only the gene's phenotype—how the genetic alteration is manifest in a person. To illustrate that the gene itself cannot be dominant or recessive, consider the mutation that causes sickle cell disease, a single nucleotide change (point mutation) at the sixth codon of the β-globin gene on chromosome 11. Sickle cell disease is a well-known autosomal recessive condition: "autosomal" because the gene involved is not on a sex chromosome and "recessive" because most people who have sickle cell disease have two copies of the mutation β^S. Individuals who are heterozygous for this mutation have only one copy of the β^S allele, and they develop clinical problems only when they become severely hypoxemic. But examination of the phenotype of erythrocytes sickling in venous blood reveals that the red cells of heterozygotes do sickle, just like the red cells of homozygotes. Thus, sickling is autosomal dominant (only one copy of the mutant allele is needed), whereas sickle cell disease is recessive. Yet both phenotypes are caused by the exact same mutation.

Most mendelian disorders are pleiotropic; that is, a single genetic mutation can produce multiple clinical manifestations. An example of pleiotropy is a defect in the LDL receptor, leading to hyperlipidemia, corneal arcus (see Color Plates), xanthelasma (see Color Plates), tuberous xanthoma, and angina. Until the molecular pathophysiology of a disorder is understood, it can be difficult to connect the seemingly unrelated pleiotropic symptoms and signs.

Figure 10.1–1 reviews the fundamental principles of mendelian genetics. There are several reasons why physicians should be familiar with the inheritance patterns of disorders caused by mutations. First, a condition that recurs in a particular pattern can give a clue to the diagnosis. For example, a bleeding disorder that affects only males in a family is more likely to be a deficiency of factor VIII or factor IX, whose genes are on the X chromosome, than a deficiency of factor V, VII, X, XI, XII, or XIII, whose genes are all mapped to autosomes. Second, rare autosomal recessive disorders are more common in patients whose parents are blood relatives (consanguineous). In highly inbred populations such as the Amish, recessive conditions can occur in multiple families or multiple generations of a family because a large proportion of the community carries a mutation that is rare in the general population. Third, documenting a mendelian condition indicates which of the patient's relatives may be at risk. This is of particular importance for relatives who are planning to have children.

Many mendelian disorders may not become evident until adulthood (Table 10.1–2). These disorders have particular implications for relatives. For example, when patients are diagnosed with hemochromatosis, all their siblings must be screened for early signs of iron accumulation. Similarly, when patients with renal failure are found to have polycystic kidney disease, the physician

must advise about the importance of screening relatives by ultrasonography for asymptomatic cysts and about the option of prenatal diagnosis through DNA linkage studies. In a number of recent adjudications, failure to provide this rudimentary level of genetic counseling has been determined to constitute medical negligence.

Factors That Confuse Pedigree Interpretation of Single-Gene Disorders

Not all single-gene mutations that cause disease behave as perfect mendelian traits. An example is "dominance." A true (complete) mendelian dominant should show the same phenotype whether the person is heterozygous or homozygous for the mutation. But in practice, when affected heterozygotes have a homozygous child, the two copies of the allele usually cause the child to have much more severe disease.

An example is familial hypercholesterolemia caused by defects of the LDL receptor. The untreated heterozygote typically has serum cholesterol values in the 300–400 mg/dL range, corneal arcus by age 30, and symptoms of coronary artery disease by age 40. The homozygote has exaggerated signs and symptoms at earlier ages: total cholesterol levels of 600–1200 mg/dL, corneal arcus before age 10, and death from myocardial infarction in the second or third decade.

Defects of the LDL receptor also reinforce the point that dominance and recessiveness are characteristics of the phenotype, not the genotype. The usual form of type IIa hyperlipoproteinemia, seen in patients who are heterozygous for LDL mutations, is a classic autosomal dominant trait. But the severe form, caused by two LDL receptor mutations, shows autosomal recessive inheritance.

Penetrance: Penetrance is important in disorders caused by mutations of single genes. Penetrance is the frequency with which a phenotype—dominant or recessive—appears when the mutant allele or alleles are present. For individuals, penetrance is an all-or-none phenomenon: The phenotype is either present (penetrant) or not present (nonpenetrant). For a family or a large population, penetrance expressed as a percentage reflects the frequency of a specific phenotypic manifestation (eg, the penetrance of dislocated ocular lenses in Marfan's syndrome is 60%) or the frequency of people with the gene who show *any* manifestation (eg, nonpenetrance in Marfan's syndrome is less than 1%). The term *variability,* not *incomplete penetrance,* should be used to describe differences in the degree to which an allele is expressed (manifested).

The most common cause of apparent nonpenetrance is insensitive methods for detecting the phenotype. Marfan's syndrome is again a good example: The characteristic dilatation of the aortic root is often missed because it is not sought with sensitive techniques like echocardiography. With disorders like this, all relatives at risk must be carefully examined before the physician develops the pedigree and gives the family genetic counseling (see "Genetic

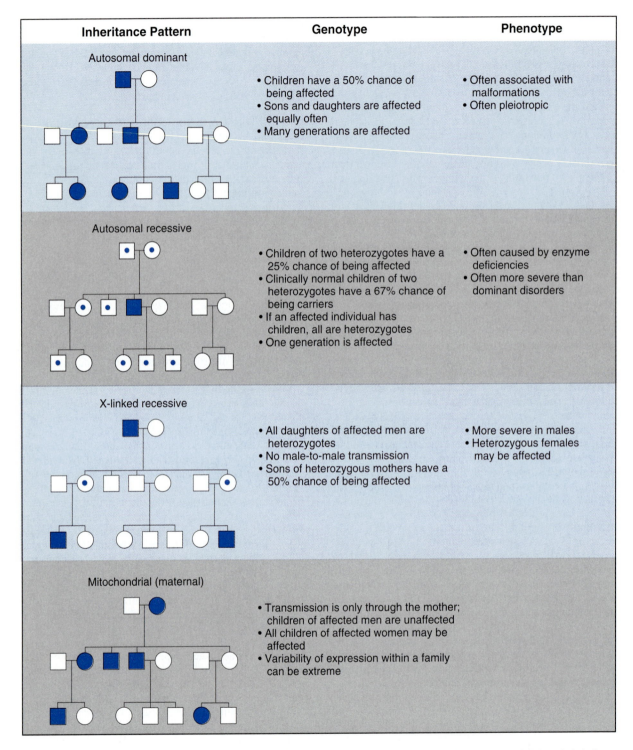

Inheritance Pattern	Genotype	Phenotype

Autosomal dominant

- Children have a 50% chance of being affected
- Sons and daughters are affected equally often
- Many generations are affected

- Often associated with malformations
- Often pleiotropic

Autosomal recessive

- Children of two heterozygotes have a 25% chance of being affected
- Clinically normal children of two heterozygotes have a 67% chance of being carriers
- If an affected individual has children, all are heterozygotes
- One generation is affected

- Often caused by enzyme deficiencies
- Often more severe than dominant disorders

X-linked recessive

- All daughters of affected men are heterozygotes
- No male-to-male transmission
- Sons of heterozygous mothers have a 50% chance of being affected

- More severe in males
- Heterozygous females may be affected

Mitochondrial (maternal)

- Transmission is only through the mother; children of affected men are unaffected
- All children of affected women may be affected
- Variability of expression within a family can be extreme

Figure 10.1–1. Pedigrees illustrating inheritance patterns. Males are designated by squares, females by circles. Solid symbols indicate individuals affected by the phenotype. Dots denote carriers. (Modified and reproduced, with permission, from Pyeritz RE: Genetics and cardiovascular disease. In: *Heart Disease: A Textbook of Cardiovascular Medicine,* 5th ed, vol 2. Braunwald E [editor]. WB Saunders, 1996.)

Table 10.1–2. Some hereditary disorders potentially undiagnosed until adulthood.

Disorder	Inheritance	Rate/100,000 Births
Sickle cell disease	Autosomal recessive	250 (among blacks)
LDL receptor defects	Autosomal dominant	200
Apolipoprotein defects	Autosomal dominant and recessive	>100
Adult polycystic kidney disease	Autosomal dominant	100
Hypertrophic cardiomyopathy	Autosomal dominant	~100
Familial Alzheimer's disease	Autosomal dominant	100?
Cystic fibrosis	Autosomal recessive	60 (among whites)
Alpha$_1$-antiprotease deficiency	Autosomal recessive	50
Neurofibromatosis	Autosomal dominant	30
Huntington's disease	Autosomal dominant	10
Marfan syndrome	Autosomal dominant	10
Hemophilia	X-linked recessive	8
Myotonic muscular dystrophy	Autosomal dominant	4
Fabry's disease	X-linked recessive	~2
Becker's muscular dystrophy	X-linked recessive	2

Counseling" below). A common cause of apparent non-penetrance in adult-onset mendelian diseases is the phenomenon of people dying before the phenotype becomes evident, but possibly after they have transmitted the mutant allele to their children. For example, Huntington's disease usually appears after the fourth decade; a person with the allele for this disease may die from some other cause without ever developing any neurologic symptoms.

Why people with the same mutant alleles express them differently and have variable phenotypes is only beginning to be understood. The same can be said of the numerous late-onset mendelian disorders, like Marfan's syndrome, polycystic kidney disease, familial polyposis of the colon, and hypertrophic cardiomyopathy. A host of biologic factors, such as hormones, imprinting (see "Imprinting" below), and the rest of the genome, affect how a defective gene product is expressed.

X-Linked Inheritance: Characteristics of X-linked inheritance (see Figure 10.1–1) depend on the severity of the phenotype, specifically how much more severely males are affected than are heterozygous females. For some disorders, affected males do not survive to reproduce. About two-thirds of these males have a carrier mother; the other third receives a mutation that arose de novo in the X chromosome (a germinal mutation). Many women who are heterozygous for X chromosome mutations that cause important diseases in their sons eventually develop signs and symptoms themselves, although at later ages than men. Furthermore, because of the vagaries of random inactivation of one X chromosome in each somatic cell, some women who are heterozygous for X chromosome mutations have a preponderance of all their cells, or at least the preponderance of cells in a crucial organ, having as their active X the one carrying the mutation. Such women develop a phenotype as severe as that in a male with the same mutation.

Imprinting: Regions of the genome are subject to imprinting, whereby a gene can be altered when it passes through the ovary, but the same gene can be altered differently when it passes through the testis. Thus, an imprintable allele inherited from the mother will be expressed differently from the very same allele inherited from the father. For example, a short region of chromosome 15 can be responsible for two distinct phenotypes, Angelman's syndrome and Prader-Willi syndrome. If only the father contributes alleles in this region, the child develops Angelman's syndrome, characterized by mental retardation, a movement disorder, and inappropriate laughter. If only the mother contributes alleles, the child develops Prader-Willi syndrome, with mental retardation and morbid obesity. If an imprinted allele causes a dominant condition, the phenotype may be less severe or otherwise distinct when inherited from only one parent. One result can be nonpenetrance and a skipped generation. Some disorders not now considered mendelian may have been misinterpreted because of the effects of imprinting.

Mitochondrial Mutations: The mitochondrion has its own small chromosome, which encodes a few of the proteins involved in oxidative phosphorylation. Mutations in this chromosome have now been linked to a number of neurodegenerative disorders, including Leber's hereditary optic neuropathy and several myopathies that produce ragged red muscle fibers. Only the mother's mitochondria are passed to the children; few mitochondria from the testes are incorporated into the fertilized egg. Thus, fathers cannot pass mitochondrial mutations to their children, but all of an affected woman's children are at risk. As a result, males and females are affected with equal frequency and severity. In a small family, this pattern may suggest autosomal dominance. Moreover, most mitochondrial disorders show marked variability, including age dependence. When the pedigree is large enough and the condition sufficiently penetrant, maternal mitochondrial inheritance can readily be distinguished from autosomal dominant or X-linked recessive mendelian patterns.

GENETIC LABORATORY TECHNIQUES AND THEIR APPLICATIONS

The genetics laboratory routinely provides the following services: assays of enzymes that are often deficient in inborn errors of metabolism; cytogenetic analysis of lymphocytes, fibroblasts, amniocytes, chorionic villi, and bone marrow; and DNA analysis for linkage studies, detection of mutations, and detection of infectious vectors. These analyses find everyday application in confirming diagnoses suspected on clinical grounds; in diagnosing, categorizing, and following neoplasia, especially leukemias and lymphomas; in screening heterozygotes for recessive and X-linked diseases and presymptomatic heterozygotes for dominant disorders; in testing carriers of infectious vectors such as human papillomavirus and HIV; and in diagnosing disease prenatally (Chapter 10.2).

Genetic Counseling

Many mendelian disorders can be detected prenatally (Table 10.1–3). The most common reason for prenatal diagnostic counseling is advanced maternal age. After about age 35, a woman faces a dramatically increased risk of bearing a child with an extra chromosome, especially trisomy 21 (causing Down syndrome), trisomy 18, or trisomy 13. Whenever a mendelian condition is detected in a family, the adults should be counseled not only about the recurrence risks but about the availability of prenatal diagnosis.

Table 10.1–3. Some disorders diagnosable prenatally.

Disorder	Detection Methods
Autosomal recessive	
Sickle cell disease	Mutation detection
Thalassemias	Mutation detection, linkage analysis
Tay-Sachs disease	Enzyme assay, mutation detection
Cystic fibrosis	Mutation detection
Autosomal dominant	
Polycystic kidney disease	Ultrasonography, mutation detection
Marfan syndrome	Linkage analysis, mutation detection
LDL receptor defects	Mutation detection
Huntington's disease	Mutation detection
Hypertrophic cardiomyopathy	Linkage analysis, mutation detection
X-linked	
Duchenne's and Becker's muscular dystrophies	Mutation detection, linkage analysis
Hemophilias	Mutation detection, linkage analysis
Fragile X mental retardation	Mutation detection
Fabry's disease	Enzyme assay, mutation detection
Aneuploidies	
Down syndrome (trisomy 21)	Karyotype, in situ hybridization

In some respects, the process of genetic counseling resembles the discussion that a physician has with any patient about the diagnosis, prognosis, and management of a disease. In both instances, the physician must convey the facts as accurately as possible, gear the presentation to the patient and family members' intelligence and medical sophistication, and pay attention to the psychological and social implications of the information as well as to the patient and family's reactions.

Genetic counseling differs from other medical advising in several important ways:

- The paramount issue may be childbearing. What are the chances that a familial condition will affect future children? What can be done to diagnose a disease prenatally? Can the risk of occurrence or recurrence be lessened?

- A number of psychological issues must be anticipated and addressed. Prospective parents have to confront how they will respond if a fetus is found to have a serious disorder. Parents and even grandparents can feel guilt, often unexpressed, over having passed a mutant allele to a child. Once a mutant allele is detected, a patient may have to face the inevitable development of a degenerative and eventually lethal disease.

- Economic concerns, always important, may carry extra weight. People identified as affected by hereditary disorders may be unable to obtain or afford health insurance. Some employers screen workers for certain hereditary susceptibilities to lessen the risk of occupational illnesses or to reduce outlays for health insurance.

- Genetic counseling often involves obtaining information about the patient's close relatives and even enlisting their cooperation. This can create problems of confidentiality, not to mention heightened family tensions over issues of nonpaternity, incest, and consanguinity.

- There is widespread agreement that genetic counseling be nondirective. That is, the counselor should provide information, ensure that the information is understood, and make available whatever testing is deemed appropriate, but allow the patient or parents to come to their own, unbiased decisions. Counselors must adhere to this principle even when the patient or family seeks direction, as by asking, "What would you do if you were in our situation?"

Counseling is thus an often lengthy, emotional process that requires training and time. At most clinical genetics units and prenatal diagnostic centers, this process is conducted by specialist genetic counselors, who work closely in a team with clinical geneticists and genetic social workers. Such counseling, provided by a trained physician or genetic counselor, will become an increasingly important part of care for both patients and their families.

SUMMARY

▶ Genes are important in the etiology of virtually all illnesses. The physician should suspect identifiable genetic factors, particularly when a patient gives evidence of disturbed homeostatic processes, when a disease of adulthood occurs at an unusually early age, or when the same condition has affected multiple relatives.

▶ With all patients, the physician should obtain a complete family history, not just that related to the present illness.

▶ Conditions that affect multiple relatives may be caused by purely environmental factors, a combination of a few genes and environmental factors, a gross disturbance of chromosomes, or the action of one specific gene.

▶ Many conditions caused by the action of one mutant gene show mendelian inheritance patterns, but small family size, incomplete family history, variability of expression, and genetic imprinting can confuse interpretation of the pedigree.

▶ The physician diagnosing a hereditary disease or predisposition must ensure that the patient receives genetic counseling and must provide for relatives at potential risk to be informed.

SUGGESTED READING

Dietz HC III, Pyeritz RE: Molecular genetic approaches to the study of human cardiovascular disease. Ann Rev Physiol 1994; 56:763.

Hoffman EP: The Evolving Genome Project: Current and future impact. Am J Hum Genet 1994;54:129.

McKusick VA: *Mendelian Inheritance in Man,* 11th ed. Johns Hopkins, 1994.

Pyeritz RE: Medical genetics. In: *Current Medical Diagnosis and Treatment 1996.* Tierney LM Jr, McPhee SJ, Papadakis MA (editors). Appleton & Lange, 1996.

Rimoin DL, Connor JM, Pyeritz RE (editors): *Principles and Practice of Medical Genetics,* 3rd ed. Churchill Livingstone, 1996.

Seashore MR, Wappner S: *Genetics in Primary Care in Clinical Medicine.* Appleton & Lange, 1996.

Clinical Applications of Molecular Genetics

George H. Sack, Jr, MD, PhD

The application of molecular genetic technology to clinical medicine is new and evolving dramatically. There are at least four reasons why understanding genetic aspects of disease is valuable.

First, it can help clarify confusion resulting from phenotypes that are indistinguishable based on clinical findings alone. For example, hemophilia A (deficiency of clotting factor VIII) generally appears the same clinically, but genetic analysis has shown a remarkable spectrum of mutations in the actual gene for factor VIII in different patients. Knowing the underlying mutation is essential for prenatal diagnosis and can help to predict the severity of clinical complications, because some mutations produce a partially functional factor VIII protein while others produce a minimally functional protein or none at all.

Second, knowing the genetic change underlying a condition may permit specific gene replacement. For example, gene therapy for adenosine deaminase deficiency provides the chance to cure an otherwise lethal immunodeficiency state.

Third, detecting genetic abnormalities can permit screening for underlying conditions or predispositions, such as the preclinical changes of familial hypertrophic cardiomyopathy, or for determining susceptibility to colon or breast cancer based on linked genetic markers or direct analysis of the responsible gene product.

Fourth, understanding the genetic basis of a disease can lead to isolating the defective gene and can permit the creation in transgenic animals of a model of a human disease. For example, transgenic mice have been produced with a single point mutation in the gene for the serum protein transthyretin; these mice develop a progressive amyloid neuropathy similar to the human disease. Such models allow researchers to study treatments in animals before trying them in humans.

The goals of this chapter are to outline how a single gene causes disease and, based on that background, to apply the quickly evolving technology of molecular genetics to clinical management decisions. Terms defined in the glossary (Table 10.2–1) are marked by an asterisk where they first appear in the text.

THE BASICS

Each human somatic cell contains about 3 billion DNA* base pairs* (bp). Detecting a single base change, such as the one responsible for sickle cell disease, requires enormous precision that has become possible only in recent years. Much of the technology of mutation analysis is ultimately based on establishing the similarities or differences between test DNA sequences (probes*) and their counterparts in an individual's DNA. Unique sequences of nucleotides* in DNA permit hybridization* studies to achieve their remarkable resolving power. These studies are based on the conventional notion of specific base pairing between two DNA strands, a specificity influenced by the local DNA base composition as well as the length of the test sequences. If a match between two complementary sequences is tested under extremely demanding conditions (high stringency*), a perfect match is required to establish stable pairing between a test sequence and an individual's DNA.

After the conditions for perfect base pairing have been established, it is possible to reduce the stringency and permit the same probe to recognize similar but not identical sequences. For example, the globin genes* are closely related, and under reduced hybridization stringency all can be detected with the same test probe. This has proved particularly valuable in analyzing different but related genes and in showing that such genes may be present in different areas of the genome.*

Common Mutations

The basic feature of any mutation, whether or not it causes disease, is a difference between one person's DNA and an established reference or normal sequence. Such differences can take several forms. By far the simplest difference is the point mutation,* which is the substitution of one DNA base pair for another. The paradigm for point mutations is sickle cell anemia. In this disease, a mutation of one of the three bases of a single triplet codon* causes an amino acid substitution (see "Sickle Cell Disease" below).

Table 10.2–1. Glossary: Terms in molecular genetics.

allele: a distinguishable copy of a gene or other DNA sequence. Identifiable alleles at a given locus can permit assignment of maternal and paternal contributions and are essential for linkage analysis.

allele-specific oligonucleotide (ASO): a short (generally about 20-nucleotide) single strand of DNA whose sequence is a perfect match for a specific allele sequence.

amplification: a local increase in the number of copies of a given DNA sequence. The sequence itself may be short, such as the trinucleotide in Huntington's disease.

base pairs (bp): structural units of double-stranded DNA. Pairing is specific (A-T or G-C).

chromosome: the visible location of DNA and associated proteins. Genes are arrayed linearly along chromosomes. The chromosomes are copied and separated during cell division and are the sites of exchanges in meiotic crossing over.

chromosome painting: use of a set of dye-labeled DNA probes specific for a certain chromosome to identify that chromosome quickly under a microscope; particularly helpful for detecting gross rearrangements and changes in chromosome number (see "fluorescence in situ hybridization" [FISH]).

codon: a group of three nucleotide bases specifying the incorporation of a specific amino acid into the encoded protein. This is the basis of the "triplet code." Some amino acids are represented by more than one codon (redundancy).

crossing over: the basis of recombination during meiosis, as DNA sequences from both parents are mixed along the final DNA strand. Crossing over can actually be seen by light microscopy as physical chromosome strand exchanges called chiasmata.

deletion: loss of nucleotides from DNA. The loss may be tiny—a single base—or large enough to be visible by light microscopic study of chromosomes.

DNA (deoxyribonucleic acid): the double-stranded helical molecule that carries genetic information in the sequence of its nucleotide building blocks.

DNA polymerase: an enzyme that extends a single strand of DNA from a primer using nucleotides complementary to a template strand.

exon: the region of a gene's DNA that will become part of the RNA after transcription and splicing.

fluorescence in situ hybridization (FISH): a method using DNA probes tagged with photosensitive dye to localize specific chromosome regions by light microscopy.

gene: the region of DNA containing the information for synthesizing an RNA or protein product. Most genes contain both introns (qv) and exons (qv).

genome: the entire DNA of an organism.

Human Genome Project: an international effort to develop detailed maps of the entire genome and ultimately to determine the complete nucleotide sequence of all human chromosomes.

hybridization: the formation of intact double-stranded DNA (or RNA) based on specific base interactions between opposite (complementary) single strands. In many studies, the assay is made between genomic DNA and a probe (qv) containing a specific sequence. The precision of the match between probe and test sequences is determined by the stringency (qv) of the hybridization conditions.

intron: the region of a gene's DNA that will be eliminated in the process of forming the RNA through splicing after initial transcription.

inversion: the physical reversal of a chromosomal DNA segment.

karyotype: the arrangement of metaphase chromosomes from an individual cell, usually distinguished by banding patterns, size, and centromere positions.

kilobase (kb): 1000 base pairs (bp); a convenient measure of length for gene studies.

linkage: the transmission together of two or more genetic markers unchanged through meiosis, at a frequency too great to be explained by chance. In general, markers that are located close to one another on a chromosome are linked tightly.

lod score: log of the **od**ds against an apparent linkage relationship existing by chance. By convention, a lod score of 3 or higher (ie, 1000:1) implies significant linkage. Since the lod score is based on a logarithm, scores from different linkage studies are additive.

locus: a specific site in the genome.

map: a linear array of specific, identifiable genetic sites. A map is usually developed for a specific chromosome or for a smaller genomic region. Maps are essential for linkage studies and are useful for isolating new genes.

marker: any testable site for which differences can be distinguished. A marker may be part of a known gene sequence, or may be an anonymous stretch of DNA, known only by its position on a chromosome.

megabase (mb): 1,000,000 base pairs (bp) or 1000 kilobases (kb); a measure of large-scale chromosome distance.

nucleotide (nt): the building block of the DNA (or RNA) polymer. The nt contains the base, sugar, and phosphate ester.

oligonucleotide: a short stretch of nucleotides; generally synthesized to be a probe (see "allele-specific oligonucleotide") or PCR primer (qv).

point mutation: a change in a single base pair in a specific DNA sequence, sometimes with deleterious consequences.

polymerase chain reaction (PCR): a method for generating multiple copies of a specific DNA region defined by site-specific oligonucleotide primers (see text and Figure 10.2–2).

polymorphism: the existence of at least two forms of a given marker (qv). The least frequent form is too common to exist by chance alone. In general, this means that the least frequent form is found in at least 5% of the population.

primer: a stretch of nucleotides that can serve as the starting point for extending a polynucleotide chain. As used in PCR (qv), the primer generally has a base sequence specific for a certain site on the genome (see Figure 10.2–2).

(continued)

Table 10.2–1. Glossary: Terms in molecular genetics. (*continued*)

probe: a stretch of DNA (or RNA) specific for a certain genomic region (target). The specificity is related to the sequence and length of the probe, the uniqueness of the target region, and the stringency (qv) of the hybridization (qv) methods used.

recognition sequence: a generally short (4–6 bp) specific nucleotide stretch that is recognized by a restriction enzyme. Most restriction enzymes make a break in the double-stranded DNA within their recognition sequence, and fail to make a break if the sequence has been changed.

repetitive sequence: a stretch of nucleotides derived by tandem duplication of a (generally) short pattern, eg, (CA). These sequences may be spread throughout the genome and may have different amounts of repetition (hence, different lengths). They thus become useful markers for specific chromosome sites. They differ from amplified (qv) sequences in being in nontranscribed regions and in not contributing to disease.

restriction fragment length polymorphism (RFLP): differences in size between DNA fragments, resulting from DNA cleavage by sequence-specific DNA cleavage enzymes. The change in cleavage usually reflects a point mutation creating or abolishing a recognition sequence for a given enzyme.

RNA (ribonucleic acid): a form of nucleic acid very similar to DNA but generally single-stranded, serving as the template upon which proteins are synthesized in the cytoplasm. RNAs used as templates in the cytoplasm contain sequence information corresponding only to exons (qv) of the corresponding chromosomal gene.

somatic mutation: a DNA change developing after the germ cell precursors have been formed; hence, a change unique to the individual and not transmissible.

Southern blot: an array of DNA fragments separated by length and captured on a binding matrix. The blot can serve as a hybridization target to identify the fragments reacting with a given probe.

stringency: a measure of the environmental conditions (eg, ionic strength, temperature) contributing to the specificity of hybridization (qv). High stringency means that the complementary base pairs in the hybridizing strands must match (usually) perfectly. Lowering the stringency of hybridization permits a probe (qv) to match up less precisely.

structural gene: the DNA region containing the actual DNA sequences needed to produce a product. In humans, many are divided into exon and intron (qv) domains.

thymidine triphosphate (TTP): one of the pyrimidine nucleotide triphosphates used in synthesizing DNA. In the DNA, thymidine (T) pairs with adenosine (A).

triplet code: see "codon."

Some amino acids are encoded by more than one triplet codon (redundancy); when one codon has mutated, the genetic machinery simply ignores the mutation, instead recognizing the other available codon(s). Thus, many base changes in genes, which, by definition, are point mutations, cause no changes in the encoded protein. For example, the change of a single nucleotide in the gene for the serum protein serum amyloid A, which can be detected by the loss of a restriction enzyme recognition site in the gene (see "Polymorphisms" below), causes no change in the corresponding amino acid of the protein. Such silent changes may, however, serve as useful genetic position markers.*

Another common type of mutation is deletion*—a loss of DNA. For example, a short deletion, involving the loss of only three bases, is the most common change in cystic fibrosis. In this mutation, all three bases of the triplet codon for phenylalanine are lost at position 508 in the protein called the *cystic fibrosis transmembrane regulator* (CFTR). Such a small deletion is invisible by microscopic study of chromosomes,* but is readily detectable by hybridization analysis.

By contrast, rare deletions may involve such long stretches of DNA that they are visible under the light microscope as chromosome changes. In addition to the problems created by the loss of DNA, these deletions can interrupt, delete, and change neighboring genes. For example, light microscopic study of stained chromosomes has shown several deletions in the large gene responsible for Duchenne's muscular dystrophy. Some patients with

these deletions have developed another X-linked immunodeficiency disorder, chronic granulomatous disease, because the responsible gene is small and is actually contained *within* an intron* of the Duchenne's gene.

Still another type of change is an increase in the number of repetitions of a small, repeating unit of DNA bases (a repeat). Such an increase is called *amplification.* Amplification events do not always produce the same number of repeats but, in the examples studied to date, amplification causes disease when the number of repeats exceeds a threshold. Such events have now been recognized in the genomes of patients with myotonic dystrophy and Huntington's disease (see "Huntington's Disease" below). Amplification may keep increasing in later generations, and the rising number of repeats can worsen the severity of the clinical manifestations. For example, in myotonic dystrophy, progressively earlier age of onset and severity of symptoms in succeeding generations parallels an increase in the repeat length of the responsible gene. In one extensive family, the grandfather had muscle weakness in his 60's, his son had early balding and muscle weakness in his 30's, and his grandson had cataracts and severe muscle disease before age 10.

Finally, the genome is occasionally subject to complex chromosome reorganizations. In addition to deletions (see above), gene sequences can undergo inversions*, in which a DNA segment actually gets turned around in the chromosome, and other gross reorganizations. Occasionally, these changes can be seen under a light microscope; even if they are not visible, they can significantly alter the involved DNA sequences. Inversions are a consequence of aberrant chromosome replication or some sort of crossing over,* but most are not completely understood at the DNA sequence level. Reorganizations are rare events, but they are most likely to be found in patients who have conditions with spontaneous mutations and in neoplasia, for example, the Philadelphia (Ph[1]) chromosome in chronic myelogenous leukemia.

Polymorphisms

A basic notion underlying genetic analysis is that there are multiple small differences between the DNA sequences in the genomes of all individuals. Occasionally, these differences are clinically detectable as mendelian traits, but most are silent, not causing any change in the phenotype. These silent mutations are nevertheless useful as markers for specific chromosomal positions in genetic analysis. A polymorphism* is a genetic difference between individuals that is found too often to exist by chance alone. Operationally, this means that a polymorphism must be present in at least 5% of the population. Some polymorphisms are common, present in 50% or more of all individuals. Different ethnic groups can have distinctive polymorphisms. Polymorphisms can be detected by many means, all serving to distinguish between specific chromosome regions. Distinctive polymorphism patterns are now being used in forensic identifications.

Particularly useful polymorphisms can be detected by

observing how a mutation affects the sizes of DNA fragments generated by restriction enzyme digestion. Restriction enzymes are bacterial proteins that create sequence-specific DNA breaks by recognizing defined DNA sequences (Figure 10.2–1). If a mutation such as a point mutation changes the DNA sequence recognized by a given enzyme, that enzyme will not break the DNA within that region. The resulting change in size of the DNA fragment produced is readily detectable. Such a pattern is a *restriction fragment length polymorphism** (RFLP). RFLPs can be detected by any sort of DNA probe; they are not limited to coding regions or known genes. RFLPs have been essential in establishing many details of the human gene map* and are fundamental to DNA-based analysis.

Another form of polymorphism that is widely distributed and diagnostically useful is based on short nucleotide patterns that may be repeated many times. An example is repeated stretches of cytosine and adenosine, written as $(CA)_n$; if n = 4, $(CA)_n$ means CACACACA. The human genome has about 50,000 stretches of $(CA)_n$ repeats. The repeats themselves are usually monotonous dinucleotide repeats and are not distinctive. Because they are flanked by unique DNA sequences, such repeats can be detected by techniques described below, and their lengths can be measured. Different lengths of dinucleotide repeats serve as important markers at specific positions throughout the genome, and are valuable in gene and disease analysis.

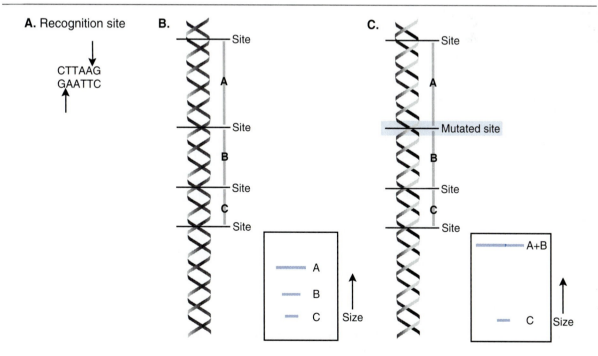

Figure 10.2–1. A: Restriction enzyme recognition site on DNA. Arrows indicate positions of phosphodiester bond cleavage. Any nucleotide change in this site prevents cleavage. **B:** Cleavage and size fractionation by gel electrophoresis. **C:** With the loss (or mutation) of a single recognition site, fragment A becomes longer (in this example, equal to both A and B) and fragment B is lost.

Gene Map and Linkage Analysis

RFLPs, $(CA)_n$ repeats, and other DNA-based markers are found on all chromosomes. These markers can be organized into a linear set of relationships that constitute the gene map. This map is developing quickly because of current cloning methods and the Human Genome Project,* the world-wide effort to identify and coordinate all mapped sites on the genome. A particularly important feature of the gene map for our concerns here is that the markers distinguish between genetic regions. This has several uses, but one that is prominent in both research and clinical applications is linkage* analysis.

The principle of linkage analysis is that although any two markers on a given chromosome may become separated by crossing over at meiosis, the likelihood of their separation rises with increasing distance between them. Thus, markers on opposite ends of a given chromosome are likely to be separated by meiosis. By contrast, markers that are close together are rarely affected by recombination.

Linkage relationships are often expressed quantitatively as "lod scores."* These are mathematical expressions of the odds against two markers appearing linked by chance alone. The score is the $logarithm_{10}$ of the **od**ds. By convention, a lod score of 3 or higher (odds at least 1000:1 against the linkage occurring by chance alone) is taken to be significant. Another useful feature of the lod score is that, because of its logarithmic basis, the scores obtained from analyzing different kindreds may be summed, permitting significant linkage relationships to be detected using multiple smaller families.

It thus becomes possible to analyze a marker that is located very close to the gene or trait of interest and to use this marker as a surrogate for studying the actual gene or trait, which may not be known or isolated. The only constraint in this method is that the marker and the trait must be close enough that they are unlikely to be separated by recombination. This becomes a statistical question as one seeks the best marker. Obviously, a large amount of recombination (genetic distance) between the marker and the trait means a low lod score of very little predictive value.

Linkage analysis is used widely to evaluate the relationship between mendelian conditions and chromosome regions that may contain the responsible gene. Of particular interest for early identification and preventive medicine are studies of genes responsible for common disorders such as colon and breast cancer. As more markers are placed on the gene map, linkage testing can define responsible gene locations more precisely. Linkage analysis has already served as the starting point for successful efforts to isolate genes responsible for some forms of colon and breast cancer. Proceeding from phenotype to a chromosome location and then to the actual gene sequence has been called *reverse genetics.*

Because humans are diploid, they have two copies of each autosomal chromosome. Small DNA differences on each member of a pair of chromosomes permit the pater- nal and maternal contributions to an individual's genome to be distinguished. Such distinctions permit tracing of linkage relationships through large kindreds and are the basis for pedigree analysis.

Polymerase Chain Reaction and Gene Study

As genetic analysis has become more useful clinically, efforts have been made to simplify the process by making the studies faster and by requiring less DNA. A particularly valuable addition to the techniques for studying gene sequences is the polymerase chain reaction* (PCR).

Based on several simple principles, PCR involves the selective amplification of a discrete, generally rather short, region of DNA (Figure 10.2–2). This region is defined by unique nucleotide sequences at its ends. To perform a PCR reaction, the examiner synthesizes short lengths of nucleotides (oligonucleotides,* generally 15–20 bp long), which are complementary to the two strands of DNA that are to be copied. Such oligonucleotides are generally made with an automatic synthesizer. When the target DNA is heated, the two constituent strands come apart. The separated DNA strands are then cooled in a mixture with the synthetic oligonucleotides, which then bind and serve as starting points (primers*) for the polymerase reaction. In the presence of a DNA polymerizing enzyme (DNA polymerase*), the primers are extended into a new complementary DNA strand. After the first round of synthesis, the DNA is again heated and the reactions are repeated. The polymerization reactions use both of the original DNA strands as templates. After several cycles, the sequence between the two primers has been amplified geometrically.

In principle, this approach permits substantial quantities of DNA to be generated from a single copy. The speed with which PCR can be performed and its broad applicability, limited only by the choice of sequences at the primer positions, have permitted PCR to become the diagnostic and analytic method of choice for many studies. Also, once the sequences of specific primers are known, the information can be transmitted to laboratories throughout the world so that new sequences can be put to use quickly.

Once PCR has amplified a gene sequence, the product can be studied either by direct sequence analysis to determine specific base changes or by other methods that may be more useful as screening tests to pick up mutations. For example, $(CA)_n$ repeat polymorphisms can be detected by amplifying the DNA between oligonucleotide primers that flank the repeat. After amplification, the products are separated by gel electrophoresis, which allows size differences to be seen easily. Another approach takes advantage of the fact that different bases change the electrophoretic mobility of single-stranded DNA. Thus, to screen for point mutations in a given region, the DNA is amplified and the products, separated into their single strands, are studied by high-resolution gel electrophoresis. Base differences often cause strands to migrate differently, thus obviating the need to determine the DNA sequence of a

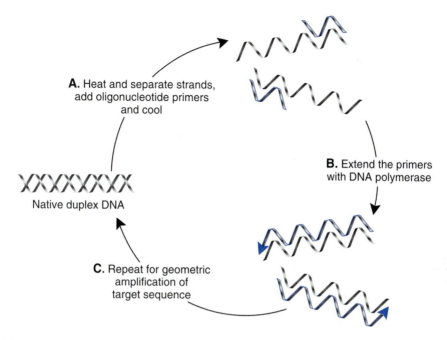

A. Heat and separate strands, add oligonucleotide primers and cool

Native duplex DNA

B. Extend the primers with DNA polymerase

C. Repeat for geometric amplification of target sequence

Figure 10.2–2. Polymerase chain reaction (PCR). **A:** The two strands of native duplex DNA are separated by heating ("melting") and then allowed to cool ("reanneal") in the presence of specific oligonucleotide primers. **B:** The primers then serve as the beginnings of new strand synthesis by the enzyme DNA polymerase. **C:** The new double-stranded DNA can then be used for a repeat reaction, leading to geometric increases in the DNA between the primers.

candidate mutation region for all study subjects. Sequencing can be confined to people for whom the test shows altered single-strand migration.

PCR is not uniquely applicable to mammalian DNA, but can be used for any DNA or RNA* substrate. Methods based on variations of PCR can be used not only for conventional DNA analysis but also to identify bacteria, parasites, and neoplastic changes.

Chromosome Studies

The basic heritable units in the cell are the chromosomes, whose number and size can readily be determined by conventional karyotype* studies. These studies involve growing the cells for some period of time, inducing and capturing a sufficient number of cells during mitosis (through mitotic arrest agents such as colchicine), and microscopic study of individual chromosomes. This approach is widely used to detect chromosome anomalies prenatally as well as in patients with mendelian disorders, neoplasms, and other conditions.

The simplest test of chromosomes is counting them. Patients with Down's syndrome have three copies of chromosome 21, for a total of 47 chromosomes. By contrast, patients with Turner's syndrome (XO) have 45 chromosomes, lacking one sex chromosome. More detailed chromosome studies involve chromosome banding, which establishes visible positions along the length of the chromosomes, based on the specific staining patterns of dyes

such as Giemsa or quinacrine. These patterns (bands) have established reference positions along the chromosomes and actually form a visible counterpart to the DNA-based marker map discussed previously; however, the two types of maps do not yet correlate precisely.

Fortunately, the relatively slow and laborious procedures of conventional chromosome analysis are also beginning to yield to faster techniques. In particular, new technology is being based on the approaches already discussed—hybridization, amplification analysis, RFLPs, mapping, linkage, PCR—all of which exploit the hybridization of specific sequences to specific regions in the genome. Since the introduction of new cloning and chromosome isolation techniques, it is becoming possible to select an entire collection of chromosome-specific sequences, which can be labeled with dye and used to hybridize to a given cell's DNA (chromosome painting*). This can rather quickly establish, for instance, whether the cell contains too few or too many copies of specific chromosomes, as in Turner's syndrome or Down syndrome. These techniques promise to speed and simplify the analysis of conditions associated with chromosome abnormalities.

Another way to analyze changes such as those of neoplasms and rare chromosome disorders is to collect DNA sequence reagents derived from certain regions of a chromosome and check them for translocations, inversions, and other reorganizations. This rapidly evolving technique uses chromosome painting and *fluorescence in situ hybridization* (FISH).* FISH will likely eliminate some conventional karyotype studies but will increase the clinical usefulness of chromosome analysis.

EVOLUTION OF CLINICAL TESTING

Following are descriptions of advances in the diagnosis of two mendelian disorders. Although all inherited disorders are not approached the same way, these examples provide models for considering other conditions.

Sickle Cell Disease

The mutation underlying sickle cell disease (Chapter 11.4) is a single point mutation in the sixth codon of the β-globin gene. Although this mutation has long been recognized, it has only recently been possible to translate the knowledge into clinical testing. The first molecular analysis of sickle cell disease was done by linkage analysis. A specific RFLP outside the structural gene* for β-globin was found to be closely linked to the sickle mutation. The restriction enzyme *Hpa* I and conventional hybridization studies permitted remarkably accurate detection of a chromosome carrying the sickle cell gene. Because this was only a linkage relationship, however, there was always the possibility that a recombination could occur between the marker and the actual gene change and separate them; this possibility limited the resolving power of the technique.

As more restriction enzymes were isolated, it was recognized that the site of the mutation in the sickle cell gene overlapped the recognition site for a restriction enzyme (Figure 10.2–3). Because restriction enzymes are sequence-specific in their recognition and cleavage, the base change of the sickle cell mutation prevented cleavage in this region by a specific restriction enzyme (in this case, *Dde* I). Thus, it was possible to study the DNA fragments revealed by *Dde* I digestion and hybridization with a β-globin gene probe. This was a direct assay for the gene change, but it was still relatively time-consuming.

A new approach for this analysis was developed that

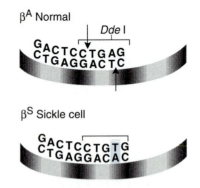

Figure 10.2–3. Sickle cell disease: A to T transversion (GAG→GTG) at position marked in blue. This transversion destroys the recognition and cleavage sequence for the restriction enzyme *Dde* I, thereby changing DNA fragment sizes after *Dde* I cleavage and distinguishing between the alleles. Arrows indicate positions of phosphodiester bond cleavage by *Dde* I.

was simpler, cheaper, and faster. It did not involve DNA cleavage or gel electrophoresis, but was based on the high specificity that can be achieved between oligonucleotide probes and their corresponding genomic DNA substrates. This method uses two allele-specific oligonucleotides* (ASOs)—one prepared with the sequence of the normal and the other with the sequence of the mutant DNA region (Figure 10.2–4). These oligonucleotides differ by a single base. Under very stringent conditions, only the oligonucleotide perfectly matched to the host sequence hybridizes. By adjusting the conditions, geneticists could hybridize either the mutant or the normal test oligonucleotide to the patient's DNA, an alternative way to study the gene.

Even more recently, PCR has been used in several new ways to detect mutations. For instance, it is possible to prepare an oligonucleotide primer for the mutant sequence; the sequence can be extended only when a critical nucleotide is added to the reaction mixture (Figure

Figure 10.2–4. Allele-specific oligonucleotide (ASO) hybridization for normal versus sickle cell genes. Two synthetic oligonucleotides are used. The hybridization stringencies are adjusted so that each oligonucleotide binds with maximum intensity to the DNA corresponding to its sequence. Each spot is a sample of DNA taken from the test or reference individual and bound to a filter. Because carriers contain one of each allele, the hybridization intensity is of intermediate intensity using either oligonucleotide. This technique does not require restriction enzyme digestion or electrophoresis.

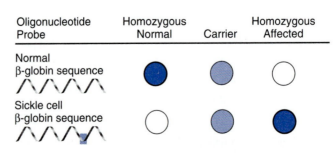

Oligonucleotide Probe	Homozygous Normal	Carrier	Homozygous Affected
Normal β-globin sequence	●	●	○
Sickle cell β-globin sequence	○	●	●

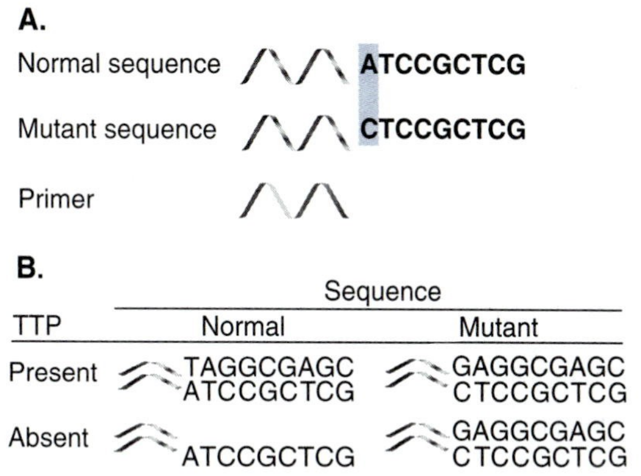

A.

Normal sequence ∧∧ **ATCCGCTCG**

Mutant sequence ∧∧ **CTCCGCTCG**

Primer ∧∧

B.

TTP	Sequence	
	Normal	Mutant
Present	TAGGCGAGC ATCCGCTCG	GAGGCGAGC CTCCGCTCG
Absent	ATCCGCTCG	GAGGCGAGC CTCCGCTCG

Figure 10.2–5. Primer extension test for a point mutation. **A:** The oligonucleotide primer is hybridized to the test DNA. The enzyme DNA polymerase is then used to lengthen the DNA strand with and without the addition of thymidine triphosphate (TTP). **B:** Without TTP in the polymerization reaction, no new nucleotides can be incorporated in the normal sequence because T is needed to pair with A in the DNA. By contrast, the mutant sequence does not need to incorporate a T as the first base (a G is used instead), and thus can be extended.

10.2–5). Thus, one can gain a quick measure of the mutation simply by performing the PCR study with and without the essential nucleotide substrate. This approach can use a very small amount of starting DNA and can yield a diagnosis promptly.

Huntington's Disease

Huntington's disease is a devastating autosomal dominant condition (Chapter 13.7). This late-onset neurodegenerative disorder is a particular problem because the symptoms may not appear until the third or fourth decade, often after an affected individual has had children. Initial work with Huntington's disease used linkage analysis, screening large kindreds with anonymous RFLP marker probes, and showed that the responsible gene was located near the end of chromosome 4. This discovery enabled all later research to be focused on that area.

After the initial mapping studies, RFLP markers were developed throughout the region implicated for the gene.

Until recently, linkage markers were used for diagnosis, although they were limited by the possibility of recombination. The biggest problem with RFLP analysis in the diagnosis of Huntington's disease has been that the region of the chromosome implicated by most mapping studies has been large—2.2 million bp (2.2 megabases* [mb], where 1 mb = 1 million bp)—and markers throughout this region were used. This long region has relatively frequent recombination. Unfortunately, markers that often recombine with the disease gene are of only limited value in linkage analysis.

After intense effort using all the techniques of reverse genetics, the gene for Huntington's disease was recently found within the predicted region of chromosome 4. This finding has proved useful both in diagnosis and in providing a new vision of disease mechanisms. Although the basic function of the gene is still unknown, the mechanism underlying its mutations is now defined. The gene contains repeats of a trinucleotide sequence (Figure 10.2–6) of which most normal individuals carry fewer than 10 copies, but affected individuals carry 20 or more. With PCR analysis using probes flanking the reiterated region, geneticists can distinguish affected and unaffected members of a kindred. It is not yet known whether the number of repeats determines the clinical severity as it does in myotonic dystrophy, a disease caused by a similar mutation.

CURRENT VIEW OF MOLECULAR GENETIC DIAGNOSIS

Molecular genetic approaches have found clinical application in studies of mendelian disorders and spontaneous mutations. It is now possible to analyze gene regions and entire chromosome reorganizations precisely. These powerful techniques are not limited to rare mendelian single gene disorders. They are also valuable in studying complex inheritance patterns in conditions like diabetes and hypertension, in which multiple genes may contribute to the phenotype, and in analyzing the molecular events of neoplastic transformation.

The ultimate result of these studies must be to clarify the molecular defects underlying diseases. This will lead to treatments based on gene replacements and, very likely, gene substitutes and novel drugs based on improved un-

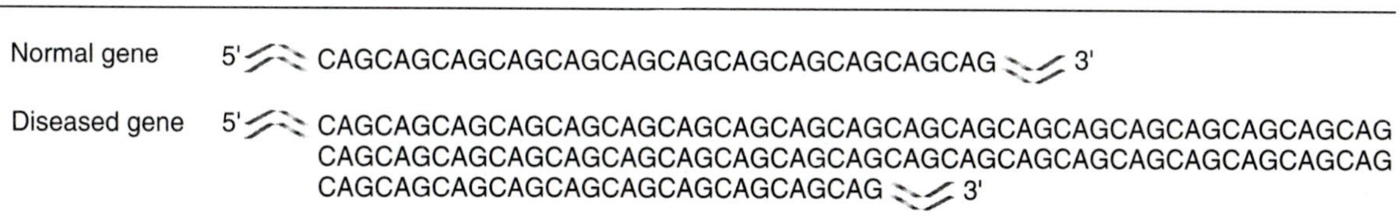

Normal gene 5' CAGCAGCAGCAGCAGCAGCAGCAGCAGCAGCAG 3'

Diseased gene 5' CAGCAGCAGCAGCAGCAGCAGCAGCAGCAGCAGCAGCAGCAGCAGCAGCAG
CAGCAGCAGCAGCAGCAGCAGCAGCAGCAGCAGCAGCAGCAGCAGCAGCAG
CAGCAGCAGCAGCAGCAGCAGCAG 3'

Figure 10.2–6. Huntington's disease. The end of the gene has an abnormally high number of (CAG) triplets. The number of triplets is not fixed, but it must exceed a threshold. There are no other changes in the gene.

derstanding of metabolism and protein structure. Identifying mutations in genes responsible for diseases can lead to developing more transgenic animal models in which new treatments can be studied. In the near future, the technology of molecular genetics will become more useful and applicable to managing many clinical conditions.

Genetic analysis also helps move clinical considerations beyond treatment and into the realm of prevention. With early identification, persons at risk for but not yet manifesting disorders such as Huntington's disease or the far more common problems of colon or breast cancer have the potential for aggressive early screening, better management, and possibly prophylactic treatment. Early testing also can assure other family members that they are not at risk for the same devastating problem. Simplified testing should eventually permit screening to improve risk assessment and management for large population groups.

Finally, improved understanding of genetic contributions to disease and population screening programs have serious ethical implications. For example, insurance policies may exclude coverage of individuals with "preexisting conditions," such as a patient who needs alglucerase enzyme replacement for Gaucher's disease or an asymptomatic child who has the mutation for sickle cell disease. Another difficulty arises as individuals either refuse screening or do not follow recommendations based on the results; some linkage studies are less useful if data from particularly important kindred members are unavailable. Finally, the growing recognition of the pervasiveness of genetic variation implies that the notion of biologic uniqueness applies to everyone. Although this certainly does not mean that each patient requires customized drugs

for hypertension, medical practice has yet to accommodate all these implications and will need to do so as the ramifications continue to broaden.

SUMMARY

▶ DNA can vary in different ways between individuals. The most common changes are point mutations, deletions, repeats, and gross rearrangements.

▶ Many DNA variations exist between individuals, but do not necessarily cause disease. They can be useful as molecular markers when their relative positions have been fixed on the gene map and if they are frequent enough to be recognized as polymorphisms. Markers near critical genes can be used in linkage analysis for clinical diagnosis as well as to help in isolating the gene itself.

▶ The polymerase chain reaction (PCR) and its variants permit detailed analysis of any region of the genome and require little starting DNA. Rapid and highly specific, PCR serves as the basis of much genetic diagnosis.

▶ Molecular hybridization techniques permit faster chromosome analysis than conventional karyotype studies and can be used in the diagnosis and interpretation of gross chromosome changes discovered both prenatally and postnatally, as well as those associated with neoplasia.

SUGGESTED READING

Caskey CT: Molecular medicine: A spin-off from the helix. JAMA 1993;269:1986.

"Molecular Medicine" (continuing series). N Engl J Med 1994; 331:315, 931, and 1995;332:45, 318, 589, and so on.

Sack GH Jr: Molecular biologic approaches to prenatal defects. Prog Clin Biol Res 1988;281:303.

Scriver CR et al: *The Metabolic Bases of Inherited Disease,* 7th ed. McGraw-Hill, 1995.

Seashore MR, Wappner S: *Genetics in Primary Care in Clinical Medicine.* Appleton & Lange, 1996.

Terwilliger JD, Ott J: *Handbook of Human Genetic Linkage.* Johns Hopkins, 1994.

Section 11

Hematology

Brent G. Petty, MD, Section Editor

Approach to the Patient with Anemia

Jerry L. Spivak, MD

Anemia is defined as a hemoglobin concentration or packed red blood cell concentration below the normal level for gender (Table 11.1–1). The cause may be excessive destruction of red cells, hemorrhage, impaired red cell production, or a combination of these. Anemia is always the consequence of another disorder that must be identified before treatment of the anemia is initiated. There is, of course, no correlation between the severity of the anemia and its underlying cause. Pursuing the cause of an anemia may lead to the diagnosis of an unrecognized underlying systemic disorder. Furthermore, because the signs and symptoms of anemia are nonspecific, anemia may be first identified during routine blood testing.

EVALUATION

History and Physical Examination

The symptoms and signs of anemia depend on its cause, extent, rapidity of onset, and the presence of other diseases (Table 11.1–2). Fatigue, headache, and exertional dyspnea are the most common symptoms. The progression of anemia, however, may be so insidious that a profound reduction in red cell mass is tolerated with few symptoms. This is frequently the situation in pernicious anemia. In chronic, compensated hemolytic anemia, a state of ill health is often appreciated only in retrospect, after the hemolytic process has been corrected.

Knowledge of previous hematologic studies or blood donation helps date the onset of anemia. Inquiry concerning medications used, environmental or occupational exposures, travel, and ethanol or drug use is mandatory. Frequently, relatives or close associates are better observers than the patient and may be able to provide important disease-related milestones with respect to the onset of pallor, jaundice, or constitutional symptoms, drug use, or toxic exposures. Unusual eating habits may suggest a cause. Pica (the unremitting craving of ice or a particular food) is pathognomonic of iron deficiency, whereas unusually restrictive diets suggest deficiency of folate or other nutrients. Jaundice or dark urine suggests hemolysis. The family history is of great importance in determining whether a blood disorder is hereditary or if a genetic predisposition to autoimmune diseases exists. African heritage increases the likelihood of sickle cell anemia, and African or Mediterranean ancestry makes thalassemia more probable.

The physical examination may reveal findings suggestive of anemia. Pallor is best evaluated from the mucous membranes, since alterations in blood flow, variations in pigmentation, and other disorders often make the determination of pallor from skin examination unreliable. As a rough guide, however, pallor of the palmar creases is not usually observed unless the hemoglobin level is 7 g/dL or less. Tachycardia is not usually observed unless the anemia is acute. Other evidence of hyperkinetic circulatory activity, however, such as a widened pulse pressure, accentuation of the first and second heart sounds, systolic flow murmurs, and a cervical venous hum, may be present with chronic anemia. Nevertheless, these symptoms are not specific, and mild anemia does not produce recognizable physical signs.

The physical examination can yield important clues to the cause of anemia (Table 11.1–3). Jaundice suggests hemolysis, and telangiectasias suggest vascular malformations elsewhere that can bleed. Petechiae, ecchymoses, or purpura suggest a bleeding disorder. Papillary atrophy of the tongue and posterior spinal column dysfunction suggest vitamin B_{12} deficiency. Lymphadenopathy, sternal or other bony tenderness, splenomegaly, and hepatomegaly may be present with lymphoma or leukemia.

A number of mechanisms are available to compensate for the decrease in oxygen transport associated with anemia. They include an increase in cardiac output, typically when the hemoglobin level falls to 7 g/dL or less, caused mainly by an increase in stroke volume without tachycardia. However, there is no correlation between the severity of the anemia and the cardiac output. For example, in patients with sickle cell anemia, the cardiac output may be elevated when the hemoglobin level is 9 g/dL, while in the elderly, severe anemia may be associated with little

Table 11.1–1. Normal hematologic values for adults.

Test	Men	Women
Hematocrit (%)	42–54 (50)	37–47 (40)
Hemoglobin (g/dL)	14.0–16.0 (15)	12.0–15.0 (14)
Red blood cell count (10^6/μL)	4.6–6.2 (6)	4.2–5.4 (5)

	Either Sex
MCV (fL)	80–100
MCH (pg/cell)	26–34
MCHC (g/dL)	32–36
RDW (%)	11.5–14.5
White blood cell count (per μL)	4,400–11,300
Platelet count (per μL)	150,000–450,000
Corrected reticulocyte count (%)	0.5–2.5

MCV, mean corpuscular volume; MCH, mean corpuscular hemoglobin; MCHC, mean corpuscular hemoglobin concentration; RDW, red cell distribution width.

change in cardiac output. On the other hand, anemia can produce circulatory congestion and fluid retention, even in the absence of cardiac disease.

LABORATORY STUDIES

In the routine complete blood count (CBC), an automated panel of tests is performed, including a combination of measured and calculated values (see Table 11.1–1). The most important results are the hemoglobin and hematocrit (or packed cell volume), which identify the presence and severity of the anemia, while mean corpuscular volume (MCV) and red cell distribution width (RDW) provide clues to the cause. If the laboratory report of a patient's anemia is unexpected, the physician should obtain a confirmatory measurement.

To complement and elucidate the automated tests, all anemic patients should have a peripheral blood smear. Although the MCV and RDW may suggest the character of a patient's red blood cells, they are not a substitute for a peripheral smear, which gives more accurate and complete information about red blood cell morphology. In addition, anemic patients should have a corrected reticulocyte count to determine whether the anemia is caused by a decrease in red cell production or an increase in red cell destruction, a urinalysis to look for hematuria and hemoglobinuria, and examination of the stool for occult blood. Positive findings serve to focus attention on certain diagnostic possibilities and the need for immediate therapeutic intervention.

Table 11.1–2. Symptoms suggesting specific causes of anemia.

Symptoms	Anemia
• Pica (craving ice or particular foods)	Iron deficiency
• Sore tongue, paresthesias	Megaloblastic anemia
• Jaundice, dark urine	Hemolysis
• Intermittent painful crises	Sickle cell disease

Table 11.1–3. Signs associated with various anemias.

Sign	Possible Diagnosis
Telangiectasia	Vascular malformations
Hepatosplenomegaly	Neoplasms, especially lymphomas
Petechiae, purpura	Bleeding disorder
Atrophic tongue, posterior spinal column dysfunction	Vitamin B_{12} deficiency
Sternal tenderness	Leukemia

Automated Tests

Three measurements are used interchangeably to quantify the concentration of circulating red cells: the red cell count, the blood hemoglobin concentration, and the volume of packed red cells (hematocrit). Once performed manually, these measurements are now routinely made with greater accuracy by electronic particle counters. The red cell count and the hemoglobin concentration are measured directly; the hematocrit is calculated from the mean red cell volume (measured directly) and the red cell count. A hematocrit determined in this fashion is always lower than one determined directly by centrifugation of whole blood in a hematocrit tube, since trapped plasma increases the apparent hematocrit in the latter instance. In both iron deficiency anemia and megaloblastic anemia, the difference between the two techniques is even greater because in those situations the red cells are more rigid than normal and more plasma is trapped. The red cell count, the blood hemoglobin concentration, and the spun hematocrit all are influenced by the plasma volume. Thus, they do not faithfully reflect just the circulating red cell mass. Nonetheless, for routine purposes, the ease with which these measurements are obtained outweighs this disadvantage.

Electronic particle counters also determine the "red cell indices": the MCV, the mean corpuscular hemoglobin (MCH), and the mean corpuscular hemoglobin concentration (MCHC) of red cells. These measurements have traditionally been used to characterize deviations from the mean in size and hemoglobin content of circulating red cells. Of the three, only the MCV is directly measured and of important discriminate value in patients with anemia; the MCH and MCHC are derived quantities and usually provide little additional information. The MCV is useful in screening for disorders producing macrocytosis (abnormally large red cells) (Table 11.1–4) or microcytosis (abnormally small red cells; Table 11.1–5). Because different disorders can produce similar alterations in the MCV, the peripheral blood smear is useful in distinguishing between them. Furthermore, the peripheral blood smear provides the only means for detecting red cell inclusions or abnormalities restricted to a portion of the circulating red cell population as well as a means of corroborating results obtained by the particle counter.

In addition to the MCV, MCH, and MCHC, electronic particle counters often provide a quantitative measurement of anisocytosis, the RDW, which is the coefficient of variation of red cell volume (also abbreviated RBC CV).

Table 11.1–4. Anemias associated with elevated MCV (macrocytosis).

Folate deficiency
Vitamin B$_{12}$ deficiency
Hemolytic anemia with high reticulocyte response
Sideroblastic anemia (usually macrocytic, but sometimes microcytic)
Liver disease
Hypothyroidism

MCV, mean corpuscular volume.

Normally, the distribution of red cell volume is Gaussian. Excessive heterogeneity of red cell volume (anisocytosis) is an early feature of disturbed erythropoiesis and is reflected by an increase in the RDW. This measurement also can be used to distinguish between thalassemia trait and iron deficiency anemia. In thalassemia trait the RDW is normal; in iron deficiency it is increased. An increase in RDW can also occur when there is a bimodal distribution of red cell volumes, as in cold agglutinin disease. In such instances, the MCV does not provide an accurate reflection of red cell volume.

Blood Smear

The peripheral blood smear represents an immediate tissue biopsy of great potential importance and, when possible, should be examined by the physician responsible for an anemic patient.

Figure 11.1–1 illustrates the type of diagnostic information that can be obtained from the peripheral blood smear that would not be provided by electronic particle counters. For example, hypersegmented neutrophils and oval macrocytes suggest megaloblastic hematopoiesis. Howell-Jolly bodies (small, dense, dark-staining spheres in red blood cells) (see Color Plates) are also seen in megaloblastic hematopoiesis and are a feature of surgical or disease-related hyposplenism. Red cell stippling (see Color Plates) may be caused by a hemoglobinopathy, a sideroblastic process, or lead poisoning, whereas spiculated red cells may be seen in patients with liver disease, hypothyroidism, and starvation. Bizarre abnormalities of red cell shape and size are a hallmark of hemolytic processes, and the type of morphologic abnormality may suggest the underlying cause of the hemolysis. Red cell fragmentation suggests mechanical intravascular destruction, which may be caused by vasculitis, a cardiac valve abnormality, metastatic tumor, or consumption coagu-

Table 11.1–5. Anemias associated with decreased MCV (microcytosis).

Iron deficiency
Thalassemia
Anemia of chronic disease (occasionally microcytic, usually normocytic)
Sideroblastic anemia (sometimes microcytic, more often macrocytic)

MCV, mean corpuscular volume.

lopathy. Sickled erythrocytes are a pathognomonic feature of hemoglobin S, whereas ovalocytosis or spherocytosis suggests underlying abnormalities of red cell cytoskeletal proteins (see Figure 11.5–1). Spherocytes may also be the consequence of antibody-mediated red cell membrane loss, whereas cold agglutinins cause red cell agglutination; rouleaux formation occurs with hyperglobulinemia, and "blister cells" occur with red cell G6PD deficiency or oxidant-induced hemolysis. Target cells may be seen with a hemoglobinopathy or obstructive jaundice.

Reticulocyte Count

The red cell count, the blood hemoglobin concentration, and the hematocrit are, of course, static measurements and reflect only the balance between production and destruction of red cells. To estimate effective red cell production, the physician can use both the presence of polychromatophilic red cells in the blood and the number of circulating reticulocytes. Polychromatophilic red cells are reticulocytes that have been prematurely released into the bloodstream before completion of hemoglobin synthesis. Normally, less than 0.1% of circulating red cells are polychromatophilic, as identified by Wright-stained blood smears. With stimulation of the marrow by erythropoietin, the number of polychromatophilic cells increases substantially and, in the absence of intrinsic disease of the marrow, can be used as an indicator of increased effective erythropoietic activity. Mature reticulocytes released into the blood can only be identified with supravital stains since they are not larger than other red cells. The reticulocyte count provides a simple means of measuring blood production and identifying anemias caused by impaired red cell production.

Since reticulocytes are enumerated in relation to the red cell number, anemia produces an apparent increase in the reticulocyte count. Furthermore, when anemia is severe, reticulocytes are released prematurely and spend a longer time in the circulation. As a consequence, the daily reticulocyte count may not faithfully reflect the actual rate of new blood production. To compensate for these effects and obtain a meaningful index of blood production, the reticulocyte count should be corrected for the degree of anemia:

$$\text{Reticulocyte count} \times \frac{\text{observed hematocrit}}{\text{normal hematocrit for gender}} = \text{corrected reticulocyte count}$$

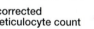

If the hematocrit is 25% or less, the "corrected" reticulocyte count should be divided by two, as an additional correction, to adjust for the prolonged maturation of the reticulocytes in the circulation. This value can be used as an index of effective erythropoiesis. If the reticulocyte count is not increased above normal in patients with anemia, there is at least an element of inadequate marrow production as a cause for the anemia or its perpetuation (Table 11.1–6).

How well does marrow respond to anemia?

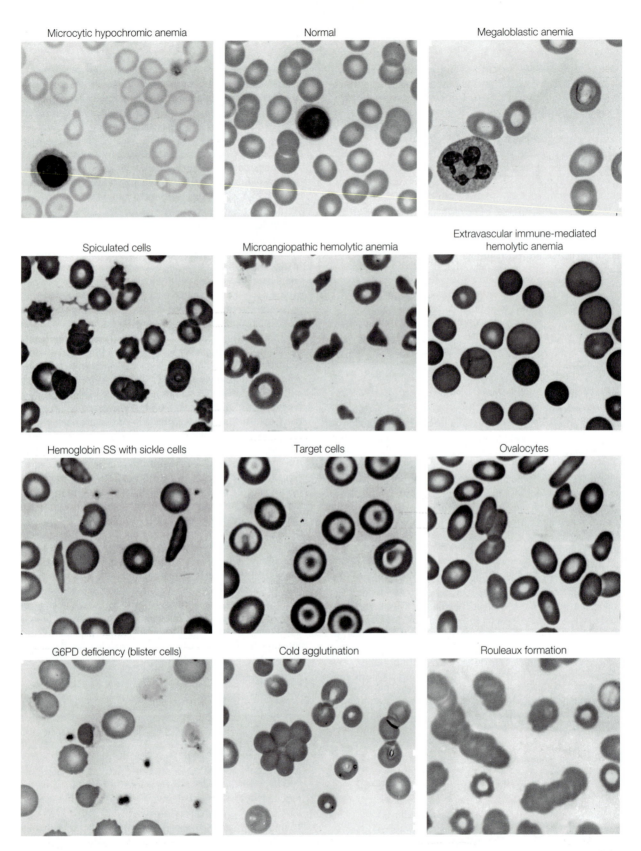

Figure 11.1–1. Normal and abnormal peripheral blood smears. (See also Figures 11.2–2, 11.4–2, 11.4–4, 11.5–1, and 11.7–1, and the Color Plates.) (All photographs in the Hematology Section were provided by Victoria E. Smith, MT(ASCP)SH.)

Table 11.1–6. Causes of hypoproliferative anemia.*

Impairment of renal function
Infection
Chronic inflammatory diseases, eg, rheumatoid arthritis
Deficiency of iron, vitamin B$_{12}$, or folic acid
Neoplasms
Drugs, toxins
Aplastic anemia
Myelofibrosis
Sideroblastic anemia
Impairment of pituitary or thyroid function
Starvation
Pure red cell aplasia

*Anemia with a low reticulocyte count.

BONE MARROW ASPIRATE AND BIOPSY

If the evaluation described thus far has not led to a diagnosis of the cause of anemia, a bone marrow aspiration may be helpful. The stained marrow aspirate permits assessment of the composition of the marrow precursor cell populations and maturation or morphologic abnormalities of these cells. A marrow aspirate is also useful in the evaluation of storage cell disorders and in the evaluation of neoplastic involvement of the marrow. It is the most reliable means for assessing marrow iron stores and provides a source of tissue for karyotypic analysis of hematopoietic cells.

In certain instances a bone marrow biopsy can provide important information not available from bone marrow aspiration. Furthermore, in the event that marrow cannot be aspirated, the physician should always obtain a bone marrow biopsy. Marrow biopsy provides the only reliable method for evaluating marrow cellularity and architecture. Bone marrow biopsy should be performed in every patient with pancytopenia, since the diagnosis of aplastic anemia can be established only by bone marrow biopsy, and in this situation the marrow aspirate can be misleading. Marrow biopsy is also useful in staging lymphomas and small-cell carcinoma of the lung. When the physician is seeking tumor infiltration of the bone marrow, bilateral biopsies increase the yield of positive results by only 15% compared with unilateral biopsy. Bone marrow biopsy may reveal granulomas, suggesting tuberculosis or sarcoidosis, where the incidence of biopsies containing granulomas is 15% and 30%, respectively.

Erythropoietin Level

Erythropoiesis is regulated by the hormone erythropoietin, which is produced in the kidneys and to a small extent in the liver. Erythropoietin interacts with erythroid progenitor cells to promote their proliferation and maintain their viability. Normally there is an inverse relationship between plasma erythropoietin and the red cell mass as defined by the hemoglobin or hematocrit. However, because of the wide range of normal for plasma erythropoi-

etin, this inverse relationship does not become apparent until the hemoglobin level has fallen below 10.5 g/dL (hematocrit 32%), unless the patient's baseline plasma erythropoietin level is known. Thus, a plasma erythropoietin measurement is not a useful diagnostic test in mild degrees of anemia. Renal disease, inflammation (eg, rheumatoid arthritis), infection (eg, AIDS), and various cancers blunt the expected increase in plasma erythropoietin for any degree of anemia. Since administration of recombinant human erythropoietin in these disorders can correct anemia, plasma erythropoietin measurements have diagnostic utility when other reversible causes of anemia are excluded and a low value would persuade the physician to recommend erythropoietin treatment.

An elevated plasma erythropoietin level in an anemic patient is an appropriate response of the kidneys to tissue hypoxia and suggests a marrow defect such as iron deficiency or an uncompensated hemolytic process as the cause of the anemia. A level greater than 500 mU/mL suggests that the marrow will not respond to exogenous recombinant erythropoietin. An inappropriately low erythropoietin level suggests that impaired erythropoietin production could be a cause of the anemia but a marrow abnormality is still not excluded. In anemic patients with renal disease (creatinine above 1.5 mg/dL), the erythropoietin response to anemia is so uniformly blunted that erythropoietin measurements are unnecessary. Of course, these patients may have additional reasons for being anemic (eg, iron or folate deficiency, chronic bleeding, hemolysis, splenic sequestration, aluminum intoxication), which must be excluded.

SUMMARY

▶ Anemia developing in an adult is a nonspecific finding and is caused by an underlying disorder, which must be identified. Prior blood counts may document the duration of the anemia.

▶ Anemia may be caused by increased red cell destruction, decreased red cell production, bleeding, or a combination of these.

▶ The reticulocyte count serves to distinguish between increased and decreased red cell production.

▶ A peripheral blood smear can give valuable clues to the cause of anemia and is an essential component of the evaluation of all anemic patients.

▶ A bone marrow aspirate is useful to evaluate the adequacy of iron stores, to document morphologic abnormalities, and to obtain tissue for cytogenetic studies. A bone marrow biopsy is mandatory if a marrow aspirate cannot be obtained or if there is pancytopenia.

SUGGESTED READING

Bessman JD, Gilmer PR Jr, Gardner FH: Improved classification of anemias by MCV and RDW. Am J Clin Pathol 1983; 80:322.

Hillman RS: Characteristics of marrow production and reticulocyte maturation in normal man in response to anemia. J Clin Invest 1969;48:443.

Payne CJ, Polk A, Eichner ER: Analysis of anemia in medical patients. Am J Med Sci 1974;268:37.

Spivak JL: Recombinant erythropoietin. Annu Rev Med 1993; 44:243.

Varat MA, Adolph RJ, Fowler NO: Cardiovascular effects of anemia. Am Heart J 1972;83:415.

Iron Deficiency Anemia

Jerry L. Spivak, MD

Iron deficiency in an adult is almost always the result of blood loss, for which the cause should be sought diligently. Although minute amounts of iron (1 mg/day) are lost by normal desquamation of epithelial cells and in the sweat, urine, and bile, these deficits are easily replenished by diet. In Western societies, inadequate dietary intake is never an acceptable cause of iron deficiency. Patients with iron deficiency anemia may present with an overt history of bleeding, or the diagnosis may be suspected from a routine complete blood count showing microcytotic erythrocytes. Once iron deficiency is detected, it is imperative to define the source of blood loss causing it.

CLINICAL FEATURES OF IRON DEFICIENCY

Only a few specific complaints can be attributed to lack of iron in an adult. The one unequivocal nonhematologic manifestation of iron deficiency is pica, an insatiable craving for a particular substance or food. Compulsive ice ingestion (pagophagia) is a common form of pica, but the craving may take more exotic forms. Patients rarely volunteer information about their dietary behavior, either because they are embarrassed by it or because they fail to recognize it as abnormal. In view of its diagnostic importance, evidence of pica should always be sought in evaluating patients with anemia. As a corollary, dietary habits such as clay ingestion may lead to iron deficiency. Starch ingestion is not uncommonly associated with iron deficiency, but starch itself does not inhibit iron absorption.

Less common manifestations of iron deficiency anemia include abnormalities of epithelial surfaces, such as glossitis, papillary atrophy of the tongue, dysphagia, and spooning of the nails (koilonychia). Contrary to previous concepts, the dysphagia-postcricoid esophageal web syndrome (Plummer-Vinson [or Paterson-Kelly] syndrome) may not have any relation to lack of iron. In contrast to experimental studies in animals, iron deficiency in adults does not produce appreciable abnormalities of either neuromuscular or cardiovascular function.

PATHOPHYSIOLOGY

The values for iron homeostasis in normal men and women are shown in Table 11.2–1. The bulk of the iron required daily for hemoglobin synthesis is provided by catabolism of senescent red cells, whereas tissue iron stores provide a reserve to maintain hemoglobin synthesis when blood loss occurs or there is a sudden demand for red cells. Dietary iron serves to replenish ordinary daily losses. The iron content of the diet is linked to caloric intake; each 1000 calories ingested contains approximately 7 mg of iron. Not all of this iron, however, is available for absorption. Dietary iron occurs in two forms, heme iron and nonheme iron, each of which is absorbed by a different mechanism. Heme compounds, primarily found in meat, are absorbed intact with high efficiency in the upper small bowel. Once absorbed, iron is released from heme within the mucosal cells by heme oxygenase. In contrast to heme iron, the bioavailability of nonheme iron is poor. This is due in part to the manner in which the iron is complexed in particular foodstuffs, such as spinach or rice, and in part to the adverse effect of other constituents of the diet on absorption of nonheme iron. Egg yolk, bran, tannates (tea and coffee), antacids, and tetracyclines inhibit nonheme iron absorption; meat, fish, and ascorbic acid enhance it.

In addition to the quantity and quality of the diet, iron absorption is affected by the gastrointestinal environment. Nonheme food iron is generally in the oxidized ferric ($3+$) form. Ferric iron is insoluble at the alkaline pH characteristic of the upper small bowel where iron absorption takes place. Chelation of ferric iron by sugars, amino acids, and ascorbic acid in the acidic environment of the stomach renders it soluble and absorbable in the small bowel.

Table 11.2–1. Normal iron balance.

	Men	Women
	(Hemoglobin 16 g/dL)	(Hemoglobin 14 g/dL)
Hemoglobin iron (mg)	2500	1900
Storage iron (mg)	1000	500
Iron intake (mg/day)	10–15	10–15
Iron absorbed (mg/day)	1.0	1–2.5
Iron loss (mg/day)	1.0	1–2.5*
		(1.0–1.5 from menstrual loss)

*This increase in menstruating women is corrected by increased efficiency of absorption; however, the menstruating woman whose iron loss increases further will become iron-deficient.

Thus, achlorhydria or loss of the gastric reservoir, as well as motility disorders or damage to the bowel wall, impair nonheme iron absorption.

Regulation of the amount of iron absorbed daily occurs at the level of the mucosal cell through mechanisms that are not well understood. The mucosa serves as a barrier to the absorption of excessive quantities of iron, which would prove toxic, but is also capable of enhancing iron absorption up to fivefold to meet increases in daily iron requirements. The most important factors that influence iron absorption are body iron stores and the rate of red cell production. Hemochromatosis represents a unique situation, characterized by excessive iron absorption in the absence of any physiologic stimulus.

Once absorbed, iron enters the circulation bound to transferrin, an α-globulin with a molecular weight of 80,000 produced by the liver. Since free iron is toxic and forms insoluble precipitates at the pH of extracellular fluids, transferrin has an essential role in iron transport. It contains two binding sites for iron that, although not biochemically equivalent, appear to function in the same fashion with respect to the delivery of iron to cells. Transferrin binds only ferric iron, and thus ferrous iron being released from cells must first undergo oxidation. This process is catalyzed by ceruloplasmin. The ferroxidase activity of ceruloplasmin may explain in part the hypochromic anemia associated with severe copper deficiency.

Normally, the binding sites of transferrin are only one-third saturated. Iron is released from the protein only at specific cell receptors, after which the transferrin is freed to repeat its cycle of iron uptake and delivery. The number of specific receptors for transferrin determines the extent of iron delivery to a particular tissue. Because of the high density of transferrin receptors on immature erythroid precursors, they receive the bulk of transferrin iron. However, when transferrin saturation falls below 16%, iron delivery to developing red cells is insufficient. Conversely, when transferrin saturation exceeds 80%, iron accumulates in other tissues, particularly the liver. The liver appears to be a passive recipient of iron, since it releases iron to the plasma when the plasma iron level falls.

Tissue macrophages, in contrast to erythroid precursors or hepatocytes, are unable to acquire iron from transferrin. Macrophage iron is obtained from the catabolism of senescent red cells taken up by the macrophage. About 75% of this iron is returned to the plasma for transport to erythroid precursors by transferrin. Since the bulk of the daily red cell iron requirement is provided by macrophages, these cells can have a profound influence on erythropoiesis. In inflammation or infection, release of iron from macrophages is retarded, plasma iron and transferrin saturation decline, and red cell production is diminished.

IRON STORAGE

Iron in excess of requirements for essential functions is stored either in ferritin or hemosiderin. Ferritin is a large and ubiquitous protein that can hold up to 4500 iron atoms. Ferritin synthesis is stimulated by iron. Iron stored in the spherical ferritin molecule is readily mobilized and also is packaged in a manner that facilitates its excretion by the cell. In addition to its intracellular role in iron storage, ferritin also circulates in the plasma. Plasma ferritin, in contrast to the intracellular form, is virtually iron-free and does not function as a transport protein.

Hemosiderin is an insoluble, paracrystalline aggregate of denatured ferritin molecules and other cell constituents, which most likely are formed within lysosomes. The iron-to-protein ratio of hemosiderin is higher than that of ferritin, and when tissue iron increases, it accumulates progressively as hemosiderin, not ferritin. Iron contained within hemosiderin is mobilized more slowly than soluble ferritin iron and represents the iron reserve that can be visualized in bone marrow aspirates by light microscopy using the Prussian blue stain.

IRON DEFICIENCY

When demands for iron for erythropoiesis exceed the capacity for iron absorption, a predictable sequence of events occurs that terminates in iron deficiency anemia if iron stores are not replenished (Figure 11.2–1). The earliest sign of iron deficiency is depletion of marrow iron stores, as determined by the Prussian blue stain. This is reflected by a decrease in plasma ferritin and subsequently an increase in plasma transferrin. When the amount of iron available for erythropoiesis falls below the minimal required level and plasma iron and transferrin saturation fall, there is an increase in free erythrocyte protoporphyrin. At first, the anemia is normocytic, but subsequently microcytic red cells begin to appear in the circulation, producing an increase in the red cell distribution width (RDW), a quantitative measure of anisocytosis, which is then followed by a reduction in mean corpuscular

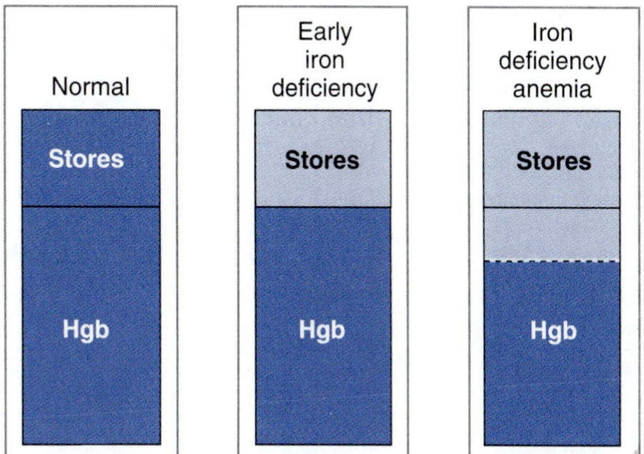

	Normal	Early iron deficiency	Iron deficiency anemia
Marrow iron	Normal	Absent	Absent
Serum ferritin	Normal	Low	Low
Serum iron	Normal	Normal	Low
Serum iron binding capacity	Normal	Normal	Elevated
Transferrin saturation	Normal	Normal	Low
Erythrocyte free protoporphyrin	Normal	Normal	Elevated

Figure 11.2–1. Sequence of changes in the development of iron deficiency. Shaded areas denote iron located in marrow stores and circulating red blood cells.

volume (MCV). If iron deficiency persists, there is a further decline in red cell production and the red cells become progressively more microcytic and hypochromic (Figure 11.2–2). Iron-deficient red cells are more rigid than normal red cells, and therefore severe iron deficiency anemia has a small hemolytic component.

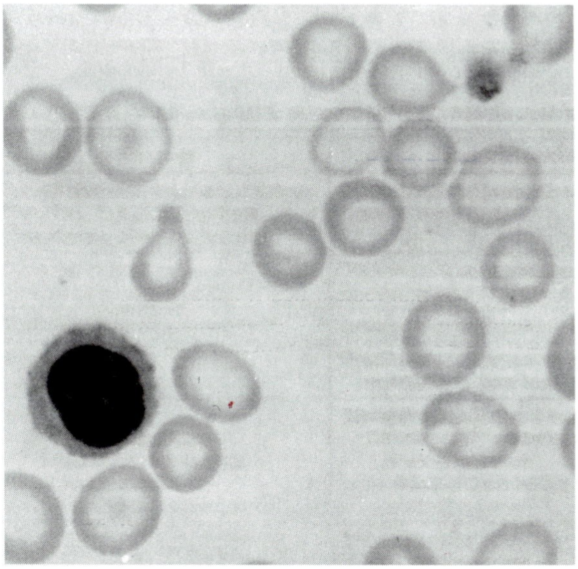

DIFFERENTIAL DIAGNOSIS OF IRON DEFICIENCY

Microcytic, hypochromic erythropoiesis is not specific for iron deficiency. Other causes include thalassemia, sideroblastic anemia, the anemia associated with systemic disease, and copper deficiency. For routine purposes, measuring plasma ferritin is the best single screening test for iron deficiency, since it more closely reflects body iron stores than the transferrin level. A ferritin level of less than 10 ng/mL in women and 30 ng/mL in men is diagnostic of iron deficiency; since ferritin is an acute-phase reactant, a ferritin level of 100 ng/mL or less in the presence of inflammation or infection suggests iron deficiency. The most reliable test for demonstrating iron deficiency is a bone marrow iron stain, provided that an adequate aspirate is obtained and carefully scrutinized. A response to a therapeutic trial of iron with increased reticulocyte count within 5–7 days is the most conclusive evidence that lack of iron is the cause of anemia, but such a trial must not be allowed to compromise the search for the cause of iron deficiency.

Figure 11.2–2. Peripheral blood smear in iron deficiency anemia.

Table 11.2–2. Representative laboratory abnormalities in microcytic and hypochromic anemias.

Test	Normal Range	Iron Deficiency	Anemia Associated with Systemic Disease	Thalassemia Trait	Sideroblastic Anemia
MCV (fL)	80–99	<80	<80	<80	<80–>100
Plasma iron (µg/dL)	65–175	<30	<30	65–175	>200
Iron-binding capacity (µg/dL)	300–360	450	200	300–360	300–360
Transferrin saturation (%)	25–50	<16	<16	25–50	>80
Plasma ferritin (µg/L)	20–250	<10♀ <30♂	20–1000	20–250	1000
Erythrocyte-free protoporphyrin (µg/dL)	27–61	180	180	27–61	180
Basophilic stippling	Absent	Absent	Absent	Usually present	Present
Marrow iron stores	Present	Absent	Present	Present	Increased

MCV, mean corpuscular volume.

The plasma iron level is not a sensitive test and even when low it is not specific for iron deficiency. A transferrin saturation below 16%, although also not specific for iron deficiency, does indicate that the quantity of iron available for erythropoiesis is inadequate. Thrombocytosis, for unknown reasons, may develop with iron deficiency and regress with iron repletion. Thrombocytosis is not, however, an invariable event and is also associated with other disorders (inflammation, infection), which themselves depress the plasma iron and transferrin saturation even with adequate iron stores. A peripheral blood smear should always be examined. Basophilic stippling and red cell fragmentation suggest that microcytosis is due to thalassemia, whereas hypersegmented neutrophils with either normocytic or microcytic red cells suggest a combined deficiency of iron and folic acid or vitamin B_{12}. The blood smear is also the only method for detecting the dimorphic red cell population of sideroblastic anemia and is an inexpensive method for evaluating the platelet count. Representative values for the laboratory studies previously described in the various microcytic and hypochromic anemias are illustrated in Table 11.2–2.

The causes of iron deficiency are many and not always evident (Table 11.2–3). Women frequently underestimate the extent of menstrual blood loss, and occult gastrointestinal blood loss can be difficult to document. Even if gastrointestinal bleeding cannot be demonstrated, men and postmenopausal women with iron deficiency should

Table 11.2–3. Causes of iron deficiency.

Impaired absorption
  Gastric surgery
  Achlorhydria
  Malabsorption syndromes
  Ingestion of clay or dirt

Increased iron loss
  Gastrointestinal hemorrhage
  Menstrual bleeding
  Pregnancy
  Lactation
  Phlebotomies
  Chronic or recurrent intravascular hemolysis
  Idiopathic pulmonary hemosiderosis

be considered to have a gastrointestinal cancer until proven otherwise. Therefore, these patients should have aggressive gastrointestinal evaluation. Not infrequently, repeated examination of the stool for occult blood and sophisticated endoscopic and radiologic techniques are required to localize the site of gastrointestinal bleeding. If gastrointestinal evaluation is unrewarding, the urine should be examined as a possible site of iron loss.

The response of patients with iron deficiency anemia is generally observed within days of starting supplemental iron. The most common preparation used is ferrous sulfate, usually given with meals. The hematocrit should show a noticeable increase within 2 weeks if the cause of blood loss is identified and treated successfully. The microcytosis and hypochromia gradually resolve. Finally, the plasma ferritin and tissue iron stores are replenished to their normal levels. After the hematocrit becomes normal, iron therapy should be continued for several months to ensure that total body iron stores have been repleted. The plasma ferritin level can serve as a guide for this. If the source of iron loss has not been established, the iron therapy should be discontinued and the patient monitored to determine whether the iron deficiency recurs.

SUMMARY

▶ Iron deficiency in an adult almost always reflects blood loss, and the bleeding site must be identified.

▶ Men and postmenopausal women with iron deficiency should be considered to have a gastrointestinal lesion until proved otherwise.

▶ Plasma ferritin measurement is the best screening test for iron deficiency; a low ferritin level is an unequivocal sign of iron lack.

▶ In patients with inflammation, infection, or cancer, the ferritin level can be elevated even when iron deficiency is present. A bone marrow aspirate can identify iron deficiency in such patients.

SUGGESTED READING

Cartwright GE, Deiss A: Sideroblasts, siderocytes, and sideroblastic anemia. N Engl J Med 1975;292:185.

Finch CA: Erythropoiesis, erythropoietin, and iron. Blood 1982;60:1241.

Lipschitz DA, Cook JD, Finch CA: A clinical evaluation of serum ferritin as an index of iron stores. N Engl J Med 1974;290:1213.

Wheby MS: Effect of iron therapy on serum ferritin levels in iron-deficiency anemia. Blood 1980;56:138.

Megaloblastic Anemia

Jerry L. Spivak, MD

Megaloblastic anemia is caused by disorders that impair DNA synthesis (Table 11.3–1). Although the effects of many of these disorders are global, they are most marked in tissues with a high rate of cell turnover, particularly the blood. The characteristic morphologic, biochemical, and proliferative changes associated with impaired DNA synthesis indicate the mechanism for the hematologic abnormalities of megaloblastic hematopoiesis but not its etiology. Most often, megaloblastic anemia is due to a deficiency of either folic acid or vitamin B_{12}. Since uncorrected vitamin B_{12} deficiency can lead to irreversible neurologic damage, it is imperative that the physician recognize megaloblastic anemia and carefully identify its cause.

Megaloblastic anemia due to vitamin B_{12} deficiency generally develops slowly, and the patient may become symptomatic only when the anemia is severe. Furthermore, the symptoms associated with a megaloblastic anemia, such as glossitis or sensory disturbances in a "stocking-glove" distribution (vitamin B_{12} deficiency only), are not specific for a vitamin deficiency state. Thus, the first clue to a megaloblastic anemia may be the discovery of macrocytosis on a routine automated blood count. The differential diagnosis of macrocytosis is wide, and the extent of the increase in the red cell mean corpuscular volume (MCV) is not helpful in distinguishing one cause from another (Table 11.3–2). In this regard, it is important to remember that blacks with megaloblastic anemia may not have macrocytosis because of the coexistence of thalassemia trait.

PATHOPHYSIOLOGY

Mammalian cells require both vitamin B_{12} and folic acid (folate) for DNA synthesis but lack the capacity to manufacture either. In megaloblastic anemia, the characteristic histologic abnormality in the red blood cell precursors is nuclear-cytoplasmic maturation dissociation, in which the cytoplasm matures faster than the nucleus. This leads to larger-than-normal red blood cells (macrocytosis), nuclei immature relative to the cytoplasm (megaloblasts), and "ineffective erythropoiesis," leading to intramedullary cell death and premature splenic sequestration of abnormal red cells and mild extravascular hemolysis (Chapter 11.5). These changes are identical, whether caused by deficiency of vitamin B_{12} or folate. Megaloblastic changes also may be seen in white blood cell precursors in the bone marrow. On the peripheral smear, the characteristic finding is hypersegmented polymorphonuclear cells (Figure 11.3–1). Disorders other than folate or vitamin B_{12} deficiency can cause pathologic changes in the bone marrow indistinguishable from those associated with these two diseases. They can be distinguished by history and laboratory investigation.

Interrelationship of Vitamin B_{12} and Folic Acid

Vitamin B_{12} is known to participate in only two metabolic processes in mammalian cells. It serves as a coenzyme for the conversion of methylmalonyl coenzyme A to succinyl coenzyme A, which accounts for the methylmalonic aciduria associated with vitamin B_{12} deficiency. The other process, which is clinically more important, is the conversion of homocysteine to methionine, for which vitamin B_{12} serves as the coenzyme. This reaction links vitamin B_{12} and folic acid, since the reaction is catalyzed by the enzyme 5-methyltetrahydrofolate-homocysteine transmethylase (Figure 11.3–2). During this reaction, 5-methyltetrahydrofolate is converted to tetrahydrofolate. Tetrahydrofolate is the immediate precursor of N^5-N^{10} methylene tetrahydrofolate, which is required for the conversion of deoxyuridylate to thymidylate. Since thymidylate is required for DNA synthesis, deficiency of either vitamin B_{12} or folic acid impairs DNA synthesis and leads to megaloblastic anemia. Essentially, vitamin B_{12} deficiency creates a folate-deficient state within the cell while N^5-methyltetrahydrofolate accumulates in the blood. This accounts for the identical morphologic mani-

Table 11.3–1. Causes of megaloblastic hematopoiesis in adults.

Folic acid deficiency
Vitamin B_{12} deficiency
Acute leukemia
Nitrous oxide inhalation
Arsenic poisoning
Cancer chemotherapy

festations of vitamin B_{12} and folic acid deficiency as well as the ability of large doses of folic acid to correct the megaloblastic abnormalities due to vitamin B_{12} deficiency. On the other hand, as would be expected, vitamin B_{12} cannot correct a folate-deficient state. In spite of the ability of folic acid initially to correct the anemia of vitamin B_{12} deficiency, macrocytosis persists, neurologic changes progress, and eventually marrow hypoplasia ensues.

Macrocytosis may be the earliest clue to a megaloblastic process, preceding anemia and other manifestations of the vitamin deficiency state by up to a year. Unfortunately, it is a clue that is frequently ignored. Careful scrutiny of a peripheral blood smear is of particular importance in the assessment of macrocytosis for several reasons. First, the macrocytes of folic acid or vitamin B_{12} deficiency differ from the macrocytes of other disorders because of their oval shape and lack of central pallor. Second, in megaloblastic anemia, there is striking red blood cell anisocytosis and poikilocytosis with microcytes, fragmented forms, and "tear-drop" cells, features not seen in other macrocytic disorders. Third, the peripheral blood smear is the only method for identifying the Howell-Jolly body (see Color Plates), a DNA remnant found in red cells in megaloblastic anemia patients or in those with hypofunction or absence of the spleen. Fourth, the peripheral blood smear is the only method for identifying neutrophil hypersegmentation, an abnormality that is pathognomonic for megaloblastic maturation. Only severe neutropenia or a marked left shift of the granulocytes will mask hypersegmentation, but it usually reappears when these abnormalities have been corrected.

Neutrophil hypersegmentation also persists for several weeks after therapy with folic acid or vitamin B_{12} has been initiated and is thus a valuable clue to the nature of the underlying anemia when therapy has been initiated

Table 11.3–2. Causes of macrocytosis.

Folic acid deficiency
Vitamin B_{12} deficiency
Liver disease
Alcoholism
Sideroblastic anemia
Aplastic or hypoplastic anemia
Hypothyroidism
Neoplasms
Hemolytic anemia
Drugs (azathioprine, cyclophosphamide, hydroxyurea, zidovudine)

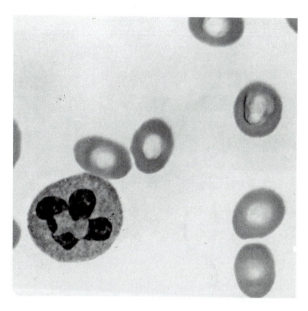

Figure 11.3–1. Peripheral blood smear in megaloblastic anemia, showing a hypersegmented polymorphonuclear cell and macrocytosis.

blindly. Hypersegmentation may also be the only clue to a vitamin B_{12} or folic acid deficiency in patients with iron deficiency, thalassemia trait, or renal disease.

Because deficiencies in folate or vitamin B_{12} are so different in their causes, associated conditions, and complications, they are considered separately in this chapter.

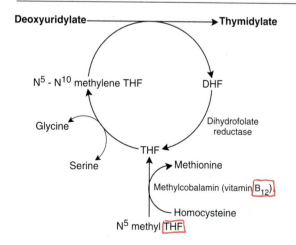

THF, tetrahydrofolate; DHF, dihydrofolate.

Figure 11.3–2. Metabolic interrelationship of vitamin B_{12} and folic acid.

Table 11.3–3. Causes of folic acid deficiency.

Inadequate intake

Defective absorption
Intrinsic bowel disease (eg, sprue)
Blind loop syndrome

Impaired utilization
Ethanol
Vitamin B$_{12}$ deficiency
Antagonists of folic acid metabolism (dihydrofolate reductase
    inhibitors) (eg, methotrexate, pyrimethamine, triamterene,
    pentamidine)
Phenytoin

Increased requirements
Pregnancy
Hemolytic anemia
Myeloproliferative disorders
Exfoliative dermatitis
Hyperthyroidism
Chronic hemodialysis

FOLIC ACID DEFICIENCY

Folic acid, also known as folate and pteroylglutamic acid, is a water-soluble, heat-labile vitamin found in green leafy vegetables, liver, kidney, yeast, and certain fruits. Absorption of folic acid takes place in the proximal third of the small intestine. The minimum daily folate requirement is 50 μg, and total body stores of folate are about 7 mg, a small quantity with respect to its turnover rate. Under normal circumstances, body stores of folic acid provide a 4- to 5-month supply of the vitamin if intake is interrupted. Folic acid deficiency can occur, however, more acutely in the setting of increased demands for the vitamin, such as pregnancy or hemolytic anemia or with ethanol abuse (Table 11.3–3). Thus, history taking should focus on signs of inadequate nutrition (including excessive cooking of green vegetables), suggestions of malabsorption (eg, steatorrhea), treatment with offending drugs (see Table 11.3–3), evidence of ethanol abuse, and conditions that require increased folic acid.

After the diagnosis of megaloblastic anemia is established, the confirmation that it is due to folate deficiency is provided by a subnormal red blood cell folate level. Measurement of serum folate is less sensitive, since serum folate may rise into the normal level with only a few balanced meals, whereas the red blood cell folate remains low until nutritionally adequate diets have been consumed for weeks to months.

Treatment for folate deficiency is dietary replacement or oral supplementation, avoidance of ethanol or offending drugs, and reversal of malabsorption when possible.

VITAMIN B$_{12}$ DEFICIENCY

Humans obtain vitamin B$_{12}$ only from foods of animal origin. Liver, kidney, eggs, and milk are rich sources. Absorption of vitamin B$_{12}$ requires the participation of intrin-sic factor, a glycoprotein produced by gastric parietal cells. Vitamin B$_{12}$ extracted from food binds in the acid environment of the stomach to B$_{12}$ binders known as R proteins because of their rapid mobility during electrophoresis. The R protein-vitamin B$_{12}$ complex is degraded in the alkaline environment of the upper small intestine by pancreatic proteases, and the free vitamin B$_{12}$ is bound by intrinsic factor. The intrinsic factor-B$_{12}$ complex attaches to specific receptors in the ileum where, in the presence of calcium and a pH greater than 6.0, the complex is absorbed.

The minimum daily requirement for vitamin B$_{12}$ is 1 μg. Body stores are large with respect to its turnover rate. Thus, in contrast to folic acid deficiency, deficiency of vitamin B$_{12}$ in an adult takes years to develop once absorption is interrupted. The disorders causing vitamin B$_{12}$ deficiency are listed in Table 11.3–4. As the table indicates, vitamin B$_{12}$ deficiency is almost always a consequence of malabsorption. Although adults who ingest vegan diets (which exclude all animal products) develop low serum vitamin B$_{12}$ levels, most evidence suggests that even these persons do not develop vitamin B$_{12}$ deficiency unless they acquire a defect in absorption.

Most patients with a vitamin B$_{12}$ deficiency have an unremarkable physical examination. In the patient with advanced disease, neurologic manifestations may be present. Otherwise, patients may complain of sore tongue and mouth, and examination may reveal a reddened tongue with smoothing of the surface caused by papillary atrophy, the result of inadequate DNA synthesis that cannot keep up with the rapid replacement of cells in the oral cavity.

Neurologic Disease Associated with Vitamin B$_{12}$ Deficiency

An important difference between folic acid deficiency and vitamin B$_{12}$ deficiency concerns the neurologic abnormalities that are associated only with vitamin B$_{12}$ deficiency and are uncorrectable with folic acid. The neurologic abnormalities are due to myelin degeneration involving the white matter of the dorsal and lateral columns of the spinal cord and the peripheral nerves (subacute combined degeneration). Its earliest manifestations

Table 11.3–4. Causes of vitamin B$_{12}$ deficiency.

Inadequate intake

Impaired absorption
Gastric abnormalities
    Pernicious anemia
    Total gastrectomy
    Lye ingestion
    Biologically inert intrinsic factor
Intestinal abnormalities
    Ileal resection or irradiation
    Granulomatous bowel disease
    Blind loop syndrome
    Fish tapeworm
    Drugs (eg, para-aminosalicylic acid [PAS])
Pancreatic insufficiency

Table 11.3–5. Evaluation of suspected folic acid or vitamin B_{12} deficiency.

Test	Result	Conclusion
Serum vitamin B_{12} level Red cell folate level	Normal Low	Folic acid deficiency
Serum vitamin B_{12} level Red cell folate level	Low Normal	Vitamin B_{12} deficiency; perform a Schilling test to determine the cause
Serum vitamin B_{12} level Red cell folate level	Low Low	Diagnosis uncertain; perform a Schilling test
Serum vitamin B_{12} level Red cell folate level	Normal Normal	If neurologic signs are present or suspicion is otherwise high, perform a Schilling test

are paresthesias in a stocking-glove distribution and loss of fine touch and vibratory sensation. As the disorder progresses, clumsiness, ataxia, weakness, and spasticity ensue. The degree of recovery depends on the duration and severity of the neurologic abnormalities. The biochemical basis for the neurologic abnormalities due to vitamin B_{12} deficiency is not well understood. Folic acid therapy can temporarily overcome and reverse the hematologic abnormalities associated with vitamin B_{12} deficiency, but not the neurologic ones. Therefore, blind treatment of megaloblastic anemia with folate is to be avoided, for if the process is caused by vitamin B_{12} deficiency, the folic acid corrects the hematologic abnormalities but permits the neurologic abnormalities to progress.

PERNICIOUS ANEMIA

The most common cause of vitamin B_{12} deficiency is pernicious anemia, a disorder of gastric function with autoimmune features in which there is malabsorption of the vitamin. The fundamental lesion in pernicious anemia is gastric atrophy with achlorhydria and failure to secrete intrinsic factor. The major manifestations of the disease, therefore, are caused by vitamin B_{12} deficiency. These patients may develop other autoimmune disorders, such as Hashimoto's thyroiditis, hyperthyroidism, vitiligo, adrenal insufficiency, and hypoparathyroidism. Patients with common variable immunoglobulin deficiency or selective IgA deficiency also may develop pernicious anemia. Antibodies to parietal cells are found in about 80% of patients,

whereas intrinsic factor antibodies are found in 50%. Both types of antibodies are present in gastric juice as well as in serum. Thyroid antibodies, lymphocytotoxins, and rheumatoid factor are also observed with an increased frequency. In black women, the disease occurs at an earlier age and with a higher incidence of intrinsic factor antibodies.

Patients with pernicious anemia have a higher incidence of gastric polyps and carcinoma than the general population. Because of this and because of its insidious onset as well as the risk of irreversible neurologic damage and the high incidence of associated endocrinologic disorders, pernicious anemia is a disorder of substantial importance to the physician.

As discussed earlier, once the diagnosis of megaloblastic anemia is established, its cause (either folate or vitamin B_{12} deficiency) must be determined. Because of the interrelationship of folate and vitamin B_{12} (see "Interrelationship of Vitamin B_{12} and Folic Acid" above), a deficiency of one vitamin often influences the level of the other. In view of this, an isolated assay for either red blood cell folate or serum vitamin B_{12} is not useful when a deficiency of either vitamin is suspected. Measurements for both must be obtained (Table 11.3–5).

Because vitamin B_{12} deficiency is almost always due to malabsorption, it is important to determine the cause of B_{12} malabsorption. The Schilling test involves administration of radiolabeled vitamin B_{12} orally after tissue and blood receptors are saturated with a parenteral dose of unlabeled vitamin B_{12} (Table 11.3–6). In normal people, at least 10% of the labeled B_{12} that is administered is excreted in the urine over the next 24 hours. If less than 10% of labeled B_{12} is excreted in the urine, it suggests inadequate absorption. This absorptive failure could be because of insufficient intrinsic factor in the stomach, intestinal mucosal dysfunction, or consumption of vitamin B_{12} by bacteria before it reaches the ileum. To distinguish among these three possibilities, a Schilling test is repeated in the patient who has an abnormal result, initially with added intrinsic factor; if the result is still abnormal, the test is repeated with intrinsic factor after a course of antibiotics to reduce bacterial overgrowth.

The mechanism for the malabsorption can be determined based on the findings of the Schilling test listed in Table 11.3–7. Since megaloblastic anemia due to vitamin B_{12} deficiency responds to therapy with folic acid, the Schilling test is of particular value in patients who have

Table 11.3–6. The Schilling test.

1. Saturation of binding sites by parenteral injection of 1 mg of unlabeled vitamin B_{12}
2. Oral administration of tracer dose of radioactive vitamin B_{12}*
3. Collection of urine for 24 hr on 2 successive days for radioactivity measurements

Normally, >9% of the administered dose is excreted in the first 24 hr

*The simultaneous administration of two different isotopes of vitamin B_{12}, one of which is combined with intrinsic factor, is not recommended because of the risk of an inaccurate and misleading result.

Table 11.3–7. Interpretation of the Schilling test.

Urinary Recovery of Labeled B_{12}*			
Without Intrinsic Factor	With Intrinsic Factor	After Antibiotic Therapy	Cause of B_{12} Deficiency
Normal	N/A	N/A	Dietary deficiency
Low	Normal	N/A	Lack of intrinsic factor
Low	Low	Low	Ileal disorder
Low	Low	Normal	Bacterial overgrowth

*Normal: ≥10% of administered dose.

been treated with folate. It is important to remember that treatment with vitamin B_{12} will not correct malabsorption of the vitamin nor compromise the Schilling test as long as vitamin B_{12} therapy is withheld during the period in which the test is performed.

Traditionally, treatment for vitamin B_{12} deficiency is monthly intramuscular or subcutaneous administration of the vitamin. For the patients whose vitamin B_{12} deficiency is due to reversible malabsorption, therapeutic supplementation of vitamin B_{12} is necessary only until those disorders are corrected.

SUMMARY

▶ Megaloblastic anemia can be caused by a variety of processes that impair DNA synthesis. Of these, folic acid deficiency and vitamin B_{12} deficiency are the most common.

▶ Vitamin B_{12} is required as a cofactor for the metabolic conversion of circulating folic acid to the form used by cells in DNA synthesis. Thus, a deficiency of either vitamin produces the same hematologic abnormalities. However, neurologic abnormalities are seen only with vitamin B_{12} deficiency.

▶ Folic acid deficiency can be due to decreased intake, malabsorption, impaired utilization, or increased requirements for the vitamin. Vitamin B_{12} deficiency is primarily due to impaired absorption, which may be due to gastric, intestinal, or pancreatic disorders.

▶ Both the red cell folate and vitamin B_{12} levels should be measured when evaluating a megaloblastic anemia.

▶ The cause of a vitamin B_{12} deficiency state should be established by a Schilling test.

SUGGESTED READING

Fairbanks VF, Wahner HW, Phyliky RL: Tests for pernicious anemia: The "Schilling test." Mayo Clin Proc 1983;58:541.

Lindenbaum J, Nath BJ: Megaloblastic anaemia and neutrophil hypersegmentation. Br J Haematol 1980;44:511.

Pruthi RK, Tefferi A: Pernicious anemia revisited. Mayo Clin Proc 1994;69:144.

Spivak JL: Masked megaloblastic anemia. Arch Intern Med 1982;142:2111.

Thompson WG et al: Evaluation of current criteria used to measure vitamin B_{12} levels. Am J Med 1987;82:291.

11.4

Hemoglobinopathies

Samuel Charache, MD

Hemoglobinopathies may be defined by the mere presence of an abnormal hemoglobin in the red blood cells of patients. A more useful and relevant definition is one in which hemoglobinopathies are considered not just biochemical findings, but disorders of hemoglobin that make people sick. In this sense, only a few of the abnormal hemoglobins produce hemoglobinopathies. The other abnormal hemoglobins are interesting because of the insights they provide into structure-function relationships in the hemoglobin molecule and into population genetics.

Because of the morbidity and increased mortality associated with sickle cell anemia and its variants, it is the most important hemoglobinopathy in the United States. Affected patients often present with symptoms that extend beyond the fatigue and pallor associated with the anemia itself. Such problems include attacks of abdominal or bone pain ("painful crises"), leg ulcers, or gallstones. An episode compatible with painful crisis in a black person should always prompt consideration of sickle cell disease in the differential diagnosis.

Although thalassemia genes usually do not produce abnormal hemoglobins, the mechanisms by which the thalassemia mutations are produced and operate are very similar to the mechanisms that produce structurally abnormal hemoglobins, and the two types of hemoglobin disorders are considered together in this chapter.

Recognizing these illnesses is important for three reasons:

1. They occasionally can be mistaken for other diseases (eg, thalassemia mimicking iron deficiency anemia).
2. Early identification allows careful monitoring (and antibiotic prophylaxis in infants with sickle cell disease).
3. Recognition facilitates family member testing and genetic counseling.

GENETIC AND BIOCHEMICAL MECHANISMS

Hemoglobinopathies and thalassemias are produced by point mutations (single base changes) in DNA sequences coding the two α- or two β-globin chains that constitute hemoglobin, as well as deletions and insertions of DNA that were probably produced by unequal crossovers between chromosomes. Substitution of one amino acid for another or deletion of one or more amino acids can distort hemoglobin structure at critical sites or permit formation of new intramolecular bonds that stabilize or destabilize the conformation of the molecule. The biochemical mechanisms that actually produce disease are listed in Table 11.4–1.

Thalassemia genes decrease the synthesis of specific globin chains; they produce anemia not only because of the resulting deficit in hemoglobin production, but because the "other" chains (α chains in β-thalassemia) are present in excess, are unstable, precipitate within red cells, and produce hemolytic anemia.

EPIDEMIOLOGY

A few abnormal hemoglobins (S, C, and E) are genetic polymorphisms, inherited conditions that are so common that they cannot have been maintained by recurrent mutation. Carriers of hemoglobin S or C make up 20–30% of some West African populations; about 8% of blacks in the United States are carriers of hemoglobin (Hb) S; and 25–54% of some Southeast Asian populations are carriers of Hb E. Thalassemia genes, which do not differ basically from the genes that produce hemoglobinopathies, can also be polymorphic. In Greece and Italy, 10% of some populations are carriers of β-thalassemia; 3–9% of Southeast Asians are carriers of other thalassemia genes; and one type of α-thalassemia is found in 25% of American blacks. Among such populations, it is thought that the heterozygous condition must confer some survival advantage. For each carrier who does not die, one abnormal gene would be saved for transmission, and the prevalence of the beneficial heterozygous condition would increase. But then more homozygotes would be born. Homozygotes are at a disadvantage, and *two* abnormal genes would be lost with each death. Depending on the magnitude of the survival advantage provided by the abnormal hemoglobin,

Table 11.4–1. Clinical disorders produced by altered hemoglobin function.

Hemoglobin Abnormality	Clinical Result
Polymerization (sickling)	Vaso-occlusion and anemia
Decreased synthesis of α- or β-globin chains (thalassemia)	Anemia, microcytosis, and hemolysis
Instability	Hemolytic anemia
Increased oxygen affinity	Polycythemia
Increased stability of Fe^{3+}	Methemoglobinemia

the incidence of the abnormal hemoglobin would rise until the advantage for gene transmission is just balanced by an increasing loss of genes from homozygotes who die before they can reproduce. It is possible that polymorphic hemoglobinopathies confer a selective advantage by providing resistance against malaria, but the mechanism of this benefit has not been clearly defined.

SICKLE CELL ANEMIA

Sickle cell anemia ("SS disease," denoting the nature of the two β-globin chains and indicating that red cells primarily contain Hb S) is a chronic hemolytic anemia associated with vaso-occlusive events caused by reduced deformability of deoxygenated red blood cells. Deformability of the cells is reduced by polymerization of deoxygenated molecules of Hb S. The vascular occlusions produce pain (painful crises) and organ dysfunction. Sickle cell anemia patients usually present in childhood or adolescence. Compound heterozygous disorders, in which a gene for Hb S is combined for a gene for another hemoglobinopathy, can produce the same clinical picture. Sickle/hemoglobin C disease (SC) and sickle/β-thalassemia (S/Thal) are the compound disorders seen most

often in the United States. They can produce any manifestation of sickle cell disease, but do so less often and usually with less severity than does sickle cell anemia; some patients are first identified in early adulthood, and a few never have symptoms referable to sickling. In those compound disorders, the red blood cells contain hemoglobins other than Hb S (Hb C in SC disease, for example). "Dilution" of hemoglobin S by that other hemoglobin reduces the tendency of red cells to become rigid and nondeformable as oxygen pressure falls.

In the United States, sickling disorders are found most frequently in blacks, but can also be seen in persons of Mediterranean, North African, Middle Eastern, and East Indian ancestry. Diagnosis requires the demonstration of Hb S in red cells, preferably by hemoglobin electrophoresis. Screening solubility tests give a positive result in all sickling disorders, but the diseases can usually be differentiated by a blood count and examination of a blood smear (Table 11.4–2 and Figures 11.4–1 and 11.4–2).

The basic mechanism in sickling disorders is polymerization of deoxygenated hemoglobin into rigid rod-like structures that make red cells resistant to deformation. Probably as a secondary phenomenon, red cells become dehydrated, bringing the Hb S molecules closer together, and thereby facilitating further sickling. A similar mechanism of erythrocyte dehydration may operate in Hb C disorders, producing enhanced sickling (SC disease) or hemoglobin crystallization (CC disease).

Anemia

SS red cells have shortened survival, but the mechanisms of hemolysis are poorly understood. Most affected adults have hemoglobin concentrations of 6–9 g/dL, with reticulocyte counts of about 7–10%. If the rate of erythropoiesis slows, as it often does with infection and vaso-occlusive crises, the hemoglobin concentration falls within a

Table 11.4–2. Comparison of common hemoglobin disorders.

Disease	Usual Hb (g/dL)	Clinical Severity	Blood Smear	Electrophoretic Pattern*	Solubility Test
SS	6–9	Usually marked	Many sickle forms, Howell-Jolly bodies, target cells, polychromatophilia, siderocytes; WBCs and platelets often increased	SFA_2 or SA_2	Positive
S/Thal	9–12	Mild to moderate	Microcytosis, target cells, poikilocytosis	$SAFA_2$	Positive
SC	9–13	Mild to moderate	Target cells, some spherocytes, occasional sickle forms	SCF or SC	Positive
S/HPFH	Normal	Asymptomatic	Normal	SFA_2	Positive
AS	Normal	Asymptomatic	Normal	ASA_2	Positive
AC	Normal	Asymptomatic	Rare target cells	AC	Negative
A/HPFH	Normal	Asymptomatic	Normal	AFA_2	Negative
A/Thal	9–12	Asymptomatic	Microcytosis, rare target cells	AA_2 or AFA_2	Negative

AC, hemoglobin AC disease; AS, hemoglobin AS disease; HPFH, hereditary persistence of fetal hemoglobin; SC, sickle/hemoglobin C disease; SS, sickle cell disease; S/Thal, sickle β-thalassemia.
*Hemoglobin components within red blood cells are listed in order of decreasing concentration, eg, ASA_2 = hemoglobin A > hemoglobin S > hemoglobin A_2.

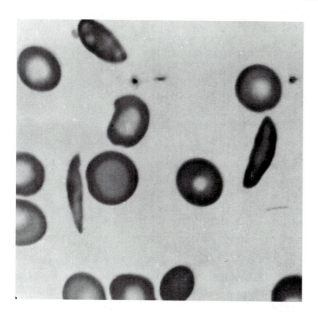

Figure 11.4–1. Peripheral blood smear in sickle cell disease (hemoglobin SS).

few days, but usually rebounds with equal speed later. Despite the severe anemia, virtually all patients can carry on activities of daily living, and some can even engage in athletics. It is important to remember that it is usually not anemia that causes disability in SS disease, but the vaso-occlusive crises.

Patients with hemolytic anemia of any type have an increased need for folic acid. The vitamin is abundant, but if foods are overcooked and vegetables omitted from the diet, intake may be inadequate. Marginal balance becomes

negative balance if a patient gets sick and will not eat, or if a woman becomes pregnant, further increasing her daily requirement. Administration of 1 mg of folic acid per day prevents these problems; since most patients are relatively young, the risk of "covering up" vitamin B_{12} deficiency is small.

Most adult patients with sickle cell anemia are essentially asplenic, the spleen having become completely infarcted because the low PO_2 and pH and the sluggish blood flow in the spleen cause repetitive microinfarctions in childhood. Nevertheless, some adults have persistent splenomegaly. They can develop "sequestration crises," with pooling of red cells in the spleen, the liver, or both. The result is increased (sometimes painful) splenomegaly, and a sudden fall in hemoglobin, sometimes associated with leukopenia and thrombocytopenia (relative to the patient's usually elevated platelet count). Adult sequestration crises are self-limited and are not life-threatening, in contrast to sequestration crises seen in children.

Aplastic crises are characterized by complete cessation of erythropoiesis. Most aplastic crises are caused by infection with parvovirus B19, an epidemic exanthem of childhood. Some form of isolation of such patients is suggested because the virus can cause hydrops fetalis in nonimmune hospital personnel who are pregnant. Other infections, and painful crises themselves, can depress erythropoiesis to a lesser degree. Sometimes the reticulocyte count stays low for several days, and the hemoglobin level can drop to less than 5 g/dL. Whether the hemoglobin falls enough to necessitate transfusion depends on the hemolytic rate, the duration of erythroid aplasia, and the patient's cardiovascular system.

Only rarely is transfusion indicated because of anemia per se. Transfusion is indicated only in patients with symptoms of oxygen lack, including older patients with angina or cerebral arteriosclerosis. Some data suggest that transfusion can speed the healing of ankle ulcers, but in general transfusion is done only for symptomatic anemia. Exchange transfusion is not used to treat anemia, but to replace sickle cells with normal erythrocytes (see "Acute Chest Syndrome" below).

Painful Crises

Acute attacks of pain, called vaso-occlusive crises, are probably caused by obstruction of small blood vessels (arterioles, capillaries, venules) by rigid sickle cells, with resultant ischemia or necrosis of tissues. Pain often develops in several sites at the same time, making it hard to understand the pathogenesis of the crisis. Bone pain is usually caused by ischemia or necrosis of bone marrow; abdominal pain can be caused by infarction of liver or spleen, but often its origin is unclear. Some precipitants of crises are recognized, but poorly documented. They include chilling, a change in the weather, emotional stress, infection, and menstruation. Flight in commercial aircraft does not usually cause problems for adult patients with SS disease (whose spleens have usually become infarcted in child-

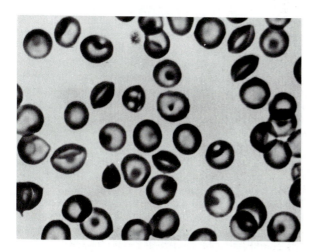

Figure 11.4–2. Peripheral blood smear in hemoglobin SC disease.

hood), but has been associated with splenic infarction in patients with Hb SC disease or sickle cell trait who were traveling in unpressurized aircraft (and a few Hb SC patients in pressurized planes).

Diagnosis: *Painful crises can be diagnosed only by exclusion of all other likely causes of a patient's pain.* Often a patient who has frequent painful crises can tell whether a particular pain is a crisis, and the physician should be guided by the patient's statements. Bone pain usually is not associated with overlying swelling or redness. Fever, probably caused by tissue necrosis, is common several days after onset of a crisis, but rarely exceeds 38.5°C (101.4°F). Chest syndrome, cholecystitis, and osteomyelitis enter into almost every differential diagnosis (see "Acute Chest Syndrome" below). It is unusual for SS patients with uncomplicated crises to have white blood counts over 25,000/μL or fevers over 39°C (102.2°F). There are *no* distinctive features of the blood count that can confirm or exclude a vaso-occlusive crisis.

Management: If other causes have been considered and ruled out, the foundations of therapy are [analgesics and fluid administration.]Oral analgesics and oral fluids are always worth trying, especially when patients feel that they can stay home. Since adult patients have an impaired ability to concentrate their urine, dehydration is a persistent threat, especially because it can probably exacerbate vaso-occlusion. Potent oral analgesics can be used for hospitalized patients, but most patients prefer parenteral administration of pharmacologically equivalent doses. There is no analgesic of choice, although meperidine is disadvantageous because its metabolite, normeperidine, can cause seizures if it accumulates in patients with renal failure. Tolerance (the need for more drug to produce the same effect) is equally likely with all potent opiates if therapy is continued for any length of time. Intravenous or subcutaneous infusion of morphine, by means of a special infusion pump controlled by the patient, may be the most effective method of narcotic administration. Parenteral nonsteroidal anti-inflammatory agents have been useful in some patients.

In general, physicians undertreat patients' pain, probably because of a fear of iatrogenic narcotic addition. Unlimited provision of strong narcotic analgesics is probably an equally bad practice. Decisions must be individualized for each patient, preferably based on prior knowledge of the patient's behavior in and out of crisis. The efficacy of treatment should be carefully noted, and drug dosage adjusted if there is evidence of respiratory depression, constipation, or inability to void.

It would seem logical to administer oxygen to patients in crisis, since it is deoxygenation that makes cells sickle, but unless the patient's hemoglobin is desaturated, only a small amount of extra oxygen can be dissolved in the plasma. Some patients insist that administration of oxygen is helpful, but there is scant experimental evidence to jus-

tify such beliefs. In contrast, if the patient's hemoglobin is desaturated, and especially if the PO_2 is less than 70 mm Hg, oxygen must be administered to try to prevent further sickling.

Acute and Chronic Organ Damage

Acute vaso-occlusive episodes cause such clinical problems as bone marrow or splenic infarction, hepatic crises, or hematuria from renal papillary necrosis. Cumulative damage over the course of years eventually leads to organ dysfunction. Aseptic necrosis of bone and renal failure are probably the most common problems, but chronic lung disease can also be a very serious problem.

Acute Chest Syndrome: Not infrequently, sickle cell patients present with acute pleuritic chest pain, fever, cough, and a new infiltrate on chest x-ray. In children, such episodes are often caused by infection by encapsulated bacteria (*Streptococcus pneumoniae* or *Haemophilus influenzae*) and may be associated with sepsis, meningitis, and early death. In adults, episodes of fever and lung disease may result from infection, infarction caused by emboli of necrotic bone marrow or aggregates of sickle cells, or primary occlusion of pulmonary blood vessels by sickled cells; a very few are caused by venous thromboemboli. The condition is termed "chest syndrome" to emphasize the inability to always define the exact cause. Treatment is often with antibiotics regardless of negative cultures of blood, sputum, and pleural fluid. In the rare instance in which thromboembolism seems likely, heparin should be used.

Whatever the cause of acute chest syndrome, any such lesion has the potential to cause sufficient arterial hypoxemia that sickling can occur throughout the body, and particularly to cause impaction of sickled cells in the lung, producing a life-threatening condition similar to adult respiratory distress syndrome. Arterial PO_2 must be measured in all patients with symptomatic vaso-occlusive disease, and oxygen must be administered to keep the PO_2 above 70 mm Hg. Repeated measurements are necessary because ventilation-perfusion defects may increase despite therapy. The frequency of such measurements depends on the clinician's evaluation of whether the patient is or is not improving. Pulse oximetry is a useful alternative to repeated arterial punctures, but the physician should initially compare its results with direct measurement of PO_2, keeping in mind the low oxygen affinity of the blood in patients with SS disease.

If the PO_2 cannot be elevated, exchange transfusion must be performed to reduce the proportion of sickle cells to less than 50% without much of an increase in blood volume. Acute partial exchange transfusion is used for treatment of severe chest syndrome, and as a measure of desperation whenever a patient becomes critically ill from any complication of sickle cell disease (when it can be life-saving). It is often used to prepare patients for general anesthesia and surgery. Chronic transfusion therapy is used to try to prevent recurrent strokes, incapacitating crises, or the calamities that sometimes befall pregnant women who have SS disease.

Hepatic Crises and Gallbladder Disease: Acute right upper quadrant pain, fever, and increased jaundice may be caused by liver infarction, hepatic sequestration of sickle cells, or acute cholecystitis. The last condition must be considered first; if gallstones are present, the bile ducts are somewhat dilated, and there is a history of recurrent discomfort after eating, patients usually require an operation. On the other hand, asymptomatic gallstones are not an indication for cholecystectomy. In cases of severe hepatic failure, presumably due to blockage of sinusoids by sickled cells and secondary interference with arterial blood flow, exchange transfusion may cause dramatic improvement. Extremely high bilirubin concentrations may be observed in hepatic sequestration because of the combination of severe hemolysis and liver dysfunction, but such hyperbilirubinemia is less significant than other measures of liver function.

Renal Disease: Loss of ability to concentrate urine is nearly universal in adult patients with SS disease, and kidney dysfunction is common. Medullary disease is probably related to facilitation of sickling by hypertonic conditions in the renal papillae, and loss of concentrating capacity and papillary necrosis are probably secondary to infarctions in that area. Hematuria from medullary infarction is not uncommon, and can be resistant to all therapeutic maneuvers. If it occurs, and no other cause is found, patients should take iron (to replace losses in the urine), drink lots of water (to keep urine flow high enough to prevent clotting within the ureters or bladder), and try to remain calm despite persistence of red urine for days or weeks. As with all other complications of sickling, more treatable disorders (infection and neoplasm) must always be considered first.

Glomerular and tubular disease are harder to explain, but certainly are part of the clinical picture in older patients with SS disease. Proteinuria and more severe anemia (the latter at least partially caused by decreased erythropoietin production) come first; azotemia and frank renal failure follow. Hemodialysis and transplantation should always be considered; if a new kidney is to be protected from sickling, chronic transfusion therapy may be necessary.

Bone Disease: Aseptic necrosis of the femoral and humeral heads is fairly common in patients with SS disease; osteomyelitis is less commonly seen in the United States. Neither condition is very amenable to treatment. Aseptic necrosis of bone is probably caused by occlusion of terminal arterioles by sickled cells; although the end result is similar, pathogenesis may be different from that of aseptic necrosis of bone in other disorders. Osteomyelitis probably reflects seeding of necrotic marrow during periods of otherwise unimportant bacteremia. Salmonella osteomyelitis is less common in patients in the United States than in developing nations, perhaps because salmonella enteritis is less common here. *Staphylococcus aureus* is the most common cause of osteomyelitis in this country for patients with or without sickle cell anemia.

Prenatal and Neonatal Diagnosis

Elegant DNA analyses permit prenatal diagnosis in very early pregnancy. The problem is not in diagnosis, but counseling: With a disease as variable as sickle cell anemia, how does one explain to prospective parents what risk their child faces? Probably because of this dilemma, utilization of prenatal diagnosis for SS disease is relatively low in the United States.

Neonatal diagnosis, on the other hand, is mandated in many states. There are real problems in handling specimens, and all questionable results must be confirmed on a second sample, but the advantages of getting affected children into the health care system as early as possible make the effort worthwhile.

Because repeated vascular occlusions in the microcirculation of the spleen lead to multiple infarctions and functional asplenia, children with sickle cell disease (SS, SC, or S/Thal) should be given prophylactic penicillin in earliest infancy. These individuals also should be vaccinated against *S pneumoniae* and *H influenzae* at an early age.

SICKLE CELL TRAIT

About 8% of black Americans are carriers of the hemoglobin S gene, and have sickle cell trait. Very few of them have any disability whatsoever. A few have hematuria, and splenic infarction has been reported in a handful of patients, but most never know they are carriers of an abnormal hemoglobin. There have been, however, disturbing reports of sudden death in Army recruits with sickle trait during basic training, in higher numbers than in black recruits without the trait. Sickle trait cells *can* sickle, and under extreme conditions it is conceivable that sickling could add to other physiologic derangements. Unexplained sudden death during exertion is a very rare complication of sickle trait, and is probably a much smaller risk than many of the hazards of contemporary urban life. As a consequence, individuals with sickle trait should not be advised to restrict their life-style except for prolonged and extreme exertion with the possibility of uncorrected dehydration.

Sickle cell trait does not cause anemia, ankle ulcers, bone pain, or chest syndrome in persons whose arterial oxygen saturation is normal. However, should severe hypoxemia be produced by advanced pulmonary disease, cyanotic heart disease, exposure to altitude above 10,000 feet, or cardiopulmonary arrest, infarction and hemolysis can be anticipated.

Although sickle cell trait ordinarily poses no threat to

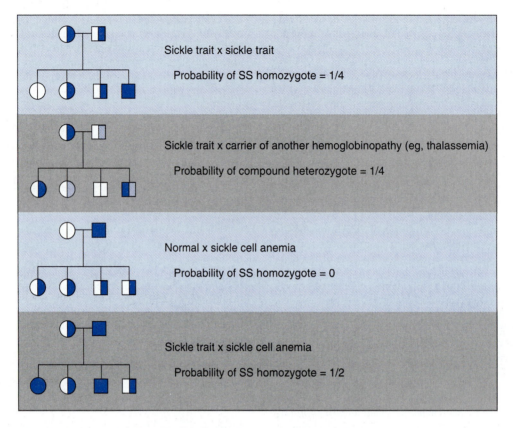

Figure 11.4–3. Inheritance of sickling disorders. The probability of having an affected child is the same for each pregnancy.

carriers, persons of reproductive age should know their risk of having a child with sickle cell anemia (Figure 11.4–3). If their blood is to be tested, education and counseling are necessary both before and after testing.

THALASSEMIA

Thalassemia syndromes are caused by decreased or absent synthesis of either α or β-globin—hence α- and β-thalassemia. Anemia in homozygous β-thalassemia (thalassemia major) can be so severe as to require regular transfusions for survival. It is a rare disease in the United States, although the carrier state is not rare.

There is a bewildering variety of thalassemia genes. The deficits that they produce in globin synthesis may be mild or severe, and combinations of different genes make classification difficult. Carriers of one type of thalassemia gene (heterozygotes) may show no clinical manifestations (silent carrier), whereas another gene may produce mild microcytic anemia (thalassemia minor) or a more pronounced anemia with clear evidence of accelerated erythropoiesis (thalassemia intermedia). Although the genes that they carry may differ, most heterozygotes do not dif-

fer clinically. In general, the effects of homozygosity can be predicted only with specific knowledge of the mutation involved.

Homozygosity for two severe genes produces thalassemia major (Cooley's anemia), but combinations of a mild with a severe gene produce thalassemia intermedia syndromes. In general, patients who need transfusions to stay alive are said to have thalassemia major; those who need only an occasional transfusion have thalassemia intermedia; and those who do not need any transfusions have thalassemia minor.

β-Thalassemia

Diagnosis of β-thalassemia is based on the demonstration of microcytosis that is not caused by iron deficiency (Figure 11.4–4), and of an elevated proportion of hemoglobin A_2 in red cell hemolysates of heterozygotes. The increase in hemoglobin A_2 is not readily explained, and may not be observed in rare instances (eg, Δ β-thalassemia). Splenomegaly and increased levels of fetal hemoglobin may be present. Iron overload and hemochromatosis are part of the disease in moderately and severely affected patients, even in those receiving relatively few transfusions. The reasons for increased iron absorption in

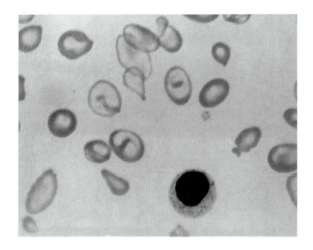

Figure 11.4–4. Peripheral blood smear in β-thalassemia (thalassemia major).

thalassemia are not well understood. At present, iron chelation therapy requires nightly subcutaneous injection of deferoxamine using a portable infusion pump; treatment is both uncomfortable and expensive. Relatively inexpensive oral chelating agents would be desirable, especially for patients in developing countries.

Because of very vigorous (but often ineffective) erythropoiesis, bone disease is also part of the clinical picture in patients with severe β-thalassemia. Today, most of the classic signs of β-thalassemia—growth retardation, the "thalassemic facies" (an almost Asian appearance produced by expansion of the marrow cavity in the facial bones), pathologic fractures, and protrusion of masses of bone marrow through the vertebral cortex into the thoracic cavity—are prevented by hypertransfusion regimens. Those transfusions keep hemoglobin concentrations at least 12 g/dL, but in turn make iron overload more of a problem.

β-thalassemia major may be the only hemoglobinopathy in which the risks of bone marrow transplantation are warranted. It is probably the treatment of choice for young children if a compatible donor is available. The increased risk of transplantation in older patients may be justified if they live in places where transfusion and chelation therapy are difficult to organize and maintain. Whether it is worth considering for patients in the United States is still debatable, but positive experience in Italy makes one consider it very seriously.

α-Thalassemia

α-thalassemia is somewhat different from β-thalassemia because there are four rather than two α-globin genes. Fetuses with four deleted or nonfunctional α-globin genes die in utero because they cannot make fetal hemoglobin ($\alpha_2\gamma_2$), which requires α globin for its synthesis. Patients with three such malfunctioning genes have "he-

moglobin H disease" (hemoglobin H is the β4 tetramer that forms because of insufficient α-chain synthesis). It is a hemolytic anemia that is not as severe as β-thalassemia major. Unlike β-thalassemia, in which the carrier state is easily diagnosed, α-thalassemia usually can be diagnosed only by excluding other causes of microcytic anemia. Two malfunctioning α-globin genes produce a condition like β-thalassemia minor, while one malfunctioning gene produces no clinical abnormality ("silent carrier").

α-thalassemia is a real problem in the developing world, but in the United States the clinical problems it causes are rare and are generally confined to children of immigrants from the Mediterranean, the Middle East, India, and Southeast Asia. Prenatal diagnosis has much to offer these parents.

UNSTABLE HEMOGLOBINS

A number of abnormal hemoglobins are unstable, precipitate within red cells, and cause hemolytic anemia in heterozygotes, probably by altering the physical properties of the erythrocyte membrane. The same drugs that cause hemolysis in glucose-6-phosphate-dehydrogenase (G6PD) deficiency can cause hemolysis in such patients (Chapter 11.5), but fever alone can cause hemoglobin denaturation. Many of these disorders are "new mutations," which bring carriers to medical attention because they produce either continuous or episodic hemolytic anemia, with jaundice and dark urine. The diagnosis is made by demonstrating in vitro that the patient's hemoglobin is less stable than normal hemoglobin; electrophoresis cannot be relied on in making this diagnosis because it may yield normal results. Patients with unstable hemoglobins should avoid the same drugs that patients with G6PD deficiency avoid.

HIGH-AFFINITY HEMOGLOBINS

Hemoglobins with high oxygen affinity do not deliver oxygen to tissues normally because they do not "unload" it at tissue PO_2. In response, more red cells are made, producing polycythemia. These very rare disorders enter into the differential diagnosis of polycythemia (Chapter 11.8). Like other patients with secondary polycythemia, patients should be managed with cautious phlebotomy so that symptoms of hyperviscosity are prevented.

SUMMARY

▶ The most important clinical disorders produced by hemoglobinopathies are sickle cell anemia and the thalassemias.

▶ Sickle cell anemia causes disease because of occlusion of blood vessels by nondeformable deoxygenated red blood cells, which leads to pain, ischemia, and infarction. Morbidity is often related to painful crises, not anemia.

▶ There is no objective test that enables us to prove that a patient does or does not have a painful crisis. One must believe what the patient says, unless there is compelling evidence to the contrary.

▶ When patients develop acute chest syndrome, which often cannot be distinguished from pneumonia, arterial oxygen pressure must be maintained above 70 mm Hg to prevent life-threatening progressive acute respiratory distress.

▶ β-thalassemia trait frequently presents with mild anemia and microcytosis, but can be distinguished from iron deficiency anemia because hemoglobin A_2 levels are increased in thalassemia.

SUGGESTED READING

Bunn HF, Forget BG: *Hemoglobin: Molecular, Genetic, and Clinical Aspects.* WB Saunders, 1986.

Embury SH et al: *Sickle Cell Disease: Basic Principles and Clinical Practice.* Raven Press, 1994.

Giardina PJ, Hilgartner MW: Update on thalassemia. Pediatr Rev 1992;13:55.

Reid CD, Charache S, Lubin B: *Management and Therapy of Sickle Cell Disease.* NIH publication 95–2117. US Public Health Service, 1995.

Serjeant GR: *Sickle Cell Disease,* 2nd ed. Oxford University Press, 1992.

11.5

Hemolytic Anemia

Thomas S. Kickler, MD

Accelerated states of red blood cell destruction are called hemolytic disorders. If the rate of red cell destruction exceeds the rate of erythropoiesis, anemia develops. Patients with hemolytic anemia may present with a wide spectrum of problems from subtle to fulminant. If the rate of red blood cell destruction is slow, patients may have only mild, nonspecific constitutional symptoms of anemia (Chapter 11.1). If the red blood cell destruction is rapid, as in autoimmune hemolytic anemia, they may have a severe illness with dark urine from hemoglobinuria, fever, tachycardia, confusion from hypoxia, and cardiac decompensation. It is important to know about hemolytic anemias for several reasons:

1. They may be associated with a serious but treatable disorder.
2. They may be caused by a genetic disorder requiring investigation of other family members and counseling about having children.
3. They may be mild disorders that have little clinical impact and primarily require reassurance.

The hemolytic anemias are either intravascular or extravascular, depending on the site of destruction. In extravascular hemolysis, red cells are destroyed in the reticuloendothelial system tissue macrophages (Table 11.5–1). The clinical manifestations of these two types of hemolysis are usually distinctive: Extravascular hemolytic disorders present with splenomegaly, whereas intravascular hemolysis produces red urine and plasma from the liberation of hemoglobin from disrupted red cells. Jaundice, gallstones, pallor, and symptoms related to decreased oxygen delivery to the tissues are common to both types of hemolysis.

CLINICAL EVALUATION

The history plays a key role in the assessment of patients who may have a hemolytic anemia. The first questions to ask are whether the anemia is new or old, and whether anemia is present in other family members. Anemia since childhood, particularly when accompanied by a family history of anemia, suggests an inherited disorder. Alternatively, the onset of hemolysis in adulthood suggests an acquired hemolytic condition. Concomitant illnesses, such as systemic lupus erythematosus or a lymphoproliferative disorder, are frequently associated with immune-mediated hemolysis, and historical features compatible with such diseases should be sought. The recent administration of a drug to a person of Mediterranean origin may suggest glucose 6-phosphate dehydrogenase (G6PD) deficiency. Hemolysis may develop in patients who have infections, who are on drugs, or who are receiving transfusions.

The physical examination may be helpful, mostly in detecting signs of concomitant illnesses that may be associated with hemolysis. Scleral icterus may develop when hemolysis presents more hemoglobin for disposition than the patient's liver can manage. Splenomegaly is characteristic of extravascular hemolysis. Certain characteristic features may be present in patients with hemoglobinopathies (Chapter 11.4).

LABORATORY TESTS

Because the hallmark of hemolytic anemia is increased red blood cell turnover, an elevated reticulocyte count is the most important clue to the presence of a hemolytic process. As described in Chapter 11.1, the reticulocyte count must be corrected for the degree of anemia. The degree of reticulocytosis increases with the severity of the hemolytic anemia, provided that adequate iron, folate, and vitamin B_{12} are available and there is not suppression of erythropoiesis as a result of drugs, renal failure, or inflammation. Hemolytic anemia is especially likely when the corrected reticulocyte count is higher than might be expected simply from the degree of anemia. Because reticulocytes are larger than mature erythrocytes, the mean corpuscular volume (MCV) may rise to over 100 fL in patients with hemolysis and a brisk reticulocytosis.

Table 11.5–1. Classification of hemolytic anemias.

Intravascular hemolysis
 Traumatic (microangiopathic) (eg, mechanical heart valve,
  disseminated intravascular coagulation, thrombotic
  thrombocytopenic purpura)
 Enzyme abnormalities
  Deficiency of erythrocyte glycolytic enzymes (eg, pyruvate
   kinase)
  Deficiency of enzymes in the pentose-phosphate pathway
   (eg, G6PD) and glutathione metabolism
 Hemoglobinopathies
 Paroxysmal nocturnal hemoglobinuria
 Infections (eg, malaria, babesiosis)
Extravascular hemolysis
 Immune hemolytic anemias
  Autoimmune diseases (eg, systemic lupus erythematosus,
   chronic lymphocytic leukemia)
  Drugs (eg, penicillin)
  Infections (eg, *Mycoplasma,* infectious mononucleosis)
 Splenomegaly from other disorders (eg, portal hypertension)
 Membrane abnormalities
  Hereditary spherocytosis
  Hereditary elliptocytosis
  Hereditary stomatocytosis
  Hereditary pyropoikilocytosis

G6PD, glucose-6-phosphate dehydrogenase.

Table 11.5–2. Peripheral smear morphologic features in hemolytic anemia.

Morphologic Abnormality	Disease
Spherocytes	Hereditary spherocytosis Immune hemolysis Extensive burns Hemoglobin C disease
Schistocytes	Thrombotic thrombocytopenic purpura Vasculitis Traumatic cardiac hemolysis Disseminated intravascular coagulation Giant hemangioma
Target cells	Thalassemia Hemoglobin C disease Liver disease
Spiculated cells	Liver disease Pyruvate kinase disease
Elliptocytosis	Hereditary elliptocytosis
Basophilic stippling	Thalassemia Lead poisoning Pyrimidine 5′-nucleotidase deficiency
Intraerythrocytic inclusions	Malaria Babesiosis
Hypochromia	Traumatic cardiac hemolysis Paroxysmal nocturnal hemoglobinuria
Sickle cells	Hemoglobin S

The peripheral smear is essential in the evaluation of hemolytic anemia, and often provides the most important data to direct further evaluation (see Figure 11.1–1). Hemolysis is suggested on a Wright-stained smear by purplish (polychromatic) red cells that are younger than the normally pink mature cells. These younger cells have retained mRNA, which stains purplish. In severe hemolysis, nucleated red cells are found because erythropoiesis is brisk and cells are released earlier in an attempt to compensate for the anemia. The specific morphologic changes of the red cells may suggest a specific hemolytic disorder (Table 11.5–2). In hemolytic anemias, the bone marrow shows erythroid hyperplasia, but is not especially helpful in confirming hemolysis as the cause of anemia or identifying the cause of hemolysis.

A number of biochemical markers are useful in documenting shortened red cell survival (Table 11.5–3). If there is intravascular hemolysis, plasma hemoglobin may be increased. This is usually accompanied by hemoglobinuria, which can cause a positive dipstick reaction for blood, but the urine microscopy examination shows no red blood cells. With chronic intravascular hemolysis, a Prussian blue stain of the urine sediment may show hemosiderin in renal tubular cells. The catabolism of hemoglobin leads to the production of various biochemical products that are useful in substantiating a hemolytic anemia. Unconjugated or indirect bilirubin is elevated in hemolysis. The serum level of "direct" or conjugated bilirubin is normal unless hepatic or biliary disease is present. Patients with significant hemolysis, whether intra- or extravascular, have low or absent serum haptoglobin levels. Red cells contain high concentrations of lactic dehy-

drogenase, the serum levels of which are typically elevated in intravascular hemolysis.

Red cell survival can be measured most directly by using isotope-labeled autologous red cells. Chromium-51 is the most widely used isotope for this purpose. To measure red cell survival, the patient's anticoagulated red cells are incubated with chromium-51 and reinjected. The radioactivity of blood samples collected over several days is counted to determine the rate of red cell destruction. Normally, 50% of the injected chromium-labeled red cells survive 29 ± 3 days. This test is not frequently required in

Table 11.5–3. Biochemical markers of hemolysis.

Laboratory Test	Result
Serum haptoglobin (serum protein that binds globin)	Reduced
Serum hemopexin (serum protein that binds heme)	Reduced in moderate-to-severe intravascular hemolysis
Serum methemalbumin	Increased in severe intravascular hemolysis
Plasma hemoglobin	Elevated in intravascular hemolysis
Hemoglobinuria	Present in intravascular hemolysis
Urine hemosiderin	Positive in chronic intravascular hemolysis
Indirect hyperbilirubinemia	Elevated
Lactic dehydrogenase	Elevated

clinical practice, but can be helpful when the rate of hemolysis is low and other parameters are not obviously abnormal.

EXAMPLES OF INTRAVASCULAR HEMOLYTIC ANEMIAS

Fragmentation Syndromes

Physical trauma to the red cells during circulation may be sufficient to cause intravascular hemolysis with hemoglobinuria and hemoglobinemia. The damaged red cells become schistocytes (fragments, helmets, or crescents), whose presence readily distinguishes red cell fragmentation syndromes from other acquired anemias.

Traumatic hemolysis may develop after placement of a prosthetic heart valve. Aortic prosthetic valves are more frequently associated with hemolysis than other valves because of the greater turbulence in flow. With contemporary valves, traumatic hemolysis is usually a sign of dehiscence. Only rarely does intrinsic valve disease (eg, aortic stenosis) lead to hemolysis. Furthermore, the hemolysis accompanying nonsurgically corrected valvular disease is rarely severe. When hemolysis and hemosiderinuria have been prolonged, iron deficiency may develop. Daily iron supplementation should be instituted if significant hemolysis is present. Reoperation may be necessary for some patients with severe hemolysis.

Red cells may also fragment in association with small artery disease. This type of hemolytic disorder is termed microangiopathic. The deposition of fibrin within the microvasculature (eg, disseminated intravascular coagulation) or severe hypertension provides the conditions for fragmentation. The diagnosis of a microangiopathic hemolytic anemia is based on the observation of schistocytes, bizarrely misshapen red cells (usually accompanied) by reticulocytosis, elevated serum lactic dehydrogenase (LDH), and reduced serum haptoglobin. Hemoglobinemia and hemoglobinuria are rarely present.

Microangiopathic hemolytic anemia may be a prominent feature of disorders associated with vasculitis. The hemolysis is rarely severe, and if the underlying disease is controlled, fragmentation ceases. When microangiopathic hemolytic anemia coexists with renal failure or neurologic deficits, vasculitis or thrombotic thrombocytopenic purpura should be considered (Chapter 11.10).

Red Cell Enzyme Defects

Glucose is the main metabolic substrate for red cells and is metabolized by the glycolytic (Embden-Meyerhof) pathway and the hexose monophosphate shunt. Inherited disorders of any enzyme in the glycolytic pathway may lead to a hemolytic anemia. The hexose monophosphate shunt protects the red blood cell from oxidative agents by the generation of glutathione. G6PD is the critical enzyme in the complex enzymatic process that recycles glutathione. G6PD functions to reduce NADP (nicotinamide-adenine dinucleotide phosphate) while oxidizing glucose

6-phosphate, thereby providing NADP in its reduced form (NADPH), a reducing agent that maintains sulfhydryl groups important in eliminating free radicals and peroxides. Of the red cell enzymopathies, G6PD deficiency is the most common worldwide.

Glucose-6-Phosphate Dehydrogenase (G6PD) Deficiency

G6PD deficiency is an X-linked disorder. Polymorphisms of the G6PD gene may lead to variants not associated with enzyme deficiency or hemolysis, other variants that cause hemolytic anemia only in the presence of chemical or physical stress, and other variants that are so functionally impaired as to produce a chronic nonspherocytic hemolytic anemia. Males with this disorder, being hemizygotes, may be markedly deficient in enzyme activity. Most females with G6PD deficiency, being heterozygotes, show low normal enzyme levels.

There are two types of G6PD deficiency. The Mediterranean form is the prototype for the G6PD deficiency states. Those with G6PD Mediterranean deficiency typically have less than 1% of the normal enzyme activity. These persons are extremely sensitive to oxidant stresses. The typical black individual with G6PD deficiency does not have any evidence of hemolysis unless challenged by oxidant drugs, infection, or noxious agents (such as the fava bean). These hemolytic episodes are self-limited. Some variants may have chronic hemolysis characterized by episodes of accelerated hemolysis. In the acute event, the hemolysis is intravascular, and abdominal or back pain may occur in association with hemoglobinuria.

During an acute hemolytic episode, polychromatophilia and nucleated red cells may be seen. A quantitative determination of G6PD establishes the diagnosis. A low normal value of G6PD with reticulocytosis may suggest the disorder. In these cases, measurement of the enzyme activity should be repeated after the hemolytic episode is over.

G6PD-deficient persons should avoid drugs such as sulfonamides or antimalarials, which may induce severe hemolysis. If hemolysis results in severe anemia, transfusions may be life-saving. Splenectomy is not beneficial in hemolytic anemia caused by G6PD deficiency.

Paroxysmal Nocturnal Hemoglobinuria

Paroxysmal nocturnal hemoglobinuria arises because of an acquired somatic mutation in hematopoietic stem cells that results in an intrinsic abnormality of all types of blood cells. An unexplained susceptibility to complement lysis leads to intravascular hemolysis. Chronic intravascular hemolysis dominates the clinical picture.

The most serious complications of paroxysmal nocturnal hemoglobinuria include thrombosis and marrow aplasia. Thrombosis of large intra-abdominal veins, especially hepatic veins, is common. Since the hemolysis is intravascular, iron deficiency may develop in patients with protracted hemolysis. Renal abnormalities may complicate paroxysmal nocturnal hemoglobinuria either as a result of thrombosis or of chronic hemoglobinuria and hemosiderinuria. Aplastic anemia may be the predominant presenting factor in patients with paroxysmal nocturnal hemoglobinuria. Occasionally, patients present with isolated thrombocytopenia. Therefore, in any patient presenting with cytopenias of obscure origin, paroxysmal nocturnal hemoglobinuria should be considered.

The red cells are frequently hypochromic and microytic because of iron deficiency, the result of chronic intravascular hemolysis and renal excretion of iron. The bone marrow characteristically shows erythroid hyperplasia with no iron stores. When pancytopenia is present, the marrow may be hypoplastic. The increased susceptibility to complement lysis constitutes the basis of the tests used in diagnosing paroxysmal nocturnal hemoglobinuria. Incubating red cells with sucrose (sugar water test), resulting in hemolysis of red cells with the paroxysmal nocturnal hemoglobinuria membrane defect, is a sensitive screening test. The acidified-serum lysis test (Ham test) should be done to confirm the diagnosis. Management is usually supportive, with red cell transfusions given to correct anemia. The condition may progress to aplastic anemia, or leukemic states may occur in some patients.

EXAMPLES OF EXTRAVASCULAR HEMOLYTIC ANEMIAS

Hereditary Spherocytosis

Red cell membrane deformability permits the red cell to traverse narrow capillary vessels. Defects in the red cell cytoskeletal proteins can cause a variety of membrane disorders that lead to hemolysis.

Hereditary spherocytosis is the most common inherited red cell membrane disorder (Figure 11.5–1). The abnormally stiff membranes lead to splenic trapping and formation of small dense red cells called *spherocytes.* There is a

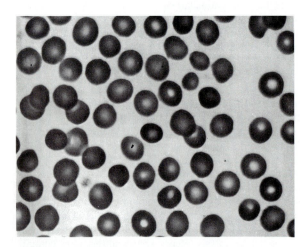

Figure 11.5–1. Peripheral blood smear in hereditary spherocytosis.

wide spectrum of severity in the anemia. Some patients are incidentally diagnosed, whereas others have severe hemolytic anemia. Unexplained splenomegaly discovered during physical examination is a common presentation. The disorder is frequently first suspected in the neonatal period because of jaundice. Biliary tract symptoms may be the presenting feature; by the third decade, over 40% of patients have cholelithiasis. Chronic leg ulcers may also complicate the disorder.

The course of the disease may be complicated by episodes of "aplastic crisis," in which erythropoiesis is suppressed but the hemolytic process continues, leading to profound anemia. These episodes of life-threatening anemia usually develop in association with parvovirus B19 infection of the hematopoietic stem cell.

Patients with hereditary spherocytosis have spherocytes and polychromatophilia on their peripheral blood smear. Spherocytes lack central pallor because of the loss of membrane surface area. The mean cell volume is normal, but the mean corpuscular hemoglobin concentration may be elevated (37–39 g/dL). The osmotic fragility test is useful in diagnosing the disorder. Because the red cells have a decreased surface-to-volume ratio, they have an increased susceptibility to lysis by hypotonic saline.

The hemolytic anemia of hereditary spherocytosis may be cured by splenectomy because this removes the principal site of abnormal red cell destruction. Transfusions are rarely necessary unless aplastic crisis occurs. Splenectomy is recommended in patients with moderate or severe hereditary spherocytosis to prevent aplastic crisis, cholelithiasis, and chronic leg ulcers. Delaying splenectomy until age 4 or 5 may reduce the risk of postsplenectomy sepsis. Prior to splenectomy, polyvalent pneumococcal vaccine should be given. Prophylactic penicillin should be given indefinitely after splenectomy to reduce the risk of overwhelming sepsis by encapsulated organisms.

Warm Autoimmune Hemolytic Anemia

Warm autoimmune hemolytic anemia is the most common type of immune hemolysis, accounting for about 70% of cases. Neoplasms of the reticuloendothelial system, collagen vascular diseases, inherited and acquired immunodeficiency states (especially HIV infections), and ulcerative colitis are diseases frequently associated with warm autoimmune hemolytic anemia.

The onset of anemia may be insidious or fulminant. Jaundice, hemoglobinuria, and fever are infrequent clinical findings. Splenomegaly is present in about 50% of patients with warm autoimmune hemolytic anemia, hepatomegaly in one-third of patients.

The hemoglobin concentration is variable, but commonly less than 7 g/dL. The blood smear shows spherocytes, polychromatophilia, nucleated red cells, and red cell clumping. Typically, the reticulocyte count is elevated. The hallmark of the disorder is a positive direct antiglobulin test (Coombs' test). This test is used to detect IgG or complement on the red blood cell membrane.

When antihuman IgG or anticomplement antibodies are added to the patient's washed red cells, microscopic agglutination is observed. In warm autoimmune hemolytic anemia, IgG is found alone or in combination with complement proteins on the red cell surface.

Initial therapy for warm autoimmune hemolytic anemia is the administration of corticosteroids. For the patient unresponsive to or unable to tolerate long-term corticosteroids, splenectomy is recommended. Transfused red cells have shortened survival, paralleling the patient's autologous red cell destruction rate. Nonetheless, if transfusion therapy is considered life-saving, red cells should not be withheld because of fear of a hemolytic reaction.

Cold Agglutinin Disease

In contrast to warm autoimmune hemolytic anemia, cold autoimmune hemolysis involves IgM antibodies. Most patients are middle-aged or elderly. Cold agglutinin disease may be associated with neoplasms, especially chronic lymphocytic leukemia, Waldenström's macroglobulinemia, and lymphoma. In addition, cold agglutinin disease is associated with mycoplasma and Epstein-Barr viral infections (infectious mononucleosis).

At cold temperatures, patients may develop hemoglobinuria. With cold exposure and resultant autoagglutination in small capillaries, blanching of the fingertips and progression to bluish discoloration (cyanosis) may be a presenting complaint. Upon warming the cooled extremity, these findings resolve.

A characteristic finding is autoagglutination of the patient's red cells following phlebotomy. Other characteristic blood smear findings are spherocytosis and polychromatophilia. The characteristic serologic results include a positive antiglobulin test due to complement on the red cell membrane. Cold-reactive IgM autoagglutinins associated with immune hemolysis are present at titers greater than 1000 when tested at 4°C (39.2°F).

Therapy is preventive: The patient is advised to avoid extreme cold exposure. Wearing gloves, hats, and warm clothing when outdoor activities cannot be avoided should be recommended. If transfusions of red cells are required, administration of the blood through a blood warmer is prudent.

Hemolysis Caused by Liver Disease

Hemolysis may accompany acute or chronic liver disease, especially alcoholic liver disease. Spur cell anemia is a hemolytic anemia found in patients with severe cirrhosis. The peripheral smear shows a predominance of acanthocytes, polychromatophilia, and nucleated red cells. Spur cell membranes contain high levels of cholesterol with normal lecithin content, reducing cellular flexibility and leading to splenic entrapment. No specific treatment is required.

SUMMARY

▶ An elevated corrected reticulocyte count is the most useful screening test for hemolysis.

▶ After establishing the presence of a hemolytic anemia, careful review of the peripheral smear may suggest the type of hemolytic anemia.

▶ Intravascular hemolysis usually presents as hemoglobinuria and hemoglobinemia, both of which are absent in extravascular hemolysis.

▶ Enlargement of the spleen is one of the most frequent clinical findings in extravascular hemolysis.

▶ G6PD deficiency can cause hemolysis when affected persons are treated with sulfonamides or antimalarial agents.

SUGGESTED READING

Ballas SK: The pathophysiology of hemolytic anemias. Transfusion Med Rev 1990;4:236.

Lux SE, Palek J: Disorders of the red cell membrane. In: *Blood: Principles and Practice of Hematology.* Handin RI, Lux SE, Stossel TP (editors). Lippincott, 1995.

Petz LD, Garratty G: *Acquired Immune Hemolytic Anemias.* Churchill Livingstone, 1980.

Valentine WN, Tanaka KR, Paglia DE: Hemolytic anemias and erythrocyte enzymopathies. Ann Intern Med 1985;103:245.

11.6

Anemia Associated with Systemic Disease

Jerry L. Spivak, MD

Systemic disease or dysfunction of a particular organ can profoundly influence blood production. Hypoproliferative anemia secondary to a systemic disease is the most common type of anemia seen in hospitalized patients; its severity does not usually correlate with the severity of the underlying disease. Since its causes are many and often correctable, the diagnostic approach must be thorough.

Whenever a patient presents with anemia, the physician must consider the diagnostic possibilities outlined in Chapters 11.1–11.5. Even when an anemic patient has a known systemic illness, it is important to consider other causes for anemia and not simply ascribe it to the systemic disease. Other concurrent events besides the known systemic illness, including the drugs used to treat the illness, should be considered. After other causes of anemia have been excluded, it is reasonable to tentatively ascribe the anemia to nonspecific marrow suppression from the systemic illness. Nevertheless, reconsideration of other causes and vigilant observation for clues suggesting another process are important obligations for the clinician.

When erythropoiesis is impaired by organ failure or systemic disease, the red cells are usually normocytic and normochromic, providing little information about the underlying disorder. Examination of a bone marrow aspirate or biopsy is often required to distinguish the nonspecific anemia resulting from inflammation, infection, or neoplasia from the anemia caused by intrinsic diseases of the marrow such as aplastic anemia, leukemia, myeloproliferative disorders, and multiple myeloma. The marrow aspirate may also reveal maturation defects caused by folic acid or vitamin B_{12} deficiency that are masked in the peripheral blood by thalassemia trait, simultaneous iron deficiency, or renal disease. Examination of the marrow is also the only way to establish red cell aplasia and the best way to evaluate iron stores in a patient with inflammation, infection, malignancy, or liver disease. Typically, in the anemia associated with systemic disease, marrow iron stores are increased. Even a normal marrow aspirate is helpful in evaluating patients with a normocytic anemia, since it reduces the number of diagnostic possibilities.

When marrow cellularity, morphology, and iron stores are normal, a hypoproliferative anemia usually has one of two causes: reduced erythropoietin production (Chapter 11.1) or end-organ unresponsiveness to the hormone.

ANEMIAS CAUSED PRIMARILY BY ORGAN FAILURE

Kidney Disease

In adults, the kidney is the major site of erythropoietin production; a small amount of erythropoietin is made in the liver, but is insufficient to sustain adequate erythropoiesis. The anemia of patients with acute renal failure usually results from the disorder that caused the renal disease (eg, thrombotic thrombocytopenic purpura, hemolytic-uremic syndrome, malignant hypertension, renal cortical necrosis, hemolytic transfusion reaction, and bacterial sepsis). In these patients, the peripheral smear shows microangiopathic red cell abnormalities and an elevated reticulocyte count. With significant chronic renal parenchymal damage, erythropoietin production is diminished, so that in chronic renal failure caused by intrinsic renal disease the red cells are usually normocytic, red cell survival is modestly decreased, the proportion of erythroid precursors in the marrow is diminished, and the reticulocyte count is low. The anemia may be modified by complications of the renal failure (inanition, bleeding, infection, and myelofibrosis caused by secondary hyperparathyroidism) or its treatment (dialysis toxins, blood loss during dialysis, dialysis of folic acid, dialysis hypersplenism, aluminum toxicity, and overtransfusion).

Although much attention has been directed toward a role for uremic toxins in the anemia of chronic renal disease, evidence is meager. The complete amelioration of anemia in patients on renal dialysis who are treated with recombinant human erythropoietin supports the contention that insufficient erythropoietin production—not uremic toxins—is the primary defect in the anemia associated with chronic renal disease. Erythropoietin treatment should be started in anemic patients with chronic renal failure who are transfusion-dependent or whose anemia causes symptoms. As treatment corrects the anemia, the quality of life improves dramatically.

Endocrine Disease

Erythropoietin is the only hormone required for red cell proliferation and differentiation, processes that may be modified directly or indirectly by other growth and developmental hormones. Androgens appear to enhance erythropoiesis directly by increasing the number of erythropoietin-responsive progenitor cells and indirectly by increasing renal erythropoietin production. Androgens are responsible for the difference in red cell mass between men and women after puberty. Lack of androgens accounts for the equalization that occurs with castration. Erythrocytosis is a complication of androgen therapy and may be a feature of virilizing tumors. Corticosteroids, growth hormone, and thyroid hormones appear to affect erythropoiesis indirectly through their influence on body metabolism and oxygen consumption. Anemia is an uncommon complication of hyperparathyroidism, seen most often in association with myelofibrosis in the secondary form of the disease in uremic patients on chronic hemodialysis.

Thyroid Disease: Anemia is a feature of both primary and secondary hypothyroidism. The anemia is generally mild, but actually may be more severe than the measured levels indicate because of a simultaneous reduction in plasma volume as a consequence of the hypothyroid state. The red cells are usually normocytic, but acanthocytes may be prominent. A small proportion of patients have macrocytosis unassociated with folic acid or vitamin B_{12} deficiency and corrected by thyroxine (T_4) therapy. Hypothyroidism caused by autoimmune thyroiditis is associated with pernicious anemia. The link between them appears to be one of autoimmunity. About 50% of patients with pernicious anemia have antithyroid antibodies, whereas 30% of patients with myxedema have antiparietal cell antibodies.

Iron deficiency is a complication of hypothyroidism. In women, menorrhagia may be the cause. Gastric achlorhydria associated with autoimmune hypothyroidism may contribute to iron malabsorption. Many hypothyroid patients without iron deficiency have a reduced serum iron and transferrin saturation, which responds to thyroxine alone. Patients with uncomplicated hypothyroidism need at least 6 months of thyroxine therapy to correct their anemia.

Liver Disease

Anemia is a common complication of liver disease and can be produced by a number of mechanisms, depending on the nature of the underlying hepatic disorder. Iron deficiency can be caused by blood loss from esophageal varices, gastritis, or peptic ulcer. Malnutrition and ethanol abuse lead to folic acid deficiency. Patients with portal hypertension often have an increase in plasma volume, which exaggerates the degree of anemia, and the associated splenomegaly can lead to red cell sequestration.

Abnormalities of red cell shape in patients with liver disease are partly due to failure of cholesterol esterification. Red cell membrane cholesterol is in equilibrium with that in the plasma, and an increase in plasma unesterified cholesterol leads to an increase in red cell membrane cholesterol. This results in redundancy of the red cell membrane and the characteristic thin macrocytes and target cells found in patients with liver disease. Patients with advanced alcoholic liver disease—and rarely patients with fulminant viral hepatitis—have acanthocytes (spur cells) and echinocytes (spiculated cells). The mechanisms responsible for these red cell changes are not entirely defined, but one study suggests that echinocyte formation in patients with liver disease is caused by red cell binding of abnormal high-density lipoproteins.

In addition to specific causes of anemia, patients with liver disease also appear to have a nonspecific depression of red cell production. The affinity of hemoglobin for oxygen is reduced and the hemoglobin-oxygen dissociation curve is shifted to the right. Thus, at any given hemoglobin level, more oxygen than normal is available to the tissues, and a normal red cell mass may not be needed. The fact that erythrocytosis develops in some patients with cirrhosis who have arteriovenous shunts suggests that the functional capacity of the marrow remains intact, at least in these patients.

ANEMIAS CAUSED BY IMPAIRED MARROW FUNCTION

Infection

Infections can produce anemia by means of a variety of mechanisms, depending on the type of infection and the characteristics of the host. Hookworm infection leads to iron deficiency and fish tapeworm infection to vitamin B_{12} deficiency if the parasite load is large. Hemolysis can be induced by direct infection of red cells (malaria [see Color Plates], bartonellosis), by toxin secretion (clostridia), or by immune mechanisms (mycoplasma, malaria, syphilis, infectious mononucleosis, and other viral infections). In patients with preexisting hemolysis, viral or bacterial infections accelerate red cell destruction by enhancing reticuloendothelial system activity. Patients with hemolytic states are predisposed to infection with organisms such as salmonella because of involvement of the reticuloendothelial system in erythrophagocytosis. In sickle cell anemia, this relative reticuloendothelial cell blockade is magnified by splenic atrophy, increasing the risk of overwhelming infection with encapsulated organisms such as the pneumococcus. In patients with red cell glucose-6-phosphate dehydrogenase (G6PD) deficiency, viral or bacterial infections induce hemolysis probably as a consequence of oxidant injury to the red cells by H_2O_2 generated in activated leukocytes.

Hematopoiesis is suppressed by infections such as osteomyelitis and HIV. Aplastic anemia is a complication of viral hepatitis and, rarely, infectious mononucleosis. Bacterial and fungal infections can produce bone marrow necrosis. Patients with chronic hemolytic anemias can also develop a transient aplastic crisis caused by infection with parvovirus B19. Although white cells and platelets as well as red cells may be involved, most often the transient aplastic crisis manifests as a rapid development of profound anemia. Although viral infections may cause a similar transient depression of hematopoiesis in normal persons, clinical evidence is only found when red cell life span is markedly reduced or the patient is chronically immunosuppressed. Consequently, when patients with chronic hemolytic anemia develop fever, their reticulocyte count should be monitored to detect a transient aplastic crisis. Another clue to transient aplastic crisis is the diminished jaundice in these habitually icteric persons.

Infiltrative Disease of the Marrow

Direct involvement of the marrow with suppression of normal hematopoiesis occurs in a variety of disorders in addition to hematologic neoplasms. These include Hodgkin's disease, non-Hodgkin's lymphomas, multiple myeloma, malignant histiocytosis, malignancies of other organs (particularly the lung, prostate, stomach, breast, and thyroid), disseminated infection with atypical mycobacteria, and Gaucher's disease. Myelofibrosis or infiltration of the marrow by tumor or granulomas may stimulate extramedullary hematopoiesis, with the appearance of nucleated erythroid and myeloid precursors and misshapen red cells (teardrop forms) in the circulation. The term *leukoerythroblastic reaction* is used to describe these abnormalities, which are not specific for invasion of the bone marrow by tumor but may be seen in such nonmalignant conditions as blood loss, hemolysis, megaloblastic anemia, drug reactions, and infections. Likewise, the absence of peripheral blood abnormalities does not exclude the possibility of tumor within the marrow. The degree of anemia seen in patients with infiltrative disease of the marrow depends on the nature and duration of the underlying disease. The extent of marrow involvement by tumor or reactive fibrosis is often not sufficient to account for the observed suppression of hematopoiesis. Other factors involved include inanition, marrow necrosis, and inhibition of hematopoietic cell proliferation by tumor products, inflammatory cytokines, or decreased erythropoietin production.

Pancytopenia or a leukoerythroblastic reaction without a discernible cause is an indication for a bone marrow biopsy. The only way to differentiate aplastic anemia from other causes of pancytopenia is with biopsy, because of its ability to evaluate marrow cellularity. A biopsy is also needed to confirm fibrosis within the marrow. Marrow fibrosis is a reactive phenomenon that is associated with acute and chronic myeloproliferative disorders, metastatic tumor, or metabolic abnormalities such as hyperparathyroidism. Although tumor cells can be identified in marrow aspirates, the incidence with which metastatic tumor is identified is increased many times when a biopsy is obtained. Overall, the prevalence of positive marrow biopsies in patients with malignant disease is about 30–40%,

depending on the type of tumor. Performing bilateral biopsies can increase the yield by 15%. In granulomatous disorders such as tuberculosis and sarcoidosis, bone marrow biopsy has a much lower diagnostic yield (15–30%) than liver, lung, or lymph node biopsy.

Anemia Associated with Chronic Disease

Although infection, inflammation, and neoplasms can cause anemia by well-defined mechanisms, more commonly the anemia observed in these conditions is nonspecific and not distinguishable on the basis of the underlying illness. The anemia is generally mild (hemoglobin levels of 10–11 g/dL), and the red cells are normocytic and normochromic, although microcytosis, hypochromia, and even severe anemia can be observed. The corrected reticulocyte count is low for the degree of anemia, and the bilirubin level is not elevated. Red cell life span is modestly reduced, but the marrow is unable to compensate even though its cellularity is normal and no evidence of maturation abnormalities is found. Serum iron and transferrin saturation are reduced. However, in contrast to iron deficiency anemia, serum transferrin is low whereas serum ferritin levels are elevated and marrow iron stores are normal or high. Erythropoietin levels are generally not appropriately elevated for the degree of anemia. Since chronic illness is often associated with a low serum T_3 level, the reduction in erythropoietin may reflect not only inflammatory cytokines suppressing its production, but also a decrease in tissue oxygen demands.

Ferrokinetic studies have also revealed a block in the release of reticuloendothelial iron to the plasma. The role in this type of anemia of agents such as endotoxin, interleukins 1 and 2, interferons, tumor necrosis factor, and prostaglandins, as well as cell-cell interactions involving lymphocytes, macrophages, and hematopoietic progenitor cells, remains undefined. Not to be overlooked, however, is the contribution of repeated diagnostic phlebotomies in a setting of limited marrow proliferative activity.

The anemia associated with chronic disease is a diagnosis of exclusion. Because this anemia may in part mimic iron deficiency anemia, diagnosis may require bone marrow aspiration. The anemia usually remits with alleviation of the underlying disease. A gradual improvement in the hematocrit is a good indicator of successful therapy of the underlying disease.

Pure Red Cell Aplasia

The syndrome of pure red cell aplasia is characterized by a normocytic, normochromic anemia, absence of reticulocytes, normal leukocyte and platelet counts, and a virtual absence of erythroblasts in the marrow, with normal myelopoiesis and megakaryocytopoiesis. An occasional patient has an increase in marrow lymphocytes and eosinophils. Pure red cell aplasia may be congenital or acquired; the acquired form can be primary or secondary (Table 11.6–1). In primary pure red cell aplasia, no underlying disease, drug, infection, or toxic exposure can be identified. Some patients with the primary form have cir-

Table 11.6–1. Causes of pure red cell aplasia.

Primary
   Antibody-mediated
   Idiopathic
   Congenital (Diamond-Blackfan syndrome)

Secondary
   Thymoma
   Other neoplasms (chronic lymphocytic leukemia, chronic
      myelogenous leukemia, Hodgkin's disease, lymphoma,
      multiple myeloma, lung carcinoma, gastric carcinoma)
   Infection (parvovirus B19)
   Renal failure
   Starvation
   Autoimmune hemolytic anemia
   Systemic lupus erythematosus
   Drugs (phenytoin, isoniazid, chlorpropamide, tolbutamide,
      phenylbutazone, azathioprine, halothane, gold, sulfonamides,
      chloramphenicol, penicillin, phenobarbital)

culating IgG that is cytotoxic to erythroid precursors; other patients show no cause for the pure red cell aplasia. In addition to antibodies cytotoxic to erythroblasts, these patients may have other immunologic abnormalities, including hypogammaglobulinemia, monoclonal gammopathy, antinuclear antibodies, and autoantibodies against red cells or platelets.

A striking feature of acquired pure red cell aplasia is its close association with thymoma. Fifty percent of patients with acquired pure red cell aplasia have a thymoma, whereas about 5% of patients with a thymoma have pure red cell aplasia. Most patients with both conditions are women, generally over age 50 years. Pure red cell aplasia never precedes the thymoma, but can develop many years after the thymoma, as well as after its resection. Thymomas are associated with other autoimmune disorders, such as systemic lupus erythematosus and myasthenia gravis. No correlation exists between the histology of the thymoma and the development of pure red cell aplasia or the other autoimmune syndromes.

The diagnosis of pure red cell aplasia is established from a marrow aspirate. If the cellularity of the aspirate is inadequate, a biopsy must be performed. Because the marrow cellularity is normal in primary pure red cell aplasia, the diagnosis is frequently overlooked. When the patient has an associated disorder such as myelofibrosis, chronic lymphocytic leukemia, or chronic myelogenous leukemia, the absence of erythroid precursors is even more likely to be missed.

After pure red cell aplasia is diagnosed, its cause must be determined. When the cause is a drug or infection, the disorder is usually self-limited. However, in immunosuppressed patients, red cell aplasia caused by parvovirus B19 infection may be persistent, and in a hemolytic anemia, parvovirus-induced red cell aplasia may cause a rapid fall in hemoglobin.

Intravenous gamma globulin is effective therapy for parvovirus B19 infection causing red cell aplasia. When aplasia complicates an autoimmune disease or neoplasm, the underlying disease must be treated to obtain remission of the red cell aplasia. When pure red cell aplasia results from a thymoma, thymectomy is usually required, since other forms of therapy are ineffective in the presence of the tumor. Rarely, radiation therapy has been effective in relieving pure red cell aplasia when the thymoma is unresectable.

When anemia does not resolve after an observation period of several months, or when thymectomy is ineffective, corticosteroid treatment should be started. If no effect is seen within 2 months, immunosuppressive therapy with either cyclophosphamide or azathioprine should be added. Cyclosporine may also be tried. Immunosuppressive agents appear to be effective, even if erythroblast antibodies are not detectable. Plasmapheresis has helped a few patients and splenectomy has been used when immunosuppressive agents have failed. Spontaneous remissions occur in pure red cell aplasia, as do relapses following drug-induced remission.

SUMMARY

▶ Anemia is a common complication of many systemic disorders and may be their presenting manifestation. Pursuing the cause of the anemia may yield the diagnosis of the systemic disorder.

▶ In most anemias associated with a systemic disorder, the anemia remits when the systemic disorder is corrected.

▶ In chronic renal failure, impaired erythropoietin production is the major cause of anemia.

▶ In patients with an inflammatory, infectious, or neoplastic disease, impaired erythropoietin production is partly responsible for the anemia.

SUGGESTED READING

Barrett-Connor E: Anemia and infection. Am J Med 1972;52:242.

Cash JM, Sears DA: The anemia of chronic disease: Spectrum of associated diseases in a series of unselected hospitalized patients. Am J Med 1989;87:638.

Clark DA, Dessypris EN, Krantz SB: Studies on pure red cell aplasia. XI. Results of immunosuppressive treatment of 37 patients. Blood 1984;63:277.

Scadden DT, Zon LI, Groopman JE: Pathophysiology and management of HIV-associated hematologic disorders. Blood 1989;74:1455.

Young N, Mortimer P: Viruses and bone marrow failure. Blood 1984;63:729.

The White Blood Cell Count

Stuart E. Selonick, MD

Whenever a patient presents with a serious illness or unexplained complaints, a complete blood count should be done, which includes a determination of the white blood cell count. This is part of the comprehensive assessment of any patient. The white blood cell count and the relative proportions of various white cell types (the differential) are important laboratory measurements because abnormalities may indicate primary hematologic disorders (eg, leukemia; Chapter 11.8) or reflect the presence or severity of underlying diseases (eg, mononucleosis, tuberculosis). Occasionally, patients have a significant blood cell count abnormality discovered incidentally on routine automated blood testing.

Determining the absolute count of each type of white cell enhances the assessment. The absolute count is calculated by multiplying the total white blood cell count by the percentage of the individual cell types; it is often reported directly on automated systems.

GRANULOCYTES

The most common abnormalities of white blood cells involve the neutrophils. In calculating the absolute number of neutrophils, one adds the bands and segmented neutrophils together, since these are the cells with normal phagocytic function. In adults, an absolute neutrophil count of less than 1800/µL constitutes neutropenia and a count of more than 8000/µL is considered neutrophilia.

Neutrophils arise from pluripotent marrow stem cells (CFU-S) that develop into cells committed to forming granulocyte colony-forming units (CFU-C), which then differentiate through the developmental phases of myeloblast, promyelocyte, and myelocyte. Further maturation results in metamyelocytes, bands, and finally polymorphonuclear neutrophils, which are released into the circulation, where they have a half-life of 4–6 hours. In the peripheral circulation, neutrophils are divided equally between a circulating and marginating pool. When the neutrophils leave the circulation, they can survive in body tissues for another 4–5 days.

Despite our knowledge of neutrophil development, the classification of neutrophil disorders is partly pathophysiologic and partly descriptive, because techniques to measure the degree of neutrophil production or destruction are not used clinically.

Neutrophilia

Although neutrophilia can result from several mechanisms (Table 11.7–1), it is usually caused by increased bone marrow proliferation. The storage pool of developing neutrophils can release up to 10 times the number of normally circulating neutrophils, but this process takes several days.

The most common cause of neutrophilia is an acute infection, especially a bacterial infection. Neutrophil production is usually stimulated enough to result in increased numbers of immature neutrophil forms, known as "a shift to the left." On the peripheral blood smear, larger-than-usual granulations (toxic granules), and bluish cytoplasmic inclusions (Döhle bodies), are further evidence of ongoing infection. Neutrophil counts of ≥40,000/µL, which might suggest an underlying leukemia but ultimately are found to be secondary to another process, are called *leukemoid reactions*. Counts may reach up to 100,000/µL and occasionally higher. The usual causes of such intense bone marrow stimulation include infections, vasculitis (Chapter 3.5), and cancers. The type of leukemia that usually needs to be differentiated from a leukemoid reaction is chronic myelocytic leukemia (Chapter 11.8). It is usually not difficult to make the distinction, because a leukemoid reaction is associated with mature neutrophils, lack of basophilia or eosinophilia, normal-sized platelets, lack of splenomegaly, and increased leukocyte alkaline phosphate staining of neutrophil granules. In contrast, chronic myelocytic leukemia is associated with a left shift of the differential, as well as eosinophilia, basophilia, enlarged platelets, splenomegaly, and poor leukocyte alkaline phosphate staining.

Table 11.7–1. Causes of elevated neutrophil count (>8000/μL).

Infections
Acute or chronic inflammation, eg, gout, myocardial infarction,
    vasculitis
Tumors
Postsplenectomy
Pregnancy
Leukemia or myeloproliferative disorders
Drugs, especially corticosteroids, epinephrine
Seizures (transient rise in neutrophils)
Hemorrhage, hemolysis
Emotional or physical stress
Chronic idiopathic neutrophilia

Neutropenia

Neutropenia can occur because of decreased production in the bone marrow, accelerated peripheral turnover, shifts of cells from the circulatory to marginal or tissue pools, or a combination of these factors (Table 11.7–2). Neutropenia may also be classified as acute or chronic, with acute reduction usually developing in a patient with increased neutrophil utilization and impaired production. Chronic neutropenia usually is caused by reduced production, but occasionally is caused by increased margination.

Persistent neutropenia requires prompt assessment. Not only does neutropenia indicate a significant disorder, but a substantial decrease makes patients vulnerable to infection. In most patients, the occurrence of infections increases only when the neutrophil count is less than 1000/μL. Patients with neutrophil counts below 500/μL are at great risk of infection. This increased risk is influenced by the duration of neutropenia as well as the cause. Disorders of bone marrow production, such as regularly accompany use of cytotoxic chemotherapy, result in the greatest susceptibility.

Many of the usual manifestations of infections may be

Table 11.7–2. Causes of isolated reduction in neutrophil count (<1800/μL).

Decreased bone marrow production
    Myelodysplastic syndrome
    Myeloma
    Leukemia
    Drugs
    Infection (viruses, tuberculosis, HIV)
    Cyclic neutropenia
    Folate or vitamin B_{12} deficiency
    Myelofibrosis
    Benign chronic neutropenia

Abnormal distribution
    Hypersplenism
    Overwhelming infection

Shortened survival
    Rheumatoid arthritis (Felty's syndrome)
    Systemic lupus erythematosus
    Autoimmune neutropenia
    Sjögren's syndrome

absent in patients with neutropenia because of the role that neutrophils play in producing the symptoms and signs of infection. For example, a perirectal abscess may have no swelling or fluctuance, a pneumonia may have only a minimal infiltrate, and pyelonephritis may lack pyuria. Fever continues to be a reliable sign even without neutrophils.

Neutropenia with anemia and thrombocytopenia is called *pancytopenia*. The approach to pancytopenia is the same as that to neutropenia, and the implication is that there is either a process affecting multiple cell lines or a primary stem cell disorder (Chapter 11.8).

The initial evaluation of a patient with neutropenia includes a careful history, emphasizing distant and recent infections, new drugs, prior illness, and toxic exposures. Obtaining old records is helpful in determining the duration of the neutropenia. Because tumors and infections can cause neutropenia, the physical examination should include particular assessment of lymphadenopathy or hepatosplenomegaly. If there is a suspicion, based on coexisting symptoms such as cough, coryza, or myalgias, that the decrease in white cell count may be temporally related to a recent viral infection (Chapter 8.11), the counts should be repeated in 1–2 weeks. The peripheral blood smear is reviewed to corroborate the low white blood cell count and assess for further clues. If the neutropenia is persistent, antinuclear antibody, rheumatoid factor, serum vitamin B_{12} level, and red blood cell folate level should be measured and serum protein electrophoresis performed to search for conditions that may cause persistent neutropenia. Measurement of antineutrophil antibody may be helpful and should be obtained if initial tests are negative or an autoimmune process is suspected. Patients who have severe neutropenia that defies explanation with these measures should have a bone marrow aspirate and biopsy performed. If there is any history of cyclic infections, serial measurements of the absolute neutrophil count are helpful.

The results of the foregoing evaluation should enable the physician to decide on the mechanisms of the neutropenia and in most cases determine the diagnosis. Suppression of granulocytopoiesis in the bone marrow is the most common mechanism of neutropenia. The possibility of drug-induced neutropenia should always be considered. Drugs may induce neutropenia by directly affecting stem cells (as in chemotherapy) or immunologic mechanisms such as hypersensitivity reactions, antibodies, or hapten-antibody complexes (Chapters 9.1 and 9.3). Neutropenia may occur with many classes of drugs, but is especially associated with phenothiazines, gold compounds, antithyroid drugs, chloramphenicol, quinidine, procainamide, phenylbutazone, sulfonamide, and penicillins.

Cyclic neutropenia is a rare condition in which patients develop malaise and mouth sores at regular intervals usually of 3 weeks, lasting 3–4 days, corresponding to cyclic decreases in neutrophil count. The disorder is inherited as an autosomal dominant disease but often is not diagnosed until adulthood. Bone marrow examination during granulocytopenia shows hypoplasia accompanied by developmental delay.

Benign chronic neutropenia is a common condition, characterized by mild chronic decrease in neutrophil count and existing in many patients dating to childhood. Patients with benign neutropenia have normal granulocyte reserve and normal bone marrow morphology. These patients do not have frequent infections and the condition is not progressive. A variant of this disorder is the so-called "ethnic neutropenia" seen in blacks and Yemenite Jews.

Hypersplenism is often associated with pancytopenia; one of the clues may be an elevated reticulocyte count. In most patients, the spleen is palpable, but occasionally assessment by ultrasonography, magnetic resonance imaging (MRI), or computed tomography (CT) is required to show the enlargement. If the patient is not thought to have liver disease or portal hypertension, bone marrow aspirate and biopsy are indicated to evaluate the cause of the enlarged spleen.

Some patients with autoimmune diseases demonstrate neutropenia secondary to decreased neutrophil survival. Felty's syndrome is the relatively uncommon association of rheumatoid arthritis and neutropenia. Splenomegaly is not always present. The degree of neutropenia may be severe, but because of normal marrow reserve, the risk of infection is not as great as with conditions that interfere with bone marrow functioning. For severe Felty's syndrome or autoimmune neutropenia, high-dose corticosteroids have proved to be useful.

In severe, self-limited episodes of neutropenia, such as those caused by chemotherapy, use of one of the genetically engineered colony-stimulating factor medications can hasten bone marrow recovery.

Eosinophilia

Although the accepted definition of eosinophilia is an absolute count greater than 500/μL, counts of 500–1000/μL are a common finding even on routine exams and often do not yield a specific diagnosis. Once the total eosinophil count is greater than 4000/μL, the underlying cause is almost always able to be defined; some patients may need a more aggressive search for parasites, vasculitis, or occult tumors (Table 11.7–3).

The evaluation of eosinophilia should include a history covering recent travel and current medications. Laboratory evaluation might include determining the IgE level, examining the stool for ova and parasites, taking a chest x-ray, and testing for antinuclear antibody. Antibodies to a number of invasive parasites can be obtained.

The hypereosinophilic syndrome is a poorly understood condition in which the absolute eosinophil count is more than 1500/μL without detectable cause. The disease is somewhat more common in men 20–50 years and has a 50% mortality rate. A variety of tissues may be damaged in the hypereosinophilic syndrome, but left heart necrosis and fibrosis may be the most significant. Oral corticosteroids and a number of chemotherapeutic agents, especially hydroxyurea, have been used as treatment.

Table 11.7–3. Common causes of eosinophil counts >500/μL.

Adrenal insufficiency
Allergic reactions
Eosinophilic pneumonitis
Hodgkin's disease, other malignancies
Hypereosinophilic syndrome
Myeloproliferative disease
Parasites
Skin diseases, eg, pemphigus
Vasculitis

LYMPHOCYTES

Lymphocytosis

Lymphocytosis is an absolute lymphocyte count greater than 5000/μL. The most common causes are listed in Table 11.7–4. Review of the peripheral smear is of paramount importance in distinguishing normal morphology from atypical lymphocytes (large cells with deep blue cytoplasm, indentation of cytoplasm by red cells) and from malignant cells. The appearance of many reactive lymphocytes suggests a viral illness. Large granular lymphocytes or very complex nuclear shapes suggests a T-cell malignancy, and many small mature-looking lymphocytes suggest chronic lymphocytic leukemia. The peripheral smear in patients with chronic lymphocytic leukemia often contains "smudge cells," which are fragile malignant lymphocytes that have ruptured (Figure 11.7–1). Bone marrow evaluation is useful in patients with lymphocytosis only when lymphoma is suspected or is being staged. If there is any question of reactive (benign) versus clonal (malignant) disease being present, cell surface markers should be obtained.

Lymphocytopenia

Lymphocytopenia is an absolute lymphocyte count of less than 1500/μL. This condition is seen in patients with acute infections and a number of other illnesses

Table 11.7–4. Causes of elevated lymphocyte counts (>5000/μL).

Normal lymphocyte morphology
  Tuberculosis
  Viral infections
  Chronic lymphocytic leukemia
  Waldenström's macroglobulinemia
  Thyrotoxicosis

Atypical lymphocyte morphology
  Infectious mononucleosis
  Cytomegalovirus
  Viral hepatitis
  Toxoplasmosis
  Drug reactions

Malignant lymphocyte morphology
  "Lymphosarcoma cell" leukemia
  Acute lymphocytic leukemia
  Sézary syndrome and other T-cell disorders
  Hairy cell leukemia
  Chronic lymphocytic leukemia

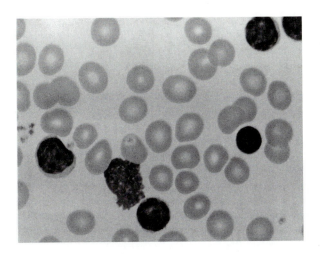

Figure 11.7–1. Peripheral blood smear in chronic lymphocytic leukemia, showing "smudge cells."

such as congestive heart failure, cancers, and vasculitis. Lymphocytopenia is commonly present in HIV infection.

MONOCYTES

Monocytosis may occur in the absence of neutrophilia. It is most often seen in patients with typhoid fever, tuberculosis, or endocarditis, or in patients recovering from an acute infection. Monocytosis may also be caused by chronic monocytic leukemia, which is a type of myelodysplastic syndrome (Chapter 11.8).

BASOPHILS

The most common cause of basophilia is chronic myelocytic leukemia. Basophils are associated with severe pruritus. Mild basophilia is also seen in some patients with polycythemia vera or myelofibrosis.

SUMMARY

▶ Neutrophilia is usually a sign of infection, inflammation, or myeloproliferative disease.

▶ Persistent neutropenia may indicate a significant condition such as a drug reaction or myelodysplastic syndrome; a neutrophil count below 500/μL predisposes to infection.

▶ The cause of mild eosinophilia is often difficult to determine, but greater increases are usually associated with an allergic reaction or parasitic infection.

▶ In evaluating lymphocytosis, the most important test is review of the peripheral smear, which assesses the morphology of the cell types that are increased.

SUGGESTED READING

Boxer LA et al: Autoimmune neutropenia. N Engl J Med 1975;293:748.

Cannistra SA, Griffin JD: Regulation of the production and function of granulocytes and monocytes. Semin Hematol 1988; 25:173.

Dale DC et al: Chronic neutropenia. Medicine 1979;58:128.

Gross R, Hellriegel KP: Drug-induced agranulocytoses. Blut 1976;32:409.

Williams WJ et al: *Hematology,* 5th ed. McGraw-Hill, 1995.

Hematopoietic Stem Cell Disorders

Alison Moliterno, MD, and Chi V. Dang, MD, PhD

Patients with stem cell disorders present with a spectrum of conditions ranging from severe anemia to erythrocytosis, from excessive bleeding to spontaneous thrombosis, from leukopenia to leukemia with overwhelming infiltration of the blood and tissues by abnormal white blood cells. The unifying feature of stem cell diseases is their clonal origin, arising from a primordial stem cell of the bone marrow. The specific presentation depends on the point of stem cell differentiation at which clonal function goes awry, the duration of disease, and host factors.

PATHOPHYSIOLOGY

Hematopoietic stem cells produce cells of the erythroid, myeloid, and megakaryocytic lineages, as well as the B and T lymphocytes. Given the relatively short life span of circulating blood cells, the bone marrow constantly produces new cells, as long as the stem cell pool maintains adequate proliferation and differentiation. Underproliferation of the stem cell population may result in failure to produce one or several cell types. Failure to differentiate may lead to the overproduction of immature forms, while unregulated proliferation may lead to the overproduction of mature forms. These disorders have often been classified according to shared clinical features, but as the implications of the disorders' genetic and molecular bases are elucidated, classification will likely change.

Through successive generations, stem cell progeny acquire the molecular, immunologic, and biochemical attributes of mature cells. With each division, hematopoietic stem cells become less pluripotential and more committed to a particular cell line. Mediators governing the proper growth and differentiation of the stem cell pool include the colony-stimulating factors, interleukins, and less specific agents such as androgens and thyroid hormone. These factors, whether produced by the stem cells themselves, by the stromal cells of the bone marrow, or by distant organs, act alone or in combination to promote differentiation, maturation, and proliferation. Growth fac-

tors may act nonspecifically across cell lines or may target cells specifically committed to one cell line.

The pathophysiology of particular stem cell disorders can be understood in terms of loss of proper differentiation, maturation, or proliferation. The frequent divisions necessary for the steady state render the stem cell population susceptible to mutagens, the results of which are expressed in all successive generations. The resulting abnormal clone may be endowed with growth advantages, maturation defects, or both (Figure 11.8–1). Mutations of the genes that encode growth factors or their receptors are specific mechanisms by which differentiation and maturation become deranged. For example, acute promyelocytic leukemia results from an alteration in retinoic acid receptors, caused by a translocation between chromosomes 15 and 17. Since retinoic acid helps promote the growth and development of certain myeloid cells, an abnormal receptor stymies maturation. Clinically, acute promyelocytic leukemia is characterized by the proliferation of cells arrested in the promyelocyte stage; the administration of all-trans retinoic acid can bring the promyelocytes to maturation and produce a clinical remission.

CLINICAL FEATURES

Presentations

By whatever mechanism, hematopoietic stem cell disorders produce abnormalities in peripheral blood counts. Too few or too many circulating cells generate characteristic symptoms and signs. The presentation and natural history of these disorders also depend on the patient's age and the maturity of the abnormal clone.

Symptoms and signs resulting from underproduction of cells relate not only to the patient's age and medical condition, but to the severity of the cytopenia (Table 11.8–1). Anemia alone usually does not cause symptoms unless the hematocrit falls below 30%. Moreover, if an anemia progresses gradually, it can become severe without causing symptoms. Symptoms of anemia can include fatigue and decreased exercise tolerance. As anemia progresses,

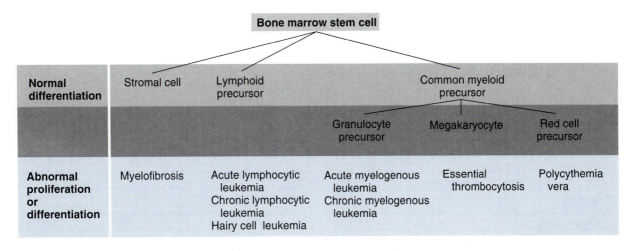

Figure 11.8–1. Hypothetical schema for hematopoietic stem cell growth and differentiation. Stem cell disorders are shown originating from normal precursors.

symptoms of coronary artery disease, peripheral vascular disease, or pulmonary disease may become unmasked or exacerbated. Signs of anemia include pallor, an increased heart rate, and a flow murmur.

Symptoms of thrombocytopenia include easy or spontaneous bruising, mucosal membrane bleeding, epistaxis, and menorrhagia. Patients typically develop symptoms when their platelet count falls below 20,000/μL. Signs include petechiae, ecchymoses, purpura, and hematomas.

The clinical features of leukopenia relate primarily to loss of immune function. Neutropenia often permits localized skin and soft tissue infections, typically in the mouth and perirectal regions. Severe neutropenia (absolute neutrophil count below 200/μL) may be accompanied by fever, sore throat, oral ulcers, and systemic infections.

The signs and symptoms of overproduction of cells are less intuitive than those of underproduction, in that they arise either from abnormal function of seemingly mature cells or from excessive cell function. For example, throm-

bocytosis caused by a myeloproliferative process does not usually produce thrombosis. Instead, despite platelet counts in the millions, patients tend to bleed, presumably because of qualitative platelet defects generated by the stem cell disorder. Overproduction of red blood cells creates toxicity by increasing blood viscosity and total blood volume. Patients complain of headaches, fullness in the face, dizziness, and tinnitus. Signs include plethora, conjunctival injection, palmar erythema, and systolic hypertension.

Finally, the symptoms of stem cell-driven leukocytoses depend on the immaturity of the clonal leukocytes. Mature lymphocytes and granulocytes generally are nontoxic, no matter what their absolute number. But immature forms are dangerous because they tend to sludge in the microcirculation of the central nervous system, heart, kidneys, and lungs. Patients with acute leukemia and elevated blast cell counts may present with leukemic strokes, myocardial infarction, renal failure, or pulmonary infarction.

Because of the smoldering course of many of the stem

Table 11.8–1. Manifestations of alterations in peripheral blood cells.

Cells	Symptoms	Signs
Erythrocytes		
Decrease	Fatigue, dyspnea, angina	Pallor, cardiac flow murmur
Increase	Dizziness, tinnitus, blurred vision, fatigue	Plethora, retinal vein engorgement
Leukocytes		
Granulocytes		
Decrease	Manifestations of infections	Fever, skin infections
Increase	Dyspnea, confusion from cerebral leukostasis	
Lymphocytes		
Decrease	Manifestations of chronic infection	Fever, signs of acute infection
Increase	Lymphadenopathy	Lymphadenopathy, splenomegaly
Platelets		
Decrease	Easy bruising, mucosal bleeds	Petechiae, ecchymoses, mucosal bleeds
Increase	Painful digits, bleeding	Embolic lesions, ecchymoses

cell disorders and the availability of automated cell counters, the diseases are often discovered through abnormalities in routine blood counts. Many of the symptoms that patients report are not specific to the disorder but rather to one of its manifestations, such as thrombocytopenia or anemia.

Evaluation

Pertinent elements of the history include toxic exposures, prior chemotherapy, and possible genetic disorders. Ionizing radiation has long been associated with all of the leukemias except chronic lymphocytic leukemia. Survivors of atomic blasts and people who have received therapeutic radiation are at increased risk for developing leukemia, with the incidence peaking 3–8 years after the exposure. Radiation also has a direct, dose-dependent toxic effect on bone marrow stem cells; massive exposure can lead to prolonged but reversible aplasia. Benzene exposure can cause aplastic anemia at the time of exposure and acute leukemia years after exposure. Chemotherapeutic drugs, particularly the alkylating agents, increase the risk of leukemia and the myelodysplastic states. Patients who received both therapeutic radiation and alkylating agents are at higher risk than those who received chemotherapy alone.

Congenital disorders that increase the risk for acute leukemia include Down's syndrome, Fanconi's anemia, and ataxia-telangiectasia. Finally, siblings of a patient with leukemia carry a lifelong increased risk for the disease.

The physical exam can tell the physician more about the nature and course of a stem cell disorder. An expanded bone marrow compartment, found in patients with chronic proliferative states or acute tumor expansion, is usually silent but can produce sternal tenderness or bone or joint pain. In normal people, the bone marrow is the only tissue that produces circulating blood cells. When the marrow fails, the liver and spleen can recapitulate their ontogeny by becoming sites of extramedullary hematopoiesis. The liver and spleen may enlarge via direct tumor invasion or extramedullary hematopoiesis. Thus, both chronic dysplastic and acute proliferative processes can present with hepatosplenomegaly. Lastly, patients with acute or chronic leukemias can have lymphadenopathy caused by invasion of cells.

Laboratory evaluation of any suspected stem cell disorder starts with examination of the peripheral blood smear. Clues from the history, physical exam, and blood smear may prompt evaluation of the bone marrow itself. Bone marrow aspirates reveal the maturity of the cells, distribution of the types of cells, and cell morphology, whereas marrow biopsies permit evaluation of the marrow's cellularity and overall architecture. Particularly when a stem cell defect is suspected, marrow karyotype may be helpful, since certain chromosome abnormalities are either diagnostic, as with chronic myelogenous leukemia, or prognostic of the clinical course or response to therapy. Additional studies include flow cytometry of cells from either the peripheral blood or bone marrow, and immunohistochemical stains, both of which allow further classification of cell types.

APLASTIC ANEMIA

Aplastic anemia develops when multipotent stem cells fail to grow and provide cells for differentiation. The result is concomitant anemia, thrombocytopenia, and granulocytopenia (pancytopenia). The pathophysiologic basis of the stem cell abnormality is heterogeneous; the disease may develop after exposure to toxins, viruses, or drugs, or may be immune-mediated.

Exposure to benzene produces a variety of hematologic disorders, with aplasia maintaining a strong dose-dependent association. Many drugs, particularly chloramphenicol and phenylbutazone, have been reported to cause aplasia. Although many cytotoxic drugs used in cancer chemotherapy produce dose-dependent cytopenias, drug-induced aplastic anemia is typically idiosyncratic. Radiation-induced aplasia is dose-related, with the bone marrow recovering within weeks after exposure.

Patients with aplastic anemia present with symptoms of anemia and thrombocytopenia. The disorder may present as acute bone marrow failure with rapid severe pancytopenia or as a chronic mild pancytopenia. Few patients have lymphadenopathy or splenomegaly. Aside from documenting the lymphocyte-sparing pancytopenia, the peripheral blood smear may look normal. The diagnosis rests on a bone marrow biopsy that shows fat replacing normal bone marrow cells. Bone marrow aspiration is often dry or produces an inaccurate assessment of the cellularity. Patients with the acquired forms have normal cytogenetics.

Prompt diagnosis of aplastic anemia is critical so that patients can be started on appropriate therapy while avoiding blood transfusions, which interfere with response to treatment. Young patients with an HLA-identical sibling have a better than 50% remission rate with bone marrow transplantation and an 80% rate if they have not received transfusions. Patients unfit for transplantation because of age or lack of a suitable donor should be given a trial of immunosuppressive therapy with cyclosporine, antithymocyte globulin, or both.

MYELODYSPLASTIC SYNDROMES

The myelodysplastic states share many morphologic abnormalities of the blood and bone marrow, and carry risk of evolving into acute leukemia. Often called "preleukemic states," the five categories of clonal disorders (Table 11.8–2) have heterogeneous clinical manifestations and prognoses.

Although the myelodysplastic syndromes are related to exposure to radiation, benzene, or chemotherapeutic drugs (particularly alkylating agents), the most important risk

Table 11.8–2. The French-American-British (FAB) classification of myelodysplastic syndromes.

Class	Peripheral Blood Findings	Bone Marrow
Refractory anemia	Macrocytosis	Megaloblastic changes
Refractory anemia with ringed sideroblasts	Normal erythrocytes + microcytes	>15% ringed sideroblasts
Refractory anemia with excess blasts (RAEB)	<5% blasts	5–20% blasts
RAEB in transformation	>5% blasts	20–30% blasts
Chronic myelomonocytic leukemia	Monocytes >1000/µL	

Modified and reproduced, with permission, from Bennett JM et al: Proposals for the classification of the myelodysplastic syndromes. Br J Haematol 1982;51:189.

factor is aging. These disorders are rare among people younger than 30; the mean age at presentation is 60. Symptoms are typically those of anemia or thrombocytopenia. Few patients have hepatomegaly, splenomegaly, or lymphadenopathy.

One or all cell lines may be reduced. The anemia is often macrocytic, with marked basophilic stippling (see Color Plates), anisocytosis, and poikilocytosis evident on the blood smear. Neutrophils are often hyposegmented and have abnormally clumped chromatin and few cytoplasmic granules. The platelets may be large and agranular. Most patients' bone marrow has normal to increased numbers of cells, although a hypocellular marrow does not rule out the syndrome. The marrow may also show small, hyposegmented megakaryocytes and erythroid hyperplasia with numerous nuclear abnormalities. Iron stain of the bone marrow aspirate may reveal ringed sideroblasts. Karyotype of the bone marrow is helpful for both diagnosis and prognosis.

The clinical course of a myelodysplastic state depends on its classification (see Table 11.8–2), the patient's age, any chromosome abnormalities and their type, a low granulocyte count, a low platelet count, and an elevated bone marrow blast count. Patients who have refractory anemia, with or without ringed sideroblasts, have a relatively good prognosis and may survive many years. Most patients with excess blasts progress to acute leukemia within 1 year. Chronic myelomonocytic leukemia carries an intermediate prognosis. Any chromosome abnormality bodes ill, and generally the more bizarre the karyotype, the worse the outlook. Some karyotypic abnormalities are typical of particular syndromes with characteristic prognoses. The 5q–abnormality is often found in patients with the "refractory anemia" subclass of myelodysplasia, and carries a good prognosis. Monosomy 7 and trisomy 8, often found in other subclasses such as "refractory anemia with excess blasts," confer a worse prognosis.

Because the myelodysplastic states are heterogeneous, no one form of therapy is appropriate for all of them. Patients who have only refractory anemia may be supported with red blood cell transfusions for years if monitored and treated for iron overload. Patients suffering from anemia with excess blasts have not benefited from attempts to promote differentiation of blast cells. Most patients whose disease progresses to acute leukemia do poorly when offered standard leukemia regimens.

In theory, bone marrow transplantation should replace the aberrant clone. This has been effective in young patients with myelodysplasia, but most patients are too old for transplantation. Patients who have severe cytopenias and cannot undergo transplantation may benefit from hematopoietic growth factors.

MYELOPROLIFERATIVE SYNDROMES

The myeloproliferative states are stem cell disorders characterized by a hypercellular bone marrow, tendency to elevated peripheral blood cell counts, splenomegaly, extramedullary hematopoiesis, and a propensity for the marrow to develop fibrosis. These are clonal disorders that generally do not involve lymphoid tissue and therefore arise from a common hematopoietic stem cell. Their classification as a group is further justified by the fact that these disorders can evolve into each other.

The myeloproliferative syndromes share a peak incidence in persons aged 50–60 years, although the age distribution is wide. Unlike the other stem cell disorders, affected patients have neither chromosome abnormalities nor a history of toxic exposures. These disorders tend to progress slowly and are much less likely than the myelodysplastic syndromes to transform into acute leukemia.

Polycythemia Vera

Although all cell lines can be involved over the course of polycythemia vera, it is the unregulated expansion of the red cell mass that is usually responsible for the clinical manifestations.

Patients with polycythemia vera may present with an incidental finding of erythrocytosis, which must be distinguished from secondary causes (Table 11.8–3). Many pa-

Table 11.8–3. Features distinguishing polycythemia vera from secondary erythrocytosis.

	Polycythemia Vera	Secondary Erythrocytosis
Red cell mass	High	Normal or high
Arterial O₂	Normal saturation	Normal or low saturation
Splenomegaly	Yes	Usually no
Platelet count	High	Usually normal
Leukocyte count	High	Usually normal
Erythropoietin level	Normal	High
Itching	Yes	No

tients present with symptoms of increased blood viscosity produced by the expanded red cell mass—headache, dizziness, a sensation of fullness in the head and face, weakness, and fatigue. Pruritus, particularly after bathing, is characteristic of polycythemia vera and helps distinguish it from secondary erythrocytosis. Patients may also present with erythromelalgia, a syndrome of intense burning, pain, and redness of the extremities. Physical signs include plethora, systolic hypertension, and splenomegaly.

The peripheral blood smear often reveals a neutrophilic leukocytosis, increased basophils, and increased platelets with large, bizarre forms; red cell morphology is usually normal. Diagnostic criteria are splenomegaly, a normal arterial oxygen saturation, and an elevated red cell mass on isotope dilution. Patients who do not have splenomegaly must have two of the following: thrombocytosis, leukocytosis, elevated leukocyte alkaline phosphatase, or elevated serum vitamin B_{12} or B_{12} binding capacity. Erythropoietin levels are generally low.

Polycythemia vera is treated with phlebotomy or cytoreductive agents to maintain the hemoglobin at 14 g/dL in men and 12 g/dL in women. The red cell mass must be controlled even if the patient is asymptomatic, because an elevated red cell mass predisposes to serious thrombotic complications, including Budd-Chiari syndrome.

Essential Thrombocytosis

Although the clonality of essential thrombocytosis is expressed in the erythroid, myeloid, and megakaryocytic lineages, it is expansion of the megakaryocytes that determines the presentation.

Most patients with thrombocytosis are asymptomatic. Those with symptoms have headache, dizziness, or visual disturbances. They may also have skin and mucous membrane bleeding, spontaneous bruising, and erythromelalgia. Despite platelet counts in the millions, bleeding is far more common than thrombotic events. Many patients have splenomegaly. The peripheral smear may show a mild neutrophilic leukocytosis and large platelets. Diagnosis rests on exclusion of the other myeloproliferative states and secondary thrombocytosis.

Asymptomatic patients do not need treatment. Erythromelalgia often responds to low-dose aspirin. The platelet count should be lowered with hydroxyurea if the patient bleeds or is facing surgery.

Idiopathic Myelofibrosis

Although "myelofibrosis" describes a pathophysiologic process, idiopathic myelofibrosis is a stem cell disorder defined by progressive, severe fibrosis of the bone marrow and consequent extramedullary hematopoiesis. Though a dominant feature of the illness, the fibrosis is a secondary phenomenon, since the clonality does not extend to the fibroblasts.

Idiopathic myelofibrosis develops de novo or evolves from a preexisting myeloproliferative process. Patients report weight loss, fatigue, weakness, dyspnea, and, occasionally, bone pain. Two-thirds of patients have hepa-

Table 11.8–4. Differential diagnosis of massive splenomegaly.

Myelofibrosis
Chronic myelogenous leukemia
Schistosomiasis
Malaria
Leishmaniasis
Lymphoma

tomegaly; virtually all have splenomegaly. Idiopathic myelofibrosis is one of relatively few diseases that can cause massive splenomegaly (Table 11.8–4). Splenomegaly can become so pronounced that patients complain of abdominal fullness or early satiety.

Diagnosis rests on finding fibrosis on bone marrow biopsy and excluding other states that can produce marrow fibrosis, such as metastatic carcinoma and disseminated tuberculosis. The peripheral smear shows teardrop forms, nucleated red cells, and a left shift of the myeloid series. Most patients have a neutrophilic leukocytosis, with the total count usually below 40,000 cells/μL. Platelets may be increased or mildly decreased. Anemia can result from increased plasma volume or ineffective erythropoiesis.

The mainstay of therapy is supportive care. Painful splenic infarcts or symptomatic splenic enlargement can be managed with either local radiation or chemotherapy. A trial of corticosteroids is warranted for patients who have antibodies to red cells or platelets. Patients tend to live with their disease for a long time. Those with rapid progression develop fever, weight loss, severe anemia, and multiple cytogenetic abnormalities.

LEUKEMIA

Acute Leukemias

Advances in general medical care, transfusion practices, and chemotherapy have transformed what were once rapidly fatal ("acute") illnesses to processes that are remittable and sometimes curable. Acute leukemias are clonal proliferations of stem cells with very little maturation and differentiation, corresponding to an arrested stage of development within either the lymphoid or the myeloid lineages. The acute leukemias are classified into acute myelogenous leukemia and acute lymphocytic leukemia. Both diseases are subclassified according to their morphologic features, cytochemical properties, immunologic reactivity patterns, and chromosome analysis.

Risk factors for these illnesses are exposures to ionizing radiation, benzene, and certain chemotherapeutic drugs. As with most cancers, the incidence of acute leukemia increases with age; affected children are more likely to develop the lymphocytic than the myelogenous form. Although genetic factors are not generally regarded as adding much to the risk of acquiring leukemia, the risk is substantially increased by trisomy 21 (Down's syndrome), Fanconi's anemia, Bloom syndrome, and ataxia-telangiectasia. The myelodysplastic states, myeloproliferative disorders, and chronic myelogenous leukemia can progress to either form of acute leukemia.

The clinical presentations of acute leukemia depend to some extent on the patient's age. Children and young adults typically have an abrupt onset of fever, lethargy, headache, and often pain in the back and legs. Many of the elderly have a slowly progressive onset marked by lethargy, anorexia, and dyspnea that can predate the diagnosis by months. Most patients present with nonspecific manifestations of anemia or thrombocytopenia. More specific to leukemia are symptoms and signs produced by leukemic cell invasion that causes gingival hyperplasia, rashes, or cranial nerve palsies. Acute lymphocytic leukemia is more likely than acute myelogenous leukemia to produce lymphadenopathy and splenomegaly.

Bone marrow aspirate and biopsy are required to confirm acute leukemia. The peripheral blood smear often shows a normochromic, normocytic anemia and thrombocytopenia. Although typical white blood cell counts are well above the normal range, some leukemias present with either normal or low white cell counts. The peripheral blood of patients with acute leukemia may contain any number of blast cells; the criterion for the diagnosis is that blasts comprise 30% of nucleated cells in the bone marrow. Auer rods (see Color Plates) in the blasts' cytoplasm signify myeloid lineage; further classification is based on immunohistochemical stains, chromosome analysis, and flow cytometry.

The natural course of acute leukemia is fulminant. Patients require urgent treatment of very high blast cell counts to reduce the risk of leukostasis in the microcirculation of the brain, lungs, heart, and kidneys. Treatment for acute leukemia begins with remission-inducing ("induction") chemotherapy, in which the majority of leukemic cells are eradicated and normal hematopoiesis resumes, followed by "consolidation therapy" to destroy any remaining leukemic cells. For patients who have acute lymphocytic leukemia, many physicians treat further with maintenance therapy to help destroy resistant cells. Specific drugs, duration of therapy, and central nervous system prophylaxis vary according to type of disease, patient age, and other drugs used.

Prognosis in acute leukemia depends on multiple factors. Risk of relapse increases with older age and a high white blood cell count at the time of diagnosis. Acute lymphocytic leukemia carries a good outlook in children but a poor outlook in adults. In acute myelogenous leukemia, very low platelet counts at diagnosis, absence of Auer rods, concomitant medical problems, and certain cytogenetic abnormalities darken the prognosis.

Chronic Leukemias

Chronic Myelogenous Leukemia: Chronic myelogenous leukemia is a clonal disorder involving the myeloid, megakaryocytic, and erythroid lineages. Frequently classified as a myeloproliferative disorder because of a benign early course characterized by overproduction of mature cells, chronic myelogenous leukemia is distinguished by its unique chromosome translocation and its inevitable transformation into acute leukemia. The pathognomonic Philadelphia chromosome is chromosome 22 after a translocation with chromosome 9. In this exchange, the breakpoint cluster region (*bcr*) on chromosome 9 moves to the c-*abl* oncogene on chromosome 22, forming a hybrid *bcr-abl* oncogene. This oncogene encodes a fusion tyrosine kinase that has increased activity and causes abnormal proliferation of hematopoietic cells.

Although chronic myelogenous leukemia affects people of many ages, it presents most often in young to middle-aged adults. The disease is strongly associated with exposure to ionizing radiation, but not with chemical exposures or familial factors. Symptoms usually develop gradually and are nonspecific; they often include fatigue, anorexia, weight loss, and excessive sweating. Most patients have splenomegaly at the time of diagnosis.

The peripheral blood smear reveals a normochromic, normocytic anemia; thrombocytosis; and a leukocytosis comprising granulocytes at all stages of maturation, with many basophils and eosinophils. This picture is often confused with the leukemoid reaction (leukocyte count over 50,000/μL) secondary to inflammatory processes, but these two types of leukocytosis have a number of distinguishing features (Table 11.8–5).

The natural history of chronic myelogenous leukemia usually has three phases: chronic, accelerated, and acute. During the chronic phase, granulocytes mature and peripheral blasts account for less than 10% of the differential. The bone marrow is hypercellular, with an increase in granulocytes compared to the erythroid and megakaryocytic elements. Definitive diagnosis is possible via both chromosome analysis (which reveals the Philadelphia chromosome in 90% of patients with the disease) and Southern blot or polymerase chain reaction analyses (which detect the gene rearrangements in nearly all patients).

Most patients enter an unpredictable accelerated phase in which the blasts increase to 15% or more of the differ-

Table 11.8–5. Features distinguishing chronic myelogenous leukemia from the leukemoid reaction.

	Chronic Myelogenous Leukemia	Leukemoid Reaction
Leukocytes >100,000/μL	Common	Unusual
Leukocyte alkaline phosphatase	Low	High
Basophilia	Common	Unusual
Philadelphia chromosome	Yes	No
bcr-abl gene rearrangement	Yes	No
Splenomegaly	Common	Unusual
Clinical course	Requires treatment	Resolves spontaneously

ential, the spleen enlarges quickly, weight loss accelerates, and anemia worsens or thrombocytopenia develops. The accelerated phase may last for 1 year or longer. Finally, the acute phase—the "blast crisis" of chronic myelogenous leukemia—is heralded by a quickly rising white blood cell count with a preponderance of blast forms that constitute at least 30% of the cells in the blood and bone marrow. The blast crisis is typically resistant to chemotherapy protocols that are effective in de novo acute lymphocytic or acute myelogenous leukemia.

Treatment with busulfan or hydroxyurea easily controls the white blood cell count and spleen size during the chronic phase; patients treated with these agents survive a median of 3–5 years. Poor prognostic factors include black race, older age, symptoms at diagnosis, hepatomegaly, and splenomegaly. Interferon-α has been shown to induce remission of the Philadelphia chromosome in many patients, but better long-term survival has not yet been shown. Younger patients should be evaluated for bone marrow transplant while they are in the chronic phase.

Chronic Lymphocytic Leukemia: The most prevalent of all leukemias, chronic lymphocytic leukemia is a clonal expansion of lymphocytes. The incidence increases with advancing age; rarely are patients younger than 30. The disease is nearly twice as common in men as women. Unlike the other leukemias, chronic lymphocytic leukemia is not associated with radiation, chemotherapeutic drugs, or benzene exposure. A genetic component is supported by a high rate of lymphoproliferative disorders among patients' relatives. Although both B- and T-lineage chronic lymphocytic leukemias exist, the T-cell form is uncommon and will not be addressed here.

B-cell chronic lymphocytic leukemia, accounting for 95% of all chronic lymphocytic leukemia, is the most prevalent lymphoproliferative disorder in older adults. Like other well-differentiated lymphoproliferative processes, this disease has a slow, often harmless course, combined with a firm resistance to cure. The clinical manifestations are peripheral lymphocytosis and extensive lymphocytic invasion of the bone marrow, liver, spleen, and lymph nodes.

Although many patients are asymptomatic, some complain of weakness, fatigue, or enlarged superficial lymph nodes. Because of their deranged immune system, patients may come to diagnosis after presenting with recurrent infections, particularly bronchitis or pneumonia. Common physical findings are splenomegaly and cervical and supraclavicular adenopathy.

Diagnosis can begin and end with the peripheral blood smear. Mature small lymphocytes constitute most of the leukocytosis, which can run into the millions without causing ill effects. Smudge cells (lymphocytes destroyed by the mechanics of processing the blood smear) (see Figure 11.7–1) litter the fields and are considered pathognomonic. Though not essential for diagnosis, bone marrow exam reveals a diffuse or patchy lymphocytic infiltration. Virtually no other process produces a lymphocytosis of this magnitude and morphology. Old blood counts usually confirm a lymphocytosis, thus sealing the diagnosis.

The course of chronic lymphocytic leukemia is less homogeneous than the morphology of its cell line. Staging classifications cite organomegaly or lymphadenopathy as marking intermediate disease, and anemia or thrombocytopenia as marking advanced disease, but clinical progression within each stage is individual. Generally, the genotype and phenotype remain stable; transformation to a prolymphocytic leukemia is uncommon, to diffuse lymphoma (Richter's syndrome) even less so, and to acute lymphocytic leukemia rare. Patients may develop hypogammaglobulinemia and progressive anemia and thrombocytopenia, as well as autoimmune hemolytic anemia and autoimmune thrombocytopenia.

Treating patients with chronic lymphocytic leukemia during the early phase of B-cell chronic lymphocytic leukemia does not improve long-term survival. Chemotherapy should be used only to reduce bulky adenopathy or splenomegaly or to control anemia or thrombocytopenia. Otherwise, the lymphocyte count should not be reduced, because the cells are far less harmful than any chemotherapeutic drug.

Hairy Cell Leukemia: Unusual morphology and encouraging therapeutic options characterize hairy cell leukemia. Also of B-cell origin, this chronic leukemia usually affects men. Classically, it presents in middle age with splenomegaly and pancytopenia; peripheral lymphadenopathy and leukocytosis are uncommon. Patients may also come to attention through bleeding or infection related to cytopenias.

Diagnosis rests on the unusual morphology and cytochemical properties of the leukemic clone. Hairy cells, named for their long cytoplasmic projections, are seen on the peripheral smear and bone marrow, and stain positively with tartrate-resistant acid phosphatase.

Patients are treated for severe cytopenias and splenomegaly, or for weight loss or fatigue. Treatment with splenectomy or alpha interferon, which benefited many patients, has now been supplanted by chemotherapy with 2-chlorodeoxyadenosine or 2′-deoxycoformycin (pentostatin), which produces a complete remission in most of the patients treated.

SUMMARY

▶ Hematopoietic stem cell disorders encompass a wide variety of illnesses, from acute, fulminating processes to chronic, indolent diseases.

▶ Despite their different pathophysiologies, the stem cell disorders cause peripheral blood count abnormalities that may produce similar clinical presentations.

▶ Highly mature clonal expansions, such as those found in polycythemia vera and chronic lymphocytic leukemia, produce more indolent but less curable illnesses than the immature clones characteristic of the acute leukemias.

▶ The patient's age determines much about the presentation, natural history, and treatment options for a particular stem cell disorder.

SUGGESTED READING

Dang CV: Myelodysplastic syndrome. JAMA 1992;267:2077.

Grignani F et al: Acute promyelocytic leukemia: From genetics to treatment. Blood 1994;83:10.

Hoffman R et al: *Hematology: Basic Principles and Practice,* 2nd ed. Churchill Livingstone, 1995.

Quaglino D, Hayhoe FGJ: *Haematological Oncology Clinical Practice.* Churchill Livingstone, 1992.

Williams WJ et al: *Hematology,* 5th ed. McGraw-Hill, 1995.

11.9

Bleeding Disorders

William R. Bell, MD

Patients with hemorrhagic disorders present with excessive or repetitive episodes of bleeding or bleeding at unusual sites. Prolonged and frequent epistaxis or gingival bleeding, menorrhagia, frank gastrointestinal hemorrhage, excessive bleeding after a tooth extraction, purpura, and bleeding into joints are situations in which the physician should consider an acquired or inherited disorder of the coagulation system. With mild forms of these diseases, the problem may be suspected when unexpectedly large volumes of blood are lost after trauma or with surgery.

The bleeding disorders can be conveniently classified as either congenital or acquired, based on etiology. Congenitally inherited abnormalities of vascular integrity, platelet function, coagulation, and fibrinolytic systems are usually single defects confined to one of these four systems. In contrast, acquired hemostatic defects more commonly result from combined disturbances of those four systems. However, both congenital and acquired defects in platelets, coagulation, or fibrinolytic functions can manifest similar symptoms. Family history and previous medical records are frequently helpful in making the distinction.

PATHOPHYSIOLOGY OF HEMOSTASIS

When a blood vessel is severed, the first response is vasoconstriction. Then, in a sequential manner, platelets, electrostatic charge, endothelial cell membranes, and circulating procoagulant glycoproteins all act cooperatively to form a hemostatic plug, preventing escape of additional blood.

In a process regulated by thrombopoietin, circulating blood platelets originate as fragments of disintegrating megakaryocytes in the bone marrow. Platelets normally have a circulating life span of 10 ± 1.5 days as anucleate structures 2–3 μm in diameter. Two-thirds of the functioning platelets are in the circulating blood and exchange with one-third that resides in the spleen. An oil immersion microscopic field of normal blood should show three to eight platelets.

When a blood vessel is injured, the alteration in endothelial membrane surface composition and charge promotes platelet adherence, cohesion, and the platelet release reaction. As platelets undergo release, the liberated substances such as adenosine diphosphate (ADP), serotonin, Ca^{2+}, K^+, platelet factors III and IV, and other biogenic amines amplify aggregation, maintain vasoconstriction, and initiate the process of coagulation.

The phenomenon of coagulation is one of proteolytic processing of inert compounds in the circulating blood to become activated, ultimately resulting in an irreversible insoluble fibrin coagulum. The process requires the integrated interaction between many different glycoproteins, proteases, phospholipids, cell membrane surfaces, and Ca^{2+}. The cooperative integration of these systems maintains vascular integrity and preserves hemostasis.

As a sequel to formation of the hemostatic plug, it is necessary that the fibrin net-like structure be removed to maintain normal vascular luminal size and permit adequate blood flow. This is accomplished by the proteolytic enzyme plasmin, which is derived by activation of the inert precursor plasminogen (synthesized by the hepatocyte) by a variety of substances present in the blood and extravascular tissues. The activity of the fibrinolytic system is modulated by 14 naturally occurring substances that circulate in the blood.

EVALUATION OF PATIENTS WITH HEMORRHAGIC DISEASE

Patient History

The patient must be questioned as to whether the problem of bleeding has been lifelong, which suggests a congenital disorder, or is of recent onset, which suggests an acquired disorder. Is the bleeding spontaneous or is trauma required for the bleeding to begin? Spontaneous bleeding without associated trauma suggests a hemorrhagic disorder. Inquire about excess bleeding with surgery (including dental extractions and tonsillectomy) and major or minor trauma. Nevertheless, not all surgical procedures uncover a bleeding disorder, and patients asymptomatically may acquire a hemorrhagic disease following their last surgical procedure.

Bleeding in the patient with cancer may result from the primary disease process, the therapy received to treat the neoplasm, or from associated diseases, infection, metabolic disorders, and nutritional deficiencies that are common in these patients. Bleeding resulting from vascular defects (eg, arteriovenous malformations) or platelet disorders usually occurs immediately after an inciting event such as trauma or surgery. In contrast, persons with congenital disorders of coagulation usually have excessive bleeding that is delayed by several hours or days.

Determine whether the patient has required transfusion of blood resulting from substantial blood loss and, if so, whether the bleeding ceased with transfusion. Resolution of bleeding with transfusion suggests disorders of coagulation deficiency. Was the bleeding localized, or confined to an area of trauma or surgery (suggesting a vascular defect)? Is the same site recurrently involved (suggesting a vascular defect), or is the bleeding widespread and migratory (suggesting a coagulation, platelet function, or fibrinolytic system defect)? An excessive time required for the indurated ecchymoses or purpura to clear without intervention, and the occurrence of delayed bleeding, suggest coagulation factor abnormalities (Table 11.9–1).

The site and type of bleeding (skin, mucous membrane, articular, periarticular, subcutaneous soft tissue, gastrointestinal, genitourinary, central nervous system) must be ascertained. Cutaneous petechiae and spontaneous mucous membrane bleeding suggest a vascular or platelet disorder. Hemarthroses are common in congenital disorders of blood coagulation (eg, hemophilia A), but are not seen in disorders of platelets. Simultaneous bleeding from multiple nonadjacent sites is most consistent with concomitant disorders of coagulation proteins, platelets, and vascular integrity such as seen in patients with disseminated intravascular coagulation or thrombotic thrombocytopenic purpura.

Most acquired hemostatic defects are associated with underlying systemic illness. Symptoms suggesting disorders of the liver, kidneys, collagen vascular system, and immune system should be sought. Abnormal bleeding may be a feature of neoplasia, infections, malabsorption,

shock, and certain complications of obstetrics such as abruptio placentae. Particular attention should be directed at a detailed history of drug intake. Direct questioning regarding use of over-the-counter compounds containing aspirin is important. Certain antibiotics may alter platelet function and adversely affect coagulation proteins. Bleeding due to surreptitious use of anticoagulants has been observed, most often in persons working in medically related occupations.

Family History

A detailed family history often is helpful by facilitating the correct diagnosis. At times, it confirms the diagnosis suggested by personal history and laboratory data. Make certain that the persons designated by the patient are actually biologic family members. If a potentially heritable bleeding disorder is found in a patient, all available blood relatives should be evaluated.

When taking a family history, knowledge of the inheritance patterns of the known hemostatic defects is essential. The most common inherited coagulation factor deficiency states involve factors VIII and IX. Factor VIII deficiency is found in two distinctly different disorders: hemophilia A (classic hemophilia) and von Willebrand's disease. Factor IX deficiency is also known as hemophilia B (Christmas disease). Of all known congenital coagulation deficiency states, only hemophilia A and hemophilia B are X-linked recessively inherited. Von Willebrand's disease is actually a spectrum of six different categories and is inherited most frequently in an autosomal dominant pattern. An autosomal dominant pattern also is observed in hereditary hemorrhagic telangiectasia, some qualitative platelet defects, dysfibrinogenemia, and congenital multiple factor deficiency states. Deficiencies of factors I, II, V, VII, X, XI, XII, prekallikrein, and high molecular weight kininogen are inherited in an autosomal recessive fashion. Usually, carriers and relatives of affected persons possess a level of about 35–50% of normal of the deficient factor. A negative family history does not eliminate the possibility of a congenital factor deficiency state because about 20–30% of newly recognized factor deficiency states appear to result from spontaneous mutations.

Physical Examination

Particular attention should be given to the site and type of bleeding. Thrombocytopenia, platelet dysfunction, and some vascular defects characteristically cause cutaneous and mucous membrane bleeding in the form of petechiae (red punctate lesions) and purpura. When these lesions progress, they become confluent and are designated as purpura. Purpura are macular, nontender, nonpruritic, and without erythematous borders, in contrast to allergic reactions. Ecchymoses (bruises) may be associated with any defect of hemostasis, but hematoma formation of cutaneous, subcutaneous, or deeper body tissues or organs is characteristic of disorders of coagulation, especially coagulation factor deficiency states.

The diagnosis of hereditary hemorrhagic telangiectasia

Table 11.9–1. Clinical features in coagulation disorders.

Platelet abnormalities
  Petechiae
  Purpura
  Mucous membrane bleeding
  Prolonged bleeding

Coagulation factor abnormalities
  Hemarthrosis
  Ecchymoses
  Prolonged bleeding

Fibrinolytic system abnormalities
  Ecchymoses
  Mucous membrane bleeding
  Prolonged bleeding with skin injury (eg, venipuncture)

and cavernous hemangioma often can be made when telangiectatic or localized hemangiomatous lesions are identified. Telangiectatic lesions, which blanch on pressure, should not be confused with petechiae, which do not blanch. Spontaneous hemarthroses are virtually diagnostic of congenital deficiency of a coagulation factor (ie, factor VIII or IX). A detailed exam for lymphadenopathy, splenomegaly, ascites, and other features of hepatic or renal disorders may provide useful clues to an underlying disorder.

Laboratory Tests

Although the history and physical exam are the most helpful and reproducibly reliable screening techniques for hemorrhagic diseases, laboratory tests are indicated in the comprehensive approach to identify a patient at risk of bleeding (Table 11.9–2).

The initial assessment of a bleeding disorder should include the following tests:

1. Platelet count and examination of peripheral blood film prepared with blood obtained directly from finger puncture to verify the platelet count and to evaluate red cell, white cell, and platelet morphology.
2. Bleeding time—using any of several different protocols—performed in a standardized manner by an experienced person to provide information regarding platelet function and blood vessels, as does a tourniquet test.
3. Prothrombin time (PT) to evaluate factors II, V, VII, and X.
4. Partial thromboplastin time (PTT) or activated partial thromboplastin time (APTT) to evaluate all the coagulation proteins and their interaction except factors VII and XIII. The test is most sensitive for factors VIII, IX, XI, and XII.
5. Thrombin clotting time (TT) to provide information on the interaction of thrombin and fibrinogen and the amount of fibrinogen.
6. Test for a circulating anticoagulant if either the PT or the APTT/PTT is prolonged.

If the above-mentioned studies do not allow precise identification of the problem, individual specific coagulation factor assays and additional special studies may be required. Hemophilia A and hemophilia B can be separated from each other only by laboratory testing. This separation is crucial because the treatment for each condition is different.

BLEEDING CAUSED BY VASCULAR DEFECTS

Vascular defects resulting in purpura without serious hemorrhage are common. Conditions or substances that result in vessel wall or endothelial damage include drugs (direct toxic damage to endothelium), scurvy (defective hydroxyproline synthesis in absence of vitamin C), infections (inducing vascular wall and endothelial cell disruption from vasculitis), Cushing's syndrome (protein wasting with excessive cortisol), Henoch-Schönlein purpura (IgA and complement disrupting the vessel wall), amyloidosis (deposition of amyloid disrupting vessel wall), simple purpura (cause unknown), senile purpura (excess estrogen in blood), Osler-Weber-Rendu (hereditary hemorrhagic telangiectasia), multiple myeloma, and heritable disorders of connective tissue in which blood loss is secondary to defects in supporting connective tissue (fibronectin) including Ehlers-Danlos syndrome, pseudoxanthoma elasticum, Marfan's syndrome, and osteogenesis imperfecta.

BLEEDING CAUSED BY THROMBOCYTOPENIA

When the platelet count declines to less than 40,000/µL, be concerned about hemorrhage, particularly if trauma has occurred. Spontaneous bleeding may occur with a platelet count of less than 20,000/µL and is common with a count below 10,000 platelets/µL.

Thrombocytopenia can result from single or multiple causes such as impaired production, increased rate of destruction, distorted distribution (sequestration), or dilution (excessive intravascular volume). Because of technical limitations or clumping of platelets (which can falsely lower an automated platelet count), verify the finding of a reduced platelet count by examination of a peripheral blood smear prepared directly from blood obtained by finger puncture. The blood smear should not be prepared from anticoagulated blood.

Table 11.9–2. Most common causes of excessive or spontaneous bleeding.

Condition	Laboratory Test Results		
	PT	**APTT/PTT**	**Platelet Count**
Acquired thrombocytopenia	Normal	Normal	Decreased
Hemophilia A	Normal	Increased	Normal
Hemophilia B	Normal	Increased	Normal
Von Willebrand's disease	Normal	Increased	Normal
Hereditary hemorrhagic telangiectasia (Osler-Weber-Rendu disease)	Normal	Normal	Normal
Disseminated intravascular coagulation	Increased	Increased	Decreased
Henoch-Schönlein purpura	Normal	Normal	Normal
Anticoagulant therapy	Increased	Increased	Normal
Fibrinolytic therapy	Normal	Normal	Normal

PT, prothrombin time; APTT, activated partial thromboplastin time; PTT, partial thromboplastin time.

Decreased Production of Platelets

Any mechanism that prevents the normal intramedullary maturation, development, and release of platelets from megakaryocytic cytoplasm results in thrombocytopenia. This may occur in association with damage by chemicals (drugs or toxins), radiation, primary or metastatic neoplasms, infections, and congenital disorders. Generally, when thrombopoiesis is impaired, platelet survival in the peripheral blood is normal.

Decreased Platelet Survival

Platelets may be released normally from the bone narrow but prematurely destroyed in the circulation. This most commonly results from spontaneous autoantibody-mediated platelet destruction, frequently induced by drugs or neoplasms. Quinidine, quinine, sulfonamides, and thiazides are the most common offenders. In addition to their abilities to induce antibodies, some drugs can directly damage the circulating platelets or marrow megakaryocyte.

Drug-Induced Platelet Damage: Whenever petechiae and purpuric lesions of the skin or mucous membranes are encountered and the platelet count is low, the patient must be questioned about the use of medications. The immunologic reaction that induces antibody and decreases platelet survival usually involves the drug or a metabolite acting as a hapten and forming a plasma protein complex that is antigenic. In other cases, the drug-carrier protein (antigen)-antibody complex may be adsorbed nonspecifically onto the platelet, which then results in prompt removal by the reticuloendothelial system. Laboratory tests to identify whether or which drug is responsible for thrombocytopenia are difficult to perform and seldom reliable. Some drugs can induce purpura without associated thrombocytopenia.

Management of thrombocytopenia mandates immediate discontinuation of as many medications as possible. If thrombocytopenia persists for longer than 2 weeks in the absence of medications, marrow examination and marrow cell culture should be performed to determine another cause. Recovery from drug-induced thrombocytopenia may be longer if the patient has hepatic or renal insufficiency or if the offending agent is excreted slowly. To avoid a recurrence of thrombocytopenia, a suitable substitute drug should be found. Since the drug-induced antibody is specific, substitute an agent of similar therapeutic utility with a different molecular structure from that of the offending agent. Purposeful readministration of the suspicious agent to confirm the diagnosis is not advisable unless there is no possible alternative and the suspected medication is essential for the patient's survival. When drugs must be reinstituted, administer one agent at a time to identify the responsible drug.

Immune Thrombocytopenic Purpura: Immune thrombocytopenic purpura (ITP) is an illness with an immunologically mediated reduced platelet count, frequently appearing in a patient with no identifiable disease or exposure to medications. This disease occurs in two forms: acute and chronic.

Acute Immune Thrombocytopenic Purpura: Acute immune thrombocytopenic purpura is found most commonly in children, equally in females and males. Usually, an immediate antecedent upper respiratory viral, and occasionally bacterial, infection is found. The patient presents with the abrupt appearance of generalized skin and mucous membrane petechiae and purpura, frequently with gastrointestinal and genitourinary bleeding. The peripheral blood film shows vastly reduced platelets; the count is usually between 10,000 and 20,000/μL. Associated fever, eosinophilia, and mild lymphocytosis are observed frequently. The acute form of the disease is self-limited, with spontaneous remission occurring in 80–90% of patients within 2–6 weeks. Usually, acute immune thrombocytopenic purpura is not associated with other immune diseases. In a small proportion of patients, remission takes longer than 2 months. Treatment is required only when frank hemorrhage accompanies a platelet count of less than 20,000/μL, wherein a short course of corticosteroids in doses of 1–2 mg/kg should be given. Intravenous gamma globulin can be used on the rare occasions when corticosteroids are ineffective. If the platelet count does not normalize in 3–4 months, splenectomy may be considered. Platelet transfusions are not helpful since transfused platelets are eliminated from the circulation in minutes.

Chronic Immune Thrombocytopenic Purpura: This type of thrombocytopenia can begin at any age and is more common in women (10–50:1 female:male ratio) aged 20–45. Usually, an asymptomatic person observes petechial lesions in the skin or mucous membranes and seeks medical attention. Occasionally, the diagnosis is first considered when an unexpected low platelet count is identified at the time of an annual medical examination or other routine blood examination. The spleen is usually not enlarged, the platelet count is reduced to 25,000–75,000/μL, and marrow megakaryocytes are increased or normal in number. Occasionally in the adult, chronic immune thrombocytopenic purpura is a part of or coexists with other immune diseases such as lymphoproliferative disorders, connective tissue diseases, systemic lupus erythematosus, thyroid disease, or autoimmune hemolytic anemia (Evans' syndrome). The cause of the thrombocytopenia in chronic immune thrombocytopenic purpura is a spontaneously appearing antibody ("ITP factor"), which damages the platelets, facilitating removal from the circulation by the reticuloendothelial system. The antibody is usually an IgG (rarely IgM) antibody, can be adsorbed by normal platelets, and probably does not fix complement, although C3 may be present on some platelets in this illness.

The diagnosis of chronic immune thrombocytopenic purpura is largely one of exclusion. Only when all possible causal agents and diseases have been excluded can the diagnosis be made with certainty. Bone marrow examination reveals a cellular marrow with increased or normal numbers of megakaryocytes. The demonstration of antiplatelet IgG on the platelet surface may be helpful, but the assay techniques required are difficult. Furthermore, the specificity of these assays has been questioned.

The medical treatment of immune thrombocytopenic purpura may include corticosteroids, high-dose intravenous gamma globulin, and immunosuppressive agents, usually tried in that order. In the menstruating woman, anovulatory agents may be helpful. Danazol may be useful in treating older women with immune thrombocytopenic purpura. Splenectomy should be used as a last resort. About 10% of adults with chronic immune thrombocytopenic purpura spontaneously enter remission, usually within 12–18 months after diagnosis.

Thrombotic Thrombocytopenic Purpura: Thrombotic thrombocytopenic purpura (TTP) is a rare but often fatal disease process that occurs abruptly in previously healthy people. It is characterized by severe thrombocytopenia with purpura, severe hemolytic anemia, fever, central nervous system disturbances, and renal disease. It occurs more frequently in females. The hemolytic-uremic syndrome that occurs in children is identical with thrombotic thrombocytopenic purpura in the adult. No single feature or test is diagnostic. The diagnosis of thrombotic thrombocytopenic purpura is made only after identifiable causes have been eliminated. Most helpful in diagnosis is the peripheral blood smear that uniformly contains striking red cell fragmentation, marked polychromatophilia, nucleated, orthochromatic normoblastic red cells, normal white blood cells, and reduced platelets. The Coombs' test is negative. Many patients have disseminated intravascular coagulation. Recently, the combined use of corticosteroids, plasmapheresis, and plasma infusion has yielded complete remissions and permanent recovery in most patients.

Traumatic Platelet Destruction: Severe thrombocytopenia is frequently observed in patients with generalized infection. This may result from direct damage to the platelet membrane from exotoxins or endotoxins released from the microorganisms. Mechanical devices placed in the vascular system such as prosthetic heart valves, Teflon septal patches, or Dacron vascular bypass grafts can damage platelet membranes, resulting in platelet removal from the circulation.

Disseminated Intravascular Coagulation: Disseminated intravascular coagulation (DIC) is a pathologic condition characterized by frank generalized hemorrhage or a tendency to bleed, associated with a severe underlying systemic illness. Disseminated intravascular coagulation is not a primary disease process. The mechanism of disseminated intravascular coagulation is complex but involves the entrance of thrombin, thromboplastin, or thromboplastic-like substances into the circulation, which activate simultaneously the coagulation and fibrinolytic systems with destruction of platelets and activation of plasma clotting factors and activation of the plasminogen system. These foreign substances may be released by neoplastic or inflammatory cells; or, these cells may release a circulating substance that causes release of thromboplastin from white blood cells (monocytes). The diagnosis can be made with appropriate laboratory studies that characteristically reveal severe thrombocytopenia, abnormal blood clot formation in a glass tube, fragmented circulating red blood cells, hypofibrinogenemia, prolonged APTT, and excessive quantities of fibrinogen-fibrin degradation products in the blood.

The fibrinogen level is reduced below baseline, but the patient may have had initial fibrinogen levels above the normal range because fibrinogen is an acute phase reactant, which increases in disorders with inflammation and neoplasms. Therefore, the fibrinogen level reduced from baseline may initially remain within normal limits or may even be slightly high. Disseminated intravascular coagulation may accompany many diseases, but most commonly is seen in patients with generalized sepsis, neoplasms, cardiopulmonary arrest, severe trauma, liver disease, and complications of obstetrics such as retained fetus, abruptio placentae, placenta previa, and septic abortion.

Successful therapy for the patient with disseminated intravascular coagulation requires early recognition and vigorous treatment of the underlying disease process. If this can be accomplished, disseminated intravascular coagulation is quickly brought under control and then disappears. The use of heparin is controversial and in reported studies has not reduced mortality. The exception is disseminated intravascular coagulation associated with malignancy (Trousseau's syndrome) in which heparin is frequently essential to sustain life.

Sequestration of Platelets

Abnormal distribution of platelets within the body is seen in patients with hypersplenism (overactive reticuloendothelial system in the spleen) and frequently gives rise to a modest reduction in the peripheral blood platelet count to 50,000–80,000/μL. Normally, about 30% of the total body platelet mass resides in the spleen; the remainder is circulating in the blood. In sequestration (hypersplenism), this distribution is reversed, with 65–75% of platelets residing in the spleen. Modest leukopenia and anemia are usually present concomitantly. Hemorrhage is unusual. The bone marrow is characteristically normal. Platelet survival is normal with a prolonged splenic transit time.

Surgery can usually be accomplished without platelet transfusions. Splenectomy may be followed by restoration of the platelet count to near-normal levels, but is rarely indicated in this disorder.

Dilution of Platelets

When patients are given excessive volume of any fluids, including blood or any of its components, they can develop thrombocytopenia with platelet counts down to 50,000/μL. Frequently, simultaneous reductions in serum electrolytes are found. In addition, copious whole blood transfusions may temporarily depress bone marrow function. Treatment consists of fluid restriction and gentle diuresis. Platelet transfusions are not indicated.

BLEEDING CAUSED BY DEFECTIVE PLATELET FUNCTION

Bleeding may occur even when the circulating platelet numbers are in the normal range if the platelets are qualitatively defective from congenital or acquired abnormalities.

Congenital Disorders

Glanzmann's Disease (Thrombasthenia): This autosomal recessive disorder is characterized by a normal platelet count, prolonged bleeding time, abnormal to absent clot retraction, and failure of platelet aggregation to ADP, epinephrine, collagen, thrombin, and arachidonic acid. Thus far, deficiencies of the platelet glycoprotein heterodimer IIb–IIIa, the fibrinogen binding receptor, have been identified in this disorder. If local hemostatic measures fail to stop bleeding, platelet transfusions may be necessary. Platelet transfusions, however, generate platelet antibodies that can substantially reduce platelet survival with subsequent transfusion. Therefore, patients with Glanzmann's disease should receive platelet transfusion only for serious bleeding.

Bernard-Soulier Syndrome: A rare autosomal recessive bleeding disorder, Bernard-Soulier syndrome is characterized by giant vacuolated platelets in the peripheral blood, prolonged bleeding time, abnormal prothrombin consumption test, abnormal aggregation to ristocetin, impaired platelet factor III binding, and deficient membrane glycoproteins Ib and Ig. Spontaneous bleeding may be life-threatening. Platelet transfusions may provide some temporary benefit but also generate platelet antibodies.

Acquired Disorders

Acquired platelet dysfunction is observed in a variety of illnesses, including myeloproliferative diseases, uremia, alcoholism, postcardiopulmonary bypass, dysproteinemias, and vitamins C and B_{12} deficiencies, as well as during the use of certain drugs. Probably the most common cause of platelet dysfunction is ingestion of aspirin or other nonsteroidal anti-inflammatory drugs. In patients with uremia, the bleeding time is prolonged in association with abnormal platelet adhesion, aggregation, and factor III release. These platelet defects may be corrected by dialysis or sometimes by infusion of fresh frozen plasma or cryoprecipitate.

Hemorrhage is frequently associated with dysproteinemic states, including Waldenström's macroglobulinemia, heavy-chain disease, μ-chain disease, or multiple myeloma (Chapter 12.7). In these diseases, the bleeding results from the platelet membrane becoming coated with the protein (thus rendering the platelet nonfunctional), increased blood viscosity, reduction in coagulation proteins, a circulating anticoagulant, or a combination of these abnormalities.

BLEEDING CAUSED BY COAGULATION PROTEIN DEFECTS

Hemorrhage associated with disorders of coagulation results from a deficiency or dysfunctional property of one or more of the plasma glycoproteins essential for normal blood coagulation or because of a circulating anticoagulant (antibody), which prevents normal interaction of these plasma proteins.

Factor VII Deficiency

Factor VII deficiency is an uncommon autosomal recessive coagulopathy associated with both abnormal bleeding and thrombotic tendencies. Homozygotes usually have less than 10% of normal factor VII activity and experience mild to severe symptoms, including hemarthroses. Heterozygotes demonstrate decreased factor VII levels but are asymptomatic. Deep venous thrombosis and pulmonary emboli have been reported in several affected homozygotes. In addition, there is a high frequency of factor VII deficiency in patients with Dubin-Johnson syndrome. Acquired factor VII deficiency is seen in the newborn, in patients on anticoagulation therapy with vitamin K antagonists, in hepatic disease patients, and in those with nutritional vitamin K depletion.

Factor VII deficiency affects the extrinsic system of clotting and is reflected by a prolonged PT with normal APTT, PTT, and TT. Immunologic detection of factor VII antigen has been described in several patients with absent biologic activity. Replacement therapy can be accomplished by infusion of stored plasma, fresh frozen plasma, or preparations of purified factor VII.

Factor VIII Deficiency

Factor VIII (antihemophilic factor, antihemophilic globin) is a circulating plasma coagulation factor composed of a large portion (called *factor VIII antigen* or von Willebrand factor or antigen) and a smaller portion (called *factor VIIIc*). Both components are required for normal function. The assay for factor VIII activity determines the functional level of the entire complex. Separate immunologic assays can detect factor VIII antigen or factor VIIIc independent of the functional activity of the proteins.

Factor VIII deficiency, classic hemophilia or hemophilia A, is inherited as an X-linked recessive disorder. It is the second most common severe congenital coagulopathy (after von Willebrand's disease). Factor VIII deficiency occurs in up to 20 of 100,000 male births. Although the disease usually clusters in families with a clear history of bleeding problems, almost one-third of cases result from a recent mutation, with no family history of a bleeding disorder. Because the severity of bleeding is related to the degree of factor VIII deficiency, hemophilia A is a heterogenous disease. Severely affected persons (factor VIII activity <1% of normal) experience repeated and often spontaneous hemorrhagic episodes. These hemorrhagic complications may become obvious shortly after birth and increase in severity and frequency with age and activity. These complications include hemarthroses (especially of the knees, elbows, hips, shoulders, and ankles), bleeding into subcutaneous and intramuscular compartments, epistaxis, intracranial bleeding, gingival bleeding, hematemesis, melena, and microscopic hematuria.

Hemophiliacs with less severe deficiencies of factor VIII activity (1–5% of normal) or mild deficiencies (5–25% of normal) rarely experience spontaneous hemorrhagic episodes, but may become symptomatic following trauma or surgery. In the absence of treatment or superimposed disease, the degree of factor VIII deficiency remains constant throughout the life of the affected person.

Hemophilia A should be suspected in any male who has unusual bleeding. It usually manifests as a prolonged APTT or PTT, unless the factor VIII activity is more than 20–30% of normal (Table 11.9–3). Whole blood clotting time is generally abnormal; PT, bleeding time, platelet count, and TT are normal. Specific assays for factor VIII activity and factor VIIIc indicate significant reductions, whereas the factor VIII antigen (von Willebrand factor), detected immunologically with heterologous antibody, is normal. Detection of female carriers of hemophilia is based on obtaining factor VIII activity intermediate to normal values. This activity serves as the numerator for a ratio constructed with the level of factor VIII antigen as the denominator. A result of less than 0.75 suggests the carrier state in family members of an established congenitally deficient patient. Although hemophilia A can occur in the daughters of a carrier female and an affected male, this is an exceedingly rare event. The diagnosis of hemophilia A in a female requires exclusion of von Willebrand's disease, a coagulopathy transmitted in an autosomal dominant manner.

The adequacy and promptness of replacement therapy in hemophilia A determine the subsequent morbidity and mortality of the disorder. For most superficial soft tissue injuries and hemarthroses, factor VIII activity should be raised to 10–20% of normal by means of fresh frozen plasma or cryoprecipitate. When factor VIII activity between 20% and 50% is required, as in major soft tissue or visceral bleeds and in minor surgical procedures, use of cryoprecipitate or lyophilized concentrates is recommended. For major surgery and documented or clinically suspected central nervous system hemorrhage, factor VIII activities of 50% are considered adequate; however, because of the great risks of intracerebral bleeding, replacement to concentrations of 100% should be attempted. This is achieved most promptly and efficiently with lyophilized concentrates.

In about 10–15% of severe hemophiliacs chronically exposed to factor VIII replacement therapy, circulating antibodies eventually develop to factor VIIIc, since it is perceived by the immune system as a foreign protein. Rarely, such antibodies have been detected in hemophilia A patients who never received transfusions. These antibodies inactivate infused factor VIII, but this inactivation can sometimes be overcome by infusions of cryoprecipitate or concentrate in high doses. When this approach fails, use of activated factors, plasmapheresis, and factor VIII concentrates of bovine or porcine origin should be considered.

Desmopressin (1-deamino-8-D-arginine vasopressin [dDAVP]) elevates factor VIII levels in plasma and is effective in treating many patients with mild or moderate hemophilia A. It increases factor VIII activity three- to fivefold in such patients, but those with severe factor VIII deficiency or circulating antibodies do not respond to desmopressin.

Von Willebrand's Disease

Von Willebrand's disease (deficiency of factor VIII antigen, designated vWF:Ag) is divided into six major types, each with several subtypes. This disease is typically characterized by nasal, sinus, gastrointestinal, and vaginal mucous membrane hemorrhage. Spontaneous hemarthroses and soft tissue bleeds are unusual.

Most patients inherit von Willebrand's disease in an autosomal dominant pattern. The degree of clinical symptomatology and laboratory abnormalities reflects heterozygous or homozygous inheritance patterns. Usually, the diagnosis is established in males and females who exhibit a mild or moderate bleeding disorder, with prolonged bleeding times and abnormal in vitro assays of factor VIII. Their family histories suggest that these are heterozygous defects. The homozygous disorder occurs much less frequently and manifests as severe bleeding and very low levels of von Willebrand factor.

Acquired von Willebrand's disease is a bleeding disorder seen in some patients who are afflicted with diseases including neoplasms, particularly lymphoma and leukemia, myeloproliferative disorders, connective tissue diseases, and dysglobulinemic states. The unique feature of some patients with this form of von Willebrand's disease is an inhibitor directed against one or more of the properties of factor VIII antigen. These patients do not experience an incremental response in circulating levels of factor VIII after transfusion of cryoprecipitate or factor VIII concentrate.

Infusion of fresh frozen plasma or cryoprecipitate corrects the defects of congenital von Willebrand's disease. Many patients respond very well to desmopressin. Specially prepared concentrates of the factor VIII antigen can also be used.

Table 11.9–3. Causes of prolonged activated partial thromboplastin time.

Hemophilia A
Hemophilia B
Von Willebrand's disease
Factor XI deficiency
Antiphospholipid antibodies
Antibodies to plasma coagulation factors
Factor XII deficiency (does not cause bleeding propensity)

Factor IX Deficiency

Congenital deficiency of factor IX (plasma thromboplastin component, Christmas factor) is known as Christmas disease or hemophilia B. It is clinically and genetically similar to hemophilia A, but it occurs less frequently. Homozygous females are rare, but symptoms may occur in females with X chromosome abnormalities such as Turner's syndrome (XO). Combined deficiencies of factors VIII and IX have been described. Hemophilia B appears to be a heterogenous group of disorders. The most common type is characterized by depressed levels of factor IX coagulant activity and normal factor IX antigen as detected by specific heterologous antibodies. Factor IX deficiency with absence of the factor IX antigen is associated with milder symptoms. A variant, designated hemophilia B$_m$, consists of an abnormal factor IX molecule that acts as a competitive inhibitor of factor VII. Plasma from B$_m$ patients manifests a prolonged APTT and PT (using bovine brain as a source of thromboplastin) despite normal levels of all coagulation factors except IX.

Factor IX levels in homozygous hemophilia B occasionally are not as depressed as factor VIII levels in hemophilia A. Activity of less than 1% of normal is less common in hemophilia B than in hemophilia A. Carriers are detected by their intermediate depressions of factor IX activity. Laboratory diagnosis of hemophilia B is a prolonged APTT and normal PT and TT. Bleeding times are usually normal. Specific factor IX assays reveal the deficiency.

Treatment of patients with hemophilia B is administration of fresh frozen plasma or prothrombin-complex concentrates. Circulating anticoagulants rarely develop. Factor IX is not present in cryoprecipitate.

Acquired factor IX deficiency occurs with administration of coumarin anticoagulants and in some patients with hepatic disease or nephrotic syndrome with proteinuria greater than 10 g/day. Combined factors IX and X deficiencies have been reported in patients with primary amyloidosis.

Circulating Anticoagulants

Acquired anticoagulants develop in three clinical situations:

1. In persons with congenital factor deficiencies (eg, factors VIII and IX) who develop antibodies to the deficient factor, usually after repeated exposure to replacement therapy. These antibodies inactivate transfused factors and increase the patient's risk of bleeding.
2. In previously healthy persons with no identifiable illness or in connection with other illnesses or associated with medications; the antibody is directed against a single coagulation factor, and those affected have excessive bleeding. Acquired anticoagulants are reported in disorders such as multiple myeloma, macroglobulinemia, asthma, ulcerative colitis, and autoimmune diseases. A curious unexplained anticoagulant of factor

VIII rarely develops postpartum. Factor VIII anticoagulants have been described with penicillin administration, and aminoglycosides have been implicated in the spontaneous development of factor V anticoagulants. An antibody against factor XIII has occurred in association with isoniazid. Drug-induced anticoagulants disappear with termination of the medication. When these antibodies are directed against factors VIII or IX, significant hemorrhage may occur, and some investigators suggest that corticosteroid plus immunosuppressive therapy should be instituted. Although the antibody may not disappear immediately, its activity may decrease.

3. In persons without preexisting coagulation abnormalities, characterized by the spontaneous appearance of antibodies that inactivate coagulation factors or interfere with the interaction of coagulation factors, platelets, or both. Although often termed "anticoagulants," this third group of antibodies is better termed "inhibitors" because they usually do not interfere with normal hemostasis. In fact, they are often associated with thrombosis (Chapter 11.10).

THE FIBRINOLYTIC SYSTEM

The central component of the fibrinolytic system is plasminogen, which is synthesized in the liver and circulates in the blood as an inert precursor or prozyme. Plasminogen is found in the euglobulin fraction of the blood in a concentration range of 12–25 mg/dL. The plasminogen-plasmin proteolytic enzyme system can be activated by proteins found in different body tissues: plasminogen activator (vascular endothelial cells), tissue activator (uterus, ovary, neoplasms), and urinary activator (renal parenchymal cells). The degree of normal fibrinolytic activity induced by these endogenous activators is minimal and inadequate to reverse thrombosis or cause bleeding.

Extremely rare inherited disorders of the plasminogen system have been recognized. Recurrent bleeding may result from excessive fibrinolysis caused by congenital absence of one or more of the 14 naturally occurring inhibitors of the plasminogen system (eg, α_2-antiplasmin, α_2-antitrypsin, α_2-macroglobulin). These deficiency states are inherited as autosomal recessive disorders. The treatment is fresh frozen plasma replacement of these missing components.

SUMMARY

▶ Prolonged bleeding or bleeding at unusual sites should raise suspicion of a bleeding disorder.

▶ The most helpful information in making the diagnosis of a bleeding disorder is a detailed personal and family history of bleeding.

▶ Mucous membrane and cutaneous petechial and purpuric lesions should signal quantitative and qualitative investigation of platelets and their function. Ecchymotic lesions suggest a disturbance of coagulation glycoproteins.

▶ Laboratory studies in patients with a suspected bleeding disorder should include platelet count, examination of peripheral blood smear, PT, APTT, and bleeding time. If any is abnormal, TT and assay of specific factor levels should be performed.

SUGGESTED READING

Furie B, Furie BC: Molecular basis of hemophilia. Semin Hematol 1990;27:270.

Furie B, Furie BC: The molecular basis of blood coagulation. Cell 1988;53:505.

Hoyer LW: Hemophilia A. N Engl J Med 1994;330:38.

Patthy L: Evolution of the proteases of blood coagulation and fibrinolysis by assembly from modules. Cell 1985;41:657.

Ruggeri ZM, Zimmerman TS: Von Willebrand factor and von Willebrand disease. Blood 1987;70:895.

Schafer AI: Approach to bleeding. In *Thrombosis and Hemorrhage.* Loscalzo J, Schafer AI (editors). Blackwell Scientific Publications, 1994.

11.10

Hypercoagulable States

William R. Bell, MD

A hypercoagulable condition should be suspected in a patient with a documented thrombotic disorder with the following presentations:

- Age below 40
- Venous thrombosis in neck, arms, abdomen, or central nervous system
- Recurrent thrombosis
- Family history of thrombosis
- Repeated thrombosis despite anticoagulation

When an otherwise healthy person younger than age 40 years has a venous or arterial thrombosis or when venous thrombosis occurs in an unusual site such as the neck, upper extremities, abdomen, or central nervous system, a hypercoagulable condition should be considered a possibility. Recurring thrombotic events or thrombosis in a patient who has a documented family history of thrombosis also merits evaluation for a hypercoagulable state. Repeated thrombosis despite therapeutic anticoagulation strongly suggests that the patient has a neoplasm with an associated hypercoagulable state. Whenever a hypercoagulable state is diagnosed, family members should be studied. In about 15–30% of all patients who present with thrombosis, some predisposing hypercoagulable condition can be recognized.

Disorders with hypercoagulability can be divided into two general categories. The first category encompasses inherited disorders for which specific defects of the natural anticoagulant mechanisms have been identified (Table 11.10–1). The second category is a heterogeneous array of diseases associated with an increased risk of thrombotic complications when compared with the risk of the general population. In contrast to the advances made in elucidating the congenital defects, the pathophysiologic mechanisms responsible for excessive coagulation in the second category have not been precisely identified.

In patients whose presentation raises the possibility of a hypercoagulable state, identification of the abnormalities usually requires a number of laboratory tests. An appropriate laboratory evaluation in this setting would include prothrombin time, activated partial thromboplastin time, Russell viper venom time, and measurement of plasma levels of fibrinogen, plasminogen, α_2-antiplasmin, and plasminogen activator inhibitor-1. One should also seek a circulating anticoagulant (Chapter 11.9), and the activity of proteins C and S and antithrombin III should be assessed. Finally, assay the patient's blood for resistance to activated protein C. Most of these tests require the expertise of a hematologist who is especially knowledgeable about these assays, the implications of the results, and the conditions that can cause hypercoagulable states.

CONGENITAL DEFECTS

The most common congenital defects leading to a hypercoagulable state are inherited in an autosomal dominant pattern with the exception of cystathionine β-synthase deficiency, which is inherited in an autosomal recessive pattern. The treatment for thrombosis in all these conditions is heparin or thrombolytic therapy, followed by oral anticoagulation, usually for prolonged periods, but not necessarily lifelong.

Antithrombin III Deficiency
Deficiency of antithrombin III (AT-III), a heparin-associated plasma protein of 56,500 daltons that inactivates the active forms of factors XII, XI, X, IX, and II and kallikrein, was first recognized in 1965 in a Norwegian family with repeated thrombotic events. Since then, numerous kindred and individuals have been identified. People with this deficiency experience repeated episodes of venous emboli (deep leg veins, iliofemoral, mesenteric, pulmonary) and rarely arterial thrombosis. Deficiency of antithrombin III rarely manifests before puberty, suggesting a hormonal influence in the expression. Three types of antithrombin III deficiency have been identified based on

Table 11.10–1. Inherited causes of hypercoagulable states.

Affected Component	Mechanism
Antithrombin III	Deficiency and dysfunction
Protein C	Deficiency and dysfunction
Factor V	Resistance to activated protein C by factor V
Protein S	Deficiency
Heparin cofactor II	Deficiency
Fibrinogenemia	Dysfunctional protein
Procoagulant factor	Deficiency
Cystathionine β-synthase	Deficiency
Plasminogen	Deficiency or dysfunctional protein
Plasminogen activator	Deficiency
Plasminogen activator inhibitor-1	Elevation

the binding characteristics of three portions of the molecule: biologic, immunologic, and heparin-binding.

Type I antithrombin III deficiency results from reduction in the synthesis of the protein. In those affected, there is equal reduction in the biologic, immunologic, and heparin-binding components of the molecule, which is attributable either to complete gene deletion or to nonsense mutations or base substitutions at splice sites. Type II results from a discrete molecular defect within the antithrombin III molecule where the biologic activity is reduced and the immunologic and heparin-binding domains are normal. Type III results from an intramolecular defect whereby the biologic and immunologic components are normal, but the heparin-binding domain is reduced or absent.

About 55% of biochemically affected patients of all three types of antithrombin deficiency experience thrombotic events. Heterozygote patients have antithrombin III levels of 25–55% of normal. The homozygous state is incompatible with life. Acquired antithrombin III deficiency may occur in the nephrotic syndrome, hepatic failure, or disseminated intravascular coagulation, or in association with oral contraceptives and L-asparaginase therapy.

Protein C Deficiency

A deficiency state of protein C, a two-chain vitamin K-dependent plasma glycoprotein of 62,000 daltons, was first reported in 1981. Since then, several kindred have been identified who have severe deficiency, with protein C blood concentrations of less than 1% of normal activity, and heterozygotes with levels of less than 50% of normal activity. Both groups show a high rate of venous thrombosis. Heterozygous deficiency of this glycoprotein has been observed in as many as 1 in 200 of otherwise healthy adults.

Two major types of protein C deficiency have been identified. Type I is characterized by a concomitant reduction in the biologic activity and immunologic concentration of protein C in the blood and results from gene deletion, gene insertion, or nonsense or missense point mutations. Type II is characterized by reduction of the bi-

ologic function of the protein, but normal concentrations when measured by an immunologic technique.

Acquired deficiency of protein C has been observed in patients with disseminated intravascular coagulation, acute leukemia, hepatic disease, warfarin anticoagulation, oral contraceptives, and elevated concentrations in the blood of protein C inhibitor. Protein C deficiency has been associated by some investigators with warfarin-induced soft tissue purpura and skin necrosis, but this association has not been confirmed by other investigators. Increased protein C levels have been observed in the nephrotic syndrome and renal transplantation.

In a patient with known protein C deficiency, warfarin anticoagulation (which may further reduce protein C levels) should be initiated only during concomitant heparin therapy. Therapeutic success in increasing the level of protein C in deficient persons has been reported with administration of danazol, desmopressin (dDAVP), stanozolol, purified protein C, and fresh frozen plasma.

Protein S Deficiency

A deficiency state of protein S, a single-chain vitamin K-dependent glycoprotein of 70,000 daltons, was first recognized in 1984 in patients with a striking history of recurrent venous thrombosis. Several families with this abnormality, associated with frequent and severe thrombotic events, have subsequently been recognized. Most affected individuals with clinical manifestations are heterozygotes with less than 40% of normal free protein S activity.

Protein S is synthesized by hepatocytes and endothelial cells under the direction of two genes on chromosome 3. It is stored in the α granule of platelets. In circulating blood, 60% of the total protein S is inert and noncovalently bound to C4b binding protein of the complement system. The remaining 40% is free and functionally interacts as a cofactor to protein C_a mediating the inhibitory effects on the coagulation system. Two types of free protein S deficiency have been identified. Type I is characterized by equal reduction in the biologically functional and immunologically reactive concentrations of protein S in the blood. Type II is recognized by decreased biologically functional activity with normal or increased immunologically reactive concentrations.

Acquired deficiency of free protein S has been observed in patients with hepatic disease, endothelial damage, disseminated intravascular coagulation, thrombotic thrombocytopenic purpura, and essential thrombocythemia, and in pregnant patients and during therapy with oral contraceptives, warfarin, and L-asparaginase.

Heparin Cofactor II Deficiency

Heparin cofactor II (HC II) is a heparin-associated plasma glycoprotein of 65,600 daltons, synthesized in the liver, which normally inhibits thrombin in the presence of heparin in a 1:1 complex. Deficiency of this glycoprotein to levels under 60% of normal has been identified in a few hundred patients. Heterozygotes are thought not to be at risk for venous thrombosis.

Acquired deficiency of heparin cofactor II has been observed in hepatic disease and disseminated intravascular coagulation. Heparin cofactor II levels are elevated in the nephrotic syndrome.

Dysfibrinogenemia

Qualitative abnormalities of the fibrinogen molecule associated with thrombotic disease were first reported in 1960. The dysfibrinogenemias are a heterogenous group of disorders that commonly are without any symptoms, but patients may experience hemorrhage and rarely thrombosis (both venous and arterial).

Acquired dysfibrinogenemia has been observed in patients with liver disease, hepatoma, and diabetes mellitus and during treatment with certain medications such as L-asparaginase.

Cystathionine β-Synthase Deficiency (Homocystinuria)

Cystathionine β-synthase deficiency, a rare disorder of transulfuration metabolism, is inherited as an autosomal recessive trait. The disease is characterized by mental retardation, ectopia lentis, skeletal abnormalities, and homocystinuria. Venous and arterial thromboembolism are a major cause of morbidity and mortality. This metabolic disorder results in sustained homocystinemia, which results in patchy venous and arterial endothelial cell damage and denudation with internal and medial fibrosis facilitating thrombosis inducing fatal myocardial, cerebral, renal, and pulmonary infarctions.

Treatment to reduce the frequency of thrombosis in patients with this deficiency is vitamin B_6, to which some of the patients will respond. Thrombus formation is treated with thrombolytic therapy, heparin, or both, followed by prolonged warfarin anticoagulation.

Disorders of the Fibrinolytic System

Inherited dysfunction of the plasminogen-plasmin proteolytic enzyme system is associated with thrombus formation. One kindred and a few individuals have been identified with dysplasminogenemia. Hypoplasminogenemia has been observed without any underlying illness and is associated with an increased frequency of venous thrombosis. A few families with increased thrombophilia have been detected with a severe deficiency of plasminogen activator. Despite stimuli, these patients cannot release tissue plasminogen activator from their endothelial cells. In other families, documented venous thrombosis has been observed in association with excessive plasma levels of plasminogen activator inhibitor-1 (PAI-1). In some patients, a strong correlation exists between plasminogen activator inhibitor-1 and elevated serum concentrations of triglycerides.

ACQUIRED HYPERCOAGULABLE STATES

The acquired hypercoagulable states consist of a diverse collection of diseases that have been associated with increased risk of thromboembolism. Although associated changes in plasma factors have been identified, specific causation has not been established.

Malignancy

The association between neoplastic disease and intravascular thrombus formation (Trousseau's syndrome) was recognized more than 100 years ago. The overall incidence of thrombus formation in patients with neoplastic disease is 5–15%. Patients with a neoplastic disease may have recurrent arterial or venous thromboembolic events or both, associated with nonbacterial endocarditis. In these patients, the neoplastic disease is sometimes difficult to identify antemortem. Even at postmortem examination tumor can be found, but the primary site frequently cannot be established. Trousseau's syndrome can be seen in association with any malignancy but is more commonly observed with neoplasms of the lung, stomach, colon, pancreas, ovaries, gallbladder and mucin-secreting tumors of all varieties. The thrombotic events may precede recognition of the neoplasm by several weeks or even many months. Recurrence of thrombotic events may occur despite therapeutic anticoagulation with warfarin. Frequently observed with Trousseau's syndrome is disseminated intravascular coagulopathy, which predisposes to simultaneous extensive hemorrhage (Chapter 11.9).

Pregnancy

An increased association of thrombotic events with the gravid state varies from 10–50% above the general population, particularly in the puerperium and the first month postpartum. A host of biochemical and hormonal changes that occur during the gravid state have been evaluated, but the precise etiology of the thrombosis remains unclear. In all pregnant patients, a significant increase, particularly in the third trimester, is found in fibrinogen and factors VII, VIII, IX, and XII, along with a decline in antithrombin III and a marked increase in plasminogen activator inhibitor-1, which depresses the activity of the fibrinolytic system. In several pregnant patients, a definite contributory problem is found to be congestion of the pelvis and direct compression by the gravid uterus of the large veins that normally return blood to the heart from the lower extremities. This compression directly predisposes to thrombus formation.

Heparin, since it does not cross the placenta, is the treatment of choice for thrombosis in pregnancy. Warfarin is teratogenic in the first trimester, and thrombolytic therapy has the potential for detaching the placenta.

Nephrotic Syndrome

Excessive loss of protein because of defects in the glomerular filtration apparatus is associated not only with renal vein thrombosis, but also systemic thrombotic events. Depending on the physical size of the glomerular defect, it is possible that almost any of the coagulation proteins or natural inhibitors may be lost into the urine. The effect of inhibitor loss appears to exceed the effect of coagulation protein loss, shifting the balance of activity favoring thrombus formation. Factors IX and XII and antithrombin III have been identified in appreciable quantities in the urine in patients with the nephrotic syndrome. Activation of platelets may occur when the serum albumin falls to exceedingly low levels, since it normally binds arachidonic acid and prevents excessive levels of thromboxane A_2 in the blood. It is interesting that proteins C and S and heparin cofactor II are elevated in the blood during the nephrotic syndrome.

Medications Predisposing to Thrombus Formation

A wide variety of medications have been recognized to be associated with an increase in thrombotic arterial and venous events. The most common are oral contraceptive agents and pure estrogen compounds. The etiology may be a combination of elevation in procoagulant proteins, a decrease in several natural occurring inhibitors, and a rise in the level of inhibitors of the fibrinolytic system. For reasons not well understood, an increased frequency of thrombosis occurs in patients receiving heparin (*white clot syndrome*), usually accompanied by thrombocytopenia.

Immobilization

Immobility is one of the most commonly recognized factors known to facilitate thrombus formation, usually of the venous system. It is postulated that venous stasis is the major contributing element, by inducing local hypoxemia with resultant endothelial cell damage and inadequate clearance of activated procoagulant proteins. Defects in the plasminogen-plasmin proteolytic enzyme system have also been recognized during the inactive state. Conditions that lead to immobility, such as cardiac disease, neoplasm, advanced age, obesity, and medications, may themselves increase the risk.

Diseases Associated with Thrombus Formation

Myeloproliferative Disease: The myeloproliferative diseases include polycythemia rubra vera, essential thrombocythemia, myelofibrosis-myeloid metaplasia, agnogenic myeloid metaplasia, megakaryocytic myelosis, and chronic myelocytic leukemia. These diseases have an increased incidence of thrombotic events—arterial and venous—with the feature that unusual anatomic sites are involved such as mesenteric, renal, splenic, portal, and hepatic (Budd-Chiari) vessels. Excellent correlation can be found between an elevated hematocrit value and blood viscosity, leading to vascular occlusive events. In patients with myeloproliferative disease who have an elevated hematocrit value, red cell mass and blood volume are greater than normal; these abnormalities should be returned to the normal range with phlebotomy.

Ulcerative Colitis and Crohn's Disease: Thromboembolic complications occur with a reported range of 5–40% in patients with inflammatory bowel diseases (Chapter 6.10). There is activation of coagulation proteins and platelets by "activators" liberated from the inflammatory process, and monocytes are hypersecretory of proteases that activate coagulation. Some data indicate that patients with inflammatory bowel disease have increased plasma levels of coagulation factors V, VIII, and I; thrombocytosis, spontaneous platelet aggregation, decreased platelet survival; and reduced levels of antithrombin III. In these diseases, about two-thirds of the thrombotic events are venous with resultant pulmonary emboli. Arterial thromboses are less common.

Behçet's Syndrome: Behçet's syndrome is a multisystem vasculitic disorder with about a 30% frequency of venous or arterial thrombosis. This syndrome is characterized by relapsing iridocyclitis, mucocutaneous oral and genital ulcers, pericarditis, arthritis, colitis, cutaneous eruption, thrombosis, and encephalopathy. The most likely problem is some immunologically mediated disruption of the vascular endothelium that initiates thrombus formation.

Intravascular Devices: Many intravascular devices are associated with thrombus formation. These devices are intracardiac valves, vessel grafts (Teflon, Dacron, Gortex), vascular stents, intravascular catheters, and peritoneovenous shunts. Thrombus formation is probably mediated by activation of the coagulation system through surface interaction of factors XII and XI, and disruptive membrane damage of the platelets and white and red blood cells. During the passage of any intravascular device for purposes of diagnosis or therapy (eg, cardiac catheterization, angioplasty, fluid infusion), many endothelial cells are damaged and sometimes large areas are denuded. When this occurs, thrombus formation takes place at the site of damage. Ascitic fluid, conveyed by peritoneovenous shunts, may contain endotoxin, cellular debris, or a variety of proteases that initiate thrombus formation when interfacing with blood.

Disseminated Intravascular Coagulation: Disseminated intravascular coagulation (DIC) is not a primary disease but is always secondary to a systemic disorder. It is characterized by a tendency to bleed and by simultaneous thrombosis. Disseminated intravascular coagulation is initiated by simultaneous activation of the fibrinolytic and coagulation systems. The latter occurs when there is entrance into the blood of a tissue thromboplastic substance, a histone, cathepsin, or protease. These substances may arise from an extravascular source or a cytokine, which induces the release of these substances from circulating monocytes. Disseminated intravascular coagulation can arise from a legion of underlying conditions, especially sepsis, neoplasms, complications of obstetrics, and severe trauma.

Hyperlipidemia: Hyperlipidemia from any cause, but in particular familial type II hyperbetalipoproteinemia, is associated with an increased incidence of thrombotic events (Chapter 4.8). This problem is characterized by premature onset of generalized atherosclerosis and superimposed thrombus.

Paroxysmal Nocturnal Hemoglobinuria: This acquired stem cell disorder results in susceptibility to complement-mediated erythrocyte lysis in vivo and in vitro and is characterized clinically by intravascular red cell lysis, pancytopenia, frequent hemorrhage, and thrombosis. The most common cause of death in affected persons is venous thrombosis with a particular but unexplained predilection for intra-abdominal veins. Those affected show a mild increase above the general population in cerebral venous thrombosis. Peripheral thrombotic events are unusual.

Thrombotic Thrombocytopenic Purpura-Hemolytic Uremic Syndrome: This rare devastating disease is characterized by the pentad of microangiopathic hemolytic anemia, severe thrombocytopenia with purpura, neurologic disease, fever, and renal dysfunction. Extensive damage of the vascular endothelium occurs in virtually all organs with microvascular thrombosis, although the liver and lungs are relatively spared. The exact mechanism of the thrombotic process is poorly understood. However, the main target for damage in thrombotic thrombocytopenic purpura-hemolytic uremic syndrome is the vascular endothelium; thus, superimposed thrombo-occlusive disease is most likely a secondary phenomenon.

Hyperviscosity Syndrome: Blood viscosity is increased when there is an elevated mass of red cells (polycythemia), increased immature adherent white cells (blastic leukemia), resistance of red cell membrane to normal deformability (sickle cell anemia), and increased globulin concentrations in the blood (plasma cell disorders). The sluggish blood flow in these conditions results in severely disturbing vaso-occlusive events, which can be fatal. Some of these disorders are associated with endothelial cell destruction. When there are excessive numbers of immature white cells, leukostasis and leuko-aggregates that obstruct vascular flow are found. These blast cells leak high concentrations of thromboplastic proteases, which also promote thrombus formation.

Antiphospholipid Syndrome: The antiphospholipid syndrome is characterized by recurrent arterial and venous thrombotic events, recurrent fetal loss, and thrombocytopenia. Neurologic manifestations are common and include transient ischemic attacks, ischemic optic neuropathy, retinal venous thrombosis, cerebral venous thrombosis, peripheral venous thrombosis, multi-infarct dementia, and stroke. In this syndrome, a gamma globulin interferes with the normal function of those procoagulant glycoproteins that act by way of associated phospholipids. These include factors II, VII, IX, and X.

A common interfering inhibitor occurs in systemic lupus erythematosus (in 5–10% of patients) and with few exceptions is usually directed toward the phospholipid of the prothrombin activator complex (factor Xa, factor V, phospholipid, and calcium). The inhibitor is usually an IgG (rarely IgM), is commonly associated with a biologic false-positive test for syphilis, and may be associated with an anticardiolipin antibody that may correlate with recurrent miscarriage. These inhibitors are called *lupus anticoagulants* because they prolong tests of coagulation, particularly the activated partial thromboplastin time (APTT) and occasionally the prothrombin time (PT).

Biologically, the lupus anticoagulants are not associated with bleeding and do not interfere with surgery, organ biopsy, or other invasive procedures. On the contrary, this circulating inhibitor is commonly associated with venous or arterial thrombosis. The mechanism whereby this inhibitor induces thrombus formation is not established but results when the IgG binds to phospholipids that are essential for the normal activation and degradative effects of protein C and protein S, thus shifting the balance in the direction of thrombus formation. The lupus anticoagulant and associated thrombotic events are seen not only in patients with systemic lupus erythematosus but in other connective tissue diseases, other diseases such as HIV, and in some persons with no discernible illness.

SUMMARY

▶ Patients with thrombotic events who should be suspected of having a hypercoagulable condition include those under 40 years old, people who experience thrombosis at unusual anatomic sites, people with recurrent thrombotic events, people with recurrent thrombotic events despite therapeutic range warfarin anticoagulation, and people with a family history of thrombosis.

▶ Most congenital defects leading to a hypercoagulable state are inherited in an autosomal dominant pattern.

▶ When a positive defect is identified, detailed family studies should be implemented.

▶ Patients with thrombotic events and a recognizable biochemical abnormality that predisposes to thrombosis should be treated with anticoagulant agents for prolonged periods but not automatically for life. People who demonstrate the biochemical abnormality but who have not had thrombotic events should not be treated with anticoagulants prophylactically.

SUGGESTED READING

Bauer KA, Rosenberg RD: The pathophysiology of the prethrombotic state in humans: Insights gained from studies using markers of hemostatic system activation. Blood 1987; 70:343.

Case 11–1990: A 38-year-old woman with abdominal pain, fever, and a rash (case records of the Massachusetts General Hospital). N Engl J Med 1990;322:754.

Guidelines on the investigation and management of thrombophilia: The British Committee for Standards in Haematology. J Clin Pathol 1990;43:703.

Joist JH: Hypercoagulability: Introduction and perspective. Semin Thromb Hemost 1990;16:151.

Nucci MR, Bell WR: Acquired hypercoagulable states. In: *Thrombosis and Hemorrhage.* Loscalzo J, Schafer AI (editors). Blackwell Scientific Publications, 1994.

Svensson PJ, Dahlback B: Resistance to activated protein C as a basis for venous thrombosis. N Engl J Med 1994;330:517.

11.11

Transfusion Therapy

Samuel Charache, MD, and Paul M. Ness, MD

The decision to use transfusion therapy involves choices between whole blood and blood products ("what?"), indications for transfusion ("when?"), calculation of requirements ("how much?"), recognition of risks ("why not?"), procedures for minimizing those risks ("how?"), and considerations of alternate means of therapy ("is there anything else?").

CHOICES AMONG BLOOD PRODUCTS (WHAT?)

Blood donations can be used most efficiently if they are separated into their components, called *blood products*. Separation of a single "unit" of whole blood creates a unit of blood product for three or four patients, who individually may need only red cells, factor VIII, other plasma proteins, or platelets (Figure 11.11–1). In other circumstances, separation into components may reduce the risk of circulatory overload (by giving red cells but not plasma), hypersensitivity reactions (by removing white cells or plasma from red cell suspensions), and alloimmunization (by removing white cells from platelet suspensions). Plasma can be separated further by chemical fractionation processes into concentrates of gamma globulin, albumin, and coagulation factors. It is much more efficient to isolate such components from large pools of plasma than from single units of blood. This greatly increases the risk of infection, however, because 1 infected unit can contaminate plasma pooled from 500 or more donors.

Because it is usually so efficient, separation of blood into components has become very prevalent—so prevalent that for a patient bleeding profusely (as after trauma), separate transfusion of red cells, plasma, and platelet components may be necessary because only limited supplies of whole blood are available. Note also that whole blood is stored under conditions that are optimal for red cells but suboptimal for platelets and labile coagulation factors, so that stored whole blood is never a complete replacement for native blood.

INDICATIONS FOR TRANSFUSION (WHEN?)

Red Cells

Red cells are transfused to restore or maintain oxygen carrying capacity of the blood. Most normal adults can lose 450 mL of blood (the actual amount lost when donating 1 unit of blood) over a short period of time with no disability, and 1000 mL can be lost without much danger or discomfort. Loss of larger volumes may require blood replacement. Initially, red cells will suffice, but if continuing blood loss approaches the normal blood volume (70 mL/kg of body weight), it may be necessary to replace platelets and plasma as well if blood coagulation is to remain normal. When transfusing 5 or more units within a matter of hours, measurement of ionized calcium, platelets, prothrombin time, and activated partial thromboplastin time should be monitored as guides for replacement of these coagulation factors. Since an accurate estimate cannot be made of the volume of acute blood lost by measuring either hemoglobin concentration or hematocrit, the patient's general condition, pulse, and blood pressure are the best criteria for whether red cell replacement has been adequate.

Transfusion for chronic anemia should be based on the patient's symptoms and the probability of alleviating them by treatment. Patients with lifelong anemias such as sickle cell anemia can engage in strenuous athletic activity with hemoglobin levels of 7–8 g/dL, because they have adapted to their anemia by alterations in blood volume, cardiac output, blood oxygen affinity, capillary density, and possibly tissue oxygen utilization. Such persons should receive transfusions for increased fatigue or breathlessness only if their hemoglobin concentration is lower than usual. If it is not, other causes should be sought. In older patients with chronic anemia, angina or cerebral dysfunction may signal the need for blood administration because of coexistent vascular disease.

No specific criterion points to a patient's need for transfusion. Therefore, patients must be evaluated individually, especially those undergoing surgery with general anesthesia. If a patient is asymptomatic at a hemoglobin level

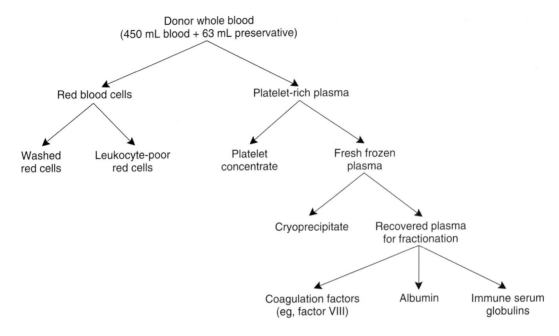

Donor whole blood
(450 mL blood + 63 mL preservative)

Red blood cells

Platelet-rich plasma

Washed red cells

Leukocyte-poor red cells

Platelet concentrate

Fresh frozen plasma

Cryoprecipitate

Recovered plasma for fractionation

Coagulation factors (eg, factor VIII)

Albumin

Immune serum globulins

Figure 11.11–1. Preparation of blood products.

below 10 g/dL, there is no reason to believe that this patient will become symptomatic when the anesthesiologist can increase the inspired PO_2 to higher than normal levels. Such a patient bleeds at surgery, but loses anemic blood; therefore, replacement need be no more vigorous than in a nonanemic person. Despite widespread belief, no good evidence supports the contention that a hemoglobin concentration of 10 g/dL is necessary for smooth anesthesia, good wound healing, and an uneventful postoperative course. Most experts believe that 7 g/dL is adequate for surgery and general anesthesia in an otherwise uncomplicated patient. In the very special case of sickle cell anemia, where not only the hemoglobin level but the abnormal red cells themselves can cause problems, no consensus exists as to the need for preoperative transfusion to raise the hemoglobin concentration or lower the proportion of sickle cells.

White Cells

In principle, white cells might be transfused to treat patients with acute neutropenia, severe bone marrow depression, or sepsis, or even to treat noninfected patients at risk for sepsis. However, neutrophils have a short life span, are difficult to harvest in significant numbers from normal donors, and can produce severe reactions in sensitized patients. As a consequence, acute neutropenia is treated only rarely and usually only in desperate situations in which antibiotic therapy has failed. In such patients, recombinant colony-stimulating factors (G-CSF, GM-CSF) may be a much more effective form of therapy than granulocyte transfusion.

Chronic neutropenia is seen in patients with bone marrow disorders and autoimmune diseases, and in some apparently normal persons. Only about 50% of available neutrophils actually circulate, and some otherwise normal persons may really have normal total body neutrophil counts. In those who do have symptoms (fever, mouth ulcers, or skin or lung infections), it is best to treat the basic disorder, rather than the blood count itself.

Platelets

Platelet counts fall because of one of two general causes: inadequate production in the bone marrow or reduced survival in the circulation. If their platelets function normally, acutely thrombocytopenic patients with inadequate production are unlikely to bleed spontaneously if their counts are more than 50,000/μL; even bleeding during surgery is unlikely if the platelet count is in this range. Severe spontaneous bleeding is a real risk in acutely thrombocytopenic patients if the count is less than 20,000/μL and is likely if the count is less than 10,000/μL. Bearing these guidelines in mind, platelets should be transfused to treat bleeding patients if the count is below 50,000/μL, and should be used prophylactically if the count is below 10,000/μL.

In contrast, thrombocytopenic patients with chronic immune thrombocytopenia may bruise and have mild gastrointestinal blood loss, but may not have serious bleeding despite counts below 10,000/μL. They usually are not given platelet transfusions because their antiplatelet antibodies destroy transfused platelets very rapidly. Treatment with prednisone or intravenous gamma globulin sometimes increases the platelet count, but severe bleeding in these patients can be very difficult to manage, even when platelet transfusions are used.

Plasma Components

Patients with deficiencies of coagulation factors usually bleed intermittently and are treated with factor transfusion only when there is evidence of hemorrhage (Chapter 11.9). Definitions of hemorrhage may differ, and minor joint aches in a patient with classic hemophilia may prompt infusion of factor VIII concentrate by some physicians, but not others. Because infusion of concentrate is not risk free, in most instances its use should be limited to patients with physical evidence of joint bleeding. In contrast, immune globulin deficiency should be treated prophylactically to prevent life-threatening infection.

CALCULATION OF TRANSFUSION REQUIREMENTS (HOW MUCH?)

It is not difficult to calculate how many milliliters of blood product are needed to correct a low hematocrit or low platelet count, but it can be very difficult to estimate whether a patient's circulatory system can handle the additional volume infused. Pulmonary edema can be produced even in young patients with normal hearts, as well as in the aged or those with recognized heart disease, if transfusions are excessive. If in doubt, go slowly, use diuretics, and monitor both fluid intake and output. Remember that salt or glucose solutions infused to "keep veins open" between bags of blood must be included in calculations and may not be excreted promptly in a sick patient.

Red Cells

In an average adult, administration of 1 unit of packed red blood cells raises the hemoglobin concentration by about 1 g/dL (or 3 hematocrit "points"). When administering a number of units to a patient with a potentially compromised cardiovascular system, note that 1 unit of packed red cells contains more than just the red cells harvested from a 500-mL bag of blood. It contains some trapped plasma, white cells, and added preservative solution, for an average total volume of about 350 mL, which is more than the 200 mL that would be expected from the separated red cells if the donor's hematocrit were 40%.

Platelets

Calculation of platelet requirements is much less precise than that of red cells. For an average adult with no antiplatelet antibodies or other clinical condition expected to decrease platelet survival, the platelets harvested from 1 unit of blood will raise the platelet count 10,000/μL per square meter of the recipient's body surface area. Thus, 6–7 units of platelets are usually pooled and would raise the platelet count for most patients by 30,000–40,000/μL. If platelet survival is markedly shortened, no increment in

the count may be found 1 hour after infusion. If survival is only slightly decreased, some increment will show at 24 hours (but less than anticipated). If there is a circulating inhibitor of platelet function (as in uremia), the count may rise, but the patient's hemorrhagic disorder will not improve. Administration of any blood product, no matter how carefully it is screened, entails some risk. Therefore, always measure post-transfusion platelet counts to avoid taking such risks in the future if the platelet count did not rise.

When transfused platelets fail to increase the patient's platelet count, it is usually because the recipient has been previously sensitized to human leukocyte antigens (HLA) on white cells that accompanied previous transfusions. The anti-HLA antibodies evoked by previous transfusions destroy not only transfused white cells, but platelets as well. Use of HLA-matched single-donor platelets (the equivalent of 6 or more units, obtained from 1 donor by pheresis techniques) might be able to retard sensitization, but without such evidence and with limited supplies, these platelets are often reserved for patients who are already sensitized. The best therapy for a thrombocytopenic patient who is refractory to routine platelet transfusions because of HLA sensitization is the use of HLA-matched platelets. This approach is not cheap or easy and frequently is unsuccessful.

Plasma Components

When using plasma to treat deficiency of coagulation factors, as in liver disease patients, or dilutional bleeding caused by overzealous administration of crystalloid solutions (eg, NaCl, Ringer's lactate), try to infuse as much plasma as possible without overexpanding blood volume. Using specific purified coagulation factors (eg, factor VIII) or cryoprecipitate (primarily containing factor VIII and fibrinogen) involves much smaller volumes; therefore, fluid overload becomes much less likely. In general, assume that some of the plasma factors infused will escape into the extravascular space; thus, administration of a dose every 6–12 hours replaces losses caused by consumption and degradation.

RISKS OF TRANSFUSION (WHY NOT?)

The risks of transfusion are related to (1) volume overload, (2) iron overload, (3) transfusion reactions, and (4) infections. Of these, the clinician has control over 1 and 2, whereas the blood bank tries to minimize (3) and (4). Volume overload and transfusion-induced pulmonary edema have already been discussed, but the importance of such preventable complications of transfusion cannot be overemphasized.

Iron Overload

Every unit of red cells contains 250 mg of iron. After it is infused, no mechanism (short of bleeding) exists for this iron to be excreted, and it initially accumulates in the cells of the reticuloendothelial system. Some frequently transfused patients seem to be able to tolerate very high iron burdens, with little or no disability at serum ferritin concentrations up to 2000 ng/mL. Others with similar ferritin concentrations develop diabetes, cirrhosis, myocardial dysfunction, and other evidence that iron is being deposited in parenchymal cells and causing injury, possibly by generating active oxygen radicals.

Iron can be removed by chelating it with parenterally administered desferrioxamine. The drug is expensive and awkward to use on a long-term basis. No good guidelines exist as to when to begin desferrioxamine therapy, but it is probably too late if cirrhosis or cardiac arrhythmias have developed. For patients with expected survival of more than a few years, with a serum ferritin level greater than 1000 ng/mL, with no suggestion that transfusion requirements will cease, and with a source of funds to purchase the drug and necessary equipment for home infusion, home chelation therapy should be instituted. Oral chelating agents are not yet available.

Transfusion Reactions

Transfusion reaction occurs because of the patient's allergy or incompatibility with the transfused material. Among transfusion reactions, allergic reactions are some of the most common and are usually no more than an annoyance to either patients or physicians. Generally, no specific allergen can be identified, and patients who have an allergic reaction once often have more. Itching and urticaria respond to oral or parenteral antihistamines, but occasionally patients develop wheezing or even laryngospasm, and epinephrine or corticosteroids may be needed to relieve symptoms. Reactions to IgA may represent the most serious type of allergic reaction and can generally be prevented by the use of washed red cells.

Febrile reactions are usually caused by some form of hypersensitivity and are important more for what they might be than for what they are. Occurring during or shortly after a transfusion, but sometimes as long as 24 hours later, febrile reactions are usually linked to the donor's white blood cells and can be eliminated by filtering or washing these white cells away from the red cells. In very sensitive patients, the extensive washing involved in deglycerolization of frozen red cells makes them the blood product of choice. Antipyretics and corticosteroids are used for serious cases.

Febrile reactions receive a great deal of attention because they can be (1) an indication of bacterial contamination of the blood product or (2) the first sign of a serious incompatibility reaction. Whenever a patient develops new fever during a transfusion, the transfusion should be stopped and the remainder of the unit sent to the laboratory for culture and Gram's stain. Organisms growing among red cells at 4°C usually are not invasive, but make trouble because of the endotoxin and other metabolites they produce. Bacterial contamination of platelets is a greater worry, since platelets are stored at room temperature and provide a more hospitable environment for bacterial growth than do red cells at 4°C. Organisms growing among platelets are familiar pathogens, often from skin flora, and may produce serious blood-borne infection.

Reactions Resulting from Incompatibility: Besides fever, transfusion reactions caused by incompatibility can occur as blood is being administered, or some days later. Immediate reactions are usually associated with intravascular hemolysis of transfused cells and may be lethal. Among the most dramatic are hemolytic reactions, which manifest as fever, backache, red urine (caused by hemoglobinuria), malaise, or hypotension. Reactions occurring in the operating room may be suspected because of hypotension or uncontrolled bleeding caused by consumption coagulopathy. In this case, the transfusion should be stopped, and the remainder of the unit returned to the blood bank. Urine and plasma should be examined for free hemoglobin. Urine output should be watched closely. Urine flow should be maintained by administration of fluid and diuretics, but since renal failure may occur, fluid balance must be monitored and dialysis may be required. Some patients escape with no morbidity, and some die.

Almost all incompatibility reactions are the result of faulty labeling of the recipient's blood sample submitted for cross-matching or faulty identification of the patient to receive the blood product—avoidable with careful attention to proper procedures.

Delayed transfusion reactions are anamnestic reactions, in which a previously sensitized patient, who has no detectable antibodies at the time of cross-matching, develops hemolytic antibodies 3–21 days after transfusion. Fever, jaundice, backache, and a fall in hematocrit may be noted, although many patients are asymptomatic. The reaction itself is almost always self-limited and needs no treatment, but the new antibody must be identified and red cells of that type avoided in the future. A wallet card or bracelet for the patient may be a good investment if future episodes are to be prevented.

Transfusion-Transmitted Infection: Febrile reactions caused by infectious agents almost always reflect contamination of a blood product during its removal from a donor. In contrast, the infectious agents that are most likely to be in donor blood usually do not cause acute febrile reactions, but constitute the major cause of transfusion-transmitted infection. These agents include hepatitis viruses, the human immunodeficiency virus (HIV-1 and HIV-2), cytomegalovirus, and, rarely, the organisms that cause syphilis and parasitic diseases.

Viral hepatitis: Viral hepatitis remains a serious complication of transfusion. The elimination of paid blood donors and screening of donor blood for hepatitis B surface antigen substantially have reduced post-transfusion hepatitis B to about 1 case in 100,000 units of blood. Nevertheless, as many as 10% of asymptomatic and anicteric recipients have developed hepatitis C (HCV), and a serologic test for the specific virus is being used in blood banks. Although prospective studies are not available, donor screening with alanine aminotransferase (ALT), anti-HBc, and anti-HCV has been demonstrated to reduce the incidence of hepatitis to less than 1 in 3300 units transfused.

Acquired immunodeficiency syndrome (AIDS): The transmission of AIDS by blood transfusion accounts for 1–2% of known AIDS cases. AIDS has also occurred in hemophiliacs treated with infected factor VIII concentrates. The availability of a screening test for HIV-1 has markedly reduced this transfusion risk. Factor VIII concentrates are now prepared by methods known to inactivate the HIV-1 virus. The remaining problem of HIV-1 transmission from blood transfusion is very small and results from the brief period in which an infected donor can have a negative HIV-1 antibody test. Since blood is not accepted from donors who have high-risk activity for AIDS, the risk of HIV-1 transmission from tested blood has been estimated to be 1 in 500,000. Because the incubation period of AIDS may be long, a detailed transfusion history should be obtained in any patient developing AIDS.

Cytomegalovirus (CMV): The potential for CMV to cause disease in transfusion recipients was first documented in cardiac surgery patients, who developed fever and splenomegaly, designated as *postperfusion syndrome.* Patients who are immunosuppressed, such as renal or bone marrow transplant recipients, are at greater risk for blood-transmitted CMV than normal recipients. To prevent CMV transmission to high-risk patients, blood products are used from donors who test negative for CMV antibodies. Because the virus appears to harbor in white cells, white cell removal by washing or special filters is another method to reduce the risk of CMV transmission from blood products.

Other infections: Syphilis transmission has been virtually eliminated by using refrigerated blood and serologic testing of donors. Malaria infection has been markedly reduced by refusing donors who have had malaria or who have traveled or lived in endemic areas in the preceding 3 years (Chapter 8.15). Any organism that infects an asymptomatic donor can cause transfusion-transmitted disease, but reports of infection by parasites, rickettsiae, or other viruses acquired through blood transfusion represent rare events.

MINIMIZING RISKS (HOW AND WHY?)

Misuse of Transfusions

As with all therapeutic interventions, transfusions should be avoided if an acceptable but less risky alternative for management can be used. For example, iron-deficient patients should be treated with iron rather than a transfusion if they have no other disease that might inhibit their erythropoietic response (eg, renal disease, cancer)

and if they are not actively bleeding. Usually, there is no indication for transfusion of only 1 unit of blood (if that's all that is needed, the patient probably didn't need it at all). Exceptions to the rule exist; that is, patients whose blood volume is already overexpanded or who have decreased cardiac function may benefit from transfusion of 1 unit, since giving more may cause unacceptable intravascular volume burdens.

Blood is not a tonic and rarely should be administered to chronically anemic patients just because they are tired and depressed—unless the hemoglobin concentration is lower than usual. Blood should never be given to a nonanemic person to improve athletic performance. The real risk of disease transmission and the potential risk of increased blood viscosity outweigh the competitive advantage that might be gained.

Therefore, the best way to minimize the risks of transfusion is not to transfuse. Iron-deficient patients can be treated with ferrous sulfate, some patients with coagulation factor deficiencies can be treated with vitamin K, and some mild hemophiliacs can be treated with agents like desmopressin (dDAVP). Patients with chronic anemia may not need treatment, but injections of recombinant erythropoietin can sometimes be useful, and other recombinant cytokines may be able to increase production of white cells and platelets.

If transfusions are used and if the donor and the donor's blood are carefully screened to try to eliminate febrile reactions and transfusion transmitted infection, the greatest single risk to the recipient is receiving incompatible blood. Labeling or clerical errors can result in a patient receiving blood cross-matched for someone else, but blood banks are extremely careful over identification of samples and blood products and such errors are unusual. Techniques to minimize risks caused by incompatibility are cross-matching of the donor's and recipient's red cell antigens and antibodies, histocompatibility testing, and autologous transfusion.

Red Cell Antigens

The antigens of the red cell membrane are glycolipids and glycoproteins, and their external carbohydrate moieties protrude into the plasma and act as epitopes during antibody formation. Some, like the Rh antigen D, are strongly antigenic, and usually lead to antibody formation if a patient is exposed to incompatible red cells. Others antigens (such as Duffy or Kidd) are much weaker and do not usually evoke an antibody response on the first exposure.

Antibodies

The antibodies of importance in transfusion therapy are usually of the IgG and IgM subclasses. Isoantibodies are the so-called "natural" antibodies, made without exposure to foreign blood cells. In some cases, they are known to be made in response to antigens found on normal bowel flora; in other cases they are assumed to result from exposure to "environmental" antigens. Anti-A or -B in persons of the opposite blood group are good examples. In contrast to IgG antibodies, which develop after exposure to a specific antibody because of pregnancy or transfusion, naturally occurring anti-A and anti-B antibodies are of the IgM subclass. Because anti-A or anti-B antibodies are universally present in the serum of patients lacking the corresponding antigens and because high levels of A and B substance are present on red cells, providing ABO-compatible blood is of critical importance in transfusion therapy.

Alloantibodies are those made after exposure to antigens on foreign red cells. Anti-D, made by a D-negative mother who has been exposed to her baby's D positive red cells, is the typical cause of Rh incompatibility, with the D antigen being the most antigenic of the Rh antigen complex (consisting of C,D,E, c,e, and a variety of lesser antigens). If a red cell antigen is nearly ubiquitous, alloimmunization to it can pose serious problems. Data suggest that some persons are more likely than others to make alloantibodies; such antibody formers may progressively make more and more new antibodies, progressively limiting their available donors to a handful of persons in a country as large as the United States. In some cases, family members may be the only compatible donors.

Histocompatibility

Ordinarily, histocompatibility is not a worry when transfusing blood products. Granulocytes are usually nonviable, and donor lymphocytes are usually destroyed by the recipient fairly quickly. But if the recipient is immunosuppressed, the transfused lymphocytes can attack the recipient, causing graft-versus-host disease. First-degree family members who share HLA antigens are also at increased risk for graft-versus-host disease. The problem is avoided by irradiating the blood to kill the donor's lymphocytes.

Autologous Transfusion

The best way to avoid risks of infection and incompatibility is to transfuse the patient's own blood (autologous transfusion). For patients who are scheduled for elective surgery and who are expected to lose significant amounts of blood intraoperatively, as much as 3–6 units of blood can be collected during the 5–6 weeks before surgery. These autologous units of blood are then given back to the patient during the operation, if necessary. This procedure prevents problems of infection and alloimmunization. Iron should be given during the period of blood collection. Erythropoietin may be useful for some patients whose anemia may limit autologous collections, and some studies suggest that erythropoietin may speed the recovery of surgical patients from anemia when administered postoperatively. Another approach is the use of intraoperative autologous transfusion, in which shed red cells are salvaged from the operative site, washed by an automated procedure, and transfused back into the patient.

ALTERNATE THERAPY (IS THERE ANYTHING ELSE?)

Artificial Blood

If it were possible to administer a synthetic nonantigenic oxygen transport agent, problems with antigen-antibody incompatibility could be avoided. If the agent were stable at room temperature and could be stored for long periods, it would have great use for victims of natural disasters, transportation calamities, and battle injuries. If the agent were derived from blood, chemical treatment could also remove the potential for transmission of infection. The one completely synthetic substance (Fluosol) used as an oxygen carrier probably has no use in transfusion therapy because it is far less efficient than red cells. Hemoglobin solutions are being evaluated as synthetic oxygen carriers, but complement activation, vasoconstriction, and nephrotoxicity remain difficult problems related to the use of these solutions.

Erythropoietin Therapy

Recombinant erythropoietin is approved for use in patients with renal failure and is being used in a variety of hypoproliferative anemias. Measurement of the serum erythropoietin level, and comparison of it with expected levels in normal persons with that degree of anemia, may be a useful guide to therapy. On the other hand, some patients with elevated endogenous erythropoietin levels have responded to the exogenous drug. Therapy is costly, but prevents not only the risk of iron overload, but transfusion-transmitted infection. Remember that a drug response is impossible unless iron is available for hemoglobin synthesis.

SUMMARY

▶ The best way to eliminate the risks of transfusion is not to transfuse. To minimize the risks, patients should be receive their own blood (autologous transfusion).

▶ Screening of blood donors through careful medical histories and infectious disease testing has substantially reduced but not eliminated transfusion recipients' risk of contracting hepatitis and HIV infection.

▶ Immediate hemolytic transfusion reactions can be fatal. Almost all such reactions can be prevented by ensuring that the pretransfusion blood sample obtained from the patient is correctly labeled, and the unit of blood brought from the blood bank is given to the correct patient.

▶ Platelets should be transfused to treat bleeding patients whose platelet counts are less than 50,000/mm^3 and are appropriately transfused to prevent bleeding in patients with counts less than 10,000/mm^3.

▶ Platelet transfusions are more effective in patients with platelet production deficits than in patients with increased platelet destruction.

SUGGESTED READING

Murphy S: Preservation and clinical use of platelets. In: *Hematology,* 4th ed. Williams WJ et al (editors). McGraw-Hill, 1990.

Ness PM, Rothko K: Principles of red blood cell transfusion. In: *Hematology: Basic Principles and Practice.* Hoffman R et al (editors). Churchill Livingstone, 1995.

Perioperative red blood cell transfusion. Consensus conference. JAMA 1988;260:2700.

Rossi EC et al: *Principles of Transfusion Medicine.* Williams & Wilkins, 1996.

Wiesen AR et al: Equilibration of hemoglobin concentration after transfusion in medical inpatients not actively bleeding. Ann Intern Med 1994;121:278.

Section 12

Oncology

Brent G. Petty, MD, Section Editor

12.1

Approach to the Patient with Cancer

John H. Fetting, MD

Cancer is not one disease, but a family of diseases, each with a unique natural history and treatment. However, cancers do share some biologic features, such as disordered cell proliferation and the ability to invade and metastasize. The management of patients with all types of cancer also shares some basic principles:

1. Diagnose cancer early.
2. Establish the diagnosis pathologically.
3. Evaluate the extent of cancer spread.
4. Define the goals of treatment.
5. Establish a partnership with patients, based on respect for their autonomy.

These principles provide a foundation on which to build more detailed knowledge of cancer biology and therapeutics. Each of these principles is elaborated in the following sections of this chapter.

DIAGNOSE CANCER EARLY

It is frustrating that common cancers are often diagnosed at an incurable stage. About two-thirds of patients with lung cancer, one-third of patients with prostate cancer, and one-third of patients with colorectal cancer have incurable disease at presentation. These numbers reflect not only the limitations of cancer treatment, but also the limited success of efforts to diagnose cancer early enough for cure. Before cancer treatment can reduce mortality, more effective treatments must be discovered or the effective treatments currently available must be applied earlier in the disease course. Fortunately, most common cancers can be diagnosed earlier, with a focused history and physical examination as well as conscientious and judicious use of screening tests.

A comprehensive medical history identifies persons who are at high risk for cancer. The family history should routinely seek evidence of potentially heritable cancer, such as relatives' cancers that occurred at multiple sites or at a younger than expected age. Special attention should be paid to cancers that cluster in families (eg, breast, colon, ovary). There is no more important part of the social history than identifying exposures to carcinogens at home and in the workplace (eg, tobacco, asbestos). Inquiry into the past medical history may reveal conditions that predispose to malignancy (eg, human immunodeficiency virus [HIV], inflammatory bowel disease, carcinoma in situ of the breast or cervix). The system review should include special attention to symptoms of common cancers and cancers for which the patient is at particular risk. For example, smokers who drink alcohol are at higher than average risk for cancers of the upper respiratory and digestive tracts, and should be questioned carefully about symptoms.

Parts of the physical examination are particularly important in diagnosing common cancers early. The skin should be inspected for skin cancer, the breasts inspected and palpated for breast carcinoma, and the rectum examined digitally for colorectal and prostate cancers.

Several screening tests should be a routine part of general medical care: screening mammography, Papanicolaou (Pap) cervical smear, and examination of stools for occult blood. All three tests have been shown to increase the fraction of cancers diagnosed at a curable stage. The prostate-specific antigen (PSA) test, which is emerging as an effective screening test for prostate cancer, may soon be routinely used as well. In contrast, chest x-rays, screening chemistry and hematology tests, and biological markers such as carcinoembryonic antigen (CEA) are not cost-effective screening tests for cancer in asymptomatic patients who have normal physical examinations. These tests may be very useful, however, in patients with symptoms or physical findings suggesting cancer.

One final point cannot be stressed too strongly. The general internist is in a unique position to educate patients on how to prevent cancer and diagnose it early. A major limitation of mass screening efforts for cancer is that many people are not motivated to take part because they are not worried about their health, much less sick. By seeking medical care, the internist's patient has already shown more motivation than the general population. The wise physician will take advantage of the opportunity to counsel patients about prevention and early diagnosis of cancer.

ESTABLISH THE DIAGNOSIS PATHOLOGICALLY

Once cancer is suspected, the physician must move decisively to establish the diagnosis by obtaining affected tissue. A cancer diagnosis can be confirmed only by cytopathologic or histopathologic examination. Cancer can be strongly suspected but never diagnosed by other means, such as CEA or PSA. A common but lamentable practice is obtaining tests to establish the extent (stage) of a suspected cancer before establishing the diagnosis. Since the type of cancer determines the type of staging evaluation (see "Evaluate Extent of the Cancer" below), tissue diagnosis should precede staging.

Obtaining a tissue diagnosis is not always a straightforward undertaking. The procedure of choice is usually the one that will establish the diagnosis with the least morbidity and cost. For example, cytopathologic examination of expectorated sputum is often a first step in diagnosing lung cancer. But some cancers require special procedures. For example, to prevent local cancer spread, inguinal orchiectomy rather than a transscrotal biopsy is indicated for a suspicious testicular mass. Increasingly, too, special studies are performed on diagnostic tissue, to help determine prognosis and treatment: Breast cancer cells are tested for receptors for estrogen and progesterone, leukemic bone marrow is tested for abnormal chromosomes, and lymphoma cells are studied for lymphocyte antigens bound to the cell surface. Many of these studies require special handling of biopsy tissues. To ensure that biopsies are performed correctly and yield as much information as possible, the physician should consult beforehand, at least informally, with cancer treatment specialists and pathologists.

EVALUATE EXTENT OF THE CANCER

Once cancer is diagnosed, the physician must assess how far it has spread ("staging"). The extent of disease predicts prognosis and directs treatment. Each cancer has its own staging system, and some cancers have more than one. The stage, most often represented as a Roman numeral (I–IV) or letter (A–D), reflects the size and extent of the primary tumor (T), regional lymph node involvement (N), and distant metastases (M)—the TNM classification. The *clinical stage* is the stage suggested by physical findings and laboratory tests; the *pathologic stage* is the stage established by pathologic examination of tissues obtained at surgery, such as axillary lymph node dissection for breast cancer. The pathologic stage more accurately predicts prognosis and may be required for treatment planning.

Rather than memorize staging systems, physicians should consider two concepts. First, the higher or more advanced the stage, the larger or more widely disseminated the cancer and the worse the prognosis. Figure 12.1–1 shows the relation between clinical stage and survival for breast cancer. Second, the stage dictates the type and goal of treatment. Local therapies such as surgery and radiation are intended to cure early-stage cancers, but may not be tried at all for more advanced stages when cure is not possible. For example, surgery usually cures breast cancer confined to the breast, but is rarely used in patients who present with metastases. Similarly, surgery may cure patients with well-localized lung cancer, but is inappropriate for patients whose disease is disseminated.

There is no universal staging or metastatic workup. Each cancer has its own staging evaluation, based on patterns and frequency of spread as well as the sensitivity and specificity of diagnostic tests. How precisely the physician stages a cancer also depends on how different degrees of spread will affect the choice of treatment. Diagnostic tests, especially radionuclide, computed tomographic (CT), and magnetic resonance imaging (MRI) scans, should be carefully selected. The physician may wish to consult with cancer treatment specialists before staging.

Two examples illustrate these concepts. The staging workup for newly diagnosed breast cancer is minimal. If, after the primary tumor has been resected, the patient has no symptoms or physical findings suggesting that the tumor has metastasized, evidence for spread is sought in the liver with tests of serum alkaline phosphatase and aminotransferases, in the lungs with a chest x-ray, and in

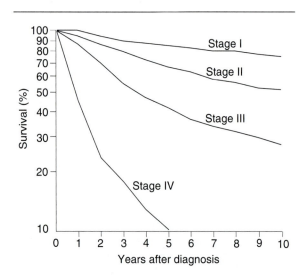

Figure 12.1–1. Relation between clinical stage of breast cancer and survival. (Modified and reproduced, with permission, from The American Joint Committee for Cancer Staging and End Results Reporting [now The American Joint Committee on Cancer], *Clinical Staging of Carcinoma of the Breast,* Chicago, 1973.)

the axillary lymph nodes with dissection. This limited workup reflects the fact that breast cancer rarely presents with overt distant metastases. Diagnostic tests in patients with a low probability of metastases have an unacceptably high false-positive rate. Another reason for this minimal workup is that more and more patients are being treated with some form of adjuvant drug therapy for presumed micrometastases, even without clinical or pathologic confirmation. Until more sensitive and specific diagnostic tests are developed that can better detect micrometastases, patients with breast cancer will need only a minimal staging workup.

In contrast to breast cancer, the staging workup for Hodgkin's disease is extensive, including thoracic, abdominal, and pelvic CT scans; lymphangiography; and bilateral bone marrow aspirates and biopsies. The principal reason for such aggressive staging is that stage determines choice of treatment. Hodgkin's disease confined to one side of the diaphragm (stage I or II) is commonly treated with radiation, whereas more widespread disease (stage III or IV) is treated with combination chemotherapy.

DEFINE TREATMENT GOALS

The goals of cancer treatment are to cure, to prolong life, or to relieve (palliate) cancer symptoms. The physician bases treatment goals on the disease stage and the predicted efficacy of treatment. In general, localized or early-stage cancers, including lung, breast, colon, prostate, and gynecologic cancers, can be cured by surgery or sometimes by radiation therapy. Increasingly, after local therapy, adjuvant drug therapy is being given to eradicate micrometastases.

Although drug therapy can palliate and prolong life, and radiation can relieve symptoms such as painful bone metastases, most patients with disseminated cancers cannot be cured. Fortunately, there are notable exceptions to the rule. Chemotherapy can cure some disseminated cancers—certain forms of acute and chronic leukemia, advanced stages of Hodgkin's and non-Hodgkin's lymphomas, small cell carcinoma of the lung, and trophoblastic and germ cell cancers.

The goal of treatment must be clearly defined after initial diagnosis and staging. The goal must be reassessed and, if necessary, changed based on the patient's response to treatment. The amount of treatment toxicity a patient can be expected to risk or withstand is justified by the goal. Intensive chemotherapy that produces considerable toxicity, including a small risk of death, can be justified for acute leukemia if the goal of treatment is cure, but it is contraindicated for metastatic pancreatic cancer, for which the goal is to palliate.

Another reason to define treatment goals is to help the physician decide how vigorously to evaluate and treat patients' intercurrent medical problems, related or unrelated to the cancer. A patient with a potentially curable lym-

phoma should receive aggressive treatment, even mechanical ventilation, for pneumonia. The same pneumonia may be treated only with supplemental oxygen and morphine to reduce air hunger in a patient with advanced lung cancer, for whom the treatment goal is palliation.

ESTABLISH A PARTNERSHIP WITH THE PATIENT

With few exceptions, cancers are life-threatening. Most patients die of or are afraid they will die of their cancer. Many cancers are also debilitating. Ironically, cancer treatment can frighten—and debilitate—patients as much as their disease. Cancer and its treatment have profound effects not only on patients but also on their families. Amid the turmoil caused by the cancer and the treatment, an effective working relationship with an empathic and knowledgeable physician is an essential source of support. Such a physician will always hold out hope for patients and their families, even if it is only to the extent of relieving pain.

The most effective doctor-patient relationships are partnerships. Establishing an effective partnership with cancer patients requires respect for their autonomy. This means that patients participate in setting treatment goals and deciding whether the toxicity of treatment is justified. For patients to participate, they must be informed. Respect for autonomy requires a readiness to keep patients informed, even if it means giving bad news. In the past, physicians routinely withheld distressing information in the name of patient welfare. This practice was criticized because physicians did not consider patients' wishes in deciding to withhold information. Surveys of patients' preferences indicate that most patients want information, even if the news is bad. Increasingly, physicians are being more candid with patients.

Respect for autonomy also requires matching the information to the patient. The physician need not tell patients everything about the cancer and its treatment at one time, but should make sure that patients understand as much as they need to at a given moment. This means identifying the relevant information and communicating it to patients in language that they can understand. There is a core of treatment information that most patients want, but some want more, some less. Some patients benefit from technical, quantitative discussions of cancer and its treatment; others have trouble grasping even the basics. Respect for autonomy requires attention not only to giving the patient accurate scientific information, but also to when and how to give it.

It is wrong to ignore the patient's psychological state in the name of telling the truth. Cancer and its treatment are distressing. Patients' anxiety and depression can interfere with their concentration, understanding, and memory. The physician must take care not to give too much information at a time when it might worsen patients' distress and thus limit their understanding.

Establishing an effective working relationship with cancer patients requires effort. Communication problems are inevitable. After all, doctors and cancer patients are often forced to make momentous decisions before they know each other well. But with sensitivity and perseverance, doctors can establish sustaining and rewarding relationships with patients and their families.

SUMMARY

▶ Diagnose cancer as early as possible, using the history, physical examination, and screening tests. Counsel patients to help them prevent cancer or allow it to be detected early.

▶ Establish the diagnosis with prompt biopsies of affected tissue for pathologic examination and special studies.

▶ After the diagnosis of cancer is confirmed, determine the stage. The stage predicts prognosis and dictates treatment.

▶ Define treatment goals: cure, prolonging life, or palliation. Treatment goals determine how much treatment toxicity is acceptable and how aggressively to manage intercurrent medical problems.

▶ Establish a partnership with patients, based on respect for their autonomy. Inform them of their condition truthfully but empathetically. Patients should take part in deciding treatment goals and options.

SUGGESTED READING

Anderson LM, May DS: Has the use of cervical, breast, and colorectal cancer screening increased in the United States? Am J Public Health 1995;85:840.

DeVita VT Jr, Hellman S, Rosenberg SA (editors): *Cancer: Principles and Practice of Oncology,* 4th ed. JB Lippincott, 1993.

Pellegrino ED, Thomasma DC (editors): *For the Patient's Good: The Restoration of Beneficence in Health Care.* Oxford University Press, 1988.

12.2

Paraneoplastic Syndromes

Brent G. Petty, MD, and Michael A. Levine, MD

Paraneoplastic syndromes are features that are observed in patients with tumors that cannot be explained by the physical or spatial characteristics of the tumor itself. Such features are produced by mediators that act "at a distance" from the original tumor. For many tumors, the mediators are never identified, so the mechanisms for their paraneoplastic effects are not understood. For other tumors, the mediators are known: These tumors have the ability to produce hormones that are not produced by the normal tissue from which the tumors arose (eg, adrenocorticotropic hormone [ACTH] production by lung cancer). This phenomenon is called *ectopic hormone secretion.*

Paraneoplastic syndromes are important because they can be the presenting manifestation of a neoplastic process and can signal the presence of a tumor months or even years before its local effects are recognized. On the other hand, paraneoplastic syndromes can develop after cancer has been diagnosed and can require specific therapy if treatment of the primary malignancy is unsuccessful. The clinician must be aware of these syndromes to recognize them as potential clues to occult cancer or as manifestations of complications during the disease course.

Table 12.2–1 lists the most common manifestations of paraneoplastic syndromes and the tumors with which they are most often associated. Whenever a patient presents with any of these signs or symptoms, the clinician must consider it as a possible manifestation of an underlying malignancy. Furthermore, the clinician should suspect that any unusual manifestation of a typical medical process may represent a paraneoplastic syndrome. This chapter outlines the most common syndromes, classified according to the affected organ system rather than the site of the primary tumor.

CONSTITUTIONAL SYMPTOMS AND VITAL SIGNS

Perhaps the most common paraneoplastic syndrome is the weight loss associated with almost all types of malignancy. This manifestation of cancer is most often mediated by tumor necrosis factor, previously known as cachectin. The patient experiences anorexia (lack of desire to eat), which leads to insufficient food consumption despite ongoing and often accelerated weight loss. The anorexia usually does not derive from an aberrant perception that food tastes bad (dysgeusia) or smells peculiar (parosmia), nor is it the result of early satiety that makes the patient feel "full" after eating only a little food. Rather, the patient is just not interested in eating. Cancer should always be considered as a cause of unexplained weight loss. On the other hand, even large or metastatic cancers may not lead to weight loss.

Unexplained fever, with or without night sweats, is another manifestation of some neoplasms, most typically lymphomas. In fact, lymphomas that produce fever have a worse prognosis than lymphomas that do not cause fever (Chapter 12.6). Fever can accompany other malignancies, such as renal cell carcinoma. Fever can also develop as a result of tissue necrosis, especially when tumor metastasizes to the liver. Malignancy is one of the three most common causes of fever of unknown origin (Chapter 8.2).

Hypertension is an uncommon manifestation of neoplasms, but patients with renal cell carcinoma or Wilms' tumor can present with new hypertension.

HEMATOLOGIC SYNDROMES

Anemia often accompanies cancer. Anemia may result from tumor infiltrating the marrow rather than from paraneoplastic causes. Anemia may also be a manifestation of nutritional deficiency (from cachexia) or "chronic disease." The most characteristic hematologic paraneoplastic syndrome associated with anemia is pure red cell aplasia, which often accompanies thymoma (Chapter 11.6). Although other conditions may cause pure red cell aplasia, it is so often a manifestation of thymoma that this tumor must always be sought as the explanation.

One of the best-recognized paraneoplastic disorders is Trousseau's syndrome, a hypercoagulable state characterized by recurrent, extensive, or unusual sites of venous

Table 12.2–1. Paraneoplastic syndromes and typically associated neoplasms.

System	Syndrome	Commonly Associated Neoplasms
Constitutional	Weight loss	Pancreatic carcinoma
	Fever	Lymphoma
Hematologic	Anemia	Many malignancies
	Hypercoagulable state (Trousseau's syndrome)	Gastrointestinal carcinomas
	Erythrocytosis	Renal cell carcinoma
	Pure red cell aplasia	Thymoma
Endocrine	Hypercalcemia	Epidermoid cancers
	Syndrome of inappropriate ADH secretion (SIADH)	Small cell carcinoma of lung
	Cushing's syndrome	Small cell carcinoma of lung
	Hyperthyroidism	Gestational trophoblastic neoplasia
Renal	Membranous glomerulonephritis	Adenocarcinoma of lung
	Minimal change glomerulonephritis	Hodgkin's disease
Musculoskeletal	Clubbing	Small cell carcinoma of lung
	Hypertrophic osteoarthropathy	Lung cancer
	Dermatomyositis	Lung cancer
Neuropsychiatric	Polyneuropathy	Lung cancer
	Myasthenia gravis	Thymoma
	Cerebellar degeneration	Lung cancer
	Lambert-Eaton myasthenic syndrome	Small cell carcinoma of lung
	Depression	Pancreatic cancer
Dermatologic	Acanthosis nigricans	Gastric cancer
	Itching	Hodgkin's disease
	Acquired ichthyosis	Lymphoma

ADH, antidiuretic hormone.

thromboses. Unusual sites include hepatic veins (Budd-Chiari syndrome) and subclavian veins. The cancers that most often cause Trousseau's syndrome are gastrointestinal adenocarcinomas. Some patients have intravascular consumption of coagulation factors without the formation of clots (disseminated intravascular coagulopathy), predisposing to bleeding.

Erythrocytosis most commonly affects patients with renal cell carcinoma, in whom erythropoietin levels are often elevated. Erythrocytosis is also seen with many other tumors, including hepatoma, pheochromocytoma, and cerebellar hemangioblastoma.

Thrombocytosis is a common hematologic manifestation of cancer. The platelet count is typically 500,000–900,000/µL.

Leukocytosis is a nonspecific abnormality noted in a small fraction of patients with cancer. The most common tumors to produce leukocytosis are Hodgkin's disease and lung cancer. Generally, the elevation is a "leukemoid reaction," with white blood cell counts rarely exceeding 40,000/µL, and with a mild left shift.

ENDOCRINE SYNDROMES

Ectopic hormone secretion is a classic paraneoplastic syndrome. A common example is Cushing's syndrome, caused by excessive secretion of ACTH from pancreatic cancer, thymoma, carcinoid, or small cell (oat cell) carcinoma of the lung. Ectopic ACTH syndromes generally produce more profound hypokalemia and subtler clinical features of Cushing's syndrome (eg, obesity, round facies, striae) than does pituitary-dependent ACTH secretion. Ectopic ACTH secretion may not be distinguishable from pituitary-dependent secretion by clinical and laboratory assessment; patients may require specialized endocrine studies such as ACTH determination in blood obtained by petrosal sinus catheterization (Chapter 4.2). Similarly, acromegaly can develop in patients with pancreatic neoplasms that secrete large amounts of growth hormone-releasing hormone. Hyperthyroidism can develop in patients with struma ovarii if the ovarian neoplasm produces large amounts of thyroid hormone. Alternatively, hyperthyroidism can appear in patients with gestational trophoblastic tumors because of the release of unusually large amounts of human chorionic gonadotropin (HCG), which has weak thyroid-stimulating activity.

Hyponatremia is the cardinal metabolic finding in patients with the syndrome of inappropriate antidiuretic hormone (SIADH) secretion. SIADH was first linked to malignancy in patients with small cell carcinoma of the lung. Since then, many other tumors have been found to cause the same syndrome.

Hypokalemia is not often caused by neoplasms, but may be produced by pancreatic tumors that secrete ACTH, or pancreatic tumors that produce vasoactive intestinal polypeptide or pancreatic polypeptide—hormones that can cause watery diarrhea.

Hypoglycemia can be caused not only by insulinomas but by hepatomas, adrenal carcinoma, or sarcomas, which may secrete insulin-like growth factors.

Hypercalcemia

Humoral Hypercalcemia of Malignancy: Humoral hypercalcemia of malignancy is a well-defined syndrome in which malignant cells produce a humoral factor that increases bone resorption, gastrointestinal calcium absorption, or both. Affected patients typically have advanced and clinically overt cancer with limited or no bone metastases. Humoral hypercalcemia of malignancy underlies about 40–80% of the hypercalcemia seen in patients with cancer. The most common solid tumors that cause humoral hypercalcemia of malignancy are squamous or epidermoid cell carcinomas of the head, neck, esophagus, and lung.

Because humoral hypercalcemia of malignancy is often accompanied by other features that are typical of excessive parathyroid hormone action (eg, hypophosphatemia, increased urinary excretion of nephrogenous cyclic AMP), patients with humoral hypercalcemia of malignancy were once thought to have "ectopic hyperparathyroidism." However, nearly all patients with humoral hypercalcemia of malignancy have been shown to have *low* serum levels of parathyroid hormone. Thus, with the exception of a few patients with small cell carcinoma of the lung or clear cell carcinoma of the ovary who have ectopic parathyroid hormone secretion, parathyroid hormone is not the cause of humoral hypercalcemia of malignancy.

In patients with humoral hypercalcemia of malignancy, the hypercalcemia usually results from the tumor secreting a novel protein called *parathyroid hormone-related protein* (PTHrP). PTHrP shares significant homology with the amino terminus of parathyroid hormone; this allows both hormones to bind and activate the same receptor (PTH/PTHrP receptor). Thus, the biochemical and histologic similarities between primary hyperparathyroidism and humoral hypercalcemia of malignancy result: Both conditions are associated with hypercalcemia, hypophosphatemia, increased urinary excretion of nephrogenous cyclic AMP, and accelerated osteoclastic bone resorption. However, serum parathyroid hormone levels are elevated in patients with primary hyperparathyroidism, but suppressed in patients with humoral hypercalcemia of malignancy. Conversely, circulating levels of immunoactive PTHrP are high in patients with humoral hypercalcemia of malignancy, but normal in patients with primary hyperparathyroidism.

Several other features can help distinguish the two conditions. Patients with humoral hypercalcemia of malignancy have more severe hypercalciuria, lower serum calcitriol levels, and depressed osteoblastic bone formation that is not functionally coupled to osteoclastic bone resorption; patients with primary hyperparathyroidism have increased osteoblastic activity that is normally coupled to accelerated osteoclastic bone resorption.

Other Humoral Mediators of Malignancy-Associated Hypercalcemia: Patients with many types of lymphoma can develop hypercalcemia. T-cell lymphomas associated with human T-cell leukemia/lymphoma virus (HTLV-1) can produce PTHrP. By contrast, many other lymphomas are associated with ectopic synthesis and release of calcitriol. Surgical or medical treatment of the lymphoma corrects the hypercalcemia and normalizes circulating calcitriol levels, confirming that the lymphoma is producing the calcitriol. The unregulated conversion of 25-hydroxyvitamin D to calcitriol in patients with lymphoma is reminiscent of the pathophysiology of hypercalcemia in sarcoidosis and other benign granulomatous diseases. Consistent with this observation, hypercalcemia and elevated calcitriol levels in many patients with lymphoma can be reversed by glucocorticoids.

Hypercalcemia Produced by Tumor Cell Invasion of Bone: Hypercalcemia can also result from direct invasion of bone by malignant cells. The tumor cells produce cytokines that activate adjacent osteoclasts to resorb bone, thereby releasing calcium into the extracellular fluid. Several substances that stimulate osteoclastic bone resorption have been implicated, including tumor necrosis factor, interleukin 1, and interleukin 6.

Direct osteolysis is also a common complication of breast and lung cancer. Tumor invasion of bone often causes intractable pain and extensive bone destruction with pathologic fractures, but leads to hypercalcemia in less than 50% of affected patients. Hypercalcemia develops as the kidneys' capacity to excrete calcium is exceeded, because of either impaired glomerular filtration or accelerated osteoclastic bone resorption.

Most patients suffering from tumor cell invasion of bone have radiographic evidence of osteolysis. This can range from osteopenia in patients with multiple myeloma to discrete osteolytic lesions in patients with breast or lung cancer. Serum alkaline phosphatase, a marker of osteoblast activity, is high in many patients who have solid tumors with extensive skeletal involvement. For similar reasons, radionuclide (eg, technetium) bone scans can be used to detect increased osteoblast activity in skeletal metastases. By contrast, osteoblast activity is not increased in patients with multiple myeloma, and alkaline phosphatase activity and bone scans are typically normal.

RENAL SYNDROMES

The nephrotic syndrome can be a manifestation of malignancy. Membranous glomerulonephritis can be caused by cancer, particularly of the lung, breast, or gastrointestinal tract. Patients with Hodgkin's disease can present with findings of minimal change glomerulonephritis. With successful treatment of the underlying disorder, these glomerulopathies resolve.

MUSCULOSKELETAL SYNDROMES

Clubbing is a common manifestation of lung cancer, primarily oat cell carcinoma of the lung, even when the patient is not hypoxemic.

One of the most characteristic paraneoplastic syndromes is hypertrophic osteoarthropathy, characterized by swelling, pain, and inflammation of bones or of the distal joints and tips of the digits. X-rays show periosteal new bone formation (Figure 12.2–1). Some patients develop pain in the long bones of the arms or legs, and they find that they are most comfortable when not standing or otherwise stressing these bones. Hypertrophic osteoarthropathy is typically associated with lung cancer, which must be sought whenever this condition is identified.

Dermatomyositis is often associated with cancer in adults but not children. Most commonly implicated are lung, breast, ovary, and gastrointestinal cancers. In contrast, patients with cancer do not have an increased incidence of polymyositis or polymyalgia rheumatica.

Other rheumatologic conditions that may be associated with malignancy are palmar fasciitis in patients with ovarian cancer, polyarteritis nodosa with hairy cell leukemia, severe arthralgias with acute leukemia, and erythromelalgia with myeloproliferative disorders.

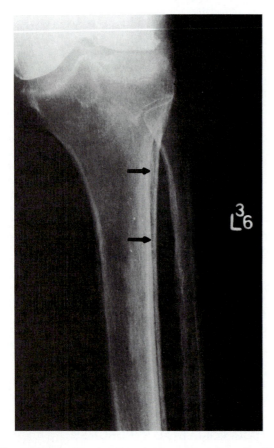

Figure 12.2–1. Hypertrophic pulmonary osteoarthropathy. The tibia shows characteristic periosteal elevation (arrows) in this patient with lung cancer. Courtesy of William W. Scott, Jr, M.D.

DERMATOLOGIC SYNDROMES

Few skin lesions are associated with internal neoplasms. One is acanthosis nigricans—velvety hyperpigmented macules on the skin of patients with adenocarcinomas of the gastrointestinal tract or, less often, other cancers. Leser-Trélat sign—new seborrheic keratoses, often associated with acanthosis nigricans and multiple skin tags—is an unusual but specific sign of internal malignancy. Palpable purpura may be seen in patients with myeloproliferative disorders. Itching in a person who does not have a metabolic disease or obvious skin condition should raise the suspicion of occult malignancy. Acquired ichthyosis (fish skin) (see Color Plates) is a rare manifestation of lymphoma.

NEUROPSYCHIATRIC SYNDROMES

The most common neurologic paraneoplastic syndrome is a symmetric sensorimotor distal polyneuropathy characterized by weakness, reduced distal deep tendon reflexes, and sensory loss. This polyneuropathy most often affects patients with lung, breast, or stomach cancer.

Myasthenia gravis can be caused by thymoma. Whenever myasthenia gravis develops, a thymoma must be sought. Thymomas should be resected if technically feasible, because their removal often eliminates the neurologic condition.

Cerebellar degeneration can afflict patients with distant cancers, most notably those arising in the lung. Cerebellar symptoms such as nystagmus, ataxia, and dysarthria may begin before conventional x-rays can detect the tumor.

Lambert-Eaton myasthenic syndrome (Chapter 13.12) is caused by antibodies to the voltage-gated calcium channels in nerve terminals. These antibodies impair the presynaptic release of acetylcholine at the myoneural junction. Patients have weakness and easy fatigue, especially of pelvic girdle and thigh muscles. The diagnosis is confirmed by an electromyogram showing a characteristic increase in amplitude on repetitive stimulation. About 70% of cases of Lambert-Eaton myasthenic syndrome are caused by cancer—50% of them small cell cancer of the lung. It is interesting that the prognosis for patients with small cell lung cancer who have Lambert-Eaton myasthenic syndrome is better than for patients without the syndrome.

Depression can be the presenting feature of cancer, most characteristically pancreatic carcinoma. The physician should keep this association in mind whenever a patient has both depression and abdominal complaints. Since depression is common and since a patient's weight loss, anorexia, and low mood can easily be ascribed to depression, the physician must remain vigilant to recognize the association between depression and cancer.

SUMMARY

▶ Newly acquired and otherwise unexplained disorders may be paraneoplastic syndromes.

▶ Paraneoplastic syndromes can be the first manifestation of cancer.

▶ Until proven otherwise, the physician should assume that conditions such as the syndrome of inappropriate antidiuretic hormone (SIADH) secretion and hypercalcemia are caused by cancer.

▶ Hypercalcemia associated with cancer can be mediated by direct bone destruction or by humoral factors (parathyroid hormone-related protein, calcitriol, or, very rarely, parathyroid hormone itself).

SUGGESTED READING

Bunn PA Jr, Ridgway EC: Paraneoplastic syndromes. In: *Cancer: Principles and Practice of Oncology,* 4th ed. DeVita VT Jr, Hellman S, Rosenberg SA (editors). JB Lippincott, 1993.

Clouston PD et al: Paraneoplastic cerebellar degeneration: III. Cerebellar degeneration, cancer, and the Lambert-Eaton myasthenic syndrome. Neurology 1992;42:1944.

Lennon VA et al: Calcium-channel antibodies in the Lambert-Eaton syndrome and other paraneoplastic syndromes. N Engl J Med 1995;332:1467.

Patel AM et al: Paraneoplastic syndromes associated with lung cancer. Mayo Clin Proc 1993;68:278.

Poole S, Fenske NA: Cutaneous markers of internal malignancy: I. Malignant involvement of the skin and genodermatoses. J Am Acad Dermatol 1993;28:1.

12.3

Breast Cancer

M. John Kennedy, MB, FRCPI, and Martin D. Abeloff, MD

Most women with breast cancer present with a painless breast nodule, discovered either by self-examination or by the physician on routine physical exam or mammography. Few women present with advanced disease, such as widely metastatic cancer or disfiguring local cancer. Breast cancer is rare in men, usually presenting as unilateral gynecomastia.

Physicians should know how to detect breast cancer early because it is second only to lung cancer in causing cancer deaths in women in the United States and because early detection and treatment improve survival. This chapter reviews the factors that put women at high risk for breast cancer, explains how to make the diagnosis, and outlines the treatment decisions that must be made based on the cancer's stage and biologic characteristics.

DIAGNOSIS AND SCREENING

About 65% of breast malignancies come to attention when the patient detects a painless lump (Figure 12.3–1). Regular breast self-exam is encouraged as a way to detect breast lumps early, although its impact on breast cancer mortality has not been well defined. In women younger than 25 years old who have no family history of breast cancer, most breast lumps are caused by benign conditions such as fibroadenomas. All new masses should be biopsied in women over age 35 and in women of any age who have a family history of breast cancer. Women aged 25–35 are in a "gray zone" in which recommendations for management are less clear.

Evaluation of a lump depends in part on the woman's age and family history, but traditionally begins with physical exam to determine the lump's consistency, size, mobility, and attachment to skin or deeper tissues. Clues that a lump is malignant include overlying skin tethering and puckering, and a mass affixed to the chest wall. Redness and heat in the overlying skin may indicate *inflammatory breast cancer,* an aggressive condition seen in about 5% of presenting breast cancers, in which tumor cells have invaded the lymphatics of the dermis. Enlarged lymph nodes in the axilla or supraclavicular fossa suggest spread beyond the breast.

Diagnostic mammography is used to characterize lumps. A mammogram should precede breast biopsy because mammography may detect occult lesions in the affected or other breast. Unfortunately, the mammogram is normal in up to 20% of patients with breast cancer. A normal mammogram does not obviate the need for a biopsy that is indicated on clinical grounds. The diagnostic procedure of choice is excisional biopsy—removal of the lump and often a ring of surrounding normal tissue. Another option is fine-needle aspiration. In able hands, this technique has an accuracy of 80%. However, because the tissue yield is small, the sample must be evaluated by an experienced cytopathologist. False-negative results do occur, and if a cytologic aspirate of a suspicious lump is negative, an excisional biopsy must still be performed. The value of needle aspiration, then, is that a positive result may lead to a recommendation for mastectomy without the intermediate step of excisional biopsy.

Screening mammography can detect breast cancer in asymptomatic patients. Before tumors can be felt or cause symptoms, mammography may reveal calcifications, masses, and architectural distortions suggesting cancer. Unfortunately, mammography remains underused. Only a minority of all breast cancers in the United States are detected by screening mammography. But regular mammographic screening combined with physical exam has been shown to reduce mortality from breast cancer. This benefit was first demonstrated in patients over age 50, but there is some evidence that regular screening may reduce deaths in women 40–50.

All authorities now recommend that women over 50 have annual screening mammography and a breast exam. Recommendations for younger women vary, mirroring controversy over the value of routine screening before age 50. The National Cancer Institute suggests that women 40–50 and their physician together decide the value of mammography, based on their individual assessment of risk. For all patients with a strong family history of breast cancer, it is generally recommended that screening begin

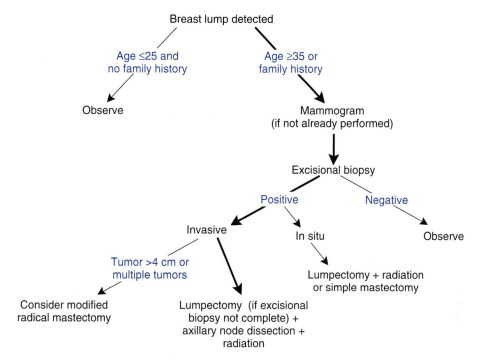

Figure 12.3–1. An approach to breast masses.

when the woman is 5 years younger than the earliest age at which a relative was diagnosed. Annual exam and mammography are also important for women who have already had breast cancer treated. This allows early detection of another tumor, for which these patients are at increased risk.

CAUSES

Heredity, hormones, and environment all contribute to the development of breast cancer (Table 12.3–1). The physician should think about breast cancer in all women, since 80% of patients have no clear predisposing family history; however, women with a family history of breast cancer are at higher risk, particularly if their mother, sister, or daughter had premenopausal bilateral disease. About 15% of patients with breast cancer have a first-degree relative who has had breast cancer; the genetic abnormalities involved are not known. The remaining 5% of patients clearly inherit a strong predisposition to breast cancer, with disease often developing early, typically between ages 30 and 50. *Hereditary breast cancer* affects families in an autosomal dominant pattern (breast cancer seen in several successive generations), as well as kindreds with a high rate not only of breast cancer but of other malignancies such as ovarian cancer or sarcomas, leukemia, and lung and adrenal cancers. In one such rare disorder, the Li-Fraumeni syndrome, affected individuals

inherit abnormalities of the p53 gene. Another gene, BRCA1, is mutated in some families with inherited breast and ovarian cancer. Intense study is being focused both on the normal function of the zinc-finger protein for which BRCA1 codes, and on how abnormalities in the gene may contribute to sporadic breast cancer.

Hormones are critical in the development of breast cancer. The disease afflicts about 100 times as many women as men; among women it is more common in those who had an early menarche or late menopause. Oophorectomy at an early age significantly reduces risk. There is some evidence that risk may be increased by prolonged use of exogenous estrogens, such as birth control pills started at an early age. It is not certain whether women who take hormone replacement therapy at or after menopause are also at increased risk. For now, estrogen treatment to prevent osteoporosis or reduce the risk of heart disease is discouraged in women who have had breast cancer.

Environmental factors also contribute to breast cancer. The disease is far less common in Asia than in western Europe and North America. Migrant studies suggest that this lower risk is partially lost in descendants of Asians who emigrate to North America. Some studies suggest that high fat and alcohol intake increase risk for breast cancer.

A number of preinvasive pathologic conditions that can be identified by excisional biopsy of a breast mass are known to increase women's risk for breast cancer. Proliferative lesions such as papillomatosis and epitheliosis in-

Table 12.3–1. Risk factors for breast cancer.

Variable	Effect
Heredity	Higher risk in women who have first-degree relatives with breast cancer, and in rare hereditary breast cancer syndromes Lower risk in Asian women
Hormone status	Higher risk in women with early menarche, late menopause, or delayed first pregnancy Possibly higher risk in women receiving exogenous estrogens
Preinvasive pathology	Higher risk in women with hyperplasias, especially cellular atypia Up to 10-fold increase in risk with carcinoma in situ
Environment	Slightly higher risk in women with high fat and alcohol intake Higher risk in women exposed to radiation, as from multiple fluoroscopies

crease the risk slightly. Hyperplasia with evidence of cytologic atypia increases risk moderately. In situ carcinomas have all the cellular attributes of malignancy, but the cells have not invaded the surrounding breast tissue. Generally, in situ ductal cancers are treated with excision and radiation therapy or simple mastectomy. Patients with isolated in situ cancers have up to 10 times the usual risk of developing an invasive cancer.

PATHOLOGY

Pathologic examination of the excised lump not only distinguishes benign from malignant lesions, but also helps predict prognosis and direct treatment (eg, by determining hormone receptor status). Increasingly, mammography reveals small lesions that turn out to be noninvasive carcinomas in situ. Although the management of these lesions remains controversial, either simple mastectomy alone or lumpectomy with radiation therapy is standard treatment when the cancer has not invaded surrounding tissue.

Invasive carcinomas derive from the mammary ductules in several pathologic patterns. About 80% of these invasive cancers are described as "infiltrating ductal." Less common histologic types include medullary, mucinous, tubular, and lobular invasive carcinomas. In general, these histologic variants of invasive carcinoma have little effect on prognosis or management.

MANAGEMENT

Primary Treatment

Surgical treatment of breast cancer has evolved substantially. In 1894, William Halsted first described radical mastectomy as a cure for breast cancer. Halsted believed that breast cancer spread from the breast to the draining lymph nodes, and only then to other sites, so that prognosis depended on the adequacy of local excision. Halsted's followers performed ever more extensive resections. But since the late 1960's, researchers have learned the real reason that breast cancer recurs: Before resection, tumor cells have spread not just to the lymph nodes, but to the blood. Thus, radical surgery offers no advantage over more conservative treatment. Removal of the tumor (inelegantly termed "lumpectomy"), with dissection of the axilla (to seek regional metastasis) and postoperative radiation therapy to the breast, affords similar survival to the modified radical mastectomy, which requires removal of the breast, pectoralis minor muscle, and axillary contents. Lumpectomy is a breast-sparing procedure that gives most patients a safe and cosmetically superior alternative to modified radical mastectomy. Lumpectomy differs from excisional biopsy only in the extent of resection: In both procedures the mass is removed, but generally in lumpectomy a larger ring of surrounding normal tissue is excised. Instead of lumpectomy, patients with very large tumors (eg, 5 cm) or multiple tumors within the breast should be considered for mastectomy.

Staging

The physician's ability to estimate whether and how much the tumor has spread by the time of surgery is crucial in determining the patient's prognosis and management. This estimate is derived from analysis of the **T**umor, draining lymph **N**odes, and **M**etastatic sites (TNM staging). Precise staging requires knowledge of tumor size, adequate axillary dissection, and laboratory tests that include a complete blood count and serum alkaline phosphatase.

The most important factor in predicting risk of relapse is the number of involved lymph nodes. At the time of diagnosis, about 40% of patients have involved nodes. These patients have only a 25% chance of cancer-free survival 10 years after diagnosis. In contrast, 75% of patients with no involved nodes are free of disease at 10 years. Within each nodal group, a larger primary tumor portends worse prognosis. A search for metastases should be confined to a careful history and physical exam, chest x-ray, complete blood count, and serum calcium and liver function tests. These tests prove normal in most patients. More sophisticated studies, such as bone scanning and computed tomography, rarely identify metastases in the asymptomatic patient.

In addition to standard TNM staging, studying the tumor's histologic, biochemical, and kinetic characteristics can be critical in identifying the 25% of patients with no involved lymph nodes who are nonetheless at high risk for relapse and are candidates for systemic adjuvant treatment (Table 12.3–2). Patients are more likely to have a recurrence if their tumor is larger than 4 cm in diameter. Patients whose tumor does not have estrogen or progesterone receptors tend to undergo relapse faster than those whose tumor has these proteins. Similarly, patients with poorly differentiated tumors tend to suffer relapse faster

Table 12.3–2. Risk factors for recurrence of node-negative breast cancer.

Tumor >4 cm in diameter
Tumor with no estrogen receptors
Tumor with poorly differentiated cells
High S-phase fraction
Expression of surface proteins, eg, cathepsin D

than those with well-differentiated tumors. Tumors that have a high S-phase fraction (ie, cells that are proliferating and making DNA) recur faster than those with a low fraction. Further efforts to define which patients with no involved lymph nodes are at high risk for relapse have focused on the tumor's expression of proteins such as cathepsin D, thought to play an important role in the mechanics of metastasis.

Adjuvant Treatment

After breast cancer has been staged, the physician decides whether the patient might benefit from systemic adjuvant therapy, and, if so, what type. Adjuvant treatment is radiation therapy, chemotherapy, hormone treatment, or a combination of these, given in an effort to eradicate occult metastases or delay their growth. Table 12.3–3 summarizes accepted indications for systemic adjuvant therapy. Combination chemotherapy reduces the annual odds of death by about 25% in premenopausal node-positive patients, and is recommended whether or not the tumor has estrogen receptors. For postmenopausal patients, chemotherapy offers only marginal benefit. However, for postmenopausal patients with estrogen receptor-positive tumors, treatment with the anti-estrogen agent, tamoxifen, appears to be as effective as chemotherapy is for premenopausal patients. The role of combined chemohormonal therapy is not yet clear for any patient group.

The exact role of adjuvant chemotherapy or tamoxifen is also uncertain in the treatment of axillary node-negative breast cancer. Most patients with no involved axillary nodes are cured by local treatments alone. However, many

Table 12.3–3. Indications for systemic adjuvant therapy of breast cancer.

Tumor Characteristics	Therapy
Axillary node-positive	
Premenopausal	Chemotherapy
Postmenopausal, estrogen receptor-positive	Hormone therapy
Postmenopausal, estrogen receptor-negative	Consider chemotherapy
Axillary node-negative*	
Estrogen receptor-negative	Consider chemotherapy for tumors >1 cm
Estrogen receptor-positive	Consider hormone therapy for tumors >1 cm

*Premenopausal versus postmenopausal status appears not to make a difference in node-negative disease.

patients receive adjuvant treatment for node-negative tumors that have features suggesting a higher risk of relapse (see Table 12.3–2). New prognostic indicators are being used in attempts to define more precisely the factors that may portend a worse prognosis for patients with node-negative breast cancer and thus identify patients who might benefit from adjuvant treatment.

Locally Advanced Breast Cancer

About 15% of patients present with tumors that are not immediately amenable to surgery. These include tumors that involve the skin of the breast, tumors or involved lymph nodes that are affixed to underlying structures, and inflammatory breast cancer. Initial resection of these tumors cannot control either local or distant disease. However, first shrinking these tumors with chemotherapy, and following up with local surgery or radiation therapy, yields long-term disease-free survival rates of up to 30%. This approach is now standard for tumors that are inoperable at presentation.

For patients who have tumors that are large but technically operable, there is increasing interest in giving systemic therapy immediately after diagnosis and before definitive surgery. The goals of this preoperative chemotherapy are to treat micrometastases as early as possible and to reduce local tumor size so as to conserve breast tissue. Whether this approach will become a real alternative to mastectomy is not yet known.

Metastatic Breast Cancer

Although a small proportion of patients are found to have metastatic breast cancer at the time of diagnosis, most patients who develop distant metastases do so at unpredictable times after primary treatment of their disease (see Color Plates). Controversy exists on how best to follow up patients who have received primary treatment and are clinically free of disease. Routine monitoring of asymptomatic patients with x-rays or serum markers may detect recurrent disease a few months earlier than checking solely for symptoms. However, the benefits of earlier detection of distant metastases are not at all clear because therapy for recurrent disease is palliative, not curative.

Breast cancer metastasizes in several characteristic patterns. Often involved are the lungs, pleura, liver, bone, brain, and nearby tissues such as the supraclavicular lymph nodes. Physicians who treat patients with a history of breast cancer should be alert to such symptoms as back or rib pain, shortness of breath, persistent cough, headaches, and unexplained anemia. Physical findings such as hepatomegaly or pleural effusions warrant prompt evaluation. Metabolic abnormalities such as hypercalcemia may be the first manifestation of recurrent disease. Bone scans are a sensitive method of looking for bone metastases. Although median time to development of metastases is about 2 years after initial diagnosis, recurrences have been recorded 30 years after mastectomy. Metastatic disease should always be considered early in the differential diagnosis when a woman has unexplained symptoms and a history of breast cancer. That possibility of recurrence, even many years after apparently successful treatment, is a large part of the emotional burden for women who have had breast cancer.

The treatment of metastatic breast cancer is palliative and should be coordinated by an oncologist. Radiation therapy should be considered for patients with isolated painful bony lesions; it also offers a good chance of controlling local or regional recurrences. Pleural effusions can be drained, and sclerosing agents such as tetracycline can prevent them from reaccumulating. Surgical stabilization may palliate pathologic fractures. Many patients with widespread disease require systemic measures to control symptoms. Patients whose tumors are estrogen receptor-positive have a 60% chance of responding to hormonal manipulations. Patients who respond to an initial hormone treatment, such as the anti-estrogen tamoxifen, but whose disease later progresses, often respond to a second hormone treatment such as progesterone. For patients whose disease is estrogen receptor-negative or has proved refractory to hormone treatments, combination chemotherapy often induces remissions. Combinations of drugs such as cyclophosphamide, doxorubicin, methotrexate, and 5-fluorouracil induce remissions in 60–70% of patients, with 10–15% achieving a complete response. Once the disease has progressed on combination chemotherapy, few patients respond to later chemotherapy. High-dose chemotherapy followed by autologous hematopoietic stem cell transplantation is the focus of intense investigation for patients with high-risk or advanced breast cancer.

SUMMARY

▶ Breast cancer is now second only to lung cancer in causing cancer deaths in women in the United States. Risk factors include a family history of breast cancer, high estrogen levels, hyperplasia of breast tissue, radiation exposure, and possibly high intake of fat and alcohol.

▶ Regular physical exams and mammography reduce mortality from breast cancer. The value of mammography in women younger than 50 is controversial.

▶ For most patients, breast-conserving treatment in the form of lumpectomy, axillary node dissection, and postoperative radiation is as effective as mastectomy.

▶ Patients at high risk of recurrence (because of large tumor, involved axillary nodes, or aggressive biochemical features) should receive systemic adjuvant therapy.

▶ For patients with metastatic disease, the primary aim of treatment is to relieve symptoms.

SUGGESTED READING

Bonadonna G: Conceptual and practical advances in the management of breast cancer. J Clin Oncol 1989;7:1380.

Chen Y et al: Aberrant subcellular localization of BRCA1 in breast cancer. Science 1995;270:789.

Fisher B et al: Eight-year results of a randomized clinical trial comparing total mastectomy and lumpectomy with or without irradiation in the treatment of breast cancer. N Engl J Med 1989;320:822.

Harris JR et al: Medical progress: Breast cancer. N Engl J Med 1992;327:319, 390, 473.

Harris JR, Morrow M, Bonadonna G: Cancer of the breast. In: *Cancer: Principles and Practice of Oncology,* 4th ed. DeVita VT Jr, Hellman S, Rosenberg SA (editors). JB Lippincott, 1993.

Malignant Tumors of the Female Genital Tract

John L. Currie, MD

Malignant tumors of the female genital tract are relatively common, but the diagnosis is often delayed or missed altogether. Given the age-specific incidence of these tumors, they will become even more common as the proportion of older members of the population continues to increase (Table 12.4–1). The astute practitioner who is aware of proper screening practices and particular symptoms compatible with these neoplasms may effect prompt diagnosis and timely treatment. Abnormal vaginal bleeding, pelvic pressure or discomfort, palpable pelvic masses, or lower abdominal pain always mandate further gynecologic investigation. Although abnormal vaginal bleeding in an otherwise healthy 30-year-old woman might be managed with a brief trial of progestational therapy for menstrual regulation, such bleeding would require invasive investigation in a 55-year-old woman. Cervical cancer can be screened successfully with periodic Papanicolaou (Pap) smears. Ovarian cancer, the leading cause of death from gynecologic neoplasms, remains a difficult problem because of a lack of effective screening techniques and the vagueness of its presenting symptoms.

Appropriate screening for gynecologic malignancies should be a high priority for primary care providers. Careful external and internal genital examination, plus Pap smear when indicated, are essential parts of the total care of a female patient. The easy availability, reliability, and relatively low cost of vaginal ultrasonography allows high-resolution imaging to augment the bimanual examination. The cost of vaginal ultrasonography should continue to decrease, and it should be used when the pelvic examination is suggestive of adnexal enlargement or uterine masses, or is technically unsatisfactory. Hence, simple and relatively inexpensive diagnostic techniques for gynecologic malignancy are readily available, and proper care of women is enhanced by their inclusion in evaluation of pelvic complaints. Such assessment will lead to earlier diagnosis and the opportunity for proper treatment.

ENDOMETRIAL CANCER

Endometrial cancer, the most common gynecologic neoplasm, is usually suggested by abnormal uterine bleeding, and proper evaluation often allows diagnosis when the disease is at an early stage. The median age at diagnosis for endometrial cancer is the early 60's, with peak age-specific incidence between 65 and 75. Although endometrial cancer is rare in young women, persistent abnormal bleeding should prompt biopsy of the endometrium at any age. In postmenopausal patients, bleeding is always abnormal and should be considered endometrial cancer until proven otherwise. Risk factors for developing endometrial cancer include exogenous obesity, multiparity, anovulation syndromes, and unopposed exogenous estrogen. Hormonal replacement therapy has been documented to lower the incidence of osteoporosis and cardiovascular disease in postmenopausal women; best practice dictates use of a progestational agent in combination with estrogen to minimize the risk of endometrial cancer.

Various office techniques are available for diagnosing endometrial cancer, including plastic tube suction biopsy, rigid tube suction apparatus, and the standard endometrial biopsy. All of these diagnostic procedures can be performed in the office without difficulty unless the patient has cervical stenosis. Dilatation and curettage in the doctor's office or a surgicenter is simple and eliminates the necessity of hospitalization. Such techniques should be in the armamentarium of anyone providing comprehensive care of the female patient, or the patient should be referred to a gynecologist. Pap smear is not adequate evaluation of postmenopausal bleeding because it cannot reliably detect endometrial cancer. After the diagnosis of endometrial cancer has been made, referral to a gynecologist or gynecologic oncologist for treating such cancers is important. Treatment usually includes surgery, but may also involve

Table 12.4–1. Age-specific incidence, risk factors, and screening for malignant tumors of the female lower reproductive tract.

Type of Cancer	Age-Specific Incidence at Peak Years	Risk Factors	Routine Screening Procedure
Endometrial cancer	110 cases/100,000 woman-yr, ages 65–75	Obesity, nulliparity, anovulation syndromes, exogenous estrogen	None
Cervical cancer	20 cases/100,000 woman-yr after age 50	Coitus early in life, multiple partners, cigarette smoking, many pregnancies, human papillomavirus infection	Pap smear
Ovarian cancer	60 cases/100,000 woman-yr, ages 70–80	Affluence, infertility, nulliparity	None

radiation or chemotherapy in patients at high risk for recurrence or with advanced disease.

Survival from endometrial cancer depends on the extent of disease and the treatment offered. For patients who have minimal or no myometrial invasion, well-differentiated tumors, and no evidence of pelvic lymph node involvement, the expected 5-year survival rate approaches 95%. Deep myometrial invasion, poorly differentiated tumors, or pelvic lymph node involvement portend a worse prognosis, with only a 60–70% 5-year survival rate. In patients who have positive periaortic nodes or evidence of more distant extrauterine disease, the 5-year survival rate is only 25–45%.

Although 95% of cancers of the endometrial cavity or of the corpus are adenocarcinomas, about 5% are uterine sarcomas. These sarcomas constitute a specialized group of neoplasms, which may derive a majority of the malignant element from both the epithelial and mesenchymal components. Such tumors are rapidly progressive, tend to affect older women, and must be treated aggressively for best survival.

OVARIAN CANCER

Cancer of the ovary constitutes about one-third of gynecologic neoplasms, but it remains the fourth most common cause of death from malignancy in women in the United States. Unfortunately, signs and symptoms of ovarian cancer are vague and the diagnosis is often made when there is advanced disease (Table 12.4–2). In such cases, treatment is disappointing. There is no satisfactory screening test for ovarian cancer, but a high sense of awareness of patients at risk as well as immediate investigation of vague but persis-

Table 12.4–2. Presenting symptoms and signs of ovarian cancer.

	% of Patients
Symptoms	
Sensation of pelvic fullness	75
Early satiety	50
Constipation	50
Pelvic pressure	50
Abdominal discomfort	50
Signs	
Adnexal mass on pelvic exam	75
Ascites	60
Palpable abdominal mass	30

tent pelvic symptoms may lead to earlier diagnosis. Ovarian cancer can strike at any age, but the incidence rises with age to a peak of 60 cases per 100,000 women between ages 70 and 80. The chances that a woman will develop ovarian cancer in her lifetime is 1 in 70.

Risk factors for ovarian cancer are upper socioeconomic class, infertility, and nulliparity. Women treated for over 1 year for infertility may be at increased risk, suggesting a potential role of ovulatory drugs. Oral contraceptives appear to be somewhat protective. Patients who have two first-degree relatives with ovarian cancer, and those with a familial syndrome of ovarian cancer or adenocarcinoma (Lynch, type 2 syndrome) are at increased risk and should be questioned carefully about ovarian cancer symptoms. Surveillance of these high-risk patients should include vaginal ultrasonography, testing for CA 125, and pelvic examination every 6 months. Although screening for ovarian cancer is probably indicated for women at high risk, the cost-effectiveness of screening low-risk, asymptomatic women has not been established. Any pelvic complaints in high-risk patients should be thoroughly evaluated immediately. Prophylactic oophorectomy in such patients is controversial, but should be performed if the patient requests this rather drastic preventive measure.

Diagnosis

The symptoms of ovarian cancer include a sense of pelvic fullness, early satiety, constipation, pelvic pressure, and vague abdominal discomfort. Although such complaints are nonspecific, they may be subtle manifestations of ovarian cancer and should remind the practitioner that a thorough pelvic examination and possibly pelvic ultrasonography are indicated. When women present with ascites or a palpable lower abdominal mass, ovarian cancer should be suspected.

Investigation for suspected ovarian cancer includes pelvic ultrasonography, computed tomography (CT) scan, or magnetic resonance imaging (MRI). Sometimes these studies are conducted for reasons unrelated to a suspicion of ovarian cancer and may reveal an asymptomatic pelvic mass. When asymptomatic masses are discovered, a positive CA 125 cancer antigen test may support this diagnosis, but CA 125 is not highly specific or sensitive. Once ovarian cancer is suspected, the diagnosis is confirmed surgically. Transabdominal needle aspiration of an ovarian cyst for diagnostic purpose is discouraged, since this may allow leakage of malignant cells into the peritoneal cavity, thereby extending the stage of disease.

Management

For patients with early disease and a well-differentiated ovarian tumor, surgery alone may be sufficient therapy. Patients who have more advanced disease may also be treated with systemic chemotherapy or intraperitoneal radioactive chromic phosphate (P32).

Most (over 80%) ovarian cancers are epithelial tumors, 60–70% of which are serous cystadenocarcinomas, and it is with this histologic type that CA 125 cancer antigen may be found in the serum. When positive in patients with ovarian cancer, following the titer of this antigen may be helpful in monitoring progress and determining extent of disease. If this marker is not positive at the beginning of therapy, it is of no future use in monitoring therapy or predicting recurrence.

Numerous chemotherapy regimens have been advocated in the treatment of ovarian cancer, but clinical trials have clearly shown that chemotherapy that includes platinum-based therapy (eg, cisplatin or carboplatin) is the treatment of choice for most epithelial, stromal, and germ cell tumors. Since its introduction into clinical trials in the late 1980's, paclitaxel (Taxol) has evolved from a much-heralded salvage chemotherapy for resistant ovarian cancer to a role as the preferred drug to combine with platinum as initial therapy of advanced disease. Including alkylating agents is traditional but controversial.

Therapy for epithelial ovarian cancer after failure with platinum-based therapy or recurrence after a lengthy disease-free interval has been disappointing. Intraperitoneal chemotherapy has been advocated and may cure some patients with low-volume disease.

Survival in ovarian cancer depends on the extent of disease at diagnosis. The 5-year survival rate for patients with early disease is 75–85%, but 60–90% of patients with advanced-stage disease succumb in 5 years. Nevertheless, aggressive treatment is mandatory if patients with advanced disease are to enjoy disease-free intervals. The data suggest that the more complete the tumor removal with the initial surgical procedure, the longer the tumor-free survival.

About 15% of patients with epithelial ovarian cancer are found to have tumors of low malignant potential. These patients often present with large abdominal masses and proliferative growth, but careful pathologic evaluation reveals a lack of frank stromal invasion and very little nuclear atypia and mitosis. Such patients do not benefit from radiation or chemotherapy, and surgical therapy usually results in long-term survival for most of those patients.

Less Common Types of Ovarian Cancer

Stromal tumors: Stromal tumors are uncommon and usually are found in older women, although they can be responsible for precocious puberty in juvenile patients as well as masculinizing symptoms at any age. Most of these are granulosa cell cancers and are treated surgically. Because only 25% of these prove to be malignant, combination chemotherapy is usually reserved for patients with advanced or recurrent disease. In addition, stromal tumors tend to have a long interval from original diagnosis to recurrence, so that a history of granulosa cell tumor should raise suspicion of recurrent disease in any patient who presents with pelvic masses or ascites.

Germ cell tumors: Germ cell tumors constitute less than 10% of ovarian cancer, although these are important neoplasms because they usually appear in young women. The average age of diagnosis is 21 years. Although germ cell tumors can be highly malignant, early evaluation and aggressive treatment with surgery and combination chemotherapy significantly increase the chances for cure. Radiation treatment for these tumors has been replaced with combination chemotherapy, which allows preservation of fertility in young women. Almost all early-stage germ cell tumors can be cured; a high response rate is likely with combination chemotherapy for advanced germ cell tumors.

Sarcomas and metastases: Ovarian sarcomas are rare, deadly tumors that spread rapidly and have a high mortality rate. These patients are treated with chemotherapy after the tumor is removed surgically.

A surprisingly common ovarian neoplasm is cancer that has metastasized from another site. The primary tumors in such cases are predominantly gastrointestinal, endometrial, or breast cancers, but virtually any malignant neoplasm can metastasize to the ovary. A previous history of cancer and pelvic mass should raise this suspicion. Treatment depends on the nature of the primary tumor.

CERVICAL CANCER

Squamous cell carcinoma is the most common histologic type of cervical cancer. Patients at high risk include those who have multiple sexual partners, coitus at an early age, and many pregnancies, and those who smoke cigarettes and have a history of sexually transmitted disease. Adenocarcinoma of the cervix, a less common variety that accounts for about 10–25% of the cases, also has definite risk factors, including upper socioeconomic class and low parity. Proper screening can detect both squamous cell and adenocarcinoma of the cervix in the preinvasive stage, but the latter is more difficult to detect on routine Pap smears.

Cervical cancer remains a near optimal example of the benefits of a screening program. The Pap smear for cervical cytology was introduced over 50 years ago, and with increased use there has been a concomitant decline in the incidence of invasive cervical cancer in developed countries. Unfortunately, as many as 30–40% of women do not have timely Pap smear screening. It is imperative that primary care physicians screen their patients for cervical cancer regularly. Pap smear is easy to obtain, and with use of endocervical brush techniques, virtually every woman can have an accurate result from a Pap smear obtained at an annual visit for health maintenance.

Among women of childbearing age, about 2–3% will exhibit the putative precursor of cancer of the cervix, which in its low-grade appearance is virtually indistinguishable from human papillomavirus (HPV) infection. Although a direct cause and effect have not been conclusively demonstrated, high-grade cervical intraepithelial neoplasia (CIN) is more often associated with HPV types 16, 18, 31, 33, and 35. It is felt that these are premalignant lesions, and high-grade CIN should be aggressively treated; low-grade CIN can be closely monitored. Laser ablation, electric loop excision, or cryotherapy are used for preinvasive disease.

Invasive carcinoma of the cervix is usually diagnosed on colposcopic evaluation of the cervix after a suspicious Pap smear is reported, or on biopsy of a lesion seen on pelvic examination. Once a diagnosis is rendered histologically, the patient should have an abdominal CT scan with contrast, chest x-ray, cystoscopy, and proctoscopy to search for advanced disease. Treatment varies with the extent of cancer spread and condition of the patient. Surgery (radical hysterectomy) is usually chosen for locally invasive disease, whereas advanced disease is usually treated with radiation, perhaps in combination with chemotherapy. The addition of chemotherapy to radiation appears to increase initial response to therapy.

The 5-year survival rate of patients with limited disease is about 90%, with survival rates in other groups falling in proportion to the extent of cancer spread.

CANCER OF THE VULVA

Cancer of the vulva is uncommon and is primarily a disease of women over age 60. Its hallmark symptom is vulvar pruritus. It is now apparent that HPV infection is associated with vulvar intraepithelial neoplasia (VIN); affected patients are usually younger and frequently have a history of sexually transmitted disease. Prompt biopsy is the cornerstone of evaluation, and all patients who have a history of vulvar pruritus should be evaluated with thorough inspection and biopsy of any suspicious lesions.

Preinvasive disease of the vulva can be treated with laser ablation, caustic chemicals, chemotherapy creams, or excision. Invasive disease requires surgical therapy and, in advanced cases, adjuvant radiation. Survival rate is high, especially when lymph nodes are not involved.

GESTATIONAL TROPHOBLASTIC DISEASE

In about 1 in 1000 pregnancies in the Unites States, abnormal fertilization can result in hydatidiform mole. The incidence is much higher in Asia and in underdeveloped countries. Most cases of this earliest form of gestational trophoblastic disease (GTD) resolve spontaneously after surgical evacuation, but in 10–30% of cases malignant sequelae can result. Once the most feared of all gynecologic neoplasms, GTD has become a highly treatable disease with chemotherapy. In fact, choriocarcinoma, the most malignant form of gestational trophoblastic disease, was one of the first solid tumors to be cured with chemotherapy. It is imperative that such patients be accurately eval-

uated and staged by a gynecologic specialist. Although these patients usually present with hydatidiform mole, occasionally hemoptysis, seizures, or hyperthyroidism may be the initial presentation. Whenever a woman of childbearing age has metastatic cancer of unknown origin, measuring serum human chorionic gonadotropin (HCG) can assess the possibility of GTD. Overall, for patients with nonmetastatic disease or minimal metastatic spread, survival rates of 100% are anticipated with appropriate chemotherapy. The survival rate for patients with extensive metastatic disease approaches 75%. These patients should be managed aggressively by a GTD expert.

VAGINAL AND FALLOPIAN TUBE CANCER

Carcinomas of the vagina and fallopian tube are extremely rare neoplasms, usually presenting in postmenopausal women. Vaginal bleeding is usually a hallmark of their presentation. Patients with vaginal cancer may complain about a mass hanging in front of the vagina or a foul discharge with pessaries. A history of CIN may lead to suspicion of vaginal carcinoma.

Beginning in the late 1940's, it was considered appropriate to treat pregnant women who were at high risk for miscarriage with diethylstilbestrol (DES), a synthetic estrogen; this practice continued until the mid-1960's, when clinical trials disproved its worth. Shortly thereafter, intrauterine exposure to DES was associated with a rare clear cell adenocarcinoma of the vagina and cervix, and to date about 400 such cases have been reported. Because of this risk (estimated at 1 in 1400 to 1 in 14,000 exposed women), such patients should have continued surveillance by a gynecologist. Vaginal cancers can be treated with surgery or radiation, alone or in combination.

Fallopian tube carcinoma is a highly malignant neoplasm that spreads in a manner similar to that of ovarian cancer. Even if aggressively treated, this type of cancer has a very high mortality rate.

SUMMARY

▶ Postmenopausal vaginal bleeding and irregular perimenopausal bleeding are caused by endometrial cancer until proven otherwise.

▶ A high index of suspicion for ovarian cancer in women with subtle symptoms leads to earlier diagnosis and improved survival.

▶ Several histologic types of ovarian cancer respond to chemotherapy.

▶ Cervical cancer is identifiable at a very early stage, and proper application of screening procedures could virtually eliminate this cancer as a cause of serious illness and death.

SUGGESTED READING

Carlson KJ, Skates SJ, Singer DE: Screening for ovarian cancer. Ann Intern Med 1994;121:124.

Currie JL: Malignant tumors of the uterine corpus. In: *TeLinde's Operative Gynecology,* 8th ed. Thompson JD, Rock JA (editors). JB Lippincott, 1996.

Hatch KD: Cervical cancer. In: *Practical Gynecologic Oncology,* 2nd ed. Berek JS, Hacker NF (editors). Williams & Wilkins, 1994.

Ovarian cancer: Screening, treatment, and follow-up. NIH Consensus Conference. JAMA 1995;273:491.

Urologic Cancers

Charles B. Brendler, MD, and H. Ballentine Carter, MD

The most common symptom in patients with cancer of the kidney, ureter, bladder, or urethra is hematuria (blood in the urine). Patients with urologic cancers can also present with fever, erythrocytosis (in renal cell carcinoma), bone pain (in metastatic prostate cancer), and an asymptomatic testicular mass. Hematuria has many benign causes, but particularly in adults it should be regarded as a symptom of malignancy until proven otherwise (Table 12.5–1).

Evaluation of hematuria is straightforward: (1) Assess the upper urinary tracts by either intravenous pyelography (IVP) or ultrasonography. (2) Examine the bladder and urethra by cystourethroscopy. (3) Perform urine cytology. These basic studies detect almost all urinary tract malignancies. If these tests are normal, the physician should search for the many benign causes of hematuria.

This chapter reviews the four most common urologic cancers: prostate, bladder, kidney, and testis. The "Suggested Reading" section covers less common urologic cancers including those of the ureter, penis, and urethra.

CARCINOMA OF THE PROSTATE

Clinical Presentation

Men with prostate cancer may present with any stage of the disease, from an asymptomatic nodule noted on routine physical examination to widely metastatic disease with bone pain and severe debility. Early prostate cancer is asymptomatic. As the disease spreads into the urethra, it may cause symptoms of urinary obstruction. If prostate cancer progresses to obstruct the ureters, the patient may present with uremia. Occasionally, the first clue to a patient's illness is an elevated alkaline phosphatase on multichannel serum chemistry tests, or an elevated serum prostate-specific antigen test as part of screening. Skeletal pain and pathologic fractures are common manifestations of metastatic disease.

Carcinoma of the prostate is the most common malignancy in men in the United States. It is the third most common cause of cancer deaths in men over age 55, with about 40,000 deaths per year. Prostate cancer is uncommon before age 40; thereafter, the incidence increases steadily with age. Of men who die from other causes after age 80, 50% are found at autopsy to have incidental prostate cancer.

Etiology and Natural History

The cause of prostate cancer is unknown. Evidence that it involves hormones comes from the facts that the disease does not occur in men who lose testicular function before puberty and that it regresses after medical or surgical castration. Benign prostatic hyperplasia (BPH) does not seem to be causally related. Environmental factors like diet may be involved: Men migrating from the Far East, where prostate cancer is uncommon, to areas where the incidence is higher are more likely to develop the disease.

The natural history of prostate cancer is unpredictable and variable. In some men, the disease progresses slowly; these patients may do well for many years without treatment. But in other men, the disease pursues a fulminant course with rapid spread and early death.

Pathogenesis

Almost all prostate cancers are adenocarcinomas. Prostate cancer usually arises in the peripheral region of the prostate, in contrast to benign prostatic hyperplasia, which arises adjacent to the urethra. Thus, early prostate cancer is asymptomatic, whereas benign prostatic hyperplasia commonly produces symptoms of urethral obstruction. Prostate cancer, however, can extend locally to obstruct the urethra, and, later, the ureter. Metastasis is to pelvic lymph nodes and then to bone. Visceral metastases occur later and are less common; the lungs, liver, and adrenal glands are the distant organs most often involved.

Physical Examination

In a patient with early prostate cancer, the physical findings are confined to the prostate. On rectal exam, prostate cancer feels firm or woody, as opposed to the rubbery texture of normal or hyperplastic prostate. Abnormal texture is more suggestive of carcinoma than is asymmetry in size between the left and right lobes of the

Table 12.5–1. Most common causes of hematuria.

Malignant
Renal cell carcinoma
Bladder carcinoma
Urethral carcinoma
Ureteral carcinoma

Benign
Urinary tract infection
Kidney stones
Instrumentation
Hemorrhagic cystitis

prostate, since the lobes are often asymmetric in benign prostatic hyperplasia. About 50% of firm areas within the prostate prove malignant; the rest are caused by prostatic calculi, inflammation, infarction, or changes after partial prostatectomy for benign prostatic hyperplasia.

Diagnosis

Early detection of prostate cancer is critical. All men over 50 should have a yearly rectal exam. There has also been considerable interest in screening with serum measurements of prostate-specific antigen (PSA), a glycoprotein that is produced exclusively by prostatic epithelial cells. About 80% of men with PSA levels above 20 ng/mL have prostate cancer, and 80% of men with levels above 50 ng/mL have metastatic disease. The problem is that PSA levels rise in both prostate cancer and benign prostatic hyperplasia; however, they rise faster in prostate cancer. In any case, PSA levels alone are not an adequate screen. PSA is more specific when combined with digital rectal exam.

Prostate cancer is confirmed by transrectal or transperineal needle biopsy of the prostate, either of which is more than 90% accurate. Prostate needle biopsies can be done on outpatients, with only topical anesthesia and minimal discomfort. Multiple cores can be obtained in a few minutes. An abnormal area within the prostate should be biopsied early. It is wrong to follow a lesion conservatively, because prostate cancer progresses subtly and may not change noticeably over successive exams.

Staging

The digital rectal exam remains the principal test for evaluating the local extent of prostate cancer. Transrectal ultrasonography, computed tomography (CT), and magnetic resonance imaging (MRI) cannot accurately detect spread beyond the capsule of the prostate or involvement of the seminal vesicles.

Prostatic acid phosphatase (PAP) is a screening test for metastatic prostate cancer. Levels are elevated in about 60% of men with metastatic disease. A radionuclide bone scan is routinely obtained in the evaluation for metastatic prostate cancer. The scan is highly accurate and far more sensitive than conventional radiography in detecting bone metastases. Imaging of pelvic lymph nodes by CT or lymphangiography has proved unreliable because these techniques are not sensitive enough to detect microscopic disease. Furthermore, they do not consistently demonstrate the obturator and hypogastric lymphatic chains, which are the primary sites of drainage from the prostate. Thus, a staging pelvic lymphadenectomy is almost always done to detect nodal metastases before radical prostatectomy.

Management

There is increasing evidence that the most effective treatment for early prostate cancer (confined to the prostate) is total prostatectomy. Survival at 15 years equals that in men of similar age who do not have prostate cancer. Until recently, total prostatectomy was not widely accepted because it left 20–30% of patients with urinary incontinence and almost all patients impotent. Recent improvements in surgical technique have drastically lessened morbidity. Now 90% of men have complete urinary control after total prostatectomy, and 8% need wear only one pad a day to control urine leaks during exercise. Only 2% have incontinence severe enough to warrant further treatment, and the condition is readily corrected with either an artificial urinary sphincter or intraurethral injection of collagen. In addition, many men retain potency. These advances have prompted patients to seek treatment at an earlier stage of disease and are making total prostatectomy the treatment of choice.

Radiation therapy is an alternative treatment for early prostate cancer. Although overall 10-year survival rates with radiation and surgery are similar, the percentage of men who die from prostate cancer within 10 years after radiation therapy is about 35%, compared with 15% for those with radical prostatectomy. In addition, after radiation therapy at least one-third of men have prostate biopsies showing residual cancer. Radiation therapy might be best reserved for patients who are at high risk for perioperative complications (Chapter 15.2).

Given these findings and the increasing attractiveness of radical prostatectomy, enthusiasm for radiation therapy has diminished. Radiation therapy in early-stage prostate cancer should still be recommended for patients who either refuse radical prostatectomy or are not good surgical candidates because of age, extent of disease, or other health considerations.

Radiation therapy is also being challenged as the preferred treatment for prostate cancer extending locally beyond the prostate but still confined to the pelvis. Here, again, survival may be equivalent with radical prostatectomy.

Patients with metastatic prostate cancer are given medical or surgical endocrine therapy. The aim is to shrink both primary and metastatic lesions by depriving prostate cells of circulating androgens. Estrogens are no longer used to treat prostate cancer because they cause cardiovascular complications. Patients can be medically castrated with luteinizing hormone-releasing hormone (LH-RH) analogs, either alone or in combination with anti-androgens such as flutamide. Although these agents are as effective as surgical removal of the testicles, they do not seem to provide any additional benefit. The mean survival after hormonal therapy is about 3 years. Nearly all men eventually relapse with hormone-resistant disease, and the mean survival after relapse is about 1 year.

Unfortunately, no effective chemotherapy is available to treat prostate cancer after failed hormonal therapy. Suramin, an antitrypanosomal agent, inhibits prostatic growth factors and is being used to treat men with advanced disease who have had relapses after hormonal therapy. Although suramin appears promising, the response has lasted a mean of only about 6 months.

CARCINOMA OF THE KIDNEY

Clinical Presentation

The clinical manifestations of renal cell carcinoma are so diverse that they can cause difficulty or delay in diagnosis. Symptoms may result from local tumor growth, paraneoplastic syndromes, and metastatic disease. Local tumor growth can produce (1) a palpable abdominal mass, (2) flank pain caused by extension into contiguous structures or tumor hemorrhage that stretches the renal capsule, and (3) hematuria caused by tumor invading the collecting system. Fewer than 10% of patients have this full triad of symptoms, but such patients are likely to have advanced disease. Tumor extending into the left renal vein or the inferior vena cava can cause a varicocele from obstruction of the spermatic vein. Extension into the vena cava can also produce manifestations of caval occlusion, such as lower extremity edema. Patients with renal cell carcinoma may become hypertensive, presumably because local tumor growth and renal ischemia spur renin production.

Paraneoplastic syndromes can produce symptoms that are not readily linked to an underlying renal cell carcinoma (Table 12.5–2). Fever, erythrocytosis, anemia, hypercalcemia, and hepatic dysfunction are the most common extrarenal manifestations of renal cell carcinoma. Erythrocytosis develops when the tumor elaborates erythropoietin. Hypercalcemia develops when the tumor produces an ectopic parathyroid hormone-like substance or prostaglandins. The etiology of the other symptoms is poorly understood.

When first seen, about 25% of patients already have ra-

Table 12.5–2. Systemic manifestations of renal cell carcinoma.

Fever
Erythrocytosis
Anemia
Hypercalcemia
Hepatic dysfunction (Stauffer's syndrome)
Weight loss
Fatigue
Thrombocytosis
Eosinophilia
Hypertension
Galactorrhea
Cushing's syndrome

diographic evidence of metastases. The most common site of metastasis is the lungs, with cough or hemoptysis often the presenting symptom. Other common sites are liver, bone, and brain.

Renal cell carcinoma is the third most common urologic cancer, accounting for 85% of all primary malignancies of the kidney. Cancers of the renal pelvis comprise another 10%, and uncommon mesenchymal tumors (eg, sarcomas), about 5%.

Etiology

Renal cell carcinoma manifests most often in patients 40–60 years old and in a male:female ratio of 2:1. The cancer arises from the proximal convoluted tubule of the kidney. The etiology is unknown, but possible factors are tobacco, obesity, and exposure to petrochemical products. Risk is higher than normal in patients with von Hippel-Lindau disease, autosomal dominant polycystic kidney disease, horseshoe kidney, and acquired renal cystic disease associated with chronic renal failure.

Diagnosis and Staging

Intravenous urography (IVU) is the technique most often used to image the urinary tract, and it is usually the first study to evaluate hematuria. Intravenous urography detects most renal masses, urothelial cancers, and stones, all of which cause hematuria. Radiographically, renal masses are cystic (usually benign) or solid (usually malignant). Most solid renal masses are renal cell carcinoma. Although intravenous urography usually indicates whether a mass is cystic or solid, sonography or CT is more reliable. On CT, the cancer is characteristically a solid mass that is less dense than the surrounding parenchyma but enhances after the patient is given intravenous contrast dye.

Patients with suspected renal cell carcinoma undergo a staging evaluation to determine the extent of the tumor. Abdominal and chest CT are used to look for spread to regional lymph nodes and other organs. CT, MRI, and venacavography can identify vena caval extension of tumor. Most patients have a bone scan to detect osseous metastases.

Management

Radical nephrectomy (removal of the kidney, surrounding fascia, ipsilateral adrenal gland, and regional lymph nodes) offers the only chance for cure in patients with renal cell carcinoma. Prognosis depends most on the surgical stage of the tumor. The 5-year survival rate for patients whose cancer is resected with surgical margins free of tumor is 50–70%, and for regionally advanced tumors (lymph nodes involved or vascular invasion), 15–35%. Patients with distant metastases have a 0–5% chance of being alive in 5 years. Radical nephrectomy is generally reserved for patients in whom all tumor can likely be excised; surgery does not prolong survival in patients with advanced disease. Partial nephrectomy is considered in an attempt to preserve some renal tissue in patients with bilateral renal cell carcinoma, patients who have only one kidney, and patients with severe renal insufficiency.

Attempts to treat metastatic renal cell carcinoma with radiation and chemotherapy have been disappointing. Immunotherapy seems to offer the most promise in treating advanced disease, since the tumor is immunogenic. Current research focuses on immunotherapy and on combinations of interferons and chemotherapeutic agents.

CARCINOMA OF THE BLADDER

Clinical Presentation

The most common symptom of bladder cancer is gross or microscopic hematuria, found in about 85% of patients. Less common are irritative symptoms like frequency of urination, urgency, and strangury (pain at the end of urination). When these symptoms are wrongly attributed to infection, the true diagnosis is delayed. Patients with irritative symptoms and a negative urine culture should be evaluated for bladder cancer.

Bladder cancer is the second most common urologic cancer, causing about 10,000 deaths per year in the United States. The male:female ratio is 3:1. The disease is more common in whites than in blacks.

Etiology

Bladder cancer was one of the first malignancies to be linked to a specific carcinogen. In 1895, Rehn found that aniline dye manufacturers had a higher than normal risk for the disease. Today, the major etiologic factor in bladder cancer is cigarette smoking. People who smoke up to two packs a day double their risk for bladder cancer; those who smoke more than three packs a day triple their risk. Other risk factors for bladder cancer include the artificial sweetener sodium cyclamate, cyclophosphamide, and schistosomiasis.

Pathogenesis

About 90% of bladder cancers are transitional cell carcinomas. Most transitional bladder cancers begin as superficial papillary lesions that invade the bladder wall and then metastasize. The rest begin as flat, insidious "ink-stain" lesions, which quickly penetrate the bladder wall. Of the two types, flat carcinomas tend to be more aggressive and have a more ominous prognosis.

The remaining 10% of bladder cancers are squamous cell carcinomas or adenocarcinomas. Squamous cell carcinoma is often associated with chronic infection and is the type of tumor seen in patients with schistosomiasis. Adenocarcinoma usually develops on either the dome or the trigone of the bladder and is also seen in patients with bladder exstrophy. Most adenocarcinomas behave aggressively and carry a poor prognosis.

Bladder cancer spreads via pelvic lymphatics and metastasizes to lung, liver, and, less commonly, bone.

Physical Examination

Early bladder cancer produces no abnormal physical findings. Advanced tumors involving the posterior wall of the bladder or urethra are palpable in only a few women on vaginal exam and a few men on rectal exam. Other abnormal findings are lymphadenopathy and hepatomegaly, both secondary to metastatic disease.

Diagnosis

Bladder cancer is usually diagnosed by cystoscopy. Cystoscopy detects all papillary tumors and reveals suspicious reddened areas that may be flat carcinoma. The diagnosis is confirmed by transurethral resection of obvious tumors and biopsies of suspicious areas. Urine cytology also accurately detects flat carcinoma. Even better than urine cytology is a bladder washing, in which the bladder is lavaged with saline, yielding many cells for analysis.

Staging

The malignant potential of a bladder tumor increases significantly after it penetrates through the lamina propria and invades the bladder's muscle wall. Transurethral surgery and topical therapy are appropriate only for patients with tumor confined to the superficial layers of the bladder. Patients with muscle-invasive disease need more aggressive treatment.

Intravenous pyelography (IVP) is helpful in staging patients with bladder cancer. IVP detects 75% of bladder tumors greater than 1 cm in diameter, as well as tumors in the upper tracts (renal pelvis or ureter) that are found concurrently in 5–8% of patients with bladder cancer. IVP also screens for other upper tract abnormalities, such as renal masses and stones.

CT enhanced by contrast dye or air in the bladder is useful in detecting bladder wall thickening, perivesical extension of tumor, and distant metastases in the abdomen and chest. CT should precede transurethral biopsy and resection, since surgery can cause bladder wall induration that may be mistaken for tumor. CT also detects local extension of disease beyond the bladder wall, but is not good at detecting pelvic lymphadenopathy.

CT and MRI are about equally accurate at staging bladder cancer. The major advantage of MRI is that it can image multiple planes, which may help determine the operability of large, bulky tumors.

Management

Superficial Disease: Transurethral resection is the initial treatment for patients with bladder tumors. In general, tumors should be resected rather than simply cauterized in order to obtain tissue for staging. When resecting the tumor, the surgeon should also take (1) muscle beneath the tumor to help stage it; (2) random biopsies adjacent to the tumor as well as from other parts of the bladder, and, in men, from the prostatic urethra, to rule out flat carcinoma; and (3) a bladder washing for cytology.

After transurethral resection, patients who are at high risk for either recurrent disease or disease progression should be given adjuvant intravesical therapy. This therapy is indicated, for example, for patients with rapid tumor recurrence, high-grade lesions, flat carcinoma, or a persistently positive urine cytology after resection of all visible lesions. Bacillus Calmette-Guérin (BCG) is the agent most often used; others are thiotepa, doxorubicin, and mitomycin C.

Muscle-Invasive Bladder Cancer: Treatment options for muscle-invasive bladder cancer include partial cystectomy, total or radical cystectomy, radiation therapy, and a combination of surgery and radiation therapy. Partial cystectomy is infrequently indicated for invasive bladder cancer because the disease is multifocal and likely to recur. Partial cystectomy should be reserved for primary, solitary tumors located away from the bladder neck and measuring less than 5 cm in diameter. Radical cystectomy in men is removal of the bladder, prostate, and pelvic lymph nodes. In women it is removal of the bladder, urethra, pelvic nodes, and genital organs, including the anterior wall of the vagina. Radical cystectomy is the most effective treatment for muscle-invasive bladder cancer. Treated patients whose tumors involve superficial muscle have a 5-year survival rate of 80%, and 50% for those whose tumors involve deep muscle or perivesical fat. Like radical prostatectomy, radical cystectomy was not widely accepted in the past because of its morbidity. Current techniques, however, allow continent reconstruction of the urinary tract to either the urethra or skin, obviating the need for an external urinary appliance; some men's potency is preserved. Radical cystectomy is now the preferred treatment for muscle-invasive bladder cancer in the United States.

External-beam radiation therapy remains popular in Europe, but in the United States, 5-year survival rates of only 20–35% make it much less satisfactory than radical cystectomy. Radiation treatment before cystectomy does not appear to increase survival.

Advanced Disease: Until 1983, there was no effective treatment for patients with advanced or metastatic bladder cancer. Since then, encouraging results have been obtained with several regimens that combine cisplatin with other agents. One frequently used combination is M-VAC (methotrexate, vinblastine, doxorubicin, and cisplatin), which produces a sustained complete response in 10–15% of patients with advanced bladder cancer. M-VAC is even more effective as adjuvant chemotherapy: Patients with involved lymph nodes or invasion of adjacent pelvic viscera who receive M-VAC after cystectomy have a 5-year survival of 30–40%, compared with only 5–10% for those not receiving adjuvant therapy. Although the timing of chemotherapy remains controversial, it appears that platinum-based combination therapy significantly enhances survival in patients with muscle-invasive and metastatic bladder cancer.

TESTICULAR CANCER

Clinical Presentation

Over 70% of testicular tumors present either as painless testicular enlargement or as a testicular mass found by the patient or his sexual partner. Occasional patients present with manifestations of metastatic disease such as retroperitoneal or supraclavicular lymphadenopathy, or hemoptysis from lung metastases. Human chorionic gonadotropin (HCG) produced by some testis tumors stimulates estradiol production by Leydig cells and causes gynecomastia in up to 5% of patients.

Testicular cancer accounts for only 1% of cancers in men. However, it is the most common solid neoplasm among men aged 20–34, and its peak incidence is between ages 20 and 40. Whites have a fourfold greater incidence than blacks, and testicular cancer is more common in higher socioeconomic groups.

Etiology

About 10% of testicular cancers occur in previously cryptorchid (undescended) testicles. The risk of testicular cancer remains high even after the testicle has been positioned in the scrotum. Furthermore, men with a history of cryptorchidism or testicular cancer have a greater risk of developing cancer in the other testis. Since hormones play a role in testicular descent, these patterns suggest that a systemic factor affects both testes. Thus, men with a history of cryptorchidism or testicular cancer should be followed carefully and encouraged to examine their testicles to detect cancer early.

Pathogenesis

Testicular neoplasms are derived from either germinal or nongerminal elements. Nongerminal tumors are usually benign, occur most often in children, and arise from Leydig cells, Sertoli cells, or testicular stroma. Almost all postpubertal testicular tumors are of germ cell origin; the exception is lymphoma of the testis, which is the most common testicular tumor after age 50. Germ cell tumors arise from a common totipotential stem cell that can give rise to a seminoma or embryonal cancer (nonseminoma). Seminoma has no potential for further differentiation (unipotential); embryonal cancer (totipotential) can differentiate to other nonseminomatous tumors (teratoma, choriocarcinoma, yolk sac tumor). Since testicular cancers arise from a common stem cell, it is not surprising that 40% of patients have several germ cell elements in the same tumor. It is important to determine whether a germ cell testicular cancer is a seminoma or nonseminoma because the two types are usually treated differently.

Diagnosis

The evaluation of a patient with testicular pain or a scrotal mass should focus on determining whether or not the pathology is in the testis. Most masses in the scrotum but outside the testicle are benign (eg, hydroceles, varicoceles, spermatoceles). In contrast, most solid masses arising within the testicle are malignant. In most patients, the physician can tell by palpation whether a scrotal lesion is intra- or extratesticular. However, testicular cancer is often confused with epididymo-orchitis because the inflammatory process in epididymo-orchitis can obliterate the normal plane between the testicle and epididymis, producing a solid mass.

One way to differentiate benign from malignant scrotal masses is to hold a flashlight directly against the posterior wall of the scrotum. Since most benign scrotal masses are cystic and fluid-filled, they are easily transilluminated. Solid lesions do not transilluminate. When the site of a mass is uncertain or testicular exam is inadequate, another way to distinguish intra- from extratesticular masses is with scrotal ultrasonography.

No radiographic technique reliably distinguishes benign from malignant solid testicular lesions. If the physician suspects an intratesticular mass on the basis of physical exam or ultrasound, orchiectomy is indicated to establish testicular cancer. The entire testicle is removed and examined histologically. If the mass is malignant, the histology guides treatment. Before surgery, the patient should have blood drawn to measure two serum tumor markers for testicular cancer: HCG and α-fetoprotein (AFP). These markers are used for both diagnosis and staging.

Staging

The staging evaluation for testicular cancers involves physical exam, measurement of serum tumor markers, and radiography. Physical exam may detect lymphadenopathy (eg, supraclavicular) and enlarged viscera (eg, hepatomegaly). Some testicular cancers produce HCG and AFP, which are important for staging. Persistent elevation of serum HCG or AFP after orchiectomy indicates residual disease. Chest and abdominal CT are used to detect spread to the lungs, abdominal organs, and retroperitoneal lymph nodes. Although the staging tests are useful, 20–30% of patients with normal serum markers and CT scans have microscopic retroperitoneal lymph node metastases found on surgical exploration.

Management

Several characteristics of testicular tumors may explain why they have higher cure rates than other solid tumors. The short doubling time of testicular tumors makes them extremely sensitive to chemotherapy. In addition, most testicular tumors spread first to the retroperitoneal lymph nodes and then to the blood. Most patients with small-volume disease localized to retroperitoneal lymph nodes can be cured if their retroperitoneal nodes are removed.

Seminoma: Specific treatment for seminoma should be given only if the tumor is pure seminoma with no other germ cell elements. Seminomas do not produce AFP. Thus, if a patient's AFP is normal and careful pathologic examination of the testis reveals pure seminoma, he should be treated for seminoma. If the AFP is high or if pathologic examination reveals other germ cell elements,

the patient should be treated for a nonseminomatous germ cell tumor.

Seminoma is a radiosensitive tumor. External-beam radiation is the recommended therapy for patients who have no evidence of disease beyond the testis and patients with involved retroperitoneal lymph nodes less than 6 cm in diameter. Over 90% of patients have been cured with this approach. Radiation therapy is not effective for patients whose seminoma involves retroperitoneal lymph nodes larger than 6 cm or for patients with metastasis extending beyond the retroperitoneal nodes. The current recommendation for these patients is chemotherapy with cisplatin plus one or two other agents. About 70% of patients with high-stage seminoma go into remission after chemotherapy.

Nonseminoma: After orchiectomy confirms nonseminomatous germ cell tumors, removal of the retroperitoneal lymph nodes is standard treatment for patients with disease localized to the testis and for patients whose retroperitoneal nodes are smaller than 6 cm in diameter by CT scan. Retroperitoneal lymphadenectomy (RPLND) is both a staging and therapeutic procedure. If no retroperitoneal disease is found on pathologic examination of the lymph nodes, patients are followed carefully without adjuvant chemotherapy. After a negative RPLND, only about 10% of patients with disease confined to the testicle relapse with metastases, almost always pulmonary. Cisplatin-based chemotherapy cures most patients who relapse. The cure rate for this approach to localized disease is over 98%.

Of patients who have normal-sized lymph nodes but microscopic metastases found at RPLND, about 25% later develop lung metastases unless they get more treatment. Nearly all of these patients are cured if given adjuvant chemotherapy either after RPLND or at the time of recurrence. Early detection of the relapse is key to these high cure rates.

In patients with retroperitoneal lymph node metastases smaller than 6 cm on CT scan, the treatment is RPLND followed by cisplatin-based chemotherapy. Nearly all these patients are cured with adjuvant chemotherapy; without it, two-thirds develop lung metastases.

Advanced nonseminomatous germ cell tumors (retroperitoneal disease greater than 6 cm on CT or metastases beyond the pelvis) are treated primarily with cisplatin-based chemotherapy and resection of residual masses. Complete remission rates for advanced disease are around 70%.

Follow-Up: Because the risk of retroperitoneal metastases is low with localized germ cell tumors, some patients with localized seminomas and nonseminomas have been treated with orchiectomy with no further treatment except check-ups (surveillance alone). About 25–30% of these patients have had relapses. Since most can be cured with chemotherapy, overall survival may be the same as for patients who get adjuvant therapy right after surgery.

Close follow-up is essential to detect early metastases, and surveillance should be used only for patients who are sure of getting regular care.

Patients who have been treated for germ cell tumors need careful periodic evaluation to detect relapses early. In general, during the first year after treatment is completed, chest x-rays and serum markers are taken monthly, with physical exam every other month. During the second year, chest x-rays and serum markers are taken every other month, with physical exam quarterly. Patients who have no evidence of disease 2 years after treatment are most likely cured.

SUMMARY

▶ Prostate cancer is the most common urologic malignancy. Early detection is critical, and all men over 50 should have a yearly rectal exam. Radical prostatectomy appears to be the most effective treatment for early disease and now can be done with very low morbidity.

▶ The lack of specific manifestations in renal cell cancer can delay the diagnosis, which should be suspected when CT shows a solid parenchymal renal mass. Surgery can save many patients with early-stage disease.

▶ Carcinoma of the bladder can cause hematuria and irritative symptoms (urgency, frequency, and pain at the end of urination) and can mimic infection. If diagnosed early (usually by urine cytology and cystoscopy), bladder cancer can be effectively treated by local endoscopic resection and topical therapy.

▶ Solid intratesticular masses are almost always malignant. They can be differentiated from benign extratesticular lesions by palpation and ultrasonography.

▶ Testicular cancer is the most common solid tumor in men aged 20–34. It is usually curable because it is sensitive to chemotherapy and it predictably metastasizes to the retroperitoneal lymph nodes, which can be resected.

SUGGESTED READING

Catalona WJ: Bladder cancer. In: *Adult and Pediatric Urology,* 2nd ed. Gillenwater JY et al (editors). Mosby-Year Book, 1991.

Chapters 20–23 on urologic malignancies. In: *Smith's General Urology,* 14th ed. Tanagho EA, McAninch JW (editors). Appleton & Lange, 1995.

Garnick MB: The dilemmas of prostate cancer. Sci Am 1994; 270(4):52.

Hesketh PJ, Krane RJ: Prognostic assessment in nonseminomatous testicular cancer: Implications for therapy. J Urol 1990; 144:1.

Loehrer PJ Sr, Williams SD, Einhorn LH: Status of chemotherapy for testis cancer. Urol Clin North Am 1987;14:713.

Walsh PC, Worthington JF: *The Prostate: A Guide for Men and the Women Who Love Them.* The Johns Hopkins University Press, 1995.

12.6

Lymphoma

Richard F. Ambinder, MD, PhD, Richard J. Jones, MD, and Eric J. Seifter, MD

Lymphomas are a heterogeneous group of malignancies that arise from cells that reside predominantly in lymphoid tissues. They are commonly divided into Hodgkin's and non-Hodgkin's lymphomas on the basis of differences in biology, histopathology, and clinical behavior. The cellular origin of the malignant cells of Hodgkin's disease is unresolved. About 90% of the non-Hodgkin's lymphomas are derived from B lymphocytes and 10% from T lymphocytes. The extent of the heterogeneity is such that even among B-cell non-Hodgkin's lymphomas some are aggressive and immediately life-threatening, whereas others are indolent with little or no impact on survival. This chapter presents a conceptual framework with which to approach questions such as when to consider a diagnosis of lymphoma, how to pursue the diagnosis, and with what urgency the patient should be treated. Prognosis and treatment are also briefly discussed.

PRESENTING MANIFESTATIONS

Patients with lymphoma commonly present with enlarged lymph nodes. These enlarged nodes may cause no symptoms or may cause organ dysfunction. For example, mediastinal or hilar nodes may compress the airway and lead to cough, dyspnea, or stridor. Hilar or mediastinal involvement can also produce the superior vena cava syndrome: facial, neck, and arm swelling with dilated veins over the chest, neck, or arms from compression of the superior vena cava. Mesenteric nodes can obstruct the intestine, and retroperitoneal nodes can obstruct the ureters. Lymphatic obstruction may lead to edema, ascites, or pleural or pericardial effusion. Involvement of lymphoid organs may manifest in other ways. Enlargement of the spleen may lead to early satiety, abdominal pain, or anemia, granulocytopenia, or thrombocytopenia. Bone marrow involvement may similarly lead to cytopenias. Alternatively, asymptomatic nodal enlargement may be detected by a radiographic study performed for other reasons.

Any organ can be involved by an aggressive lymphoma; however, the gastrointestinal tract (representing about 40% of all primary extranodal lymphomas), skin, and bone or bone marrow are the most common extralymphatic sites. The sinuses, lungs, pleura, pericardium, meninges, spinal cord, brain, stomach, and intestines all may be involved.

Finally, patients may present with constitutional symptoms. Generally attributed to the production of a variety of cytokines by tumor cells, these symptoms may include fever, night sweats, weight loss, pruritus, and fatigue. Fever and night sweats are most common in Hodgkin's disease, but are also associated with particular subsets of non-Hodgkin's lymphoma such as peripheral T-cell lymphoma arising in the setting of angioimmunoblastic lymphadenopathy with dysproteinemia.

The patient's age and background may provide important clues to the pathologic diagnosis. Several lymphomas have well-recognized and distinctive population distributions. Children in equatorial Africa are at high risk for developing diffuse small non-cleaved cell (Burkitt's) lymphoma. These tumors carry the Epstein-Barr virus (EBV) in each tumor cell and are referred to as endemic Burkitt's lymphoma. In Western countries, tumors with this histology have a low incidence, only occasionally carry EBV, and are referred to as sporadic. The incidence is dramatically increased in patients with HIV. The role of the retrovirus in their pathogenesis seems to be indirect, since these tumors never carry HIV (and only occasionally EBV). Regardless of the geography or presence or absence of EBV or the association with HIV, these tumors carry one of a family of characteristic chromosomal translocations that juxtapose the c-myc gene on chromosome 8 with an immunoglobulin locus, usually the heavy-chain locus on chromosome 14.

Patients from Japan, the Caribbean basin, and occasionally the southeastern United States are at risk for developing adult T-cell lymphoma-leukemia, a disease that is extraordinarily rare in other settings. This geographic distribution corresponds to that of infection with the HTLV-I, a retrovirus, and the viral genome is integrated into tumor cell DNA. It should be noted, however, that less than 1% of persons with HTLV-I infection develop this lymphoma, and on the average more than 40 years passes between the time of infection and the time the tumor is diagnosed, suggesting that factors other than viral infection play a decisive role in the pathogenesis.

A higher than normal incidence of B-cell lymphomas is found in patients with immunodeficiency. Diffuse large cell, diffuse immunoblastic, and Burkitt's lymphomas all occur with increased frequency in these patients. Many of these tumors are EBV-associated.

Many other lymphomas have characteristic age-incidence curves. Adolescents and young adults, particularly young men, develop lymphoblastic lymphoma. Hodgkin's disease is most common between ages 15 and 45 or after the age of 60. In the younger adult group, Hodgkin's disease is most likely to affect women. Indolent B-cell lymphomas occur almost exclusively in adults, and their incidence rises with age. Etiologies other than those related to infection or immunosuppression are not well established. However, this is an area of intense epidemiologic investigation because it appears that the worldwide incidence of lymphoma has been rising about 1–2% per year since the 1950's.

DIAGNOSTIC EVALUATION

Lymphadenopathy may be a manifestation of infection, drug reaction, or another nonneoplastic disorder. Categories of nonneoplastic causes of lymphadenopathy and examples of each are listed in Table 12.6–1. Investigations to exclude these nonneoplastic disorders should be focused by the clinical context. Thus, a young adult with cervical lymphadenopathy, a history of recent pharyngitis, and hepatosplenomegaly should be evaluated for infectious mononucleosis. Other systemic infections that can cause lymphadenopathy include HIV, tuberculosis, syphilis, toxoplasmosis, and cytomegalovirus. Drug reactions and acute and chronic infections of the extremities or throat may also cause lymphadenopathy. Splenomegaly without lymphadenopathy is an uncommon presentation of lymphoma and should prompt consideration of infection or myeloproliferative disease such as chronic myelogenous leukemia.

Few clinical characteristics distinguish neoplastic from benign nodes, although tender, inflamed nodes are more common in association with local infection and nodes that are hard and fixed to underlying tissue suggest metastatic carcinoma rather than lymphoma. In general, lymphomatous nodes are firm and nontender; the overlying skin is not red. There may be normal palpable nodes up to 2 cm in diameter in the inguinal region and smaller nodes elsewhere. However, even small supraclavicular, epitrochlear, and scalene lymphadenopathy suggests malignancy. As a general rule, the enlargement of a node or nodes to greater than 1 cm persisting for more than 3 weeks without explanation warrants excisional biopsy.

The pace and extent of evaluation for Hodgkin's and non-Hodgkin's lymphoma should be dictated by the clinical manifestations. Evidence of spinal cord compression, tumor lysis syndrome, or superior vena cava syndrome indicates the necessity for immediate therapeutic intervention, even if a histologic diagnosis has not yet been firmly established. On the other hand, history of a small cervical node that has remained unchanged for several months and is not accompanied by systemic symptoms demands attention and workup, but not on an emergent basis. Nodes involved by lymphoid malignancy can remain stable for many months or can wax and wane in size, with spontaneous regression being particularly common in the indolent lymphomas and Hodgkin's disease.

CLASSIFICATION OVERVIEW

Histopathologic appearance by light microscopy is the basis for diagnosing lymphomas. An excisional lymph node biopsy is crucial to proper histopathologic classification. Architectural features defining a follicular or diffuse process are much more difficult to discern by needle biopsy, extranodal sampling, or organ biopsy. However, diagnosis is sometimes assisted by more specialized techniques like cell surface marker or immunoglobulin/T-cell receptor gene rearrangement analyses. These techniques are particularly useful in distinguishing lymphoma from undifferentiated carcinoma. Hodgkin's disease is distinguished from non-Hodgkin's lymphoma by the recognition of characteristic multinucleated malignant giant cells known as Reed-Sternberg cells. Hodgkin's disease is unique among malignancies in that the malignant cells generally constitute substantially less than 1% of the cells in a tumor mass.

Hodgkin's disease is considered separately from the non-Hodgkin's lymphomas because of its distinctive mode of contiguous nodal spread and remarkable curability with radiation therapy, chemotherapy, or both. Hodgkin's disease has traditionally been subdivided into four histologic categories: nodular sclerosis, mixed-cellularity, lymphocyte-predominant, and lymphocyte-depleted (Table 12.6–2). Although the histopathologic subclassification of Hodgkin's disease has some clinical correlates, histologic subtype per se is not an independent prognosticator in appropriately treated patients; Hodgkin's disease of any histology should be regarded as potentially curable.

In general, non-Hodgkin's lymphomas tend to be clini-

Table 12.6–1. Differential diagnosis of nonlymphomatous lymph node enlargement.

Category	Examples
Viral	Infection with Epstein-Barr virus (infectious mononucleosis), HIV, cytomegalovirus
Bacterial, fungal, parasitic	Streptococcal infection, histoplasmosis, toxoplasmosis
Metastatic	Lung cancer, breast cancer, Kaposi's sarcoma
Miscellaneous	Drug reaction, sarcoidosis, dermatopathic lymphadenitis

Table 12.6–2. Hodgkin's disease subclassification.

Type	Clinical Features
Nodular sclerosis	Especially common in young women; often manifests in the cervical, supraclavicular, and anterior mediastinal nodes
Mixed cellularity	Often disseminated
Lymphocyte-predominant	Usually localized
Lymphocyte-depleted	Often disseminated

Table 12.6–4. Diseases that may manifest as leukemia, lymphoma, or both.

Blood and Bone Marrow Involvement Predominates		Lymph Node and Solid Organ Involvement Predominates
Acute lymphoblastic leukemia (T cell)	↔	Lymphoblastic lymphoma
Acute lymphoblastic leukemia (B cell)	↔	Diffuse small non-cleaved cell lymphoma
Chronic lymphocytic leukemia	↔	Diffuse small lymphocytic lymphoma

cally indolent or aggressive (Table 12.6–3). The indolent lymphomas share characteristics of slow growth, a tendency to widespread involvement including bone marrow involvement, long median survivals (ranging from 4 to 12 years), and responsiveness to gentler forms of therapy such as oral chemotherapy. However, indolent lymphomas are also essentially incurable, with inevitable relapses, declining durations of response, and a tendency to convert to more aggressive disease. The aggressive lymphomas are characterized by rapid—in some instances, explosive—growth, but about one-third are curable with combination chemotherapy. Not included in Table 12.6–3 is a very aggressive lymphoma, adult T-cell lymphoma-leukemia caused by HTLV-I, which, in contrast to other aggressive lymphomas, responds very poorly to therapy and is rarely, if ever, cured.

Non-Hodgkin's lymphomas involve lymph nodes in diffuse or follicular patterns. Diffuse lymphomas may be either indolent or aggressive, and their clinical behavior in general corresponds to the lymphocyte morphology (size and nuclear shape). Diffuse small non-cleaved cell lymphomas and diffuse large cell lymphomas are aggressive, whereas diffuse small lymphocytic lymphomas and diffuse small cleaved cell lymphomas are indolent (see Table 12.6–2). Follicular lymphomas, in general, tend to be indolent, and lymphocyte morphology is much less important, although it is still included in most classification schemes. Most follicular lymphomas have the associated chromosomal abnormality t(14;18) involving the immunoglobulin heavy-chain locus and the *bcl*-2 gene and are of B-cell origin.

In several instances, the terms "lymphoma" and "leukemia" do not designate distinct disease entities, but rather arbitrary divisions of a continuous spectrum of nodal and blood (and marrow) involvement (Table 12.6–4). Patients with these leukemia-lymphomas may present with involvement of the blood, lymph nodes, or both, or may progress from involvement of one compartment to involvement of the other compartment. Whether classified as leukemia or lymphoma, these diseases behave similarly in terms of aggressiveness, responsiveness to therapy, and curability or tendency to relapse.

STAGING

Staging of lymphomas is useful for determining the prognosis and a plan of treatment. Originally developed for Hodgkin's disease, the Ann Arbor classification has been widely applied to the non-Hodgkin's lymphomas as well. However, as a consequence of the orderly pattern of spread, staging the extent and locus of tumor in Hodgkin's disease has been much more important than in non-Hodgkin's lymphoma.

Staging of Hodgkin's disease begins with a history and an assessment of constitutional symptoms, several of which have been shown to adversely affect prognosis in Hodgkin's disease. These are fever, night sweats, and weight loss. Collectively, they are referred to as B symptoms. History should include details of these constitutional symptoms. Thus, it must be determined whether the fever was, or is, unexplained or attributable to an infection or other cause. Only unexplained fevers higher than 38°C (100.4°F). occurring on three or more consecutive nights qualify as B symptoms. Similarly, night sweats have prognostic importance only if they are "drenching," that is, requiring a change of sheets or bedclothes and occurring on three or more consecutive nights. Finally, weight loss must be unexplained and amount to 10% or more of body weight to be considered significant. The staging classification is summarized in Table 12.6–5.

Physical examination should focus on all nodal sites, including Waldeyer's ring (pharyngeal) and the epitrochlear nodes. Computed tomography (CT) scans of the neck, chest, abdomen, and pelvis, and bone marrow biopsy complete the basic staging. At some centers, lymphangiography or gallium scanning, and diagnostic laparotomy with splenectomy, open biopsy of left and right lobes of the liver, and nodal sampling are a part of routine

Table 12.6–3. Pragmatic grouping of non-Hodgkin's lymphomas.

Aggressive-curable
  Diffuse small non-cleaved cell (Burkitt's, diffuse undifferentiated)
  Diffuse large cell or immunoblastic
  Lymphoblastic

Indolent-relapsing
  Follicular lymphomas
  Diffuse small lymphocytic
  Diffuse small cleaved cell
  Mycosis fungoides (cutaneous T-cell lymphoma)

Table 12.6–5. Lymphoma staging.*

Stage	Description
I	Involvement of a single lymph node region (including a single localized extralymphatic site)
II	Involvement of ≥2 lymph node regions (including a single localized extralymphatic site) on the same side of the diaphragm
III	Involvement of lymph node regions (including localized involvement of 1 extralymphatic site, spleen involvement, or both) on both sides of the diaphragm
IV	Diffuse involvement of ≥1 extralymphatic organs (bone marrow, liver, lungs)

Constitutional symptoms

A	No symptoms
B	Fever, drenching sweats, weight loss

*Patients with Hodgkin's disease are commonly assigned both clinical and pathologic stages. The clinical stage is based on physical exam and noninvasive studies. The pathologic stage is based on biopsies for different sites, including laparotomy. Localized extralymphatic disease is designated "E."

evaluation for patients with clinical early-stage disease. The extent and invasiveness of the diagnostic evaluation depend largely on therapeutic philosophy (see below). Liver involvement is rare in the absence of splenomegaly.

Hematologic abnormalities, including leukemoid reaction, monocytosis, and lymphopenia are all common. Erythrocyte sedimentation rate, serum copper, and a variety of other acute-phase reactants have been used to monitor disease activity. Their usefulness in clinical practice is limited by their nonspecificity.

For the non-Hodgkin's lymphomas, staging involves distinguishing between localized disease (stage I and in some cases contiguous stage II) or more widespread involvement. Thoracic, abdominal, and pelvic CT scans and bone marrow biopsy are usually adequate. For aggressive lymphomas, the serum lactic dehydrogenase should also be checked, because this is an important prognostic variable and also has value as a marker to follow the course of the disease. A serum protein electrophoresis may be helpful for following the disease in the uncommon patient whose lymphoma produces a monoclonal immunoglobulin.

INDOLENT LYMPHOMAS

Indolent lymphomas increase in incidence with age, being rare in childhood and uncommon in young adults. These lymphomas occur almost exclusively in lymph nodes and in lymphoid organs. Most patients have stage IV disease; yet only 10–20% present with constitutional symptoms (fever, night sweats, weight loss). Indolent lymphomas usually grow slowly, often waxing and waning in size for months or years.

With treatment, and sometimes without treatment, some patients with indolent lymphomas survive for more than a decade. Spontaneous regressions that may last from a few months to several years are not uncommon. However, remissions are almost inevitably followed by relapse. Patients can relapse after a few months or after many years. Some older patients die *with* rather than *from* their disease.

About one-third of indolent lymphomas evolve into aggressive lymphomas, usually diffuse large cell lymphomas. This transformation is often heralded by constitutional symptoms and rapid tumor growth, sometimes in spleen or extranodal sites not previously involved by the indolent lymphomas. Patients with tumors that have transformed have particularly poor survival rates, with less than 20% surviving 2 years after conventional therapy.

Although radiation therapy often cures localized indolent lymphomas, more than 90% of indolent lymphomas are too advanced at presentation for radiation therapy with curative intent. For these advanced-stage patients, standard therapy involves consideration of a "watch-and-wait" approach, with treatment only when symptoms or laboratory abnormalities indicate that therapy may yield a specific benefit such as relief from constitutional symptoms, resolution of cytopenias related to marrow infiltration, or shrinkage of a mass obstructing lymphatic drainage. This approach is based on studies that show no better long-term survival for patients treated at the time of original diagnosis than for those treated only when there was a specific indication. When therapy is required, modalities to be considered include local radiation therapy, single-agent chemotherapy (eg, oral cyclophosphamide), and combination chemotherapy (eg, cyclophosphamide, vincristine, and prednisone, with or without doxorubicin). The choice of chemotherapy is based on the extent of systemic disease, the toxicities of therapy, and the importance of a rapid response.

AGGRESSIVE LYMPHOMAS

The aggressive lymphomas may present with nodal or extranodal disease. Anterior mediastinal involvement is characteristic of lymphoblastic lymphoma. About 20% of patients have bone marrow involvement; this is particularly common in lymphoblastic lymphoma and diffuse small non-cleaved cell lymphoma. This same subset of lymphomas is also especially likely to involve the central nervous system. Aggressive lymphomas usually grow rapidly, and without effective chemotherapy, survival can usually be measured in months. When other considerations preclude therapy, as is sometimes the case in patients with AIDS who have a compromised hematologic status and active opportunistic infections, lymphoma is almost inevitably the cause of death. However, when patients with aggressive lymphomas achieve complete remissions with therapy, the remissions are often sustained. Relapses usually occur within the first several years after therapy. Most patients who do not relapse within this period are cured.

Among patients with aggressive lymphomas, about 20% have stage I disease. Despite some controversy regarding the optimal approach, these patients have an excellent prognosis, with an expected cure rate of over 70%. Patients in whom the disease is not localized require combination chemotherapy, such as cyclophosphamide, doxorubicin, vincristine, and prednisone. Intrathecal chemotherapy to treat or prevent meningeal involvement is used for diffuse small non-cleaved cell and lymphoblastic lymphomas. These regimens produce a 20–55% cure rate in various aggressive lymphomas, with the patient's age, performance status, size and location of tumor mass or masses, and bone marrow involvement being important prognostic factors. Patients with aggressive lymphomas who relapse are rarely cured with conventional chemotherapy or radiation, but may be cured with high-dose therapy and autologous or allogeneic bone marrow or peripheral stem cell transplantation.

HODGKIN'S DISEASE

Patients with Hodgkin's disease usually present with nodal disease, most commonly involving the cervical, supraclavicular, and mediastinal nodes. Nodular sclerosis very commonly is seen as a mediastinal mass in young women. About one-third of Hodgkin's patients have constitutional symptoms.

Chemotherapy cures more than 50% of patients with advanced-stage disease and an even higher fraction of patients with early-stage disease. The first curative combination chemotherapy was the MOPP regimen of nitrogen mustard, vincristine (Oncovin), procarbazine, and prednisone. This regimen caused short-term toxicities (nausea, vomiting, alopecia, myelotoxicity) and long-term toxicities (sterility, acute nonlymphocytic leukemia). For many years, MOPP was the gold standard against which all other regimens or approaches were compared. More recently, combination chemotherapy regimens such as the ABVD regimen (doxorubicin [Adriamycin], bleomycin, vinblastine, and dacarbazine) have achieved better results with less long-term toxicity.

Hodgkin's disease is also very sensitive to radiation therapy, and radiation cures more than 90% of patients with stage I disease. Patients with stage II and even some with stage III disease may be cured with appropriate radiation fields. In comparison with MOPP, early toxicities are less severe with radiation therapy, leukemia is not a long-term complication, and sterility can generally be avoided if the gonads are not within the radiation port. Thus, when MOPP was the chemotherapy of choice, whenever possible, patients were treated with radiation therapy rather than chemotherapy. With the demonstration that other chemotherapy regimens are at least as effective as MOPP, and recognition of the long-term complications of radiation therapy—including a dramatically increased risk of second nonhematopoietic malignancies within or adjacent to radiation ports—many centers are reevaluating the relative risks and benefits of radiation and chemotherapy. The decision as to whether radiation therapy is likely to be curative in a particular patient, and exactly what tissues should be irradiated, depends on a detailed knowledge of the extent of the disease.

To fully define the extent of disease, physicians in the past often undertook staging laparotomy. Discovery of abdominal disease, particularly lower abdominal disease, liver disease, or extensive splenic disease indicated the need for chemotherapy. The availability of CT and magnetic resonance imaging (MRI) has improved the quality of information available without laparotomy at the same time that alternatives to radiation therapy have become more palatable. As a result, the role of staging laparotomy is controversial. However, there is universal agreement that such an investigation should be undertaken only if the results will be used to guide therapy.

Combination chemotherapy given for about 6 months is standard for advanced-stage Hodgkin's disease (III, IV). These regimens produce a 50–90% cure rate. High-dose cytotoxic therapy, followed by autologous or allogeneic bone marrow or peripheral stem cell transplantation, is often recommended for patients who relapse after a short remission.

SUMMARY

▶ The indolent lymphomas share characteristics of slow growth, long median survival, inevitable relapse or progression, and risk of conversion to an aggressive lymphoma.

▶ The aggressive lymphomas are characterized by rapid growth and short survival without therapy. About one-third are curable with combination chemotherapy.

▶ Hodgkin's disease is distinguished by its contiguous pattern of spread and high curability.

SUGGESTED READING

Ambinder RF: Lymphomas. In: *The Molecular Basis of Medicine.* Dang CV, Feldman AM (editors). BC Decker, 1995.

Fisher RI et al: Comparison of a standard regimen (CHOP) with three intensive chemotherapy regimens for advanced non-Hodgkin's lymphoma. N Engl J Med 1993;328:1002.

Jones RJ, Ambinder RF, Seifter EJ: Non-Hodgkin lymphoma. In: *The Fundamentals of Clinical Hematology,* 3rd ed. Spivak JL, Eichner ER (editors). Johns Hopkins, 1993.

A predictive model for aggressive non-Hodgkin's lymphoma: The International Non-Hodgkin's Lymphoma Prognostic Factors Project. N Engl J Med 1993;329:987.

Urba WJ, Longo DL: Hodgkin's disease. N Engl J Med 1992; 326:678.

Plasma Cell Dyscrasias

Richard L. Humphrey, MD

The plasma cell dyscrasias are usually characterized by uncontrolled proliferation of a clone of plasma cells and excessive production by these cells of a homogeneous immunoglobulin (monoclonal gammopathy) (Figures 12.7–1C and 12.7–4). The plasma cell dyscrasias customarily are classified according to the type of monoclonal immunoglobulin (sometimes called an M component) produced. Multiple myeloma, the most common malignant plasma cell dyscrasia, involves monoclonal production of IgG, IgA, IgD, IgE, or free monoclonal light chain, either kappa or lambda. When only monoclonal light chain (Bence Jones protein) is produced, the process has also been called light-chain disease (Figures 12.7–2C and 12.7–4). A plasma cell dyscrasia producing a monoclonal IgM is called Waldenström's macroglobulinemia (Figure 12.7–5). Rarely, only a fragment of an immunoglobulin heavy chain is made, leading to the designation of heavy chain disease.

In amyloidosis, the chief problem is deposition of a fibrillar protein in tissues, causing organ dysfunction. A plasmacytoma is a localized collection of plasma cells, which presents as a mass with or without detectable monoclonal immunoglobulin; the mass may be inside (osseous) or outside bone (extramedullary). Plasma cell leukemia results when the excessive proliferation of plasma cells involves the peripheral blood, where an absolute number of plasma cells above 500/µL in a differential count confirms the diagnosis. Finally, in the condition known as *monoclonal gammopathy of undetermined significance*, a monoclonal immunoglobulin is produced in excess without any apparent tissue destruction, organ dysfunction, or progression over time.

Patients with plasma cell dyscrasias are usually in their sixth decade or older. The clinical manifestations encountered most often result from bone marrow failure (eg, anemia, bleeding from thrombocytopenia), destruction of the skeletal system (eg, bone pain, pathologic fractures, hypercalcemia, osteoporosis), progressive nephropathy, hyperviscosity, and increased susceptibility to infection.

Some patients are asymptomatic, and their diagnosis is suspected only because they are found coincidentally to have either hyperglobulinemia on a multichannel chemical analysis or proteinuria on screening urinalysis, leading to the discovery of a monoclonal gammopathy.

HYPERGAMMAGLOBULINEMIA

Whenever elevated serum globulins are reported on patient blood testing, follow-up serum protein electrophoresis and immunoglobulin quantitation are imperative. Exaggerated production of heterogeneous immunoglobulins is polyclonal gammopathy (see Figure 12.7–1D), which is not a plasma cell dyscrasia. Polyclonal gammopathy must be distinguished from monoclonal gammopathy.

Polyclonal Gammopathy

Polyclonal gammopathy is seen in many disorders, such as chronic infections (especially HIV), sarcoidosis, rheumatic diseases, and many liver diseases. In most instances, the polyclonal gammopathy is clinically silent, although rarely the immunoglobulin level rises so high (over 4 g/dL) as to cause hyperviscosity syndrome (see "Hyperviscosity Syndrome" below).

Monoclonal Gammopathy

Although monoclonal immunoglobulins usually are composed of intact molecules that are structurally normal, about 25% of patients with multiple myeloma have excess (unbalanced) synthesis of light chains (see Figure 12.7–4). In another 25% of patients with myeloma, only light chains are produced by the plasma clone. Because light chains have low molecular weight (about 22 kD), they are readily filtered by the glomerulus; if the concentration exceeds the catabolic capacity of the renal tubular epithelium, they appear as a homogeneous protein in the urine (see Figures 12.7–2C and 12.7–4, "Unbalanced Synthe-

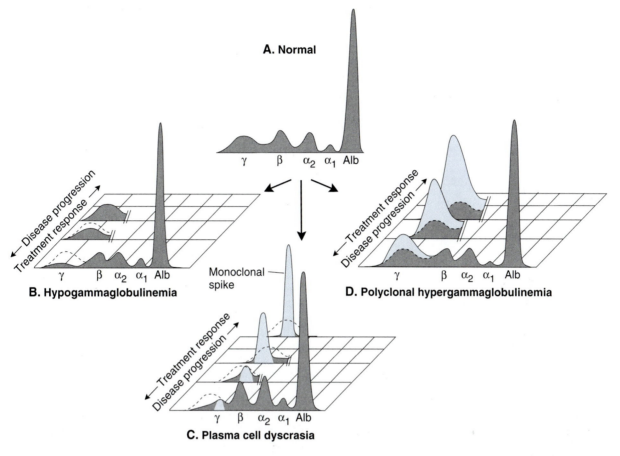

Figure 12.7–1. Common serum protein electrophoretic patterns. (Abnormalities are shown in blue.) **A: Normal pattern. B: Hypogammaglobulinemia.** The dotted line shows progressive loss of the gamma region as disease worsens. **C: Plasma cell dyscrasia.** Normal immunoglobulins are suppressed. With disease progression, the "spike" generally increases; with effective treatment, it decreases. **D: Polyclonal hypergammaglobulinemia** (polyclonal gammopathy).

sis"). These monoclonal light chains are called *Bence Jones proteins,* to honor the first person who described them.

Rarely, only a fragment of the heavy chain (eg, gamma, alpha, mu) is synthesized (heavy chain disease). These polypeptide chains are only 50–75% of the length of their normal counterparts. Since they are larger than light chains but smaller than intact immunoglobulins, they can often be detected in both serum and urine.

Monoclonal Immunoglobulin Identification: Monoclonal gammopathy is detected by serum protein electrophoresis (see Figure 12.7–1C). In the presence of an M component, immunoglobulin quantitation often reveals elevation of a single immunoglobulin class, with a reduction in concentration in one or both of the two other main classes. For example, IgG might be markedly increased whereas serum IgA and IgM are below normal. Immunofixation electrophoresis further reveals the mono-

clonal nature of the homogeneous band, demonstrating that it contains a single light-chain type (either kappa or lambda).

Light-chain or Bence Jones proteinuria is often missed by a dye-impregnated strip (dipstick), which detects albumin but not immunoglobulin. Sulfosalicylic acid (SSA) detects both. Definitive identification of Bence Jones proteinuria is best accomplished by urine protein electrophoresis and immunofixation electrophoresis (see Figure 12.7–2C).

Occasionally, the serum and the urine are entirely normal, quantitatively and by protein electrophoresis (see Figures 12.7–1A and 12.7–2A). Under these circumstances, a low-concentration monoclonal gammopathy, if present, can be detected by the use of immunofixation electrophoresis (IFE) which is a great deal more sensitive and specific than serum or urine protein electrophoresis.

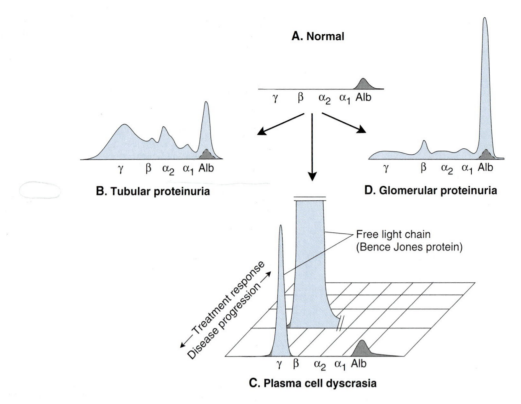

A. Normal

B. Tubular proteinuria

D. Glomerular proteinuria

Free light chain
(Bence Jones protein)

Treatment response →
← Disease progression

C. Plasma cell dyscrasia

Figure 12.7–2. Common urine protein electrophoretic patterns. (Abnormalities are shown in blue.) **A: Normal pattern.** Normal urine has either no detectable protein or only trace amounts of albumin. **B: Tubular proteinuria.** When the renal tubular epithelium is compromised, normally filtered low molecular weight proteins such as light chains and lysozyme are not reabsorbed and catabolized, and they appear in the urine. **C: Plasma cell dyscrasia.** When immunoglobulin synthesis is "unbalanced" (see Figures 12.7–4 and 12.7–5) and excess free light chain is produced, it easily passes the glomerulus and appears in the urine as a monoclonal spike. **D: Glomerular proteinuria.** When the glomerular filtration apparatus is compromised, serum proteins of intermediate molecular weight pass into the urine. The electrophoretic pattern resembles that of serum except for the decreased amount of very large proteins such as α_2-macroglobulin and IgM.

IFE should be considered when a plasma cell dyscrasia is suspected and neither the serum nor the urine shows a characteristic monoclonal "spike."

MONOCLONAL GAMMOPATHY OF UNDETERMINED SIGNIFICANCE

Occasionally, the serum or urine or both of an otherwise normal individual contains an M component, particularly among the elderly. According to some series, this occurs in up to 10% of the population over age 60 years. Whether such persons will develop other evidence of a progressive disorder or remain stable for years cannot be reliably predicted, regardless of the magnitude of the protein spike. Therefore, they should be followed up every few months to observe for any evidence of progression, such as anemia or skeletal disease. When stable over time,

this condition previously was called benign monoclonal gammopathy, but now is designated monoclonal gammopathy of undetermined significance (MGUS). The latter term is preferable, since the former presupposes knowledge about the future biologic behavior of the abnormal clone. About 25% of such patients progress to a malignant process over 15 years.

When a monoclonal gammopathy is detected, the physician must answer two questions. (1) Does the patient have a malignancy, or is the process best considered provisionally as MGUS? (2) Does the patient now have any symptoms or findings that require treatment?

The diagnosis of a malignant disorder depends on the demonstration of organ system damage or dysfunction. Whether to treat may depend in part on the physiologic abnormalities caused by the monoclonal protein itself. For example, symptomatic hyperviscosity requiring treatment can result from a very high concentration of the monoclonal immunoglobulin.

MULTIPLE MYELOMA

Multiple myeloma has an incidence of about 5 per 100,000, increases with age, and is extremely rare in children and adolescents. Mean age and median age in most series are about 60 years. Men and women are affected equally, but blacks are more susceptible and have an earlier age of onset. Radiation exposure (eg, Hiroshima survivors, radiologists) and exposure to certain chemicals (eg, pesticides, petroleum products, asbestos) are associated with an increased incidence of myeloma.

Clinical Presentation

The onset and early course of multiple myeloma are usually insidious. Common initial complaints are tiredness, weakness, and anorexia with accompanying weight loss (Table 12.7–1). In more advanced cases, pain caused by bone involvement, anemia, renal insufficiency, neurologic deficits, and repeated bacterial infections may become increasingly prominent.

Skeletal Lesions: Bone pain is related to osteolytic lesions produced by focal accumulations of plasma cells. The margins of these lesions are often sharply demarcated on radiologic examination and result in the common descriptive term of "punched out." They may be located in any part of the skeletal system but are seen most often in the red marrow-bearing areas of the skeleton, such as the skull, spine, ribs, and pelvis (Figure 12.7–3). This bony destruction is related to the production of cytokines (eg, interleukin-1β [IL-1β]) and tumor necrosis factor (TNF), which have osteoclast activating factor activity.

Diffuse demineralization (generalized osteoporosis) may occur in the absence of discrete lytic lesions. Pathologic fractures of ribs, pelvis, and weight-bearing long bones are common. Collapse of demineralized vertebral bodies may produce nerve root or spinal cord compression. Hypercalcemia is frequently encountered in patients with multiple myeloma and, when severe, can be a life-threatening problem requiring prompt treatment. Some patients have no demonstrable skeletal lesions initially, and a few patients never develop any skeletal abnormalities. Failure

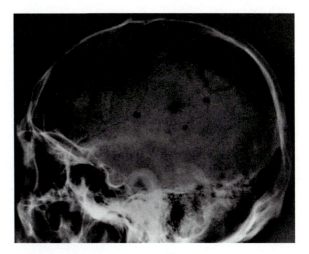

Figure 12.7–3. Lateral skull x-ray of a patient with multiple myeloma. The numerous "punched-out" lytic lesions are typical of multiple myeloma.

to appreciate this fact may obscure the diagnosis of multiple myeloma. Bone scans, which detect new bone formation but not bone destruction, are inferior to plain films in diagnosing skeletal lesions in multiple myeloma. Magnetic resonance imaging (MRI) scans can be helpful in establishing both skeletal destruction and marrow involvement.

Nephropathy: Renal impairment can be either acute or chronic. The acute form is almost always seen in patients with Bence Jones proteinuria, which is often complicated by hypercalcemia or dehydration. Correction of volume depletion and hypercalcemia often reverses this acute renal failure. Hemodialysis may be required for temporary support.

Chronic renal insufficiency is common in multiple myeloma with light-chain proteinuria. Biopsy shows eosinophilic lamellated casts in the renal tubules, and renal tubular epithelial cell atrophy (myeloma kidney). The renal tubular epithelium is the principal site for catabolism of free light chains, and toxic damage results from the reabsorption and catabolism of some Bence Jones proteins. Why some Bence Jones proteins are nephrotoxic and others are not is unclear; lambda light chains tend to be somewhat more nephrotoxic than kappa chains.

Neuropathy: Many patients with myeloma develop neurologic signs and symptoms, which can be caused by (1) skeletal destruction allowing compression of nerve roots or the spinal cord itself, (2) amyloid deposition damaging peripheral nerves, or (3) antibody activity of the M component producing demyelinating syndromes.

Bacterial Infections: Patients with myeloma can come to medical attention because of repeated infections such as pneumonia or urinary tract infections. Susceptibility to

Table 12.7–1. Common clinical presentations of multiple myeloma.

Symptoms
Weakness and loss of energy
Loss of appetite and weight
Skeletal pain
Recurrent infections (eg, pneumonia, urinary tract infections)
Bleeding (eg, bruising, epistaxis)
Numbness, paresthesias

Physical findings
Pallor
Cachexia
Skeletal tenderness, fractures
Bleeding (petechiae, purpura)
Neurologic abnormalities (eg, nerve root and spinal cord
    compression)

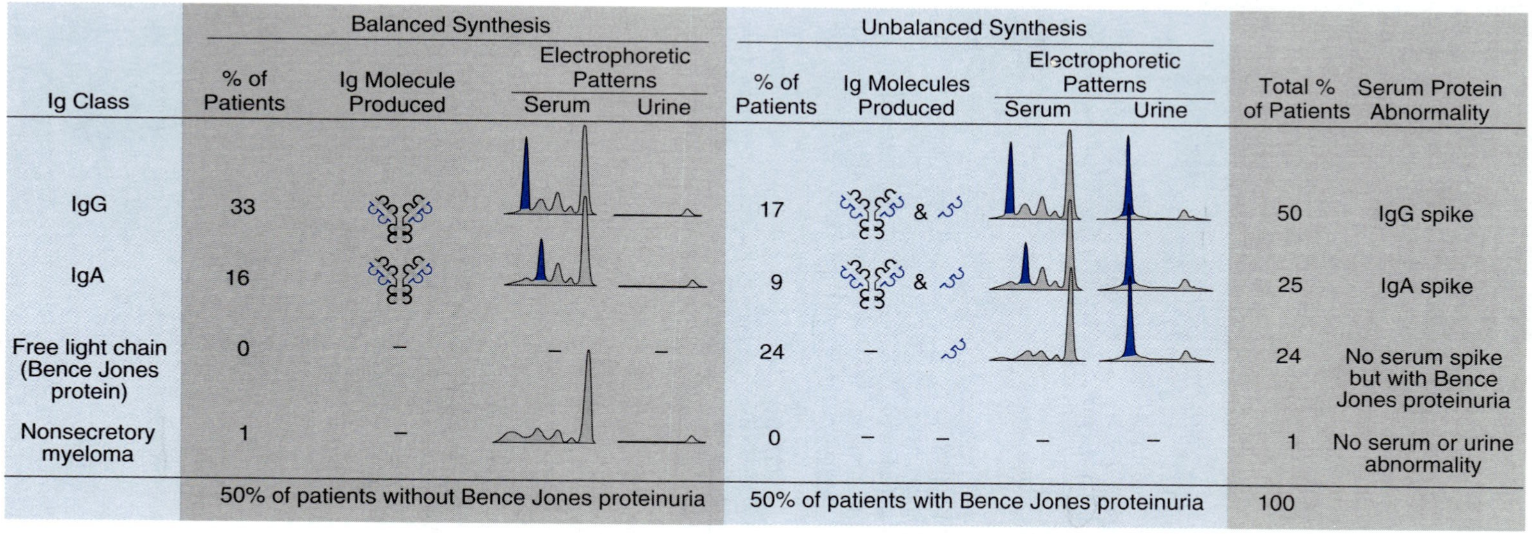

Ig Class	Balanced Synthesis: % of Patients	Balanced Synthesis: Ig Molecule Produced	Balanced Synthesis: Electrophoretic Patterns, Serum	Balanced Synthesis: Electrophoretic Patterns, Urine	Unbalanced Synthesis: % of Patients	Unbalanced Synthesis: Ig Molecules Produced	Unbalanced Synthesis: Electrophoretic Patterns, Serum	Unbalanced Synthesis: Electrophoretic Patterns, Urine	Total % of Patients	Serum Protein Abnormality
IgG	33				17	&			50	IgG spike
IgA	16				9	&			25	IgA spike
Free light chain (Bence Jones protein)	0	–	–	–	24	–			24	No serum spike but with Bence Jones proteinuria
Nonsecretory myeloma	1	–			0	–	–	–	1	No serum or urine abnormality
	50% of patients without Bence Jones proteinuria				50% of patients with Bence Jones proteinuria				100	

Figure 12.7–4. Common patterns of immunoglobulin synthesis in multiple myeloma. **Balanced synthesis:** When plasma cells produce a complete, intact IgG or IgA immunoglobulin molecule with no excess light-chain production, the abnormal spike appears in the serum and the urine is normal. **Unbalanced synthesis:** When light chain is produced alone or in excess of what is assembled into the complete immunoglobulin molecule, Bence Jones protein is detectable in the urine. About 25% of patients with myeloma produce only a Bence Jones protein (light-chain disease); if they have hypogammaglobulinemia, this is their only serum abnormality and they do not show a spike. About 1% of patients with myeloma produce neither an intact immunoglobulin nor a free light chain; their disease is described as "nonsecretory." Altogether, about 50% of patients have a Bence Jones protein, and about 75% of patients have a serum spike.

Ig Class	Balanced Synthesis				Unbalanced Synthesis				Total % of Patients	Serum Protein Abnormality
	% of Patients	Ig Molecule Produced	Electrophoretic Patterns		% of Patients	Ig Molecules Produced	Electrophoretic Patterns			
			Serum	Urine			Serum	Urine		
IgM	90	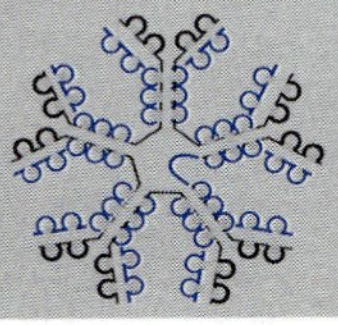	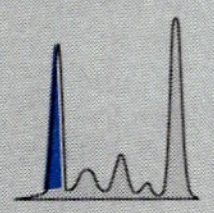	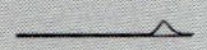	10	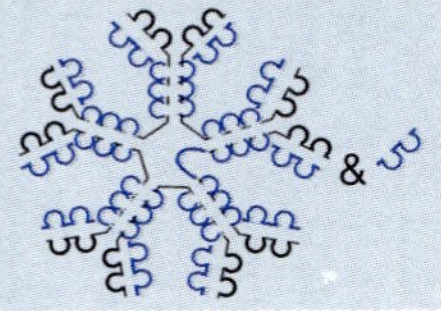	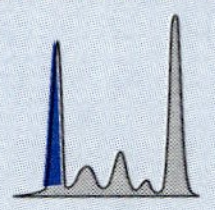	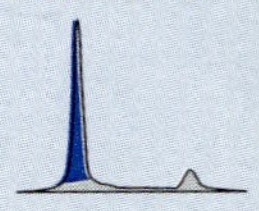	100	IgM spike

Figure 12.7–5. Common patterns of immunoglobulin synthesis in Waldenström's macroglobulinemia. **Balanced synthesis:** When the plasma cells produce a complete, intact IgM molecule, a spike is seen in the serum and the urine is normal. **Unbalanced synthesis:** When light chain is produced in excess, Bence Jones protein is found in the urine, in addition to the spike in the serum.

807

bacterial infections, especially encapsulated organisms like *Streptococcus pneumoniae,* is related to decreased ability to synthesize normal amounts of specific antibody following antigenic exposure. Even though myeloma patients may be chemically hypergammaglobulinemic, they should be thought of as functionally hypogammaglobulinemic and immunodeficient, since the M component does not provide any useful antibody protection and the normal polyclonal immunoglobulins are often markedly suppressed.

Hematologic Abnormalities: A normochromic normocytic anemia is an almost invariable accompaniment of multiple myeloma, and complaints related to anemia often bring patients to the physician. Rouleaux formation (red cells clumping like a stack of coins) on peripheral blood smear and an elevated sedimentation rate may provide early clues to the diagnosis of myeloma. Plasma cell proliferation in the marrow may also result in leukopenia and thrombocytopenia.

Occasional plasma cells can be found in the peripheral blood, especially if buffy coat is examined. If sufficiently numerous (absolute plasma cell count greater than 500/μL), the diagnosis is plasma cell leukemia. At presentation, this usually indicates very aggressive disease. Plasma cell leukemia may also be seen as a late or preterminal event in the course of more typical myeloma.

Occasionally, the M component has the property of gelling or precipitating at a temperature lower than body temperature (cryoglobulinemia). Patients so affected may present with purpura, Raynaud's phenomenon, or even localized areas of necrosis and gangrene (eg, ears, fingers, and toes).

Rarely, the monoclonal immunoglobulin has detectable antibody activity. If such antibody activity is directed against a normal body constituent, binding to its antigen may cause symptoms. (For example, the M component binding to a factor in the clotting cascade results in a bleeding diathesis.)

Natural History and Prognosis

Median survival with untreated multiple myeloma is about 12 months. Patients who are bedridden or have hematocrit below 30% have a median survival of only 6–8 months. Other factors that also predict for shortened survival include hypoalbuminemia (less than 3 g/dL), thrombocytopenia (less than 20,000/μL), leukopenia (less than 1000/μL), renal insufficiency, amyloidosis, plasma cell leukemia (more than 500 plasma cells/μL), failure to respond to treatment, or relapse after an initial response. Other factors that correlate with a poor prognosis are advanced age and elevated serum β_2-microglobulin, C-reactive protein, IL-6, and plasma cell labeling index. Patients without these factors have median survival expectancy of about 2 years, even without a response to treatment.

Another important determinant of survival is the tempo or pace of the disease. This is often difficult to assess by the features of the disease at the time of presentation and becomes apparent only as the patient is followed. Although multiple myeloma advances with varying degrees of rapidity in different patients and may seem to remain static for prolonged periods, complete spontaneous remissions virtually never occur and progressive disease is always an indication for treatment. Treatment significantly prolongs survival and improves quality of life.

Management

The major problems in the management of patients with myeloma include bone pain, structural defects of the skeleton, hypercalcemia, progressive renal insufficiency, recurrent bacterial infections, and bone marrow failure with refractory anemia, leukopenia and thrombocytopenia. Supportive treatment of these abnormalities is basic to optimal patient care. The maintenance of ambulation helps to forestall bone demineralization and hypercalcemia. In the management of renal insufficiency, the benefits of adequate hydration cannot be overstated. Depending on the status of the underlying disease, peritoneal dialysis or hemodialysis can be justified, and in some patients renal function has been restored with renal transplants.

In view of the known immunosuppression of patients with multiple myeloma, replacement therapy with intravenous gammaglobulin preparations has proved to be of some use in patients with recurring infections. Febrile patients with monoclonal disorders should be treated promptly with broad-spectrum antibiotics while awaiting specific identification of the causal organism and antibiotic sensitivity studies. This is particularly true if the patient is also neutropenic.

Systemic treatment with a variety of agents can induce partial remissions in 60–80% of patients. Complete remissions, including the recovery of normal levels of polyclonal immunoglobulins and recalcification of bony lesions, are rare. Intermittent administration of melphalan and prednisone remains the most common initial therapy. Other effective agents include cyclophosphamide, BCNU, vincristine, doxorubicin, and α-interferon.

Responses are characterized by relief of symptoms, reduction in bone marrow plasmacytosis, decrease in light-chain proteinuria, decrease in the serum M component, and improvement in hematocrit, white blood cell count, and platelets. Median survival in responding patients is extended by 3 or 4 years. Bone marrow transplantation, especially allogeneic, has proved to be curative for some patients.

VARIANTS OF MULTIPLE MYELOMA

Light-Chain Disease (Bence Jones Proteinemia and Proteinuria)

In about 20% of patients with multiple myeloma, immunoglobulin synthesis by the malignant plasma cell is deranged, and light chain alone is produced. In these cases, the serum abnormality is often that of hypogamma-globulinemia (see Figure 12.7–1B). Overlooking the fact that myeloma may be a cause of hypogammaglobulinemia constitutes a common diagnostic error. An important clue is the monoclonal light chain (Bence Jones protein) in the urine (see Figure 12.7–2C). Occasionally, with severe renal impairment or a large tumor burden, the free light chain can be found in the serum (Bence Jones proteinemia), especially by immunofixation electrophoresis.

Nonsecretory Myeloma

Rarely (fewer than 1% of cases), a plasma cell neoplasm is observed that is not accompanied by an M component in either serum or urine (see Figure 12.7–4). Some cases are marked by the cells' inability to secrete the M component after synthesis in the cytoplasm, whereas others represent an inability to synthesize an immunoglobulin molecule or fragment.

Solitary Plasmacytoma

A single mass in a bone, composed of plasma cells, with no evidence of generalized spread in bone marrow, is called a solitary osseous plasmacytoma. If treated by means of surgical resection followed by local radiation therapy, some patients with solitary osseous plasmacytoma may survive for many years, but most osseous plasmacytomas eventually disseminate. In contrast, most patients who have a mass composed of plasma cells in soft tissue outside the bones (extramedullary plasmacytoma) can be cured by surgery followed by radiation therapy.

WALDENSTRÖM'S MACROGLOBULINEMIA

Macroglobulinemia is a relatively rare disorder characterized by an uncontrolled proliferation of a clone of cells that synthesizes a homogeneous IgM. In a sense, it is "IgM myeloma," but is given a separate diagnostic category in honor of the man who first described the disease and in recognition of its unique clinical features. It is usually observed in persons over the age of 50; its incidence peaks in the sixth and seventh decades and is twice as common in men as in women.

Clinical Presentation

Macroglobulinemia may be a coincidental laboratory discovery before the onset of symptoms presenting as a monoclonal gammopathy of undetermined significance. The common complaints of weakness, lassitude, headache, weight loss, and mild exertional dyspnea are not distinctive and may be insidious in onset. Many of the distinctive clinical features are related to serum hyperviscosity (Table 12.7–2).

Diagnosis

The diagnosis of Waldenström's macroglobulinemia is based primarily on the coexistence of high serum concentrations of monoclonal IgM (more than 3000 mg/dL) as-

Table 12.7–2. Common clinical presentations of Waldenström's macroglobulinemia.

Symptoms
Weakness and loss of energy
Loss of appetite and weight
Bleeding, epistaxis
Headache
Impaired vision
Dyspnea
Numbness, paresthesias
Fever without infection

Physical findings
Pallor
Cachexia
Retinal hemorrhages and venous congestion
Lymphadenopathy
Hepatosplenomegaly
Neuropathy

sociated with abnormal accumulations of plasmacytoid lymphocytes in the bone marrow and other tissues. Amyloidosis has been associated with macroglobulinemia but is uncommon (less than 5% of cases). In contrast to myeloma, skeletal destruction with Waldenström's macroglobulinemia is uncommon.

Hyperviscosity Syndrome

The IgM molecule is large and asymmetric, with a high intrinsic viscosity (see Figure 12.7–5). Plasma viscosity levels many times those of normal plasma may result when IgM is present in high concentrations. The clinical features resulting from high blood viscosity have been termed the hyperviscosity syndrome.

Blood flow in capillaries is compromised, with resulting anoxic damage and tissue hemorrhage. Spontaneous bleeding from the mucous membranes and at the sites of minor trauma occurs. Visual disturbances and even blindness can result from intraocular hemorrhage. The workload on the heart is significantly increased because of the blood's resistance to flow. When severe, the hyperviscosity syndrome is life-threatening, leading to coma, convulsions, and fatal cerebrovascular accidents.

Although symptoms from hyperviscosity are not usually found when relative viscosity of plasma is below 3.0 (normal range, 1.5–1.9), the level of plasma viscosity at which symptoms arise varies from individual to individual. However, in a given individual it is reasonably reproducible. This has been termed the "symptomatic threshold," and therapeutic measures (plasmapheresis or chemotherapy or both) that maintain viscosity below this level prevent the development of symptoms.

Management

The supportive care of patients with Waldenström's macroglubulinemia is similar to that of patients with multiple myeloma. Dramatic relief from neurologic symptoms, ocular disturbances, overt bleeding diathesis, and heart failure results from lowering plasma viscosity.

Since most of the M component is within the vascular space (about 80% for IgM compared with 25% for IgG and IgA) and since viscosity increases exponentially with increasing concentrations of IgM, plasmapheresis is an effective way of controlling hyperviscosity. Modest reduction of IgM concentration can result in clinically important reduction in blood viscosity. Some patients can be managed for prolonged periods by plasmapheresis alone. Survival of patients with Waldenströms macroglobulinemia is similar to that of patients with multiple myeloma.

Alkylating agents, such as chlorambucil and cyclophosphamide, have been helpful in the long-term treatment of patients with Waldenström's macroglubulinemia. Reports of the use of nucleoside analogs (eg, fludarabine, cladribine) are encouraging. Responses include a decrease in neoplastic tissue mass, a reduction of organomegaly, a lowering of serum macroglobulin concentration, reduced plasmapheresis requirement, an improvement in anemia, a related improvement in the patient's symptoms, and improved survival.

AMYLOIDOSIS

Amyloidosis is a rare disorder characterized by accumulation of extracellular proteinaceous fibrils in various tissues, frequently causing organ dysfunction. There are four major types of amyloidosis: (1) primary amyloidosis—occurring in the absence of any other identifiable disease; (2) myeloma-associated amyloidosis—occurring as a complication of an overt plasma cell dyscrasia; (3) secondary amyloidosis—occurring as a result of a chronic inflammatory condition (eg, osteomyelitis); and (4) familial or hereditary amyloidosis—comprising a variety of syndromes and a number of biochemically distinct forms of amyloid. In addition, there are a number of minor forms of amyloidosis, each with their own unique biochemistry and clinical expression.

Amyloid is not starch, as the name implies, but rather a complex protein mixture dominated by a fibrillar component. There are several specific ways to identify amyloid. With light microscopy, using hematoxylin and eosin staining, amyloid is characterized by an amorphous, extracellular, eosinophilic material infiltrating tissues and organs. The amyloid material is further identified by its pink-staining reaction with alkaline Congo red, which undergoes a brilliant yellow-orange to apple-green birefringence when examined with polarized light. When examined by electron microscopy, the amorphous material consists of a felt-like mat of fibrils of about 80 angstroms in diameter.

Amino acid sequence studies of the fibrillar component of amyloid from different patients have identified two major distinct biochemical forms. In the primary and myeloma-associated forms of amyloid, the fibrillar component was found to be the variable end of immunoglobulin light chain or intact light chain. These forms of the disease are therefore a type of plasma cell dyscrasia and together make up about 85% of all cases of amyloid in the United States. In contrast, in the secondary and some of the hereditary forms of amyloid (eg, familial Mediterranean fever), the amyloid fibril (called *amyloid A,* or AA) is the same from patient to patient and is unrelated to immunoglobulin. The hepatocyte synthesizes the serum precursor of amyloid A, called *serum amyloid A* (SAA). SAA behaves like C-reactive protein and other acute-phase reactants and is found in serum in increased amounts in inflammatory conditions.

Clinical Presentation

The extent and location of the amyloid deposits determine the presenting symptoms (Table 12.7–3). Especially susceptible to amyloid deposition and subsequent dysfunction are heart, kidney, and peripheral nerves. Therefore, restrictive cardiomyopathy predominates in some patients, while the nephrotic syndrome or peripheral neuropathy predominates in others. Postural hypotension caused by autonomic nerve damage can be very severe and difficult to manage. Carpal tunnel syndrome may be a presenting condition. A sprue-like syndrome can result from amyloid deposition in the small bowel. Constitutional symptoms are often nonspecific and insidious in onset, but fatigue and weight loss are prominent.

Physical findings of amyloidosis include hepatomegaly and, less frequently, splenomegaly and adenopathy. Macroglossia with fixed indentations on the tongue margins caused by pressure of the teeth is almost pathognomonic. Purpura is sometimes prominent, especially in areas subjected to trauma or increased hydrostatic pressure. Periorbital purpura from coughing, vomiting, or rubbing the eyes may be dramatic. The skin may be so fragile as to mimic epidermolysis bullosa or may be infiltrated with nodules or plaques resembling xanthelasma.

Table 12.7–3. Common clinical presentations of amyloidosis.

Symptoms
Weakness and loss of energy
Loss of appetite and weight
Diarrhea
Swelling
Dyspnea
Light-headedness, syncope
Voice change
Difficulty in swallowing
Bleeding
Numbness, paresthesias

Physical findings
Cachexia
Edema
Orthostatic hypotension
Macroglossia
Periorbital purpura, epistaxis
Pinch purpura (minor trauma)
Carpal tunnel syndrome
Hepatosplenomegaly

Diagnosis

Once amyloid is suspected, the diagnosis is confirmed histologically by biopsy. The choice of which tissue to biopsy is determined by the site of clinical derangement. Sutton's law applies here: "Go where the money is." Biopsy material is obtained more conveniently from the rectum (mucosa and submucosa), gingiva, tongue, abdominal fat pad aspiration, or biopsy of a clinically involved area of skin. Biopsy of the stomach or small bowel, or needle biopsy of the bone marrow, kidney, or liver, may reveal the amyloid deposits. Endomyocardial biopsy via catheter has been of growing importance in establishing amyloid as the etiology in patients who present with otherwise unexplained restrictive cardiomyopathy. Bleeding after biopsy can be a problem in patients with amyloidosis, and the choice of a biopsy site should be governed partly by the ease with which bleeding can be recognized and controlled.

Primary Amyloidosis: Primary amyloidosis (ie, amyloidosis not associated with another illness) is rare before the age of 40. Peak incidence is in the middle 60's, with males outnumbering females. With the demonstration of the immunoglobulin nature of the amyloid fibril, it is easy to understand why the symptoms and laboratory features of patients with primary amyloidosis resemble those of patients with myeloma-associated amyloidosis. Discrimination between primary amyloidosis and myeloma-associated amyloidosis is based on the lack of skeletal destruction and the lesser degree of marrow replacement by the plasma cells in primary amyloidosis.

Possible laboratory findings are glomerular proteinuria (see Figure 12.7–2D), sometimes in massive amounts, as well as Bence Jones proteinuria (see Figure 12.7–2C), a serum M component (see Figure 12.7–1C), anemia, bone marrow plasmacytosis, and evidence of renal failure. Serum albumin may be low and alkaline phosphatase elevated, but liver function, even with massive infiltration, usually is well preserved. Compared with myeloma patients, in whom kappa light chain predominates (2:1—kappa:lambda), this ratio is reversed in patients with amyloidosis. Hence, lambda light chain seems to be more amyloidogenic.

The prognosis for patients with primary amyloidosis is poor. Cardiac failure and renal failure are prominent causes of death, but a progressive failure to thrive and malnutrition from tongue and bowel involvement can also play a role.

Treatment of patients with amyloid has been largely supportive, but there are scattered reports of remissions induced with alkylating agents such as melphalan. Corticosteroids given alone do not seem to help these patients. Chronic hemodialysis and peritoneal dialysis have been of value in some patients, and a few patients have benefitted from kidney transplantation.

Myeloma-Associated Amyloidosis: The 5–15% of patients with myeloma who develop amyloidosis suffer the relentless damage from amyloid deposition and also are subject to the difficulties related to the progressive proliferation of the plasma cells themselves. Survival is accordingly less favorable than with either myeloma alone or primary amyloidosis, and if no response to therapy is achieved median survival is about 5 months. The general principles of management are the same as for multiple myeloma.

Secondary Amyloidosis: Amyloidosis secondary to chronic inflammatory conditions accounts for 8–16% of amyloid cases. In former years, tuberculosis led the list of associated diseases, but with the development of effective antituberculosis therapy, rheumatoid arthritis has become the most common associated disorder, with osteomyelitis second. The incidence of amyloidosis among patients with rheumatoid arthritis ranges from 5% to 26%, and amyloidosis should be suspected if otherwise unexplained proteinuria develops in such a patient. Other associated conditions are bronchiectasis, pyelonephritis, lepromatous leprosy, paraplegia, and various malignancies. The clinical patterns seen in patients with secondary amyloidosis include the nephrotic syndrome, malabsorption, neuropathy, and amyloid deposition causing enlargement of the liver, spleen, and lymph nodes.

Management of secondary amyloidosis consists of treatment and resolution of the underlying disease process. If this can be accomplished, the amyloidosis can be stabilized or even partially resolve.

Familial or Hereditary Amyloidosis: There are a number of other biochemically distinct varieties of amyloid, inherited in both autosomal recessive and dominant modes. In familial Mediterranean fever (FMF), the amyloid is the AA form. Its deposition is systemic, involving primarily the kidneys, liver, spleen, and adrenal glands. In this setting, proteinuria is often observed to progress to the nephrotic syndrome and eventually to increasing renal failure. Colchicine therapy reduces the frequency and severity of the periodic attacks of fever and sterile peritonitis that characterize the disease. This therapy helps to prevent and delay the deposition of amyloid, with corresponding extension of survival.

A single amino acid substitution (mutation) in precise locations in some normal proteins is sufficient to lead to amyloid formation. This is perhaps best illustrated in the group of disorders known as the familial amyloidotic polyneuropathies (FAP). In different kindreds, there are different single amino acid substitutions in the transthyretin molecule (formerly known as prealbumin), which result in somewhat different clinical expressions of amyloidosis.

Another form of amyloidosis develops in some patients on chronic hemodialysis in which the fibril is composed of B_2-microglobulin. Other forms of amyloidosis result from the deposition of various prohormones or still other proteins whose normal counterpart or biochemical function is unknown (eg, β protein in the inherited form of Alzheimer's disease).

SUMMARY

▶ The plasma cell dyscrasias share the common features of clonal proliferation of a lymphoid/plasmacytoid cell that usually produces a homogeneous (monoclonal) immunoglobulin molecule or fragment.

▶ Malignant plasma cell dyscrasias (multiple myeloma, Waldenström's macroglobulinemia) differ from monoclonal gammopathy of undetermined significance (MGUS) by demonstrating progression and by producing organ system damage.

▶ Responses achieved by systemic therapy (chemotherapy, bone marrow transplantation) result in major improvement in quality of life and extension of survival.

▶ A plasma cell dyscrasia should be considered when an elderly or middle-aged patient presents with an ill-defined, insidious failure to thrive, combined with subtle and often nonspecific multisystem symptoms.

▶ Amyloidosis is characterized by the deposition of abnormal proteinaceous material as fibrils in tissues with subsequent organ dysfunction.

SUGGESTED READING

Alexanian R, Dimopoulos MA: Management of multiple myeloma. Semin Hematol 1995;32:20.

Baldini L et al: Role of different hematologic variables in defining the risk of malignant transformation in monoclonal gammopathy. Blood 1996;87:912.

Gobbi PG et al: Study of prognosis in Waldenström's macroglobulinemia: A proposal for a simple binary classification with clinical and investigational utility. Blood 1994;83:2939.

Klein B: Cytokine, cytokine receptors, transduction signals, and oncogenes in human multiple myeloma. Semin Hematol 1995;32:4.

Kyle RA: Monoclonal gammopathy of undetermined significance. Blood Rev 1994;8:135.

Seiden MV, Anderson KC: Multiple myeloma. Curr Opin Oncol 1994;6:41.

Tan SY, Pepys MB, Hawkins PN: Treatment of amyloidosis. Am J Kidney Dis 1995;26:267.

Section 13

Neurology

Brent G. Petty, MD, Section Editor

Approach to the Patient with a Neurologic Disorder

Hamilton Moses III, MD

Neurologic diseases, especially stroke, Parkinson's disease, epilepsy, multiple sclerosis, and chronic pain, account for more long-term disability than all other conditions combined. Every physician has many patients with headache, dizziness, back or neck pain, weakness, or insomnia. These symptoms may or may not be associated with significant underlying abnormalities of the nervous system. Thus, it is essential that all physicians have an organized approach for evaluation of neurologic symptoms and familiarity with neurologic diseases.

Important advances have been made in the prevention and treatment of neurologic diseases. The incidence of stroke, particularly hypertensive hemorrhage, has shown dramatic and sustained decline over the past two decades, probably caused by changes in the American diet and vigorous control of hypertension. The incidence of thrombotic stroke has likewise decreased. Conversely, the incidences of glioblastoma multiforme and Guillain-Barré syndrome appear to be increasing.

New neurologic therapies include riluzole for amyotrophic lateral sclerosis, sumatriptan for migraine, plasmapheresis and immune globulin for Guillain-Barré syndrome, and a proven role of β-interferon for relapsing-remitting multiple sclerosis. Conversely, controlled trials have cast doubt on the usefulness of some therapies that were formerly considered standard, such as external carotid–internal carotid bypass surgery for ischemic stroke and corticosteroids for optic neuritis. Although in the past neurology was considered a field with only limited therapeutic options, today one may observe dramatic success of medical therapy in epilepsy, Parkinson's disease, migraine, subarachnoid hemorrhage, myasthenia gravis, and certain peripheral neuropathies.

THE NEUROLOGIC EXAMINATION

The ability to make clinical observations and assemble them into an understandable pattern requires conscious effort, familiarity with the nervous system, knowledge of the disease process, and proficiency in examination. Although this principle is true for all medical disciplines, it is especially true in neurologic diagnosis. The goals of neurologic evaluation are: (1) define the anatomy of the lesion, (2) discern in what way normal physiology is altered, and (3) judge what the etiology is likely to be. Only after information about these three areas has been obtained by history-taking and neurologic examination can proper studies be undertaken and therapy prescribed. In reaching a tentative diagnosis, the history is of prime importance, the examination second, and ancillary studies clearly third. Experienced neurologists estimate that about two-thirds of all diagnoses can be reached by information supplied primarily in the history, that the examination adds about one fourth, and that ancillary studies add only a small increment to defining a neurologic problem.

Neurologic History

The aim of the neurologic history is to document the abnormalities noticed by the patient (or other observers), together with the circumstances under which they developed. Following are guidelines for history-taking:

1. What is the pattern of disease? Many disease processes result in similar neurologic manifestations and disabilities, in part because dysfunction of a particular region of the nervous system leads to predictable symptoms. However, the timing, rate, and

pattern of progression are usually distinctive. Several examples of the patterns of disease are given in Figure 13.1–1.

2. Can we bracket the lesion? That is, what is the highest (rostral) and what is the lowest (peripheral) point in the nervous system that can account for the dysfunction? Do the symptoms suggest a single lesion or multiple lesions?

3. Where should the physician's efforts be focused? A detailed examination of all possible neurologic func-

tions is lengthy, dull, and unrewarding. Proper interpretation of the history should steer the physician to the parts of the neurologic examination that require greater attention. For instance, memory loss or hallucinations indicate more detailed examination of the mental state, while paresthesias or numbness suggests that sensory examination should be emphasized.

4. Is the patient aware of the dysfunction? In many instances of acute disease such as strokes or seizures, the patient is totally unable to report what has happened. In

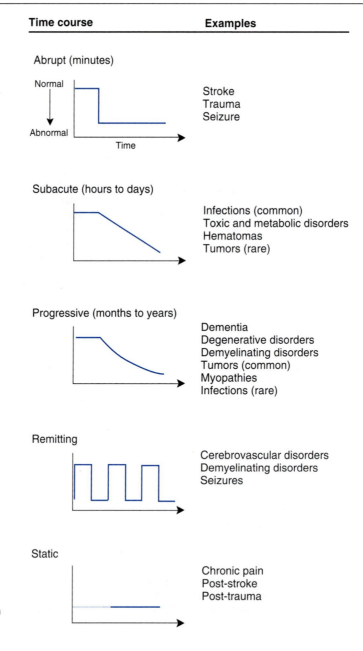

Figure 13.1–1. Patterns of progression of neurologic illness.

these circumstances, important observations about the onset and pattern require the report of another person. In eliciting this outside information, one should be aware that sudden disruption of neurologic function can be an extremely frightening event for witnesses. Thus, witnesses' comments on subjects such as the duration or degree of unresponsiveness should be interpreted cautiously.

5. Is there an underlying disease? Many treatable conditions affecting the nervous system are manifestations of systemic illnesses. Thinking of the nervous system in isolation from the rest of the body can lead to serious errors in diagnosis and management. For instance, overlooking a subtle nodule in the breast when an intracranial mass is obvious can cause one to miss the diagnosis of metastatic breast cancer. This principle applies to all underlying diseases, but patients with neoplastic, metabolic, toxic, connective tissue, and cardiac diseases are particularly likely to present with neurologic manifestations.

Information about occupation and hobbies is important in taking the history of patients with neurologic disease, because both toxic exposures and trauma may predispose to certain disorders (eg, seizures or polyneuropathy) and because neurologic dysfunction may jeopardize the patient's safety at work or at home.

The patient's family history is also of importance, since many inherited conditions that have neurologic implications are easily overlooked. This is especially true of abnormalities that begin in adolescence or early adulthood, but it is also true of many that manifest in middle or late life. For example, proper diagnosis of Huntington's disease, which usually begins in midlife, largely depends on the discovery of other family members with characteristic psychiatric or neurologic abnormalities, followed by definitive genetic testing. Also, after a neurologic diagnosis has been established, the implications for the family should be considered, both when the condition is familial and when it is not. For instance, many families fear that they or future generations will be at risk for epilepsy, Parkinson's disease, or stroke, even when inherited factors and risks are few.

Neurologic Examination

Assessment of a patient begins at the moment of first meeting the physician. The patient may betray an aphasia or dysarthria when saying "hello." Physical signs can be observed during the course of taking the history: A tilt of the head may suggest an ocular motor paresis, or the physician may see facial weakness with the first smile. The patient may not try to smile and may have difficulty arising from a chair or climbing onto the examining table, thus displaying two of the cardinal elements of parkinsonism. The patient may limp, showing weakness or pain in the leg, or may make a double foot slap, which occurs with distal weakness from polyneuropathy.

ANCILLARY NEUROLOGIC TESTS

The physician should know what each procedure can and cannot do, the relative risks of each procedure, and the most effective and efficient sequence of tests for a particular clinical problem. In addition, the physician should clearly communicate what diagnostic question needs to be answered, since the technique often needs to be varied depending on the type of information sought.

When possible, the most specific test for a clinical problem should be performed first, since less specific tests may thereby be avoided. In general, one should proceed from the simpler examinations, which have little risk or discomfort, to more complex tests, which often have greater risk. The sequence of tests is often very important, because certain procedures make the performance or interpretation of subsequent procedures more difficult. For instance, a lumbar puncture should be deferred in a patient being considered for myelography, because the tear in the arachnoidal membrane may allow myelographic contrast material to escape from the subarachnoid to the subdural space.

Examination of the Cerebrospinal Fluid

Cerebrospinal fluid is formed within the ventricular system by secretion from the choroid plexus and transudation of cerebral interstitial fluid. This fluid circulates through the ventricular foramina, down over the surface of the spinal cord and roots, and up through the basal cisterns to sites of reabsorption over the surface of the brain. Lumbar puncture reveals intracranial pressure and provides a sample of cerebrospinal fluid for microscopic, microbiologic, and chemical analysis.

Areas of Usefulness: Changes in the cerebrospinal fluid may be diagnostic of intracranial infections or subarachnoid hemorrhage. Unless there is clear contraindication (coagulopathy or evidence of increased intracranial pressure), the cerebrospinal fluid should be examined in patients suspected of having meningitis, patients with a positive serologic test for syphilis, and those suspected of having neurosyphilis. Examination of the cerebrospinal fluid is also important in determining whether the central nervous system is involved in leukemia or lymphomas, certain solid tumors, systemic vasculitis, and opportunistic infections. Changes in the cerebrospinal fluid are also important for diagnosing many primary diseases of the nervous system, including multiple sclerosis, inflammatory neuropathies, and many inherited and degenerative diseases. Often, normal spinal fluid is an important negative finding, such as in the diagnosis of Alzheimer's disease, metabolic encephalopathy, and idiopathic epilepsy, and in those with altered mental status who are HIV-positive. Stroke may cause red cells or xanthochromia, which indicates past intracranial bleeding, but normal cerebrospinal fluid findings do not exclude thrombosis, embolism, parenchymal intracranial hemorrhage, or epidural and subdural hematoma. Intracranial masses produce either elevated protein or increased pressure, but lumbar puncture has no role in evaluating most masses, since primary diagnosis is more directly and safely made by computed tomography (CT) or magnetic resonance imaging (MRI) scans.

Technique: Cerebrospinal fluid is usually sampled from the lumbar subarachnoid space, and proper positioning of the patient is essential for easy entry. The patient should lie on the side, with the neck flexed and head supported by a pillow. The thighs should be flexed on the abdomen, with the plane of the back flush with the mattress and perpendicular to the top surface of the bed. The L4–L5 interspace may be identified just inferior to an imaginary line connecting the iliac crests. After the skin is cleaned with iodine and after the antiseptic has been removed with alcohol, the skin and intraspinous ligament are infiltrated with a local anesthetic and the lumbar puncture needle advanced. The stylet should always be in place inside the needle as it is advanced, to avoid introduction of cutaneous tissue that can produce an intraspinal epidermoid inclusion cyst many years later. The needle should be kept parallel with the top surface of the bed, with the bevel turned upward to pass through the longitudinally running fibers of the dura. There is usually a distinct "pop" as the dura is penetrated. Nevertheless, the stylet should be withdrawn periodically after the needle is advanced, to determine whether cerebrospinal fluid is flowing.

After the needle has entered the subarachnoid space, particularly with an anxious or uncooperative patient, it is wise to remove a few drops of fluid for cell count before moving the patient. The patient is then allowed to extend the neck and thighs slowly to avoid spurious increase in the pressure measurement. After removal of appropriate fluid for studies, a final pressure is determined and the needle withdrawn.

If the pressure is unexpectedly high, there will be enough fluid within the manometer for cell count, culture, and chemistries. It is important in this situation that no excess fluid be removed. Jugular compression (manometrics) may be useful to demonstrate spinal subarachnoid block, but its use has decreased as imaging techniques have improved.

The patient should be instructed to lie prone for 3 hours after lumbar puncture to allow the dural rent to close. Consuming fluids liberally may hasten replacement of the cerebrospinal fluid that has been removed.

Risks:

Headache: The incidence of headache after lumbar puncture used to approach 25%, but newer techniques (especially with the use of 22- or 25-gauge small spinal needles) have lowered the rate to about 10%. The size of the dural rent best predicts loss of cerebrospinal fluid and subsequent headache. The headache is usually generalized, often bifrontal and temporal, occasionally strictly occipital, and rarely unilateral. Nausea is occasional and

vomiting rare. Usually, all symptoms disappear within a few hours, but they may persist for several days. Persistence for longer than 1 week suggests continuing cerebrospinal fluid leak and requires further investigation. Pathophysiology of headache in this setting is presumed to be irritation of the basal meninges and blood vessels caused by "sagging" of the brain following removal of cerebrospinal fluid.

Pain and paresthesias: Radicular pain and paresthesias occur at the time of lumbar puncture in 10–15% of persons but persist in about 0.1%, usually resolving within 1 year. Cranial nerve palsies, especially of the abducens, may immediately follow lumbar puncture or may appear after several weeks; they are thought to be caused by stretching of the long intracranial sixth nerve. Arachnoiditis occurs very rarely unless foreign materials (iodine, anesthetic agents, or adulterants) have been inadvertently introduced into the spinal subarachnoid space.

Cerebral herniation: This is the most dreaded complication of lumbar puncture. Similarly, compression of the spinal cord can be precipitated by removing cerebrospinal fluid below a block. Both complications can be prevented by excluding intracranial mass or spinal lesion with a CT or MRI scan before the procedure. Clinical deterioration is a threat both when a mass is known to exist and when a mass can be expected to evolve rapidly, as in the stage of cerebritis before brain abscess. The risk of herniation is 10–20% when a mass is known to exist. Rapidly evolving lesions (brain abscess, parenchymal hemorrhage, and malignant tumors with extensive edema) and those in the posterior fossa are most likely to deteriorate, while slowly progressive lesions (small benign tumors, chronic subdural hematomas) are less likely to deteriorate. Occasionally, when meningitis is thought to coexist with a mass, lumbar puncture may be unavoidable. Alternatively, empiric treatment with antibiotics may be justified when a mass is large. Lumbar puncture with a known mass requires expert judgment, and consultation with a neurologist or neurosurgeon is mandatory.

Findings: Normally, the fluid is crystal clear, contains at most 5 mononuclear cells/μL, and has a protein content of 45 mg/dL or less, of which 14% or less is gamma globulin. The glucose concentration is greater than 50% of the concurrent blood glucose, and the pressure is less than 180 mm H_2O.

Certain examinations should always be performed on the cerebrospinal fluid, including cell count and protein determination, as well as a description of its appearance. Bacterial culture and glucose determinations are indicated when a white cell pleocytosis is found or infection otherwise suspected. Simultaneous blood sugar should also be obtained for comparison with cerebrospinal fluid glucose. When infection, cerebrospinal fluid inflammation, or subarachnoid hemorrhage is suspected, cell count should be performed within 15 to 30 minutes, since cells may rapidly lyse, causing ambiguities in interpretation.

Special studies of the cerebrospinal fluid are indicated

in certain circumstances: for example, cytologic examination in a patient with cancer or certain fungal infections; myelin basic protein assay in a patient with multiple sclerosis and degenerative diseases of white matter; oligoclonal banding of IgG in multiple sclerosis, vasculitis, and infections; and syphilis serology when serum serology is positive or when suspicion is high.

Neuroradiology

Indications for various neuroradiologic procedures are given in Table 13.1–1.

Skull Films: Skull films are used to evaluate the integrity of the cranial bones and skull anatomy. These x-rays may also show the location of normally calcified structures, such as the pineal and choroid plexus, or the presence of abnormal calcification. Although skull films have a role in cases of direct trauma to the skull, they have been largely replaced by CT and MRI scans for this indication and for most other neurologic conditions.

Computed Tomography: Images of the skull, cerebrospinal fluid, and the different densities of white and gray matter in the brain parenchyma are easily, quickly, and safely obtained by CT. Herniations, ventricular size, and the nature of other intracranial structures can be seen at once, with the etiology—infarct, hemorrhage, edema, abscess, or tumor—usually easily determined. The integrity and distribution of the vasculature can be demonstrated by "enhancement," which is obtained by performing a CT scan after intravenous injection of an iodinated x-ray contrast dye.

Risks: The patient is exposed to a radiation dose about equal to that of a skull series. Anaphylaxis after intravenous iodinated dye is the major concern. As with all investigations, physicians should be suspicious about reported abnormalities that do not correspond to the patient's neurologic signs and symptoms. Artifacts do occur on CT scans and can best be checked by repeating the procedure or by subsequent MRI. False-negative CT scans occur with small lesions near the base of the skull; in the orbits, the parasellar region, and the posterior fossa; and at the craniocervical junction. When conditions in these locations are suspected, the radiologist can recommend special views that minimize false-negatives.

Magnetic Resonance Imaging: Clinically useful images of extraordinarily high quality can be obtained by MRI. Inside the scanner, the patient is surrounded by a high-strength magnetic field through which pulses of radiofrequency radiation are projected, thereby exciting the nuclei of hydrogen, phosphorus, oxygen, or other elements. Coils within the scanner are placed close to or on the patient's body and serve as antennae for the altered radiofrequency signal that is produced as the nuclei relax after stimulation. Computer manipulation of the data thus acquired produces a clinically useful image. By varying the strength of the magnetic field, the frequency and energy of the radiofrequency stimulation, and the timing of the stimulation pulses, selected images of many biologic materials can be discerned in the living patient. In particular, differences between white and gray matter, lesions within white matter, structures of the brain that are in close proximity to bone (such as the skull base and within

Table 13.1–1. Value of neuroradiographic procedures.

	Skull X-Ray	CT Scan	MRI Scan	Angiogram	Isotopic Scan	SPECT/PET
Skull fracture	+					
Bone density	+	+	±			
Bone erosion	+	±	±			
Intracranial calcification	+	+				
Ventricular system						
Size		+	+	±		
Displacement		+	+	±		
CSF dynamics			+		+	
Brain substance						
Atrophy		+	+	±		
Masses		+	+	±	+	
Infarction		+	+			
Hematoma		+	+	±	±	
Vascular pattern						
Patency		±	+	+		
Displacement				+		
Malformation		±	+	+	±	
Aneurysm				+		
Blood flow			+	±	±	+
Cerebral metabolism						+

CSF, cerebrospinal fluid.

the spine), and the distinction among cerebral infarction, edema, and neoplasm all are aided by MRI.

Areas of usefulness: MRI is the imaging modality of choice for the diagnosis of multiple sclerosis and the early detection of cerebral infarction and intracranial neoplasms. MRI has replaced CT for the diagnosis of many intracranial conditions—although CT continues to be important for staging many intracranial diseases—and for evaluation of the spine. CT or MRI scan has replaced pneumoencephalography, arteriography, and isotopic brain scanning as the primary diagnostic procedure for investigation of patients with acute or chronic intracranial processes.

Risks: In MRI, the patient receives no ionizing radiation, and the magnetic and radiofrequency fields used have not been shown to have any biologic effects. MRI is therefore recommended when repeated examinations in a single patient are required and when the patient is pregnant. Metallic intracranial clips (because of the risk of displacement) and cardiac pacemakers are the only absolute contraindications to MRI, although magnetic materials in other parts of the body, such as certain prosthetic cardiac valves or orthopedic prostheses, may represent risk because of heating. Consultation with the radiologist prior to a study is advisable when these materials are present.

Radionuclide Brain Scanning: Cisternal scans are used to demonstrate the patency of pathways of cerebrospinal fluid flow and reabsorption. Radioactive material is injected in the lumbar subarachnoid space, and serial scans of the head are performed at periodic intervals for up to 72 hours. Normally, little isotope enters the ventricles, the majority of it going over the convexities of the cortical surface as cerebrospinal fluid is reabsorbed. In communicating hydrocephalus secondary to a block in reabsorption of cerebrospinal fluid, the isotope enters the ventricular system to an abnormal degree and may persist for 24 to 72 hours (ventricular stasis). Cisternography is also useful for detecting the site of a cerebrospinal fluid leak in patients with recurrent meningitis or after head injury.

Angiography: Cranial angiography is usually performed by retrograde insertion of a catheter in the femoral artery, through which injections may be directed into the carotid arteries, either vertebral artery, or the aortic arch. Radiographic images are sequentially obtained. Digital imaging has replaced conventional film screen techniques, allowing reduction in the amount of injected dye, a particular attraction in patients who require multiple injections or who have significant cardiovascular or renal disease. Intravenous digital subtraction angiography (with injection of a large volume of iodinated contrast material) is useful for imaging the great vessels and major intracerebral branches, although it provides considerably less detail (and possibly no less risk) than intra-arterial injections. Digital technology has made angiography a faster, safer, and more pleasant procedure than in the past. Radiologic

consultations should be sought to select the optimal procedure.

Areas of usefulness: In subarachnoid hemorrhage, careful angiography is essential for demonstrating the site of bleeding, whether from aneurysm or from arteriovenous malformation. Correct assessment of surgical feasibility depends on careful coordination among neurologic, neurosurgical, and neuroradiologic personnel. Special views are often required to demonstrate the exact shape and position of an aneurysm. Balloon occlusion and embolization by catheter play an increasing role in the definitive treatment of arteriovenous malformations, large congenital vascular anomalies of the skull and brain, and acquired carotid cavernous fistulas.

Risks: Most large series of angiography cite a 0.5% risk of serious neurologic complications and a 5–7% risk of transient reversible neurologic signs or symptoms. In patients with cerebrovascular disease, the risk may be two to three times higher, but it may be decidedly lower in the young. Angiography requires meticulous technique, coordination between the primary physician and the neuroradiologist, and clear indications for performing the study. Hematoma or vascular spasm at the site of injection is usually self-limited. The most serious complications are emboli, either produced from the end of the catheter or dislodged from the vessel wall; dissection of an artery; and hypersensitivity reactions to the dye. In elderly patients with known arteriosclerotic vascular disease, the increased risk of angiography should be weighed against the feasibility and efficacy of possible later treatments, such as carotid endarterectomy.

Single Photon Emission Computed Tomography (SPECT) and Positron Emission Tomography (PET): SPECT and PET are investigational tools that have not yet become routinely available clinically. Along with electroencephalography, PET scanning is one of the few modalities that indicate the physiologic function of the brain. Radioactive energy substrates, such as glucose or oxygen, or ligands of neurotransmitters are injected into an awake patient. Images are obtained from positrons that are emitted from the brain while radioactive material binds or is consumed within the parenchyma. Both the rate of consumption (or binding) and the location can thereby be deduced. Selection of appropriate substrates or ligands allows imaging of specific tissues, such as dopaminergic neurons, or areas that use abnormally high amounts of energy, such as epileptogenic regions. Although PET is currently an investigational tool, it plays an important role in the delineation of seizure foci, the distinction of normal brain from neoplastic tissue, and the elucidation of the border zone of ischemia that surrounds areas of cerebral infarction. SPECT permits imaging of cerebral blood flow; this is valuable in the evaluation of ischemic stroke, diagnosis of dementia, and planning of therapy for neoplasms. Both PET and SPECT have been used as adjunctive tests in judging prognosis of coma and the persistent vegetative state.

Electroencephalography

The electroencephalogram (EEG) records electrical activity generated near the surface of the cerebral cortex. Newer techniques, including EEG telemetry, prolonged ambulatory EEG monitoring, and combined video EEG monitoring, are important in the evaluation of syncope and seizures.

Areas of Usefulness: The EEG is the only widely available technique for determining the physiologic activity of the brain. Most of the alterations to which the cerebral cortex is predisposed cause focal or generalized disruption of the normal rhythms of the awake and sleeping brain. For instance, general metabolic derangements that result in delirium, stupor, or coma reliably produce generalized slowing of the EEG, whereas withdrawal from depressant drugs commonly activates it. The EEG is especially useful for characterizing epileptic disorders. Discrete sharp waves and spikes are seen with focal seizure discharges, while three-per-second spike and wave abnormalities suggest subcortical discharges, as does bilateral symmetric frontal activity. However, seizure activity, particularly that coming from the deep temporal lobes, may not be reflected as an abnormality in scalp recordings. Sleep deprivation, hyperventilation, photic stimulation, and special nasopharyngeal electrodes may make certain seizure discharges more evident.

Although the EEG may detect intracranial masses (owing to the appearance of slow delta waves) or subdural hematoma (locally decreased amplitude), CT and MRI are far superior. A normal EEG by no means excludes an intracranial mass lesion.

The EEG is commonly used for ongoing physiologic monitoring of the state of the brain during anesthesia, in cardiac and intracranial surgery, and for ongoing assessment of the state of drug intoxication, metabolic encephalopathies, diffuse infections, and severe trauma. The EEG may show abnormalities in the temporal lobe; this can help in assessing patients suspected of having herpes encephalitis. An electrically silent ("flat") EEG has become an almost universal criterion for the diagnosis of brain death.

Technique: The electroencephalographer must know which medications the patient is taking and the nature of the diagnostic problem, because these influence the techniques that will be used and the interpretation of the result. For example, if temporal lobe seizures are suspected, recordings during sleep or with specially placed electrodes may be required.

No significant risks are associated with EEG, although the patient who receives sedation for the recording should not drive for several hours afterward.

Cortical Evoked Potentials

Stimulation of the visual, auditory, or somatosensory pathways produces transient potentials that can be recorded by electrodes along the sensory pathways, especially electrodes applied to the scalp. These potentials that are time-locked to the stimulus may be recorded by an electroencephalograph and averaged by computer. The resulting evoked potentials have a highly reproducible amplitude, latency, and waveform. Each peak or wave corresponds to a particular sensory relay, and alterations of the timing or amplitude of the wave reflect an abnormality at a certain anatomic site.

Visual evoked potentials were discovered first and are the most easily recorded. A flashing light or alternating light and dark pattern is displayed to the patient, who fixates on the object with one eye alternately covered. The evoked potentials are recorded over the occiput. Visual evoked potentials give information about the optic nerve, lateral geniculate, and occipital cortex, but are most useful for abnormalities of the optic nerve itself. The detection of asymptomatic lesions in multiple sclerosis, evaluation of visual acuity in the very young or the retarded, and the distinction of blindness from malingering are particular indications.

Brain-stem auditory-evoked responses are recorded over the scalp after a tone or click is introduced unilaterally into an earphone. The pathways measured include the auditory nerve itself, cochlear nucleus, olivary lateral lemniscus, inferior colliculus, thalamus, and auditory radiations of the temporal lobe. In practice, information about the peripheral auditory apparatus and brain stem may be derived from analysis of the potentials. Brain-stem auditory-evoked responses are particularly useful in the assessment of eighth nerve tumors, further characterization of audiometric abnormalities, the assessment of lesions located ventrally in the pons and medulla (which include brain-stem tumors), plaques in multiple sclerosis, and trauma to the brain stem.

Somatosensory-evoked potentials are produced by stimulation of a peripheral nerve and recorded over the neck and scalp. Relays include the spinal cord, thalamus, and somatosensory cortex. The technique is most useful for disorders of the spinal cord and brain stem. Somatosensory potentials are now routinely recorded during orthopedic and neurosurgical operations to ensure integrity of the spinal cord or brain stem while it is manipulated. Maintenance of evoked potentials may be of prognostic value in cases of spinal trauma. They are also useful in following the progress of patients with a variety of intraspinal abnormalities, particularly syringomyelia, intramedullary tumors, and spinal vascular malformations.

Neuropsychological Assessment

Techniques derived from cognitive and sensory psychology may be applied to patients with neurologic disease. Patients who complain of failing memory, intellectual deterioration, spatial disorientation, a variety of sensory alterations, aphasia, agnosia, and apraxia may have their abnormalities characterized by careful neuropsychological study. The examinations themselves are complex and must be administered by an experienced psychologist, neurologist, or psychiatrist who has intimate knowledge of the patterns of neurologic disease. Unless the examination is tailored to the precise question being considered, misleading findings usually result. Neuropsychological assessment is frequently helpful in determining unsuspected cognitive abnormalities and may also provide reassurance for the patient or physician who fears an abnormality in the cognitive sphere when none actually exists.

Projective and nonprojective personality tests are helpful in the evaluation of patients who have neurologic symptoms that do not have a clear origin. In hysteria, in somatization disorders (hypochondriasis), with the "worried well," and in conditions causing chronic pain, personality testing may indicate the roots of the problem and provide a fruitful rationale for therapy.

Biopsy

Brain biopsy is used for the definitive diagnosis of brain tumor and for certain types of inflammatory, degenerative, and infectious diseases. Peripheral nerve biopsy, usually of the sural (a purely sensory) nerve, is valuable in specific diagnosis of familial, inflammatory, and certain metabolic defects of nerve, for example, metachromatic leukodystrophy and amyloidosis. Muscle biopsy is a routine, simple, and often essential part of the evaluation of patients with weakness. Fibroblasts derived from the conjunctiva or skin may be used to assay for specific enzymes and are used for the diagnosis of a variety of metabolic diseases in children and adults.

SUMMARY

▶ Prompt and accurate diagnosis of neurologic disorders is important because many are now treatable.

▶ The proper use of sophisticated and expensive neurologic diagnostic testing depends on the thoughtful clinician gathering accurate information from the patient's history and physical examination.

▶ Computed tomography and magnetic resonance imaging have vastly expanded the sensitivity and timeliness of neurologic diagnosis.

▶ Lumbar puncture remains an essential diagnostic test for patients with central nervous system infection, carcinomatous meningitis, and, in some cases, subarachnoid hemorrhage.

SUGGESTED READING

Adams RD, Victor M: *Principles of Neurology,* 5th ed. McGraw-Hill, 1993.

Bannister R: *Brain and Bannister's Clinical Neurology,* 7th ed. Oxford University Press, 1992.

Brazis PW, Masdeu JC, Biller J: *Localization in Clinical Neurology,* 2nd ed. Little, Brown & Company, 1985.

Greenberg JO: *Neuroimaging.* McGraw-Hill, 1995.

Haerer AF: *DeJong's The Neurologic Examination,* 5th ed. JB Lippincott, 1992.

Joynt RJ (editor): *Clinical Neurology.* JB Lippincott (looseleaf with annual updates), 1995.

Medical Research Council (UK): *Aids to the Examination of the Peripheral Nervous System.* Baillière-Tindall, 1995.

13.2

The Unconscious Patient

Robert S. Fisher, MD, PhD

How the physician approaches the diagnosis and management of an unconscious patient can make the difference between a full recovery and a disastrous outcome. Because the unconscious patient cannot give a history—the usual mainstay of diagnosis—the clinician must use clues from observers, family members, physical examination, and laboratory studies.

When the physician sees an unconscious patient, the order of thinking should be medical stabilization, history and examination, categorization of the type of coma, determination of etiology, and treatment of causal factors.

LEVELS OF CONSCIOUSNESS

Consciousness is an awareness of self and environment. Unconsciousness can range from sleep to coma (Table 13.2–1). A person in coma may breathe and move spontaneously, but does not alter behavior in response to noise or painful stimuli such as sternal rub, supraorbital pressure, or pinching of a limb. The Glasgow coma scale is a commonly used means of assessing consciousness (Table 13.2–2). The physician should record each type of stimulus and response to give a precise picture of the patient's condition.

When describing a patient in stupor, the physician should be specific about the degree of responsiveness. Alertness and level of mental function usually fluctuate over a period of minutes to hours. Delirious patients may be agitated or quiet. Delirium must be distinguished from dementia (Chapter 14.2), which is a chronic, progressive decrease of cognition in full alertness.

"Vegetative state" and "coma vigil" are among the terms that have been used to describe persons who appear to be awake and alert, or who cycle through apparent wakefulness and sleep, but who show no ability to respond to voice or gestures or to provide for their own basic needs. An important cause of the vegetative state is widespread destruction of neocortex by global hypoxia or hypoglycemia. The examining physician must distinguish vegetative state from the "locked-in state," in which the patient is completely aware, but cannot speak or move. Causes include neuromuscular conditions (eg, poisoning with curare, advanced motor neuron disease, severe Guillain-Barré syndrome) and pontine strokes that destroy corticospinal and corticobulbar tracts. Patients in the locked-in state may still be able to blink and move their eyes voluntarily or in response to command.

ANATOMY OF LOSS OF CONSCIOUSNESS

Consciousness is mediated by the cerebral hemispheres. Even though the left and right hemispheres specialize in different cognitive functions, either can support consciousness. Patients subjected to hemispherectomy on either side remain awake and alert. Another structure critical to consciousness is the reticular activating system, which appears to bias the cortex toward attention and alertness. The reticular activating system remains imprecisely mapped; it traverses medulla, pons, midbrain, and portions of the diencephalon near the ventricular system.

There are two ways to impair consciousness: by diffuse injury or dysfunction of cortex and by lesions of the reticular activating system. Cortical dysfunction can be caused by many processes. Fainting causes loss of consciousness because of transiently decreased blood flow to the whole brain. Prolonged anoxia, ischemia, or hypoglycemia can lead to coma by diffusely damaging cortex, since the substrates for neuronal metabolism and survival are glucose and oxygen, each delivered by the circulatory system. Generalized seizures induce loss of consciousness by temporarily disrupting cortical electrical function. In stroke, consciousness is lost when the posterior circulation cannot maintain an adequate blood supply to the reticular activating system. The mechanisms of loss of consciousness in concussion are uncertain; shear and stretch of brain-stem reticular activating system fibers may be a factor. Distortion of the brain stem by tumors or compression can also cause coma.

Table 13.2–1. Commonly used terms relating to consciousness and unconsciousness.

Consciousness: awareness of self and environment
Unconsciousness: lack of consciousness
Coma: unarousable unresponsiveness
Sleep: arousable unresponsiveness
Stupor: unresponsiveness except by vigorous stimuli
Obtundation: same as stupor
Delirium: fluctuating disorientation and cognition while not fully alert
Dementia: chronic, progressive decrease of cognition while alert
Vegetative state: apparent alertness, but without cognition
Locked-in state: paralysis, but alert and aware

CAUSES OF UNCONSCIOUSNESS

Unconsciousness has been classified in many ways. The simplest classification scheme is "unconsciousness associated with diffuse signs" versus "unconsciousness with focal signs." These are spoken of as diffuse coma versus focal coma, or as metabolic versus structural coma.

Diffuse Coma

Diffuse coma can be produced by any condition that interferes with oxygen or glucose delivery to the brain. Diffuse coma usually results from a general derangement of brain function, such as that caused by hypoglycemia, subarachnoid hemorrhage, meningitis, or a postictal state (Table 13.2–3).

The most common cause of unexpected loss of consciousness is syncope, resulting from a transient decrease of blood flow to the entire brain (Chapter 1.9). The ordinary faint is called vasovagal syncope because the auto-

Table 13.2–2. Glasgow Coma Scale.

Category	Response	Score
Eye opening	Spontaneous	4
	To speech	3
	To pain	2
	None	1
Best verbal response	Oriented	5
	Confused	4
	Inappropriate	3
	Incomprehensible	2
	None	1
	(If intubated)	(T)
Best motor response	Obeys commands	6
	Localizes pain	5
	Flexion-withdrawal	4
	Decorticate (flexion)	3
	Decerebrate (extension)	2
	None	1

By number or in words, the examiner should record each level of response to stimuli. Although physicians often combine the section scores and record the total, interpretation of total scores is difficult because the scale is nonlinear.
Modified and reproduced, with permission, from Teasdale G, Jennett B: Assessment of coma and impaired consciousness: A practical scale. Lancet 1974;ii:81. © by The Lancet, Ltd.

Table 13.2–3. Major causes of diffuse loss of consciousness.

Deficient metabolism
  Syncope
  Hypoxia
  Hypoglycemia
Toxins
  Exogenous (drugs)
  Endogenous (uremia, hepatic encephalopathy)
Fluid or acid-base disorders
  Hyponatremia
  Hypercalcemia
  Alkalosis
Severe sepsis
Hypothermia (<32°C [89.6°F])
Endocrine conditions
  Hypothyroidism
  Adrenal insufficiency
  Pituitary apoplexy
Meningeal syndromes
Trauma
Postictal states
Psychiatric conditions

nomic nervous system shunts blood to muscle and away from brain. Vasovagal syncope characteristically occurs in a setting of emotional distress, such as blood drawing, pain, or shocking news. People usually feel lightheaded, nauseated, and clammy before losing consciousness and generally regain consciousness spontaneously within minutes.

Hypoxia can lead to loss of consciousness, and if continued for longer than about 10 minutes, to diffuse cortical injury. Hypoglycemia can cause diffuse coma because the brain is absolutely dependent on glycolytic metabolism. Hypoglycemia has many causes, including prolonged fasting, an inappropriately large insulin surge in response to a carbohydrate load, and excessive exogenous (treatment for diabetes) or endogenous (insulinoma) insulin (Chapter 4.7). Vitamin B_1 (thiamine) is a required cofactor for glucose metabolism as well as for several other metabolic processes. In alcohol abusers and other nutritionally deprived persons, thiamine deficiency can lead to Wernicke's encephalopathy, with eye movement abnormalities (nystagmus or ophthalmoparesis), and mental status changes ranging from confusion to coma.

Intoxication is the most common cause of diffuse coma encountered in modern emergency rooms. Frequently implicated exogenous toxins are both illicit drugs and prescription medications, including alcohol, benzodiazepines, barbiturates, antidepressants, and opiates. Patients can develop endogenous intoxication from the accumulation of metabolic products in renal or hepatic failure. Water intoxication can produce hypo-osmolar coma. Metabolic abnormalities, including hyperosmolar states such as non-ketotic hyperglycemia, can lead to coma. Hypercalcemia with total serum calcium above 15 mg/dL produces stupor. Severe acidosis and sepsis may lead to stupor or coma. It is a common, although poorly understood, experience to find a treatable pneumonia or urinary tract infection in an elderly person with impaired consciousness; the patient's cognition improves when the infection is successfully treated. Hypothermia, with core temperatures below 32°C (89.6°F), induces a reversible stupor or coma (Chapter 15.3). Endocrine conditions, including hypothyroidism (myxedema coma), pituitary failure, and Addison's disease, present in part with altered consciousness.

The meninges and subarachnoid fluid are in contact with large areas of cortex. Infection or irritation from blood, intrathecal chemotherapy, or neoplastic cells can produce headache, stiff neck, and decreased consciousness. Trauma is a well-known cause of both diffuse and focal coma. A person who comes to medical attention during the postictal period after a generalized seizure may present in coma. Most postictal patients return to awareness within minutes, although some patients take as long as a few hours. Patients with psychiatric conditions account for a small percentage of those with diffuse coma; psychogenic coma may be difficult to diagnose unless the physician maintains a high index of suspicion.

Focal Coma

Focal coma usually results from a structural brain stem injury, such as vertebrobasilar stroke or brain-stem compression (Table 13.2–4). Brain-stem ischemia, infarction, or hemorrhage affecting the reticular activating system leads to loss of consciousness. In over 95% of patients, the examiner can detect other brain-stem signs or symptoms, such as dysarthria, visual changes, diplopia, tinnitus, ataxia, numbness, or weakness in the neurologic history or examination.

Brain Herniation Syndromes: These syndromes are important causes of focal coma, calling for immediate recognition and treatment. The brain herniates as a consequence of increased intracranial pressure. The brain can herniate in five locations: (1) mesial temporal uncus through the tentorium (uncal herniation); (2) midline thalamus through the tentorium (central herniation); (3) medulla and cerebellar tonsils through the foramen magnum (tonsillar herniation); (4) out of a craniotomy defect; and (5) cingulate gyrus under the falx in the midline. Uncal, central, and tonsillar herniation syndromes can be fatal unless recognized and treated promptly. Craniotomy and cingulate herniation are very serious, but not necessarily fatal.

The major causes of brain herniation (see Table 13.2–4) are examples of acute mass lesions or decompensated hy-

Table 13.2–4. Major causes of focal coma.

Brain-stem infarction or hemorrhage
Brain-stem trauma
Herniation secondary to:
Subdural hematoma
Hemispheric hemorrhage
Hemispheric infarct and edema
Hemispheric abscess
Hemispheric tumor ± hemorrhage or edema
Decompensated chronic hydrocephalus

drocephalus. A lesion with anatomic asymmetry and rapid onset is more likely to produce herniation than is a slow-onset, symmetric lesion.

The uncal herniation syndrome usually presents with a third-nerve palsy as the uncus compresses the third nerve. An early clinical sign of third-nerve compression is ipsilateral pupillary dilation. Disruption of the third nerve leaves only lateral (sixth nerve) and downward (fourth nerve) eye movement. If not treated, this condition may progress to contralateral hemiparesis (because of corticospinal tract compression at the midbrain) and coma. Central herniation results from bilaterally symmetric increases in intracranial pressure, such as those caused by hydrocephalus or a midline hemorrhage. The supratentorial structures herniate straight down through the tentorium onto the midbrain. Both pupils become fixed and dilated; decerebrate posturing and coma ensue. Herniation of the cerebellar tonsils through the foramen magnum is usually lethal because the tonsils compress cardiorespiratory centers in the medulla. This syndrome typically accompanies uncal or central herniation, a cerebellar hematoma or infarct with edema, or a posterior fossa tumor.

Brain herniation syndromes are emergencies. The goal of medical therapy is to buy the staff a few hours to organize definitive treatment, usually neurosurgical (see "Management of the Comatose Patient" below).

EXAMINATION OF THE UNCONSCIOUS PATIENT

Since unconscious patients are unable to give a history (although information should be sought from family or bystanders), the physical examination is very important (Table 13.2–5). Coma is a life-threatening emergency. Accurate and frequent monitoring of vital signs is imperative. The patient's overall level of alertness should be described specifically or assessed in terms of the Glasgow coma scale (see Table 13.2–2). The purposes of the physical exam are to seek focal neurologic findings and to detect correctable metabolic etiologies such as hypotension, hypoxia, hypoglycemia, intoxication, and sepsis.

During the general exam, the physician should look for signs of trauma, such as boggy scalp hematomas, blood behind the ear (Battle's sign of basilar head trauma), and blood behind the tympanic membrane. Until proven otherwise, the examiner must assume that the traumatized patient's neck is broken. Neck stiffness, as an index of meningitis, may be masked in coma, since patients do not feel the pain of meningismus. A patient with central nervous system trauma likely has other traumatized organs that may require immediate attention.

Breathing

The patient's breathing pattern can give a clue to the level of a lesion causing coma. Cheyne-Stokes respiration, a breathing pattern of cyclically increasing and decreasing respiration amplitude, indicates either widespread cortical

Table 13.2–5. Examination of the comatose patient.

Finding	Significance
Fever	Sepsis
Hypothermia	Sepsis, hypothyroidism
Abnormal pulse or blood pressure	Cardiovascular causes
Responsiveness	Favorable prognosis
Spontaneous eye opening	
Good verbal response	
Good motor response	
General exam	
Bruises	Trauma, seizure
Malodorous breath	Ketosis, alcohol, uremia
Pale, clammy skin	Hypoglycemia, uremia, hypotension
Jaundiced skin	Liver failure
Neck stiffness	Meningitis, subarachnoid hemorrhage
Bruits	Risk for vascular disease
Respiratory pattern	
Cheyne-Stokes	Diffuse cortical or brain-stem lesion
Hyperventilation	Acidosis, midbrain lesion
Irregular breathing	Medulla or pons lesion
Hiccough	Systemic toxicity, brain-stem lesion
Pupils	
One fixed and dilated	Herniation, third-nerve lesion
One small and reactive	Horner's syndrome
Both fixed mid-position	Midbrain lesion, drugs
Pinpoint	Pontine lesion, opiate overdose
Both fixed large	Anoxia, ischemia, drugs, death
Eye movements	
Conjugate deviation (can cross midline)	Hemispheric lesion or seizure
Conjugate deviation (cannot cross midline)	Lateral pontine lesion or below
Dysconjugate movements	Brain-stem lesion
Funduscopic exam	
Papilledema	Increased intracranial pressure
Hemorrhages and exudates	Hypertensive crisis
Retinal blood lakes	Subarachnoid hemorrhage
Interruption of blood columns	Circulatory sludging, eg, hyperviscosity
Motor exam	
Movements	Favorable prognosis
Hemiparesis	Focal coma
Unilateral Babinski's sign	Focal coma

dysfunction or a brain-stem (pons, midbrain) lesion. Cheyne-Stokes breathing can also follow cardiorespiratory arrest without a primary neurologic disorder. Hyperventilation may reflect a midbrain lesion (in which case it is called *central neurogenic hyperventilation*) or metabolic acidosis. Irregular breathing signals dysfunction in the low brain stem, and is a poor prognostic sign. Hiccough is usually a trivial breathing aberrancy, but in a comatose patient, hiccough is an ominous sign indicating severe damage to the brain stem.

Pupils

Examination of the pupils can help distinguish structural (focal) from metabolic (diffuse) coma, since in most cases of metabolic coma the pupils remain equal and reactive. Certain toxins and drugs (eg, anticholinergic agents) may paralyze the pupils, but the pupils remain symmetric. Unequal pupils imply structural coma. A large, unreactive pupil in an eye also deviated down and out indicates an ipsilateral third-nerve palsy (Figure 13.2–1). Such a lesion can occur with uncal herniation, aneurysm of the posterior circle of Willis, or peripheral third-nerve injury, as with trauma or meningitis.

A small reactive pupil suggests an ipsilateral Horner's syndrome, characterized by ptosis, miosis, and anhidrosis. Horner's syndrome can result from damage to any part of the sympathetic system. Possible sites of injury are the hypothalamus, brain-stem reticular formation, intermediolateral column of the cervical cord, and in the sympathetic chain, superior cervical ganglia, or sympathetic fibers near the carotid arteries. Central herniation syndrome or overdose with certain drugs can produce midposition, fixed pupils. Pinpoint reactive pupils occur with pontine lesions or opiate overdoses. Bilateral, fixed large pupils may result from anoxia, ischemia, certain drugs, or death. The examiner should not dilate a comatose patient's pupils with mydriatic drugs, since dilation obliterates their usefulness in serial neurologic examinations.

Eye Movements

An understanding of eye movements is useful in evaluating patients in coma. The cortex has multiple "gaze centers" for pursuit (smooth tracking) movements and saccadic (step) movements. The most important saccade center lies in the frontal lobe; when activated, it steps the eyes conjugately in the opposite direction. The most important smooth pursuit center lies in the parietal lobe; when activated, it moves the eyes conjugately to the same side. Cortical gaze centers are activated with physiologic functioning, during focal frontal or parietal seizures, or in rare cases of hemorrhage (irritative lesions). A destructive lesion of the left frontal lobe, such as an acute stroke, causes the eyes to deviate conjugately to the left, because of unbalanced input from the healthy right frontal lobe. A left frontal seizure deviates eyes laterally to the right and conjugately during the seizure and to the left in the postictal "exhausted" state. Parietal lesions produce less consistent effects on resting gaze, but usually impair pursuit eye movements toward the side of the lesion.

Cortical neurons connect to contralateral eye movement centers in the brain stem, which execute the cortically generated eye movement commands. Lateral eye movements require a signal generated in the lateral pons, activating the ipsilateral VIth nerve (lateral rectus), and the contralateral third nerve (contralateral medial rectus). Stimulation of the left lateral gaze center in the pons drives the eyes conjugately to the left, and stimulation of the right lateral gaze center drives gaze to the right. De-

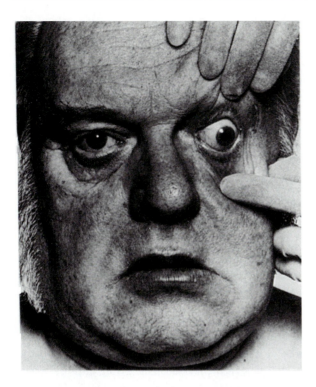

Figure 13.2–1. A right third cranial nerve palsy, showing eye deviated out and down, and a dilated pupil. (Reproduced, with permission, from Spillane JD, Spillane JA: *An Atlas of Clinical Neurology,* 3rd ed. Oxford University Press, 1982.)

structive lesions of the lateral pons have the opposite effect from that of stimulation. Therefore, a patient with, for example, a left conjugate gaze preference, could have either a left frontal lobe lesion or a right pontine lesion. Lesions of the oculomotor system distal to the dorsolateral pons cause dysconjugate gaze and eye movements.

The physician can examine eye movements by quickly turning the patient's head from side to side after first making certain by a neck x-ray that the neck is stable (if the patient has suffered trauma). In a normal person, a vestibulo-ocular reflex attempts to stabilize the eyes in space when the head moves, a phenomenon called the *doll's eyes reflex.*

A stronger stimulus for the vestibulo-ocular reflex is ice water placed in the external auditory canal (the physician should look in the canal first to rule out perforation of the tympanic membrane). The cold inactivates the ipsilateral vestibular input to the eye movement center and normally produces slow deviation toward the irrigated ear. If the patient is not in coma, contralateral saccades also appear, with a corrective fast phase beating away from the cold stimulus. Fast phases are more sensitive to brain-stem depression than are slow phases, so they disappear first as coma progresses. Dysconjugate eye movements in re-

sponse to the doll's eyes maneuver or ice water calorics suggests a structural lesion distal to the lateral pons. Full loss of vestibulo-ocular reflexes indicates severe structural or metabolic depression of the brain stem. With cortical lesions, the deviating eyes can be made to cross the midline of the gaze field by activating the vestibulo-ocular reflex with the doll's maneuver or ice water calorics. If the pontine lateral gaze centers are impaired, the deviating eyes cannot be returned across the midline with the doll's or ice water maneuvers.

Funduscopy should be performed in all unconscious patients. Retinal hemorrhages and exudates may point to severe hypertension or diabetes. Large uniform regions of hemorrhages, called *retinal blood lakes,* suggest subarachnoid hemorrhage. Intravascular emboli are sometimes visible. Sludging of blood from hyperviscosity can appear as "boxcars" (interruption of a continuous blood column) in retinal vessels. Papilledema presents as blurring of disk margins, loss of normal venous pulsations, and later as hemorrhages and exudates. Papilledema indicates increased intracranial pressure, but may lag behind an acute rise in intracranial pressure by 24 hours. Therefore, its absence is not proof of normal intracranial pressure.

The examiner performs a motor exam on a comatose patient to look for focal findings. Motor exam in this setting usually includes evaluation of spontaneous movements, power of withdrawal to pain, hemiparesis, tone, muscle stretch (tendon) reflexes, and search for Babinski's sign. Focal findings suggest structural lesions in hemispheres or brain stem. Nonfocal exams increase the likelihood of a metabolic cause of coma.

MANAGEMENT OF THE COMATOSE PATIENT

Coma is a medical emergency. The physician's immediate task is to stabilize the patient; the cause of coma can be analyzed later (Table 13.2–6).

Treatment begins with ABC: airway, breathing, and circulation. The airway should be cleared. Patients who are breathing poorly or having trouble with respiratory secretions should be intubated. Blood pressure and pulse should be checked. Intravenous access should be estab-

Table 13.2–6. Emergency treatment of coma.

ABC: Airway, Breathing, Circulation
Establish IV access
Draw blood for serum glucose
Do other laboratory studies (eg, serum electrolyte panel, toxicology screen) as indicated
Give naloxone IV
Give thiamine IV
Consider giving glucose bolus
Give normal saline ± dextrose for circulatory impairment
Stabilize neck
Obtain CT or MRI scan
Observe for herniation; treat as needed
Determine cause

lished, but before fluids are given, blood should be drawn for a baseline serum glucose and other studies. If trauma is a possibility, the neck should be stabilized until cervical spine films rule out an unstable fracture.

When the physical exam (see "Examination of the Unconscious Patient" above) shows focal signs, an urgent brain computed tomographic (CT) or magnetic resonance imaging (MRI) scan is indicated. If a herniation syndrome is suspected, the physician should elevate the head of the bed 30 degrees (unless the patient is hypotensive), intubate, hyperventilate to an arterial PCO_2 of less than 30 mm Hg, give intravenous mannitol and dexamethasone, and follow urinary output. The physician should not perform a spinal tap in patients with focal coma. If the exam and neuroradiographic studies suggest a potentially remediable structural cause of coma, such as hemispheric or cerebellar mass lesion or hydrocephalus, neurosurgeons immediately should be consulted.

When the exam shows no focal signs, diffuse (metabolic) coma is likely. The opiate antagonist naloxone should be given intravenously. Naloxone wears off faster than many opiates, so the patient with opiate overdose requires ongoing observation and may need repeated naloxone doses. Intravenous thiamine is given before a glucose bolus; the thiamine provides a necessary cofactor for glycolytic reactions and thereby avoids precipitation of Wernicke's encephalopathy. The specific benzodiazepine antagonist flumazenil can be tried if benzodiazepine overdose is life-threatening. The patient who needs circulatory support should be given normal saline, with or without dextrose. An electroencephalogram (EEG) is useful in the diagnosis of nonconvulsive status epilepticus. If the cause of diffuse coma is not evident after the previously mentioned actions, neuroradiographic studies should be done to rule out atypical mass lesions and signs of brain trauma or hemorrhage.

SUMMARY

▶ The many causes of coma can be divided into two broad categories: structural lesions, which tend to produce unconsciousness with focal findings, and metabolic lesions, which produce unconsciousness without focal findings.

▶ The most common causes of loss of consciousness are syncope, seizures, trauma, brain anoxia-ischemia, toxins, and hypoglycemia.

▶ Physical examination, with attention to level of responsiveness, breathing patterns, eye findings, and motor exam, often points to the site of a lesion.

▶ Emergency treatment consists of assuring the airway, breathing, and circulation, and giving dextrose, opiate antagonists, and any necessary circulatory volume expanders.

▶ The outcome of coma depends primarily on the underlying cause and the effectiveness of prompt treatment.

SUGGESTED READING

Diringer MN: Early prediction of outcome from coma. Curr Opin Neurol Neurosurg 1992;5:826.

Hamel MB et al: Identification of comatose patients at high risk for death or severe disability. SUPPORT Investigators. Understand Prognoses and Preferences for Outcomes and Risks of Treatments. JAMA 1995;273:1842.

Medical aspects of the persistent vegetative state. 1. The Multi-Society Task Force on PVS. N Engl J Med 1994;330:1499.

Persistent vegetative state and the decision to withdraw or withhold life support. Council on Scientific Affairs and Council on Ethical and Judicial Affairs. JAMA 1990;263:426.

Samuels MA: The evaluation of comatose patients. Hosp Pract (Off Ed) 1993;28:165.

Turner BH, Knapp ME: Consciousness: A neurobiological approach. Integr Physiol Behav Sci 1995;30:151.

Spells: Seizures, Dizziness, and Other Episodic Disorders

Peter W. Kaplan, MB, FRCP

A spell is an event that begins suddenly and usually ends quickly; it may affect awareness, behavior, speech, or motor function. Patients may have subjective complaints such as malaise, dizziness or light-headedness, or poorly definable sensations of anxiety or dissociation. Spells are difficult to evaluate and manage because they are hard to describe and recall, and many go unwitnessed by others. Often the clinician must formulate a working diagnosis using fragments of information, much as an archeologist uses shards of pottery to obtain an idea of the whole. And sometimes the first impression is wrong.

During and after spells, patients may be alarmed as well as impaired and may not be able to give objective accounts of the event's duration, sequence, and other details. If episodes impair consciousness, the patient may be the last person to know about them. The sensations experienced are often novel, and the patient may lack adequate words to describe them. The description of a fleeting, alarming experience may be fraught with the same inconsistencies as the account of a public accident: The variations in the testimony of subjects and witnesses are legion. Blood or imaging tests are often unhelpful, and extended monitoring of brain activity or heart rhythm and rate are costly and, when ordered indiscriminately, of low yield. For example, transient changes in behavior may not reflect structural abnormalities, yet patients are subjected to computed tomography (CT) of the head. Conversely, a physician may request an electroencephalogram (EEG) several days after a seizure-like event, at which time the EEG may be normal, providing little information. However, if the EEG is performed just after, or, when possible, during an event, the diagnostic value increases substantially.

There are no hard-and-fast rules regarding when it is appropriate to investigate a spell, but some general guidelines can be offered. A single, brief, mild dizzy spell need not be evaluated. Most episodes of isolated dizziness do not represent serious disease, and resolve spontaneously. Investigation is warranted for most events that lead to serious injury (eg, broken bones) or are associated with palpitations or chest pain. The decision to evaluate means considering (1) the probability that a particular test will confirm or exclude a diagnosis, (2) whether a particular diagnosis is serious enough to warrant confirmation or exclusion, and (3) the potential risks of the procedure itself (eg, angiography potentially causing nephrotoxicity or stroke). There is also the risk that a false-positive result could lead to unnecessary testing or treatment. Tests should be used to confirm carefully formulated, probable diagnoses rather than to exclude rare and unlikely ones.

Although most spells are caused by seizures, syncope (Chapter 1.9), inner ear disorders, or psychological problems, many arise from other medical and neurologic conditions and from prescription or recreational drugs and alcohol (Table 13.3–1).

HISTORY

The history is of paramount importance in diagnosing spells. The physician should encourage patients to describe a sensation in their own words and should try to understand what patients mean when they describe a symptom.

Dizziness is a common complaint that often defies accurate definition. After much discussion, a patient may still say, "Doctor, I can't describe it. I feel just plain dizzy." To different people, "dizziness" may mean light-headedness, unsteadiness or imbalance, generalized weakness, malaise, or a sensation of rotation. More specific is *vertigo,* a perception of spinning or tilting in space, usually when the person is in the horizontal plane; vertigo most often suggests problems of the inner ear or brain stem. Many people use *light-headedness* to describe a

Table 13.3–1. Frequent causes of spells.

Syncope
Migraine
Seizures
Transient ischemic attacks
Hypoglycemia
Alcohol or drug-related syndromes
Vestibular or inner ear disease
Delirium
Panic attacks and hyperventilation
Hysteria, conversion disorders, malingering
Sleep disorders

feeling of fullness, tightness, or pressure in the head, with a sensation of swaying or floating, graying-out of vision, and faintness. *Presyncope* is also used to describe a sensation of near-fainting but without loss of consciousness, while *disequilibrium* connotes a sensation of imbalance or falling while upright. These entities have overlapping features: All may be associated with at least momentary nausea, sweating, pallor, tachycardia, and unsteady gait.

The history must include a full description of the context of each episode, preceding events, precipitating factors, symptoms, observed behavior, pattern, course, duration, and resolution. Spontaneous descriptions by the patient or witnesses are best; this avoids "leading the witness." When the patient or witnesses do not volunteer relevant information, the examiner should ask questions that will amplify the account of events and support a particular diagnosis. For example, the clinician should try to learn from witnesses whether the patient had preserved or impaired consciousness; an increase or decrease in body tone; limb, head, or body movements; urinary or fecal incontinence; and "postspell" confusion or an immediate return to alertness.

Certain initial symptoms may be common to several types of spells. For example, malaise with light-headedness or vertigo may precede a fall with either a seizure or

syncope. The examiner should ask whether the episode included tongue biting or was followed by drowsiness, confusion, and aching muscles, all of which suggest a tonic-clonic seizure. Conversely, preceding light-headedness, a sensation of spinning, nausea, perioral numbness, fading of vision, a brief loss of consciousness, and an immediate or early return to alertness suggest ischemia of the posterior cerebral circulation with syncope.

The patient's history often differs from that given by a witness. A lapse in attention may go unnoticed by the patient, but not by a family member; hence, the importance of seeking out an observer. "Did the patient stop all activity, stare, smack or lick his lips, pick at his clothing, look dazed or confused, or stop speaking?"—typical of a complex partial seizure. "Did the patient become stiff, look and turn her head sideways, show jerking movements, fall to the ground, and then appear confused or stuporous?"—features of a secondarily generalized tonic-clonic seizure. "Was the patient drinking alcohol or drunk before or during the event?"—suggesting an alcoholic blackout, hypoglycemia, or seizure. All these inquiries may lead to differing diagnostic possibilities (Table 13.3–2).

The physician should always be wary of prepackaged diagnoses. A patient may believe that the event was a "faint" or a "seizure," sometimes because of a previous medical opinion, sometimes to steer the doctor in a certain direction, or often because of what friends, family, or witnesses have said. The examiner should base the diagnosis on available clinical features, not a previous diagnostic label, which may be outdated or wrong.

The clinician must use tact in establishing the features of the patient's spells. It can be frustrating for the patient to have to describe to yet a third physician, a fifth witness, or an entourage of unhelpful faces, an experience of which he may be only dimly aware. Furthermore, a question or remark that seems unsympathetic may make a patient defensive or close-mouthed, further obscuring the account.

Table 13.3–2. Differentiating features among common types of spells.

	Syncope	Tonic-Clonic Seizure	Psychogenic "Seizure"	Complex Partial Seizure	Migraine
Premonitory symptoms	Light-headedness, dim vision	Sometimes an aura (with partial onset only)	Varied	Sometimes an aura	Malaise, visual symptoms
Onset	Gradual	Sudden	Variable	Sudden	Gradual
Repeating pattern of features	Yes	Yes	Variable	Yes	Yes
Posture at onset	Usually standing	Any	Any	Any	Any
Progression and duration	Brief	Usually brief	Often prolonged	Brief	Prolonged
After the event	Normal	Confusion, lethargy	Normal	Confusion	Normal
Tonic-clonic movements	Fairly common	Common	Common	None	Never
Accidental trauma related to spell	Uncommon	Common	Rare	Uncommon	Never
Incontinence	Rare	Common	Rare	Rare	Never

Modified, with permission, from Blume WT: Differential diagnosis of epileptic seizures. In *Clinical Neurophysiology of Epilepsy: Handbook of Encephalography and Clinical Neurophysiology,* revised series, vol 4. Wada JA, Ellingson RJ (editors). Elsevier, 1990.

One of the most important issues to be addressed is whether the episodes are organic (real) or psychogenic. When events appear to be triggered by a reproducible physiologic mechanism such as hyperventilation or standing up, they should be reproduced in the physician's presence. But if the purported trigger is bizarre or highly variable, the spells may be psychogenic. Although a minority of spells are purely psychogenic, up to 40% may have a psychiatric component.

The history suggests a working diagnosis, which a careful, directed physical examination and laboratory tests can help to confirm.

PHYSICAL EXAMINATION

The exam is most useful when it is directed at finding evidence to confirm a suspected diagnosis. An irregular heart rate, cardiac murmurs, or a postural drop in blood pressure may support syncope; atrial fibrillation or carotid bruits may correlate with transient ischemic attacks; a bitten tongue or cheek lends credence to a generalized seizure. In patients with seizures, focal neurologic findings such as hemiparesis suggest that the cause is a focal central nervous system disorder. Unfortunately, the physical exam often reveals few if any relevant abnormalities.

INTERPRETATION OF SPELLS

Diagnoses are often based on the constellation of symptoms given by the patient and signs described by witnesses. The multiplicity of clinical features and their combinations has led to a myriad of syndromes. Since patients come to the doctor with signs and symptoms, not diagnostic categories, the rest of the chapter will outline some of the more common syndromes.

Spells Predominantly with Subjective Complaints

Many dizzy patients have vestibular problems, although many others have psychiatric disturbances, presyncope, or disequilibrium. Isolated vertigo or light-headedness rarely suggests serious neurologic illness. Light-headedness can be seen with hypoglycemia, disturbances of the posterior brain circulation, or psychological dysfunction, while vertigo signals middle ear dysfunction, drug effects, migraine, or disturbances of the posterior circulation. Both vertigo and light-headedness can be features of many other conditions and are rarely sufficient to indicate a particular diagnosis.

True vertigo with unsteady gait and nausea suggests problems with vestibular structures of the ear. If the examiner quickly changes the patient's position from sitting to lying, with the head back and to the side (Hallpike maneuver), the onset of jerky eye movements (nystagmus) and reproduction of the symptoms confirms vestibular dysfunction. Further tests of vestibular dysfunction are available in clinics that specialize in these disorders. Ringing in the ears (tinnitus) and deafness suggest disease of the cochlea or auditory nerve, and a combination of vertigo, nausea, tinnitus, and deafness builds a case for middle or inner ear disease. Vertigo and tinnitus occasionally precede seizures; the diagnosis is strongly supported by subsequent confusion, semipurposeful movements, or convulsions.

When light-headedness without sustained tinnitus or deafness is associated with a sensation of malaise, fading of vision, perioral numbness, sweating or faintness (presyncope), or loss of consciousness (syncope), the likely cause is brain-stem ischemia. Such cerebral ischemia is often accompanied by apprehension, anxiety, and faintness. Witnesses may describe patients as being pallid and sweaty, and patients may feel an urge to urinate or defecate. As symptoms progress, patients may sit or lie down; if unable to do so, they may collapse and lose consciousness. If they then have convulsive syncope with jerking limb movements, they may be given a mistaken diagnosis of epileptic seizures.

The combination of sweating, malaise, nausea, and weakness can also be seen with hypoglycemia. Causes include excess insulin from exogenous or endogenous sources, as well as liver disease, alcoholism, excessive intake of oral hypoglycemic medication, and gastrojejunostomy. Hypoglycemia occasionally triggers tonic-clonic seizures.

When patients have light-headedness, malaise, anxiety, and digital tingling, the clinician should consider hyperventilation or panic attacks (see "Psychogenic Spells" below).

Spells with Subjective and Objective Complaints: Seizures and Epilepsy

Seizures are a common cause of spells. A seizure is an abnormal, hypersynchronous or excessive, acute neuronal discharge originating in the brain and with clinically observable expression, often including changes in behavior. The term "epilepsy" is the chronic condition of recurrent unprovoked seizures. The varying spread and degree of epileptic discharge produces a wide spectrum of clinical expression. The clinical features may therefore vary from the entirely subjective (eg, a bad smell in a simple partial seizure) to the entirely objective (eg, immediate impairment of consciousness, staring, and fidgeting that the patient does not remember, in a complex partial seizure). Many seizures have elements of both subjective and objective disturbance.

The diagnosis of a tonic-clonic seizure is usually straightforward, based on the history of a patient falling to the ground, unresponsive, with body stiffness, tonic-clonic jerks, and urinary or fecal incontinence. Most difficulties in diagnosis involve seizures with few or no convulsive (jerking) elements or with purely subjective complaints or amnesia.

Key features of a patient's spell allow the diagnosis of a particular seizure type (Table 13.3–3) and have therapeutic and prognostic implications. For example, absence

Table 13.3–3. Common types of seizures.

Type	Characteristics
I. Partial (focal) seizures	
A. Simple partial seizures (with preserved awareness)	
1. Motor	Focal movements
2. Sensory (old name: aura)	
Somatosensory	Tingling and numbness
Visual	Light flashing
Auditory	Buzzing
Olfactory	Bad smell
Gustatory	Bad taste
Vertiginous	Vertigo and dizziness
3. Autonomic	Sweating, pallor, flushing
4. Psychic	Dream-like states, fear, hallucinations
B. Complex partial seizures (with impaired awareness) (old name: psychomotor or temporal lobe seizures)	
1. Simple partial onset, with impaired consciousness	
a. Without automatisms	
b. With automatisms (staring, lip smacking, fidgeting, picking movements)	
2. Impaired consciousness at onset	
a. Without automatisms	
b. With automatisms (staring, lip smacking, fidgeting, picking movements)	
C. Partial seizures evolving to secondarily generalized seizures	
1. Simple partial evolving to generalized seizures	
2. Complex partial evolving to generalized seizures	
3. Simple partial evolving to complex partial, then to generalized seizures	
II. Generalized seizures	
A. Absence (old name: petit mal)	Staring, inattention, blinking
B. Myoclonic	Quick repetitive jerks
C. Tonic	Stiffness, flexion
D. Tonic-clonic (old name: grand mal)	Convulsions followed by lethargy
E. Atonic	Drop attacks with unconsciousness

Modified and reproduced, with permission, from The Commission on Classification and Terminology of the International League Against Epilepsy: Proposal for revised clinical and electroencephalographic classification of epileptic seizures. Epilepsia 1981;22:489.

seizures (part of absence epilepsy, a genetic condition) require an EEG for diagnosis, but no head CT scan. Treatment is usually with drugs directed at primary generalized seizures. By contrast, when people first develop partial seizures after age 40, whether or not the seizures generalize, the physician should assume an underlying cause such as stroke or tumor and should seek it with a head CT or MRI scan.

Simple partial seizures (which do not impair attention or consciousness) may cause recurrent familiar or unfamiliar perceptions (déjà vu and jamais vu); frightening or pleasant sensations; distortions of vision (objects appear larger, smaller, closer, or farther away than they really are); distortions of smell, hearing, and sensation; jerking movements on one side of the body; or even sweating, pallor, and palpitations. The seizures occur in parts of the brain that subserve these functions.

Complex partial seizures impair attention or consciousness through focal seizure activity. These seizures are characterized by staring; most patients also have other features like blinking, lip-smacking, unresponsiveness with semipurposeful automatic picking or hand rubbing movements (automatisms), confused behavior, and amnesia.

Absence seizures (previously called "petit mal") are also characterized by motionless staring, often with blinking, but are caused by generalized seizure activity. In contrast to complex partial seizures, absence seizures usually last less than 20 seconds, briefly interrupt ongoing activity, can occur frequently throughout the day, and do not leave the patient confused or lethargic. These seizures begin in childhood and usually regress in adulthood. Absence seizures are often brought to the physician's attention by parents or school teachers who have noticed the child to be staring and inattentive.

Tonic-clonic seizures (convulsions) are characterized by stiffening of the body, upward rolling of the eyes, clenching of the teeth, grunting, tongue or cheek biting, urinary incontinence, clonic limb jerks, and unconsciousness. There are two types of generalized seizures: (1) primary generalized, in which seizure activity occurs symmetrically and synchronously in both hemispheres of a structurally normal brain, and (2) secondarily generalized, in which seizure activity begins focally in one abnormal part of one hemisphere and then spreads to involve the whole hemisphere as well as the contralateral hemisphere.

Myoclonic seizures are bilateral rapid limb jerks, often with preserved consciousness; they may be seen in juvenile myoclonic epilepsy. Most patients also have other seizure types, such as generalized tonic-clonic or absence seizures. Myoclonic seizures with coma are often seen after prolonged cardiorespiratory arrest with a severe anoxic or ischemic brain insult.

A seizure is usually diagnosed from the history, but short of capturing an event on EEG, there is no absolute diagnostic test. The examiner may be able to confirm absence seizures by inducing them with photic stimulation (flickering light) and hyperventilation (rapid breathing while stationary), both done during EEG recording. Many patients with primary generalized seizures, whether absence, myoclonic, or tonic-clonic, have "telltale" generalized spike-wave (epileptiform) bursts on routine EEG, even between seizures. Focal seizure disorders (simple partial or complex partial seizures) are less likely to have epileptiform discharges; these discharges appear focally.

It is important to remember that isolated epileptiform discharges on the EEG do not confirm that a particular spell was epileptic, since patients may have spells of other causes. Nonetheless, epileptiform discharges correlate highly with seizure disorders.

Uncertainty in Diagnosis: If the diagnosis of seizures is in doubt, repeated outpatient EEGs or, if necessary, inpatient video and EEG monitoring may capture a typical spell for analysis and confirm the diagnosis. A spell of "unconsciousness" during which the EEG is normal indicates a nonepileptic cause.

The physician should resist applying a label like "epileptic seizures" or "epilepsy" to patients whose diagnosis is in doubt. Such a label can cause patients to lose their job and driving privileges, and cause other financial and social problems. Rather than risk making a false diagnosis of "epilepsy," the physician is better advised to obtain more information, reassure the patient, explain the diagnostic process, and await further spells.

A common nonepileptic cause of subjective discomfort, impaired consciousness, and behavioral disturbance is intoxication with prescription drugs, recreational drugs, or alcohol. Depending on the substance, the clinical features can vary widely, but a toxic cause may be revealed when a suspicious physician inquires about timing of spells in relation to dosing of prescription medicines, and, if necessary, urine or blood screening for drugs and toxins (also see "Delirium" below).

Spells Predominantly with Falls or Limb or Body Movements

Sudden falls to the ground, often with little warning (drop attacks), are diagnostic challenges. Falls with unconsciousness often occur with complex partial seizures, but patients with gradual vertebrobasilar ischemia can experience light-headedness, pallor, a feeling of faintness, and collapse, also with loss of consciousness (Chapter 1.9). In middle-aged and elderly women, sudden falls without warning are also thought to be caused by vertebrobasilar ischemia; the only thing of which these patients are unaware is the fall itself. Children with atonic seizures suddenly collapse and lose consciousness. An infrequent

cause of drop attacks is seizures that induce a slow heart rate (bradycardia), which is momentarily insufficient to sustain brain circulation and results in unconsciousness. The rare colloid cyst tumors of the third ventricle can cause severe headache and suddenly obstruct cerebrospinal fluid outflow, causing unheralded falls with or without loss of consciousness.

Narcolepsy is a sleep disorder characterized by somnolence and frequent falling asleep; cataplexy (a sudden loss of tone, often with falls, and brought on by emotion); hallucinations just before sleep (hypnagogic) and on awakening (hypnopompic); and momentary inability to move on wakening (sleep paralysis). During cataplectic attacks—unlike syncope or seizures—patients remain conscious. Each patient may not have all the clinical features of narcolepsy; the only constant element is sleepiness. Sleep-monitoring studies confirm the diagnosis.

Focal motor seizures (simple partial seizures) cause jerking limb movements, which occasionally appear to move or march proximally up a limb (jacksonian march); the patient remains aware. The epileptic nature of these events is suggested by the fact that patients have jerky flexor movements (in the arm) that they cannot voluntarily suppress; some of these seizures may be triggered by movement.

Unilateral, flinging limb movements (hemiballismus) are not seizures, but a movement disorder brought on by small basal ganglia strokes. These movements typically do not recur.

Periodic limb movements of sleep (nocturnal myoclonus) are a nonepileptic cause of leg kicks in adults, often arousing them from sleep and causing waketime sleepiness. The leg kicks are slower than those of epileptic myoclonus, and patients are responsive immediately after the kicks. The diagnosis may be confirmed with overnight sleep-monitoring studies.

Sleepwalking and frightening dreams may cause alarming nocturnal spells of which the patient is unaware. Sleepwalking episodes (lasting up to 30 minutes) usually occur during the first 2 hours of sleep. They are characterized by their often elaborate, coordinated, and sustained semipurposeful behavior, but, in distinction to complex partial seizures, without automatisms such as lip smacking or picking at clothes. Children with *night terrors* are suddenly aroused with great fright and screaming from early deep sleep.

Occasionally, patients purposely or subconsciously produce limb movements or states of unresponsiveness that resemble seizures. The bizarre, nonstereotyped nature of these events should alert the physician to the possibility of psychogenic seizures (see "Psychogenic Spells" below).

Spells Predominantly Causing Impaired Consciousness

Delirium is characterized by a waxing and waning of responsiveness, often with periods of excitation, agitation, hallucinations, and somnolence (Chapter 14.2). Delirium is often seen in the elderly, in patients with dementia, and in postoperative patients. The cause may be metabolic disturbances or drug toxicity, which must be fully investigated and treated. Common drug groups implicated are corticosteroids, theophylline, and antidepressants. The diagnosis is based on fluctuating confusion with lethargy, agitation, and sleep-wake disturbances; further support comes from a finding of diffuse slowing on the EEG.

Spells with Gradual-Onset Visual, Sensory, or Motor Complaints

Migraine is readily diagnosed when the patient develops classic symptoms of unilateral headache, visual warning signs (auras), photophobia (avoidance of bright light), phonophobia (avoidance of loud sounds), and nausea (Chapter 13.5). Some migraine variants have a more gradual onset of visual, sensory, or motor problems, without headache. Migraine auras can include visual and auditory distortions and sensory or motor symptoms. Few patients have impaired speech, memory, and consciousness, causing confusional states. Other features distinguishing migraine from seizures are migraine's gradual progression of symptoms, absence of tonic-clonic movements and tongue biting, and usual preservation of consciousness.

Psychogenic Spells

Some of the most difficult spells to diagnose are psychogenic. These spells include a number of paroxysmal disturbances of behavior involving decreased responsiveness, wandering, seizure-like episodes, and sensory or motor disturbances—all of which may resemble organically based spells. Psychogenic spells are precipitated by reactions to stress or anxiety or by a need to escape unwanted situations or seek sympathy or disability. Most psychogenic spells are characterized by illogical anatomic involvement and a social context with identifiable psychiatric components or secondary gain for the patient (Chapter 14.6). Psychogenic events can have a great variety of signs and symptoms, constituting one of the "great imitators" of clinical medicine. A high index of suspicion should direct the physician toward "volitional" anomalies that differentiate psychogenic conditions from similar physiopathologic disorders like syncope, seizure, and transient ischemic attacks.

Hyperventilation: Hyperventilation often affects patients with anxiety or depression. Their deep respiratory efforts lower the PCO_2, causing tingling of the hands and around the mouth, confusion, light-headedness, further anxiety, malaise, pallor, and, rarely, unconsciousness. Although the features of hyperventilation are not epileptic, hyperventilation may trigger absence seizures in predisposed young people. Reassurance can terminate hyperventilation attacks, but has no effect on seizures.

Panic Attacks: Panic attacks are characterized by acute, intense anxiety or fear, sweating, palpitations, and numbness. Often seen with hyperventilation, panic attacks may cause light-headedness and tingling of the hands and lips. The lack of automatisms, the preservation of consciousness, longer duration, and response to β-blockers help distinguish panic attacks from seizures.

Pseudoseizures and Fugue States: Psychogenic pseudoseizures are nonepileptic events that look like seizures but are triggered subconsciously by patients who seek attention. Pseudoseizures may be a reaction to stress or a way for the patient to win sympathy or deliberately avoid undesired situations, obligations, or work (malingering).

Characteristically, pseudoseizures resemble some seizure types but last longer than syncope or true seizures and often lack their exact stereotypy. Inconsistent behavior can be exemplified by seizures that are triggered by emotional situations, with a gradual increase in truncal rigidity and, often, purposeful movements. During the spell, breathing is often deep and purposeful, accompanied by emotional reactions and meaningful speech. The observer of a questionable seizure should watch for retained consciousness, thrashing (rather than jerky) limb movements, and pelvic thrusting. Verbal instruction does not halt a true tonic-clonic seizure, but may arrest a factitious one. When there is doubt, video-EEG monitoring may reveal normal waking activity and no seizure discharges.

Dissociative periods (fugues) are states in which a patient may wander aimlessly for hours to days (unlike seizures or postictal states, which are much briefer). Many patients have previously had psychiatric symptoms. During attacks, patients appear awake and have a normal waking EEG.

SUMMARY

▶ A careful history of a spell must detail the context, pattern, duration, responsiveness, and recovery phases. The patient and witnesses should be questioned on each of these points.

▶ The constellation of signs and symptoms of a spell suggests particular diagnoses. Common causes of spells are seizures, vestibular dysfunction, vertebrobasilar insufficiency, hypoglycemia, drugs, alcohol, migraine, and psychological problems.

▶ The physical exam and laboratory tests should be directed toward confirming the suspected diagnosis and not merely be a fishing expedition. Routine "battery" workups of spells are often not cost-effective.

▶ When the diagnosis is uncertain, the physician should not apply a label like "epilepsy," but should obtain more information, reassure the patient, explain the diagnostic process, and await further spells.

SUGGESTED READING

Brodie MJ, Dichter MA: Antiepileptic drugs. N Engl J Med 1996;334:168.

Brodtkorb E et al: Hyperventilation syndrome: Clinical, ventilatory, and personality characteristics as observed in neurological practice. Acta Neurol Scand 1990;81:307.

Gates JR et al: Ictal characteristics of pseudoseizures. Arch Neurol 1985;42:1183.

Kroenke K et al: Causes of persistent dizziness: A prospective study of 100 patients in ambulatory care. Ann Intern Med 1992;117:898.

Porter RJ: Recognizing and classifying epileptic seizures and epileptic syndromes. Neurol Clin 1986;4:495.

Sleep Disorders

David W. Buchholz, MD

One out of three people responding to surveys reports chronic difficulty with sleep or wakefulness. Most have insomnia—trouble getting to sleep or staying asleep. Many have excessive waketime sleepiness—inability to stay awake when they should. Others have abnormal behaviors related to sleep.

These common problems with sleep are underreported, underdiagnosed, and undertreated. In one study, only 15% of those with sleep disturbances had sought medical help. Even fewer receive it. In part, this reflects a lack of awareness of sleep disorders. Moreover, physicians tend to underestimate the impact of these problems on their patients' life satisfaction and health. Data indicate that sleeping less than 7 hours daily is associated with increased mortality from ischemic heart disease, stroke, and cancer. Excessive daytime sleepiness not only impairs performance and mood but also predisposes to accidents. For example, sleepiness has been reported to contribute to 27% of traffic accidents and was implicated in 83% of traffic deaths. It has been estimated that 2–4% of middle-aged workers have sleep apnea syndrome.

Although sleep disorders centers are available for consultation and formal sleep studies, most sleep problems, especially insomnia, can be effectively diagnosed and managed by primary care physicians.

INSOMNIA

Usually, insomnia is assumed to have a psychological basis. Although this is often true, insomnia may also be due to numerous physical causes (Table 13.4–1). Also, insomnia is frequently regarded as being frustrating to treat, and hypnotic medications are often inappropriately prescribed. For the educated clinician, knowledgeable diagnosis and treatment of insomnia, using largely behavioral techniques, make it a rewarding rather than annoying complaint to address.

Insomnia takes three forms, each of which has diagnostic implications: (1) difficulty initiating sleep, which usually implies a psychological problem such as anxiety or learned insomnia; (2) difficulty maintaining sleep, which suggests that a physical disorder may be disrupting sleep; and (3) early morning awakening, which strongly suggests depression.

Causes

Chronic insomnia typically has two components: a primary cause and learned behavior. Any of the following causes may be the precipitating or underlying factor that provides the opportunity for insomnia to become a learned behavior. This in turn can become a self-perpetuating problem, which persists even after the initial cause has resolved.

Everyone sleeps poorly from time to time because of situational anxiety, such as on the night before an important examination. Similarly, febrile illness may be accompanied by difficulty in sleeping. These natural occurrences are transient and of little significance, except that they can set the stage for learned insomnia.

Environmental Stress: People sleep best in conducive settings such as dark, cool, quiet places. Simple measures such as wearing ear plugs or obtaining dark window shades may create a better sleep environment, thereby promoting sleep. Since part of the function of sleep is thermal regulation, most people don't sleep well when it is too warm. The value of simple measures such as fans and air conditioners should not be underestimated.

Alcohol: Although alcohol may relax or intoxicate people and thereby help to induce sleep, it is a poor "sleeping pill." Alcohol causes sleep disruption, making sleep difficult to maintain after drinking alcohol close to bedtime. One reason for sleep disruption is that alcohol is a short-acting drug, and withdrawal, accompanied by a surge of catecholamines, occurs several hours after consumption. Also, alcohol exacerbates several conditions that may interfere with sleep, including restless legs syndrome, gastroesophageal reflux, and sleep apnea.

Table 13.4–1. Differential diagnosis of insomnia.

Situational stress
Environmental stress
Alcohol and illegal drugs
Medications (eg, adrenergic agonists, β-blockers, xanthines)
Physical disorders
   Conditions exacerbated by lying flat (eg, gastroesophageal
     reflux, congestive heart failure)
   Painful disorders (eg, carpal tunnel syndrome)
   Endocrine disorders (eg, hyperthyroidism)
   Sleep apnea
Restless legs syndrome and periodic movements in sleep
Sleep-wake schedule disorders
Psychiatric disorders
Learned insomnia

Medications: Drugs (and dietary items) containing caffeine are likely to contribute to insomnia. Adrenergic agonists such as decongestants and theophylline may interfere with sleep. β-blockers, especially propranolol, sometimes cause sleep difficulty and nightmares. Similar problems arise with corticosteroids such as prednisone and dexamethasone, especially at high dosage. Insulin and oral agents to treat diabetes can cause nocturnal hypoglycemia followed by a catecholamine response and nocturnal awakening. Serotonin reuptake inhibitors for depression, such as fluoxetine and sertraline, often produce insomnia. Chronic use of hypnotic medications is more likely to aggravate than relieve insomnia.

Physical Disorders: Conditions that are exacerbated by lying flat may cause arousal from sleep. Examples are gastroesophageal reflux and congestive heart failure. Pain problems such as arthritis and carpal tunnel syndrome, which may become exacerbated at night, can prevent comfortable sleep. Hyperthyroidism is associated with insomnia. Sleep apnea occasionally produces repetitive nocturnal awakenings without apparent cause, although more typically sleep apnea results in subconscious arousals that silently fragment sleep and cause excessive waketime sleepiness rather than insomnia (Chapter 2.6).

Restless Legs Syndrome and Periodic Movements in Sleep: Restless legs syndrome is the disturbing sensation of restlessness, tension, or discomfort in the legs that is brought on by rest—especially lying in bed at night while trying to fall asleep—and is momentarily relieved by moving or rubbing the legs. Periodic movements in sleep are repetitive flexions of the legs that occur every 30 seconds or so during sleep. These conditions are closely related, and they occur in up to 5% of persons, especially the elderly. The numerous causes of these conditions are uremia, pregnancy, tricyclic antidepressant medication, and neurologic disorders, but most cases are idiopathic and many are familial. Restless legs syndrome and periodic movements in sleep produce not only insomnia but also excessive waketime sleepiness as a result of sleep deprivation and fragmentation. Carbidopa-levodopa and opiates are effective treatments for both of these conditions.

Sleep-Wake Schedule Disorders: To best understand these problems, it is important to realize that people have internal clocks with a daily cycle length of about 25 hours. Consequently, the natural inclination is to fall asleep later and wake up later every day. This tendency is more evident on weekends and during vacations. External forces such as clocks, work schedules, and sunlight help people to conform to the 24-hour solar day length. Sunlight or a bright lightbox can be used therapeutically to adjust sleep-wake schedules. One hour or so of bright light exposure in the early morning helps patients to fall asleep earlier at night, whereas bright light exposure later in the day delays sleep onset.

Delayed sleep phase syndrome occurs in persons who have daily cycle lengths that are even longer than the normal 25 hours and therefore cannot easily adjust to the 24-hour convention. These "night owls" habitually fall asleep too late and wake up too late to be able to keep normal work schedules. Teenagers are prone to this problem, which can be perpetuated in a permissive environment such as living at college. Conversely, elderly people tend to be "larks," preferring to go to sleep early and wake up early, because the daily cycle length shortens with aging.

Unfortunately, some elderly people go to bed much too early and find themselves awake several hours before sunrise. These persons should postpone bedtime so that their duration of sleep carries them through to the morning. In addition, many patients doze and nap during the day, which results in fragmentation of their daily sleep-wake schedules. It is best to remain awake and active throughout the day and preserve the sleep need for nighttime.

Time zone changes produce "jet lag," which is more of a problem traveling eastward than westward. This is because of the natural inclination to fall asleep later each day than the day before, which is what happens when traveling westward. However, falling asleep ahead of schedule is difficult, as expected when traveling eastward. It helps to be well rested when traveling westward and somewhat sleep deprived when traveling eastward. Alcohol (as a hypnotic agent) and caffeine (as a stimulant) are not effective drugs to help adjust to time zone changes, but a short-acting hypnotic medication may help to induce sleep and thereby readjust the sleep-wake schedule after eastward travel.

Twenty-five percent of the population of the United States works rotating shifts, and these people often suffer chronic insomnia and excessive waketime sleepiness. Shift changes should be made infrequently, if possible, such as every month rather than every week, to allow resynchronization of the sleep-wake schedule and other bodily rhythms with each shift change. Also, shift changes are best made in a clockwise direction, conforming to our natural tendency to fall asleep later and wake up later every day.

Psychiatric Disorders: Many psychiatric problems are associated with insomnia, including anxiety disorders, obsessive-compulsive tendencies, and mania. The most common is depression, which characteristically produces early morning awakening. Psychotherapy and antidepressant medication, especially sedating tricyclic agents, are highly effective treatments.

Learned Insomnia: This is the most common basis for chronic insomnia, but it usually coexists with or follows one of the other causes of insomnia previously listed. Learned insomnia occurs especially in those who are anxious, pessimistic, and somatically preoccupied and who tend to respond to any cause of poor sleep by anticipating recurrent nights of poor sleep. This anticipation leads to emotional arousal in the form of anxiety or even panic, and the anticipation thereby becomes a self-fulfilling prophecy. Counterproductive sleep habits develop, such as sleeping late in the morning or napping during the day to compensate for lack of sleep at night. Fortunately, there are ways to interrupt this vicious cycle of insomnia.

Management of Insomnia

A number of behavioral measures, collectively known as *sleep hygiene,* can be very useful in promoting better sleep (Table 13.4–2). Treatment for insomnia starts with sleep hygiene.

Persons with overwhelming situational stress or anxiety disorders may have the symptom of insomnia as part of more pervasive lifestyle or psychological problems. In these persons, attention should be focused on the underlying psychological issues, using techniques such as relaxation exercises, stress management, and formal psychotherapy.

The patient with difficulty initiating sleep can often be helped by the simple method of *sleep restriction.* The person is instructed to remain out of bed and awake until the usual time of falling asleep in bed, which may be hours after the person's normal bedtime. This accomplishes two things: first, the patient's preoccupation is shifted from difficulty falling asleep to difficulty staying awake; and, second, the patient becomes sleep deprived. Conse-

quently, when the patient finally gets into bed, sleep comes fairly quickly. After the patient has learned that he or she is capable of falling asleep shortly after getting into bed, the bedtime is adjusted very gradually toward the desired hour, proceeding in small increments of 15 or 30 minutes at a time and stabilizing at each new bedtime before advancing the bedtime again.

Note that sleeping pills (hypnotics) are adjunctive therapy for short-term insomnia. It may be appropriate to prescribe hypnotic medication to a person experiencing insomnia in the setting of situational stress such as during hospitalization, but these agents should not be used on a chronic basis and should be avoided, if possible, in the elderly. Insomnia in the elderly often has specific medical and psychiatric causes that should be dealt with directly. Furthermore, hypnotic medication is more likely to have adverse effects in elderly people.

Over-the-counter sleeping pills contain antihistamines and have limited efficacy. Among prescription medications, benzodiazepines or zolpidem are the drugs of choice for nondepressed persons with situational insomnia. Short-acting agents are generally preferable to long-acting agents because they are less likely to exert a prolonged drug effect and cause daytime sedation.

For a patient who has been taking hypnotic medication on a nightly basis, gradual drug withdrawal is recommended, whether or not insomnia is a persistent complaint. After nightly use has been eliminated, a reasonable compromise may be to allow the patient to take hypnotic medication every third night following consecutive nights of poor sleep.

Insomnia, especially in the form of early morning awakening, is often a presenting or prominent symptom of depression. Patients with insomnia due to depression are better treated with antidepressant medication such as a sedating tricyclic or trazodone, rather than a benzodiazepine.

EXCESSIVE WAKETIME SLEEPINESS

Most people require 8–10 hours of sleep per day to be maximally alert. Few get enough sleep and as a result are habitually sleepy. This explains why many tend to fall asleep in permissive situations, such as boring lectures with the lights turned down. The level of sleepiness is determined by two factors: duration of prior wakefulness and phase of the sleep-wake cycle. The longer the period of wakefulness, the more sleepiness ensues, suggesting the accumulation of a sleep-promoting substance during wakefulness and its clearance during sleep. Presumably, this sleep-promoting substance would be the ideal hypnotic medication, but it has not been identified. People also are naturally sleepy at two phases of the daily sleep-wake cycle: night-time, when most have prolonged sleep, and midafternoon, at which time people in many cultures wisely respond by taking naps (although naps should be avoided by those with night-time insomnia).

Table 13.4–2. Principles of sleep hygiene.

1. Sleep in a cool, quiet, comfortable place.
2. Keep a regular sleep-wake schedule, especially a regular waketime.
3. When having trouble sleeping at night, avoid daytime naps. Find time to exercise during the day.
4. Avoid caffeine, alcohol, and food within several hours of bedtime.
5. Make bed a restful haven for sleep and sex. Do not perform waketime activities in bed.
6. If unable to sleep because of preoccupation with something in your life, write down your mental concerns in 1 or 2 sentences and return to bed temporarily unburdened of these concerns.
7. Try changing your sleep environment, such as sleeping in a different bedroom or moving the location of your bed.
8. If unable to sleep after 30 minutes in bed, get up and do something relaxing. Return to bed when you feel sleepy.
9. Don't worry about not getting enough sleep. Be assured that insomnia, although unpleasant, is not harmful. Worrying only makes it worse.

Beyond these factors, numerous conditions constitute a differential diagnosis of excessive waketime sleepiness: inadequate sleep duration, sleep fragmentation (eg, sleep apnea and periodic movements in sleep), physical illnesses (eg, hypothyroidism), central nervous system depressant substances (eg, medications, alcohol, and illegal drugs), and central nervous system disorders (eg, narcolepsy).

Causes

In approaching the excessively sleepy patient, physician should first consider the possibility of chronic inadequate sleep duration. If average sleep duration is less than 8 hours, a trial of sleep extension to 8 hours or more per night for at least several weeks should be advised. If excessive sleepiness persists, general medical evaluation should be performed, looking for problems such as hypothyroidism, anemia, kidney and liver disease, pulmonary insufficiency, and diabetes. Medications should be reviewed, because drugs such as antihypertensives, antihistamines, sedatives, and long-acting hypnotic agents may be responsible for waketime sleepiness. Alcohol abuse and illicit drug use should be considered contributing causes.

If a patient's excessive waketime sleepiness remains unexplained despite attention to the issues mentioned above, the patient probably has a primary sleep disorder. Such patients should be referred to a sleep disorders center for expert consultation and sleep studies.

Sleep Apnea: The most common primary sleep disorder causing excessive waketime sleepiness is sleep apnea (Chapter 2.6). Sleep apnea should be suspected in sleepy middle-aged men and postmenopausal women who have been noted to snore loudly and breathe irregularly during sleep, especially if they are overweight.

Narcolepsy: This central nervous system disorder has a partial genetic basis and causes excessive sleepiness beginning in teenage or early adult years and persisting throughout life. Many narcoleptics have cataplexy, which is brief episodic loss of muscle strength without loss of consciousness, usually triggered by emotional stimulation. A minority of patients with narcolepsy experience vivid nocturnal hallucinations and sleep paralysis, which is the inability to move while drifting off to sleep or beginning to be aroused from sleep.

Narcolepsy is not a rare disorder; its prevalence is 10% of that of epilepsy. Many cases remain undiagnosed because physicians mistakenly presume that narcolepsy causes dramatic sleep attacks in the middle of waking activities. More typically, patients with narcolepsy drift off to sleep when they are unstimulated. The diagnosis is confirmed by sleep studies showing an absence of nocturnal sleep pathology combined with a tendency to fall asleep and enter rapid eye movement (REM) sleep too quickly during the day.

The neurochemical details of narcolepsy remain unclear, but conceptually narcolepsy can be understood as a disorder of unbridled REM sleep. Patients with narcolepsy tend to enter REM sleep or experience aspects of REM sleep inappropriately during what should be wakefulness. Episodes of cataplexy and sleep paralysis represent limb muscle paralysis that normally accompanies REM sleep, and the nocturnal hallucinations of narcolepsy are dreams, which normally occur during REM sleep, taking place in an awake brain.

Narcolepsy is managed with a combination of proper sleep habits and medication. Patients should get at least 8 hours of sleep per day and may benefit from "preventive naps" lasting 10–15 minutes every few hours throughout the day. Stimulant medications such as pemoline or methylphenidate are usually effective in controlling excessive sleepiness in patients with narcolepsy, and agents such as tricyclic antidepressants and fluoxetine are helpful in managing cataplexy.

ABNORMAL SLEEP-RELATED BEHAVIORS

A wide variety of peculiar activities can occur in association with sleep, the most important of which are discussed below.

Abnormal Arousal from Slow-Wave Sleep

Slow-wave sleep, which includes the deepest stages of non-REM sleep, tends to occur during the first 1 or 2 hours of sleep and is especially prominent in children. Accordingly, disorders related to abnormal arousal from slow-wave sleep occur during the early portion of sleep and mainly in children. These conditions are sleepwalking, night terrors, and enuresis; all are related and often occur together within an individual or a family.

Sleepwalking: Sleepwalking takes place when a person becomes aroused from deep slow-wave sleep but fails to make a normal transition into lighter stages of non-REM sleep. The sleepwalker enters into a peculiar state in which motor activities are intact but arousal and memory are impaired. Sleepwalking is most likely to occur after sleep deprivation or with stress, and its occurrence beyond childhood often indicates psychopathology. Sleepwalkers should be gently guided back to bed and should be protected from injury using measures such as window locks, bedroom door alarms, and stair gates.

Night Terrors: Night terrors are different from nightmares. Nightmares are frightening dreams that occur during REM sleep and are recalled after awakening. Night terrors are episodes during which the person appears awake and terrified, accompanied by screaming, crying, and signs of profound anxiety; later, the person retains no memory of the event. Accordingly, the experience is disturbing primarily to those who witness it. Treatment is not usually necessary, although benzodiazepines can be used to help suppress night terrors by reducing not only the depth of slow-wave sleep but also arousals from it.

SUMMARY

▶ The complaint of insomnia should be carefully evaluated, with consideration of a broad differential diagnosis, rather than an assumption of a psychological basis.

▶ Difficulty in falling asleep is usually due to a psychological problem; difficulty in staying asleep suggests a physical disorder; early morning awakening suggests depression.

▶ The primary treatment for insomnia consists of behavioral approaches; hypnotic medication should be considered as short-term adjunctive therapy for insomnia.

▶ Excessive waketime sleepiness that cannot be corrected with sleep extension should be investigated first with general medical evaluation, including review of medications and assessment for sleep apnea, narcolepsy, or periodic movements in sleep.

SUGGESTED READING

Everitt DE, Avorn J, Baker MW: Clinical decision-making in the evaluation and treatment of insomnia. Am J Med 1990; 89:357.

Gillin JC, Byerley WF: The diagnosis and management of insomnia. N Engl J Med 1990;322:239.

Kryger MH, Roth T, Dement WC (editors): *Principles and Practice of Sleep Medicine,* 2nd ed. WB Saunders, 1994.

O'Keeffe ST: Restless legs syndrome: A review. Arch Intern Med 1996;156:243.

Parkes JD: *Sleep and Its Disorders.* WB Saunders, 1985.

Young T et al: The occurrence of sleep-disordered breathing among middle-aged adults. N Engl J Med 1993;328:1230.

13.5

Headache

David W. Buchholz, MD

Headaches afflict almost everyone at one time or another. They can be a manifestation of a disorder as serious as subarachnoid hemorrhage or, more frequently, they arise as a benign, self-limited process. The accurate assessment of the cause of headaches can be very satisfying for the clinician and reassuring for patients, who often fear the worst (eg, brain tumor) as the cause of their headaches. Treatment of headaches has become more successful, not only because of emphasis on prevention but also because of better acute remedies. This chapter reviews the diagnosis and management of headaches, from the ordinary (eg, "hangovers" and caffeine withdrawal) to those due to serious disorders that the physician cannot afford to miss.

When a patient presents with a complaint of headache, the first and foremost question is, "Is this headache due to a serious condition?" The history and physical examination are essential as the first screen for serious disorders and for deciding when to do additional tests, such as brain imaging (computed tomography [CT] or magnetic resonance imaging [MRI] scan) or lumbar puncture (Table 13.5–1). The onset of the headache, previous history of similar episodes, associated symptoms (eg, fever, photophobia, neurologic deficits), family history of headaches, and concomitant known illnesses (eg, previously diagnosed cancer, recent injury, immune deficiency) all are important historical features. Severe hypertension, nuchal rigidity, papilledema, retinal hemorrhages and exudates, and neurologic deficits are key elements in the physical examination.

SERIOUS DISORDERS PRESENTING WITH HEADACHE

A patient with subarachnoid hemorrhage classically presents with the sudden onset of an unusually severe headache, often described as "the worst headache of my life." Headache associated with unexplained fever, nuchal rigidity, papilledema, or new neurologic deficits should prompt aggressive evaluation to rule out meningitis, encephalitis, idiopathic intracranial hypertension, and hemorrhage into a tumor. Patients with brain tumors usually present with symptoms such as seizures, altered mentation, or focal deficits rather than with headache.

Giant Cell (Temporal) Arteritis

Inflammation of temporal arteries causing headache tends to occur in persons over the age of 55 years and is characterized by temporal artery tenderness, jaw claudication, and a markedly elevated sedimentation rate (Chapter 3.5). Blindness may result from ophthalmic artery involvement; therefore, confirmation of the diagnosis by temporal artery biopsy and treatment with corticosteroids are urgently indicated.

Idiopathic Intracranial Hypertension

Also known as pseudotumor cerebri, idiopathic intracranial hypertension is a poorly understood disorder, which tends to occur among obese young females. It is characterized by markedly increased intracranial pressure and consequent headaches, papilledema, and sometimes visual symptoms including diplopia, visual field loss, and blindness. This condition is suspected when head CT or MRI imaging is normal but lumbar puncture reveals substantially elevated opening pressure. Treatment involves serial lumbar punctures to lower the pressure, medications including acetazolamide and corticosteroids, and in extreme cases surgery such as lumboperitoneal shunting and optic nerve sheath fenestration to prevent blindness due to ischemic optic neuropathy.

NEUROVASCULAR HEADACHE

Pathophysiology

In recent years, a major revision of headache diagnosis and treatment has taken place. What used to be regarded as muscle contraction, "stress" or "tension" headache is

Table 13.5–1. Serious disorders presenting with headache.

	Clinical Clues	Evaluation
Infections		
Meningitis	Fever, nuchal rigidity	LP
Encephalitis	Fever, disorientation	MRI, LP, EEG
Brain abscess	Fever (in 50% of patients), focal neurologic signs, seizures	MRI or CT
Increased intracranial pressure		
Neoplasm	Uncommonly presents solely with headache unless complicated by hemorrhage; usually presents with seizures, altered mentation, or focal deficits	MRI or CT
Idiopathic intracranial hypertension	Papilledema, obese patient	MRI or CT to rule out mass lesion; then LP
Cerebrovascular disorders		
Subarachnoid hemorrhage	Sudden onset of "worst headache of my life," nuchal rigidity	CT, LP, arteriogram
Cerebral venous or venous sinus thrombosis	Seizures, focal deficits, often postpartum	MRI
Hypertensive encephalopathy	Severe hypertension, retinopathy, cardiac and renal failure, altered mentation	MRI or CT
Giant cell arteritis	Elderly patient, temporal artery tenderness, jaw claudication	Erythrocyte sedimentation rate, temporal artery biopsy

LP, lumbar puncture.

now considered to be one aspect of a continuum of headaches that includes migraine and is related to an underlying neurovascular disturbance. In fact, most headaches arise from a neurovascular mechanism, which is centered in the brain and, when activated, culminates in extracerebral vasodilatation and inflammation and intracranial vasoconstriction. These changes can produce a broad spectrum of headaches and a wide variety of neurologic symptoms.

This neurovascular mechanism involves a cascade of events that is activated in response to a variety of trigger factors. Examples of these trigger factors are hormones (especially fluctuations in hormone levels during the menstrual cycle), chemicals such as tyramine and nitrates derived from foods and beverages, emotional distress, disturbance of the sleep-wake cycle, and sensory stimuli such as bright light and strong odors.

The trigeminal nucleus caudalis plays a central role in linking trigger factor input to the vascular changes that generate headaches and associated neurologic symptoms. Outside the brain, in the meninges, scalp, and sinus mucosa, vasodilatation and inflammation occur, causing headache. When the trigeminal nucleus caudalis is activated, vasoactive substances such as substance P and calcitonin gene-related peptide (CGRP) are released by perivascular branches of the trigeminal nerve. Serotonin modulates the release of these vasoactive neuropeptides, and selective serotonin agonists such as sumatriptan are able to inhibit vascular dilatation and inflammation by binding to presynaptic receptors at the level of the nerve-vessel interface. Within the brain, reversible vasoconstriction occurs, causing transient neuronal ischemia and dysfunction.

Symptoms

The most widely recognized form of headache that arises from this neurovascular mechanism is traditionally labeled *migraine* and defined as a severe, episodic, unilateral throbbing headache associated with nausea, photophobia, and visual or neurologic symptoms. The headaches generated by this neuromuscular mechanism may also be mild, chronic, and nonspecific in character. Occasionally, the neurologic symptoms predominate or even occur without headache. The neurologic symptoms vary according to the region of the brain affected but may include scintillating scotoma or other visual changes (occipital lobe), vertigo and ataxia with nystagmus (brain stem or cerebellum), or paresthesias (parietal lobe). More profound problems such as hemiparesis, syncope, seizure, and stroke infrequently occur. In addition, autonomic functions, which are controlled by the hypothalamus, become disordered. Examples are disturbances of gastrointestinal motility (vomiting, diarrhea, and constipation) and cutaneous vasomotor regulation (pallor, sweating, and flushing).

Management

The most effective approach for controlling neurovascular headaches and neurologic symptoms is prevention, which involves two strategies: avoidance of headache trigger factors and elevation of the headache threshold by means of prophylactic medication. Trigger factor avoidance focuses on the chemical factors that are most easily avoided, especially common dietary and medicinal items (Table 13.5–2).

Prophylactic medication is indicated if neurovascular headaches or neurologic symptoms remain problematic

Table 13.5–2. Neurovascular headache trigger factors.

Dietary
Caffeine
Chocolate
Cheese (especially aged), yogurt, sour cream
Monosodium glutamate
Processed meats (with nitrites and nitrates)
Alcohol
Nuts
Citrus fruits and juices
Fresh-baked, yeast-risen bread products

Medicinal
Caffeine-containing agents
Decongestants
Oral contraceptives
Estrogen replacement therapy
Ergotamines and isometheptene (if used regularly)
Adrenergic agonists for asthma
Nitrates

for several days or more per month despite avoidance of trigger factors. These agents include calcium channel blockers (verapamil, diltiazem), tricyclic antidepressants (nortriptyline, amitriptyline), β-blockers (propranolol, nadolol), cyproheptadine, valproate, and methysergide. Each agent is generally safe, and about 50–70% of patients derive satisfactory relief from any one of these drugs, with additional benefit when used in combination.

Analgesic medication, such as acetaminophen or ibuprofen, is appropriate for acute relief of headaches that break through preventive treatment. The most effective approach for relief of severe vascular headaches involves selective serotonin agonists such as sumatriptan, which blocks perivascular neuropeptide release and thereby inhibits the neurovascular inflammatory process that leads to painful extracerebral vasodilatation.

CLUSTER HEADACHE

Cluster headache is pathophysiologically and symptomatically related to ordinary neurovascular headache, but cluster headache is much less common and has certain distinctive clinical features. It tends to occur in young men on a periodic basis with "clusters" lasting several weeks to months during which headaches occur once or more daily, often at night, separated by headache-free intervals of months. A less common chronic form of cluster headache causes daily cluster-type headaches without headache-free intervals. Individual headaches are excruciating, unilateral, and periorbital and last up to 1 hour. Accompanying symptoms include ipsilateral conjunctival injection, lacrimation, and nasal stuffiness.

Preventive management of cluster headaches involves medications such as prednisone, verapamil, methysergide, valproate, or lithium, prescribed at the onset and for the duration of the cluster period. Effective abortive approaches include sumatriptan and inhalation of 100% oxygen.

FACIAL PAIN

Bacterial Sinusitis

Acute purulent bacterial sinusitis can cause localized pain and tenderness over the affected sinus, associated with fever and purulent discharge. Biting, chewing, or bending over at the waist can increase the pain of maxillary sinusitis.

Trigeminal Neuralgia

Severe electric shock-like pain radiating across the face characterizes this distinctive form of facial pain, representing irritation of one or more branches of the trigeminal nerve. Most often affected are the elderly, probably because of contact of a tortuous blood vessel against the trigeminal nerve root as it enters the brain stem. The pain is typically triggered by stimulation of the sensory field of the involved nerve, such as by touching the face or brushing the teeth, and it can be controlled by either antiseizure medication (such as carbamazepine or phenytoin), glycerol injection into the region of the trigeminal nerve root, or microvascular decompression of the nerve root by way of posterior fossa craniotomy.

Dental Disease and Other Causes

Occult dental abscesses should be diligently sought as the potential cause of unexplained facial pain. Temporomandibular joint syndrome is characterized by localized pain at one or both joints, along with locking or dislocation of the joints and difficulty opening the jaw. Use caution in ascribing facial pain to ill-defined entities such as "chronic sinusitis" without clear-cut evidence for such a diagnosis. More likely, the mechanism of neurovascular headaches is the basis for facial pain that remains unexplained despite careful evaluation, and a standard neurovascular headache treatment approach is usually effective.

SUMMARY

▶ Sudden onset of severe headache suggests subarachnoid hemorrhage.

▶ Patients whose headaches are associated with unexplained fever, nuchal rigidity, papilledema, or new neurologic deficits should be evaluated aggressively.

▶ Most headaches as well as a wide array of neurologic symptoms are caused by activation of a neurovascular mechanism by trigger factors, resulting in extracerebral vasodilatation and inflammation and intracranial vasoconstriction.

▶ Avoidance of trigger factors and use of prophylactic medication such as tricyclic antidepressants, calcium channel blockers, and β-adrenergic blockers can effectively control recurrent headaches in most cases.

SUGGESTED READING

Moskowitz MA: The neurobiology of vascular head pain. Ann Neurol 1984;16:157.

Olesen J: The ischemic hypotheses of migraine. Arch Neurol 1987;44:321.

Raskin NH: *Headache*, 2nd ed. Churchill Livingstone, 1988.

Sacks OW: *Migraine*. University of California Press, 1992.

Welch KM: Migraine: A biobehavioral disorder. Arch Neurol 1987;44:323.

13.6

Cerebrovascular Disorders

Barney J. Stern, MD, Constance J. Johnson, MD, and Thomas J. Preziosi, MD

Patients with symptoms from cerebrovascular disease present with sudden loss of neurologic function because of impaired blood flow within the brain. If the loss of function lasts only a few minutes or up to 24 hours, and then normal function returns, the event is called a *transient ischemic attack* (TIA). If loss of function persists for longer than 1 day, the patient has suffered a stroke. The loss of function may be hemiparesis, reduced sensation, aphasia or dysarthria, or altered cognition or consciousness. Stroke syndromes can be heralded by an abrupt, severe headache.

The first step in evaluation is to determine whether the problem is an ischemic or hemorrhagic disorder or another disease presenting as if it were a stroke (Table 13.6–1). Ischemic strokes are caused by arterial occlusion, whereas hemorrhagic strokes are caused by intracranial bleeding. This distinction is occasionally difficult to make on clinical grounds alone; therefore, all patients suspected of having a stroke should have a brain computed tomographic (CT) scan. Of those patients who suffer a stroke, 80% have ischemic strokes and 20% have hemorrhagic strokes (Table 13.6–2). Evaluation should include repeated neurologic assessments, especially over the first few hours, to determine whether the patient's condition is unchanging, improving, or deteriorating, since this will influence both diagnostic considerations and management. Finally, the clinician must determine whether the condition is related to a systemic disease and whether it is treatable, with medications, surgery, or both.

ISCHEMIC DISORDERS

Typical patients with ischemic cerebrovascular disease are elderly and have atherosclerotic cardiovascular disease associated with hypertension, diabetes mellitus, hypercholesterolemia, or a smoking history. It is with regard to these predisposing factors that measures can be taken to reduce the risk of strokes. In fact, the steady reduction in stroke rates over the past decade is attributed to improved control of hypertension. The presentation of ischemic

strokes varies somewhat, depending on whether the patient's problem is the result of an embolus from the heart or proximal artery, or a thrombus, which can be associated with atherosclerotic lesions. A clot can also be related to an underlying hematologic or systemic disorder.

Cardiogenic Embolism

Patients with an embolus arising from the heart, accounting for 20% of ischemic strokes, may or may not have a previously known cardiac problem. The history of any patient presenting with a sudden loss of neurologic function should include inquiry about causes of cardiogenic embolism, including atrial fibrillation, recent myocardial infarction, dilated cardiomyopathy, akinetic ventricular segment, infectious endocarditis, mitral stenosis, artificial valve, nonbacterial thrombotic endocarditis, and myxoma. A "paradoxical" embolism, arising in the venous circulation and bypassing the lungs to reach the systemic arterial tree, can result from a patent foramen ovale or atrial septal defect.

Typically, the patient is neurologically intact until the embolus lodges in an artery and causes loss of function referable to the region of brain supplied by the blocked vessel. Depending on where the embolus lodges, the patient can suffer an extensive deficit from infarction of a large portion of a cerebral hemisphere or a critical portion of a smaller area. For example, a contralateral (opposite side from damaged brain) hemiparesis could develop in a patient with a large infarction of the motor cortex in the frontal lobe, or by a much smaller infarction in the internal capsule. In the smaller infarction, however, one would not expect to see the associated sensory abnormalities that typically accompany a large cortical infarction. There may be a more selective loss of function if only a small volume of a particular part of the brain is damaged (eg, infarction of Broca's area causing an expressive aphasia). The patient may suffer transient and completely reversible dysfunction (TIA) if the embolus only briefly obstructs blood flow. An embolus that has completely interrupted blood flow to a region of the brain, leading to infarction of brain tissue, may lyse within hours to days. Then, the infarcted territory supplied by the

Table 13.6–1. Differential diagnosis of sudden loss of neurologic function.

Stroke or transient ischemic attack (TIA)
Seizure
Tumor
Subdural hematoma
Hypoglycemia
Intoxication
Psychiatric disturbance
Migraine
Demyelination

blocked artery can be once again perfused, but vascular integrity in the area is reduced, allowing blood to potentially escape from the vascular tree. In this way, a hemorrhagic stroke can follow an ischemic stroke as blood leaks out of damaged vessels. Patients with infarcts that involve a large volume of brain are at particularly high risk for such hemorrhage. If severe bleeding occurs, the hematoma can compress or displace brain tissue (mass effect) and worsen the patient's already compromised neurologic status.

Evaluation and Management: If a cardiogenic embolism is suspected, a brain CT scan should be obtained to make sure that there is no hemorrhage or mass lesion. Recombinant tissue plasminogen activator (t-PA) has been found to improve the outcome of cardiogenic embolic stroke when given within 3 hours after stroke onset. In the management of cardiogenic embolism, one must weigh the risk of recurrent emboli, which is about 1% daily during the first 2–3 weeks following the stroke, against the relatively unlikely, but potentially catastrophic, risk of a large hemorrhagic infarction. If the patient has relatively minor neurologic deficits and no contraindications to anticoagulation (eg, gastrointestinal bleeding or a systolic blood pressure above 180 mm Hg), intravenous heparin should be given to elevate the activated partial thromboplastin time to 1.5 times control. Patients who have been treated with t-PA should not be started on anticoagulation for 24 hours. If the patient has an extensive neurologic deficit (eg, hemiplegia and sensory loss with a homonymous hemianopia and global aphasia or neglect), anticoagulation should be deferred. After 5–7 days, if the patient is not moribund and if a repeat brain CT scan does not demonstrate a substantial hemorrhagic infarction, heparin therapy can be started. If the underlying cause of the cardiogenic embolism cannot be corrected, the patient should be given chronic warfarin treatment to achieve an international normalized ratio (INR) of 2–3.

Patients who do not have known cardiac disease and, on the basis of their clinical presentation, are suspected of having suffered a cardiogenic embolus should have a transthoracic echocardiogram. Such clinical presentations include sudden onset of symptoms, age below 45 years, persons without clinical evidence of arterial disease (see below), and patients with no obvious explanation for their stroke. If a transthoracic echocardiogram is unrevealing and the clinical suspicion of cardiogenic embolism is high, a transesophageal echocardiogram should follow, if available, to obtain a better view of the heart and aorta, another potential source of emboli. Continuous electrocardiographic (Holter) monitoring should be performed if the echocardiogram and a routine electrocardiogram are normal. Holter monitoring occasionally reveals an episodic arrhythmia, such as paroxysmal atrial fibrillation, which may be a cause of emboli.

Table 13.6–2. Types of strokes.

	Typical Hosts	Percent of Strokes	Distinguishing Features
Embolism			
Cardiogenic	Patients with known cardiac disorders; age <45	15	Sudden onset of maximal symptoms
Artery-to-artery (extracranial artery disease)	Men, whites; neck bruit, hyperlipidemia, coronary or peripheral artery disease	10–30	Prior TIAs in a single vascular territory; moderate sensory, motor, or cognitive deficits
Thrombosis			
Large-sized artery disease (eg, origin of internal carotid artery)	Similar to artery-to-artery embolism	10–30	Extensive sensory, motor, and cognitive deficits
Medium-sized artery disease ("named vessel," eg, middle cerebral artery)	Blacks, Asians	5	Stereotyped TIAs
Intracranial small-sized artery disease (penetrating arteries, eg, lenticulostriates)	Hypertension, diabetes	15	Discrete motor or sensory deficits typical
Hemorrhage			
Subarachnoid hemorrhage	More common with increasing age; women; coagulopathy	10	Sudden onset of "worst headache ever"
Intraparenchymal hematoma	Hypertension, vascular malformations, trauma	10	Headache, quick evolution of clinical deficits

TIA, transient ischemic attack.

Artery Disease

Large extracranial artery disease usually leads to neurologic symptoms by serving as a source of emboli to a more distal artery and by causing reduced perfusion, predisposing to thrombosis at a stenotic lesion (Figure 13.6–1). Many patients with carotid artery disease present with transient ipsilateral (same side as damaged brain) monocular blindness (amaurosis fugax) and contralateral hemiparesis or hemisensory loss, or aphasia, depending on the hemisphere involved. Brain tissue is particularly at risk for infarction in "watershed" or "border zone" areas—areas at the margins of territories supplied by major arterial branches, such as between the parieto-occipital regions (between the territories of the middle and posterior cerebral arteries). In these

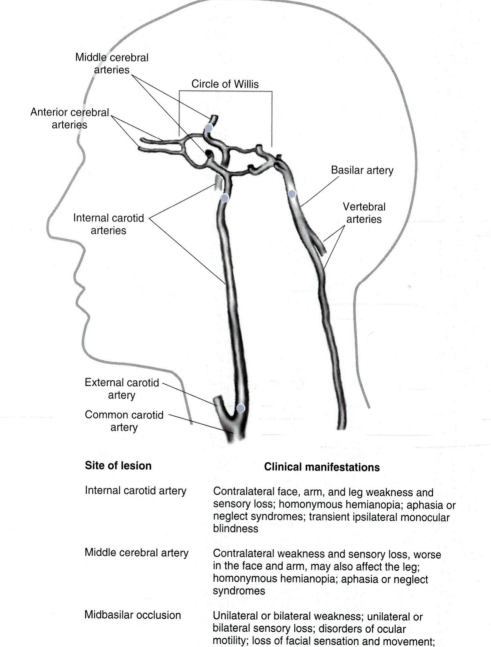

Site of lesion	Clinical manifestations
Internal carotid artery	Contralateral face, arm, and leg weakness and sensory loss; homonymous hemianopia; aphasia or neglect syndromes; transient ipsilateral monocular blindness
Middle cerebral artery	Contralateral weakness and sensory loss, worse in the face and arm, may also affect the leg; homonymous hemianopia; aphasia or neglect syndromes
Midbasilar occlusion	Unilateral or bilateral weakness; unilateral or bilateral sensory loss; disorders of ocular motility; loss of facial sensation and movement; ataxia

Figure 13.6–1. Common sites of cerebral artery obstructive lesions.

areas, circulation may be adequate under normal circumstances but becomes insufficient with hypotension or with proximal stenosis or occlusion. Vertebrobasilar artery disease causes bilateral visual disturbances, diplopia, ataxia, bilateral weakness, ipsilateral facial numbness or weakness with contralateral limb numbness or weakness, vertigo, or impaired consciousness.

The most common cause of artery disease is atherosclerosis. Other causes are arterial dissection, fibromuscular dysplasia, and vasculitis. Although the following discussion primarily addresses atherosclerotic disease, the principles presented are relevant to the other pathologic processes as well.

Evaluation and Management: Patients may be suspected of having extracranial artery disease as a basis for their sudden neurologic dysfunction if they have risk factors for atherosclerosis, a past history of transient ischemic events in the same arterial territory, or a cervical bruit (suggesting stenosis at the internal carotid artery origin). A brain CT or magnetic resonance imaging (MRI) scan should be obtained to exclude other conditions (such as a tumor or subdural hematoma masquerading as a stroke), to document the absence of a hemorrhagic event, and possibly to document the extent of the stroke. Because brain MRI is more sensitive than CT in detecting an ischemic stroke, it should be used if the CT is normal, the clinical suspicion of stroke remains, and better anatomic localization is needed to identify whether the anterior or posterior vascular territory is involved.

Extremes of blood pressure should be avoided. In particular, a special effort should be made not to lower the blood pressure excessively, since doing so can compromise blood flow through otherwise marginally perfused brain and worsen the stroke. Hypertensive patients need not have their systolic blood pressure acutely lowered to less than 180–200 mm Hg unless there is another indication for doing so. Also, hyperglycemia should be avoided since this may worsen cerebral lactic acidosis through increased anaerobic glycolysis and impair neuronal function; normal saline is often recommended for hydration, rather than an infusion containing 5% dextrose.

A complete blood count, including platelets, should be obtained to rule out an underlying predisposing hematologic disorder. Syphilis serology should be obtained to rule out lues or assess the possibility of biologic false-positives associated with collagen vascular disease or the lupus anticoagulant. An elevated erythrocyte sedimentation rate might also suggest a concomitant systemic illness. Prothrombin time and partial thromboplastin time may be helpful to look for coagulopathy and to guide initial anticoagulant therapy. Risk factors for atherosclerosis should be identified and treated. Patients with atherosclerosis at the internal carotid artery origin are at risk for coronary artery disease; efforts should be made to identify clinically silent, but potentially lethal, cardiac disease using stress tests, if necessary.

Recombinant tissue plasminogen activator (t-PA) has been found to improve outcome for all types of ischemic strokes, as shown by a higher proportion of treated than untreated patients with minimal or no disability at 3 months. t-PA must be given intravenously within 3 hours after the onset of an ischemic stroke, with strict adherence to guidelines (see National Institute of Neurological Disorders and Stroke rt-PA Stroke Study Group reference in "Suggested Reading") to prevent hemorrhagic complications.

To guide further management, it is important to identify clinically which arterial system—the carotid or the vertebrobasilar—is likely to be responsible for the patient's complaints. This is important because established surgical options are confined to carotid disease. It is also helpful to determine whether the problem is extracranial carotid artery disease or intracranial disease because intracranial disease is inaccessible to the surgeon. Magnetic resonance angiography can noninvasively provide a view of the extracranial and intracranial blood vessels and is especially helpful if it shows no significant stenosis (ie, there are few false-negatives). A duplex ultrasound study can define noninvasively the extent of disease at the internal carotid artery origin. A transcranial Doppler examination can noninvasively characterize blood flow patterns in the large arteries at the base of the brain and identify occlusion or stenosis. Nonetheless, traditional angiography remains the best technique for defining vascular anatomy. One might insist on angiography when the risk of the test is low, and the risk is outweighed by the benefit of the improved detail provided by the study. This would be the case in a young patient, when there is a suspicion of vasculitis rather than atherosclerosis, and when surgery is likely if the anatomy is amenable.

Extracranial carotid artery disease: Patients with a transient ischemic attack or minor stroke ipsilateral to a 70–99% stenosis at the internal carotid artery origin have less of a chance of having a future stroke if they undergo a carotid endarterectomy. Patients with a less severe stenosis should be treated with aspirin because it reduces the risk of platelet-mediated emboli. If such patients continue to have symptoms on aspirin, the aspirin dose can be increased or the patient can be treated with ticlopidine, another platelet inhibitor, which is more expensive than aspirin and associated with somewhat more adverse side effects, including leukopenia, diarrhea, and rash.

Intracranial artery disease: Therapeutic guidelines for stroke patients with severe stenosis or occlusion of a large intracranial artery are not well defined. Some physicians anticoagulate such patients for several months and then substitute aspirin or ticlopidine if the patients are doing well. Other physicians begin treatment with an antiplatelet agent, and advocate anticoagulation only if the patient is having continuing symptoms.

Patients with small artery disease (small vessels that penetrate into the substance of the brain) often present with discrete neurologic deficits such as pure motor or sensory loss. Multiple small strokes or isolated, strategically placed lesions can cause more complex syndromes such as ataxic hemiparesis, or cognitive or behavioral deficits. Most small artery occlusions reflect damage from chronic hypertension; normotensive patients may have an underlying inflammatory or hematologic disorder. Hypertension should be treated. Aspirin is commonly prescribed.

The deteriorating patient: The physician must address several questions when faced with a patient who has progressively deteriorating neurologic function: Is the blood pressure so low that marginally perfused brain is being compromised? Is cerebral edema developing, shifting brain tissue, or causing a rise in intracranial pressure? Has the ischemic infarct become hemorrhagic? If the patient is being treated with heparin, is the intensity of anticoagulation sufficient or has the patient developed heparin-associated thrombosis, thereby extending the injury?

If there is no ready explanation for the patient's decline (eg, hypotension), many physicians begin heparin treatment on the assumption of intra-arterial clot propagation or artery-to-artery emboli. Unfortunately, rigorous evidence supporting a beneficial response to anticoagulation in this setting is lacking. It is particularly important to identify the cause of stroke in these patients to guide future management.

The Asymptomatic Patient: Patients with an asymptomatic carotid bruit should have noninvasive vascular testing to define the degree of atherosclerosis at the internal carotid artery origin. Occasionally, vascular studies performed for other indications reveal internal carotid artery disease. Patients with a 60–99% stenosis have an 11% 5-year risk of stroke if managed medically compared with a 5.1% risk with carotid endarterectomy. Since surgery conveys only a 1% per year advantage over medical management, careful consideration needs to be given to surgical intervention, especially if perioperative complications could exceed 3%. Risk factors for atherosclerosis should be modified and the patient evaluated for coronary artery disease.

Hematologic and Systemic Disorders

Sickle cell anemia causes ischemic stroke through microinfarcts or large vessel disease; polycythemia vera causes ischemic stroke through increased viscosity. Recently, conditions leading to increased blood coagulability have been identified and implicated as causes of stroke. Antiphospholipid autoantibodies, including the lupus anticoagulant and anticardiolipin, are associated with large and small artery thrombosis, cardiac valvular vegetations, and venous thrombosis. Thrombosis can also be caused by deficiencies of proteins S or C and antithrombin III and by abnormalities of fibrinolysis (Chapter 11.10). Other conditions associated with hypercoagulability are pregnancy, malignancy, paraproteinemia, and nephrotic syndrome. Patients with stroke who have no obvious cause for cardiac or arterial disease should be evaluated for an underlying hypercoagulable state.

HEMORRHAGIC DISORDERS

Intracranial hemorrhage can involve bleeding into the subdural, epidural, and subarachnoid spaces, into the brain, or into the ventricles. The clinical presentation, physical exam, and CT scan allow the physician to differentiate these conditions.

Subarachnoid Hemorrhage

Leakage from a berry (congenital) aneurysm is the most common and important cause of nontraumatic subarachnoid hemorrhage, but other causes include arteriovenous malformation, drug abuse, coagulopathy, vasculitis, and mycotic aneurysm. History and diagnostic studies usually define the pathogenesis. Because aneurysmal subarachnoid hemorrhage is fatal in almost 50% of patients, it will be discussed in detail.

Aneurysm: Most berry aneurysms arise at the bifurcations of the arteries forming the circle of Willis. They are more common in patients with polycystic kidney disease, coarctation of the aorta, fibromuscular dysplasia, moyamoya disease, Ehlers-Danlos and Marfan syndromes, pseudoxanthoma elasticum, and polyarteritis nodosa, as well as in patients with a family history of aneurysms.

Before rupture, an aneurysm may cause symptoms by compressing a portion of the brain or a cranial nerve. For example, an aneurysm of the posterior communicating artery occasionally compresses the oculomotor nerve, causing ptosis, mydriasis, and ophthalmoplegia. Rarely, aneurysms at other sites are large enough to produce focal neurologic signs or headache. Unfortunately, the first evidence of most aneurysms is rupture.

It is particularly important to recognize a "heralding bleed," a small, self-limited hemorrhage that occurs in about 40% of patients who later have a severe subarachnoid hemorrhage. The clinical picture is the abrupt onset of a new or atypical generalized or focal headache that cannot be explained by any obvious process such as migraine or sinusitis. The neurologic exam is normal, as may be a CT scan, but lumbar puncture reveals blood in the spinal fluid. Discovery of a heralding bleed allows patients to be treated before they suffer neurologic injury.

Virtually every patient with an aneurysmal rupture has an abrupt, excruciating headache, "the worst headache of my life." On exam, most patients have meningismus and some have preretinal hemorrhages. Since most aneurysms rupture into the subarachnoid space and only infrequently into the brain itself, patients usually show few if any focal neurologic signs.

CT is the preferred imaging technique to look for intracranial hemorrhage of any sort. Most patients with subarachnoid hemorrhage have subarachnoid blood in the basal cisterns or over the cerebral convexities. Less often, patients have associated intraventricular or intracerebral blood. If blood is seen on CT scan, lumbar puncture is not needed.

Once subarachnoid hemorrhage is confirmed, the patient should be placed on strict bed rest. General care includes stool softeners, mild sedation if the patient is anxious, analgesia for headache, and phenytoin to prevent seizures. Extremes of blood pressure should be avoided. The serum sodium concentration should be checked daily and fluids given to maintain normal serum sodium with normovolemia.

As soon as possible after a subarachnoid hemorrhage is confirmed, patients should have an angiogram. More than 90% of patients are shown to have an aneurysm. Since they can have multiple aneurysms, angiography should include views of all intracranial vascular territories.

Complications of subarachnoid hemorrhage include recurrent bleeding, increased intracranial pressure, hydrocephalus, cerebral vasospasm, hyponatremia, and cardiac ischemia and arrhythmias. Intracranial pressure is increased by both extravasated blood and hydrocephalus caused by blocked cerebrospinal fluid flow. If worsened headache or lethargy leads to suspicion of intracranial hypertension, the intracranial pressure is evaluated, and treated if elevated.

About 10–20% of patients with subarachnoid hemorrhage have more bleeding, most often within a few days after the first bleed. Therefore, efforts to seal off the aneurysm as soon as possible are justified. Neurologic deterioration from a rebleed is often abrupt, but changes from increased intracranial pressure, hydrocephalus, hyponatremia, vasospasm, or sedating medications are more gradual. Repeat CT scan, and occasionally repeat cerebrospinal fluid examination, are needed to confirm rebleeding.

Most cerebral aneurysms are surgically accessible. Early surgical intervention to "clip" the neck of the aneurysm is recommended, thereby eliminating the risk of subsequent hemorrhage. Interventional neuroradiologic techniques are occasionally used to obliterate an aneurysm, but are limited by technical considerations such as the character of the neck of the aneurysm.

Vasospasm typically begins 5–9 days after hemorrhage and characteristically produces gradually progressive focal neurologic signs. The resulting ischemic infarction can contribute to intracranial hypertension. Vasospasm is difficult to treat. Nimodipine, a calcium antagonist, can decrease the incidence of delayed ischemic events by one-third. Maintaining a euvolemic state may help prevent ischemic stroke. If the aneurysm has not been surgically clipped and vasospasm is suspected, normotensive hypervolemic therapy can be started. Following successful clipping of the aneurysm, hypertensive hypervolemic treatment is often effective in improving neurologic deficits. Angioplasty of vasospastic arteries or intra-arterial papaverine infusion can also be used to treat symptomatic patients who are not responding to medical intervention.

Hyponatremia, a common complication of subarachnoid hemorrhage, is caused by the syndrome of inappropriate antidiuretic hormone secretion (SIADH), diuretic therapy, hypotonic fluid overload, or a centrally mediated salt-losing process (cerebral salt wasting).

Parenchymal Hemorrhage

If an artery ruptures into the substance of the brain rather than one of the intracranial spaces, the resulting hematoma (the collection of blood from a hemorrhage) enlarges over minutes to hours. Hematomas can cause deceptively mild neurologic signs or can be catastrophic. The patient typically complains of headache. Bleeding into one of the cerebral hemispheres can produce hemiplegia, hemisensory loss, aphasia, visual loss, neglect syndromes, and difficulties with ocular motility. Patients with pontine hemorrhage usually present with early loss of consciousness, gaze palsy, facial palsy, and quadriplegia.

Cerebellar hemorrhage may present cryptically but is especially important to recognize because quick intervention may save the patient's life. Although the classic triad consists of nausea/vomiting, headache, and ataxia, the neurologic findings may be mild, beginning only with ataxia of the trunk and an impairment of balance. Later, the limbs become incoordinate. If the brain stem is compressed, the patient becomes sleepy, with paralysis of lateral gaze and progressive motor signs. These signs may appear rapidly in a patient who at first did not seem very ill. Further compression of the cerebral aqueduct or the fourth ventricle can cause hydrocephalus, rapid deterioration, and death.

Intraparenchymal hemorrhage is easily diagnosed by CT scan. The hemorrhage appears as a high-density mass within the brain substance. The scan also identifies brain edema as well as displacement and distortion of the ventricles. Lumbar puncture is rarely indicated in patients with an intraparenchymal hematoma and is contraindicated if CT scan identifies a large intracerebral mass.

Although historically ascribed to the damaging effects of chronic hypertension on small penetrating arteries, deep hemorrhage is not always linked to chronic hypertension, and in 50% of patients no predisposing hypertension is identified. Hemorrhage may also be caused by trauma, coagulation deficits, vascular malformations, arteritis, brain tumors, drug abuse, and an acute increase in perfusion of normal or infarcted ischemic brain.

Elderly patients with lobar hemorrhage may have cerebral amyloid angiopathy. This can lead to repeated hemorrhages at varying sites. These patients typically are not hypertensive, or only mildly so. The diagnosis can be confirmed only by brain biopsy. Since vessels containing amyloid are prone to bleed, surgical diagnosis or treatment, though feasible, is rarely pursued.

Immediate management of parenchymal hemorrhage is general medical support. Particular attention should be devoted to controlling blood pressure, to avoid both extreme hypertension and relative hypotension. Although surgery for cerebellar hemorrhage can save lives, the indications for surgery for hemorrhage at other sites remain controversial. A reasonable approach is to consider surgical evacuation of a hematoma if it is in the nondominant hemisphere, if the patient is worsening, if intracranial hypertension cannot be controlled by medical means, and if the hematoma is surgically accessible. Surgical approaches include craniotomy as well as stereotactic techniques.

If a cause other than chronic hypertension is suspected, CT or MRI can help identify an arteriovenous malformation or neoplasm, especially when performed after the hematoma has resolved. Angiography can further define an associated vasculopathy such as arteritis.

Vascular Malformations

Vascular malformations include cavernous angiomas, venous angiomas, and arteriovenous malformations (AVM). Malformations should be suspected as a source of hemorrhage in young, normotensive individuals. An AVM can present with a seizure, hemorrhage, fluctuating neurologic deficit, or headache. Since malformations lie within the substance of the brain, their rupture often causes focal neurologic deficits. MRI almost always identifies an AVM. Management is anticonvulsant therapy for seizures, and surgical resection, embolization, and stereotactic radiation therapy, often in combination. The risk of bleeding from an untreated AVM is 2–3% per year.

Cavernous angiomas are usually clinically silent, although they can bleed or cause seizures. They are readily visualized by MRI. Venous angiomas are usually asymptomatic.

Extra-Axial Hematoma

Epidural and subdural hematomas are usually caused by trauma. They cause brain compression and herniation syndromes.

Epidural hematomas result from arterial bleeding, most commonly from injury to the middle meningeal artery after a skull fracture. Immediately after injury, the patient transiently loses consciousness, but promptly regains it. Several hours later, the patient suddenly begins a rapid deterioration caused by an enlarging hematoma and increasing intracranial pressure. Prompt surgical evacuation of the hematoma can be life-saving.

Subdural hematomas result from venous bleeding. The hematoma can be small, causing little neurologic deficit, or life-threatening if large or fast-growing. Although most subdural hematomas are caused by severe head trauma, they can be produced by trivial trauma in the elderly or patients receiving anticoagulation therapy and can also occur spontaneously. Presentations include focal neurologic deficits, seizures, and cognitive deficits. Management often includes surgical drainage of the hematoma, but a small, chronic subdural hematoma may be left to resolve on its own if the patient is stable. Surgical intervention of a chronic subdural hematoma may lead to rebleeding with worsening of the clinical state, especially in the elderly.

REHABILITATION

For a patient with a persistent neurologic deficit after stroke, rehabilitation is essential. Measures should be taken in the immobile patient to prevent decubitus ulcers; these measures include padding of bony prominences, keeping the skin clean and dry, and frequent turning. Physical therapy should begin during the first days of paralysis to prevent contractures. The patient with difficulty swallowing should be positioned to avoid aspiration. A formal swallowing evaluation with counseling can help decrease the risk of aspiration. Bladder hygiene is essential, and an indwelling catheter should be avoided. Thrombophlebitis is a constant threat; measures should be instituted to decrease the likelihood of venous thrombosis in the legs such as sequential compression devices or minidose subcutaneous heparin. Patients should be warned about orthostatic hypotension when they arise and should be taught to get up gradually. Emotional problems, especially depression, are common after stroke, and, if unrecognized or untreated, can hamper recovery.

SUMMARY

▶ In patients presenting with a stroke, a CT scan should be performed to determine whether the stroke is ischemic or hemorrhagic.

▶ Causes of ischemic stroke are cardiogenic embolism, artery disease, and hematologic and systemic disorders.

▶ Treatment options for ischemic stroke include thrombolysis, antiplatelet agents, anticoagulation, and carotid endarterectomy. Coronary artery disease and risk factors for atherosclerosis should be treated.

▶ Subarachnoid hemorrhage should be diagnosed rapidly and neurosurgical consultation promptly obtained for patients with ruptured berry aneurysm.

▶ Supportive measures and possibly surgery are important for treatment of parenchymal hemorrhage.

SUGGESTED READING

Adams HP Jr et al: Guidelines for the management of patients with acute ischemic stroke: A statement for healthcare professionals from a special writing group of the Stroke Council, American Heart Association. Stroke 1994;25:1901.

Barnett HJM, Eliasziw M, Meldrum HE: Drugs and surgery in the prevention of ischemic stroke. N Engl J Med 1995;332:238.

Feinberg WM et al: Guidelines for the management of transient ischemic attacks. From the Ad Hoc Committee on Guidelines for the Management of Transient Ischemic Attacks of the Stroke Council of the American Heart Association. Stroke 1994;25:1320.

Mayberg MR et al: Guidelines for the management of aneurysmal subarachnoid hemorrhage: A statement for healthcare professionals from a special writing group of the Stroke Council, American Heart Association. Stroke 1994;25:2315.

Moore WS et al: Guidelines for carotid endarterectomy: A multidisciplinary consensus statement from the Ad Hoc Committee, American Heart Association. Stroke 1995;26:188.

National Institute of Neurological Disorders and Stroke rt-PA Stroke Study Group: Tissue plasminogen activator for acute ischemic stroke. N Engl J Med 1995;333:1581.

Movement Disorders

Stephen G. Reich, MD

Movement disorders reflect disease of the basal ganglia and are often called "extrapyramidal disorders" to distinguish them from diseases of the pyramidal tract. The clinical manifestations of movement disorders range from a paucity of voluntary motor activity, such as the slowness seen in Parkinson's disease, to an excess of involuntary motor activity characterizing tremor, dystonia, choreoathetosis, motor tic disorders, and myoclonus.

The basal ganglia are large paired nuclei situated at the base of the brain, made up of the putamen, caudate, and globus pallidus. The basal ganglia have rich connections with almost all brain regions—the cortex, thalamus, brainstem, and cerebellum. In addition to their prominent role in normal and abnormal motor activity, the basal ganglia are involved in oculomotor control, language, behavior, mood, and cognition, accounting for the diffuse clinical manifestations of many movement disorders.

PARKINSON'S DISEASE

Parkinson's disease is one of the most common movement disorders, affecting up to 1% of persons over age 60 years. The cause is unknown. Pathologically, Parkinson's disease is characterized by loss of the pigmented dopaminergic neurons in the substantia nigra of the midbrain. These neurons project to the basal ganglia. The cytologic hallmark of Parkinson's disease is the Lewy body, an eosinophilic, intracytoplasmic inclusion whose function is unknown.

Symptoms and Signs

Patients with Parkinson's disease present around age 60, and the diagnosis is made on clinical grounds. Parkinson's disease typically begins unilaterally, in either an arm or a leg. Little has been added to James Parkinson's original 1817 description from his *Essay on the Shaking Palsy*:

> . . . involuntary tremulous motion, with lessened muscular power, in parts not in action and even when supported; with a propensity to bend the trunk forward, and to pass from walking to a running pace.

The diagnosis of Parkinson's disease rests on finding at least two of the three cardinal signs: rest tremor, cogwheel rigidity, and bradykinesia.

Tremor is the most common presenting sign, although not all patients have tremor. The tremor is of low frequency (3–6 Hz) and is most prominent when the limb is at rest. The movement has a "pill-rolling" morphology—abduction-adduction at the thumb and flexion-extension at the fingers. Cogwheel rigidity is characterized by a ratchety feeling, perceived by the examiner, with limb movement; it is best felt with flexion and extension of the wrist, elbow, or neck. Bradykinesia (slowness of movement) is the sine qua non of Parkinson's disease. Patients notice that it takes longer to carry out day-to-day activities, particularly when performing fine motor tasks such as buttoning, applying makeup, fastening jewelry, or shaving; walking is also slower.

Additional signs of Parkinson's disease include micrographia (small handwriting), diminished arm swing while walking, a stooped posture, shuffling gait, impaired balance, diminished blink rate and facial expression (hypomimia), and a soft monotone voice (hypophonia). Nonmotor signs of Parkinson's disease include increased facial oiliness, seborrhea, and mild dysautonomia. Dementia affects at least 15% of patients with Parkinson's disease, typically late in the disease, but should not be viewed as an inevitable consequence. As many as 50% of patients develop depression.

Although most patients who present with this constellation of signs have idiopathic Parkinson's disease, as many as 20% have one of the several mimickers of idiopathic Parkinson's disease, collectively called "parkinsonian syndromes" (Table 13.7–1). Clues that a patient has a parkinsonian syndrome rather than idiopathic Parkinson's disease are little or no response to treatment with levodopa, young age at onset, early-onset dementia, rapid progression over several years to severe debility, prominent and early dysautonomia, early falling, impaired ocular motility, or lower motor neuron, cerebellar, pyramidal, or sensory signs. The most important of the parkinsonian syndromes to recognize is drug-induced

Table 13.7–1. Differential diagnosis of parkinsonism.

Toxins
Manganese
Carbon monoxide
Carbon disulfide
Cyanide
Methanol
MPTP (1-methyl-4-phenyl-1,2,3,6-tetrahydropyridine)

Drugs
Neuroleptics
Metoclopramide

Multisystem degeneration
Progressive supranuclear palsy
Diffuse Lewy body disease
Shy-Drager syndrome ("multisystem atrophy")
Olivopontocerebellar atrophy
Striatonigral degeneration
Corticobasal degeneration

Primary dementing illness
Alzheimer's disease
Creutzfeldt-Jakob disease

Genetic disease
Wilson's disease
Juvenile Huntington's disease

Multi-infarct state

Calcification of the basal ganglia
Idiopathic calcification
Hypoparathyroidism

parkinsonism, since it is reversible, but it may take 6–12 months to resolve after the offending medication is stopped.

Management

Even though Parkinson's disease is progressive, with treatment almost all patients have a normal life span. The goal of treatment is to use the least amount of medication possible to help the patient function at an adequate level, rather than to attempt to abolish all symptoms and signs. The rationale for treatment is based on the loss of dopamine in the basal ganglia, leading to a relative excess of acetylcholine. Although anticholinergic agents reverse this defect, the mainstay of treatment is levodopa, the precursor of dopamine, since dopamine does not cross the blood-brain barrier. Levodopa is metabolized to dopamine by dopa decarboxylase in the substantia nigra. Since this conversion is not limited to the central nervous system, levodopa is combined with carbidopa, a peripheral decarboxylase inhibitor, to limit the peripheral conversion to dopamine.

Levodopa typically improves symptoms within several weeks, and most patients do well for the first 5 years, sometimes longer. However, with time, the beneficial response to levodopa tends to wane, and many patients develop periods with limited mobility alternating with periods of near-normal functioning. As the therapeutic window narrows, the threshold is lower for levodopa toxicity, which produces excessive involuntary movements known as *dyskinesias*. Dyskinesias take the form of

chorea or dystonia (see Dystonia below), affecting various and often multiple parts of the body. They may appear when levodopa is peaking (about 90–120 minutes after a dose) or randomly, seemingly unrelated to the timing of medication. Additional long-term complications of levodopa may include orthostatic hypotension, hallucinations, confusion, and psychosis.

Additional antiparkinsonian agents are direct-acting dopamine agonists such as bromocriptine and pergolide, and the antiviral agent amantadine, which has both anticholinergic and dopaminergic activity. The monoamine oxidase B inhibitor selegiline (Deprenyl) potentiates the effect of levodopa by blocking the catabolism and reuptake of dopamine. Selegiline may have a separate prophylactic effect in slowing the progression of early Parkinson's disease.

TREMOR

Tremor is a rhythmic oscillation of a body part. Tremors are classified by the position of maximal activation noted during clinical examination. A slow tremor at rest, with a pill-rolling morphology, is characteristic of Parkinson's disease. A tremor maximally activated during maintenance of a posture is characteristic of essential tremor, and a tremor maximally activated during movement (a kinetic or intention tremor) generally indicates cerebellar disease.

Essential tremor is one of the most common movement disorders. The cause is unknown. Essential tremor most frequently affects the upper limbs and may also affect the head or voice. Unlike Parkinson's disease, in which the tremor is accompanied by other neurologic signs, patients with essential tremor have an otherwise normal neurologic exam.

In practice, almost all patients presenting with tremor prove to have either essential tremor or Parkinson's disease. A few key features of the history and physical exam can usually separate the two (Table 13.7–2). Although most Parkinson's disease is sporadic, essential tremor is often familial, with autosomal dominant inheritance. Alcohol suppresses essential tremor in at least 60% of patients, but only rarely affects a parkinsonian tremor. The tremor of Parkinson's disease typically begins unilaterally, whereas essential tremor is almost always bilateral, although it may be asymmetric.

The two most effective medications for essential tremor are propranolol and primidone. For the small percentage of patients who have disabling essential tremor that responds poorly to medications, stereotactic thalamotomy is a safe, effective, and underused treatment. Thalamotomy is also useful for a kinetic (cerebellar) or parkinsonian tremor.

Enhanced physiologic tremor, a fine postural tremor resembling essential tremor, is seen in many settings (Table 13.7–3). Unlike essential tremor, which is permanent, enhanced physiologic tremor resolves when the offending drug, toxin, illness, or metabolic derangement is reversed.

Table 13.7–2. Differentiation of a parkinsonian tremor from essential tremor.

	Parkinson's Disease	Essential Tremor
Age at onset	60	Variable, more common after 50
Duration of symptoms prior to seeking medical attention	Weeks–months	Months–years–decades
Family history	No	Autosomal dominant inheritance (≥60%)
Response to alcohol	Rare	Yes (≥60%)
Position of maximal activation	Rest	Maintenance of a posture
Frequency	3–6 Hz	6–12 Hz
Side affected at onset	Unilateral	Bilateral
Body parts affected	Upper limb>lower limb>lip=chin	Upper limbs>head>voice>chin
Associated neurologic signs	Yes	No

DYSTONIA

Dystonia is a syndrome of sustained muscle contractions producing twisting and repetitive movements or abnormal postures. Dystonia may involve any part of the body and is classified by the body regions involved, the mode of inheritance, or, when possible, the etiology. Adults tend to have focal dystonias, involving a single region of the body, typically the craniocervical musculature. With rare exceptions, the adult-onset focal dystonias are idiopathic rather than the result of an underlying structural or metabolic abnormality, and they are usually sporadic.

The most common focal dystonia is *blepharospasm*—

Table 13.7–3. Differential diagnosis of enhanced physiologic tremor.

Situational
Anxiety
Fright
Fatigue
Exercise or postexercise

Endocrine
Thyrotoxicosis
Hypoglycemia
Pheochromocytoma

Drugs
Sympathomimetics
Caffeine
Theophylline
Valproic acid
Lithium
Tricyclic antidepressants
Phenothiazines
Butyrophenones
Withdrawal from alcohol or sedative-hypnotic drugs

forceful, involuntary bilateral eye closure. This may be infrequent and asymptomatic or so sustained as to cause functional blindness. When blepharospasm coexists with dystonia of the oromandibular region, it is called Meige's syndrome.

The second most common focal dystonia in adults is *torticollis* (cervical dystonia), characterized by sustained abnormal head postures. The head is usually rotated to one side, but may deviate in any direction. In addition to sustained (tonic) deviation, many patients with torticollis have superimposed head jerks (clonic movements).

Adductor spasmodic dysphonia (laryngeal dystonia) produces involuntary adduction of the vocal cords during phonation. This produces irregular breaks in sentences and words, and a strained quality to the voice. Dystonia of the muscles of mastication causes involuntary jaw closure (trismus), jaw opening, or lateral deviation.

Dystonic writer's cramp is often misdiagnosed. It is a task-specific movement disorder—dystonia occurs only during certain tasks—whereas other uses of the limb are normal. Dystonic writer's cramp is manifested by involuntary posturing of the hand when the patient tries to write. Handwriting is slow, laborious, and often illegible. The cramp component is misleading, since it is often painless; this should not be confused with the local pain that most people feel after sustained writing.

Hemidystonia involves the ipsilateral arm and leg. Unlike the other focal dystonias, hemidystonia is often caused by a structural lesion of the contralateral basal ganglia.

Management

Since the cause of dystonia is unknown, treatment is empirical. Commonly prescribed drugs include anticholinergics, benzodiazepines, muscle relaxants, and anticonvulsants. With such treatment, alone or in combination, less than 50% of patients improve. A major breakthrough has been the introduction of local injections of botulinum toxin into the overactive muscles. Botulinum toxin inhibits release of acetylcholine at the neuromuscular junction, thereby weakening overactive muscles. Within 3–6 months, muscle strength returns and additional injections are required.

CHOREA

Chorea consists of rapid, nonrhythmic, nonstereotyped (ie, each one is different) distal movements that flow inconsistently from one body region to another. It often coexists with slower, writhing movements known as athetosis (choreoathetosis). In its most extreme form, choreoathetosis is called ballismus and is characterized by violent, flinging proximal movements.

The prototypic choreiform disorder is Huntington's disease (see below). Chorea may be drug-induced, typically from neuroleptics or antiparkinsonian agents, or it may be the result of toxins such as carbon monoxide. Additional causes of chorea are hyperthyroidism, polycythemia vera, systemic lupus erythematosus, Sydenham's chorea, cerebral palsy, and Wilson's disease. Although most disorders causing chorea develop insidiously, chorea may present acutely, typically unilaterally (hemichorea), caused by an infarct involving the subthalamic nucleus.

The classic triad of Huntington's disease (Chapter 10.2) is chorea plus dementia and an autosomal dominant inheritance pattern. Patients with Huntington's disease usually present in the third or fourth decade with chorea or dementia. Patients live an average of 15 years after onset. The gene for Huntington's disease is on the short arm of chromosome 4; the genetic defect is an expanded repeat of three nucleotides: cytosine, adenosine, and guanine.

MYOCLONUS

Myoclonus is similar to chorea but much faster, manifested by very rapid (lightning-like), random, nonrhythmic muscle jerks. Physiologic myoclonus is a common normal event that happens as a person drifts off to sleep. Pathologic myoclonus is generally seen in patients with a metabolic, hypoxic-ischemic, or toxic encephalopathy, with a degenerative neurologic syndrome such as Creutzfeldt-Jakob or Alzheimer's disease, or with epilepsy.

Related to myoclonus is asterixis. Sometimes called "negative myoclonus," it consists of brief lapses of posture (flapping) of the dorsiflexed hands, caused by inhibition of the wrist extensors. Asterixis is characteristic of a metabolic encephalopathy, and was originally described with hepatic failure, the classic "liver flap."

TICS

Motor tics may be either simple, such as a repetitive shoulder shrug, or complex. The movements are characterized by their erratic appearance in different body parts, usual onset in childhood or adolescence, lack of rhythmicity (as differentiated from tremor), and association with vocalizations (occasionally profanities) and behavioral disturbances. Unlike other movement disorders, tics are often preceded by a buildup of inner tension that subsides after the tic. Tic disorders have a wide spectrum, from benign, transient tics of childhood through severe cases of Tourette's syndrome, a combination of motor and vocal tics, frequently associated with a behavioral disturbance, such as obsessive-compulsive disorder; onset is before age 21. Monosymptomatic tics, such as repetitive throat clearing, a rapid head jerk, or shoulder shrug, may be the most common of all movement disorders.

DRUG-INDUCED MOVEMENT DISORDERS

All the movement disorders mentioned in this chapter can be caused by medications (Table 13.7–4). The prototype drug-induced movement disorder is tardive dyskinesia, characterized by choreoathetosis of the buccolingual

Table 13.7–4. Drug-induced movement disorders.

Parkinson's disease
Antipsychotics
Metoclopramide
Methyldopa
Amiodarone
Reserpine

Dystonia
Antipsychotics
Metoclopramide
Levodopa

Tremor
Lithium
Antipsychotics
Valproic acid
Corticosteroids
Tricyclic antidepressants
β-adrenergic agonists

Chorea
Phenytoin
Levodopa
Antipsychotics
Estrogens

Myoclonus or asterixis
Almost any drug at toxic doses
Meperidine (especially in patients with renal insufficiency)

Tics
Antipsychotics
Amphetamines
Levodopa
Carbamazepine

muscles. While most drug-induced movement disorders resolve when the drug is discontinued, tardive dyskinesia may be permanent.

WILSON'S DISEASE

Almost any movement disorder in a young person can be the presenting sign of Wilson's disease, an autosomal recessive disorder associated with a deficiency of ceruloplasmin, the copper-binding protein, and an accumulation of copper in multiple tissues. The gene has been localized to chromosome 13 encoding a copper-transporting ATPase whose deficiency allows the intracellular accumulation of copper. In addition to movement disorders, Wilson's disease can present with hepatic dysfunction (Chapter 7.4) or psychiatric abnormalities, ranging from a mild behavioral disturbance to a drop-off in school performance, a change in personality, depression, mania, and psychosis.

SUMMARY

▶ Movement disorders, suggesting disease of the basal ganglia, are characterized by either a paucity of voluntary movement or excessive involuntary movement.

▶ Parkinson's disease is caused by loss of dopamine-producing cells from the substantia nigra in the midbrain. The goal of treatment is to use the least amount of medication possible to help the patient function at an adequate level, rather than to attempt to abolish all symptoms and signs.

▶ Essential tremor differs from Parkinson's disease in that it is often familial, begins bilaterally, is maximally activated with maintenance of a posture, and often attenuates with alcohol.

▶ Any movement disorder may be drug-induced. Although most drug-induced movement disorders resolve when the offending medication is stopped, tardive dyskinesia may be permanent.

▶ Any movement disorder in a young person should prompt an evaluation for Wilson's disease.

SUGGESTED READING

Gusella JF et al: Molecular genetics of Huntington's disease. Arch Neurol 1993;50:1157.

Hallett M: Classification and treatment of tremor. JAMA 1991; 266:1115.

Marsden CD: Parkinson's disease. J Neurol Neurosurg Psychiatry 1994;57:672.

Marsden CD, Quinn N: The dystonias. Br Med J 1990;300:139.

Shoulson I: On chorea. Clin Neuropharmacol 1986;9(Suppl 2): S85.

13.8

Multiple Sclerosis

Justin C. McArthur, MB, BS, MPH

Multiple sclerosis is a disease of young adults, characterized by recurring attacks of neurologic dysfunction. The cardinal lesion is a *plaque,* an area of inflammation and myelin breakdown in the brain or spinal cord. Because the neurologic deficits can be subtle and often involve the sensory system more than the motor system, the early stages of multiple sclerosis can be mistaken for neuropathy, hyperventilation, or hysteria. The diagnosis usually becomes clearer over time, as patients suffer more attacks involving widely disparate portions of the central nervous system with no chronologic pattern. The typical features are best summed up as "lesions disseminated in time and place." Multiple sclerosis should be considered in any young person who has episodic neurologic deficits. The course of disease of some patients is steadily progressive rather than showing defined episodes, but the pathophysiology seems to be identical.

It is important to know the features of multiple sclerosis because it is a fairly common disease that may be confused with other neurologic disorders, because few tests are needed to make the diagnosis in patients who present with compatible clinical histories, and because it now appears possible to slow the disease's progression and reduce the duration and frequency of attacks.

PATHOPHYSIOLOGY

Multiple sclerosis is caused by an immunologically mediated attack on myelin in the central nervous system. Other organ systems are not affected. The plaques that result from this damage can appear anywhere in the central nervous system, although they are densest in white matter, particularly around the ventricles and in the optic nerves, brain stem, and spinal cord. Symptoms and signs often correlate poorly with the distribution and number of plaques seen radiographically or at autopsy.

The demyelinating plaques disturb normal conduction of electrical impulses within the central nervous system. A partially demyelinated axon may continue to conduct impulses, but less effectively. With complete demyelination, electrical transmission ceases.

Multiple sclerosis is by far the most common of the demyelinating diseases. These are disorders in which the primary abnormality is myelin breakdown, with neurons and axons relatively spared. Some less common demyelinating diseases are the leukodystrophies, which are inherited defects in myelin metabolism impairing either the synthesis or maintenance of myelin lipids or proteins. Demyelinating disease can also be caused by infections, such as progressive multifocal leukoencephalopathy (PML) in patients with AIDS and other immunodeficiency states, and subacute sclerosing panencephalitis (SSPE) after measles. Although all these diseases share demyelination, they differ in their typical clinical presentations.

EPIDEMIOLOGY

About 90% of patients with multiple sclerosis develop their first symptoms between ages 20 and 40. Multiple sclerosis is the third most common cause of disability among adults under age 40, after trauma and rheumatologic conditions. The fatality rate is extremely low; the disease only slightly shortens life expectancy.

The prevalence of multiple sclerosis in northern Europe and the northern United States is 30–80 per 100,000; in southern Europe and the southern United States, 6–14 per 100,000; and in the tropics, less than 1 per 100,000. People who migrate after age 15 years seem to carry with them the prevalence rate of their country of origin, while those migrating in early childhood assume the risk of their new home. There have also been local clusters or "epidemics" of multiple sclerosis, as in the Faeroe Islands after British occupation in World War II, and in Key West, Florida. These epidemiologic clues suggest that exposure to some extrinsic factor, possibly an infectious agent, during the first 15 years of life is an important determinant of multiple sclerosis in adulthood.

The rate of multiple sclerosis is 15–20 times higher in first-degree relatives of patients than in the general population. The risk is 3% for a patient's children, 4% for siblings, and 20–30% for an identical twin. Patients of European ancestry have a high incidence of the HLA histocompatibility antigens A3, B7, Dw2, and Dr2.

Currently, the most plausible explanation for multiple sclerosis is that an individual with susceptible immune response genes is exposed during childhood to certain exogenous trigger factors, possibly viruses, and develops multiple sclerosis after a latent period of 10–30 years.

CLINICAL FEATURES

Up to 80% of patients with multiple sclerosis present with a relapsing-remitting pattern (Figure 13.8–1). Typical patients suddenly develop a neurologic deficit (Table 13.8–1) that begins over a few hours or days and lasts for about 2–6 weeks. Over the next weeks or months, patients recover completely or almost completely (remission). Months to years later, they have another attack (a relapse or exacerbation), which may resemble the original event or, because the disease is multifocal, may be completely different. New symptoms and signs must persist for more than 48 hours to be classified as a relapse.

A patient who presents with what looks like a first attack may have forgotten an episode that happened years earlier, so the physician must inquire about past events. A remission can last months or years, but is followed at variable and unpredictable intervals by other relapses. With each episode, permanent neurologic deficits may accumulate.

During the first 5 years of multiple sclerosis, patients have relapses on the average of every 6–12 months, but the frequency varies greatly. After 5 years, the frequency

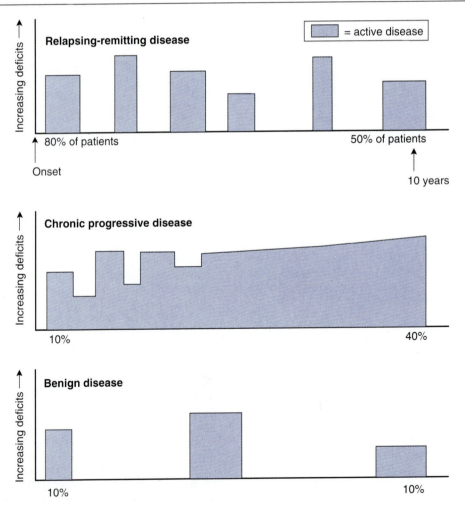

Figure 13.8–1. Possible courses of multiple sclerosis. About 80% of patients have relapsing-remitting disease at onset, 10% have progressive disease from onset, and 10% have infrequent relapses. By 10 years after diagnosis, about 30% of patients who began with relapsing-remitting have changed to progressive disease.

Table 13.8–1. Common presenting features of multiple sclerosis.

	% of Patients
Symptoms	
Paresthesias	40
Gait difficulty	35
Leg weakness	20
Visual loss	20
Arm weakness	10
Double vision	10
Bladder urgency	10
Vertigo	5–10
Signs	
Hyperreflexia	80
Leg ataxia	60
Bilateral Babinski's sign	50
Decreased vibration sense	50
Optic neuritis	40
Nystagmus	35
Spasticity	20
Paraparesis	20
Cerebellar dysmetria	20
Internuclear ophthalmoplegia	10
Cerebellar truncal ataxia	10

Modified and reproduced, with permission, from Matthews WB: Symptoms and signs. In: *McAlpine's Multiple Sclerosis,* 2nd ed. Matthews WB et al (editors). Churchill Livingstone, 1991.

may decline. But by 10 years after diagnosis, about 30% of patients who started with a relapsing-remitting course have changed to a steadily progressive course (secondary progressive multiple sclerosis).

About 10% of patients have a chronic progressive pattern from the outset, without remissions (primary progressive multiple sclerosis). The final 10% of patients have benign multiple sclerosis, with infrequent, mild attacks that leave little or no residual deficit.

DIFFERENTIAL DIAGNOSIS

Systemic diseases such as vasculitis, sarcoidosis, and Lyme disease can affect the central nervous system and produce relapsing and remitting neurologic symptoms. These conditions are usually readily distinguished from multiple sclerosis by their systemic involvement. For example, most patients with systemic vasculitis have constitutional symptoms—fever, hematuria, weight loss, and an elevated erythrocyte sedimentation rate.

Disorders such as leukodystrophies and vitamin deficiencies can produce progressive neurologic syndromes, principally affecting the spinal cord. Adrenoleukodystrophy is an X-linked recessive disorder characterized by central nervous system demyelination and adrenal insufficiency and is identified by an accumulation of long-chain fatty acids. The spinal forms of multiple sclerosis can be confused with an adult form of adrenoleukodystrophy (adrenomyeloneuropathy), which typically begins in the third decade and causes a spastic paraparesis and cognitive impairment. A single structural lesion at a critical place, such as the foramen magnum, might affect several neurologic systems and mimic multiple sclerosis. Adrenomyeloneuropathy is distinguished by the inheritance pattern, the biochemical finding of excess long-chain fatty acids, adrenal insufficiency, and peripheral neuropathy, none of which are seen in multiple sclerosis.

Spinal arteriovenous malformation can cause relapsing spinal cord symptoms, but often also produces back pain and an abrupt onset of neurologic symptoms. Cervical spondylotic myelopathy, a common cause of gait dysfunction in the elderly, is unusual in persons aged 20–40. Psychological conditions—hypochondriasis, somatoform disorder, and anxiety—are often difficult to distinguish from mild forms of multiple sclerosis in patients who have predominantly sensory complaints and few physical findings. Here neurodiagnostic tests may be useful.

COMMON PRESENTATIONS

Optic Neuritis

Optic neuritis presents as a loss of vision, usually in one eye, without redness but usually with some pain on eye movement. Patients describe a loss of central vision, "like looking through cellophane" or "a smear on my glasses." Funduscopic exam may be normal or show papillitis (a pink, swollen optic disc) without retinal hemorrhage or uveitis (inflammation in the anterior chamber). After recovery, the disc may be pale, chalky white. Color vision testing is often abnormal. The patient may also have an afferent pupillary defect (Marcus-Gunn pupil) and a central scotoma. Between 25% and 40% of all patients with multiple sclerosis develop symptomatic optic neuritis at some time; another 30% have optic neuritis that is detectable only by electrophysiologic testing with visual evoked potentials. About 30% of patients with isolated optic neuritis (occurring by itself) go on to develop multiple sclerosis. But multiple sclerosis is not the only condition that isolated optic neuritis can herald; it can also be caused by postinfection demyelination, systemic lupus erythematosus, sarcoidosis, and syphilis.

Spinal Cord Involvement

Another common presentation of multiple sclerosis is spinal cord involvement, which can cause either a slowly progressive myelopathy or an acute transverse myelitis. Transverse myelitis presents with a relatively abrupt onset of spinal cord dysfunction, affecting the cord bilaterally (hence, "transverse"). As with optic neuritis, transverse myelitis can herald multiple sclerosis or can be an isolated monophasic illness after a viral infection. Sensory symptoms include numbness below a sensory level, and paresthesias. The legs may be weak, with spasticity, clonus, and increased reflexes indicating upper motor neuron involvement. An affected bladder can cause hesitancy, retention, or incontinence, and an affected bowel can cause constipation or fecal incontinence.

Brain Stem

Multiple sclerosis often involves the brain stem white matter tracts in characteristic patterns. In a young person, these patterns should raise a suspicion of multiple sclerosis. One picture is new-onset diplopia, which may represent internuclear ophthalmoplegia, a characteristic eye movement abnormality of conjugate gaze resulting from a plaque in the medial longitudinal fasciculus, the white matter tract linking the third and sixth nerve nuclei. Patients with internuclear ophthalmoplegia have sluggish or no adduction of the eye opposite to the direction of lateral eye movement. For example, if patients are asked to look to the right, the left eye does not move normally past the midline and toward the nose. However, convergence remains normal: When patients look at the tip of their nose or an examiner's finger brought toward their nose, both eyes move medially (cross-eye). Patients also show nystagmus in the abducting eye. Other eye movement abnormalities are so common in multiple sclerosis that if a patient has *normal* eye movements, the diagnosis is suspect. The abnormalities range from jerky (saccadic) pursuits to sixth cranial nerve weakness with impaired lateral gaze.

Other common brain stem syndromes in multiple sclerosis are facial pain from trigeminal neuralgia caused by a demyelinating plaque close to the trigeminal nucleus; slurred speech from incoordination or weakness of the palate and tongue; and dysphagia from disturbance of swallowing mechanisms. Some patients have spells of vertigo, caused by involvement of the vestibular system in the lower brain stem.

Cerebrum and Cerebellum

Many patients with multiple sclerosis present with hemiparesis or hemisensory symptoms caused by plaques within the centrum semiovale and cerebral white matter, or with truncal ataxia and limb incoordination caused by plaques within the cerebellar white matter or peduncles. Many patients have dysmetria (incoordination of the limbs), which is brought out by "finger-nose" or "heel-knee-shin" testing. The speech may become incoordinated, too, with excessive variation in pitch and volume, so-called "scanning" speech. Some patients develop a coarse tremor of the head and trunk (titubation), which can also be seen in patients with parkinsonian syndromes and essential tremor (Chapter 13.7). A small proportion of patients with multiple sclerosis develop significant cognitive impairment, usually personality change and memory loss. Seizures are uncommon and should suggest other diagnoses such as vasculitis and central nervous system infection.

Other common nonlocalizing symptoms in patients with multiple sclerosis include fatigue or lack of endurance, heat sensitivity, and Lhermitte's phenomenon. *Lhermitte's phenomenon* consists of electric shock sensations radiating down the spine, produced by neck flexion. *Heat sensitivity* is the provocation or unmasking of neurologic symptoms, such as paresthesias, when core body temperature is elevated by fever or external heat, such as a bath or shower. These transitory symptoms do not represent a true relapse, but result from transient conduction impairment in areas of previously damaged myelin.

COURSE AND PROGNOSIS

Although multiple sclerosis is unpredictable and the outlook uncertain, several clinical points help in prognosis (Table 13.8–2). As a general rule, persons who develop multiple sclerosis between the ages of 20 and 35 have less long-term disability than those diagnosed before 20 or after 50. Frequent relapses early in the disease increase the chance of disability. Patients who present with cerebellar, cognitive, or progressive motor symptoms fare worse and become more disabled than patients with only visual or sensory complaints. Patients who achieve complete remissions after each relapse, with full resolution of neurologic symptoms and signs, have a better prognosis than patients who accumulate deficits after each relapse. A steadily progressive course from onset implies little likelihood of remission and high risk for disability.

About 50% of patients with multiple sclerosis need to walk with a cane or walker by 10 years after disease onset, and 70% by 30 years. The more optimistic view of these numbers is that *not everyone* with multiple sclerosis becomes physically limited.

Multiple Sclerosis and Pregnancy

Women with multiple sclerosis have a lower risk of relapse during pregnancy, probably because of the natural immunosuppression afforded by progesterone, α-fetoprotein, and the other hormones of pregnancy. But during the 3 months after delivery, women may have an increased risk of exacerbation. On aggregate, pregnancy has minimal effect on the course of multiple sclerosis. Similarly, multiple sclerosis has little effect on the course of pregnancy. Most women with multiple sclerosis have normal pregnancies and are able to deliver normally; epidural anesthesia does not seem to provoke relapses. There is no increase in birth defects.

Table 13.8–2. Prognostic factors in multiple sclerosis.

	Good Prognosis	Poor Prognosis
Age at onset	20–35	<20 or >50
Presenting symptom	Visual or sensory	Cerebellar, cognitive, or motor
Remission	Complete	Accumulating deficits
Early relapses	Few	Many
Course from onset	Relapsing-remitting	Progressive

Modified and reproduced, with permission, from Swanson JW: Multiple sclerosis: Update in diagnosis and review of prognostic factors. Mayo Clin Proc 1989;64:577.

DIAGNOSIS

Multiple sclerosis is diagnosed primarily on clinical criteria (Table 13.8–3). Laboratory and imaging studies can be corroborative and can help in excluding other conditions (see "Differential Diagnosis" above), but cannot replace a detailed history and exam. *Definite* multiple sclerosis requires a description of at least two episodes of neurologic symptoms affecting discrete areas of the central nervous system and evidence of white matter involvement in at least two areas. If the patient's symptoms and signs suggest only a single lesion, ancillary studies may help to disclose subclinical disease elsewhere in the central nervous system.

Table 13.8–4 outlines some of the conditions that may be misdiagnosed as multiple sclerosis, and Table 13.8–5 lists some of the clinical features that would make multiple sclerosis unlikely. Since the mimicking conditions are uncommon, have different neurologic symptoms and signs from multiple sclerosis, or have systemic features, most patients can be diagnosed with reasonable certainty by just a careful history and exam.

Ancillary studies should be chosen carefully to minimize morbidity and cost. Only those tests required to corroborate the clinical diagnosis are indicated; serial studies are rarely justified. All patients with suspected multiple sclerosis should have magnetic resonance imaging (MRI) of the brain (Figure 13.8–2), spinal cord (Figure 13.8–3), or both, depending on symptom sites. MRI is so sensitive in defining demyelinating lesions in brain and cord as to render computed tomography (CT) and myelography unnecessary. MRI with gadolinium contrast can even differ-

Table 13.8–4. Conditions mistaken for multiple sclerosis.

Relapsing-remitting multifocal central nervous system disease
Vasculitis
Sarcoidosis
Lyme disease
Syphilis
Systemic lupus erythematosus

Progressive multifocal central nervous system disease
Vitamin B_{12} or E deficiency
Leukodystrophies (eg, adrenoleukodystrophy)
Neurodegenerative conditions (eg, olivopontocerebellar degeneration)

Single central nervous system lesion
Spinal cord or foramen magnum tumor
Spinal arteriovenous malformation
Cervical spondylitic myelopathy

Nonorganic disorders
Hypochondriasis
Anxiety
Somatoform disorders

entiate brightly enhancing active new plaques from nonenhancing chronic plaques (see Figure 13.8–3). Brain imaging can also pick up "silent" plaques that are not causing any symptoms. If MRI is unavailable, a CT scan with contrast can detect demyelinating lesions within the brain, but CT does not allow good visualization of the brain stem and spine.

The typical MRI findings in patients with multiple sclerosis are the demyelinated plaques, which appear as multiple bright round or oval lesions scattered around the ventricles or in the brain stem. The long axis of oval lesions sits perpendicular to the ventricles, because the plaques form along the radially arranged veins. On a T_2-weighted MRI, a plaque is difficult to distinguish from cerebrospinal fluid space, because both look bright. They are better distinguished by proton-weighted images, in which plaques remain bright while cerebrospinal fluid looks gray. A typical radiographic feature of multiple sclerosis is "notching" of the corpus callosum on sagittal T_1-weighted images.

In people who do not have multiple sclerosis or any neurologic disease, MRI sometimes shows artifacts termed "unidentified bright objects" (UBOs). Although UBOs look similar to demyelinated plaques, they may

Table 13.8–3. Diagnosis of multiple sclerosis.

	Findings
History	Relapsing-remitting (80% of patients) or progressive (10%) symptoms
Examination	Multifocal central nervous system involvement
Brain MRI + gadolinium contrast	Multiple plaques, particularly periventricular, that enhance with gadolinium; discrete lesions within the spinal cord
Evoked potential studies (visual, brain stem, somatosensory)	Evidence of central conduction delay (useful for detecting subclinical lesions)
Cerebrospinal fluid	
Cells	Mononuclear pleocytosis (10–20/μL)
Protein	Slightly elevated (40–60 mg/dL)
IgG index	Elevated in 70% of patients with clinically definite multiple sclerosis
Oligoclonal bands	In 80–90% of patients with clinically definite multiple sclerosis
Myelin basic protein	Elevated during acute attacks; a nonspecific indicator of disease activity

Table 13.8–5. Features casting doubt on a diagnosis of multiple sclerosis.

No optic nerve involvement or oculomotor abnormalities
No clinical remission, especially in a young patient
Unifocal disease
No sensory findings
No bladder involvement

Modified and reproduced, with permission, from Rudick RA et al: Multiple sclerosis: The problem of incorrect diagnosis. Arch Neurol 1986;43:578. © 1986 American Medical Association.

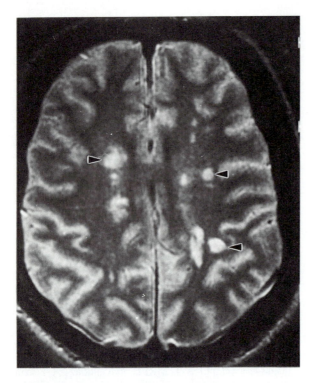

Figure 13.8–2. Cranial magnetic resonance scan in a patient with multiple sclerosis. Multiple plaques (arrowheads) are seen in the periventricular white matter. The increased signal (on T_2-weighted scan) represents increased water in inflammatory lesions.

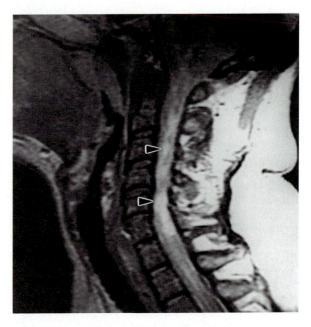

Figure 13.8–3. Sagittal cervical spine magnetic resonance scan in a patient with multiple sclerosis. Two plaques (arrowheads) within the cord enhance with gadolinium, reflecting active inflammation within the plaques.

represent overlarge—but normal—perivascular spaces. Thus, bright round lesions on MRI should not necessarily be interpreted as representing demyelination, especially in persons who have no neurologic symptoms or signs. In patients with cerebrovascular risk factors such as diabetes mellitus or hypertension, most white matter lesions reflect small areas of infarction.

Few patients need cerebrospinal fluid analysis, particularly not those who have a characteristic history and neurologic abnormalities and an abnormal MRI. Cerebrospinal fluid analysis should be reserved for atypical cases, patients presenting after age 55, and patients with confounding illnesses such as malignancy or possible infection. About 70% of patients with clinically definite multiple sclerosis have an elevated cerebrospinal fluid IgG level, reflecting immune overactivity. The increased IgG comes from plasma cells derived from B-cell clones within the brain and spinal cord. It is not known against which antigens these immunoglobulins are directed. Subfractions of this IgG have specific oligoclonal bands, which are found in 80–90% of patients with definite multiple sclerosis. The bands persist between acute attacks and perhaps for life. But oligoclonal bands have also been found in 7% or less of patients with other neurologic conditions, such as Guillain-Barré syndrome, viral meningoencephalitis, HIV infection, tumors, and even stroke.

Myelin basic protein, a component of myelin, appears in the cerebrospinal fluid during acute exacerbations and may be a useful, albeit nonspecific, indicator of disease activity. Myelin basic protein may also be elevated after head trauma or stroke or with inflammatory conditions such as systemic lupus erythematosus.

MANAGEMENT

There is no proven cure for multiple sclerosis and as yet no therapy proven to improve progressive disease or stimulate remyelination. Patients are best managed by an interdisciplinary team of neurologist, primary care giver (if not a neurologist), rehabilitation specialist, urologist, and social worker. Critical treatment elements include education, counseling, empathy, and encouragement. Especially patients with severe disease are helped to maintain function and independence by rehabilitation services: physical and occupational therapy, assistive devices (eg, canes, walkers, wheelchairs), vocational training, and home modification (eg, rails, ramps, easy-to-open doorknobs).

Treatment of symptoms is important in maintaining and improving patients' quality of life. For example, clonazepam can be given to suppress cerebellar tremor. Patients with bladder incontinence should be treated promptly for bladder infections and given intermittent bladder catheterization rather than an indwelling catheter. A drug such as propantheline or oxybutynin can improve continence by reducing bladder urgency and increasing bladder capacity. Patients with marked limb spasticity or flexor spasms can benefit from an antispasticity drug like baclofen or diazepam.

Chronic administration of β-interferon by subcutaneous or intramuscular injections has reduced the frequency of relapses and the appearance of new lesions on MRI. For the first time, we may have an agent that can alter the natural history of multiple sclerosis and prevent exacerbations. β-interferon is expensive and causes flu-like symptoms, and it has not yet proven effective for chronic progressive disease.

Relapses appear to be shortened by glucocorticoids such as prednisone and methylprednisolone, which are less expensive than adrenocorticotropic hormone (ACTH) and lack some of its mineralocorticoid effects. Short courses of corticosteroids are also widely given, although they have not yet been definitively proven to alter the natural history. Corticosteroids' side effects argue against their long-term use.

There have been promising results in the treatment of chronic progressive multiple sclerosis, which has the worst long-term prognosis. Studies suggest that the disease can be stabilized by courses of high-dose intravenous cyclophosphamide plus ACTH or cyclosporine, although at the cost of serious side effects. Methotrexate given once a week has shown some benefit in stabilizing progressive disease.

SUMMARY

▶ Multiple sclerosis is a central nervous system disorder that usually affects young people and causes attacks of neurologic symptoms separated by long remissions.

▶ A typical attack lasts several weeks and causes sensory disturbance, weakness and incoordination, eye movement abnormalities, and painless loss of visual acuity.

▶ The primary lesions are multiple foci of inflammation and demyelination affecting the white matter in brain, optic nerves, and spinal cord.

▶ Magnetic resonance imaging, the most sensitive neurodiagnostic study, shows scattered white matter lesions around the ventricles, brain stem, or spinal cord.

▶ Immunosuppressive agents such as glucocorticoids may shorten acute exacerbations, and β-interferon reduces the frequency of attacks.

SUGGESTED READING

Cook SD (editor): *Handbook of Multiple Sclerosis.* Alan Dekker, 1990.

Duquette P et al: Interferon beta-1b in the treatment of multiple sclerosis: Final outcome of the randomized controlled trial. Neurology 1995;45:1277.

Goodin DS: The use of immunosuppressive agents in the treatment of multiple sclerosis: A critical review. Neurology 1991; 41:980.

Goodkin DE et al: Low-dose (7.5 mg) oral methotrexate reduces the rate of progression in chronic progressive multiple sclerosis. Ann Neurol 1995;37:30.

IFNB Multiple Sclerosis Study Group: Interferon beta-1b is effective in relapsing-remitting multiple sclerosis. I. Clinical results of a multicenter, randomized, double-blind, placebo-controlled trial. Neurology 1993;43:655.

Miller DH et al: Guidelines for the use of magnetic resonance techniques in monitoring the treatment of multiple sclerosis. Ann Neurol 1996;39:6.

Poser CM et al: New diagnostic criteria for multiple sclerosis: Guidelines for research protocols. Ann Neurol 1983;13:227.

Sibley WA: *Therapeutic Claims in Multiple Sclerosis,* 3rd ed. Demos, 1992.

13.9

Neuro-Oncology

Stuart A. Grossman, MD

About 75% of tumors of the brain, meninges, and spinal cord are metastatic from systemic cancers. These metastases are becoming more common as therapies for systemic cancers improve and survival is prolonged. The remainder consists of primary tumors of the nervous system. Patients with neoplasms of the nervous system can present with new-onset seizures, sudden neurologic deficits as with strokes, or more slowly progressing neurologic deficits. This chapter reviews the diagnosis and treatment of primary neoplasms of the central nervous system, neurologic complications of systemic cancer, and cancer pain.

Although patients with tumors of the nervous system are frequently treated by subspecialists, primary care physicians have a critical role in the management of these patients. Tumor must be distinguished from other causes of neurologic dysfunction, tissue may be needed for diagnostic purposes, and drugs to control seizures and edema in the brain or spinal cord may be required urgently. Prompt diagnosis and therapy of these disorders usually result in improvement or stabilization of neurologic function and prevention of severe, irreversible disabilities.

PRIMARY BRAIN TUMORS

Clinical Manifestations of Intracranial Tumors

Brain tumors produce symptoms by raising intracranial pressure or by compressing or infiltrating normal brain. Increased intracranial pressure caused by expansion of tumor and peritumoral edema within the confines of the skull is often associated with progressive signs and symptoms. Headaches are common, especially with rapidly growing tumors. These headaches are typically worse in the morning, gradually increase in severity as the disease course progresses, and eventually awaken the patient at night. Many patients experience changes in mental status, ranging from irritability to forgetfulness, dementia, lethargy, and coma. These deficits may not be recognized by family members and colleagues until they are substantial. Focal or generalized seizures occur in over one-third of patients, while papilledema is seen in less than 25%. Nausea and vomiting are particularly prominent in infratentorial tumors. Vasomotor and autonomic changes and signs of herniation are late signs of increased intracranial pressure.

Focal manifestations of these tumors depend on their location within the brain. These signs usually develop slowly but occasionally occur with stroke-like rapidity. Patients with tumors in the frontal lobes may be relatively asymptomatic until they present with seizures, altered mentation, apathy, lethargy, or urinary incontinence. Dysphasia and motor weakness suggest involvement of the speech areas and motor cortex in the frontoparietal region. Masses in the temporal lobes are associated with seizures, personality changes, thought disorders, and altered sleep patterns. Contralateral superior quadrant visual field defects can be seen in deep temporal lesions. Many patients with left-sided parietal lesions present with a receptive aphasia and a contralateral hemianopia, while those with right-sided lesions are more likely to manifest spatial disorientation, constructional apraxia, and a left homonomous hemianopia. Brain-stem and cerebellar lesions lead to cranial nerve palsies, abnormalities of coordination, and rapid increases in intracranial pressure and hydrocephalus if cerebrospinal fluid (CSF) flow pathways are compromised.

Evaluation

The clinical presentations described in the previous text provide information about the location but not the histology of an intracranial lesion. Contrast-enhanced computed tomography (CT) and magnetic resonance imaging (MRI) are the primary modalities used to evaluate patients with suspected intracranial tumors. These scans enable detection of most lesions over 0.5 cm in diameter. If no abnormality is found, a repeat scan in 4–6 weeks often is revealing.

The differential diagnosis of enhancing lesions includes abscess, recent cerebral infarction, plaques from multiple sclerosis, and vascular abnormalities with or without hemorrhage. MRI is particularly useful for lesions at the base of the skull, brain stem, and spinal cord.

A histologic diagnosis can be obtained by biopsy or surgical debulking. A biopsy can be performed through an open craniotomy or by CT-guided stereotactic techniques. Surgical debulking of nonresectable lesions may provide a tissue diagnosis, improvement in neurologic signs and symptoms, and a decompression that provides ample time for radiation therapy and chemotherapy to be administered. An attempt to totally resect the tumor is indicated in some patients with primary or metastatic brain tumors. Surgery may also be indicated to alleviate increased intracranial pressure that results from obstruction of CSF flow pathways.

Histology and Management

Primary tumors of the central nervous system are the most common nonhematologic malignancies of childhood. In adults, the incidence of primary brain tumors steadily increases with age. Increases in the age-adjusted incidence of high-grade astrocytomas in the elderly and geographic and familial clusters of these tumors suggest environmental or infectious exposures as possible etiologic factors. A wide variety of cell types within the nervous system are capable of transforming into tumors. Many primary brain tumors are histologically mixed, suggesting that astrocytomas, oligodendrogliomas, and ependymomas arise from a common progenitor cell.

The most common primary brain tumors in adults are astrocytomas. Even if they are diagnosed early, these tumors are virtually never cured with aggressive local therapies such as surgery and radiation therapy. Tumor cells appear to be carried by the flow of extracellular fluid to distant portions of the brain early during the course of the illness. Astrocytomas are classified by grade (I–IV), depending on cellularity, mitoses, endothelial proliferation, and the presence of necrosis. Grade I and II astrocytomas (commonly referred to as astrocytomas) usually do not enhance on CT or MRI scans, are most common in young adults, and are associated with a more favorable prognosis. Grade III (*anaplastic astrocytomas*) and grade IV astrocytomas (*glioblastoma multiforme*) are associated with considerable peritumoral edema and contrast enhancement on neuro-imaging studies.

Prolonged survival of patients with primary brain tumors is associated with young age, good performance status, and low-grade tumors. Surgery provides a definitive diagnosis and reduces tumor burden and mass effect. Radiation therapy prolongs survival, whereas standard chemotherapeutic agents generally provide little added benefit in the treatment of most brain tumors. An exception is in treatment of anaplastic oligodendrogliomas, which may be particularly responsive to chemotherapy.

NEUROLOGIC COMPLICATIONS OF SYSTEMIC CANCER

Epidural Cord Compressions

Epidural metastases are a common and potentially devastating complication of systemic malignancies. About 5–10% of all patients with cancer develop spinal cord or cauda equina compressions. These are most common in patients with lung, breast, prostate, and lymphatic tumors but also occur in patients with leukemias and other solid tumors. Although they are most frequently seen in patients with widespread malignancies, epidural metastases can be the first manifestation of cancer.

Patients with cancer develop epidural cord compressions by two distinct mechanisms (Figure 13.9–1). (1) A vertebral body metastasis can erode through the cortical margin and extend into the epidural space compressing the spinal cord. (2) Alternatively, a paravertebral tumor can traverse the intervertebral foramina to reach the epidural space. Eighty-five percent of spinal cord compressions in patients with solid tumors and 25% of compressions in patients with lymphomas arise from vertebral body metastases. These are usually accompanied by a positive bone scan and abnormal spinal x-rays at the time of diagnosis. Seventy-five percent of patients with lymphomas and 15% of patients with solid tumors develop epidural metastases from a paravertebral lesion. In these patients, bone scans and spinal x-rays can be normal despite advanced neurologic signs and symptoms from epidural cord compressions.

Symptoms and Signs: The symptoms and signs of epidural cord compressions are identical, regardless of the pathogenesis. Pain is the most common symptom, occurring in more than 90% of patients. This usually begins as a local discomfort in the area overlying the tumor. Radicular pain often follows the local pain, but may precede it or occur alone. The discomfort is typically worse at night, may be aggravated by movement or Valsalva maneuvers, and is usually present for weeks to months prior to the development of other neurologic signs and symptoms. The interval between the onset of pain and neurologic disabilities depends on the tumor's growth rate.

Neurologic deficits, such as motor weakness or bowel and bladder dysfunction, result from compression of the spinal cord or cauda equina by tumor or collapsed vertebrae or interruption of the vascular supply to the spinal cord. When these begin, they may progress rapidly, and patients with only pain can become permanently paraplegic in hours or days. For this reason, an epidural cord compression is usually considered a medical emergency.

Diagnostic Studies: Many laboratory tests are available to facilitate the evaluation of patients suspected of having epidural metastases. A definitive diagnosis requires a radiologic study demonstrating a mass impinging on the thecal sac. Myelography or MRI is the procedure of choice. High-

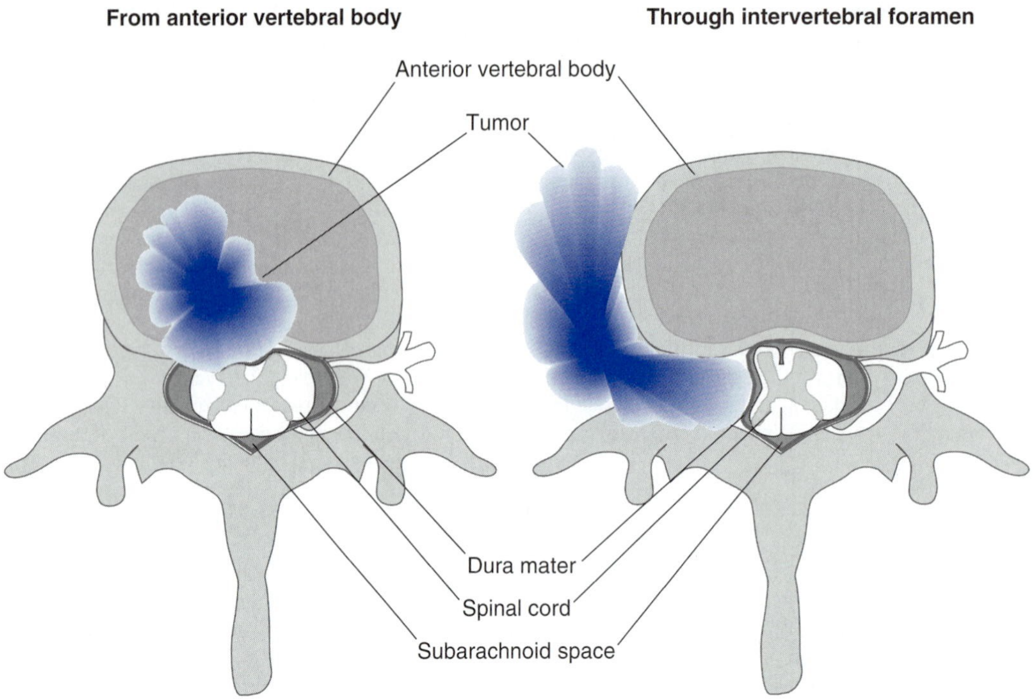

Figure 13.9–1. Mechanisms of epidural cord compression. (Modified, with permission, from Grossman SA: Management of epidural cord compressions. The Johns Hopkins Medical Grand Rounds [slide-tape series] 1983;10[2]:9.)

resolution images of the epidural space, adjacent bone, and subarachnoid space are obtained when intrathecal water-soluble contrast agents are used in conjunction with CT. Excellent resolution is also obtained noninvasively with MRI of the spine. CT scans without intrathecal contrast do not provide direct information on the epidural space but can delineate the extent and location of tumor within vertebrae or the paravertebral region.

Spinal x-rays are exceedingly useful in determining which patients are at high risk for epidural metastases. Bone scans, which may identify very small vertebral lesions, do not predict epidural extension. Examination of CSF is rarely helpful because leptomeningeal involvement by tumor is infrequent with epidural metastases.

Over 75% of patients with cancer, back pain, and a myelopathy or radiculopathy have epidural tumor, and all should be studied with myelography or MRI. Patients with a plexopathy should also be carefully evaluated, since epidural extension of tumor is present in about 30% of these patients. Documentation of the caudal and rostral extent of epidural tumor is needed to treat the entire tumor mass. Spinal x-rays are pivotal in the evaluation of patients with cancer, back pain, and a normal neurologic examination (Figure 13.9–2). If the x-rays reveal vertebral body collapse, pedicle loss, or lytic lesions, a greater than 60% probability exists that a myelogram will demonstrate epidural tumor. Epidural tumor may be present with normal spinal

x-rays in patients with small vertebral body metastases or with paravertebral lesions that extend into the epidural space. A CT scan through symptomatic regions can determine which patients with normal spinal x-rays are at high risk for epidural extension of their tumors.

Management: The responsiveness of the tumor to radiation and the patient's neurologic status are important factors associated with treatment outcomes. Treatment of ambulatory patients usually results in excellent pain relief and preservation of neurologic function. Unfortunately, most patients with epidural tumor are incontinent and unable to walk by the time the diagnosis is established. These neurologic disabilities usually do not reverse even with appropriate therapy.

Corticosteroids, radiation therapy, surgery, and chemotherapy all have roles in the treatment of epidural metastases. Glucocorticoids can provide excellent pain relief and improve or stabilize the patient's neurologic status while antineoplastic therapy is initiated. Radiation is the mainstay of therapy for most patients, whereas surgery is usually reserved for patients with an unestablished diagnosis, neurologic progression during radiation therapy, recurrence in a previously irradiated area, or spinal instability. Chemotherapy can be used in patients with tumors responsive to these agents when radiation and surgery are not feasible.

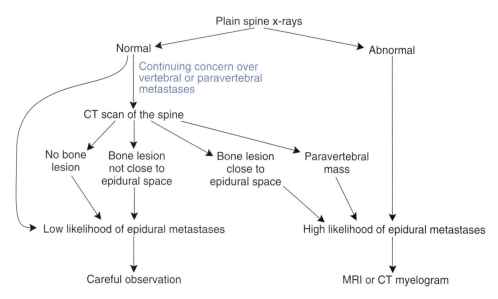

Figure 13.9–2. Evaluation of patients with cancer, back pain, and a normal neurologic exam. A patient with normal spine x-rays is considered to be at low risk for epidural metastases if the physician has no clinical concern that the plain films have missed a small vertebral body lesion or a paravertebral mass that could compress the epidural cord. (Reproduced, with permission, from Grossman SA, Lossignol D: Early diagnosis and treatment of epidural metastases. Medical Rounds 1989;2[4]:175.)

Brain Metastases

Intracranial metastases occur in about 25% of all cancer patients and represent the most common neoplasms in the brain. Most reach the brain by hematogenous routes. Although melanoma has the greatest propensity to spread to the brain, breast and lung cancers—because of their prevalence—represent the most common sources of brain metastases. Lung, gastrointestinal, and urinary tract tumors account for 80% of brain metastases in men, whereas breast, lung, and gastrointestinal tumors and melanoma account for 80% in women. About 80% of parenchymal metastases are supratentorial and 15% are cerebellar. Clinical and autopsy studies have shown that most patients have multiple rather than single metastases, and over 50% of patients with brain metastases also have lung lesions. Eighty percent of brain metastases occur in patients with a known antecedent primary tumor, and the remainder are diagnosed at the same time that the systemic tumor is identified (synchronous) or while the primary tumor remains occult.

Symptoms and Signs: Symptoms and signs in patients with brain metastases are not notably different from those in patients with other intracranial mass lesions. Headache, weakness, cognitive or affective changes, and seizures are the most common presenting symptoms. CT and MRI usually demonstrate a contrast-enhancing lesion with associated peritumoral edema and mass effect.

The weakness and alterations in cognitive function associated with brain metastases have a disproportionate effect on quality of life, and treatment is indicated in virtually all patients to prevent or repair serious neurologic dysfunction.

Management: Glucocorticoids repair the blood-brain barrier dysfunction associated with brain metastases and can result in dramatic symptomatic improvement in 24–72 hours. Dexamethasone is commonly prescribed at doses of 16 mg daily, but some patients who do not improve on this dosage respond to dosages as high as 100 mg/day. Radiation therapy is generally used in all patients with brain metastases. Because of the high incidence of multiple gross or microscopic intraparenchymal tumor foci, radiation therapy is usually administered to the whole brain. Many dose fractionation schedules have been studied. Shorter treatment programs appear to have equal efficacy but less expense and inconvenience, and are often indicated in this patient population.

Brachytherapy and stereotactic radiosurgery, which provide high doses of radiation to localized regions of the brain, can be useful in selected patients. Surgery is indicated to obtain a pathologic diagnosis, decompress a mass lesion, or relieve an obstruction to the flow of CSF. Patients with solitary brain metastases, limited systemic disease, a significant interval from the diagnosis of the primary tumor to development of brain metastases, and good performance status should be considered for surgical resection followed by radiation therapy. Studies suggest that this approach improves neurologic status and survival in such patients. Chemotherapy can also be beneficial in the treatment of brain metastases in responsive neoplasms.

The disrupted blood-brain barrier in the region of the intraparenchymal lesions permits these agents to enter the brain metastases. Regimens that are effective for the systemic tumor should be considered in the treatment of the brain metastases.

Neoplastic Meningitis

Multifocal seeding of the leptomeninges by malignant cells is referred to as neoplastic meningitis. Although they were once thought to be rare and were uncommonly diagnosed before death, metastases to the leptomeninges are being noted more frequently. This probably results from a heightened index of suspicion, better diagnostic tests, and improved therapy for systemic metastases. Leptomeningeal metastases occur most commonly in patients with known and progressive systemic cancer. Autopsy studies demonstrate that 20% of patients with neurologic complications from cancer have meningeal involvement. In some malignancies, such as small cell lung cancer and melanoma, nearly 20% of patients develop clinical evidence of leptomeningeal involvement, whereas in those with other malignancies this is rare.

Pathophysiology: Malignant cells gain access to the subarachnoid space by migration through arachnoid vessels or the choroid plexus, by extension from preexisting tumors in the central nervous system, or by following nerve roots. After the tumor reaches the meninges, it spreads along the surface of the brain and spinal cord and sheds cells that are carried by the flow of CSF to distant regions of the central nervous system. This results in the development of new metastatic deposits along the meningeal surface, which commonly involve the basilar cisterns, posterior fossa, and cauda equina.

Diagnosis: A high index of suspicion is required to make an early diagnosis of leptomeningeal involvement. Obstruction of normal CSF flow pathways by focal tumor deposits can result in signs and symptoms of increased intracranial pressure. Parenchymal invasion, direct involvement of nerves traversing the subarachnoid space, and occlusion of penetrating pial blood vessels produce focal neurologic abnormalities or seizures. Alternatively, interference with normal central nervous system metabolism, which results in a diffuse encephalopathy, may be the primary presenting syndrome. Headache, changes in mental status, cranial nerve palsies, back or radicular pain, incontinence, lower motor neuron weakness, and sensory abnormalities are common findings at presentation. The diagnosis should be considered when the patient's signs and symptoms suggest involvement of multiple anatomic sites in the central nervous system.

Examination of the CSF is the most useful laboratory test for the diagnosis of neoplastic meningitis. A completely normal lumbar puncture is distinctly uncommon in patients with leptomeningeal metastases. Elevations in opening pressure and CSF protein, reductions in CSF glucose, and a pleocytosis are nonspecific abnormalities that

can be associated with neoplastic meningitis. Positive CSF cytology is found in about 50% of patients with this disorder on the initial lumbar puncture and in 85% after three samplings of CSF. Other CSF markers are of limited usefulness. Contrast-enhanced CT or MRI brain scans may reveal multiple subarachnoid masses, contrast enhancement of the basilar cisterns or cortical convexities, or hydrocephalus without an apparent mass lesion.

Management: Treatment of neoplastic meningitis is designed to improve or stabilize neurologic status and to prolong survival. Without therapy, the median survival is 4–6 weeks, and death usually results from progressive neurologic dysfunction. In general, fixed neurologic deficits, such as cranial nerve palsies, do not resolve with therapy, whereas an encephalopathy may respond dramatically. Therapy must encompass the entire central nervous system because tumor cells are disseminated throughout the neuraxis. Standard therapy has evolved to include radiation to sites of bulk and symptomatic disease, intrathecal chemotherapy, and optimal treatment of systemic disease. With prompt and appropriate therapy, local control of the leptomeningeal symptoms is likely, and patients are more apt to die from systemic than from leptomeningeal tumor progression.

Patients who are most likely to benefit from aggressive treatment of neoplastic meningitis are those with good performance status, few fixed neurologic deficits, and either no evidence of systemic tumor or slowly progressive systemic cancer that is likely to respond to treatment.

CANCER PAIN

About 75% of patients with cancer require narcotic analgesics to control pain. Pain is the earliest symptom that prompts many patients to seek medical attention. In advanced cancer, pain results from direct tumor involvement of bones, neural structures, soft tissues, or hollow viscera. It also occurs with diagnostic procedures and with a variety of antineoplastic therapies (Table 13.9–1).

Table 13.9–1. Cancer pain syndromes.

Associated with direct tumor involvement
Invasion of bone
Invasion of mucous membranes
Invasion or compression of nerves
Invasion or compression of viscera
Invasion or compression of blood vessels

Associated with cancer therapy
Postoperative pain syndromes
Postchemotherapy pain syndromes
Postradiation pain syndromes

Associated with cancer
Paraneoplastic syndromes
Myofacial pain syndromes
Debility syndromes

Numerous studies document the undertreatment of patients with pain. About 70% of cancer patients receive inadequate treatment for their pain in spite of evidence suggesting that such pain can be well controlled using conventional approaches. Many reasons for these therapeutic inadequacies have been proposed. Table 13.9–2 provides general guidelines for the effective management of cancer pain.

Defining Pain Intensity: The tendency for clinicians to treat "cancer pain" as a unique entity without further defining the cause of the discomfort can lead to inappropriate treatment. Studies suggest that patients and their health care providers often have divergent impressions of the amount of pain that patients experience. However, since pain is an entirely subjective experience and its intensity can be sensed only by the patient, physicians and nurses must carefully ascertain pain intensity from patients, accept patient reports of pain, and treat accordingly. Many medical personnel are excessively concerned about narcotic tolerance, toxicities, and addiction. Lack of knowledge regarding narcotic equivalencies and pharma-

Table 13.9–2. Guidelines for effective treatment of cancer pain.

View relief of pain as an important responsibility
Determine the cause of a patient's pain and apply specific therapy when possible
Continually solicit the patient's assessment of the severity of pain and treat accordingly; if possible, allow the patient to control the dispensing of analgesia
Avoid undue concerns about opiate addiction, tolerance, and toxicities
Understand basic opiate pharmacology
Avoid undue concern over drug regulatory agency investigation for opiate prescribing

cology also hampers effective pain treatment (Figure 13.9–3). In addition, increased federal and state drug enforcement initiatives have led some physicians to perceive themselves at risk for investigation for prescribing narcotic analgesics to cancer patients.

Management: Narcotic analgesics are the most commonly prescribed treatment for cancer pain. The World Health Organization has proposed an "analgesic ladder,"

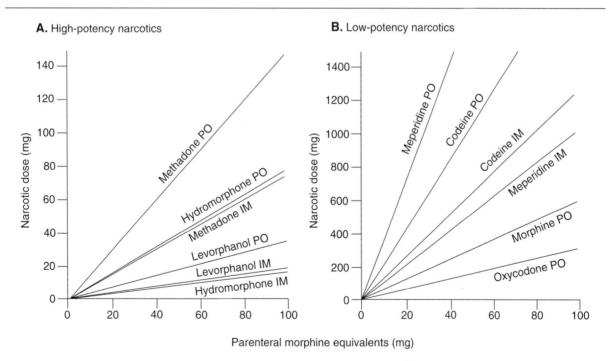

Figure 13.9–3. Narcotic conversion nomogram for high-potency narcotics (**A**) and low-potency narcotics (**B**). The nomogram is designed to facilitate the conversion from one narcotic analgesic (or route of administration) to an approximately equal dose of another. It incorporates generally accepted information on the pharmacology of narcotics, but does not take into account chronic dosing, alterations in absorption, or abnormalities of renal and hepatic function that may affect the half-life of some narcotics. Considerable controversy surrounds many of the oral:parenteral conversion ratios. (For example, values for morphine range from 6:1 to 2:1. This nomogram uses a 6:1 ratio.) Intravenous, intramuscular, and subcutaneous doses of narcotic analgesics are considered equivalent. For these reasons, the nomogram should be used only to estimate dose equivalency. It is often easiest to make conversions using total milligrams of drug administered per day. (Reproduced, with permission, from Grossman SA, Sheidler VR: An aid to prescribing narcotics for the relief of cancer pain. World Health Forum 1987;8:525.)

which begins with nonopiates or mild analgesics (aspirin or acetaminophen) for mild pain. The weak opiates (codeine, oxycodone, propoxyphene) are added for moderate pain not controlled by mild analgesics. In patients with severe pain, strong opiates (morphine and related compounds) are recommended alone or with other agents. Proper application of this therapeutic strategy will control pain in nearly 85% of patients with cancer pain. In general, opiates with short half-lives are used initially to rapidly escalate doses and control pain. Longer-acting agents, such as the sustained-release oral morphine preparations, can be substituted later to simplify drug administration schedules.

Although most patients with cancer pain can be successfully managed with oral narcotics, more sophisticated techniques are available. Patient-controlled analgesia allows patients to titrate their pain relief and narcotic side effects. Continuous intravenous and subcutaneous opiate infusions minimize fluctuations in drug levels and can yield improved analgesia with fewer side effects. Narcotics have also been administered into epidural, subarachnoid, and intraventricular sites to minimize their systemic toxicities. These approaches require special catheters and delivery pumps but can be useful in carefully selected patients. A potent, lipid-soluble narcotic, fentanyl, has been introduced as a transdermal patch for patients with cancer pain. The use of these high technology approaches to the treatment of cancer pain are often invasive and costly and are not indicated until more conventional approaches have had an adequate trial.

Other pharmacologic agents, including nonsteroidal anti-inflammatory agents, glucocorticoids, antidepressants, anticonvulsants, anxiolytics, phenothiazines, and amphetamines can be useful adjuncts in the treatment of cancer pain. Transcutaneous nerve stimulation, local anesthetic and neurolytic blocks, and neuro-ablative procedures also provide excellent palliation in some patients. Biofeedback, hypnosis, relaxation, and imagery should be considered in the therapeutic armamentarium.

Patients with cancer pain can also greatly benefit from conventional antineoplastic therapies. For example, 90% of patients treated with radiation therapy for symptomatic bone metastases have significant improvement in pain and over 50% experience complete pain relief. Surgery is likely to provide optimal palliation for a pathologic fracture or an obstructed viscus, and tumor reduction from effective chemotherapy can also provide dramatic pain relief.

SUMMARY

▶ Central nervous system tumors are usually metastatic and are becoming more common as primary tumors are better controlled.

▶ Seizures, weakness, incontinence, headache, and changes in cognitive function are frequent presentations.

▶ A high index of suspicion and early diagnosis and treatment optimize comfort, preservation of neurologic function, and sometimes even survival in these patients.

▶ Health care providers should become skilled in the management of cancer pain so that no patient suffers unrelieved discomfort.

SUGGESTED READING

Foley KM: Controversies in cancer pain: Medical perspectives. Cancer 1989;63:2257.

Gilbert MR, Grossman SA: The incidence and nature of neurologic problems in patients with solid tumors. Am J Med 1986; 81:951.

Grossman SA, Moynihan TJ: Neoplastic meningitis. Neurol Clin North Am 1991;9:843.

Grossman SA et al: Correlation of patient and caregiver ratings of cancer pain. J Pain Symptom Manage 1991;6:53.

Lesser GJ, Grossman SA: The chemotherapy of adult primary brain tumors. Cancer Treat Rev 1993;19:261.

13.10

Diseases of the Spine and Spinal Cord

James N. Campbell, MD

Any bony disease can lead to pain and loss of mobility. Bony diseases of the spine, however, can cause further dysfunction because of their effects on the spinal cord and nerve roots. As part of the central nervous system, the spinal cord is subject to many of the diseases that affect the brain. Thus, patients with diseases of the spine or spinal cord can present not only with pain and loss of mobility but with neurologic dysfunction. Because many patients present to their internist with these disorders, physicians must be familiar with them.

PRINCIPLES OF LOCALIZATION

A satisfying aspect of assessing spinal cord disease is that, in a high percentage of patients, the history and physical examination tell the clinician where the disease is located, and often the nature of the disease. The physician must be able to recognize the sequelae of injury to different parts of the spinal cord and to each of the nerve roots.

Upper versus Lower Motor Lesions

The major motor pathway for voluntary control of movement in the arms and legs is the corticospinal tract, located in the dorsolateral portion of the spinal cord. Below the foramen magnum, the tract is ipsilateral to the extremity in question. The corticospinal tract terminates on the anterior horn cells, which in turn give rise to motor axons of the nerve roots and peripheral nerves. The corticospinal tract and associated pathways exert a net inhibitory effect on the anterior horn cells and deep tendon reflexes. Thus, lesions of the spinal cord that affect motor function lead to spasticity and an increase in the deep tendon reflexes. In contrast, lower motor neuron lesions, caused by damage to the anterior horn cells and the associated peripheral nerve fibers, lead to flaccid loss of motor control.

The motor exam readily reveals whether the patient has an upper or lower motor neuron problem (Table 13.10–1). In upper motor neuron disorders, patients have an increase in muscle tone. Efforts to move the joints passively are met with resistance. The gait may look wide-based and

scissoring. The more severe the lesion, the greater the reflexes. The patient may have clonus at the ankle (alternating plantar flexion and relaxation evoked by abrupt dorsiflexion of the foot) and ultimately Babinski's sign (dorsiflexion of the great toe and fanning of the remaining toes, evoked by stroking the plantar surface of the foot). The muscle remains innervated by the anterior horn cells, so there is little or no muscle atrophy.

With lower motor lesions, the patient's lack of voluntary control of muscles is associated with decreased muscle resistance on passive motion. Reflexes are decreased or absent. Early on, the patient may have fasciculations (visible slight local muscle contractions). With time, the muscle atrophies.

Thus, the motor exam is essential in helping to define the level of spinal column lesions. The spinal cord ends at the L1 spinal column level. Lesions above L1 lead to a spastic paralysis of the legs, and lesions below L1 lead to a flaccid paralysis.

The Sensory Examination

Patients develop what is termed a "sensory level" at the position where the spinal cord is severed. A patient whose spinal cord is severed at T6 (sixth thoracic vertebra) has a T6 sensory level. To determine the sensory level at the bedside, the examiner strokes a pin down the trunk on both sides, front, and back (then disposes of the pin). The physician should recall that the area just below the clavicle is innervated by the cervical plexus and corresponds to dermatomal levels C3–4. Therefore, a patient who has sensation in this area may still have a lower cervical spinal cord injury.

Determination of Level of Injury

Lesions at the thoracolumbar junction may injure the conus medullaris (terminal part of the spinal cord). Here, in addition to doing the usual motor and sensory exam, the physician should check the anal wink reflex—a contraction of the external anal sphincter when the anus is stroked with a pin. This reflex distinguishes whether lesions are above (when reflex is present) or below (when reflex is

871

Table 13.10–1. Characteristics of upper and lower motor neuron lesions.

	Upper Motor Lesions	Lower Motor Lesions
Reflexes	Increased	Decreased
Atrophy	No	Yes
Muscle tone	Spastic	Flaccid
Fasciculations	No	Yes

absent) the termination of the conus medullaris. Urinary difficulties are often the earliest manifestation of cauda equina compression, particularly if the lesion is near the conus medullaris.

When the hands or arms are involved in the paralysis along with the legs, the patient is said to be quadriplegic (a patient with some function in the legs is said to be quadriparetic). Patients are categorized according to the most rostral paralyzed motor root. Thus, a patient with paralyzed legs and intrinsic hand muscles has a C8 quadriplegia; a patient with paralyzed triceps and wrist extensors has a C7 quadriplegia.

Injuries or diseases of the spinal cord may affect only a portion of its width rather than the entire structure. There are two common forms of partial cord dysfunction: Brown-Séquard's syndrome and central cord syndrome. All patients with hemiparesis require a careful sensory exam to distinguish these conditions.

Brown-Séquard's Syndrome: Loss of function on one side of the spinal cord leads to Brown-Séquard's syndrome. This is a distinctive entity in which the patient loses pain and temperature sensation on the side opposite the spinal cord lesion, but develops paralysis ipsilateral to the lesion. Tactile sensibility remains intact in the region where pain and temperature sensibility is lost. This condition is termed a *dissociated sensory loss.*

The primary afferent fibers concerned with pain and temperature sensation ascend several levels in Lissauer's tract (a tract posterolateral in the spinal cord) before synapsing with the dorsal horn neurons that give rise to the spinothalamic tract. Thus, the spinal cord lesion is several segments above the level where the patient loses pain and temperature sensation.

Central Cord Syndrome: Central cord lesions also produce distinctive neurologic problems. These lesions may arise from acute trauma, tumors, or syringomyelia (see "Tumors" below). Anterior horn cell dysfunction at the level of the lesion leads to segmental loss of motor function with a lower motor neuron pattern of deficit. For example, a patient with a central cord lesion at the cervical spinal cord level typically has weakness in the hands but none in the legs. Because the spinothalamic tracts cross the midline within the core of the spinal cord, they are reliably affected by central lesions. Thus, the patient has a dissociated sensory loss at segments in the region of the lesion. With a lesion of the cervical spinal cord, the patient loses both pain and temperature function in the hand (especially on the ulnar side), but retains proprioception, touch, and vibratory sense. Pain and temperature sensation in the legs is unaffected.

Other Patterns of Spinal Cord Dysfunction: Additional patterns of spinal cord dysfunction accompany specific diseases. For example, disorders such as Guillain-Barré syndrome and polio selectively affect the anterior horn cells; the patient has a flaccid paralysis (lower motor neuron) in the affected myotomes, with little or no sensory involvement. Amyotrophic lateral sclerosis (ALS) (Chapter 13.12) involves the anterior horn cells and the corticospinal tract, leading to a pattern of mixed upper and lower motor neuron signs, again without sensory symptoms.

Radicular Disease

The passage of nerve roots from the thecal sac to the neural foramina is a precarious one. This is primarily because of the narrowness of the neural foramina and the tendency of compressive lesions such as bone spurs and disk prolapse to compromise the passage further. Compression of a nerve root, as by a herniated disk, leads to a radiculopathy. The most common radiculopathies in the cervical area involve the fifth, sixth, and seventh nerve roots (Table 13.10–2). In the lumbar spine, the most common sites are the fourth and fifth lumbar roots and the first sacral root.

Remembering the innervation of the muscles helps in diagnosing root syndromes. Most muscles are innervated by more than one root. Nevertheless, the most important innervation to the shoulder muscles is from the C5 root, and the muscles that move the elbow get primary innervation from the C6 root. The most important innervation of the wrist muscles and triceps muscle is from the C7 root, and the intrinsic muscles of the hand are innervated by the C8 and T1 roots. Leg innervation is also easy to remember. The hip flexors derive innervation from L2-3. The knee extensors are innervated by L4. Ankle dorsiflexion is L5 and ankle plantar flexion is S1.

Skin is also innervated by more than one root. In fact, findings of dense sensory loss (cutaneous anesthesia) can-

Table 13.10–2. Functional impairment caused by radiculopathy.

Nerve Root Affected	Site of Weakness
C5	Shoulder abduction
C6	Elbow flexion
C7	Elbow extension, wrist flexion and extension, hand grip
C8	Hand grip, hand intrinsic muscles
L2-3	Hip flexion
L5-S1	Hip extension
L3-4	Knee extension
L4-5	Knee flexion, ankle dorsiflexion
L5-S1	Ankle plantar flexion

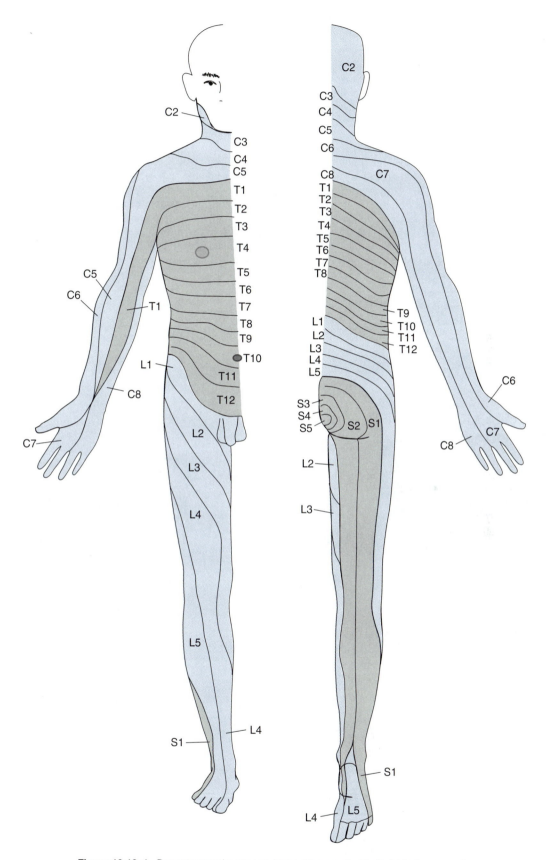

Figure 13.10–1. Dermatomes: the sensory innervation supplied by individual nerve roots.

873

not be explained by a lesion of a single nerve root, and typically denote more distal peripheral nerve involvement. Bearing this in mind, the physician must recall the following general sensory distributions (Figure 13.10–1). The C6 root innervates the thumb and index finger. The C7 root innervates the index, middle, and ring fingers. The C8 root innervates the ring and little fingers. The T4 root innervates the nipple; T10 innervates the umbilicus. The L5 root innervates the top of the foot, and S1 innervates the side of the foot.

To understand radicular disease, the physician must keep in mind some confusing anatomic relationships. The first cervical root exits above C1 (the atlas). Thus, in the cervical area, the name of the nerve root is based on the vertebra just below, and a disk herniation affects the nerve root at that level. For example, the sixth nerve root exits between the fifth and sixth cervical vertebrae and may be affected by any mass lesion, such as a herniated disk, at the C5–6 level (Figure 13.10–2).

This relationship changes at the cervicothoracic junc-tion because there are eight cervical roots (the eighth cervical root exits between C7 and T1). The root affected by a disk herniation at the T6–7 junction is the T6 root, not T7. This relationship persists throughout the lumbar spine. Accordingly, the fifth lumbar root exits between the fifth lumbar vertebra and the sacrum.

However, the lumbar vertebrae are much taller than the thoracic vertebrae. The nerve root exits the spinal canal just beneath the pedicle, and as it passes distally the nerve root is very far lateral by the time it is at the level of the disk. Thus, a herniated disk in the lumbar area typically has no effect on the nerve root that passes through the neural foramen at that level; instead, the nerve root below is affected. A herniated disk at L4–5 affects the L5 root, and a herniated disk at L5-S1 affects the S1 root. In the lumbar area, therefore, the name of the nerve root is based on the vertebra above, but the root affected (as in the cervical area) has the same name as the vertebra below.

Table 13.10–3 summarizes the features of the most common radiculopathies.

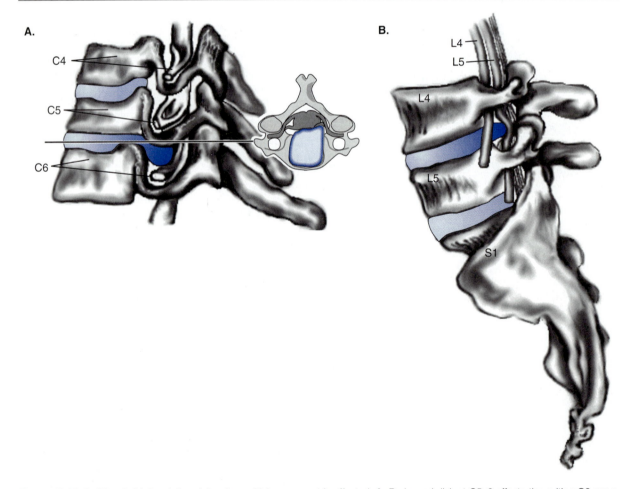

Figure 13.10–2. Site of disk herniation determines which nerve root is affected. **A:** Prolapsed disk at C5–6 affects the exiting C6 nerve root. **B:** Prolapsed disk at L4–5 affects the L5 nerve root, even though the L5 root exits the spine between L5 and S1.

Table 13.10–3. Common nerve root lesions.

Nerve Root	Sensory Supply	Sensory Loss	Area of Pain	Reflex Arc	Motor Deficit
C5	Lateral border of upper arm	Lateral border of upper arm	Lateral border of upper arm, medial scapular border	Biceps jerk	Deltoid, supraspinatus, infraspinatus, rhomboids
C6	Lateral forearm; hand, including thumb	Lateral forearm; hand, including thumb	Lateral forearm; hand, especially thumb and index finger	Supinator jerk	Biceps, brachioradialis, brachialis, pronator teres, supinator
C7	Over triceps, midforearm, and middle finger	Middle fingers	Middle fingers and medial scapular border	Triceps jerk	Latissimus dorsi, pectoralis major, triceps, wrist extensors, wrist flexors
C8	Medial forearm; hand, including little finger	Medial forearm; hand, including little finger	Medial forearm; hand, including little finger	Finger jerk	Finger flexors, finger extensors, flexor carpi, ulnaris (thenar muscles in some patients)
L4	Across knee to medial malleolus	Medial leg	Down to medial malleolus	Knee jerk	Inversion of the foot
L5	Side of leg to dorsum and sole of foot	Dorsum of foot	Back of thigh, lateral calf, dorsum of foot	None	Dorsiflexion of toes and foot
S1	Behind lateral malleolus to lateral foot	Behind lateral malleolus	Back of thigh, back of calf, lateral foot	Ankle jerk	Plantar flexion and eversion of foot

Modified and reproduced, with permission, from Patten J: *Neurological Differential Diagnosis.* Springer-Verlag, 1977.

The physician must often distinguish between lesions of the nerve root and lesions of the peripheral nerve more distally. For example, does a patient with a foot drop have an L5 radiculopathy or a lesion of the common peroneal nerve? The following general principles can aid in making these kinds of distinctions. Most muscles are innervated by more than one nerve root. A given area of skin typically has representation in more than two roots. Thus, if a single root is cut, patients are unlikely to have a dense sensory or motor deficit. But the deficit becomes more profound if the lesion is more distal. Cutting the C7 nerve root causes a trivial amount of wrist weakness, but cutting the radial nerve prevents wrist extension. Thus, a profound sensory and motor deficit in one extremity suggests a peripheral nerve lesion rather than a root lesion.

The compound sensory nerve action potential, obtained by recording the potential evoked by stimulation of a sensory nerve, also helps to distinguish between nerve root and peripheral nerve disorders. This potential, recorded as part of nerve conduction studies, is normal only if the nerve fibers are functionally connected to the cell body in the dorsal root ganglion. Cutting the nerve root proximal to the dorsal root ganglion leaves the sensory nerve action potential intact. But cutting the peripheral nerve eliminates the sensory nerve action potential, which is recorded distally. Most radiculopathies that arise from disease in the spinal canal affect the nerve root proximal to the dorsal root ganglion. A herniated disk, for example, rarely affects the sensory action potential.

Myelopathy Caused by Mass Lesions

When spinal cord function is disrupted caudal to a particular level, such as T4, the physician should consider the possibility of a mass lesion. A mass lesion at T4 is suggested by weakness in the legs and decreased sensation below the level of the nipples. A mass lesion may affect the spinal cord or cauda equina from one of three sites: extradural, intradural-extramedullary, or intradural-intramedullary (Chapter 13.9).

When a patient presents with a myelopathy (literally, a disorder of the spinal cord), the physician should first try to determine a level. Having identified the involved region of spinal cord, the physician orders magnetic resonance imaging (MRI) of the area to determine whether the myelopathy results from a mass lesion and to determine what compartment is affected.

Then the differential diagnosis becomes easy (Table 13.10–4). The most important extradural diseases that affect the spinal column are spondylosis and disk disease, metastatic cancer, and, much less frequently, epidural abscess. The most important intradural-extramedullary diseases are tumors; meningiomas and neurofibromas are most common, although in a patient with another central nervous system malignancy, metastatic disease would be most likely. A multitude of lesions can affect the spinal cord itself (intradural-intramedullary) (see below). However, if consideration is limited to mass lesions, the possible diagnoses are few. The most common offenders are tumors (most often a glioma, ependymoma, or hemangioblastoma) and syrinx. Rarely, the culprit is an abscess or sarcoid.

Although radiographic studies determine in which of the three compartments a mass is located, the neurologic exam also provides strong hints. Extradural compression of the spinal cord by a midline lesion leads to a symmetric spastic paresis. Intradural-extramedullary lesions often present from one side and so produce a Brown-Séquard's syndrome and segmental signs. Intramedullary lesions present with a central cord syndrome.

Table 13.10–4. Differential diagnosis of mass lesions affecting the spinal cord.

Extradural
Spondylosis and disk disease
Metastases
Epidural abscess

Intradural-extramedullary
Meningioma
Neurofibroma

Intradural-intramedullary
Glioma
Ependymoma
Hemangioblastoma
Syrinx

SPECIFIC DISEASES OF THE SPINE AND ASSOCIATED STRUCTURES

Diseases of the spinal axis may be distinguished by whether the disorder arises in the spine or the nervous system.

Degenerative Disorders of the Spine

Degenerative disorders of the spine include some of the most common problems in medicine. In a sense, the spine serves three roles: to protect the nervous system, to provide structural support, and to confer flexibility. These roles are to some extent at odds with one another. A completely rigid spine might serve the first two goals, but at complete sacrifice of the third. Too much bone pursuant to the second goal (eg, formation of bony spurs to compensate for disk degeneration) may lead to compression of the nervous system and thus be at odds with the first goal.

Spondylosis: Spondylosis is the most common degenerative disorder of the spinal axis and is increasingly prevalent with age (Figure 13.10–3). Spondylosis is a triad of degenerative changes: disk degeneration (usually with some protrusion), ligament hypertrophy, and formation of bone spurs. These changes most often affect two areas of the spine that are mechanically precarious—the lower cervical spine and the lower lumbar spine. With age, disks degenerate, putting stress on contiguous structures, in particular the ligaments and facet joints. The ligaments, facet joints, and structures surrounding the disk respond to the added stress by undergoing hypertrophy. The ultimate consequence is spinal stenosis, with compression of the thecal sac and nerve roots.

Spondylosis is the most common cause of extradural compression. Patients may present with axial pain in the neck or low back, and many have radicular pain. Cervical stenosis can cause myelopathy, and lumbar stenosis can cause a cauda equina syndrome (neurologic dysfunction produced by bilateral involvement of the lumbar and sacral nerve roots).

The neurologic exam is not good for detecting lumbar spinal stenosis. The first abnormality is a decrease in the ankle jerk reflex, but this happens late in the disease. A common symptom is neurogenic claudication. As with vascular claudication, pain develops in the legs as the patient walks. Most patients with pain also complain of weakness. Patients may say that their legs give out after they walk a specific distance.

Sometimes vascular claudication and neurogenic claudication present similarly. Several features suggest neurogenic claudication: First, patients note that they can walk farther if they lean forward. Second, many patients develop weakness at the same time as pain, and weakness may be their chief symptom. Third, back pain favors a neurogenic mechanism. Fourth, patients develop pain when both standing and walking. One feature suggests vascular claudication: Only with vascular claudication do the symptoms start sooner when patients walk up an incline than when they walk on level ground. When the distinction remains ambiguous, it may be clarified by noninvasive vascular tests and imaging studies of the spine.

Spondylolysis (see Figure 13.10–3) is a particular structural weakness in the lumbar spine, not to be confused with spondylosis. Spondylolysis is a defect in the pars interarticularis. Four spinal elements converge on the pedicle: the transverse process, the lamina, and the inferior and superior articular processes. Significant mechanical forces converge on the junction between the inferior articular process and the pedicle. A defect here usually results from trauma or repeated stress or is a complication of surgical laminectomy. Bilateral pars defects (bilateral spondylolysis) significantly weaken the spine and can ultimately lead to *spondylolisthesis* in which the vertebra above slips forward in relation to the vertebra below (see Figure 13.10–3). Spondylolisthesis can also develop simply from loss of overall structural stability of the spine. Because this is a complication of degenerative disease, it is called *degenerative spondylolisthesis*. Spondylolisthesis can be associated with severe pain and can lead to cauda equina and nerve root compression.

Acute Disk Herniation: Spondylosis develops insidiously over years. But a disk can rupture acutely into the spinal canal with—or, commonly, without—coincident spondylosis. A weakness develops in the annulus that normally contains the disk in the intervertebral space, and the disk material either protrudes through this defect into the spinal canal or forces the weakened annulus against the thecal sac or nerve root. If the disk ruptures laterally, it produces an acute monoradiculopathy. If the disk ruptures in the midline, the patient may present with sudden onset of a myelopathy in the cervical area or a cauda equina syndrome in the lumbar area.

Acute disk rupture generally causes severe pain. In the cervical area, many patients have pain in the neck and arm according to the radiculopathy. The C5, C6, and C7 roots are most commonly involved. In the lumbar area, patients may have back pain along with pain in the leg, again according to the root involvement. The L5 and S1 roots are most commonly involved; impingement on these struc-

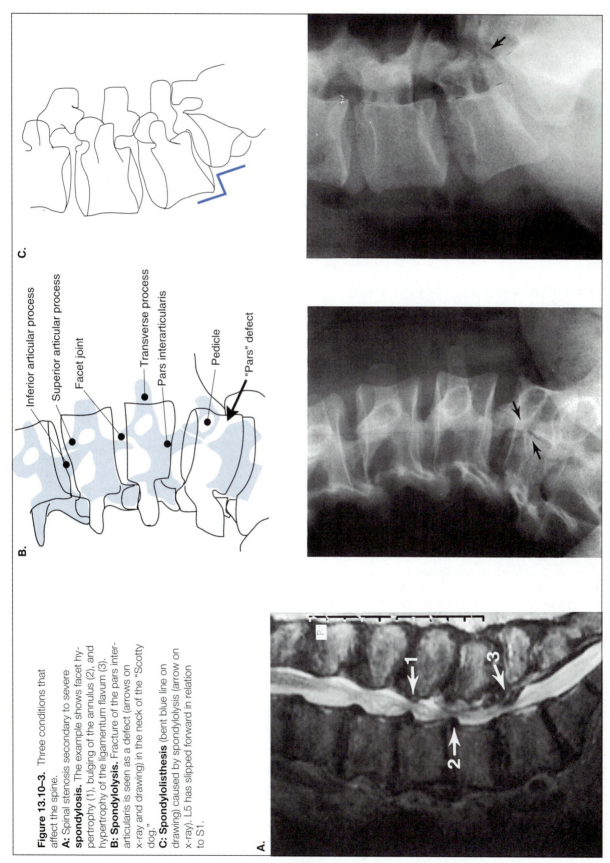

Figure 13.10–3. Three conditions that affect the spine.

A: Spinal stenosis secondary to severe **spondylosis.** The example shows facet hypertrophy (1), bulging of the annulus (2), and hypertrophy of the ligamentum flavum (3).

B: Spondylolysis. Fracture of the pars interarticularis is seen as a defect (arrows on x-ray and drawing) in the neck of the "Scotty dog."

C: Spondylolisthesis (bent blue line on drawing) caused by spondylolysis (arrow on x-ray). L5 has slipped forward in relation to S1.

Inferior articular process
Superior articular process
Facet joint
Transverse process
Pars interarticularis
Pedicle
"Pars" defect

877

tures often causes sciatica (pain radiating down the posterior or posterolateral side of the leg to the foot).

Physical exam can help to determine the neurologic involvement. For the lumbar area, the most useful muscles to examine are the extensor hallucis longus (extensor of the great toe), the extensor digitorum brevis (a small, easily visualized muscle on the dorsolateral side of the foot that extends the digits), and the toe flexors. Patients with a ruptured disk can contract these muscles without increasing their back and leg pain. The more proximal muscles are more difficult to examine because contraction may increase pain. Weakness that reflects decreased effort by the patient so as to avoid pain is called *antalgic weakness.*

Provocative maneuvers greatly aid diagnosis. Patients with symptomatic cervical disease have a worsening of pain if they hyperextend their neck or tilt it toward the symptomatic side. A useful maneuver for a ruptured L4-5 or L5-S1 disk is the straight leg raising test: When the leg is flexed at the hip with the knee kept straight, the roots of the sacral plexus are brought forward against the disk. If the disk is herniated, the patient has pain. The examiner records how many degrees of flexion are needed to reproduce the symptoms; for example, pain with hip flexion up to 45 degrees strongly suggests lumbar disk herniation. As a useful control, hip flexion with a flexed knee does not cause pain in a patient with disk herniation, but might in a patient with hip disease.

Inflammatory Disorders

Infections can affect the spine, meninges, or spinal cord itself. Infection of the meninges (meningitis) is covered in Chapter 8.3. The infections most likely to affect the spinal cord directly include such viral syndromes as poliomyelitis, coxsackievirus, rabies, and herpes zoster. In rare patients, the spinal cord is the site of a bacterial abscess or tuberculoma.

Infectious Disorders of the Spine: Epidural abscess, diskitis, and osteomyelitis all can affect the spine. These are challenging disorders to diagnose and treat. The disk space is a particularly prevalent focus for bacterial infection. Diskitis resembles spinal metastases in that both destroy bone; however, tumor preferentially involves the vertebral body, whereas infection tends to involve the disk space. An exception is tuberculosis of the spine (Pott's disease), which typically concentrates around the disk and presents with involvement of several vertebral bodies.

The combination of severe pain, an elevated erythrocyte sedimentation rate, and marked percussion tenderness over the affected area of the spine points strongly to bacterial diskitis. The organism is identified by blood culture, aspiration of the disk, or biopsy of the disk space. Epidural abscesses present similarly, but neurologic deficits develop earlier.

Noninfectious Inflammatory Disorders of the Spine: The spine may be involved in a number of inflammatory diseases, which are grouped under the name "spondy-

loarthropathies." A prominent condition in this group is ankylosing spondylitis (Chapter 3.7). The hallmarks are bone erosion and ankylosis. Early in the disease, erosion begins at places where ligaments insert into bone. With time, the junction of the annulus fibrosis and the vertebral end plates fuses (syndesmophytes). Initially, the facet joints are inflamed; many patients learn to lean forward to relieve the pressure on the facets. In uncontrolled ankylosing spondylitis, the spine characteristically fuses in this kyphotic position, and the patient gradually assumes a bent-over posture and walks looking at the ground. Patients should be suspected of having ankylosing spondylitis if they have a triad of the insidious onset of persistent back pain before age 40, morning stiffness, and improvement with exercise. Many patients are positive for the human leukocyte antigen HLA-B27.

Three other spondyloarthropathies are worth noting. The spine, particularly the sacroiliac joints, may be involved in Reiter's disease. The spinal involvement is generally self-limited and does not cause long-term disability. Patients typically are HLA-B27-positive. Arthritis complicates psoriasis in about 7% of patients; about 20% of patients with psoriatic arthritis have spine involvement. Inflammatory bowel disease can also be associated with spinal arthritis.

Although rheumatoid arthritis primarily affects the peripheral joints, it can also affect the synovium-lined joints in the cervical spine (Chapter 3.3). By destroying the joint and making important ligaments lax, inflammation of the synovium destabilizes the spine. This is a particularly important problem at the C1-2 junction, where involvement of the transverse ligament leads to atlantoaxial subluxation (anterior displacement of C1 with respect to C2). The C2-3 and C3-4 levels may also be involved, as may more caudal levels.

SPECIFIC DISEASES OF THE SPINAL CORD

Tumors

As noted above, the clinician gains considerable insight into the nature of a mass lesion affecting the spinal cord simply by knowing the compartment that the tumor occupies. Almost all extradural tumors are metastases. Among the more common extradural metastatic tumors are lung, breast, and prostate cancers. One exception to the rule is hemangiomas: Most hemangiomas are extradural, but they are benign tumors of the vertebral body. They give the vertebral body a vertical striated appearance on plain lateral spine x-ray. Hemangiomas are extremely vascular and can pose significant challenges to the unwary surgeon. Although usually of no clinical significance, they can produce mass effect on the spinal cord and can lead the vertebral body to collapse.

Also as noted earlier, meningiomas and neurofibromas account for nearly all intradural-extramedullary tumors. These benign tumors are generally cured by surgical resection.

Intramedullary tumors of the spinal cord are uncommon. Glial cells can give rise to low-grade tumors (astrocytomas) or less commonly to the highly malignant glioblastoma multiforme. Ependymal cells can form ependymomas, most of which are low-grade malignancies. Hemangioblastomas, a distant third in frequency, are benign tumors that are sometimes associated with cyst formation.

Syringomyelia is not truly a neoplastic disorder, but may nevertheless present as a mass. This cystic lesion of the spinal cord develops insidiously over many years, generally in patients with the Arnold-Chiari malformation. The Arnold-Chiari malformation is a congenital hindbrain anomaly in which ectopic cerebellar tissue exists below the foramen magnum, causing impaction at the foramen magnum and blocking cerebrospinal fluid flow. Because of the obstruction to spinal fluid flow, pressure waves from events such as Valsalva's maneuvers are directed to the spinal cord's central canal. Over years, these pressure waves lead to a cystic dilatation of the cervical spinal cord. Because of the insidious development, some patients present only after considerable neurologic deterioration. Because of selective loss of pain sensation, patients may have scars on their hands from burns and other injuries. Patients have intrinsic weakness of the hand muscles, and no reflexes in the arms.

Neurodegenerative and Genetically Related Disorders

A number of disorders in this category are dominated by spinal cord manifestations. Motor neuron diseases are disorders primarily involving the anterior horn cells of the spinal cord (Chapter 13.12). These disorders present distinctively: Patients lose motor function and develop lower motor neuron signs, but their sensory function is spared. The motor neuron diseases include amyotrophic lateral sclerosis (ALS) and Guillain-Barré syndrome. Symptoms of Guillain-Barré syndrome progress faster than those of ALS; the cerebrospinal fluid protein is elevated in Guillain-Barré but not in ALS. The corticospinal tract is typically involved in ALS but not in Guillain-Barré; therefore, patients with ALS present with upper as well as lower motor neuron findings.

Multiple sclerosis, the prototype demyelinating disorder, often affects the spinal cord white matter, causing patients to present with upper motor neuron findings or vague sensory complaints (Chapter 13.8). The diagnosis is strongly suggested by neurologic signs or symptoms pointing to lesions in disparate areas of the neural axis.

Signs and symptoms of spinal cord involvement are the most common neurologic manifestations of vitamin B_{12} deficiency (combined system disease). Posterior column involvement leads to loss of vibratory and position sense. The lateral columns and peripheral nerves may also be involved, leading to upper and lower motor neuron signs.

Spinocerebellar degeneration constitutes a group of degenerative disorders, many of which have a well-established genetic basis. These diseases, which typically begin in childhood or early adulthood, are characterized by slowly progressive ataxia and some degree of sensory and motor involvement. Degeneration of the spinocerebellar tracts contributes to the ataxia. After many years, patients may develop skeletal deformities and muscle atrophy.

Vascular Disease

Three main forms of vascular disease affect the spinal cord: vascular occlusion (thrombosis or embolism), arteriovenous malformations, and arteritis. Vascular occlusion is caused principally by involvement of feeding vessels. Any embolic disease, such as atrial fibrillation and endocarditis, can affect the spinal circulation. One particularly vulnerable vessel is the artery of Adamkiewicz. This vessel can originate from any of the left lower intercostal arteries. It varies from person to person in size and importance. When it is occluded, as from embolic disease, the patient may suffer an extensive infarction of the anterior half of the spinal cord from T6 down to the conus medullaris. Thus, patients have a T6 sensory level for pain and temperature sensation along with a flaccid paralysis (flaccid because the anterior horn cells are involved), but preservation of touch, vibratory, and position sense.

Spinal cord arteriovenous malformations assume many forms. The most common is a dural arteriovenous fistula. The fistula is likely an acquired anomaly, most often affecting men and developing in the neural foramen. The result is dilated, tortuous, coiled pial vessels with marked venous engorgement, typically located on the dorsal surface of the spinal cord. Patients with arteriovenous malformations may present with the sudden onset of severe spinal cord dysfunction, or, more commonly, with a progressive myelopathy. Segmental (radicular) pain can be an initial symptom. The diagnosis may be suggested by spinal myelography or MRI and confirmed by angiography.

SUMMARY

▶ Many diseases that affect the brain affect the spinal cord in the same way.

▶ Spinal column disease can be caused by degeneration, trauma, infections, and many systemic bone and joint diseases.

▶ Lower motor neuron involvement leads to flaccid paralysis. Upper motor neuron involvement leads to spastic paralysis.

▶ Physical examination must test pain and temperature sensation, which is controlled by a different part of the spinal cord from touch and proprioception.

▶ A first step in diagnosis is determining by magnetic resonance imaging whether a myeloradiculopathy is caused by extradural, intradural-extramedullary, or intradural-intramedullary disease.

SUGGESTED READING

Asbury AK, McKhann GM, McDonald WI (editors): *Diseases of the Nervous System: Clinical Neurobiology,* 2nd ed. WB Saunders, 1992.

Frymoyer JW et al (editors): *The Adult Spine: Principles and Practice.* Raven Press, 1991.

Wilkins RH, Rengachary SS: *Neurosurgery,* 2nd ed. McGraw-Hill, 1996.

13.11

Peripheral Neuropathies

John W. Griffin, MD

Disorders of the peripheral nervous system, termed *peripheral neuropathies,* are among the most frequently encountered neurologic diseases. In some instances, these diseases are slowly evolving, and at the outset patients may be asymptomatic for long periods, as in those with diabetic neuropathy. At the other extreme are the fulminant, life-threatening neuropathies such as the Guillain-Barré syndrome. Although the peripheral and central nervous systems share the same categories of disease (metabolic, vascular, toxic, immune-mediated, heritable, and infectious etiologies), in the peripheral nervous system the spectrum of pathologic and clinical manifestations is more restricted. It is important to understand peripheral neuropathies because (1) they are frequently a manifestation of a systemic illness, (2) they may be cured or at least slowed in progression, and (3) proper management does much to enhance the patient's quality of life.

SYMPTOMS AND SIGNS OF NEUROPATHY

The symptoms of neuropathy are weakness and alterations in sensation, varying in severity according to the cause. The cardinal findings that suggest a peripheral neuropathy on physical examination are decrease or loss of tendon reflexes at one or more sites, muscle weakness and wasting, and loss of sensibility. These elements are not in themselves sufficient to diagnose a neuropathy. The likelihood is increased when the patient exhibits the distal distribution of involvement that is characteristic of most neuropathies. The changes in sensation, strength, and reflexes are usually first seen in the feet and lower legs. Typically, sensory abnormalities are greatest in the toes. Weakness is first seen in extension of the toes and dorsiflexion of the foot at the ankle, and the tendon reflexes are usually first lost at the ankle, even when they are still present at the knees and in the arms. This pattern defines a *distal symmetric polyneuropathy,* which is the most frequently encountered pattern of neuropathic involvement. This pattern reflects the length-dependent vulnerability of peripheral nerve fibers in most types of peripheral neuropathy: in general, long nerve fibers tend to be affected before shorter ones. A few neuropathies can produce patchy, global, or even predominantly proximal involvement.

Alterations in Sensibility

Patients with neuropathy use a remarkable variety of descriptions to communicate their sensory symptoms, and their analogies are often evocative and precise. While "numbness" may cover a host of meanings, phrases such as "it feels as if I were walking on cotton wool" or "it's like walking on coals" cannot be misunderstood. Common complaints are *paresthesia*—tingling, "pins and needles"; *dysesthesia*—unpleasant perceptions of normally innocuous stimuli; and *hyperpathia*—a markedly painful experience of tactile or thermal stimuli. *Hypesthesia* describes an elevated threshold to perception of a stimulus; for example, a patient may appreciate the sharp or painful quality of a pinprick only when the pin is applied with greater pressure than is normally required. *Hyperesthesia* is a seemingly heightened sensibility, in that faint stimuli are experienced intensely. Careful testing often reveals that the threshold stimulus is elevated above normal, but that when the threshold is reached, an unusually intense perception is experienced. Occasional patients show profound deficits in sensibility on examination, with few sensory symptoms and little functional deficit.

Simple bedside tools are used to examine sensation: disposable pin, tuning fork, and cotton wisp. Because of the length dependency of most neuropathies, most effort is concentrated on determining sensory thresholds in the toes and fingers. Many patients have deficits in all sensory modalities—pain, temperature, light touch, vibration, and joint movement (proprioception)—but it is helpful to look for selective loss because it may suggest a specific diagnosis. Patterns to identify are selective loss of pain and temperature sensibility, implying loss specific to small fibers, and selective loss of joint position sense and vibratory sensibility, suggesting large-fiber disease.

Motor Changes

Disease of the motor fibers in the peripheral nerves produces flaccid weakness and, after the first few weeks of denervation, atrophy of the affected muscles. The distribution of weakness and atrophy is essential to accurate diagnosis, and individual muscle testing is required to determine this. In asymmetric nerve diseases, particularly those involving only one extremity, it is necessary to determine whether the lesion is of a nerve root (radiculopathy), a nerve plexus (brachial or lumbosacral), or a nerve. For example, injury to the C5 root may produce marked weakness of the deltoid, supraspinatus, and infraspinatus muscles, as well as some weakness of the brachioradialis. On the other hand, weakness of the opponens, short abductor, and short flexors of the thumb would suggest median nerve damage rather than a nerve root lesion. A convenient guide to individual muscle testing and the innervation patterns of muscle is *Aids to the Investigation of Peripheral Nerve Injuries* (see "Suggested Reading").

In most neuropathy, the weakness is greatest distally. Early manifestations often include weakness of dorsiflexion of the toes and ankles. Atrophy may be seen in the short extensor of toes and in the anterior tibialis. In the hands, atrophy often involves the intrinsic muscles, including first thenar and hypothenar eminences and first dorsal interosseous muscles.

Loss of Tendon Reflexes

Tendon reflexes, elicited by percussion over the Achilles, patellar, biceps, brachioradialis, and triceps tendons, are reduced in peripheral nerve disease because of abnormalities in the afferent (sensory) limb or the efferent (motor) limb of the monosynaptic reflex. In neuropathies, tendon reflexes are typically lost first at the ankle, again reflecting the disease's length dependency.

Autonomic Abnormalities

Because symptomatic involvement of the autonomic nervous system is unusual and is seen mainly in a small group of peripheral nerve diseases, autonomic dysfunction has differential diagnostic importance. Autonomic dysfunction can often be suggested by the history. For example, is there orthostatic light-headedness (in the absence of hypotensive drugs)? Are there changes in the sweating pattern (particularly a loss of sweating over the feet and legs)? In males, is there impotence or a change in sexual function? Bedside screening involves testing for orthostatic hypotension, for sinus arrhythmia with respiration, and for slowing of the pulse rate at release of Valsalva's maneuver. Pupil reactivity and the distribution of sweating should be sought. Individuals with loss of sweating in the legs or trunk often complain of excessive sweating over the face and scalp.

DIFFERENTIAL DIAGNOSIS OF NEUROPATHY

Neuropathies are clinically grouped as follows: disorders that affect individual peripheral nerves, such as the ulnar, median, or peroneal (mononeuropathies); disorders that involve several individual nerves, such as the ulnar on one side and the peroneal on the other, and in which progression is usually stepwise (multiple mononeuropathies or mononeuritis multiplex) (Figure 13.11–1); and disorders that produce *polyneuropathies,* which are typically symmetric, with distally predominant involvement and a pattern that moves to involve more proximal regions with time. Mononeuropathies most often result from pressure or chronic compression, from local trauma, or from small-vessel disease (such as diabetes). Multiple mononeuropathies are even more suggestive of small-vessel involvement, with diabetes and vasculitis being the most common causes.

Polyneuropathies have the longest list of possible etiologies and the most extensive differential diagnosis. So numerous are the conditions causing polyneuropathy that the goal of the history and the physical examination is to limit the diagnostic possibilities. The five keys to differential diagnosis of polyneuropathies at the bedside are (1) age at onset, (2) rate of progression, (3) selectivity of functional involvement (motor, sensory, or autonomic), (4) distribution of involvement (distal, proximal, or global), and (5) associated neurologic or systemic diseases. To these clinical assessments, the use of electrodiagnostic testing is often an essential adjunct.

Electrodiagnostic testing suggests the type of underly-

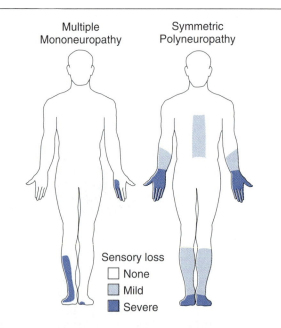

Figure 13.11–1. Difference of distribution of sensory loss in multiple mononeuropathy and distal symmetric polyneuropathy. Multiple mononeuropathy affects discrete nerve distributions, eg, right superficial peroneal, left ulnar, left deep peroneal. This involvement of several individual nerves contrasts with the distally predominant symmetric sensory loss in polyneuropathy. (Reproduced, with permission, from Griffin JW: Diabetic neuropathies. The Johns Hopkins Medical Grand Rounds 1985;12[1]:20.)

ing cellular pathology in the nerves. Normal nerve function depends on the integrity of both the axons and the myelin sheaths that surround and insulate the axons, and abnormalities of either interrupt nerve function (Figure 13.11–2). Some processes affect mainly the nerve cell body (axon), resulting in axonal degeneration, as seen in most drug-induced neuropathies, such as that induced by alcohol or vincristine. Other disorders, such as Guillain-Barré syndrome, selectively affect Schwann cells or myelin, resulting in demyelination. In many of the most common metabolic and heritable neuropathies, both axonal degeneration and demyelination are evident, reflecting the mutual interdependence among the cellular elements of the peripheral nervous system.

The age at onset and the rate of progression obtained from the history must be interpreted cautiously (Table 13.11–1). Often patients give specific and recent times of onset; such dates are precise and valuable in the acute neuropathies, but in more chronic neuropathies they often represent the time at which a longstanding progressive process finally became overtly symptomatic. In heritable neuropathies, the patient and the family may have been unaware of mild neuropathic features while the patient

was young, yet they remark that the affected individual never kept up with his or her peers in races and was always chosen last for sports teams. High-arched feet (pes cavus) with hammer toe deformities are important indicators of childhood onset, because they are the consequence of longstanding imbalances of distal muscles.

Selective functional involvement is particularly helpful in making a diagnosis (Table 13.11–2). Most neuropathies have both sensory and motor abnormalities, with sensation more severely affected than strength. Some neuropathies are predominantly motor, including the inflammatory neuropathies (such as the Guillain-Barré syndrome), the heritable motor-sensory neuropathies (such as Charcot-Marie-Tooth disease), porphyric neuropathy, and those neuropathies caused by certain toxins, particularly lead. Disorders with primarily sensory involvement and little motor involvement, such as diabetes, amyloidosis, and leprosy, can be separated into those with loss of all modalities (global loss), those with loss of pain and temperature sensibility but little loss of vibratory sensation (small-fiber neuropathies), and those in which associated loss of proprioception and vibratory sensibility predominates (ataxic neuropathies).

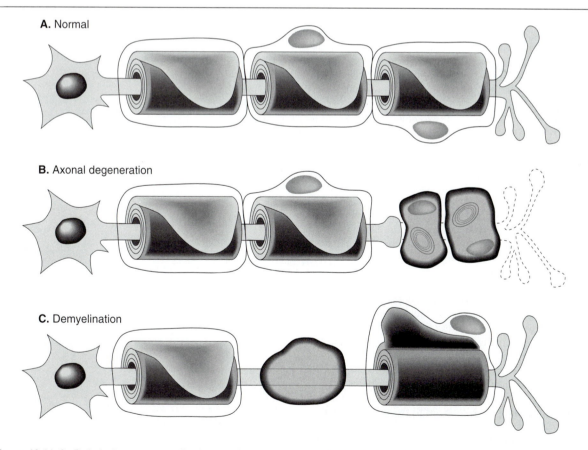

Figure 13.11–2. Pathologic processes affecting peripheral nerve fibers. **A:** Normal. **B:** Distal axonal degeneration. **C:** Demyelination. The second segment has demyelinated. The third segment shows unraveling of the myelin sheath.

Table 13.11–1. Differential diagnosis of polyneuropathies: Onset and course.

Acute onset monophasic (days)
Guillain-Barré syndrome*
Porphyric neuropathy
Diphtheritic neuropathy

Subacute onset (weeks)
Many toxins*
Nutritional neuropathies*
Carcinomatous neuropathies
Uremic neuropathy

Relapsing
Relapsing inflammatory neuropathy
Refsum's disease

Chronic (many months or years)
Diabetic sensorimotor neuropathy*
Chronic inflammatory neuropathies

Lifelong, slowly progressive
Heritable motor-sensory neuropathies (Charcot-Marie-Tooth disease)

*Most common causes.

Table 13.11–2. Differential diagnosis of polyneuropathies: Selective involvement of nerve fiber types.[†]

Sensorimotor polyneuropathies
Diabetic polyneuropathy
Alcohol
Toxin
Nutritional deficiency
Metabolic disorder
Inflammatory neuropathies

Predominantly motor polyneuropathies
Guillain-Barré syndrome
Relapsing and chronic inflammatory neuropathy
Acute intermittent porphyria
Lead neuropathy
Heritable motor-sensory neuropathies (Charcot-Marie-Tooth)

Predominantly sensory polyneuropathies
Global loss
Diabetic polyneuropathy*
Paraproteinemia and cryoglobulinemia
Tabes dorsalis
Primarily loss of pain and thermal sensibility ("small-fiber" pattern)
Diabetic polyneuropathy*
Amyloidosis
Hereditary sensory neuropathies
Lepromatous leprosy
Primarily loss of joint position and vibration sensibility (ataxic neuropathies)
Carcinomatous sensory neuropathy
Acute idiopathic sensory neuropathy
Sensory ganglionitis associated with Sjögren's syndrome
Cisplatin
Metronidazole
Vitamin B_6 overdose
Subacute combined degeneration
Friedreich's ataxia

Autonomic neuropathy
Diabetic polyneuropathy*
Amyloid polyneuropathy*
Acute, chronic, and relapsing pandysautonomia
Dysautonomia (Riley-Day)

*Most common causes.
[†]Most polyneuropathies produce both sensory and motor disturbances.

The development of a rapidly evolving, ataxic sensory neuropathy in an adult may be a remote manifestation of an underlying malignancy. The process underlying carcinomatous sensory neuropathy is an immune-mediated inflammatory destruction of dorsal root ganglion cells (ganglioradiculitis), reflecting shared epitopes on the tumor cells and the neurons. This syndrome is among the most distinctive of the malignancy-related neurologic syndromes and mandates a thorough search for a tumor.

Typically, neuropathy causes distal signs and symptoms. When the pattern of involvement is proximal instead, a short list of diagnoses should come to mind (Table 13.11–3).

Neuropathies with prominent autonomic involvement may present with impotence, urinary hesitancy, constipation, or symptoms of orthostatic hypotension. Often autonomic neuropathies coexist with spontaneous pain and the "small-fiber" pattern of sensory loss, with decreased pain and temperature sensibility but preserved strength, vibration, proprioception, and tendon reflexes. This picture is one of the manifold presentations of diabetic neuropathy, as well as of systemic amyloidosis.

Special Diagnostic Studies

Electrodiagnostic studies evaluate the physiology of both nerve and muscle. Nerve conduction studies stimulate individual nerves at two points, usually by surface electrodes. The amplitude of the evoked response and the velocity of nerve conduction are measured. Sensory and motor components of nerve are assessed independently. These special diagnostic studies are not necessary when the cause of neuropathy is obvious, as in persons with longstanding diabetes with painful sensory neuropathy, but they are fundamental to the evaluation of neuropathy of unknown cause. These data can determine whether or not the patient has a significant neuropathy, indicate

Table 13.11–3. Differential diagnosis of polyneuropathies: Distribution of deficits.*

Proximal weakness
Guillain-Barré syndrome
Porphyria
Carcinomatous neuropathy with proximal weakness ("carcinomatous neuromyopathy")
Spinal muscular atrophies

Proximal sensory loss
Porphyria
Tangier disease (analphalipoproteinemia)

Temperature-related distribution
Lepromatous leprosy

*Most polyneuropathies produce distal involvement.

whether it is predominantly sensory or motor, and suggest the nature of the underlying pathophysiology (Figure 13.11–3). On electrodiagnostic testing, axonal degeneration is characterized by relatively preserved velocities of conduction but reduced evoked amplitudes. Conversely, studies indicative of demyelination have reduced nerve conduction velocity but relatively normal evoked amplitudes. Because nerve conduction studies can only test the large myelinated fibers, they are insensitive to diseases of the small unmyelinated autonomic and pain fibers.

Electromyography, the recording of spontaneous and voluntary muscle activity through needle electrodes inserted into muscle, can aid in confirming that weakness is caused by denervation and in delineating the distribution of involvement. It is a useful adjunct when the cause of weakness—nerve, muscle, or spinal cord disease—is uncertain. Similarly, muscle biopsy can confirm a denervating process rather than a primary muscle disease (Chapter 13.12).

In selected patients, nerve biopsy can yield a specific diagnosis or can determine the type of lesion (acute demyelination, recurrent demyelination, axonal degeneration with large- or small-fiber loss), thereby focusing further diagnostic evaluation. Its usefulness, however, is limited. First, the tissue must be specially processed to provide maximum information. Second, only a sensory nerve (usually the sural at the ankle) can be biopsied, so that biopsy provides a very small "window" into a disease process whose severity usually differs regionally and changes with time. Third, few neuropathies produce specific pathologic changes; this lack of specificity reflects the limited types of pathologic responses possible in the peripheral nervous system. Specific diagnoses, including amyloidosis, sarcoidosis, vasculitis, leprosy, and some inherited metabolic disorders such as metachromatic leukodystrophy, may be made by nerve biopsy. However, often laboratory tests or biopsy of other tissues would more easily establish the diagnosis.

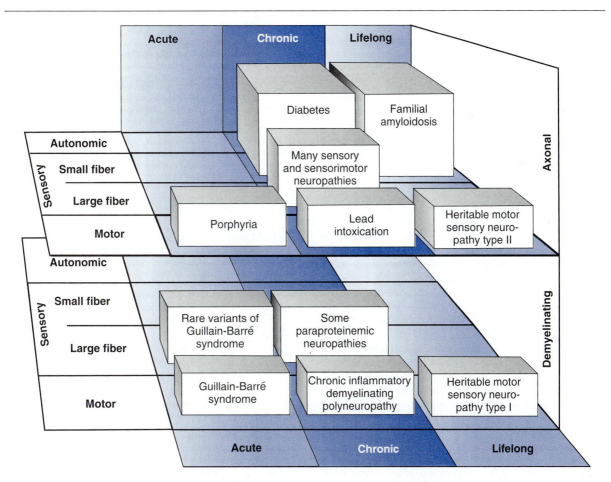

Figure 13.11–3. Important forms of peripheral neuropathy, classified by time course, pathophysiology (demyelinating versus axonal, as assessed by electrophysiology), and selective functional involvement.

SPECIFIC NEUROPATHIES

Diabetic Neuropathy

The various manifestations of the diabetic neuropathies cover by themselves nearly the full spectrum of peripheral nerve disease (see Table 13.11–2). Diabetic mononeuropathies and multiple mononeuropathies indicate vascular insufficiency or infarction in nerve, presumably caused by small blood vessel disease. Their onset is often abrupt and painful, with cranial nerves III and VI, the femoral nerve, or other major nerves of the extremities commonly affected. Involvement of the lumbosacral plexus can lead to diabetic amyotrophy, a syndrome that can be confused with intraspinal disease. The clinical picture of this disorder is asymmetric weakness of the hip girdles with little sensory loss. Although the initial manifestations may be incapacitating, the prognosis for eventual recovery in diabetic multiple mononeuropathies is usually good.

The most prevalent neuropathic complication of diabetes is diabetic polyneuropathy, which causes distal sensorimotor or predominantly sensory neuropathy. In many instances, the sensory abnormalities include small-fiber dysfunction, with spontaneous neuropathic pain in the feet, elevated pain perception thresholds, and associated autonomic dysfunction with impotence and pupillary abnormalities. This complex is an important cause of morbidity and disability in diabetes and contributes to the likelihood of painless diabetic foot lesions.

As with many other diabetic complications, no definitive treatment exists for the diabetic neuropathies. Increasing evidence suggests that prolonged hyperglycemia, even at relatively low levels, may contribute to the development of the polyneuropathy, either by metabolic effects on nerve fibers or by promoting small-vessel disease. It is prudent to strive for the lowest levels of blood glucose that can be safely achieved.

Small-fiber involvement produces particularly difficult medical and psychologic problems. The diminished pain sensibility can lead to painless injuries (eg, Charcot joints caused by painless trauma) and contribute to skin ulcers, osteomyelitis, and, ultimately, spontaneous or surgical amputation. Prevention through education is paramount. Foot care, avoidance of trauma and pressure to anesthetic extremities, and prompt attention to early lesions are mandatory. The spontaneous neuropathic pain of diabetic polyneuropathy may respond to anticonvulsants such as phenytoin or carbamazepine, or tricyclic antidepressants such as nortriptyline. Full therapeutic doses are required, and the dose must be raised slowly to minimize side effects such as dizziness. Opiates are contraindicated because of their potential for addiction.

Toxic Neuropathies

The toxic neuropathies most often seen in medical practice are those caused by drugs (Table 13.11–4). In most toxic neuropathy, the lesion is degeneration of the distal regions of the longest or largest axons, so that early clinical involvement may involve blunting of sensation in the toes, loss of the Achilles tendon reflex, and weakness of

Table 13.11–4. Drugs that most commonly produce peripheral neuropathies.

Alcohol
Amiodarone
Cisplatin
Colchicine (causes neuromyopathy)
Dapsone
Didanosine
Dideoxycytidine
Disulfiram
Furantoins
Gold salts
Isoniazid
Metronidazole
Paclitaxel
Penicillamine
Perhexilene
Phenytoin
Suramin
Vincristine

the intrinsic muscles of the foot. With some agents, including vincristine, amiodarone, dideoxycytidine, and didanosine, neuropathy is an expected side effect of potentially life-sustaining therapy, and dosage schedules are devised to minimize nerve damage. For most drugs, including isoniazid, nitrofurantoin, amiodarone, and cisplatin, dosage schedules have been refined to make neuropathy an uncommon complication. Preexisting nerve disease, including heritable neuropathies, predispose the patient to more severe damage induced by neurotoxic drugs. Most of these agents produce a distally predominant sensorimotor neuropathy of the axonal type. Paresthesia or neuropathic pain is troublesome in some toxic neuropathies, including those caused by dideoxycytidine, didanosine, and vincristine. The specific therapy for most toxic neuropathies, when medically possible, is withdrawal of the agent. Because recovery occurs by axonal regeneration, it can be a prolonged process.

The list of industrial and environmental agents that can injure peripheral nerves is growing. Industrial exposure is suggested when the history reveals that workers besides the index patient have developed similar syndromes. Careful occupational and recreational history, and in some instances visits to the home or place of work, may uncover neurotoxins. Metal poisoning by lead, mercury, thallium, and arsenic are among the few neurotoxic agents that can be detected by laboratory measurements. Although environmental and workplace neurotoxicities are of widespread concern, most ingested neurotoxins either are iatrogenic (from prescribed medications) or reflect personal habits. An example is the ingestion of neurotoxic amounts of vitamin B_6 (over 50 mg per day) by health food enthusiasts.

Alcohol and Nutritional Neuropathies

Several types of substance abuse, including glue sniffing and "huffing" of solvents, produce nerve disease. By far the most prevalent is alcohol. Although alcohol itself may have some neurotoxic properties, the neuropathies seen in alcoholics are caused or amplified by associated nutritional inadequacy. Often, there is burning discomfort in the feet and hyperesthesia, associated with elevated thresholds to vibratory stimuli and loss of tendon reflexes in the ankles. There is typically a mild degree of weakness in the feet and ankles, but severe motor involvement is uncommon. Multivitamin therapy, adequate protein-calorie intake, and treatment of the underlying alcoholism are the cornerstones of therapy.

Inflammatory Demyelination Neuropathies

The inflammatory neuropathies are a group of related disorders classified by time course as acute, chronic, or relapsing. They are immunologically mediated and share the pathologic features of demyelination of spinal roots and peripheral nerves, with variable degrees of macrophage-mediated myelin stripping and mononuclear cell infiltration within nerve. All produce predominantly motor involvement with reduced nerve conduction velocities and, in most patients, elevated spinal fluid protein without pleocytosis. In these ways, these disorders are a clinical counterpart of experimental allergic neuritis, a disorder produced by immunizing susceptible animals against peripheral nerve myelin or its constituents. Although these disorders most likely represent a spectrum of a single process, they are considered separately because of the differing approaches to treatment.

Acute Inflammatory Neuropathy (Guillain-Barré Syndrome): Since the eradication of polio, this disorder has become the most common cause of acute flaccid paralysis. In 60% of patients, the condition follows an event such as infection (especially herpesviruses and *Campylobacter jejuni*), parturition, surgery, or immune dysfunction (as seen in HIV infection, Hodgkin's disease, and pharmacologic immunosuppression). Because of the alarming speed with which weakness and respiratory insufficiency can develop, Guillain-Barré syndrome should always be regarded as a potential medical emergency. Back pain and leg pain with paresthesias are a common presenting manifestation, and at this stage trivial viral infections or functional complaints are often suspected. A clue to the potential gravity of the complaint is often the finding of depressed or absent reflexes. In most cases, weakness rapidly becomes the predominant problem. Weakness is generally symmetric and may have an ascending pattern, but it can involve any distribution, including cranial nerves. Proximal as well as distal muscles are usually affected.

The diagnosis of Guillain-Barré syndrome is supported by demonstration of reduced conduction velocities, compatible with demyelination, at some level of the peripheral nervous system. These changes may be detectable only in very distal nerve regions or within spinal roots. An elevated spinal fluid protein also supports the diagnosis and may reach dramatic levels; however, the rise in protein level may follow onset of neuropathy by many days, so that a normal protein at the time of presentation is common. The possibility of acute intermittent porphyria

should be excluded because of the implications for management. One viral syndrome associated with Guillain-Barré syndrome, infectious mononucleosis, should be considered as an antecedent factor.

Patients with Guillain-Barré syndrome should be hospitalized and their respiratory status closely monitored. Autonomic involvement is a major contributing factor to complications and death and may be manifested by flushing, orthostatic hypotension, or heart rhythm changes. The keystone of therapy is early and expert critical care, including good pulmonary toilet, prevention of thrombophlebitis, prevention of corneal ulcerations in patients with facial weakness, and, when necessary, ventilator support.

Plasmapheresis and intravenous immunoglobulin are remarkably beneficial in the treatment of Guillain-Barré syndrome. Because of the suspicion that relapses are more frequent following intravenous immunoglobulin therapy, many groups favor plasmapheresis when the required intravenous access can be safely achieved. When performed on patients unable to walk unassisted and during the first 30 days of illness, plasmapheresis increases the extent of recovery at 1 month, shortens the time on a respirator, and shortens the time to independent walking.

Although about 30% of patients require respirator assistance, modern intensive care has reduced the mortality rate to 2–3%. The nadir of the clinical course of Guillain-Barré syndrome is usually reached within 2–4 weeks of onset, and improvement can be dramatic. In a severely affected patient, however, recovery may be very prolonged, and 15% of patients have substantial residual deficits.

Chronic and Relapsing Inflammatory Neuropathies: These autoimmune disorders, sometimes called "chronic Guillain-Barré syndrome," are among the most common neuropathies that are referred for intensive evaluation because of diagnostic confusion. The suspicion is usually raised by the finding of a predominantly motor neuropathy with reduced conduction velocities and elevated spinal fluid protein. Because their onset and progression can be insidious, the inflammatory neuropathies must be carefully distinguished from the heritable motor-sensory neuropathies described in the text that follows. The establishment of diagnosis is important because these are among the most treatable of the peripheral nerve disorders. Initial therapy is with adrenal corticosteroids. In patients with contraindications to corticosteroids, plasmapheresis, infusions of human immune globulin, and immunosuppression are efficacious. Patients with chronic inflammatory neuropathies who improve either spontaneously or in response to treatment are at risk for subsequent relapse. With this caution, the prognosis in steroid-responsive patients is good.

Hereditary Neuropathies: There are many inherited disorders of the peripheral nervous system; hereditary motor-sensory neuropathy (Charcot-Marie-Tooth disease) is the most common. Because of the chronicity of the symptoms and their slow evolution, many patients do not realize they have peripheral nerve disease until middle or old age. Weakness, particularly footdrop and hand weakness, is the most severe manifestation in most patients and may be associated with the high-arched feet and hammer toes described previously, as well as marked thinness of the calf and anterior tibial muscles (stork legs). Most patients with Charcot-Marie-Tooth disease have a demyelinating neuropathy, with recurrent demyelination and remyelination, resulting in redundant Schwann cell processes called "onion bulbs," which occupy space and contribute to a visible and palpable enlargement of nerves (hypertrophic neuropathy) in many individuals.

The diagnosis of an hereditary neuropathy can usually be established by a history of childhood onset and examination of family members. Mildly affected individuals may have only foot deformities or slowed conduction velocities. Nerve biopsies showing marked onion bulb formation strongly suggest a heritable etiology. The disorder is dominantly inherited, and many persons with this phenotype have a triplication of a region of chromosome 17q, altering expression of the myelin protein PMP-22. This phenomenon allows definitive diagnosis of this group of patients with Charcot-Marie-Tooth disease. Reassurance about the slow rate of progression, as well as physical therapy and rehabilitation measures including ankle bracing, are the bases of therapy.

Monoclonal Gammopathies

Monoclonal gammopathies cause a diverse group of neuropathies. Whether the gammopathy is a "monoclonal gammopathy of unknown significance" appearing in elderly persons, or frank myeloma or Waldenström's macroglobulinemia, nerve damage can occur (Chapter 12.7). In some of these gammopathies, the monoclonal immunoglobulin reacts with identified constituents of peripheral nerve. For example, a predominantly sensory neuropathy occurs with IgM monoclonal antibodies that "see" a particular sulfated glycoconjugate epitope found in some nerve glycolipids as well as in a specific glycoprotein, the myelin-associated glycoprotein (MAG). These anti-MAG antibodies are clearly the cause of nerve damage. In most patients with paraproteins, immunoglobulin-mediated nerve damage is suspected, but the specific epitopes involved have not been determined.

Most of the time, monoclonal gammopathies evolve slowly, often worsening imperceptibly over years. Serum electrophoresis and immunoelectrophoresis or immunofixation are essential diagnostic tests in patients with undiagnosed neuropathies. Therapies such as plasmapheresis and cytotoxic drugs for neuropathy caused by monoclonal gammopathy are expensive, hazardous, and of limited benefit. Thus, the majority of patients benefit most from physical therapy and, when necessary, gait training.

Vasculitic Neuropathies

Vasculitis associated with any of the underlying rheumatologic disorders (eg, polyarteritis nodosa, Sjögren's syndrome) can produce nerve damage, and in some patients peripheral nerve involvement is the presenting and predominant problem. Vasculitis characteristically produces a multiple mononeuropathy, with a stepwise progression and asymmetric involvement. The differential diagnosis may include diabetic multiple mononeuropathy. Although serologic testing may be consistent with underlying rheumatologic disease, definitive diagnosis is histologic; biopsy of muscle for or in addition to nerve has increased the yield of positive diagnoses. Similarly, identification of skin or other organ involvement may provide an appropriate site for biopsy.

The therapy is that of the underlying rheumatic disease (Chapters 3.4 and 3.5).

Neuropathies Associated with HIV Infection

HIV infection is associated with a daunting list of peripheral nerve complications. Many are stage-specific. For example, early in the course of HIV infection, usually before the development of AIDS, there is an increased incidence of inflammatory demyelinating neuropathies, and Guillain-Barré syndrome has been described at the time of seroconversion. A vasculitis can develop in association with AIDS-related complex and produce multiple mononeuropathy. As AIDS supervenes, cytomegalovirus can directly infect the cauda equina, producing a dramatic syndrome of multiple lumbosacral radiculopathy associated with polymorphonuclear leukocytosis in the spinal fluid, or it can produce a more indolent multiple mononeuropathy reflecting multifocal infection of endothelial cells and other cells in the peripheral nervous system.

The most prevalent neuropathic complication of HIV infection is the predominantly sensory neuropathy of AIDS. This affects about 30% of patients with AIDS and in a significant proportion is characterized by severe neuropathic pain in the feet. The pathogenesis of this complication has not been established, and only symptomatic therapy is available. Note that the neurotoxic syndrome produced by the antiretroviral agents, dideoxycytidine and didanosine, closely resembles the picture produced by the sensory neuropathy of AIDS itself, but the neuropathic pain can be alleviated by discontinuation of these agents.

Trigeminal Neuralgia (Tic Douloureux)

Trigeminal neuralgia is a common cause of facial pain. It is characterized by paroxysmal flashes or shocks of pain severe enough to cause patients to wince and to interrupt other activities. It usually involves the maxillary and mandibular distributions of the trigeminal nerve. The paroxysms of pain are triggered by touch, temperature change, or other stimuli in the affected region. There is no objective evidence of sensory loss in the Vth nerve distribution, and other physical findings and laboratory studies are normal; therefore, the diagnosis is made by history.

Medication provides effective pain relief in most individuals. Carbamazepine is the drug of choice, but phenytoin and baclofen are useful in some individuals. In a minority of patients in whom medical therapy is ineffective, subcutaneous injection of the ganglion with glycerol provides relief and can be repeated if necessary.

Idiopathic Facial Nerve Palsy (Bell's Palsy)

Bell's palsy is a syndrome characterized by abrupt onset of VIIth nerve paralysis, resulting in weakness of the facial muscles, difficulty with eye closure, and in some patients hyperacusis and loss of taste. The disease can begin at any age. The cause and pathogenesis are not known, but in over 80% of patients there is good spontaneous recovery. The disorder produces degeneration of facial nerve axons. If after 5 days, electrical stimulation of the facial nerve produces facial movement, a relatively good prognosis can be anticipated. However, nerve regeneration and reinnervation of facial muscle may result in aberrant reinnervation (misregeneration). In this setting, eye closure may produce movements of muscles around the mouth, or conversely, opening the mouth may produce movements in the upper face.

"Crocodile tears" describe a syndrome caused by misregeneration of autonomic fibers subserving taste and lacrimation, so that gustatory stimulation results in tearing. In patients with Bell's palsy, very early treatment with a short course of high-dose corticosteroids is frequently advocated in an attempt to prevent extensive axonal degeneration and improve the prognosis. An important aspect of management is protection of the eye from corneal abrasion.

SUMMARY

▶ Peripheral nerve disease produces varying degrees of sensory loss or weakness associated with muscle atrophy and reflex loss; in most neuropathies, these findings are distally predominant, involving the feet and hands.

▶ Similar clinical pictures can be produced by the two major pathophysiologic mechanisms—axonal degeneration or demyelination. Electrodiagnostic studies are a valuable way to assess the contribution of each of these processes. Only a few nerve diseases produce demyelination, so identifying demyelination shortens the list of diagnostic possibilities.

▶ The differential diagnosis of peripheral neuropathies begins with placing the individual patient's problem in a matrix defined by age of onset, rate of progression, distribution of involvement, selective functional involvement, and associated medical diseases or exposures.

▶ Diabetes is the most prevalent cause of peripheral nerve disease in the developed world; the varieties of diabetic nerve involvement include mononeuropathies, multiple mononeuropathies, and distal symmetric polyneuropathies.

SUGGESTED READING

Dawson DM: Current concepts: Entrapment neuropathies of the upper extremities. N Engl J Med 1993;329:2013.

Dyck PJ et al (editors): *Peripheral Neuropathy,* 3rd ed. WB Saunders, 1993.

Griffin JW, Cornblath DR: Diseases of the peripheral nervous system. In: *Comprehensive Neurology.* Rosenberg RN (editor). Raven Press, 1991.

Griffin JW, Cornblath DR: Peripheral nerve. In: *Neurobiology of Disease.* Pearlman AL, Collins RC (editors). Oxford University Press, 1990.

Medical Research Council: *Aids to the Investigation of Peripheral Nerve Injuries.* London, 1984.

Schaumburg HH, Thomas PK, Berger AR: *Disorders of Peripheral Nerves.* FA Davis, 1992.

13.12

Diseases of the Motor Unit

Ralph W. Kuncl, MD, PhD

There are four general categories of neuromuscular diseases, based on anatomy of the motor unit: motor neuron disorders (eg, amyotrophic lateral sclerosis), peripheral neuropathies (Chapter 13.11), disorders of neuromuscular transmission (eg, myasthenia gravis), and myopathies. Diseases of the motor unit are discussed together here because they all share a cardinal manifestation—weakness.

APPROACH TO THE PATIENT

A directed history followed by a hypothesis-testing physical examination is most important in recognizing a specific disease or disease category. Failure to arrive at a testable hypothesis at the bedside usually leads to inaccuracy and confusion after laboratory testing. Nevertheless, serum creatine kinase activity, electromyography, and muscle or nerve biopsy can play an essential role in certain diseases.

History

Delineating true weakness in the history demands knowing exactly what the patient means by "weakness." The physician should define weakness as the reduction of a specific motor function, in order to distinguish it from nonneurologic symptoms such as physical fatigue, expressed in terms of tiredness or loss of stamina, and from mental fatigue (neurasthenia), couched in terms of lassitude, low energy, or depression. Pressing patients to define what they mean by weakness in terms of activities of daily living not only adds diagnostic specificity but also is a useful gauge of severity and progression. The physician assesses arm muscle strength by asking patients whether they have problems with hair brushing, opening jar lids, buttoning, and handwriting. For truncal strength, the physician asks whether patients have difficulty sitting up or rolling over in bed. For leg strength, the physician asks whether patients have difficulty arising from a chair or commode or climbing stairs without a banister, and whether they trip and fall while walking. The context of the weakness is important: If it is accompanied by a sensory or autonomic disturbance, peripheral neuropathy is more likely.

Pain is rarely a part of the diseases of the motor unit considered here. True muscle cramp (charley horse) or radiating pain is most often associated with peripheral neuropathy and radiculopathy. Muscle pain (myalgia) is more commonly associated with systemic disease than with myopathy. Nevertheless, some metabolic myopathies have exercise-related pain, and occasionally inflammatory myopathies and toxic myopathies have prominent myalgia. Therefore, when patients have muscle pain, it is helpful to establish whether it occurs with normal strength, whether it persists, and whether it is exercise-related.

Examination of Strength

To assess weakness, the physician should not get lost in a ritual exam of every muscle. What is important is pattern testing. Most diseases can be discerned by examining the eyelids, extraocular muscles, face, neck, and a few proximal and distal limb muscles. The physician then decides the patient's pattern of weakness. A semiquantitative assessment of strength should be recorded with the British Medical Research Council (MRC) scale (Table 13.12–1). Individual muscle strength is best quantified with a hand-held dynamometer or by timed testing (eg, of gait or swallowing) to judge objectively the changes in strength over time or following therapy. Functional testing is also a useful grading technique. All weak patients should be tested for how well and how fast they can rise from the floor, hop on one foot, rise from a squat, climb stairs, and rise from a chair with arms folded.

It is often difficult to differentiate true weakness from inadequate effort or feigned weakness. The latter are characterized by absence of smooth recruitment on gradually increasing effort and by a "give-way" quality when resistance is broken. Hysterical weakness is often characterized by co-contraction of agonist-antagonist pairs.

Other Signs

In developing a bedside hypothesis, the physician should note the relationship between weakness and muscle wasting. Weakness precedes wasting in myopathy, correlates with wasting in denervation, and lags far behind the weight

Table 13.12–1. Manual motor testing: MRC Scale.

Grade	
5	Normal strength
4	Active movement, against gravity and resistance (slight, moderate, and strong resistance indicated by 4–, 4, and 4+)
3	Active movement, against gravity only
2	Active movement, with gravity excluded
1	Flicker of muscle contraction
0	No muscle contraction

MRC, Medical Research Council of Great Britain.
Modified and reproduced, with permission, from *Aids to the Examination of the Peripheral Nervous System.* Baillière Tindall, 1986.

loss and wasting of cachexia. Focal muscle atrophy is an important early sign of a lower motor neuron disorder or focal neuropathy. Mild wasting is a late concomitant of some myopathies. A generalized decrease in body bulk, reflecting loss of nonmuscle subcutaneous tissues, but without significant weakness, is not a sign of neuromuscular disease but indicates cachexia from a process like impaired nutrition, neoplasm, or severe kidney or liver disease.

Fasciculations may indicate a disorder of the lower motor neuron, most notably amyotrophic lateral sclerosis, but they are not pathognomonic of amyotrophic lateral sclerosis. Fasciculations on contraction or in a cold room are common and normal. Even fasciculations at rest may be benign. But fasciculations in a rested, weak, wasted muscle usually indicate denervation from lower motor neuron disease, radiculopathy, or, less often, peripheral neuropathy.

Deep tendon reflexes should be used to confirm the hypothesis that the physician has been developing in the history and physical exam. At first, reflexes should answer the question, "Is this disease of the motor unit primarily affecting the upper motor neurons (pathologically brisk reflexes), the lower motor neurons (hypoactive or absent reflexes in neuropathy; hypoactive or normal reflexes in myopathy), or both?" The amplitude of reflexes should be carefully defined; a traditional scale of 0–4+ is useful. The broad range of physiologic reflexes, from sluggishness to jumpiness caused by anxiety or caffeine, is all defined as 2+. Reduced deep tendon reflexes are defined as 1+ when reinforcement (enhancement of the reflex, eg, by having the patient contract the muscle being tested) is needed to obtain them, and as 0 when they cannot be elicited even with reinforcement. Pathologically brisk reflexes are defined as 3+ when contraction spreads to other muscle groups outside the reflex arc; 4+ is sustained clonus.

DIFFERENTIAL DIAGNOSIS

The differential diagnosis of diseases of the motor unit is made primarily on the basis of the pattern of weakness and the temporal course.

What is the pattern of weakness? The brief, directed exam of muscle strength (see "Examination of Strength" above) will have determined a general pattern of weakness, such as proximal weakness in myopathy or distal weakness in neuropathy. The physician need make only a slight refinement of that pattern of weakness to define a more specific diagnosis (Table 13.12–2).

What is the temporal course? After the physician establishes that the patient is having problems with weakness, the first branch point in the differential diagnosis of weakness depends on the temporal course. The clinician must determine whether the disorder is steadily progressive (eg, amyotrophic lateral sclerosis, polymyositis), episodic (eg, hypokalemic periodic paralysis, hysteria), abrupt in onset (Guillain-Barré syndrome), or characterized by diurnal variation (eg, myasthenia gravis). Weakness beginning in the second decade and slowly progressing over decades would be typical of an inherited disease like facioscapulohumeral dystrophy or acid maltase deficiency.

What role does the family history play? A complete understanding of a neuromuscular disease sometimes re-

Table 13.12–2. Clues to interpreting patterns of weakness.

Pattern	Diagnosis
Limb muscles	
Proximal weakness	Myopathy
Distal weakness	Neuropathy
Arms weaker than legs	Facioscapulohumeral dystrophy
	Porphyric neuropathy
	Lead neuropathy
Legs weaker than arms	Polymyositis
	Steroid myopathy
	Duchenne's muscular dystrophy
Triceps weakness >> biceps weakness	Myasthenia gravis
	C7–C8 radiculopathy
Cranial muscles	
Bilateral facial weakness	Sarcoidosis
	Myotonic dystrophy
	Myasthenia gravis
	Guillain-Barré syndrome
Facial weakness + lid ptosis	Myotonic dystrophy
	Oculopharyngeal dystrophy
	Myasthenia gravis
Prominent dysphagia	Oculopharyngeal dystrophy
	Myasthenia gravis
	Amyotrophic lateral sclerosis
	Polymyositis
Truncal muscles	
Head ptosis	Amyotrophic lateral sclerosis
	Myasthenia gravis
	Cervical spondylosis
Presentation with respiratory failure	Amyloid myopathy
	Polymyositis
	Acid maltase deficiency
	Myasthenia gravis
	Guillain-Barré syndrome
	Amyotrophic lateral sclerosis

quires a detailed family history and even examination of family members. Muscular dystrophies are by definition genetic disorders of muscle. Many forms of spinal muscular atrophy are inherited as autosomal recessive traits. The physician should ask whether any members of the extended family were weak as children, required orthopedic aids like crutches or wheelchairs, or have traits similar to the patient's. However, it is important to realize that autosomal dominant diseases are notorious for variable penetrance and expressivity (Chapter 10.1). A floppy baby may be the index case in a family that has had many generations of people with mild facial weakness, frontal balding, early cataracts, or hand stiffness—individually minor medical problems, but essential to the bedside diagnosis of myotonic dystrophy. Similarly, a family photograph showing lid ptosis in the members may be all that the physician needs to diagnose oculopharyngeal dystrophy in an elderly woman who presents with dysphagia. In such dominantly inherited disorders, the physician should not accept a patient's report of "no family history of weakness," but should evaluate as many primary relatives as is feasible.

What other signs give clues? Other physical findings play a secondary role unless they are specific to a particular disease. But some signs are so characteristic and so helpful to diagnosis that they deserve special mention (Table 13.12–3). An important example is muscle pseudohypertrophy (replacement of muscle by fat and connective tissue) and contracture of muscles in Duchenne's and Becker's muscular dystrophy.

Table 13.12–3. Interpreting signs other than weakness.

Hypertrophy
  True hypertrophy
    Myotonia congenita (Herculean appearance)
    Childhood hypothyroidism
    Syndrome of continuous muscle fiber activity
      (Isaacs' syndrome)
    Chondrodystrophic myotonia (Schwartz-Jampel syndrome)
  Pseudohypertrophy
    Duchenne's and Becker's muscular dystrophy
    Acid maltase deficiency
    Amyloid myopathy
    Cysticercosis
    Radiculopathy (rare)

Macroglossia
  Amyloid myopathy
  Cytochrome oxidase deficiency (with the de Toni-Fanconi-
    Debré syndrome)

Congenital absence of a muscle
  Facioscapulohumeral dystrophy

Short stature
  Kearns-Sayre syndrome
  Debrancher enzyme deficiency
  Schwartz-Jampel syndrome

Contractures
  Duchenne's and Becker's muscular dystrophy
  Emery-Dreifuss (humeroperoneal) muscular dystrophy
  All types of congenital muscular dystrophy

LABORATORY TESTS

Serum Enzymes

A very sensitive screening tool in neuromuscular diseases is measuring the activity of the serum enzyme creatine kinase (CK). CK is often elevated in myopathies, but is not pathognomonic (Table 13.12–4). How far the CK exceeds the upper limit of normal is of some diagnostic significance. CK is highest in necrotizing and dystrophic processes (increased up to 50-fold or more). It is modestly elevated, only one- to threefold, in about one-third of patients with amyotrophic lateral sclerosis, spinal muscular atrophy, and some other denervating diseases. CK is usually normal in most neuropathies and neuromuscular junction disorders. There are important exceptions to the rule that CK is elevated in myopathy (see Table 13.12–4). It is also important to note that, although the CK-MB fraction is a cardiac isoenzyme, immature skeletal muscle fibers contain CK-MB, so any myopathy marked by regeneration elevates the MB fraction as well.

Other serum enzymes are not as helpful as the CK. Traditionally, physicians have tested for myopathies by measuring the serum aldolase, but this is not useful because in almost every myopathy the aldolase is less likely to be elevated than is the CK. Lactic dehydrogenase (LDH), often obtained incidentally, is also less sensitive. Aspartate aminotransferase (AST) and alanine aminotransferase (ALT) are not only liver enzymes, but are elevated whenever CK activity is increased more than three- to fivefold for any reason. In muscle necrosis, the serum enzymes are usually elevated in this order: CK>>LDH>AST>ALT.

Electromyography

Electromyography (EMG) can be used to confirm a diagnosis of myopathy or neurogenic weakness. EMG is a sampling technique that is directed by the neurologic exam and is therefore an extension of it. This is a subjective test, dependent on the examiner's skill. The test should be designed and performed by a trained physician, not a technician.

Table 13.12–4. Interpretation of serum creatine kinase elevation.

Causes of creatine kinase elevation that do not imply neuromuscular disease
  Hemolysis of specimen
  Intramuscular injection
  Trauma, bruise
  Abscess or cellulitis near truncal muscles (perinephric, psoas,
    retroperitoneal)
  Seizure, especially status epilepticus
  Psychosis, especially manic-depressive illness
  Exercise
  Compression, crush

Myopathies with usually normal serum creatine kinase activity
  Hyperthyroid myopathy
  Steroid myopathy
  Myopathies of glycogen or lipid metabolism causing exercise
    intolerance or myoglobinuria (between attacks)
  Periodic paralysis (unless many attacks)

In EMG, concentric needle electrodes record spontaneous electrical discharges and motor unit potentials, which are the summated action potentials from all the muscle fibers making up an individual motor unit. In myopathy, the total number of motor units available is not decreased, but death of scattered individual myofibers within motor units reduces their amplitude and duration on EMG. In neurogenic disorders, whole motor units are lost and the remaining units fire rapidly. Denervated myofibers show spontaneous discharges called *fibrillations* and *positive sharp waves*; the remaining motor unit potentials become long in duration and large in amplitude because of regenerative sprouting of axons as they adopt muscle fibers orphaned by previous denervation.

In the myotonias, spontaneous or stimulus-sensitive muscle fiber potentials fire at an abnormally fast rate, characteristically waxing and waning in both amplitude and frequency. Myotonia (involuntary delayed relaxation after a contraction) is related to abnormal sodium or chloride channels in skeletal muscle membranes, resulting in abnormal sodium and potassium ion fluxes; myotonia can be seen in various heritable myotonic disorders, acid maltase deficiency, and occasionally other myopathies.

Muscle Biopsy

The principal uses of muscle biopsy are in (1) distinguishing myopathy from neurogenic causes of weakness; (2) recognizing morphologically distinctive muscle diseases (eg, central core disease); (3) diagnosing systemic disorders, including vasculitic (eg, polyarteritis nodosa), infiltrative (eg, amyloid), and parasitic (eg, trichinosis); and (4) identifying specific metabolic disorders of muscle (eg, carnitine deficiency, myophosphorylase deficiency) and central nervous system disorders that may be reflected in muscle (eg, mitochondrial encephalomyopathy with lactic acidosis and stroke).

Muscle biopsy may suffer from sampling error, since only a small portion of tissue is assessed at a single site at one moment. Furthermore, biopsy is limited largely to structural and biochemical rather than physiologic analysis. Modern muscle biopsy technique requires cryosection histology and histochemistry. Standard paraffin sections have limited usefulness; they are best at identifying inflammation (eg, polymyositis) or organisms (eg, pyomyositis). Proper biopsy procedure requires detailed knowledge of the case by a pathologist skilled in histochemistry of muscle, appropriate selection of a minimally weak muscle (usually MRC grade 4+), and avoiding sampling muscle that is affected by a trivial or unrelated process (eg, needle trauma of EMG, nerve root compression).

Muscle biopsy can distinguish myopathy from neurogenic atrophy. Most limb muscles are a mosaic of approximately equal numbers of fatigue-resistant type I myofibers (poor in "fast" myosin ATPase but rich in lipids, mitochondria, and oxidative enzymes) and fast-contracting, fatigue-prone type II myofibers (rich in fast myosin ATPase, glycolytic enzymes, and glycogen). In muscle disease caused by denervation, this mosaic is replaced by small groups of angular atrophic fibers, which indicate acute or ongoing denervation, and by fiber-type grouping, which indicates more chronic reinnervation. By contrast, myopathy is usually characterized by (1) increased variability in myofiber diameter, caused by both atrophy and compensatory hypertrophy; (2) scattered myofiber necrosis and regeneration; and (3) other reactive changes such as fibrosis or vacuolation.

PRINCIPLES OF MANAGEMENT

The most important neuromuscular disorders for which genetic testing is available are listed in Table 13.12–5. Genetic testing is most advanced for Duchenne's muscular dystrophy. It is possible to predict the risk that a person has the carrier state; identify specific gene deletions; distinguish the disease from the milder allelic disorder, Becker's muscular dystrophy; and make the diagnosis in utero.

Management of many of the chronic neuromuscular diseases may require orthopedic and occupational therapies. Exercise programs involving active resistance training have proved effective in surprisingly few muscle disorders (one being acid maltase deficiency), although, within limits, exercise is not harmful. Analysis of a patient's activities of daily living by an occupational therapist becomes the basis for prescription of some of the numerous adaptive devices available to aid almost any household or occupational activity, whether it is shaving, typing, writing, eating, bathing, or communicating by computer. Spinal fusion can correct progressive scoliosis, which affects many patients with spinal muscular atrophy and some of the muscular dystrophies; this surgery helps patients to maintain ventilatory capacity, keep upright posture, and fit comfortably into a wheelchair. Custommolded, articulated ankle-foot orthoses made of lightweight plastic are essential for safety and improved gait in patients with footdrop, such as develops in motor neuron diseases, muscular dystrophies, and neuropathies.

Because many chronic neuromuscular diseases affect the respiratory muscles, respiratory management is an important issue. Pulmonary function should be assessed regularly. The most important test of neuromuscular respiratory impairment is vital capacity, which can be easily measured by spirometry (a hand-held spirometer is convenient). The other important measure is negative inspiratory force. This value begins to decline by a measurable amount when the vital capacity falls below 1.5 L or, more precisely, 50% of the patient's predicted baseline. The negative inspiratory force is a useful indicator of respiratory *muscle* status (with contributions from the intercostal muscles, diaphragm, and accessory muscles of respiration), exclusive of parenchymal lung disease. Arterial blood gas tests are rarely useful in such diseases as myasthenia gravis, amyotrophic lateral sclerosis, and muscular dystrophy, because significant hypoxia or hypercarbia is only a late predictor of respiratory muscle failure.

Table 13.12–5. Selected genetic disorders causing diseases of the motor unit.

Disorder	Inheritance Pattern	Gene Mutation*
Motor neuron syndromes		
Familial ALS	AD	21q22.1–22.3 (Cu-Zn superoxide dismutase)
Spinal muscular atrophy, acute (Werdnig-Hoffmann) and chronic (Kugelberg-Welander)	AR	5q11.2–q13.3 (survival motor neuron protein; neuronal apoptosis inhibitory protein)
Muscular dystrophies, congenital myopathies, and ion channel disorders		
Duchenne's and Becker's muscular dystrophy	XR	Xp21.2 (dystrophin)
Facioscapulohumeral dystrophy	AD	4q35-qtr
Myotonic dystrophy	AD	19q13.2–q13.3 (myotonin-protein kinase)
Myotonia congenita	AD, AR	7q35 (muscle chloride channel)
Nemaline myopathy	AD	1q21-q23 (α tropomyosin)
Central core disease	AD	19q13.1 (ryanodine receptor)
Malignant hyperthermia	AD	19q13.1 (ryanodine receptor)
Hyperkalemic periodic paralysis	AD	17q13.1-q13.3 (sodium channel)
Paramyotonia congenita	AD	17q13.1-q13.3 (sodium channel)
Hypokalemic periodic paralysis	AD	1q31-q32 (calcium channel [dihydropyridine receptor])
Metabolic myopathies		
Type II glycogenosis (Pompe's disease)	AR	17q23 (acid maltase)
Type V glycogenosis (McArdle's disease)	AR	11q13 (muscle-type phosphorylase)
Carnitine palmityltransferase deficiency	AR	1p11–p13 (carnitine palmityltransferase)
Mitochondrial disorders		
Kearns-Sayre syndrome	Sporadic	Single large deletion or duplication
Progressive external ophthalmoplegia	Sporadic	Single large deletion or point mutation
Myoclonic epilepsy with ragged red fibers	Maternal	Point mutation (tRNA lysine)
Mitochondrial encephalomyopathy with lactic acidosis and stroke-like episodes	Maternal	Point mutation (tRNA leucine and others)

ALS, amyotrophic lateral sclerosis; AD, autosomal dominant; AR, autosomal recessive; XR, X-linked recessive.
*Gene product, if known, is listed in parentheses.

Patients with acute respiratory insufficiency are managed with chest physiotherapy, intermittent positive-pressure breathing, and treatment of acute respiratory infections. Patients with chronic progressive respiratory insufficiency may be able to use a home ventilator; these people may also benefit from discussion about living wills, so the physician knows how aggressively they wish to be treated. Patients may do well with short-term intermittent or night-time use of a negative pressure ventilator. Those with marginal respiration may need bilevel positive airway pressure through a nasal mask. Low-flow supplemental oxygen (1–3 L/min) can be used, particularly at night to combat the hypoxia associated with the supine hypoventilation typical of these diseases. Patients with a flaccid diaphragm have better ventilation if they sleep with their trunk elevated 30–45 degrees. Ultimately, when such temporary measures no longer help, portable positive pressure ventilators can be adapted to the wheelchair or home for total ventilator support, given a cooperative family and the many necessary resources.

Aspiration of food is a risk in neuromuscular diseases such as amyotrophic lateral sclerosis and myasthenia gravis. Patients who aspirate often or have difficulty clearing secretions should be prescribed portable suction machines, and the family should be trained in the Heimlich maneuver and cardiopulmonary resuscitation. When a patient's diet provides inadequate nutrition, the alternatives are nasogastric feeding tubes and feeding gastrostomy.

MOTOR NEURON DISEASES

Motor neuron diseases are system degenerations; that is, they cause a slow decline in the number or function of motor neurons, but not other types of neurons (selective vulnerability).

Types

Motor neuron diseases are usually classified according to whether they affect upper motor neurons in the motor cortex, lower motor neurons in the brain stem and spinal cord, or both. *Amyotrophic lateral sclerosis* (ALS) is by far the most common acquired motor neuron disease. Both lower and upper motor neurons are involved. ALS must be distinguished from other chronic acquired motor neuron diseases that mimic it, because they may differ in both prognosis and management. For example, in idiopathic ALS, the cerebrospinal fluid protein is usually normal or only minimally elevated; however, a cerebrospinal fluid protein above 75 mg/dL or oligoclonal bands make paraproteinemia (as determined by immunofixation electrophoresis), lymphoma, or macroglobulinemia more likely. When patients with such disorders have an associated motor neuron disease, treatment should be directed at their underlying immunologic disorder. *Primary lateral sclerosis* is a degeneration of unknown cause, affecting upper motor neurons exclusively; this disorder progresses more slowly than ALS. *Lathyrism* is also an exclusively upper motor neuron disease, probably caused by β-*N*-oxalylamino-L-alanine in the chickling pea, a staple food in the Third World. *Spinal muscular atrophy* affects lower motor neurons exclusively. *Multifocal motor neuropathy,* manifested as progressive lower motor neuron disease with weakness and wasting and characterized by persistent electrophysiologic conduction block and often high-titer serum antiglycolipid antibodies, may mimic other motor neuron diseases or chronic inflammatory demyelinating polyneuropathy. Multifocal motor neuropathy is important because it can be treated. Although it does not respond well to corticosteroids, it is very responsive to cyclophosphamide or intravenous immunoglobulin.

The inherited motor neuron diseases are important to recognize because their diagnosis may allow genetic testing and counseling. *Familial ALS,* which accounts for 5% of all ALS, is an autosomal dominant disorder that differs little from idiopathic ALS in age of onset, presentation, and prognosis. The two diseases are so alike that sporadic ALS must share some basic mechanisms with familial ALS, and the discovery of the causes for the familial disorder certainly would bear on the etiology of the more common form. A mutation in the gene for the Cu-Zn isoform of superoxide dismutase has been shown to account for the familial ALS in 20% of pedigrees. *Childhood spinal muscular atrophy* is autosomal recessive, and its highly variable age of onset and rate of progression have fueled a longstanding dispute about its genetic heterogeneity. The discovery of the gene location for the disease has shown that both acute and chronic forms are probably allelic variants of one defect on chromosome 5. *Hexosaminidase A deficiency* can also cause a motor neuron disease; although the gene for hexosaminidase is on chromosome 5, the hexosaminidase defect does not cause the childhood spinal muscular atrophies also linked to chromosome 5. *Kennedy's syndrome,* a bulbospinal muscular atrophy syndrome associated with gynecomastia, is caused by an X-linked defect of the androgen receptor.

Amyotrophic Lateral Sclerosis

The diagnosis of ALS requires a history of weakness, with observed progression, in a patient who has no sensory, bowel, or bladder abnormalities. Exam shows a combination of lower motor neuron signs (focal weakness, focal wasting, and fasciculations) and unequivocal upper motor neuron signs (eg, extensor plantar response, or incongruously overactive tendon reflex in a weak, wasted muscle). Since this is a *system* degeneration of *motor* neurons, significant dementia and unexplained peripheral neuropathy exclude the diagnosis. The physician should exclude systemic disorders that might explain the weakness, such as combined cervical and lumbar spondylotic amyotrophy, plasma cell dyscrasias, polymyositis, diabetic amyotrophy, spinal cord arteriovenous malformation, syringomyelia, neoplasia, lead intoxication, hyperthyroidism, and hyperparathyroidism.

There is no test for ALS. Rather, the physician rules out mimicking disorders. Electrodiagnostic testing is essential in excluding such mimics as multifocal motor neuropathy, chronic inflammatory demyelinating polyneuropathy, and multiple radiculopathies. Sensory conduction studies are always normal; motor conduction studies are normal except for reduced amplitude of the compound muscle action potentials. EMG shows widespread denervation potentials; a myopathic EMG would exclude the diagnosis. The cerebrospinal fluid is acellular.

Incidence of ALS increases with age; the mean age at onset is about 60 years, and less than 1% of patients are diagnosed before age 35. The male:female ratio is about 1.5:1. The course is one of inexorable progression, with an average 3-year survival rate of 50% and a 10-year survival rate of 10%. There is remarkably little geographic or racial variation worldwide in incidence of ALS. One notable exception was a 20- to 80-fold higher prevalence before World War II on the island of Guam, in some regions of the Kii peninsula of Japan, and in certain villages of southwest New Guinea. This endemic form of ALS has led to speculation that dietary excitotoxins (eg, cycad nuts), mineral deficiencies, excess trace metals, and viruses might play a role in the pathogenesis. But no risk factors have been confirmed in adequately controlled studies. Many theories of pathogenesis have been considered, but three popular hypotheses with some experimental support are that ALS may be (1) a slow degeneration caused by endogenous excitotoxins (such as the neurotransmitter glutamate) acting on motor neurons, (2) the result of chronic oxidative stress (see Table 13.12–5), or (3) an unconventional autoimmune disorder.

There is no cure for ALS. Riluzole can slightly prolong survival, and insulin-like growth factor I can slow somewhat the progression of weakness. Physiotherapy, exercise, and adaptive aids can alleviate problems related to weakness and loss of autonomy, swallowing, communication, and respiratory function. Placebos and fraudulent therapies abound for any such disease with uniformly poor prognosis. Patients should be encouraged to participate in valid, controlled clinical research. Information about current clinical trials is available from the Muscular Dystrophy Association.

Spinal Muscular Atrophy

Spinal muscular atrophy (SMA) is characterized by weakness, muscular atrophy, and often scoliosis, without involvement of the corticospinal tracts. SMA affects younger people than does ALS, has a longer course (except the infantile form), and is hereditary (usually autosomal recessive) rather than sporadic. Intellect and sensation are spared. The disease can be distinguished from myopathy by EMG and muscle biopsy, which show denervation. Neuropathologically, SMA is characterized by extensive neuronal loss limited to the large motor neurons of the spinal cord. The adult-onset form of spinal muscular atrophy has a slow, protracted course and must be differentiated from muscular dystrophies and other myopathies. Patients are managed as outlined above in "Principles of Management."

Poliomyelitis

The polio enterovirus induces cytopathic changes selectively in motor neurons of the spinal cord and brain stem. These changes lead to acute weakness, paralysis, and sometimes death. Vaccine programs have almost eradicated polio from most developed countries. Poliovirus does not predispose to ALS, but some patients develop new, progressive, disabling muscle weakness and atrophy 20–50 years after recovering from acute paralytic poliomyelitis. This syndrome of progressive postpolio amyotrophy is not caused by reactivation of the poliovirus, is not a form of ALS, and is not caused by new depletion of anterior horn cells in the spinal cord. The cause is thought to be increased susceptibility to later (possibly age-related) degeneration in the periphery of enlarged motor units. Postpolio amyotrophy is important to recognize because it may at first be misdiagnosed as ALS, but the amyotrophy progresses more slowly and is not life-threatening.

NEUROMUSCULAR JUNCTION DISORDERS

Disorders affecting the neuromuscular junction deserve special emphasis because myasthenia gravis is a model for all other autoimmune diseases and because revolutionary progress has been made in its treatment.

Myasthenia Gravis

Myasthenia gravis used to be disabling or fatal for the majority of patients, but with modern immunotherapy most patients can be restored to full, productive lives. The basic abnormality in myasthenia gravis is a deficit of available acetylcholine receptors at neuromuscular junctions, caused by autoantibodies to those receptors.

The reduction in junctional acetylcholine receptors accounts for most if not all of the clinical and physiologic abnormalities in myasthenic gravis. The basic principle is that the amplitude of end-plate potentials depends on the number of interactions between presynaptically released acetylcholine molecules and postsynaptic acetylcholine receptor molecules. In myasthenia gravis, the decrease in receptors limits the number of interactions, dropping the amplitude of end-plate potentials below the threshold needed to trigger muscle action potentials. Thus, neuromuscular transmission fails. When transmission fails at many junctions, the whole muscle loses power, and the clinical manifestation is weakness.

Neuromuscular fatigue is the single most characteristic feature of myasthenia gravis. The patient cannot sustain or repeat forceful muscle contractions. Electrophysiologically, fatigue is seen as a progressive drop in the amplitude of muscle responses evoked by repetitive stimulation of motor nerves. It is normal for acetylcholine release to decline after the first few repeated stimulations of motor nerves; in people with too few acetylcholine receptors, repeated stimulation causes fatigue.

The neuromuscular abnormalities in myasthenia gravis are caused by serum anti-acetylcholine receptor antibodies, which are found in 80–90% of patients. These autoantibodies reduce the number of junctional acetylcholine receptors by at least three mechanisms:

1. Accelerated endocytosis and degradation of acetylcholine receptors. In about 90% of patients with myasthenia, autoantibodies cross-link receptors, causing enhancement of their endocytosis and subsequent degradation in lysosomes.
2. Functional blockade of acetylcholine receptors. In many patients, antibodies can block the ligand-binding site of acetylcholine receptors.
3. Damage to receptors. Electron microscopy of patients' neuromuscular junctions reveals complement deposition and simplification of postsynaptic folds.

The absolute concentration of circulating anti-acetylcholine receptor antibodies correlates poorly with the clinical severity of myasthenia gravis. But a large change (more than 50%) in a patient's antibody concentration generally correlates with a change in clinical status.

Immune dysregulation may play a role in the development and maintenance of myasthenia gravis. About 75% of patients with myasthenia have thymic abnormalities; of these, 85% show germinal center formation (hyperplasia), and about 15% have thymomas. The disease has been reported in association with many other autoimmune diseases, including Hashimoto's thyroiditis, Graves' disease, pernicious anemia, rheumatoid arthritis, polymyositis, systemic lupus erythematosus, pemphigus, Lambert-Eaton myasthenic syndrome, and idiopathic thrombocytopenic purpura.

The incidence of myasthenia gravis is age- and sex-related, with two peaks—one in the teens and 20's, mostly in women, and the other in the 50's and 60's, mostly in men. Because myasthenia is a disease of the nicotinic acetylcholine receptor, only the motor system is impaired. The cardinal features are weakness and fatigability of skeletal muscles. Sensation, reflexes, cognition, and other neural functions remain normal. The history includes weakness, usually in a characteristic distribution involving elevators of the eyelids and extraocular muscles (ptosis and diplopia), and often affecting the neck extensors (head drooping) and proximal limb muscles. When the muscles of expression, phonation, articulation, and chewing are affected, patients may have a characteristic facial "snarl" and nasal, dysarthric speech, and they may need to prop their jaw closed. Most patients give a history of fluctuation and diurnal variability in the weakness and fatigability—worse in the afternoon, worse with repeated activity, improved by rest. If the weakness has a vague and variable pattern, it may be misinterpreted as being of psychogenic origin. In women, weakness may worsen premenstrually. Infants born to mothers with myasthenia may have transient weakness.

On physical exam, the findings are limited to the motor system; patients have no loss of reflexes or change in sensation or coordination. The physician should document patients' baseline strength with a survey of motor power; this allows later evaluation of the results of treatment. The deltoids, triceps, and iliopsoas are the most frequently involved limb muscles. Measures of motor function should include timed forward arm abduction, vital capacity, and dynamometry of selected muscles and grip.

Since immunotherapy is often lifelong, treatment should not be started until the diagnosis has been confirmed objectively by laboratory tests, best done in this order:

- Edrophonium test. If muscle strength definitely improves after administration of the short-acting cholinesterase inhibitor edrophonium, the test is positive. Only weak muscles that can be measured objectively should be assessed. An initial test dose of 2 mg is given intravenously, and if there is no change, the patient is given an additional 8 mg and reassessed.

- Repetitive nerve stimulation of weak or proximal muscle groups

- Anti-acetylcholine receptor antibody assay

- Single-fiber EMG

When myasthenia gravis is confirmed, patients should have computed tomography or magnetic resonance imaging of the mediastinum to search for a tumor or enlargement of the thymus. They should also have thyroid function tests and spirometry. Conditions that may worsen myasthenia gravis include hyper- and hypothyroidism, occult infection, and certain medications, including but not limited to antiarrhythmic agents and aminoglycoside antibiotics. Disorders that may interfere with immunosuppressive therapy include tuberculosis (a skin test should always precede immunotherapy), other chronic infections, diabetes, peptic ulcer, occult gastrointestinal bleeding, and hypertension.

The prognosis for patients with myasthenia gravis has improved strikingly as a result of advances in treatment. The most important current treatments are anticholinesterase agents, thymectomy, immunosuppressive drugs, and plasmapheresis.

Anticholinesterase agents enhance neuromuscular transmission by prolonging the action of acetylcholine released at the neuromuscular junction. The most widely used drug is pyridostigmine bromide. Its action begins within 10–30 minutes, peaks at about 2 hours, and then declines gradually. The usual initial dose is 60 mg every 4 hours during the day; it is then adjusted according to the patient's response. Although anticholinesterases benefit most patients, the improvement is often incomplete, and most patients require further measures.

Thymoma is a universally accepted indication for surgery, since the tumor may spread locally and become invasive, although it rarely metastasizes. If the whole tumor cannot be removed, patients should be given postoperative radiation. Whether or not the thymus gland is enlarged, thymectomy is also indicated for all patients with generalized myasthenia gravis between puberty and about age 50 who have not improved enough on an anticholinesterase alone. The optimal surgical technique is a maximal transsternal approach with exploration of the neck, designed to remove as much thymus tissue as possible. Up to 85% of patients improve after thymectomy; of these, about 35% achieve drug-free remission. However, benefit from thymectomy is delayed, rarely appearing before 6 months and often requiring up to 2–5 years.

Prednisone, azathioprine, and cyclosporine are now considered first-line drugs for chronic immunosuppressive therapy in myasthenia gravis. Immunotherapy is indicated when either generalized weakness or eye symptoms are not adequately controlled by cholinesterase inhibitors and are sufficiently disabling to the patient that they outweigh the risks of the drugs' possible side effects. Prednisone or cyclosporine usually takes a few weeks to start working, and the patient may not receive maximal benefit until 3–6 months into treatment. Azathioprine can take 3–12 months to start working, and the peak effect may require 1–2 years. Cyclophosphamide is potent but highly toxic and so is reserved for rare patients who do not respond to other therapies. Plasmapheresis or intravenous immunoglobulin is often useful for short-term management of acute problems, or as pre- or postoperative therapy; but these measures give only transient benefit, and they are extremely expensive.

Lambert-Eaton Myasthenic Syndrome

Lambert-Eaton myasthenic syndrome is an autoimmune disorder of the presynaptic nerve terminals. The affected patient usually presents with symmetric proximal weakness without atrophy (mimicking myopathy) and variable, fluctuating (hence, myasthenic) weakness of the legs and arms. Lambert-Eaton myasthenic syndrome differs from myasthenia gravis in several ways: Cranial muscles are affected only mildly, if at all; patients may have mild ptosis, but no ophthalmoplegia; respiratory function is usually unimpaired; diurnal variation is less common; strength rarely fatigues on continuing muscle activity and may even improve; distal deep tendon reflexes are often absent; and patients have autonomic symptoms (dry mouth, pupil abnormalities). Lambert-Eaton myasthenic syndrome can be distinguished from myopathy and myasthenia gravis by electrophysiologic studies. Repetitive nerve stimulation reveals a progressive increase in amplitude of muscle responses after brief exercise or high-frequency stimulation.

The disease is caused by IgG antibodies directed against voltage-gated Ca^{2+} channels in motor nerve terminals, resulting in impaired quantal release of acetylcholine and consequent muscle weakness. In two-thirds of patients, the disease is associated with small cell lung cancer, in which autoantibodies triggered by tumor Ca^{2+} channels cross-react with nerve terminal Ca^{2+} channels. The remaining one-third of patients have the disease in association with other autoimmune disorders, or in isolation. Because the disease may precede by years the recognition of small cell tumor of the lung, gastric cancer, or renal cancer, all patients with the syndrome should have a careful search for neoplasms at regular intervals, at least once a year.

Immunotherapy succeeds variably, best with prednisone or plasmapheresis. Controlling the underlying cancer with surgery, radiation therapy, or chemotherapy may bring a partial or, rarely, a complete remission. Patients respond modestly at best to cholinesterase inhibitors, but giving 3,4-diaminopyridine to enhance presynaptic acetylcholine release is of proven benefit.

Botulism

The toxin of *Clostridium botulinum* blocks the release of acetylcholine from motor nerve terminals, thereby producing an acute syndrome that shares many features with Lambert-Eaton myasthenic syndrome. Cranial and limb muscles are affected in a descending pattern that develops over hours to days. The earliest symptoms are usually visual blurring or diplopia, dysphagia, and dysarthria. Many patients have autonomic symptoms such as dry mouth, constipation, and urine retention. Fatal respiratory paralysis is averted by early recognition and intensive care.

Sources of the toxin are inadequately sterilized food that contains the toxin and organisms contaminating a wound (wound botulism). In infants, *C botulinum* itself can grow in the gastrointestinal tract, allowing chronic absorption of small amounts of toxin. Botulism is diagnosed by distinctive electrophysiology showing a presynaptic neuromuscular transmission defect (as in Lambert-Eaton myasthenic syndrome) and by identifying the toxin in the stool or wound.

Trivalent antitoxin is used to prevent progression of botulism. Antibiotics are ineffective. 3,4-Diaminopyridine improves strength by enhancing acetylcholine release. Most survivors of botulism recover fully.

MYOPATHIES

"Myopathy" describes disorders that produce weakness by affecting muscle fibers without interfering with their nerve supply or neuromuscular junctions. The myopathies are a large, heterogeneous group of disorders classified by both etiology and temporal course. The myopathies to be discussed are muscular dystrophies and myotonias, metabolic myopathies, inflammatory myopathies, mitochondrial multisystem disorders with myopathy, myopathies related to systemic diseases and drugs, episodic muscle disorders, and congenital myopathies as they apply to adults.

How can these heterogeneous disorders be recognized? Most myopathies present similarly, with symmetric proximal muscle weakness. Patients may have little or no atrophy; severe atrophy almost always appears long after the weakness (unlike denervation, in which atrophy is an early sign). The remainder of the neurologic exam, including sensation, is normal. Tendon reflexes can usually be obtained until weakness is advanced. The pattern of weakness looks similar in most myopathies, so other clinical and laboratory features must be used to distinguish one myopathy from another.

The most important diagnostic clue is weakness, as defined by impaired function. Patients may report arm weakness as difficulty keeping their arms abducted, as when brushing their hair, carrying heavy objects, or putting things on high shelves. They report proximal leg weakness as difficulty with running, climbing stairs, or rising from a low chair or from the bathtub. Stair climbing and gait may be waddling because hip extensor weakness makes the pelvis tilt from side to side. Pain and muscle tenderness are generally *not* presenting features, except rarely in toxic or inflammatory myopathies. When pain or tenderness is the only or the most prominent symptom, the physician should not suspect myopathy. Polymyalgia rheumatica, polyarteritis nodosa, and psychogenic disorders are much more likely to produce severe pain.

Although it is a useful rule of thumb that proximal muscle weakness suggests myopathy, there are important exceptions (Table 13.12–6). Sometimes diseases of the central nervous system that affect the corticospinal tracts cause apparent proximal muscle weakness. Negative findings in myopathy—the absence of extensor plantar responses, fasciculations, and sensory findings—also distinguish it from other diseases of the central or peripheral nervous system.

Muscular Dystrophies

Muscular dystrophies are by definition primary muscle diseases that are inherited and progressive. Dystrophies are classified by unique phenotypic and genetic features.

Duchenne's and Becker's Muscular Dystrophies: Duchenne's muscular dystrophy is an X-linked myopathy that causes progressive necrosis as a result of the absence of the sarcolemmal protein dystrophin. The disease is characterized by muscle pseudohypertrophy (especially in the calf), tendon contractures, progressive weakness beginning at the toddler stage, and progression to death from respiratory muscle paralysis or cardiomyopathy in the

Table 13.12–6. Proximal weakness is not equivalent to myopathy.

Proximal weakness that is not myopathic
Lambert-Eaton myasthenic syndrome
Myasthenia gravis
Guillain-Barré syndrome
Porphyric neuropathy
Chronic inflammatory demyelinating polyneuropathy

Myopathies with prominent distal weakness
Myotonic dystrophy
Scapuloperoneal muscular dystrophy
Inclusion body myopathy

Asymmetric or "skip" patterns of weakness in myopathies
Facioscapulohumeral dystrophy (spares deltoids)
Inclusion body myopathy (involvement of forearm flexors and quadriceps may be severe)

teens or 20's. It is the adult respiratory and cardiac problems that internists are asked to manage. All patients have markedly elevated serum CK activity and an absence of dystrophin by immunoblot and immunocytochemistry of biopsied muscle; on DNA analysis, two-thirds of patients have an out-of-frame deletion of the dystrophin gene (a deletion that causes misreading of triplet codes). Treatment involves physiotherapy and tendon lengthening for disabling contractures, bracing to prolong ambulation, and temporary corticosteroid treatment, which is known to delay the loss of ambulation.

Becker's muscular dystrophy is a far milder allelic "dystrophinopathy." The muscle hypertrophy, contractures, and patterns of weakness are similar to the more severe allelic form, but most boys with Becker's dystrophy can still walk independently in their late teens or even their 20's and 30's, and most survive longer than boys with Duchenne's dystrophy. In this disease, dystrophin is usually shortened in length or reduced in amount (because of in-frame deletion), rather than absent as in Duchenne's dystrophy. A significant proportion of patients have cardiomyopathy or muscle cramping. In fact, the mildest variants may present with these features alone and so present a diagnostic challenge to the internist. Management is similar to that for Duchenne's dystrophy.

Facioscapulohumeral Muscular Dystrophy: This disorder is autosomal dominant and highly variable in expressivity. The patient standing with arms outstretched laterally has a pathognomonic appearance: bilateral facial and shoulder girdle muscle weakness, with characteristically high-riding superior scapular margins, giving a double-humped appearance to the outline of the trapezius. Curiously, there are "skip" patterns of weakness, so that, for example, the supraspinatus and biceps may be weak but the neighboring deltoids are unaffected. Muscle biopsy shows myopathic changes and sometimes inflammation. Surgical fixation of the scapulae to the rib cage may greatly improve shoulder girdle function.

Oculopharyngeal Muscular Dystrophy: This form of muscular dystrophy typically begins in the 40's or later, with progressive lid ptosis, weakness of eye muscles, and eventually dysphagia. Because of this presentation, the disorder is often confused with myasthenia gravis. Inspection of family reunion photographs for hereditary ptosis is often diagnostic. The muscle biopsy is distinctive, showing not only the expected myopathic findings, but numerous autophagic vacuoles and intranuclear filamentous inclusions. There is no specific management, and repair of ptosis by plicating the eyelids never lasts.

Myotonic Dystrophy: Myotonic dystrophy, the most prevalent inherited neuromuscular disease in adults, is a multisystem disorder characterized by progressive wasting and weakness of distal muscles and myotonia. Many patients can be recognized instantly by their characteristic frontal balding, long face, ptosis, glasses with aphakic lenses for cataracts, hollowing of the masseter and temporalis muscles, slackened mouth, facial weakness, and thin neck and limbs. Other features include intellectual impairment, testicular atrophy, excessive daytime somnolence, insulin resistance, and cardiac conduction defects. The important finding on exam is myotonia—involuntary delayed relaxation following a contraction, such as after sustained handgrip. However, patients complain of weakness, not the myotonia. This autosomal dominant disease is highly variable in severity and age of onset; it exhibits "anticipation," the phenomenon of increasing severity of inherited disease in successive generations of an affected family.

The genetic defect is amplification (Chapter 10.2) of an unstable trinucleotide CTG repeat located in an untranslated region of the gene for myotonin-protein kinase on chromosome 19. The number of CTG repeats may run from about 50 in mildly affected individuals to thousands of copies in severely affected patients. Amplification of the CTG repeat is the molecular basis for genetic anticipation. When myotonic dystrophy presents at birth (congenital myotonic dystrophy), weakness is severe and mental retardation is the rule. Paternal inheritance of very large CTG repeats is genetically inhibited, accounting for maternal inheritance of the congenital form.

Myotonic dystrophy is diagnosed by recognizing the syndrome, supported by findings of myotonia on EMG and multihued speckled cataracts on slit-lamp exam. When troublesome, myotonia can be treated with phenytoin or other drugs, but few patients request this. Distal weakness causing footdrop is treated with ankle-foot orthoses.

Other Myotonic Disorders: Myotonia congenita causes muscle stiffness, especially during rest after exercise, but little or no weakness. EMG displays the myotonia. The myotonia, which may be disabling, can be treated with acetazolamide, procainamide, tocainide, phenytoin, mexiletine, or other drugs.

In paramyotonia congenita, muscle hyperexcitability and myotonia are provoked more by cold exposure than by rest or activity. Patients do not have fixed weakness. Many patients require no treatment other than modification of exercise and avoidance of cold, but tocainide and mexiletine are effective for the myotonia.

Inborn Errors of Muscle Metabolism

Defects Presenting with Exercise Intolerance: Several disorders of glycolysis can present similarly, with fatigue and pain starting during the first few minutes of strenuous exercise. In the classic disorder, myophosphorylase deficiency (McArdle's disease), patients develop painful contractures (electrically silent contraction of muscle) soon after exercise, as the brief intramuscular carbohydrate supply is exhausted but glycolysis cannot make new fuel. Patients are generally normal on exam, without detectable weakness or wasting, and the usual laboratory tests (serum CK, EMG, and muscle biopsy) are unrevealing unless the biopsy is stained with a specific histochemical reaction for myophosphorylase. The physician should consider the diagnosis if the forearm exercise test (refer to Brooke in "Suggested Reading") fails to cause a normal three- to fourfold elevation in lactate during the first 3 minutes after exercise. Rare patients have myoglobinuria in addition to their exercise intolerance. Inherited deficiencies of phosphofructokinase, phosphoglycerate kinase, phosphoglycerate mutase, and LDH can present similarly.

By contrast, deficient carnitine palmityltransferase makes a person unable to use fatty acids as fuel in endurance exercise (20–30 minutes into exercise). The deficient enzyme normally is responsible for linking long-chain fatty acids to carnitine, this process being necessary to transport fuel across the mitochondrial membrane for oxidation. Patients have muscle pain or fatigue or weakness, but they can tolerate brief (anaerobic) exercise. Attacks may be severe enough to include myoglobinuria. The most telling feature is that the attacks follow prolonged exercise or fasting, which causes muscle to depend on fatty acid metabolism. Physical exam is generally unrevealing, and patients have normal bulk and strength. Laboratory tests—CK, EMG, and muscle biopsy—are generally unrevealing unless the biopsy specimen is analyzed biochemically for carnitine palmityltransferase. Management is avoiding fasting and exercise that is strenuous or lengthy enough to provoke pain.

Defects Presenting with Weakness: Carnitine, the transporter of fatty acids for oxidation by muscle mitochondria, may itself be deficient. Because 98% of the body's carnitine is in muscle, the chief feature of carnitine deficiency is myopathy, manifested as slowly progressive muscle weakness. Fasting may exacerbate it. Patients may also present with cardiomyopathy. Myoglobinuria is rare. EMG shows myopathy, and muscle biopsy shows distinctive accumulation of excess lipid droplets within muscle fibers. The diagnosis is established by measurement of carnitine in serum or muscle. The disorder can be treated by carnitine supplements of 2–4 g per day and avoidance of fasting. Patients can also become weak when carnitine is depleted systemically secondary to hemodialysis, cirrhosis, Reye's syndrome, certain drugs, or β-oxidation defects with organic aciduria. In some of these disorders, carnitine replacement has improved muscle weakness.

Inflammatory Myopathies

Rheumatologic aspects of the inflammatory myopathies are covered in Chapter 3.6. This discussion stresses these diseases' neuromuscular features.

Polymyositis and Dermatomyositis: The proximal weakness in polymyositis and dermatomyositis is more pronounced in the legs than the arms and usually evolves over months. Twenty percent of patients have dysphagia. Respiratory muscles can be affected, and rare patients present with respiratory insufficiency. It is important to note that only 25% of patients with polymyositis or dermatomyositis have significant muscle pain or tenderness. Serum CK activity is a sensitive, but nonspecific, test for polymyositis and dermatomyositis, with elevated levels in more than 85% of patients. Levels can reach 50 times normal. A normal CK does not exclude the diagnosis.

Polymyositis has a characteristic but not pathognomonic EMG showing fibrillations or positive sharp waves at rest, as well as myopathic motor unit potentials (brief, small, and polyphasic). The same EMG is seen in dermatomyositis, inclusion body myopathy, acid maltase deficiency, and necrotizing or lysosomal myopathies induced by drugs. Muscle biopsy shows autoreactive T lymphocytes and macrophages surrounding and invading muscle fibers, with resultant necrosis and regeneration.

Dermatomyositis is not polymyositis with a rash. The two disorders have distinct clinical and pathophysiologic features (Chapter 3.6). The pathologic findings of dermatomyositis are perifascicular myofiber atrophy, necrosis, and regeneration. Muscle capillaries are reduced in number and complement membrane attack complex is deposited within the microvessels, indicating an immune-mediated vascular pathogenesis.

When initial treatment with corticosteroids fails, or for steroid-sparing when steroids are too toxic, patients with polymyositis or dermatomyositis are given immunosuppressive therapy such as azathioprine, methotrexate, cyclosporine, or human immunoglobulin. The degree of weakness—and, to a lesser degree, the serum CK elevation—guides the duration and amount of immunotherapy.

History and muscle biopsy must distinguish conditions that mimic polymyositis and dermatomyositis clinically. These are drug-induced myopathies, sarcoid myopathy, HIV-associated inflammatory myopathy, inclusion body myositis, pyomyositis, viral and parasitic inflammatory myopathies, eosinophilic fasciitis, metabolic myopathies such as acid maltase deficiency, and rarely myasthenia gravis or muscular dystrophies with inflammation. To exclude these mimics, the physician should try to confirm polymyositis or dermatomyositis pathologically before immunotherapy.

Polymyositis, and even more, dermatomyositis, have a definite though infrequent association with malignancy. The diagnosis of cancer can precede or follow polymyositis or dermatomyositis by years. Adult patients should be evaluated for malignancy with, at a minimum, stool for occult blood, mammography, pelvic exam, and chest computed tomography.

Inclusion Body Myopathy: Like polymyositis, this disorder has cytotoxic T cells infiltrating muscle, but the morphology is distinctive for two kinds of inclusion bodies: numerous autophagic vacuoles and both cytoplasmic and intranuclear inclusions of intermediate filaments

(15–20 nm in diameter). The vacuolar and filamentous inclusions can be recognized by electron microscopy or immunocytochemistry for amyloid or ubiquitin, which are bound to the filaments.

Most patients with inclusion body myopathy are older men. The disease seems to affect patients who have had polymyositis for a few years. Some researchers believe that inclusion body myopathy is a sequel to typical polymyositis. But the pattern of weakness occasionally differs from polymyositis in that more patients have asymmetric and distal muscle weakness (typically, forearm flexors). There is no pain. An important distinguishing feature is that inclusion body myopathy does not respond to corticosteroids.

HIV-Associated Inflammatory Myopathy: An inflammatory myopathy clinically indistinguishable from polymyositis is associated with HIV infection. Because of the therapeutic implications, the physician must distinguish HIV inflammatory myopathy from zidovudine-induced myopathy, which typically begins about 1 year after patients start zidovudine therapy. All patients with zidovudine-induced myopathy have high serum CK activity, most are weak, and many have myalgia. Biopsy is essential because it may be the only way to differentiate the two conditions. The distinguishing morphologic feature of HIV-associated inflammatory myopathy is so-called primary inflammation surrounding and invading nonnecrotic myofibers; in contrast, the "bystander" inflammation sometimes seen in zidovudine myopathy is only interstitial.

The response to a change in therapy can help make the distinction. In some patients, HIV inflammatory myopathy responds to corticosteroids or human immune globulin; more potent cytotoxic drugs are not generally used because of the risks of immunosuppression. By contrast, zidovudine myopathy responds to reducing or stopping the drug. The physician best documents remission by graphing the serum CK activity weekly and correlating it with measurements of strength. CK returns to normal, and strength recovers in 4–8 weeks. Some patients can then restart therapy on 50% of the previous dose. Virtually no one with an immune-mediated inflammatory myopathy has such an early remission.

Mitochondrial Myopathies

Mitochondrial cytopathies are multisystem neurologic disorders that can include myopathy, chronic progressive external ophthalmoplegia, encephalopathy, retinal pigment degeneration, cardiomyopathy, sensorineural deafness, polyneuropathy, and even gastrointestinal disorders. Mitochondrial cytopathies can begin at any time from childhood to the 50's. The disorders are clinically and genetically heterogeneous and overlapping, but some syndromes imply a specific mutation (see Table 13.12–5).

These mitochondrial disorders have several clinicopathologic correlations that distinguish them from other inherited myopathies: (1) maternal inheritance implicates a mutation of mitochondrial DNA (Chapter 10.1); (2) the great reliance of skeletal muscle and the central nervous system on mitochondrial ATP accounts for the high frequency of disease in these tissues; (3) the mutation rate of mitochondrial DNA is high and increases with age, in part because of injurious free radicals generated within mitochondria, lack of protective mitochondrial histones, and limited mitochondrial DNA repair.

What links the symptoms of mitochondrial myopathies is their tendency to involve skeletal muscle mitochondria, producing giant mitochondria with inclusions and mitochondrial proliferation. These abnormalities are recognized on muscle biopsy as "ragged red" muscle fibers by their distinctive histochemical appearance on modified Gomori trichrome stain. Important diagnostic clues are elevations of the serum lactate:pyruvate ratio and the cerebrospinal fluid protein. Many of the mitochondrial myopathies share abnormal muscle activity of cytochrome C oxidase, a huge and essential mitochondrial enzyme with 13 subunits, of which 10 are encoded and regulated in autosomes, and 3 are encoded in the mitochondrial gene.

The mitochondrial disorders have fanciful acronyms. In myoclonic epilepsy with ragged red fibers (MERRF), the seizures are most prominent, but severely affected patients have dementia, ataxia, and mitochondrial myopathy. Mitochondrial encephalomyopathy with lactic acidosis and stroke-like episodes (MELAS) is characterized by weakness, episodes of headache or vomiting associated with lactic acidosis, and stroke-like focal brain lesions predisposed to developing in the occipital and parietal cortex. The Kearns-Sayre syndrome presents as chronic progressive external ophthalmoplegia, weakness, retinal degeneration, short stature, ataxia, dementia, and deafness; many patients die of heart block. Patients with mitochondrial disorders may also have syndromes of isolated cardiomyopathy, chronic progressive external ophthalmoplegia, or recurrent myoglobinuria with exercise intolerance.

Management of the patient with a mitochondrial disorder is symptomatic: fluids and bicarbonate for lactic acidosis, pacing for heart block, and anticonvulsants for seizures. Many patients have been given antioxidants in the hope of preventing mitochondrial depletion caused by ongoing oxidative damage, plus cofactors (such as ubiquinone) to "bridge the gap" in mitochondrial electron transport; only occasional patients respond.

Myopathies and Neuromuscular Disorders Related to Systemic Disease

The metabolic myopathies associated with hyper- and hypothyroidism, hyperparathyroidism, Cushing's disease, and Addison's disease generally cause only mild proximal weakness. Serum CK activity is usually normal; the exception is a mild elevation in hypothyroidism. EMG is often normal or nonspecific, and muscle biopsy generally shows only type II myofiber atrophy and mild nonspecific myopathic changes. In fact, it is the *lack* of significant laboratory evidence in a patient with proximal weakness that may first suggest a metabolic myopathy. All the metabolic myopathies are reversible with treatment of the underlying metabolic disorder.

Skeletal muscle involvement in systemic diseases like sarcoidosis, polyarteritis nodosa, and Wegener's granulomatosis may or may not cause symptoms. Most affected patients have asymptomatic involvement, which explains the "blind" muscle biopsies taken to diagnose these disorders. Symptomatic myopathy—far less common—is usually an indolent process with proximal muscle weakness and wasting. When the diagnosis has been confirmed by muscle biopsy, patients are treated first with corticosteroids.

Amyloid myopathy, associated with AL (amyloid light chain) amyloidosis and usually IgG κ-paraproteinemia, is a rare but distinctive cause of weakness, muscle pseudohypertrophy, macroglossia, and respiratory insufficiency.

Patients with neuromuscular diseases may first present

Table 13.12–7. Cardiomyopathy in neuromuscular disease.

Muscular dystrophies
  Duchenne's muscular dystrophy (ECG changes are common early in course; pathology is universal at autopsy)
  Becker's muscular dystrophy
  Myotonic dystrophy (two-thirds of patients have conduction disturbance)

Myopathies
  Drug-induced myopathies (see "Drug-Induced Myopathies" in text)
  Type II glycogenosis (acid maltase deficiency) (infantile form [Pompe's disease] may be fatal)
  Type III glycogenosis (debranching enzyme) (all patients have hypertrophy; 40% have congestive failure)
  Carnitine deficiency

Neuropathies
  Beriberi (thiamine deficiency)
  Alcoholism
  Diabetes mellitus
  Amyloidosis
  Fabry's disease (ceramide trihexosidase deficiency) (painful autonomic neuropathy, cutaneous manifestations, cardiomyopathy, cardiac and cerebral infarcts)
  Refsum's disease (phytanic acid storage disease) (hypertrophic neuropathy, deafness, retinitis pigmentosa, cerebellar ataxia, cardiomyopathy)

Other
  Friedreich's ataxia (hypertrophic cardiomyopathy in 90% of patients)
  Mitochondrial diseases, especially Kearns-Sayre syndrome (heart block)

Systemic disorders (manifestations in both heart and nerve or muscle; nerve and muscle involvement is not necessarily symptomatic)
  Polyarteritis nodosa
  Sarcoidosis
  Systemic lupus erythematosus

to the cardiologist, gastroenterologist, pulmonary specialist, or intensive care specialist. Cardiomyopathy or a cardiac conduction disturbance is often an important clue to unrecognized neuromuscular disease (Table 13.12–7). Gastroenterologists may see patients for dysphagia that turns out to be an early manifestation of neuromuscular disease (see Table 13.12–2). Although many chronic neuromuscular disorders eventually affect the respiratory muscles, a few can actually present with respiratory failure (see Table 13.12–2).

Steroid Myopathy: Prolonged use of high-dose corticosteroids can cause impressive muscle atrophy and weakness (steroid myopathy), especially when patients take divided doses or suffer another muscle insult such as protein malnutrition, alcohol abuse, or denervation. Most steroid myopathy affects patients taking daily doses equivalent to at least 25 mg of prednisone.

Steroid myopathy produces proximal weakness, with legs weaker than arms—identical with the pattern in nearly all patients with polymyositis. CK is usually normal or unchanged from baseline. In patients who are taking corticosteroids to treat polymyositis, steroid myopathy may be difficult to distinguish from the polymyositis itself. In fact, the two may coexist. A therapeutic trial of dose reduction or dose escalation may resolve the confusion. In steroid myopathy, a major dose reduction improves the patient's strength, usually within 2–4 weeks and always within about 8 weeks.

Drug-Induced Myopathies: Toxic myopathies are underrecognized. Drugs alone rarely cause myopathy, but require a second risk factor. Chronic renal insufficiency is the key risk factor for clofibrate and colchicine myopathies. When patients with reduced creatinine clearance take these drugs, the physician must monitor their serum CK and muscle strength carefully to prevent a potentially disabling disease. The nephrotic syndrome is an additional risk factor in clofibrate myopathy, since the drug is strongly protein bound.

Fasting is the risk factor for myonecrosis and myoglobinuria from ethanol. Ipecac myopathy is seen in patients with bulimia or anorexia.

Drug interactions can also be a risk factor. For example, lovastatin can produce a necrotizing myopathy and myoglobinuria. The risk increases 5- to 30-fold when the drug is given concomitantly with cyclosporine or gemfibrozil, both of which are bile-excreted, like lovastatin.

Toxic myopathies often coexist with neuropathy or cardiomyopathy that can overshadow the myopathy. Many of the drugs that produce systemic toxicity are amphophilic; that is, they contain both hydrophobic and hydrophilic regions. This property allows such drugs to enter cell membranes in nerve, muscle, heart, lung, and liver, where they cause necrosis or lysosomal lipid storage. In a patient with myopathy, the finding of a concurrent axonal neuropathy sharply limits the diagnostic possibilities. Drugs that can cause both conditions include amiodarone, chloroquine, clofibrate, colchicine, vincristine, doxorubicin, ethanol, hydroxychloroquine, organophosphates, perhexiline, and tryptophan. Probably the most common nondrug causes of neuromyopathies are uremia, collagen vascular disorders, AIDS, and paraneoplastic syndromes. Cardiomyopathy with myopathy can be caused by drugs such as ethanol, emetine, doxorubicin, and chloroquine. For nondrug causes, see Table 13.12–7.

Infections: Pyomyositis is a treatable bacterial abscess usually limited to a few contiguous muscles, but in rare patients it causes a progressive generalized inflammatory myopathy. The affected muscle is hot, swollen, and painful, worsening with movement. *Staphylococcus aureus* causes more than 85% of cases, and tuberculosis and streptococci the remainder. Pyomyositis is most common in the tropics, but has been recognized increasingly in temperate climates. Diagnosis by Gram's stain and culture of homogenized muscle permit appropriate antibiotic therapy.

Parasitic infections of muscle include trichinosis, toxoplasmosis, and cysticercosis. Still common worldwide, trichinosis is contracted by eating pork or feral meat containing the encysted larvae of the nematode *Trichinella spiralis*. Trichinosis is characterized by diarrhea, malaise, fever, myalgia, severe myositis, and sometimes periorbital edema. Almost all patients have an eosinophilic leukocytosis and a modest rise in CK activity, but hypergammaglobulinemia makes the erythrocyte sedimentation rate low. Diagnosis is by muscle biopsy and *Trichinella* serology, both most likely to detect the organism during the third week of infection. Mebendazole or thiabendazole, with or without prednisone, is effective treatment.

Many types of viral infections, such as influenza and coxsackievirus, can cause transient inflammatory myopathies that are treated symptomatically.

Periodic Paralysis

Periodic paralysis is a rare syndrome characterized by spells of severe weakness in the limb muscles. The spells last minutes to hours. Cranial muscles are rarely involved, and the respiratory muscles are almost never involved. The syndrome can be subdivided into hyper-, hypo-, and normokalemic types. The hyperkalemic type is caused by defective inactivation of sodium channels, leading to changes in potassium flux across muscle membranes. By contrast, the hypokalemic form is caused by a calcium channel defect (see Table 13.12–3). In rare patients, hypo- or hyperkalemia causes a complicating cardiac arrhythmia. An acquired form of hypokalemic periodic paralysis is associated with thyrotoxicosis, most commonly in young Hispanic and Asian men. Acute attacks of hypokalemic periodic paralysis respond to potassium salts. Acetazolamide can help prevent further attacks of all but the thyrotoxic form, which requires specific antithyroid therapy.

The hyperkalemic form of periodic paralysis may be associated with paramyotonia congenita (cold-induced weakness and stiffness), another allelic disorder of sodium channels. In this disorder, spells of weakness are rarely severe and may respond to oral glucose. Prophylaxis against further attacks requires thiazide diuretics.

Congenital Myopathies

The congenital myopathies are marked by congenital floppiness and a usually benign, nonprogressive limb and facial weakness. These disorders are defined by the distinctive muscle morphology for which they are named: central core disease, nemaline (rod) myopathy, myotubular myopathy, and congenital fiber type disproportion. Muscle biopsy histochemistry is therefore diagnostic. Although occasional patients have malignant variants with severe, disabling lifelong weakness or early death, most patients have a normal life span and may even present as weak adults. Associated signs can include a long face, high arched palate, pes cavus, and kyphoscoliosis.

Myoglobinuria

Rhabdomyolysis is acute widespread muscle necrosis that sends myoglobin, CK, creatine, potassium, phosphate, amino acids, and uric acid into the blood. Myoglobin is a small protein that is filtered through the renal glomeruli. When muscle is severely damaged, myoglobinuria develops; the urine looks brown if it contains more than 1 g of myoglobin per liter. The major complication of myoglobinuria is acute renal failure from tubular necrosis, the mechanism of which is unknown. Many patients with rhabdomyolysis develop life-threatening hyperkalemia.

The symptoms of rhabdomyolysis are severe muscle pain, swelling of the extremities, and pigmenturia. Urgent diagnosis is required. The swelling can cause compartment syndromes with peripheral nerve compression and ischemic contracture; patients with these syndromes require prompt fasciotomy. The extremity and trunk muscles become weak and painful, but cranial muscles are rarely involved. Early in rhabdomyolysis, myoglobin turns the urine dark (red to brown), but later the myoglobinuria disappears. Myoglobinuria is missed completely in 50% of patients with rhabdomyolysis, especially when the onset is protracted, as when caused by a toxin. The differential diagnosis of myoglobinuria includes other causes of pigmenturia, such as hemoglobinuria.

Laboratory tests in patients with rhabdomyolysis show a severe increase in serum CK activity, usually more than 200-fold. The physician should first screen the urine for myoglobin by looking for a positive dipstick orthotolidine reaction in erythrocyte-free urine. For confirmation and serial follow-up, urine myoglobin can be quantitated by radioimmunoassay. The serum potassium and phosphate may be high because of cellular necrosis. Patients may have a secondary decrease in calcium, linked to hyperphosphatemia. EMG and muscle biopsy are usually unnecessary. If the intent of muscle biopsy is to search for a predisposing, underlying neuromuscular disease (especially an enzyme deficiency), the biopsy must be delayed for 6–12 weeks to allow the acute degeneration and regeneration to pass.

The innumerable known causes of myoglobinuria can be organized according to mechanism. By far the most common causes are trauma (crush syndrome), ischemia (from a prolonged tourniquet, disseminated intravascular coagulation, or lengthy coma with ischemic muscle crush), exercise-induced rhabdomyolysis (from exercise by untrained persons, status epilepticus, or status asthmaticus, especially when patients are given β-adrenergic receptor agonists), and many drugs that can induce rhabdomyolysis (eg, ethanol, lipid-lowering agents such as clofibrate and lovastatin). Less common causes of myoglobinuria are systemic diseases that alter thermal regulation or demand great energy expenditure (eg, heat stroke, malignant hyperthermia, severe sepsis), and preexisting polymyositis or dermatomyositis. Primary myopathies like metabolic myopathies (eg, myophosphorylase deficiency, carnitine palmityltransferase deficiency) and muscular dystrophies are still less common causes, unless myoglobinuria is recurrent or familial. In a large minority of patients, myoglobinuria seems to be idiopathic.

Since renal failure and cardiac arrhythmias are the major complications of rhabdomyolysis, all patients presenting with this syndrome should be considered for critical care. Life-threatening hyperkalemia should be corrected with sodium bicarbonate, glucose-insulin infusions, or dialysis. Patients need sufficient hydration and alkalinization of the urine. Serum CK, creatinine, and electrolytes are monitored serially until stable. Potentially toxic agents and drugs should be removed immediately. If renal failure progresses, patients require hemofiltration or hemodialysis. Patients with malignant hyperthermia or the neuroleptic malignant syndrome are treated with dantrolene, other muscle relaxants, or bromocriptine.

SUMMARY

▶ Weakness is the cardinal manifestation of all diseases of the motor unit. Urging patients to define what they mean by "weakness" in terms of their activities of daily living not only adds diagnostic specificity but is a useful gauge of severity and progression.

▶ Muscle pain is much less likely to be caused by myopathy than by neuropathy, radiculopathy, or systemic disease.

▶ The diagnosis of amyotrophic lateral sclerosis (ALS), a degeneration of motor neurons, requires a history of progressive weakness and a combination of lower and upper motor neuron signs in a patient with no significant sensory, bowel, or bladder abnormalities.

▶ Myasthenia gravis, marked by weakness and fatigability, is caused by autoantibodies producing a deficit of acetylcholine receptors at neuromuscular junctions. This formerly disabling or fatal disease is now fully treatable with immunotherapy.

▶ In myopathies, proximal muscle weakness usually predominates; however, some myopathies are distal, and some denervating diseases can be proximal. The pattern and temporal course of weakness sort out the differential diagnosis.

SUGGESTED READING

Brooke MH: *A Clinician's View of Neuromuscular Diseases,* 2nd ed. Williams & Wilkins, 1986.

Caroscio JT (editor): *Amyotrophic Lateral Sclerosis: A Guide to Patient Care.* Thieme, 1986.

Dalakas MC: Polymyositis, dermatomyositis, and inclusion-body myositis. N Engl J Med 1991;325:1487.

Drachman DR: Myasthenia gravis. N Engl J Med 1994; 330:1797.

Engel AG, Franzini-Armstrong C (editors): *Myology,* 2nd ed. McGraw-Hill, 1994.

Griggs RC, Mendell JR, Miller RG: *Evaluation and Treatment of Myopathies.* FA Davis, 1995.

Section 14

Psychiatry

Paul W. Ladenson, MD, and Thomas A. Traill, FRCP, Section Editors

Approach to the Patient with a Suspected Psychiatric Disorder

Paul R. McHugh, MD

Doctors suspect a psychiatric disorder when a patient's complaints are accompanied by emotional intensity or incoherence of thought. However, like other patients, those with psychiatric disorders may also come to attention through some chief complaint—"I'm depressed," "I'm anxious," "I'm in pain"—or through the concerns of others—"he's forgetful," "she's drinking too much." Much psychiatric care can and should be given by internists. How physicians confirm the suspicion that their patient has a psychiatric problem and how they move to identify the disorder and its best management are the subjects of this chapter and the remaining chapters in this section.

Psychiatric disorders express themselves through a person's thoughts, moods, or behavior. These disorders can be grouped into four categories: (1) expressions of diseases of the brain; (2) expressions of difficulties in life management arising from psychological characteristics such as intelligence, degree of introversion or extroversion, and emotional stability; (3) behaviors expressing a drive, hunger, appetite, or addiction; and (4) expressions of distress provoked by some past or present life encounter (Table 14.1–1).

Disorders within and across these four categories can share symptoms, but each category has a different fundamental cause and nature, and each requires different treatment and carries a different prognosis. The goal of evaluation is to place patients' problems in one of the categories by gathering evidence from their history and their presenting mental and physical states. For example, a person who has had recurring depression and has a strong family history of a similar mood disorder likely shares that condition. This person must be managed differently from a person whose low mood has been provoked by grief in response to a life event, for example, loss of a loved one (Chapter 14.3).

Acknowledgment: Patricia B. Santora, PhD, contributed to the writing of this chapter.

EVALUATION

As psychiatric disorders become better understood and more treatments become available, evaluation can become systematic and standardized, enabling the physician to classify patients and treat them correctly. The components of a systematic evaluation are the patient's life history (Chapter 14.7), the mental status examination, and, when indicated, a physical examination. For many patients, the assessment must be done in stages, not just in one sitting, because mentally disturbed patients may at first find it difficult to recount their past history and present circumstances. Much information must be sought from family and friends who can describe the patient's past behavior, attitudes, life setting, and overall personality.

The first encounter lays the foundation for every later meeting. From the outset, the physician must make patients as comfortable as possible and win their cooperation. It is helpful at the start to explain to patients what information is needed and to say that some questions may seem irrelevant to the presenting complaint, but all will prove helpful in management. At first, the discussion must focus on patients' immediate distress; this should reassure them that the physician recognizes the importance of their presenting problem and will deal with it. Then the focus can shift to the history; this is often when the therapeutic relationship emerges between patient and physician, whose interest is evidenced to the patient by thoroughness and depth of concern.

History

The patient's history provides a background for understanding the presenting complaint. It is useful to explain to patients that some aspects of their presenting problem are best understood in the context of their history and personality and that this history is best approached chronologically.

Table 14.1–1. The four categories of psychiatric disorders.

Category	Examples
Brain diseases	Dementia Delirium Korsakoff's psychosis Manic-depressive (bipolar) disorder Schizophrenia
Personality traits with psychiatric significance	Mental retardation Unstable extroversion Unstable introversion
Behavior disorders	Alcoholism Drug addiction Sexual paraphilias Anorexia nervosa Hysteria
Disorders related to life events	Grief Demoralization Situational anxiety

The history is structured in two levels. The first and simpler level of inquiry reveals the basic elements of every person's life—birth, family, development, schooling, occupations, sexual emergence and marital or other life commitments, habits, legal encounters, medical illnesses, and abiding personality characteristics. Within this "sketch," the physician notes the patient's burdens, recurring problems, and strengths. Patients should be asked about prior psychiatric problems and treatments.

The second level of assessment goes beyond simply writing a biography. This phase is the search for themes that permit the physician to classify the presenting problem. The physician compares the patient's past and present histories for similarities and differences in mental state and behavior, trying to discern whether the present problem is new or whether it is a current expression of longstanding difficulties that earlier in life may have taken the form of problems with schooling, interpersonal relationships, and career development. This distinction between new and longstanding problems is fundamental to psychiatric assessment and management, because it distinguishes between a disorder that is manifesting for the first time in mental life and behavior, and the recurrence of a lifelong disturbance. For example, an attack of mania typically appears "out of the blue" as a disruption of a person's thoughts, emotions, and behavior. In contrast, a person who has a dramatic and self-preoccupied personality may present with demoralization that will have been presaged by similar reactions to demanding past life circumstances, such as arguments with schoolteachers or inability to get along with a spouse or cooperate with coworkers.

Mental Status Assessment

The mental status assessment is the psychiatric exercise that corresponds to the physical exam in internal medicine. The mental status exam is an assessment of patients at the present moment—a "cross-section" of the contents and capacities of their conscious mind and their behavior during the exam.

Principles: The principal aim of the mental status exam is to discern whether patients' thoughts, moods, and interests are organized in a comprehensible way, and, if not, exactly how they are deranged. The physician can usually get a sense of how well the elements of a patient's mental life are integrated, even if the patient is quite distressed. In many patients with psychiatric disorders, derangements are obvious from the start.

The physician must help patients through the unfamiliar exercise of reviewing their thoughts and moods. Patients are usually reassured when the doctor says, "I'm going to ask you a number of questions about yourself and about problems that some people have. By asking you these questions, I'm not suggesting that you've had any of these experiences." The doctor should also explain that one purpose of the interview is to find out how patients are feeling right now; at the same time, the doctor must remember to observe now and interpret later.

The mental status exam must address the patient's presenting complaint, but the physician must also be thorough. The patient determines how much ground can be covered in one session and to what extent the doctor must individualize the exam. For example, patients may have such suppressed consciousness (drowsiness, lethargy) that the doctor cannot hold their attention. For these patients, the exam should focus on determining degree of consciousness—from alertness to coma—and assessing their ability to answer simple questions about who and where they are. Other patients want to talk only about hallucinatory visions they see or voices they hear, or they reveal that they are dominated by delusions—false, idiosyncratic, incorrigible ideas. Patients may even have delusions about the physician. For example, they may refuse to talk to the physician because they believe that the police are depriving them of their wealth and freedom and that the doctor is in on the plot. Here, the mental status exam must be channeled into winning patients' cooperation to proceed.

The physician must also tailor the exam for patients who are overcome by depression, with its tendency to retard their responses to questions, or by manic excitement, with its flighty distractibility. Patients with a mood disorder may well try to make sense of their emotions by tying them to their life circumstances. Then, when the physician asks, "Do you feel low today?," patients may shift the focus away from their mood by answering, "How would *you* feel if you were in my place?" A physician who takes the patient's explanation out of context from the rest of the exam can mistake one mental disturbance for another, such as diagnosing demoralization when the real problem is major depression (Chapter 14.3).

Procedures: A physician who suspects that a patient has a psychiatric disorder conducts the mental status exam in three systematic parts. First, the doctor must study patients' appearance and behavior, noting their dress and general demeanor as well as their speech and activity during the interview. For example, is it easy or difficult to win the patient's cooperation? Does the patient respond to questions directly and coherently, or vaguely and disjointedly? It is important to write down verbatim the patient's answers to such questions as "How is your mood?" or "What has you worried?" Recording these quotes helps to illustrate the patient's way of speaking and thinking.

The second part of the exam explores the contents of patients' conscious mind, to discern whether they are experiencing hallucinations, holding delusional beliefs, or being subject to intrusive thoughts that recur, frighten, or preoccupy them against their will. At this stage, the physician must ask patients directly, "Please describe your mood. How do you feel about yourself? How hopeful do you feel about the future?" The physician can introduce these questions amiably by saying that they are intended to explore patients' possible thoughts, but do not imply that the patients must harbor such thoughts. In this way, a physician can even ask whether patients are hearing voices of people who are not present and whether they believe that they are the focus of some threatening plot. The range of questions should allow the examiner to assess whether patients are depressed and self-blaming, or, at the other extreme, excited, overconfident, or delusional.

The third part of the exam evaluates patients' cognitive capacities. Patients should be assessed for alertness, responsiveness, adequacy in answering orientation questions ("What's your name? Where are you? What day is this?"), capacity to remember ("What did you eat at your last meal?"), and ability to use language properly and follow commands ("Hold up your right hand. Close your eyes."). The examiner tries to detect conditions like delirium and dementia. These are often overlooked when patients' cognition is not directly tested, but assumed to be intact simply because they seem cooperative. The Mini-Mental Status Examination is a reliable and valid tool for assessing cognitive ability (Chapter 14.2).

Interpretation

To be useful, the information derived from the history and mental status exam must be formulated so that it relates the patient's condition to the four categories of psychiatric disorders. Knowledge of the patient's condition guides decisions about further studies (eg, physical exam, psychological testing) and, eventually, a treatment plan. Although the differential diagnosis and treatment of many psychiatric disturbances are covered in later chapters, the four categories are briefly described here.

CATEGORIES OF PSYCHIATRIC DISORDERS

Diseases

Physicians' usual concern is to make sure that patients are not suffering from some brain disease that might render them unable to cooperate with treatment. Patients with dementia can be recognized by a history of declining mental capacity; on the mental status exam, patients are conscious but impaired in memory, language, and abstract reasoning. Patients with delirium caused by toxic states (eg, kidney or liver failure) are drowsy and difficult to arouse, with impaired cognitive powers such as memory. These patients need a careful review of their general physical condition and of all medications that they are taking, in case they are intoxicated (Chapter 14.2).

Among the most common psychiatric diseases—and one that often afflicts patients who have other concurrent illnesses—is major depression (Chapter 14.3). Patients' consciousness comes to be dominated by disturbances of mood and by distressing beliefs in their own worthlessness and hopelessness. If an internist's patients begin to withdraw from treatment for some medical condition and complain that perhaps the treatment is being wasted on them, the internist should suspect major depression and promptly refer them to a psychiatrist.

The most problematic disease of mental life is schizophrenia. This disease causes disruption of thought, perception, and behavior that the internist may recognize through a patient's bizarre presentation or report of hallucinations or delusions. A crucial rule is that schizophrenia is a diagnosis of exclusion and should not be made until other conditions such as delirium, dementia, and mood disorders have been excluded. These conditions, too, can severely disrupt thought, perception, and behavior. They must be distinguished from schizophrenia because they often signal some acute physical condition that requires prompt management.

Personality Traits

Some patients become disturbed in ways that have afflicted them at difficult times in the past. A common example is individuals of subnormal intelligence who become discouraged and depressed when challenged by school or a demanding occupation.

Individuals vary in other ways. For example, extroverts tend to have brisk emotional responses to life stresses, whereas introverts' responses are slow, persisting, and unrelieved. Either type of reaction can cause difficulties in situations that require emotional stability. The internist who knows patients well may be able to predict which circumstances they will find burdensome and either help guide them or recommend psychotherapy.

The mental status exam should allow the physician to make the crucial distinction between a troubled personality and a disease such as major depression, but an experienced psychiatrist may be needed to confirm the diagnosis.

Behaviors

Some patients seek help from an internist because they are overwhelmed by hungers and drives to pursue unhealthy or socially unacceptable activities. They may complain of trouble with sleep, excessive hunger for food, problems of too much or little sexual interest, or manifestations of addiction. Psychiatrists and internists must collaborate in searching for diseases that may provoke these behaviors and in developing treatments to alleviate them.

The most common behaviors for which patients need medical help are addictions—alcoholism and drug abuse

(Chapter 14.4). Most often, patients present to a physician under the pressure of one of the four "L's": loved ones, law (eg, charges of driving while intoxicated), liver (ie, all the physical disorders that alcohol or drugs can produce), and livelihood (eg, the possibility of losing one's job). When patients seek care because of one of these pressures rather than because they recognize their own need for help, the physician's task in both evaluation and treatment becomes more complicated.

Life Encounters

Many people develop mental distress because of a life event that would be disruptive to anyone. The prototypic event is the loss of a loved one. People suffer a stereotyped period of demoralization, the severity of which depends, for example, on the closeness of the relationship, whether or not the death was expected, and the person's personality and outside support. Internists who differentiate such grief-stricken persons from those with true depression can do much to help them. They can offer sedation during acute, overwhelming grief. They can offer counsel, explain the stages of grief, and assure patients that their distress is normal and not a medical concern. They can watch to ensure that the grieving process is following its usual course and not developing into an illness such as major depression.

Likewise, other life circumstances can be understood as the source of a person's state of discouragement. A teenager's academic or social failure, a discovery of betrayal in marriage, a distressing encounter with the legal system, or being a crime victim can cause demoralization and need for counseling. If demoralization is accompanied, as it often is, by physical aches and pains (eg, muscle tension, gastrointestinal distress), the internist is most likely to be the professional whose advice is sought first, and often the person who can help the most in advising and comforting the patient.

MANAGEMENT

Assigning a patient's psychiatric disorder to one of the four categories enables the physician to approach management rationally. Patients with diseases such as delirium or depression may need medical treatment for their underlying condition, for example, hyponatremia or hypothyroidism. When the disease cannot be treated, they need relief from their more distressing symptoms. Many old and new psychopharmacologic drugs can help patients with panic attacks, depression, mania, and schizophrenia.

Patients with personality difficulties such as mental retardation or an unstable emotional temperament need guidance. The physician can help these patients and their families by spelling out how they become vulnerable under certain circumstances and by recommending vocational and psychological counseling.

Patients with a disruptive behavior need help to stop it and reorganize their life so that they can eliminate it. In particular, alcoholics must be helped to acknowledge their difficulty. Internists can point out to drinkers the toll that alcohol has already taken on their body. Then a program of group therapy, which might involve such groups as Alcoholics Anonymous, can be developed to help the patient live without drinking.

Patients suffering reactions to life events need support and help in adjusting. Here psychotherapeutic support includes acknowledging the naturalness of patients' response to the distressing events and counseling about successful ways to overcome their problems. At the same time, patients should be helped with any related physical symptoms.

Beyond reaching a diagnosis, the physician must determine whether patients need protection. Ideally, during the evaluation the physician recognizes patients who are at risk for suicide, and decides how much supervision they need (Chapter 14.3). This can range from telling relatives and friends to be watchful, to admitting patients to the hospital and instituting suicide precautions.

SUMMARY

▶ Psychiatric disorders can be grouped into four categories: those caused by (1) nervous system disease, (2) personality characteristics, (3) abnormal behavior, and (4) distress provoked by life encounters.

▶ The history and the mental status and physical examinations are essential to categorize the patient's disorder, define proper treatment, and predict prognosis.

▶ Management comprises healing diseases, guiding individual temperaments, stopping destructive behaviors, and modifying responses to life events.

▶ Much psychiatric care can and should be given by internists.

SUGGESTED READING

Frank JD, Frank JB: *Persuasion and Healing: A Comparative Study of Psychotherapy,* 3rd ed. Johns Hopkins, 1991.

McHugh PR: A structure for psychiatry at the century's turn: The view from Johns Hopkins. J R Soc Med 1992;85:483.

McHugh PR, Slavney PR: *The Perspectives of Psychiatry.* Johns Hopkins, 1986.

Disorders of Cognition: Dementia and Delirium

Marshal F. Folstein, MD, and Susan E. Folstein, MD

Dementia is a syndrome, or cluster of signs and symptoms, defined as deterioration of multiple cognitive functions in clear consciousness. It differs from delirium, which is defined as a deterioration of multiple cognitive functions in the presence of *clouded* consciousness. Dementia is differentiated from mental retardation and learning disabilities, which are lifelong cognitive impairments. It is also distinguished from cognitive deteriorations that affect single functions out of proportion to others, amnestic syndromes, and aphasia. Dementia, delirium, and mental retardation are not mutually exclusive; a patient with mental retardation can become demented or delirious.

DEMENTIA

In a community sample in Baltimore, one-third of patients with dementia were diagnosed with Alzheimer's disease and one-third with multi-infarct disease. The remaining one-third included patients with vascular disease, trauma, and factors related to alcoholism. Most dementing diseases begin gradually and progress. Few are reversible, with exceptions being the dementia that accompanies major depression or the dementia caused by neurosyphilis and hypothyroidism. Dementia after trauma is sudden and can be static, whereas dementia after stroke can begin acutely, worsen, and then improve over the course of months. Causes of dementia are listed in Table 14.2–1.

CORTICAL AND SUBCORTICAL DEMENTIA

The cognitive impairments of dementia occur in two different patterns: cortical and subcortical. The cortical pattern is more common and is characterized by amnesia, aphasia, apraxia, agnosia, and delusions. A typical patient, for example, with Alzheimer's disease, has profound memory deficit and fluent aphasia yet remains moderately attentive and normally responsive to questions. In contrast, the subcortical dementia pattern, so-named because it is usually associated with disease of the basal ganglia, is characterized by slowly responsive thought and action, reduced activity, and inattention. This is the type of dementia seen in patients with Huntington's disease, AIDS dementia complex, supranuclear palsy, and occult hydrocephalus. Patients have a nonfluent dysarthria but fully comprehend speech and have only a mild memory disorder.

In contrast to patients with cortical dementias who become unable to recognize their family members and surroundings, patients with subcortical dementia comprehend their setting and its requirements, but they have great difficulty in exercising good judgment, in planning, and in changing from one task to another. Although patients with cortical dementia have few motor signs until late in the illness, patients with subcortical dementia usually present with a motor disorder that produces an abnormal movement and gait. In addition, patients with subcortical dementia are more likely than those with cortical dementia to have a depressive syndrome.

NONCOGNITIVE SYMPTOMS ACCOMPANYING DEMENTIA

The common noncognitive symptoms that accompany dementia are abnormalities of mood, such as depression, anxiety, aggression, and apathy; delusions and hallucinations; and abnormal behaviors, such as increased activity, failure to eat, sleep disturbance, aggression, and altered sexual behavior.

Table 14.2–1. Causes of dementia.

Cause (Prevalence)	Comments
Alzheimer's disease (50%)	By far the most common cause (see text for symptoms; other causes should be excluded using the rules given in the text); treatable causes particularly important to consider in differential diagnosis; risk factors—apo E4, head trauma, family history
Lewy body dementia (5%)	Alzheimer's features, with prominent hallucinations and sensitivity to neuroleptic agents; extrapyramidal motor signs much more prominent than in Alzheimer's disease
Stroke (10–30%)	If stroke alone causes dementia, it is either in right hemisphere or multiple large strokes
Alcohol dementia (10%)	The additive effects of vitamin deficiency, head trauma, and liver disease in severe alcoholics
Major depression (7%)	Dementia common in elderly persons with severe depression; MMSE usually above 16 or 17
Huntington's disease (3–5%)	Depression, abnormal movements, family history
Brain tumor (3–5%)	Motor signs may be subtle or even absent
Hydrocephalus (3–5%)	Gait disturbance and urinary incontinence
AIDS (varies by hospital)	CD4+ count <400/μL; prominent apathy and psychomotor retardation; trouble with executive function
Vasculitis, autoimmune (<1%)	Increased erythrocyte sedimentation rate, muscle aches
Hypothyroidism (<1%)	Slow, cold; high thyroid-stimulating hormone level
Cushing's syndrome (<1%)	Moon facies; mood disturbance
Nutritional deficiency (<1%) Niacin, thiamine, B$_{12}$	Peripheral neuropathy, rash, diarrhea, anemia
Chronic brain infection (<1%) Syphilis, cryptococcosis	Headache, abnormal spinal fluid, increased erythrocyte sedimentation rate
Wilson's disease (rare)	Liver disease and extrapyramidal signs, low ceruloplasmin
Demyelinating diseases (<1%)	Although demyelinating diseases not rare, dementia seen only in the end stage; prominent motor signs; multiple large white matter lesions on scans
Progressive multifocal leukoencephalopathy (rare)	Associated with lymphomas and AIDS
Lipid storage diseases (rare)	Tay-Sachs, Kufs' disease
Prion diseases (<1%)	Subacute course with cortical dementia; motor signs and sharp waves in EEG
Progressive supranuclear palsy (<1%)	Dementia occurs early relative to extrapyramidal signs; abnormal eye movements
Parkinson's disease (5–10%)	Dementia in late stages after severe motor signs are present
Brain trauma (<1%)	Prominent deficits in executive function; dementia caused by contusion, subdural hematoma, and hydrocephalus
Pick's disease (<1%)	Early behavioral disorder, frontal-temporal atrophy on scan, EEG often normal

MMSE, Mini-Mental State Examination.

Mood Disorders in Dementia

A sustained depressive syndrome occurs in 30–60% of patients with subcortical dementia and 10–20% of patients with cortical dementia. This depressive syndrome has the characteristic features of affective disorder and responds to treatment with antidepressants and electroconvulsive therapy (ECT). Pathologic laughter or crying occurs when the dementia syndrome is caused by bilateral corticobulbar lesions as, for example, in multiple strokes or multiple sclerosis. Such laughter or crying is often prompted by a meaningful psychological stimulus, such as a conversation or even music. The outbursts are pathologic because they are experienced as a compulsion. That is, the emotion is expressed against the resistance of the patient, who does not always feel sad or happy.

Irritability and explosiveness are other abnormal mood states seen with dementia, especially the dementia of Huntington's disease. These outbursts are also prompted by meaningful stimuli, but are inappropriately intense and prolonged; they are different from the "catastrophic reactions of Goldstein"—excessive emotional outbursts in settings of task failure often seen in patients with cortical dementia.

Anxiety appears in several contexts in patients with dementia. Patients with cortical and subcortical dementia become fearful and restless in the following situations: when separated from their caregivers, in response to delusions and hallucinations, in relation to depression, or as part of a reaction to failure or unexpected changes in routine.

Apathy means a lack of feeling and activity. Patients sit in one spot and stare ahead blankly until encouraged to participate in an activity. Although apathetic patients also suffer from a failure of their planning capacities, they express no sense of boredom or distress at their inert state. Apathy may also be seen as a feature of depression, but in this case, the patient has a dysphoric mood.

Delusions and Hallucinations in Dementia

Delusions occur in 20–40% of patients with cortical dementia. Patients believe that their property has been stolen, that their spouse is unfaithful or is an imposter, that their house is not their home, or that deceased relatives are alive. Sometimes patients act on these ideas and become violent. Hallucinations are less common and are likely to be visual or olfactory, rather than auditory or tactile.

Although their prevalence is unknown, delusions and hallucinations certainly occur in subcortical dementia. Some depressed patients with Huntington's or Parkinson's disease develop depressive delusions like believing that they have cancer, that they are dead in a coffin, or that they are poverty-stricken. Parkinsonian patients often have visual hallucinations caused by the disease or by treatment with dopaminergic agents.

Abnormal Behaviors in Dementia

Three types of abnormal behavior are seen in patients with dementia. All types may be seen in the same patient at the same time or at different times during the illness. Some of the abnormal behaviors seem to be physiologically driven and are not related to the patient's premorbid personal attributes. These include overeating and undereating, disturbed sleep, very high or low activity levels, and inappropriate sexual behavior. Some patients with Alzheimer's disease spend all day rummaging through drawers and moving their (and other people's) belongings from place to place. Rummaging is not seen in those with subcortical dementia.

Other abnormal behaviors, particularly aggressions, seem to arise in response to hallucinations and delusions. Patients with Alzheimer's disease who have misidentification delusions may attack family members whom they believe are intruders, or they may try to escape from their own home, which they believe is a strange place.

Aggression can also occur in response to actual upsetting events such as irritable caregivers, changes in routine, or inability to communicate effectively. Many patients with dementia become aggressive quickly and remain upset and touchy for a long time after the irritative event has passed.

CAUSES OF CORTICAL DEMENTIA

Alzheimer's Disease

Alzheimer's disease is a clinically and etiologically heterogeneous group of disorders that share a cortical dementia syndrome and characteristic pathology of the cerebral cortex and its connections to the limbic system and brain stem. The dementia syndrome begins insidiously with memory loss and progresses to involve language and motor skills. Ten percent of patients with Alzheimer's disease develop seizures. Gait, fine motor coordination, and primary sensation are preserved until late in the disease, when the patient becomes unable to move. The average duration of the disease from onset to death is 8 years. On average, cognitive decline is steady, about 2–3 points per year on the Mini-Mental State Examination score (see below).

When a patient's cognitive decline accelerates, the physician should look for a complicating medical condition such as a urinary tract infection, drug intoxication, or depression.

Diagnosis and Diagnostic Criteria: The diagnostic evaluation of patients with Alzheimer's disease is based on the history and on repeated mental status examinations that establish the expected progression of symptoms. The

Table 14.2–2. NINDS criteria for Alzheimer's disease.

Criteria for probable disease
1. Dementia syndrome established by clinical examination and documented by the MMSE, Blessed Dementia Scale, or some similar examination, and confirmed with neuropsychological tests
2. Deficits in two or more areas of cognition
3. Progressive worsening of memory and other cognitive functions
4. No disturbance of consciousness
5. Onset between 40 and 90 years of age, and most often after 65
6. No systemic disorders or other brain diseases that could account for the progressive deficits in memory and cognition

Criteria for possible disease
1. Dementia syndrome without other neurologic, psychiatric, or systemic disorders sufficient to cause dementia, and with variations in onset, presentation, or clinical course
2. A second systemic or brain disorder sufficient to produce dementia but not considered to be the cause of the dementia
3. A single, gradually progressive, severe cognitive deficit without other identifiable causes

Definite Alzheimer's disease
• Clinical criteria for and histopathologic features of Alzheimer's disease on a biopsy or autopsy examination

NINDS, National Institute for Neurological Disorders and Stroke; MMSE, Mini-Mental State Examination.

criteria in Table 14.2–2 allow three levels of diagnosis: possible Alzheimer's disease, probable Alzheimer's disease, and definite Alzheimer's disease. The clinical examination, along with laboratory studies to exclude other causes of dementia, is accurate in 80–90% of cases verified by autopsy.

Course of Illness: The course of Alzheimer's disease can be divided into three stages based on the spread of the disease through the brain. The earliest symptoms of the *limbic phase* appear in the first 2–3 years after onset and involve the olfactory system with anosmia and odor amnesia. As the cognitive impairment worsens, the olfactory threshold rises, suggesting progressive disease in the olfactory system and its connections in the limbic system. Anterograde and retrograde amnesia for explicitly learned events, pictures, and words also occurs early. Patients cannot remember facts learned minutes earlier. Eventually, patients with Alzheimer's disease lose the ability to recall events from long ago. In this early limbic stage, patients retain the capacity to perform tasks implicitly learned, such as playing cards.

In addition to anosmia and amnesia, 17–20% of patients in the limbic stage become depressed. Risks for depression include a previous history and a family history of depression. Depression carries a poor prognosis; patients with depression are more often institutionalized and, when institutionalized, have higher mortality rates than other patients with Alzheimer's disease. Patients with depression have greater neuronal degeneration of the locus caeruleus, the brain-stem nucleus of norepinephrine neurons that project to widespread cortical areas.

The *parietal phase* occurs 3–6 years after onset of

symptoms. Patients lose comprehension of spoken language but remain fluent, like a patient with fluent aphasia. They have difficulty naming pictures of common objects; this can be scored to follow progression. A second aspect of the parietal phase is apraxia, the inability to perform previously learned motor skills such as dressing, bathing, and, eventually, eating. Patients develop visual and auditory agnosia, the inability to recognize common visual and auditory stimuli. These symptoms lead to misinterpretation of the environment; patients may not recognize their caregivers or even their own reflections. Delusions of identification and visual and auditory hallucinations can occur in the limbic phase, but are more common as cognitive impairment worsens, suggesting that they are manifestations of the parietal phase. Delusions of this type may reflect a decreased capacity to comprehend the environment because of aphasia and agnosia.

The *late frontal stage* occurs 6–8 years after onset of symptoms. Motor disturbances, primitive reflexes, and seizures appear. Patients become unable to walk, or even, eventually, to move. These motor signs are attributable to concurrent Parkinson's disease in some patients, but in others, who have grasping and sucking reflexes, gait disorder is related to frontal lobe disease. In the end, patients have difficulty in swallowing, with subsequent aspiration and death.

Even in late frontal stage Alzheimer's disease, primary sensory function is preserved. Thus, patients can detect pain, touch, and other sensations even though the illness is far advanced. Communication with patients can be enhanced by using their remaining sensory modalities. For example, patients might be able to recognize a caregiver by the sense of touch after they are unable to recognize her by vision or hearing.

Electroencephalography and Brain Imaging Characteristics: Electroencephalogram (EEG) frequencies eventually become slow and correlate in severity with measures of cognitive decline. Magnetic resonance imaging (MRI) and computed tomography (CT) scans demonstrate cortical atrophy with enlargement of ventricles, Sylvian fissure, and suprasellar cistern. Quantitative measurements of areas of the CT scan such as the suprasellar cistern are sensitive indicators of Alzheimer's disease. Positron emission tomography (PET) and single photon emission computed tomography (SPECT) scans may demonstrate decreased blood flow and metabolism of glucose in the temporal and parietal lobes.

Pathology: On postmortem examination, the brain of a person with Alzheimer's disease is found to be small and atrophic with neuronal loss. Many of the remaining neurons contain a remarkable accumulation of intracellular neurofibrillary tangles. In the neuropil are found extracellular neuritic plaques whose cores consist of a beta-pleated sheet of beta-amyloid protein. This protein is coded by the amyloid preprotein gene on chromosome 21. Embedded

in the amyloid mass are bits of neurons derived from the cholinergic and adrenergic systems. Amyloid is also deposited in blood vessels. The composition of the neurofibrillary tangle is under investigation, but some evidence indicates that it consists of an amyloid fibril "decorated" with a variety of proteins including ubiquitin and tau.

The distribution of these cellular changes in the brain is not random. Limbic and parietal areas are most affected. The findings support the suggestion that the distribution of pathologic changes in Alzheimer's disease follows spread of the disease from neuron to neuron along defined sets of cortical fiber connections that include the olfactory system and its connections in the limbic system and parietal cortex.

Etiology: At least 50% of all cases of Alzheimer's disease are familial, and several genetic loci have been demonstrated. Loci on chromosomes 14 and 1 and three rare mutations on chromosome 21 have been identified in families with Alzheimer's disease in whom the onset is early (40–60 years of age). In numerous families with late-onset (65 years or over) disease, affected members are more likely to have alleles 3 or 4 of the apolipoprotein gene (apo E). Some asymptomatic persons in families with the apo E4 allele have PET glucose metabolic patterns that are similar to those seen in early Alzheimer's disease. However, the apo E4 allele is common in the general population and on its own is not a powerful predictor of Alzheimer's disease. Also, not all late-onset families have the apo E4 allele. Suspected environmental risk factors include repeated head trauma and aluminum in water supplies and air.

Ten to fifteen percent of cases of Alzheimer's disease will be complicated by prominent extrapyramidal signs and often early psychosis—*Lewy body dementia.* This variant has a more rapid course than straightforward Alzheimer's disease and is more sensitive to the side effects of neuroleptics. On autopsy, in addition to the characteristic changes of Alzheimer's disease, the brain shows inclusions called Lewy bodies in cortical and sometimes subcortical neurons. These inclusions have the same appearance as those found in the substantia nigra in Parkinson's disease.

The Prion Diseases

Prion diseases are rare causes of dementia. For every 100 cases of Alzheimer's disease, the clinician might see one case of prion disease. Jakob-Creutzfeldt disease (JCD) (also known as Creutzfeldt-Jakob disease), Gerstmann-Sträussler-Scheinker disease, and kuru all are prion diseases. Only one patient in the literature of familial Alzheimer's disease was subsequently determined to have prion disease. All of these disorders are characterized by a subacute course. Symptoms of cortical dementia appear and progress to severe dementia over weeks to months, occasionally lasting years. A prodromal state of anxiety and behavioral change are common. In addition, motor signs such as myoclonus and ataxia appear as the disease progresses. The EEG sometimes shows characteristic waveforms. Brain scans show cortical atrophy. The pathology of the brain is a characteristic brain atrophy with microscopic spongiform degeneration without plaques and tangles.

The cause of these diseases is complex, since the prion is a particle of protein that can be infectious. Thus, the prion can be transmitted from human to human when infected material of one human is ingested by another, as in kuru, or when it is injected as part of pituitary replacement or corneal transplantation in the case of JCD. Prions can also be transmitted in the germline and thus appear hereditary. Ten percent of JCD is distributed in families like an autosomal dominant trait.

Frontal Dementias

Pick's Disease: Pick's disease is characterized by a slowly progressive cortical dementia syndrome with prominent behavioral and frontal features. The presenting symptoms are often odd behaviors that the patient adopts early in the illness when cognitive impairment is mild. After several years, the patient with Pick's disease becomes less talkative; most become mute. The EEG is often normal, but brain scans show a frontal or temporal lobar atrophy or both. The pathology consists of neuronal death without plaques and tangles but with the presence of intracellular inclusions called *Pick bodies*. The etiology is sometimes hereditary.

Frontal Dementia or Hippocampal Sclerosis: Up to 10% of autopsy series of Alzheimer's disease show a clinical and pathologic pattern similar to that of Pick's disease but without Pick's inclusion bodies. Such cases are now called frontal dementia or hippocampal sclerosis.

CAUSES OF SUBCORTICAL DEMENTIA

Diseases causing subcortical dementia include Huntington's disease, hydrocephalus, supranuclear palsy, Parkinson's disease, multiple sclerosis, AIDS, hypothyroidism, and depression. Subcortical vascular diseases are multi-infarct dementia, lacunar dementia, and Binswanger's disease.

Multi-Infarct Dementia

Multi-infarct dementia describes a dementia syndrome associated with prominent infarctions of the brain—in some cases estimated to be larger than 50 mL—which can have a variety of causes. Hypertension and atrial fibrillation are the most common associations. The clinical diagnosis of multi-infarct dementia is based on a history of episodic and sudden worsening of the patient's mental state, usually associated with asymmetric motor signs and CT or MRI signs of several cerebral infarcts. The natural history of the disease is not well described. Claims have been made that its course may be altered by vigorous treatment of hypertension. Multi-infarct dementia can also be caused by inflammation of cerebral vessels with subsequent infarctions in the territory of small vessels. This picture occurs in patients with neurosyphilis and autoimmune cerebral vasculitis.

Binswanger's Disease

Binswanger's disease is a subcortical white matter degeneration associated with hypertension. The lesions are visible on CT and MRI scans, and biopsies show vessels with a variety of abnormalities.

Parkinson's Disease

Parkinson's disease is characterized by the triad of akinesia, rigidity, and tremor, associated with degeneration of the dopaminergic neurons of the substantia nigra (Chapter 13.7). In recent years, cases of Parkinson's disease have been divided into two types: those associated with the neuritic plaques and tangles of Alzheimer's disease and those with a pure substantia nigra degeneration.

Parkinson's disease is associated with a clear dementia syndrome. A high proportion of patients also develop depressive disorders. The treatment of the depressed parkinsonian patient often includes levodopa (L-dopa), and antidepressant therapy or ECT, which is effective in alleviating the motor, cognitive, and mood features of the disorder. Delusions and hallucinations are also commonly found in patients with Parkinson's disease.

Huntington's Disease

Huntington's disease is an autosomal dominant disorder characterized by chorea and a prominent subcortical dementia syndrome, usually beginning between ages 35 and 50, with a course of illness of about 16 years. Neurons are gradually lost in caudate nucleus and putamen and eventually other striatal nuclei. Cortical atrophy is sometimes seen, but there is little neuronal loss except in deep layers. The cause of the disease is a gene on chromosome 4p, which contains an expanded trimeric repeat sequence. Although the function of the gene is unknown, there is marked loss of glutamate receptors in striatum. It is possible that an abnormality in the glutamate system leads to excessive excitation of the striatal neurons by incoming excitatory glutamatergic fibers from the cortex. Glutamatergic excitation would lead to cell death through calcium influx, kinase activation, and eventually oxygen-free radical accumulation.

Dementia of Depression

Severe depression in the elderly causes a cognitive impairment that clears with treatment of the depression. Some affected patients suffer relapse and have permanent cognitive deterioration, but others remain well. These patients present with a cognitive syndrome that includes disorders of mood, cognition, and movement.

AIDS Dementia

HIV infection is associated with both primary and secondary infections of the central nervous system. In patients with primary central nervous system HIV infection, which presents as a subcortical dementia, two types of pathology occur: a progressive white matter degeneration and an encephalitis with multinucleated giant cells. Thirty to fifty percent of all patients diagnosed with AIDS have central nervous system HIV infection.

Multiple Sclerosis

Multiple sclerosis (MS) is a demyelinating disease with lesions clearly visualized by MRI, dispersed in the nervous system (Chapter 13.8). Two forms are described: (1) relapsing and remitting, and (2) chronic progressive. Cognitive changes in MS occur late in the disease, typically with a subcortical pattern.

Hypothyroidism

Hypothyroidism is well recognized as a cause of cognitive impairment, but few case series describe the pattern of symptoms. One report describes a well-documented subcortical dementia pattern.

Occult Hydrocephalus

Occult hydrocephalus, a more typical subcortical disorder, is characterized by a triad of dementia, ataxia, and urinary incontinence associated with a large dilatation of the cerebral ventricles with relatively mild cerebral atrophy. The disorder is caused by the defective drainage of cerebrospinal fluid usually due to a blockage of reabsorption sites secondary to head trauma, previous hemorrhage, or infection. A proportion of these cases respond to surgical drainage of cerebrospinal fluid; thus, diagnosis is critical.

Nutritional Deficiency

Deficiency of vitamin B_{12} or niacin can cause a dementia syndrome. Deficiency of thiamine causes Wernicke-Korsakoff syndrome.

ASSESSMENT OF THE PATIENT WITH DEMENTIA

The approach to a patient with impaired cognition begins with the history and examination, on which the physician bases a formulation that includes four distinct perspectives on the patient's illness: (1) the disease perspective that includes diagnosis; (2) the dimensional approach, in which impairment and disability are quantified; (3) the behavior perspective; and (4) the life story perspective. Because many patients have impaired memory, another person who knows the patient well must be interviewed. Often the time spent in finding adequate informants is more valuable than sophisticated laboratory tests. Important clinical observations of cognitively impaired patients come from the physical and neurologic examina-

tions and the examination of the patient's present mental state. The patient should be examined alone to avoid family members' prompting and to avoid embarrassing the patient when deficits are elicited.

Information from the history, mental status examination, and physical examination serves to identify the likely syndrome and to focus the medical evaluation in the search for pathology and causes:

1. Is cognitive impairment present? History and mental status examination are the methods used to determine this. Mini-Mental State Examination score (see below) lower than age and education norms is expected. Twenty-seven is the median score for an adult with a high school education.
2. If cognitive impairment is present, has there been a decline from a previous level? If yes, then mental retardation is ruled out as a cause of the present illness. Clearly, mentally retarded persons can also suffer from disorders that cause deterioration in cognition; for example, persons with trisomy 21 (Down's syndrome) may grow up mentally retarded and then develop Alzheimer's disease after age 40.
3. Is there a disturbance in the level of consciousness? If yes, then delirium is the diagnosis. The most useful laboratory test to confirm delirium is the EEG, which is diffusely slow and differentiates delirium from depression and schizophrenia. (A slow EEG can also be found in some disorders causing dementia; see "Alzheimer's Disease" and "The Prion Diseases" above). Agents that cause delirium include ingestion of prescribed or illicit drugs, epilepsy, systemic or cerebral infections, and metabolic disorders such as electrolyte disturbances. These are sought using appropriate blood tests and lumbar puncture. If there is no disturbance in level of consciousness, the remaining differential diagnosis consists of a dementia syndrome, an amnestic syndrome, and an aphasic syndrome.
4. Are there multiple cognitive defects? If yes, the diagnosis of dementia is made. If memory is affected out of proportion to other deficits, a diagnosis of amnestic syndrome is made. If language is affected out of proportion to other deficits, the diagnosis of an aphasic syndrome is made.
5. Is the dementia associated with prominent motor signs and a gait disorder from the outset? If so, the clinical features are those of a subcortical syndrome, and the differential diagnosis should include multi-infarct dementia, neurosyphilis, Parkinson's disease, subdural hematoma, hydrocephalus, MS, Huntington's disease, severe depression, AIDS dementia, severe nutritional deficiencies (eg, vitamin B_{12}), and metabolic disorders (eg, hypothyroidism).

   If no focal motor signs or gait disorder is present, the diagnosis is likely to be one of the cortical dementias, Alzheimer's disease, Jakob-Creutzfeldt disease, or Pick's disease.
6. Is the onset rapid or insidious? The pathogenesis and

etiology of the dementia syndrome are suggested by the onset and course of symptoms. Dementias developing over days to weeks are likely to be related to tumors, infections, vascular disease, nutritional or metabolic abnormalities, or trauma. Dementias developing over months to years are likely to be caused by primary neuronal loss, as in Alzheimer's disease, Parkinson's disease, or Huntington's disease.

7. Is the course relapsing and remitting or a steady-state decline? A relapsing and remitting course usually implies vascular disease or MS. A downhill course evolving over weeks and months suggests Jakob-Creutzfeldt disease, tumors, or chronic infections such as HIV and fungus. A course evolving over years usually implies primary neuronal degenerations such as Alzheimer's disease, Parkinson's disease, or Huntington's disease.

The pathologic diagnosis of a patient with dementia is confirmed by laboratory tests. Blood tests and lumbar puncture are used to rule out vasculitis, vitamin deficiencies, metabolic disorders, and infections. An EEG is performed to confirm lateralization of signs, to assess the potential for seizures, and to differentiate depression (the EEG is normal) from Alzheimer's disease (the predominant frequencies are slower than normal). Finally, a brain CT or MRI scan is obtained to rule out focal lesions (tumors, stroke, hematoma) and to quantify the extent of neuronal loss by measurement of ventricular size and cortical volume.

Measuring Impairment in Cognitively Impaired Patients

Psychological tests that quantify impairment and disability have three purposes for the evaluation and care of the cognitively impaired patient: assessing severity, assessing the effect of cognitive impairment on social functioning, and assessing outcomes of interventions.

The Mini-Mental State Examination: The Mini-Mental State Examination (MMSE) is useful in screening for cognitive impairment and in monitoring the course of illness, because it is quick, it can be administered at the bedside, and it has normative values for various levels of age and education (Figure 14.2–1). For the common conditions causing dementia, it is a sensitive and specific measure of cognitive impairment.

The MMSE begins by assessing orientation. The patient is asked 10 questions to determine whether he or she is oriented to time and place. The capacity to remember is then tested by two tasks: (1) registration and (2) attention and calculation. Registration is tested by asking the patient to repeat the names of a group of three unrelated objects (eg, a pony, a quarter, and an orange). Concentration and calculation are then tested: The patient is asked to subtract 7 from 100 and continue subtracting 7 from each subsequent remainder up to five subtractions. The serial 7's task is given not only as a test of attention and calcula-

tion but as a distractor before the patient is asked again to recall the three words. Only if the patient refuses to attempt this task should he or she be given the option to spell the word "world" backwards.

The examination continues with questions on language function (see Figure 14.2–1); these questions distinguish it from other brief screening batteries. The median score for the adult population is 27; 95% of the population scores higher than 23. The scores of individual groups of patients vary according to their age and education. Elderly persons and those with little education score lower.

The MMSE concludes with rating the patient's level of consciousness on an analog scale from comatose to fully alert. The rating of consciousness can be performed reliably and is a measure of the patient's level of alertness, responsiveness, and accessibility to the examiner. Patients who have cognitive impairment and an altered level of consciousness have delirium.

Measuring Disability: Disability is defined as impairment of mental or physical function caused by a medical condition that leads to difficulty in performing a socially defined behavior such as working or living independently. A disease (eg, Alzheimer's disease) may cause a particular impairment, such as memory loss, which leads in turn to a particular failure of social function, such as the inability to work. Disability can be assessed at the bedside by an interview with the patient and an informant using standard scales that measure impairment along four dimensions: mobility, the capacity to walk to the store or up a flight of steps, or to use public transportation; activities of daily living, the ability to cook, bathe, dress, and use the toilet; communication, the ability to use the telephone and talk to friends; and upper extremity function, the capacity to use the arms and hands to reach and carry objects.

Laboratory Tests of Cognitive Impairment:

The Wechsler Adult Intelligence Scale: Bedside examination of cognitive impairment often reveals the necessity for detailed quantification of cognitive function to confirm the clinical opinion and to educate the patient about current strengths and weaknesses. The best-known measure of cognitive function is the Wechsler Adult Intelligence Scale. This 1–2-hour test battery includes tests of comprehension of social situations, mental arithmetic, conceptual similarities, digit span, and vocabulary, and various nonverbal "performance" tests; it is a useful predictor of performance in school and work. Although the Wechsler Adult Intelligence Scale was originally designed for measurement of intellect in the normal population, it has come to be used to estimate the severity of impairment produced by disease. The problem with this application is that scores do not always reflect the extent of disability attributable to cognitive decline. An IQ cutoff of 70 as designating mental retardation is not always appropriate to define a dementia. Patients with Alzheimer's disease with higher IQs may be disabled by severe memory

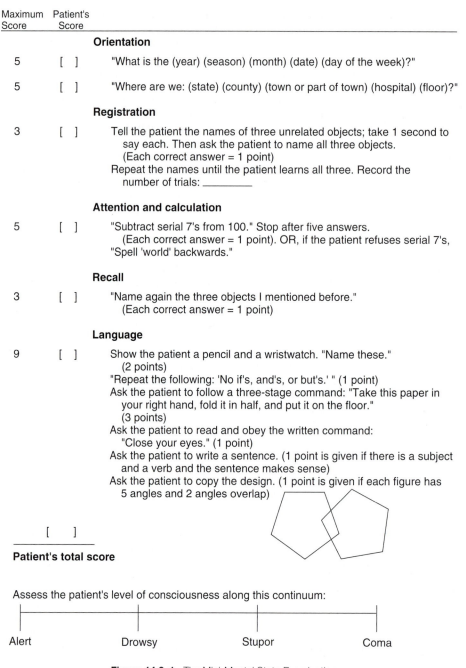

Maximum Score	Patient's Score	
		Orientation
5	[ ]	"What is the (year) (season) (month) (date) (day of the week)?"
5	[ ]	"Where are we: (state) (county) (town or part of town) (hospital) (floor)?"
		Registration
3	[ ]	Tell the patient the names of three unrelated objects; take 1 second to say each. Then ask the patient to name all three objects. (Each correct answer = 1 point) Repeat the names until the patient learns all three. Record the number of trials: _____
		Attention and calculation
5	[ ]	"Subtract serial 7's from 100." Stop after five answers. (Each correct answer = 1 point). OR, if the patient refuses serial 7's, "Spell 'world' backwards."
		Recall
3	[ ]	"Name again the three objects I mentioned before." (Each correct answer = 1 point)
		Language
9	[ ]	Show the patient a pencil and a wristwatch. "Name these." (2 points) "Repeat the following: 'No if's, and's, or but's.' " (1 point) Ask the patient to follow a three-stage command: "Take this paper in your right hand, fold it in half, and put it on the floor." (3 points) Ask the patient to read and obey the written command: "Close your eyes." (1 point) Ask the patient to write a sentence. (1 point is given if there is a subject and a verb and the sentence makes sense) Ask the patient to copy the design. (1 point is given if each figure has 5 angles and 2 angles overlap)

[   ]
_____

Patient's total score

Assess the patient's level of consciousness along this continuum:

Alert   Drowsy   Stupor   Coma

Figure 14.2–1. The Mini-Mental State Examination.

loss. In Huntington's disease, performance on an IQ test bears little relation to cognitive performance in a work situation.

Tests of specific cognitive functions: In addition to the Wechsler Adult Intelligence Scale, particular cognitive dimensions have been defined by separate test batteries. These include tests for memory, attention, language, motor skill, and problem solving.

Assessing Abnormal Behavior

The cognitively impaired patient often needs help with specific problem behaviors. Examples are aggression, activity level, wandering, shadowing caregivers, repetitive talk and actions, catastrophic reactions, resistance to care, incontinence, and suicide attempts. The approach to assessment includes constructing an inventory of problem behaviors focused on what the patient does, rather than on interpretations of the likely reasons for its occurrence. As a second, separate step, each behavior is assessed to decide whether it is likely to be physiologically driven, whether it represents a response to an abnormal experience, or whether it is likely to result from antecedent causes and consequent rewards that occur in the patient's environment. Motivated behaviors such as eating, sleeping, and sexual behavior can be disrupted in their pattern, force, and consummation because of memory loss, as when the patient with dementia eats many meals because of forgetting that he or she has just eaten. Appetite and sleep may also be reduced, perhaps because of physiologic changes in brain-stem nuclei. On the other hand, aggressive behavior can be precipitated by an antecedent cause, such as physical restraint, or it may be a response to a hallucination.

MANAGEMENT OF DEMENTIA

Patients with dementia are best managed through the coordinated efforts of physicians, nurses, social workers, psychologists, nutritionists, physical therapists, dentists, and others. Ideally, the same team manages the patient through all stages of the illness, whether at home or in a nursing home. Quality of life for both patient and family is improved by maintenance of physical and mental health. Thus, the patient should have good routine medical and dental care, and the noncognitive complications of dementia should be treated. Families of a patient with dementia often suffer depression, anxiety, and exhaustion, and the physician must be prepared to detect and manage emotional disorder in family members as well as in the patient. Almost all caregivers become exhausted by the care of a chronically ill patient and can be helped by amplifying social supports such as home helpers, day care, respite care, nursing home placement, or hospice care.

Reversible conditions such as malnutrition, endocrine disorders, depression, tumors, and infections can be treated as they would be in any medical patient. Complications such as delirium from drugs and other conditions to which the patient with dementia is particularly susceptible can usually be prevented by close medical surveillance and cautious use of medication. Falls from unsteady gait and automobile accidents can usually be prevented by helping the family to plan and institute restrictions at the appropriate times.

Patients with dementia remain calmer and less anxious in environments with a minimum of stress and uncertainty. Mobility and morale should be maintained by visits to occupational and physical therapy. Patients seem more alert during the day and sleep better at night if activities are provided. Tasks and life activities must be regular and predictable. Although all activities must be planned, they can be simple, such as a morning walk, regular meals, or regular visits from familiar family members. New or unexpected variations in routine lead to serious emotional distress in patients with dementia.

Treatment should address the noncognitive symptoms that often accompany dementia. Depression and its accompanying sleeplessness are treated with tricyclic antidepressants, titrated to a dose sufficient for a normal night's sleep. Delusions and hallucinations can be treated with low doses of neuroleptic agents, but with care to identify the side effect of delirium, which often occurs 5–6 weeks after the patient has been started on medication. Abnormal behaviors can often be stopped if the underlying cause is understood. For example, a patient who is wandering in response to hallucinations stops wandering if the hallucinations are treated with neuroleptics. A patient who is wandering because of restlessness and anxiety due to depression usually stops if treated with an antidepressant.

Long-term management of patients with dementia requires the physician to establish an empathic relationship with the patients and caregivers. The physician should spend time alone with the patients to hear their concerns, complaints, and hopes. The physician should ask patients what they want to know about their condition, test results, and prognosis. As the cognitive impairment worsens, and the patient develops language difficulties, the physician must try to maintain the same relationship with the patient, even though communication will have become difficult. This is important for the patient's self-esteem, even though the information that the patient provides requires confirmation by a family member. By the same token, it is important to maintain an attitude of interest and respect for the patient during discussions with family members.

DELIRIUM

Delirium is the syndrome of altered consciousness described also as acute confusional state, encephalopathy, acute brain syndrome, or sundowning. Delirium is the most common serious mental disorder seen in general hospitals. Especially common in the elderly, patients with structural brain disease, and those taking multiple medications, delirium occurs in 10–20% of hospital admissions. In addition, every patient recovering from general anesthesia goes through a period of delirium.

Defining Features

The defining features of the syndrome of delirium are an alteration of consciousness and cognitive impairment. Alteration of consciousness can be subtle or severe. The patient may report feeling groggy and may be easily aroused in response to the examination or may fall asleep during the interview and be difficult to arouse. The alertness of patients with delirium can vary from drowsy to hypervigilant. On the basis of this variation in consciousness, delirium can be classified as *somnolent delirium* (also called acute confusional state) or *vigilant delirium,* as in delirium tremens. Cognitive impairment of either somnolent or vigilant delirium is characterized by slowed perception and marked inability to fix attention or sustain concentration. Patients are disoriented and unable to learn new material. Most of the events and experiences of the delirious episode are forgotten after recovery, although islands of memory may remain. Delirious patients are typically apraxic and have difficulty in writing.

Noncognitive Features

Although disorders of consciousness and cognition are the defining features of delirium, most delirious patients also suffer mood disorders, delusions, hallucinations, behavior disorder, and autonomic and motor disorders. Since the cognitive impairment can be subtle and elicited only by careful examination, delirious patients often draw the attention of physicians because of their noncognitive features. For example, delirious patients are frequently anxious and depressed; however, they can be distinguished from other patients with disturbed mood, because, in addition to anxiety and depression, they reveal an altered level of consciousness and cognitive impairment.

Delusions and hallucinations, particularly visual hallucinations, are common. These are vivid and often the source of the patient's unusual behaviors. The patient may be agitated and pacing around the room or remain in bed immobile, barely responsive to the environment. Suicidal behavior can be a product of depressive thoughts, and misinterpretations of the environment can lead the patient to become aggressive toward the staff. The patient's sleep is always disrupted, often with reversal of the sleep cycle. Delirium leads to incompetence in making decisions, including consenting to medical procedures or giving advance directives.

Autonomic abnormalities include sweating and fever. Disturbances of the motor system may be seen, such as a flapping tremor when the patient is asked to sustain a fixed posture. Myoclonus, dysarthria, and ataxia may also be present. Difficulties with gait can lead to falls, particularly in elderly persons.

Causes of Delirium

The common causes of delirium are cerebral injury and ingestion of or withdrawal from drugs or alcohol. Particularly at risk are elderly patients or those with preexisting neurologic disease such as stroke or dementia. Less common precipitants are systemic infection, metabolic disturbances (especially hyperglycemia), endocrine disturbances, and seizures (Table 14.2–3).

Cerebral Injury: Patients with structural central nervous system damage are prime candidates for developing delirium, whether the injury takes the form of stroke, Alzheimer's disease, or head trauma. The same patients may suffer from seizures, which themselves can cause delirium, either after a single seizure or during a flurry of attacks. Delirium can be caused by meningitis or encephalitis of bacterial, viral, or fungal origin, and a lumbar puncture is therefore necessary as part of the evaluation of the delirious patient.

Table 14.2–3. Causes of delirium.

Predisposing causes
Age
Underlying structural brain disease (eg, Alzheimer's disease or stroke)
Epilepsy
Hypoalbuminemia

Precipitating causes in patients seen in the community
Multiple causes: usually several interacting causes such as Alzheimer's disease with a urinary tract infection or stroke with drug toxicity
Drug intoxication: drugs with anticholinergic effects, such as atropine, neuroleptics, antidepressants, and analgesics; patients may be taking small amounts of several such drugs
Endocrine diseases: mainly diabetes; occasionally thyroid disease

Precipitating causes seen in hospitalized patients
Drug intoxication: see above
Drug withdrawal: most commonly from alcohol, benzodiazepines, and other sedatives (not usually cocaine and opiates)
Infections: CNS infections; also non-CNS disorders such as pneumonia and typhoid; minor infections in predisposed persons; gangrene
Metabolic/endocrine/electrolytes: any disturbance of oxygen, glucose, water, or electrolytes; dehydration probably the most common
Postoperative: caused by residua of intraoperative events, such as anoxia or anesthesia—even after adjustment of drugs, electrolytes, and oxygen; particularly the elderly (may remain delirious for days to weeks)
Vascular: particularly strokes in right hemisphere
Epilepsy: seizures, postictal states, or anticonvulsant intoxication
Trauma: usually seen initially or on awakening from coma
Brain tumor or abscess: from effects of brain displacement, edema, or local effects of the tumor

Drug-Related Delirium States: Drugs can cause delirium when ingested or when withdrawn after chronic ingestion. The mechanism by which drugs produce delirium is often their capacity to block brain cholinergic receptors—hence the potential for confusion after treatment with anesthetic agents, antispasmodics, antidepressants, neuroleptics, and atropine, all of which have anticholinergic properties. Withdrawal syndromes are seen after discontinuing heavy alcohol intake, barbiturate use, or benzodiazepine use (Chapter 14.4). Delirium tremens can begin within hours after the last dose of alcohol or drug, with tremor, agitation, and seizures. In the first 2 days, a hallucinatory state in clear consciousness may develop, which sometimes becomes chronic and indistinguishable from schizophrenia. Two or three days after withdrawal, patients develop a hypervigilant state with disorientation, attentional deficits, memory loss, vivid hallucinations, delusions, anxiety, and depression. Also present are tachycardia, sweating, fever, and sleeplessness.

Management of Delirium: The treatment of delirium involves removing the cause and preventing known complications, treating specific manifestations such as giving low-dose neuroleptics to treat hallucinations, and giving empathic appreciation of the patient's individual situation. Prevention of complications includes treating infections, reducing the levels of drugs, maintaining adequate nutrition, and mobilizing measures to prevent stasis and venous thrombosis. Empirical treatment with low doses of haloperidol (given by mouth, intramuscularly, or intravenously) is often helpful. Benzodiazepines are useful in treating withdrawal from alcohol or benzodiazepines and may need to be administered in large doses.

The empathic approach is very important in dealing with patients with delirium. Patients are disoriented and apparently out of touch, and easily misinterpret procedures and staff requests. They are very sensitive to perceived unkindness and need to be reassured. The care of the patient with delirium can be greatly aided if family members are instructed to stay with the patient and assist the nursing staff. In this way, physical restraints can be avoided, and medication use can be minimized. The family members involved in the care of a patient with delirium are themselves in the midst of a crisis, and it is essential that the physicians and medical staff develop a supportive relationship with them, taking time to explain test results and procedures and discussing possible outcomes.

SUMMARY

▶ Alzheimer's disease is the most common form of progressive dementia and typifies the pattern of cortical dementia; the cognitive deficit is characterized by profound memory loss, fluent aphasia, and delusions, with motor involvement occurring only in the final stages.

▶ Subcortical dementia, seen in multi-infarct dementia, AIDS, and Huntington's disease, causes slowness of thought and action and depression, and is accompanied by early gait and movement disorders. Memory disturbance is characteristically mild.

▶ Assessing cognitive impairment includes measuring severity with the bedside Mini-Mental State Examination or laboratory tests of cognitive function and quantifying disability in terms of mobility, activities of daily living, communication, and upper extremity function.

▶ Delirium is altered consciousness with cognitive impairment; its most common causes are cerebral injury—acute or chronic—and ingestion of or withdrawal from drugs and alcohol.

SUGGESTED READING

Adams R, Victor M (eds): *Principles of Neurology,* 5th ed. Mc-Graw-Hill, 1994.

Crum RM et al: Population-based norms for the Mini-Mental State Examination by age and educational level. JAMA 1993; 269:2386.

Int Psychogeriatr 1991;3(2), entire issue devoted to discussion of delirium.

Terry RD, Katzman R, Bick KL (eds): *Alzheimer Disease.* Raven Press, 1994.

14.3

Depression

J. Raymond DePaulo, Jr, MD

Of all the patients a physician sees, at least one in three is feeling depressed. Two-thirds of these "depressed" patients have a low mood as a normal but intense response to a stressful life event such as a serious medical illness. But the remaining one-third are suffering from major depression, which requires specific medical intervention. About 5–10% of Americans suffer one or more periods of major depression in their lifetime.

The internist is usually the first health professional to see a depressed person. In the worst case, a patient is brought in after a suicide attempt. More commonly, patients seek help for their low mood or for symptoms (fatigue, poor sleep, or somatic complaints) that they do not recognize as being related to depression. Primary care providers can—and should—diagnose and treat most depressed patients without needing to refer them to a psychiatrist.

Accurate diagnosis is crucial. Much suffering and many suicides can be prevented only by treatment directed at the right condition. Major depression can exist alone or be a feature of another serious disease such as hypothyroidism, stroke, Parkinson's disease, or pancreatic cancer. Although most major depression affects genetically predisposed persons, psychiatric and medical disorders frequently coexist, so the physician cannot assume that patients with a confirmed depressive disorder have no other medical conditions. Since many of depression's symptoms and signs are nonspecific (eg, insomnia, fatigue, anorexia, and weight loss), it is crucial that the differential diagnosis of all patients who present with these features include depression. On the other hand, the physician should not conclude from a normal physical or laboratory evaluation that a patient has depression—or any other psychiatric illness—unless the person displays some of that disorder's classic features.

Only 50% of clinically depressed patients seek help, and only 50% of those who do are correctly diagnosed and treated. Most doctors and patients misread depressive symptoms as normal reactions to stressful life events. The majority of people, if asked, will recite a litany of stressors that could explain or explain away depressive symptoms. The problem with these explanations is that they may distract both patient and doctor from clear signs and symptoms of major depression, which requires treatment. Four in five patients with major depression have a triggering event. Yet, it is not the distressing event that determines whether a person's sadness is depression, but rather the persistence and severity of the mood change and its accompanying features.

CLINICAL FEATURES

Although every person's depression is different, the condition has characteristic features. A major depression is a syndrome of persistently low mood, lowered self-esteem, and loss of physical and mental energy. Depressed people have a low mood, although many describe it less as sadness than as anxiety, numbness, or a deadening of emotion. Mood may be worst in the morning. Self-confidence can fall dramatically. Depressed people have decreased feelings of self-worth and may feel as if they have never been good at anything. They may have unrealistic fears, for example, about their health and financial prospects. Although they may try to hide what they see as their incompetence, they are sure that it is obvious to the onlooker. They may have irrational guilt feelings.

Patients typically feel that they have lost mental and physical capacity. Their thinking is slow and confused, and they cannot concentrate. They feel tired; they may

Acknowledgments: Parts of this chapter are derived, with permission, from earlier chapters and a book by the author: (1) Affective disorders. In: *Principles of Ambulatory Medicine*, 4th ed. Barker LR, Burton JR, Zieve PD (editors). Williams & Wilkins, 1995; (2) Depression. In: *Current Therapy in Neurologic Disease*, 3rd ed. Johnson RT (editor). BC Decker, 1990; (3) DePaulo JR Jr, Ablow KR: *How to Cope with Depression: A Complete Guide for You and Your Family.* Fawcett Crest, 1989.

Paul R. McHugh, MD, contributed to the section on preventing suicide.

move and speak slowly. They may be left exhausted by opening the mail. Balancing the checkbook may suddenly be beyond their ability. Patients with the severest forms of depression may develop hallucinations, such as hearing the voices of dead relatives, and delusions, such as feeling personally responsible for all the evil in the world.

Many patients experience changes in their basic drives. They have trouble falling asleep and awaken too early in the morning, or else they sleep too much. They lose their appetite (and weight) or they overeat. They lose their libido. They withdraw from friends and family and may become afraid to go to work or even leave home. They lose interest in the things that used to bring them pleasure (anhedonia), and they see nothing to look forward to in the future. This hopelessness can lead to thoughts of suicide.

In addition to the characteristic features of depression, most patients have at least a few aches or pains related to real but nondisabling medical conditions, and these symptoms worsen whenever the patients become depressed. Such symptoms may be the presenting complaint for patients who are more aware of the physical than the psychological aspects of their condition. In fact, patients who experience their depression primarily somatically are more likely to seek care from their family physician than from a psychiatrist.

Depression is usually episodic. An episode can last for weeks, months, or years. Patterns of severity, duration, and frequency of relapses vary widely. One-third of patients have only one depressive episode in their lifetime; two-thirds have recurrences. In patients with bipolar (manic-depressive) disorder, depression can alternate with mania (see "Differential Diagnosis" below). Atypical forms of depression may be hard to diagnose because they are milder and tend to be chronic rather than episodic, leading others to dismiss the person's unhappiness as moodiness. During depressive periods with these milder forms, people tend to overeat and oversleep and to have more prominent anxiety than patients with typical depression. Symptoms wax and wane, often worsening during the fall and winter, or, in women, premenstrually.

DIAGNOSIS

Primary care physicians can diagnose depression in patients who present complaining of depression, as well as in those whose presenting complaint appears unrelated to depression or who are not aware that they are depressed. The tools are the history and mental status exam (Chapters 14.1 and 14.2); laboratory tests offer little help.

During routine comprehensive evaluations, the physician should assess patients' mood by asking: "How are your energy and concentration lately? How is your mood? Do you ever get depressed? How are you sleeping? How is your appetite? How is your sex drive? Have any of these changed recently?"

Even when a patient's mood appears normal, the physician should be suspicious if the person reports other symptoms that match those of depression. Most depressed patients complain to their doctor not of low mood but of worsening of their customary mild aches and pains (ranging from headaches to irritable bowel syndrome, anxiety, or fatigue). When asked about their mood, most depressed patients acknowledge that they feel depressed or apathetic. If patients are obviously feeling low, the physician should try to learn how depressed they are, to determine what treatment they need and whether they are at risk for suicide (see "Preventing Suicide" below). The clinician should also observe any changes in a patient's grooming, appearance, movement, speech, and emotional reactions to sad or funny comments and should ask the patient's family and friends to corroborate and add to the patient's report.

DIFFERENTIAL DIAGNOSIS

Major depression is but one of several "affective" (mood) disorders. Less severe than major depression is "adjustment disorder with depressed mood"—a depressed mood that is an understandable but unusually intense reaction to a distressing life event. Patients are demoralized but not medically ill. They come to medical attention because their reaction causes them suffering or problems in everyday functioning. Their distress may reflect the severity of the provoking event but may also arise in part from their personality vulnerabilities. The goals of professional intervention are to help assess the loss and to teach that it need not be devastating. But the clinician must reassess patients if their problems are unusually persistent or severe or if the characteristic symptoms of major depression emerge.

Major depression can also resemble—and coexist with—grief. The grief response to the loss of a loved one has somewhat predictable elements. Most bereaved persons first go through a short period of numbness or shock, and then, less predictably, a longer phase of intense sadness and loneliness, a period of withdrawal and disorganized efforts to pull their life together, and finally a period of reorganizing and rejoining society.

Although sadness is a prominent feature of both grief and depression, they differ in the nature and duration of symptoms. Americans have general ideas of what is a "normal" response to distressing life events like the death of a spouse, divorce, or being jilted, laid off, bankrupted, maimed, or given a diagnosis of a serious illness. The intensity and duration of these responses vary according to people's temperaments and circumstances. Because sympathetic clinicians expect a patient to feel sad at these times, they do not always look carefully enough for signs that the loss has triggered something beyond the expected grief. Physicians should be suspicious when someone's grief seems to continue unrelieved for too long.

Recurrent major depression is the *unipolar* mood disorder. In *bipolar* disorder, depression alternates with its opposite, *mania.* Manic patients are abnormally elated or irritable, with hyperactivity, rapid speech, less-than-usual need for sleep, overconfidence, and a loss of financial, social, and sexual judgment. Perhaps one-third of patients who have major depressive episodes also have attacks of mania or a milder form of mania called *hypomania.*

CAUSES

Evidence is strong that major depression is a disease, not a weakness of personality. Major depression is often referred to as a "biochemical imbalance," because antidepressant medications such as monoamine oxidase (MAO) enzyme inhibitors and reuptake inhibitors have such powerful effects on specific neurotransmitter (eg, serotonin, norepinephrine) pathways. Supporting the disease argument is the fact that major depression is seen in many patients with clear neuropathologies such as Parkinson's disease, multiple sclerosis, and stroke. The strongest link is in patients with left frontal stroke, 60% of whom develop a major depression; the risk is especially high if the lesions involve the left basal ganglia and the associated orbital frontal cortex. Studies using positron emission tomography also show left frontal abnormalities in depressed patients who do not have signs of brain injury.

Most patients with major depression have no clear neuropathology; their tendency to affective disorders is inherited. Twin and adoption studies strongly support a genetic basis for most recurrent major depression and bipolar disorder. However, family studies do not show a simple mendelian pattern.

Many cases of major depression that are not clearly neuropathologic or genetic are caused by endocrine disorders (eg, hypothyroidism, Cushing's syndrome) or medications (eg, corticosteroids, reserpine).

MANAGEMENT

Most depressive episodes remit spontaneously or respond to specific therapies. However, so little is known about the pathophysiology of the mood disorders that their management must still be based on empiric drug treatment and psychological therapy. Most people can be treated as outpatients.

Antidepressant Drugs

The best-studied drugs are the tricyclic antidepressants, which have been widely used since the early 1960's. The easiest tricyclics for patients to tolerate—and the safest—are nortriptyline and desipramine. They are less sedating and less anticholinergic than their parent compounds, amitriptyline and imipramine. Nortriptyline has the added advantage of causing less orthostatic hypotension than the other tricyclics. In addition to orthostatic hypotension, the major serious side effects of the tricyclics are sedation, falls, and delirium. More common but less problematic side effects are dry mouth and constipation.

When a patient achieves a steady-state tricyclic blood level after 2 weeks on a stable dose, the clinician should obtain a drug blood level and adjust the dose to achieve a blood level within the range proven to give the best antidepressant effect. After 2 months on an adequate tricyclic dose, 65–80% of depressed patients are well. Patients tend to do less well on any antidepressant if they have had symptoms for 2 years or longer or if they have a delusional or incapacitating depression.

A new group of drugs, the selective serotonin reuptake inhibitors (SSRIs), has surpassed the tricyclics as the most widely prescribed antidepressants. The major SSRIs are fluoxetine, paroxetine, sertraline, and fluvoxamine. Although these drugs are no more effective than the tricyclics, they generally cause less sedation, dry mouth, constipation, and orthostatic hypotension. Because they are better tolerated and require less dosage titration, these drugs are more likely to be prescribed and taken at therapeutic doses. The SSRI's most common side effects, usually lasting 1–4 weeks, are nausea, insomnia, and nervousness or anxiety.

If after 6–8 weeks of therapy patients are not much better, lithium carbonate may be added to their antidepressant regimen. The effectiveness of this combined treatment should be noticeable within 2 weeks. If the combination is working, it should be continued; if not, both drugs should be stopped. Patients can then be tried on bupropion or a MAO inhibitor such as phenelzine. These drugs are also alternatives for patients who cannot take or do not improve on a tricyclic or SSRI.

Patients who have not responded after two adequate medication trials should be referred to a psychiatrist. Many patients are reluctant to see a psychiatrist, and, when referred, fear that their own physician does not want to see them anymore or that their condition is hopeless. Thus, their physician should explain the referral and see them again after the first psychiatrist visit to reinforce the positive expectation. In addition, patients who are seriously suicidal or who have hallucinations, delusions, or profound slowing of their thoughts and actions should be referred for immediate psychiatric consultation. Such patients may recover only with hospitalization and electroconvulsive therapy (brief electrical stimulation of the brain to induce a modified seizure).

Electroconvulsive therapy (ECT) is a highly effective short-term treatment for severe major depressive or manic episodes. ECT is used when patients require a very quick response because of suicide risk or severe medical compromise, when patients have delusional depressions (which are unlikely to respond to medications), when antidepressants cannot be safely given, when antidepressants have failed, and when patients request it. The treatment, given under brief general anesthesia, takes only a few minutes. The current is passed for ≤2 seconds, and the modified seizure usually lasts 20–60 seconds. The major risks are those of the brief anesthesia, headaches and muscle aches, and memory impairments that generally resolve within 1–3 months after the last treatment.

Depression poses special management problems when it arises from a primary neurologic disorder like stroke or Parkinson's disease. Neurologically impaired patients may be less responsive to usual antidepressants but more likely to respond to ECT. They must have their antidepressant drug therapy monitored with special care because they are at higher risk than other depressed patients for delirium and other drug toxicity.

Drug treatment has further pitfalls. Patients may need to try several classes of antidepressants before they find one that works. Even if the antidepressant could be effective, the dose may be too low. Even if the dose is right, some patients stop taking their medicine before it has a chance to work. This is a particular problem during the first 2 weeks of treatment, when a drug's side effects are worst and the benefits have not yet appeared. The physician should strongly encourage patients to keep taking their drug, explaining that they will need at least 2 (and up to 8) weeks on the right medication at the right dose to begin to see improvement in their energy, concentration, sleep, and appetite; they may need 8–12 weeks to recover these functions fully and to have more self-confidence and self-esteem.

The manic phase of bipolar disorder is treated with lithium, often combined with a neuroleptic drug, such as haloperidol or fluphenazine. This treatment should be supervised by a psychiatrist. Lithium and tricyclics are often given together for several weeks during the acute depressive phase of bipolar disorder, even though tricyclics can trigger manic attacks.

Duration of Medical Treatment: Most patients should be treated for a single depressive episode for 12 months after their symptoms remit. This is a period of high risk for relapse. Patients who have frequent severe depressions should continue a well-tolerated, effective antidepressant for at least 2 years, or perhaps much longer. Long-term maintenance can reduce the frequency and severity of later episodes. In the 30 years that tricyclics have been in use, no long-term complications have been reported.

Manic-depressive patients should be maintained indefinitely on lithium or another mood stabilizer and should take intercurrent antidepressants only briefly, as noted above.

When a recovered patient stops an antidepressant, the dose should be tapered by 25%/wk. There are two reasons for tapering. First, many patients have relapses of depression within days to months after they stop treatment. These recurrences are more easily controlled with a tapering schedule than with a complete halt. Secondly, sudden cessation of tricyclics causes perhaps 10% of patients distressing "cholinergic rebound" symptoms of nausea and vomiting. Reasons for stopping a drug quickly are that the patient has developed toxicity or is being switched to another, similar antidepressant.

Psychological Management

Psychological treatments focus on easing the ill person's suffering, rather than eradicating the causes of the disease. For patients who have moderate-to-severe depression, psychotherapy alone is less valuable than medication alone, but the two treatments combined are of substantial benefit. Every facet of medical care can contribute to psychological healing. In particular, a physician who takes a complete history, does a thorough exam, and explains the diagnosis, prognosis, and treatment plan in a reassuring way can give enormous relief and hope to a depressed person.

Many depressed patients believe that their problems are too complex to allow a simple diagnosis or a straightforward treatment plan. Many are convinced that their prognosis is hopeless. The clinician can reassure patients by explaining depression. It often helps to say that depression is caused by an as yet undefined brain disorder but that with treatment, the prognosis for recovery is excellent. The clinician should contact patients every 2 weeks to ask how they are feeling, give encouragement, check for suicidal thoughts, and make any necessary medication adjustments. The doctor should advise depressed patients not to make any major life decisions during the 2-month acute treatment period, except the decision to seek and accept treatment. Many depressed patients, assuming that their problem is environmental, try to "fix" it by changing locations, jobs, or spouses.

Preventing Suicide

Major depression is the most powerful predictor of suicide. Other important predictors in depressed patients are delusional ideas, alcohol abuse, and male sex. Of patients with major depression or manic-depressive illness, 15% eventually kill themselves. Many more think about it, plan it, or try it. Risk is highest when depressed patients develop delusions or when patients are beginning to recover and have the energy to make a suicide attempt before an improved self-attitude reemerges to prevent it. These patients should be given no more than a 1-week supply of medication. Overtly suicidal and delusional patients should be referred to a psychiatrist.

The physician should ask all possibly depressed patients their thoughts about self-injury and suicide. The first questions should be general; if warranted, questions should become specific. The physician should begin by simply trying to open a conversation about self-injury: "Sometimes when people feel down-hearted, they think they might be best off dead. Do you ever have thoughts like this?" Most patients say, "No, I'm not that depressed," or "My thoughts are not that morbid." But some patients respond with a tentative, "Yes, I think about ending my life." This answer should prompt the physician's next question: "Have you thought about how you do it?" Again, most patients answer, "It's only a thought, not a plan," or repeat, "I'm not that depressed." But some patients say that they have thought about an overdose of pills, or gas, or cutting themselves. "Yes" answers indicate higher risk and call for more questions: "Have you gotten the pills to carry out your plan?" "Do you have the knife that you would use?" A reassuring answer would be, "These are just fleeting thoughts, not plans." But if patients say that they have the means of attempting suicide, they need to be protected.

Finally, the physician should ask, "Have you ever tried taking an overdose?" ". . . cutting yourself?" ". . . inhaling carbon monoxide?" Patients who answer yes must be kept under supervision, and the physician must assume responsibility for their immediate care.

When patients are not delusional but are having persistent suicidal thoughts that they cannot dismiss, a clinician must make a management plan with them and their family. Although each plan is individual, its two purposes are to minimize the suicide risk and to ensure that the clinician is alerted promptly if the patient needs protection or hospitalization. Most patients who have suicidal thoughts do not want these thoughts and do not want to act on them. Patients generally cooperate with and are grateful for help in working out a clear plan for reporting increasing suicidal thoughts and seeking short-term protection with family or friends, or, if necessary, in the hospital. Successful management depends on regular contact between clinician and patient, as well as the willingness and helpful participation of family and friends until the suicidal ideas remit or the patient can resist them easily.

SUMMARY

▶ Depression is a usually remitting and relapsing syndrome of low mood, lowered self-esteem, and loss of physical and mental energy. Depression may alternate with mania, a syndrome of abnormally high mood, self-esteem, and energy.

▶ Major depression is the main predictor of suicide. Patients must be carefully monitored for suicidal thoughts.

▶ Most mood disorders are probably caused by genetic factors. Depression is also linked to some neurologic conditions, particularly left frontal stroke, and to hypothyroidism and some medications.

▶ Most patients respond to antidepressant drugs, with tricyclics or selective serotonin reuptake inhibitors the drugs of choice.

▶ Suicidal patients and patients who have not responded to two antidepressant drugs should be referred to a psychiatrist.

SUGGESTED READING

Goodwin FK, Jamison KR: *Manic-Depressive Illness.* Oxford, 1990.

Robins LN et al: Lifetime prevalence of specific psychiatric disorders in three sites. Arch Gen Psychiatry 1984;41:949.

Robinson RG, Szetela B: Mood change following left hemispheric brain injury. Ann Neurol 1980;9:447.

Stine OC et al: Evidence for linkage of bipolar disorder to chromosome 18 with a parent-of-origin effect. Am J Hum Genet 1995;57:1384.

Wells KB et al: The functioning and well-being of depressed patients: Results from the Medical Outcomes Study. JAMA 1989;262:914.

Alcohol and Drug Dependence

Alan J. Romanoski, MD, MPH

At any given moment, 10% of adults in the United States are experiencing clinical and social problems related to their use of alcohol and drugs; more than 20% have problems at some point in their life. High as these figures are, they do not take into account the misery that alcohol and drug users inflict on the people around them. Clinical problems often go unaddressed until users develop such a blatant syndrome as cirrhosis or major withdrawal. The fact that most drinkers and drug users appear healthy, appropriately dressed, and coherent at routine medical visits, coupled with the high prevalence of these conditions, demands that physicians always maintain a high index of suspicion. The only clues may be seemingly innocuous findings such as a finger accidentally cut by a kitchen knife, liver function test abnormalities on routine lab screening, a healed rib fracture on chest x-ray, or a worried loved one.

Alcohol and drug use disorders are persistent behavioral patterns that focus on acquiring and self-administering substances whose effects increase the likelihood of their continued use. These behaviors—everything from recurrent use in hazardous situations (eg, drinking and driving) to a full dependence syndrome—predispose users to physiologic, psychological, behavioral, social, and occupational consequences. In lay terms, "alcoholism" and "drug abuse" mean repeatedly drinking or using drugs when one should not; alcohol or drug "dependence" means that use has become an integral part of one's daily life.

ELEMENTS OF DEPENDENCE SYNDROMES

Narrowing of the pattern of use: The manner and timing of drinking or drug taking become increasingly stereotyped (Table 14.4–1). For example, persons who once varied the amount and type of alcoholic beverage they drank in accordance with social circumstances begin to drink the same amount of the same beverage prepared in the same way and at the same time, whether on holidays, weekends, or weekdays, or with friends, colleagues, or alone.

Preoccupation with drink- or drug-seeking: The priority given to acquiring and using the drug increases, and unpleasant consequences progressively fail to deter further use. Over time, drinking- and drug-related activities compete more successfully against others that were once more important—career advancement, leisure pursuits, social standing, child care responsibilities, personal hygiene, keeping one's marriage or job, protecting a fetus, avoiding HIV infection, or bleeding to death from esophageal varices.

Increased tolerance: Doses of alcohol or drug once sufficient to disinhibit, elate, intoxicate, stupefy, or cause coma progressively fail to do so. Mechanisms inducing tolerance include increased hepatic clearance and the proliferation of substance-specific receptors that require ever-higher synaptic drug concentrations to exert the same neuronal effect. Many persons in whom the drug causes brain injury or advanced liver disease eventually lose their tolerance.

Repeated withdrawal symptoms and substance use to relieve or avoid them: Abstinence after months to years of sustained use often produces drug-specific symptoms, which range from mild discomfort to life-threatening physiologic derangements. Many people who discover that self-prescribed "replacement therapy" provides prompt relief get caught in a vicious cycle of increasing use and worsening withdrawal. As an extreme example, some withdrawing alcoholics who vomit back their drinks steadfastly continue drinking until the emesis stops. More often, alcoholics drink in the morning to relieve a hangover, keep a drink at bedside to stave off withdrawal, or never stop drinking long enough to experience severe withdrawal.

Awareness of a compulsion to use: The repeated urge to use can be felt as a craving or manifested by maneuvers to ensure that the drug will always be available, such as hiding "stashes" or "pre-drinking" (drinking before attending an event where access to alcohol might be limited). Many persons impose measures on themselves to

Table 14.4–1. Elements of alcohol and drug dependence syndromes.

Narrowing patterns of use
Preoccupation with seeking the substance
Increased tolerance
Repeated withdrawal symptoms
Use to relieve or avoid withdrawal
Craving or compulsion to use
Reinstatement of full syndrome after resumption of use

Modified and reproduced, with permission, from Edwards G, Gross M: Alcohol dependence: Provisional description of a clinical syndrome. Br Med J 1976;1:1058.

help them resist these urges, such as not keeping alcohol at home, avoiding "drinking buddies," and restricting access to cash so as not to buy cocaine on impulse.

Reinstatement of the full syndrome after relapse: Abstinence does not extinguish dependence syndromes. No matter how long they have been off a drug, most dependent people who resume use reacquire all elements of the syndrome within days to weeks. The mechanisms include neural memory, habituation, and behavioral conditioning (see "Sustaining Factors" below). It is this phenomenon that prompts many to regard alcoholism as a disease and to hold that abstinent alcoholics are "recovering" but never fully "recovered," and thus must never take their "first drink."

Denial is a person's failure to acknowledge the full scope of the syndrome. Denial encompasses disbelief, limited grasp, rationalization, embarrassment, defensiveness, identification with "normal" peers who exhibit the same behaviors, and, occasionally, lying.

ETIOLOGY AND PATHOGENESIS

The pathogenesis of alcohol and drug use disorders can be understood as interactions among agent (drug), host (user), and environment. The reasons why a person begins to drink or take drugs (initiating factors) are often unrelated to the reasons why the person continues use (sustaining factors).

Initiating Factors

Agent: Cocaine, amphetamines, marijuana, nicotine, ethanol, opioids, barbiturates, and benzodiazepines all have self-reinforcing properties—effects that increase the likelihood that the drug will be taken again. But these drugs differ in their "abuse liability," the relative strength of their self-reinforcing effects. Cocaine's abuse liability is so high that many laboratory animals offered the choice between cocaine and food die of starvation by persistently opting for cocaine. By comparison, benzodiazepines have little abuse liability.

Host: Multiple dispositional, psychological, and genetic factors predispose a person to alcoholism and drug use disorders. For example, extroverted people are at high risk

for alcohol and drug misuse because they are prone to seek excitement, adventure, and immediate gratification, and are unlikely to dwell on unpleasant consequences of their behavior.

For unknown reasons, the state induced by these agents is more rewarding to some persons than others. Many cocaine users liken the drug state to sexual orgasm, while others dislike the "jittery" feeling that cocaine gives them. Similarly, innumerable drinkers profess to have known from their first drink that they were "hooked" on alcohol, while others take years to acquire a "taste" for alcohol.

Identical twins are significantly more concordant for alcoholism than fraternal twins. Men have three times the risk of women. Children of alcoholic parents have three to five times the risk, even if adopted at birth and raised in a nonalcoholic household. Tolerance to alcohol is a heritable trait that increases the odds that people will drink again, by sparing them the common pitfalls of early drinking experiences—sloppy drunkenness and hangover. Conversely, inherited *in*tolerance, such as occurs in people with inherited acetaldehyde dehydrogenase variants (see "Alcohol-Related Medical Sequelae" below), can protect against alcoholism by causing discomfort after even minimal drinking.

Environment: A person's environment can either enhance or override the rewards of early experiences with alcohol and drugs. The younger the age at which people have repeated exposures to and intoxications with alcohol and drugs, the higher their risk for becoming dependent. Vulnerable people may be encouraged if the agents are available and affordable, and if peer and social attitudes are positive. The psychological state that alcohol and drugs can induce, their inherent abuse liability, and social reinforcement all promote accelerated use, which, in turn, facilitates increased tolerance. The individual becomes more motivated to manipulate the environment so as to ensure ready access to alcohol, drugs, and the positive reinforcement and social acceptance that their use brings. Friendships and associations change and other patterns of behavior adjust, so that use gradually follows a routine (habituation).

Sustaining Factors

Agent: Alcohol and drugs have inherent but differing capacities to induce tolerance and cause withdrawal symptoms—properties independent of their abuse liability. Drugs differ from one another in their "withdrawal potential"—their relative ability to cause physiologic withdrawal symptoms after cessation of sustained use. Cocaine and cannabis have high abuse liability but low withdrawal potential compared with opioids and benzodiazepines, which can produce severe withdrawal symptoms. Although repeated use to relieve withdrawal is a strong reinforcer of opioid and benzodiazepine dependence, there is no clear evidence that people maintain excessive cocaine, cannabis, or alcohol intake to avoid withdrawal.

Host: Alcohol and drugs often reward users for reasons other than their inherent self-reinforcing effects. For example, alcohol's anesthetic properties temporize not only physical pain but also distressing moods and anxiety states, thus rendering drinkers with these afflictions particularly vulnerable to alcohol dependence. Dependence syndromes are particularly common among people with mental diseases such as schizophrenia and major mood disorders. Similarly, many people drink to numb the demoralization that accompanies adversities such as physical disability, separation, divorce, widowhood, and financial worry. Many dependent people find themselves in a downward vortex in which further use and adversity fuel one another.

Environment: Some lonely people go to bars looking for companionship, but the companionship that they find centers around drinking. The pairing of positive experiences with drinking and drug taking is a potent sustaining force. Tolerance, withdrawal, and craving can be also sustained as conditioned responses to environmental cues. For example, many opioid addicts, after years of abstinence while incarcerated, report experiencing opioid withdrawal and craving when they return to their home environment.

Jobs in the hotel and restaurant trade, advertising, and entertainment, as well as unskilled, seasonal, or day labor, are conducive to sustaining drinking and drug use.

Habit: A habit is a stereotypic sequence of behaviors that, with each repetition, becomes more fixed and requires less conscious attention to perform. Many persons drink or smoke today because they did yesterday. Habits are easily sustained through classic conditioning. When alcohol or drug taking grows to fill one's "disposable time"—time not earmarked for fulfilling responsibilities—boredom can sustain its use.

Dependence Syndromes: Motivated Behaviors or Diseases?

Alcohol and psychoactive drugs can spur proliferation of specific central nervous system receptors, a process implicated in the development of tolerance. Thus, repeated exposures to these agents cause structural and functional changes that literally become embodied in the person and induce an internal craving—a psychobiologic drive experienced as a hunger—distinct from an external attraction. It is this neurophysiologic embodiment that distinguishes dependence syndromes from other potentially rewarding, goal-directed behaviors that some people find extremely difficult to resist, such as gambling.

Alcohol and drug dependence syndromes are like "motivated" behaviors in that they create an appetite similar to that for eating, sleeping, and sex, but differ in that they are acquired and lack the internal self-regulation normally inherent in the natural drives. Somnolence or physical incapacity, not satiety, ends a dependent person's round of drinking or drug use. Drug hunger, coupled with other internal and environmental sustaining factors and the agents' own self-reinforcing properties, makes it progressively more difficult for people to deny themselves.

Heated controversy exists as to whether dependence syndromes should be considered diseases. If diseases, they would be the only ones in which the host actively continues to seek out the pathogen. Strengths of the disease model are its recognition that psychoactive drugs have the unique ability to alter brain anatomy and chemistry, that people differ in their susceptibilities to developing these neuronal changes, and that these changes may not be reversed simply by abstinence. However, many behaviors important to sustaining the disorder lie outside the domain of drugs' chemical actions. Procuring, preparing, inhaling, ingesting, and injecting these agents are not reflexes but complex, integrated, purposeful activities. The choice to resist further use remains with the user.

Advantages of the disease model are that it legitimizes allocation of resources for prevention and treatment, acknowledges that recovery usually requires more than sheer determination and strong character, and permits the person to assume the patient role with less blame and shame. A major disadvantage is any inference that dependent persons are not fully accountable for their behavior, its consequences, and their role expectations. In clinical practice, uniformly invoking or debunking the disease model can confuse patients and vex families. The disease model is best reserved for encouraging demoralized but highly motivated patients.

MEDICAL CONSEQUENCES OF ALCOHOL AND DRUG USE DISORDERS

Alcohol

Intoxication: Beverage alcohol (ethanol) is completely absorbed by the gut and reaches peak blood concentrations 30–90 minutes after ingestion. Ethanol is a central nervous system depressant that alters membrane fluidity, perturbs ion transport, and augments gamma-aminobutyric acid (GABA)-mediated synaptic inhibition. Ethanol may also be able to bind to benzodiazepine receptors, as suggested by benzodiazepine antagonists' ability to block specific effects of ethanol intoxication. At high concentrations, ethanol depresses all central nervous system functions.

At blood ethanol levels of 30–50 mg/dL, most nontolerant persons have a slowing of reaction time, diminished fine motor control, and changes in their judgment and affective responsiveness. Blood levels greater than 150 mg/dL usually correlate with gross intoxication: lethargy, dysarthria, ataxia, inattention, slowed comprehension, impaired judgment, labile mood, and disinhibition of aggressive and sexual impulses. Except in highly tolerant persons, ethanol blood levels of 300–500 mg/dL can cause obtundation, respiratory depression, and death.

Withdrawal Syndromes: Alcohol withdrawal symptoms can appear within hours after a big drop in blood alcohol level, even if the person is still drinking. The severity and duration of withdrawal symptoms directly correlate with the intensity and duration of recent drinking, the degree of concurrent medical and surgical morbidity, and the number and dosage of other drugs being taken. A long period of abstinence does not protect heavy drinkers from getting full withdrawal symptoms within days after they resume heavy drinking, if they then allow their blood alcohol level to fall.

Many persons have predictable patterns of withdrawal symptoms. For example, a person who has had withdrawal seizures in the past is likely to have them in future withdrawals.

Minor withdrawal: The earliest and most common minor withdrawal symptoms are disturbed sleep, night sweats, appetite loss, anxiety, dysphoria, and irritability. Morning gagging and retching often cause people to skip breakfast or not brush their teeth. Autonomic overactivity, which can be caused by a sudden cessation of alcohol-induced GABAergic inhibition, is manifested as sweating, palpitations, tachycardia, high blood pressure, hypervigilance, and mydriasis (dilated pupils). Autonomic overactivity and tremulousness are most prevalent 48–72 hours into withdrawal, but can continue for as long as 2 weeks. Patients' consciousness remains clear, and their cognition relatively intact.

Although alcohol is an obvious temporary antidote to withdrawal, sedatives with longer half-lives attenuate it much more safely. Medium- to long-acting benzodiazepines (eg, oxazepam, lorazepam, diazepam, chlordiazepoxide) are the agents of choice because the wide therapeutic window between their pharmacologic and toxic effects affords great latitude for safe dosing. Patients should be weaned off benzodiazepines at doses and rates appropriate to their half-lives, adjusting, if necessary, for reduced hepatic clearance. Even though withdrawal dysphoria, irritability, and sleep disturbance can persist for months, people are less likely to relapse into drinking if they stop rather than continue taking benzodiazepines.

Major withdrawal: During early withdrawal, disturbed REM sleep can cause nightmares and misperceptions of visual and auditory stimuli, especially while the person drifts in and out of sleep. Even when fully conscious, people can have frank visual hallucinations, frequently of persons or vermin, as well as auditory hallucinations that are threatening or derogatory (Figure 14.4–1). Hypervigilant drinkers, frightened by these unexpected experiences, often act on them and seriously harm themselves or others.

Hallucinations require immediate intervention. The treatment of choice is an intravenous or oral benzodiazepine. Patients should be kept in a calm milieu with minimal stimulation, moderate lighting, predictable and systematized staff contact, frequent reorientation and reassurance, and, if needed, constant observation to prevent self-injury. About 10% of patients with auditory hallucinations continue having them for weeks to months after other withdrawal symptoms have abated; these people may be helped by a neuroleptic medication, particularly haloperidol.

Within the first 48 hours of withdrawal, drinkers can suffer tonic-clonic seizures that are not preceded by an aura. Unlike patients with idiopathic or post-traumatic epilepsy, most of those with withdrawal seizures have a normal interictal electroencephalogram (EEG). Focal seizures suggest an underlying central nervous system lesion and warrant further evaluation. Although alcohol withdrawal seizures are self-limited, it is usually wise to halt them with intravenous diazepam or lorazepam. These agents should then be tapered gradually and stopped when all withdrawal symptoms have ended. Phenytoin and other anticonvulsants not only fail to control alcohol withdrawal seizures, but increase the risk of delirium. Patients with preexisting epilepsy, however, are at high risk for seizures during withdrawal or even after short bouts of heavy drinking, and should be given loading and maintenance doses of anticonvulsants.

Delirium can begin suddenly, without warning (Chapter 14.2). Delirium is most likely to occur 2–5 days into withdrawal. Delirium tremens ("DTs"), a potentially lethal syndrome, consists of delirium, psychomotor agitation,

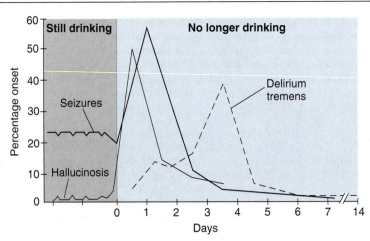

Figure 14.4–1. Major alcohol withdrawal syndromes: Percent distribution of onset, in relation to time of last drink. For example, of all drinkers who develop seizures, about 20% have their first seizure while still drinking; another 50% have their first seizure about 1 day after they stop drinking. (Modified and reproduced, with permission, from Victor M, Hope JM: The phenomenon of auditory hallucinations in chronic alcoholism. J Nervous Mental Dis 1958;126:451.)

tremulousness, autonomic overactivity, and other cognitive impairment. Many people have a mild fever (37.5°C [99.8°F] or above), many have hallucinations, and one-third have seizures. All patients should be given intravenous benzodiazepines every 5–15 minutes until they are calm, and then should be weaned gradually. Serum electrolytes and hydration must be closely monitored; most patients need intravenous fluids. Many patients require constant observation and restraints to prevent self-injury.

Alcohol withdrawal syndromes can be eased or prevented by quickly controlling concurrent illnesses, closely attending to the patient's metabolic state and hydration, replacing depleted minerals such as potassium and magnesium, giving benzodiazepines, minimizing the numbers and doses of other medications being given, and maintaining a calm environment.

Alcohol-Related Medical Sequelae:

Metabolic syndromes: Most systemic ethanol is oxidized in the liver to acetaldehyde and then to acetyl CoA by alcohol dehydrogenase and aldehyde dehydrogenase. Inhibition of aldehyde dehydrogenase by drugs such as disulfiram, metronidazole, tolbutamide, isosorbide dinitrate, and chlorpropamide can cause acetaldehyde buildup, which at low concentrations produces vasodilatation, deep flushing, headache, nausea, and dyspnea. Most hangovers are mild forms of this syndrome. At high concentrations, acetaldehyde can cause severe hypotension, heart failure, and shock. The antidote for this "acetaldehyde syndrome" is vitamin C, given intravenously, together with oxygen by nasal cannula or face mask. The weak activity of aldehyde dehydrogenase isoenzymes in most Asian populations helps to explain their lesser ability to oxidize acetaldehyde, their poor tolerance of alcohol, and their low prevalence of alcoholism.

Oxidation of large quantities of alcohol favors the reduction of pyruvate to lactate, the shunting of acetyl CoA into synthesis of cholesterol and fatty acids, and the development of "fatty liver" (Chapter 7.3). Lactate accumulation inhibits renal excretion of uric acid and can lead to hyperuricemia and gout (Chapter 3.8).

Heavy drinkers who substitute alcohol for food or who vomit repeatedly may have excess catabolism of fatty acids to acetate derivatives, leading to a nondiabetic ketoacidosis. Large amounts of alcohol inhibit hepatic gluconeogenesis. This inhibition, when coupled with decreased glycogen stores in a diseased liver, can result in hypoglycemia, especially in poorly nourished drinkers. Thus, the physician should suspect hypoglycemia in obtunded patients who appear intoxicated.

Nutritional deficiency syndromes: Heavy drinkers develop nutritional deficiencies by drinking instead of eating real nutrients. Moreover, alcohol interferes with absorption, metabolism, storage, and retention of vitamins and minerals. Heavy drinkers are especially vulnerable to nutritional deficiencies when they have genetic abnormalities in enzymes whose cofactors depend on these vitamins and minerals.

Thiamine deficiency can lead to beriberi, peripheral neuropathy, optic neuritis, and Wernicke's syndrome, which is the triad of ophthalmoplegia, cerebellar ataxia, and short-term memory loss. This triad's amnestic component, also known as Korsakoff's syndrome (Chapter 14.2), leads many people to confabulate, that is, to fill in memory gaps with manufactured material. Transketolase activity, which requires thiamine pyrophosphate as a cofactor, is low in both Wernicke's and Korsakoff's syndromes. Intravenous thiamine given at the onset of either syndrome can completely reverse it, but if treatment is delayed, the deficits can become permanent. Thiamine replacement should be continued indefinitely, since deficits may resolve over weeks or months. The physician should always give thiamine before starting glucose-containing solutions, to prevent glucose from precipitating these syndromes by acutely depleting patients' limited thiamine reserves.

Poorly nourished heavy drinkers are susceptible to pyridoxine deficiency. Acetaldehyde from excessive alcohol catabolism displaces pyridoxal phosphate from albumin binding sites, leaving it vulnerable to enzymatic degradation. Pyridoxine deficiency can contribute to the development of peripheral neuropathies (Chapter 13.11) and sideroblastic anemia (Chapter 11.2). Folate deficiency, common among poorly nourished heavy drinkers, can cause megaloblastic anemia (Chapter 11.3).

Neurotoxicity: Ethanol directly causes axonal degeneration and demyelination beyond that resulting from poor nutrition. Alcoholic polyneuropathy is characterized by numbness, paresthesias, and weakness in the distal extremities. Symptoms usually begin insidiously in the legs and progress proximally. Asymptomatic patients may have minimal or no ankle jerks. Patients with advanced disease develop severe burning dysesthesias, sensory loss in a "stocking-glove" pattern, and distal muscle weakness and wasting (Chapter 13.11). Ethanol toxicity can also cause cerebellar atrophy, which presents much like the cerebellar dysfunction of Wernicke's syndrome. Recovery from these neurotoxic syndromes takes months to years and is often incomplete even with total abstinence, good nutrition, and vitamin B therapy.

Myotoxicity: Ethanol and acetaldehyde have direct toxic effects on muscle. After protracted binges, drinkers can have acute rhabdomyolysis (dissolution of muscle), presenting as the sudden onset of tenderness, pain, cramps, and proximal muscle weakness. Drinkers can also develop an irreversible dilated cardiomyopathy, manifested by elevated creatine kinase levels, arrhythmias, and heart failure. Myoglobinuria is a common complication that can lead to hyperkalemia, kidney failure, and death.

Chronic skeletal myopathies are usually painless and more often affect the legs than arms. How much a person drinks seems to correlate with the severity of these skeletal myopathies, which often improve after months of abstinence.

Reproductive dysfunction: Alcoholic men with cirrhosis can develop hypogonadism and gynecomastia. Alcohol's toxic effects on Leydig's cells and seminiferous tubules can reduce serum testosterone levels and sperm production. Even prolonged abstinence may not reverse impotence if alcohol has damaged autonomic nerves that control erectile function.

Heavy alcohol use disrupts menstrual function and significantly increases risks for infertility and spontaneous abortion. One in three infants born to alcoholic mothers has the fetal alcohol syndrome: retarded growth and development, congenital physical anomalies, and brain dysfunction ranging from hyperactivity to mental subnormality.

Other sequelae: Chronic heavy drinking is particularly damaging to the gastrointestinal system, primarily the liver (Chapter 7.3). Heavy drinkers have a high incidence of gastritis, gastrointestinal bleeding, pancreatitis, hepatitis, and cirrhosis, as well as cancers of the liver, colon, and esophagus.

Chronic heavy drinking can suppress all bone marrow elements. The most common problem, thrombocytopenia, usually responds quickly to abstinence. The mean corpuscular volume can be high, even without folate deficiency.

Cocaine and Other Nervous System Stimulants

Cocaine is a central nervous system stimulant that increases synaptic concentrations of dopaminergic and noradrenergic neurotransmitters by inhibiting their re-uptake, thus potentiating sympathetic nerve stimulation.

Cocaine hydrochloride can be injected intravenously, crystallized from aqueous solution and "snorted" in the nose, or treated with alkali to form an un-ionized "free base," which in its solid form is called *crack*. Crack cocaine vaporizes at low enough temperatures to be smoked. *Free-basing* is smoking the highly volatile vapors produced by heating a solution of cocaine's un-ionized base in organic solvent. The absorption of intranasal cocaine is limited by vasoconstriction and surface area, but huge volumes of cocaine vapors can be absorbed quickly through the lungs. Cocaine quickly concentrates in the brain and has a 1- to 2-hour serum half-life. Tolerance can become established within hours of repeated use.

The immediacy, intensity, short duration, and rapidly acquired tolerance to cocaine's euphoric effect lead users to repeat dosing at ever-shortening intervals, up to several times per hour. This can cause nausea, vomiting, hypertension, tachycardia, tremulousness, muscle twitching, and fever. Vasoconstriction, inhibited noradrenergic re-uptake, and release of adrenal catecholamines can cause myocardial ischemia, arrhythmias, and myocardial infarction, even in healthy young persons with no history of cardiovascular risk factors or injury. Central nervous system effects include agitation, suspiciousness, paranoid delusions, hallucinations, delirium, and seizures. Cerebrovascular spasm can cause transient ischemic attacks and stroke.

Cocaine withdrawal symptoms are the precipitous onset of drug craving and a depression that often is indistinguishable from major depression (Chapter 14.3). This depressive syndrome usually subsides within days but can persist for weeks to months. The syndrome carries a high mortality, not from physiologic perturbations, but from suicide. For many, cocaine withdrawal cravings and depression respond quickly to tricyclic antidepressants.

Amphetamines and other centrally active sympathomimetic amines have actions and toxic manifestations that, apart from their longer duration, resemble those of cocaine. Withdrawal usually causes depression, anhedonia, lack of energy, and hypersomnolence.

Opioids

The pharmacology of morphine is prototypic of that of other opioids. Heroin (diacetylmorphine) is quickly metabolized to morphine. The mechanism by which morphine produces euphoria and tranquility is not known, but its wide spectrum of central nervous system effects is explained by its affinity for many types of opiate receptors.

The psychopharmacologic effects of opioids outlast their analgesic effects. Tolerance to opioids becomes established within days to weeks of sustained use, so that patients who are administered increasing doses of opioids to keep pace with their growing analgesic requirements can quickly become toxic.

Mild opioid toxicity is characterized by miosis (contraction of pupils), decreased gastrointestinal motility, flaccid muscles, and urine retention. Severe intoxication produces hypotension, hypoventilation, noncardiogenic pulmonary edema, and cyanosis. Central nervous system effects range from sedation, delirium, and seizures to coma. Opioid toxicity can be reversed within 1–2 minutes by intravenous naloxone, an opiate antagonist. There are no specific contraindications to naloxone, so treatment should be repeated if the patient does not respond. Because naloxone has a half-life of only about 1 hour, adequate naloxone levels must be maintained or the full toxic syndrome recurs.

The withdrawal potential of opioids is extremely high: After only weeks of sustained use, people can suffer severe physiologic withdrawal. Repeated use to avoid withdrawal is the most potent reinforcer of opioid dependence. Withdrawal symptoms and signs appear 8–12 hours after abrupt cessation of opioid use, reach peak intensity at 48–72 hours, and last 4–5 days. Acute withdrawal is typified by intense muscle cramping, nausea, vomiting, diarrhea, sweating, rhinorrhea, tearing, dilated pupils, restlessness, insomnia, fever, and, occasionally, mild delirium; the piloerection (gooseflesh) seen in many victims spawned the term "going cold turkey" to describe this state. Although withdrawal is miserable, it is rarely life-threatening unless it worsens some preexisting condition, eg, triggers bronchospasm in a person vulnerable to asthma.

Withdrawal provokes such an intense craving for opioid that many patients resort to dramatic measures to procure more drug. Opioid-dependent patients who legitimately need opioid analgesia often go undermedicated if caregivers feel manipulated or otherwise put off by patients pleading for more drug. Caregivers should consider that highly opioid-tolerant patients may require unusually high doses to achieve analgesia or prevent withdrawal.

Methadone, with its slow onset of action, minimal euphorigenic effects, and 24-hour half-life, is the agent of choice for detoxification or for stabilizing opioid addicts who are admitted to the hospital for other reasons. A useful adjunct for relieving acute withdrawal is clonidine, which reduces sympathetic activity by acting on presynaptic α_2-adrenergic receptors to down-modulate norepinephrine release from peripheral nerve endings.

Chronic opioid withdrawal is characterized by weakness, anergy, irritability, and dysphoria. This syndrome can persist for 6 months after cessation of use and responds poorly to nonopioid drug treatment.

Chronic opioid-induced spasm of the sphincter of Oddi can increase common bile duct pressure, as reflected by elevations in plasma amylase, lipase, and liver function tests. Chronic opioid use can also cause anemia, leukocytosis, and abnormal glucose tolerance.

Sedative, Hypnotic, and Anxiolytic Drugs

Barbiturates are central nervous system depressants with sedative, anxiolytic, and disinhibitory effects. These drugs can produce withdrawal syndromes nearly identical to those of alcohol, but lasting longer because of their longer half-lives. The fact that most people begin taking barbiturates as prescribed medicine rather than for "recreation" makes their initial self-reinforcing properties stronger than those of alcohol. Tolerance and susceptibility to withdrawal can develop in weeks to months, so dependence syndromes are common among regular users. After people abruptly stop barbiturates, they can have major withdrawal syndromes persisting for weeks and minor withdrawal for months. Phenobarbital, with its long half-life, is the treatment of choice for stabilization and detoxification.

Benzodiazepines are more widely used than barbiturates and other sedatives because benzodiazepines have a broader range between their therapeutic and toxic levels; thus, high doses are much less likely to cause the motor impairments characteristic of other sedatives. Benzodiazepines also have less abuse liability than other sedatives, and benzodiazepine users generally take months to years longer to develop tolerance and susceptibility to withdrawal. Nonetheless, the potential for benzodiazepine withdrawal is relatively high. Most benzodiazepine withdrawal syndromes are similar to but less life-threatening than those of barbiturates.

Other Agents

Cannabinoids: Most of the actions of marijuana and hashish are attributable to L-delta-tetrahydrocannabinol, which has high abuse liability. Low doses produce euphoria, paroxysms of spontaneous laughter, heightened sensory awareness, distorted time perception, and inability to execute sequential tasks. Higher doses can cause severe anxiety, perceptual distortions, and hallucinations. Acute toxicity is best managed with calm reassurance and benzodiazepines. Tolerance develops easily. Contrary to pop-

ular folklore, tetrahydrocannabinol can provoke a minor withdrawal syndrome lasting as long as several days, with sleep disturbances, dysphoria, headaches, impaired concentration, restlessness, and irritability. Chronic use produces a peculiar apathetic state characterized by severe impairment in initiating and sustaining tasks; people can continue in this state for weeks to months after stopping use.

Chronic marijuana smoking carries three to four times greater risk for asthma and lung cancer than tobacco smoking. Chronic use is associated with reduced testosterone levels in men and with anovulatory menses, shortened pregnancies, and increased risk of teratogenicity in women.

Phencyclidine (PCP): PCP is a dissociative anesthetic (one that blocks not pain but the sense of being bothered by the pain) that has high abuse liability but produces relatively few physiologic withdrawal symptoms. PCP is usually smoked, although it is occasionally taken by mouth or injected. Low doses produce euphoria and disinhibition and often instill a great sense of physical strength and invulnerability. High doses cause perceptual distortions, hallucinations, hypervigilance, extreme belligerence, and generally the most unpredictable and dangerous behavior of any psychiatric patient. Toxic manifestations also include nystagmus, ataxia, mild hypertension, muscle twitching, seizures, and coma. This toxic state can last as long as 48 hours. Removing patients from nearly all environmental stimulation is crucial for safe management, and moderate to high doses of benzodiazepines are helpful. Postintoxication states mimicking mania and schizophrenia often persist for weeks and respond only partially to neuroleptics.

LSD-25, Mescaline, and Psilocybin: All these agents have high abuse liability, but produce few withdrawal symptoms. They produce a mild delirium that lasts for several hours. Toxicity can usually be managed by a calm milieu and mild sedation with benzodiazepines.

Tobacco: Nicotine inhaled through smoking causes mild euphoria lasting 1–3 minutes. The rapid onset, short duration, and quickly acquired tolerance to this euphoric effect lead to frequent dosings. Repeated use produces nausea, dizziness, cough, tachycardia, and a rise in blood pressure. Abrupt cessation of chronic smoking produces an abstinence syndrome of intense craving for tobacco, plus fatigue, nausea, headache, anxiety, and impaired psychomotor performance. The syndrome usually lasts 3–14 days, but some symptoms can continue for months or years.

Detoxification with slow-release nicotine preparations (nicotine-containing chewing gum or transdermal patches), in combination with education and counseling, enables many smokers to quit smoking (Chapter 15.1). Most of the 30% of smokers who quit permanently have multiple

Table 14.4–2. Screening for alcoholism: The CAGE questionnaire.

Have you ever felt a need to **C**ut down on your drinking?
Have people **A**nnoyed you by criticizing your drinking?
Have you ever felt bad or **G**uilty about your drinking?
Have you ever had a drink (**E**ye-opener) first thing in the morning to steady your nerves or get rid of a hangover?

> Two or three "yes" answers are highly suggestive of alcohol dependence

Modified and reproduced, with permission, from Ewing JA: Detecting alcoholism: The CAGE questionnaire. JAMA 1984;252:1905. © 1984, American Medical Association.

relapses along the way, speaking to the long-term need for patience, ongoing counseling, and even multiple courses of detoxification.

DIAGNOSIS OF DEPENDENCE SYNDROMES

Alcohol and drug dependence syndromes can be reliably and accurately diagnosed by history. The alcohol history should include the CAGE screening test (Table 14.4–2). Similar inquiries should be made about all other classes of psychoactive drugs. Physicians should always ask significant others for their observations or concerns about the patient's alcohol and drug use.

Physicians should be suspicious when they smell beverage alcohol on a patient's breath in any clinical setting. Hand-held devices that screen for ethanol in expired air are readily available "bedside" tools for quickly confirming or refuting the suspicion. Physical findings that warrant further inquiry include facial or digital "puffiness" or edema, unexplained bruises or abrasions, cigarette-stained fingers, spider nevi or angiomas (caused by pooling of blood in the peripheral vessels), gynecomastia, small testicles, hypertension, tachycardia, and hepatomegaly. Many heavy drinkers have thrombocytopenia, a high mean corpuscular volume, and elevations of serum uric acid, aspartate aminotransferase, and gamma-glutamyltransferase. All these findings suggest alcoholism, but none is pathognomonic or even sensitive.

Symptoms and signs of withdrawal are clear evidence of physiologic dependence on a drug, if not a full dependence syndrome. Weight loss, restlessness, and scarring or necrosis of the nasal septum suggest cocaine use. Keloids on the forearms or legs often indicate subcutaneous or intravenous drug use. The physician should follow up a suspicion of drug use with a urine toxicology screen; inexpensive tests are available for all classes of psychoactive drugs.

PRINCIPLES OF MANAGEMENT

No treatment uniformly applied to all patients for alcoholism or any other drug use disorder has ever been shown to be more effective than any other, or particularly effective in its own right. Treatments must address the specific interactions among the agent (alcohol, drug, or both), the vulnerable patient, and the environment.

A few medicines can block the effects of psychoactive substances. For example, a single oral dose of the opiate antagonist naltrexone can completely block the effects of injected opiates for up to 72 hours. However, in clinical practice, only 20% of unselected heroin addicts stay in naltrexone treatment. Even if medicines were developed that could completely block the "rewarding" effects of other psychoactive drugs, such medicines would probably be insufficient to manage the behavioral aspects of dependence.

Thus, treatments must focus on modifying patients' behavior within their environment and on identifying and managing "sustaining factors," intercurrent illnesses, and other conditions that render them more vulnerable to drinking or drug-taking.

The First Encounter

First and foremost, the physician should tell patients their diagnosis of an alcohol or drug syndrome, explain what it means in terms that they can grasp, and provide objective evidence based on their behavioral patterns and physical and mental findings, rather than on the consequences of their use. For example, patients are less defensive about admitting to morning drinking to calm their shakiness, than about connecting their drinking with an automobile accident, poor job evaluation, or family friction. Also, patients who are "in denial" cannot be expected to believe their diagnosis just by virtue of the doctor's authority. Pronouncing to patients that they "abuse" alcohol or have a drug "problem" may only make them incredulous, defensive, or angry. It is far more persuasive to explain how seldom people have their symptoms (eg, blackouts) and behaviors (eg, "pre-drinking") *without* having the diagnosis, and to outline host (eg, family history) or environmental (eg, repeated intoxication before or during adolescence) factors that may have conspired to render them vulnerable. Denial is best countered with facts, logic, and a sympathetic smile.

Having agreed on the diagnosis, patient and physician should immediately close on a coherent, stepwise treatment plan. Involvement of immediate family members and significant others is important at this point and at every other treatment stage.

Many persons with dependence syndromes are either unaware of the strength of their drug-seeking drive or so strongly motivated to seek the drug that they pursue it despite knowing that further use is irrational and potentially injurious. These persons can be protected from irreversible physical, psychological, social, or occupational harm only by a formal "intervention." This is essentially an artificial crisis, fabricated by others to whom the patient has strong emotional or motivational ties; the patient's agreeing to accept treatment becomes the best way to resolve the conflict. Interventions should always led by an expert who rehearses all participants in advance.

Treatment Steps

Stop the behavior: Total abstinence is the goal, even though it is not always achieved in practice. Of people who misuse alcohol and drugs but do not have full-blown dependence syndromes, few can learn to drink appropriately or take licit drugs under supervision. People with full dependence syndromes cannot be permitted to try to "cut down" on their drinking or drug taking. They must halt it abruptly, lest the agent's "rewarding" aspects reinforce its continued use. Patients who are likely to get withdrawal symptoms require detoxification. Patients' environment must be "sanitized" to eliminate exposure to alcohol and drugs. Some patients need to be sequestered early in treatment, with hospitalization if they are seriously ill or in severe withdrawal, residential treatment if social supports are inadequate, or boarding with supportive friends or family who are willing to become involved.

Neutralize factors that sustain the behavior: Many patients, families, and health care providers want to believe that treatment is complete after a few days or weeks of abstinence. However, with abstinence, factors that provoked or sustained the behavior become more evident. Withdrawal syndromes emerge. Intercurrent illnesses, including psychiatric syndromes, become easier to identify. In general, depressive and anxiety symptoms that improve within days after quitting a drug are epiphenomena of withdrawal, but if these symptoms worsen with time, they usually signify an underlying psychiatric condition. Patients should be treated to relieve any psychopathologic symptoms and should be asked about and prepared to cope with stressful situations. Caregivers should give advice, counter demoralization, provide encouragement and countermotivation, and mobilize social supports. However, patients must bear full responsibility for any social or legal consequences of their alcohol- or drug-related behavior.

Psychotherapy aimed at giving patients insight into the causes of their drinking or drug-taking behavior is doomed to failure. If given, psychotherapy instead must remind patients of the consequences of their behavior and arm them with constructive ways to cope. The patient-doctor interaction should be individualized to accommodate patients' dispositional differences. For example, a "tough love" approach helps to engage many extroverted patients, but it is guaranteed to alienate those with an introverted temperament. Introverted patients respond better to frequent encouragement, praise for accomplishments, and relative inattention to shortcomings.

Extinguish the habit: behavior modification: The behavioral aspects of alcohol and drug dependence are treated much like any disorder of motivated behavior. Patients should be given education and a structured treatment plan with concrete steps to follow. Programs like Alcoholics Anonymous and Narcotics Anonymous provide such structure. Group membership provides peer support, lessening of embarrassment, and a larger reservoir of encouragement than can be given in individual therapy alone. Recovering patients and group leaders can serve as role models. Patients should be reminded of the bad consequences of their drinking and drug taking by listening to others' stories and recounting their own.

Patients and staff must catalog situations that used to be cues for drinking and drug taking, plan specifically how to navigate them, and make contingency plans for managing relapses. Patients must fill any "disposable time" with therapeutic activity directed at recovery and leisure pursuits not formerly associated with drug use. Strict adherence to daily and weekly schedules helps patients to avoid unexpected situations that might trigger drinking or drug use. Patients' progress should be monitored for an indefinite period, by objective measures such as breath alcohol tests, urine toxicology screens, and follow-up of abnormal physical and laboratory findings.

With treatment, patients gradually learn to assume greater autonomy in limiting their environmental exposures to alcohol and drugs by seeking new friendships, places, and activities. The general tone of treatment should be positive reinforcement of achievements, minimizing of setbacks, and relative inattention to weaknesses.

Disulfiram (Antabuse), naltrexone, and methadone are adjunctive medicines that deserve mention. Supervised use of disulfiram, a potent noncompetitive inhibitor of aldehyde dehydrogenase, can help deter drinking. When a patient premedicated with disulfiram drinks alcohol, the buildup of the intermediate metabolite, acetaldehyde, causes unpleasant flushing, headache, sweating, palpitations, chest pain, and vomiting. Disulfiram slows the hepatic metabolism of warfarin, anticonvulsants, and neuroleptics. Patients who are taking these agents should not take disulfiram. Neither should patients with serious heart or liver disease, because the acetaldehyde syndrome can cause profound hypotension and coma.

Naltrexone, which blocks the action of opioids on opiate receptors, is useful in treating opioid dependence. Naltrexone can also reduce craving for and consumption of alcohol by heavy drinkers. Increased brain levels of acetaldehyde, alcohol's principal metabolite, have been linked to increased production of specific endogenous opiates in the brain; naltrexone may work by blocking receptors for these opiates.

The goal of methadone maintenance programs is not abstinence, but reduction of the personal and social chaos caused by the constant drug-seeking behavior of opioid-dependent persons. Patients substitute a single daily dose of the long-acting opioid methadone for their usual, and most likely short-acting and illicitly obtained, opioid of choice. All decisions about starting, maintaining, or discontinuing methadone maintenance management are best left to specialty clinics.

Disulfiram, naltrexone, and methadone have little benefit if taken alone, but they can be helpful when their administration is witnessed and monitored and is part of an overall treatment program.

Relapse

Relapse is an integral part of the dependence syndrome and does not necessarily indicate lack of patient motivation or compliance. Relapse may mean that treatment was incomplete or otherwise ineffective or that a contingency was not properly anticipated. Some relapses are totally unrelated to factors that had previously helped initiate or sustain drinking or drug use. Relapse requires intervention within days, to abort reinstatement of the full dependence syndrome. Patients should be restored to normal social roles as quickly as possible. As patients recover, relapses become shorter and less frequent.

SUMMARY

▶ Alcohol and drug dependence syndromes are acquired disorders of motivated behavior that are distinct from other illnesses in that, once established, the host (pa-

tient) actively manipulates the environment to gain more access to the pathogen (alcohol or drug).

▶ The severity, course, and prognosis of withdrawal syndromes and the frequency of complications are closely related to accompanying medical or surgical problems, a history of withdrawal, and other medicines being taken. Major withdrawal syndromes are medical and psychiatric emergencies that must be managed aggressively.

▶ Most major and minor withdrawal syndromes can be prevented by proper drug prophylaxis, prompt control of concurrent illness, minimizing of polypharmacy, and a calm milieu. Withdrawal is best managed before signs become evident.

▶ No single treatment for alcoholism or drug use disorders works for all patients.

▶ The three treatment steps are to stop the alcohol or drug use behavior, identify and neutralize all physical and psychological factors that sustain it, and prescribe a behavioral program to extinguish habits that reinforce it.

SUGGESTED READING

Bebbington P (editor): Psychiatry and the addictions. Int Rev Psychiatry 1989;1:3.

Brady JV: Animal models for assessing drugs of abuse. Neurosci Biobehav Rev 1991;15:35.

Brady JV: A biobehavioral research perspective on alcohol abuse and alcoholism. Public Health Rep 1988;103:699.

Edwards G, Gross MM: Alcohol dependence: Provisional description of a clinical syndrome. Br Med J 1976;1:1058.

O'Brien CP, Jaffe JH (editors): *Addictive States.* Raven Press, 1992.

14.5

Eating and Weight Disorders

Arnold E. Andersen, MD

Abnormal eating behaviors are typically caused by a combination of factors, including social norms promoting thinness, personality vulnerabilities, distortions of perceived appearance, overvaluing the benefits of weight or shape change, and dieting itself, especially at critical stages of development. Together, these forces can lead to self-sustaining eating disorders, primarily anorexia nervosa and bulimia nervosa. Abnormal eating behaviors that begin as a response to calorie restriction gradually become coping mechanisms for problems in self-esteem, interpersonal relationships, and mood regulation. These behaviors are sustained by a determined pursuit of thinness and an irrational fear of fatness.

Physicians must be able to recognize eating disorders and understand their potential complications, which can include death from severe malnutrition, and suicide in depressed patients. The earlier an eating disorder is diagnosed, the better the patient will do. The first clue to anorexia or bulimia nervosa may be subtle (Table 14.5–1). For example, women may present with amenorrhea from hypothalamic dysfunction caused by weight loss, with fractures from estrogen deficiency-related osteopenia, or with esophagitis or loss of tooth enamel from repeated vomiting. When patients present with weight loss, the physician must consider disorders such as hyperthyroidism, diabetes mellitus, malabsorption, and malignancy. However, the excessive and unrealistic fear of fatness in patients with anorexia nervosa differentiates it from other psychiatric and medical conditions causing weight loss.

Overweight is a risk factor for many important disorders, including hypertension, hypercholesterolemia, diabetes mellitus, and, in women, endometrial carcinoma. Morbid obesity, a weight greater than twice normal, can lead to potentially fatal cardiopulmonary disease (Chapter 2.6). Obesity is typically multifactorial: In addition to excessive eating, common contributing factors are genetic predisposition, social class norms, nutrient availability and density, basal and exercise-dependent energy expenditure, and, occasionally, underlying medical, neurologic,

or psychiatric disorders. In general, the more severe the weight abnormality and the earlier it manifests, the more likely genetic or medical factors are involved.

EATING AND WEIGHT REGULATION

The search for freedom from starvation has characterized much of human history; paradoxically, the availability of plentiful food in modern industrialized cultures can provoke extreme reactions. Especially since the 1950's, Western industrialized nations have increasingly defined attractiveness in terms of artificial norms for thinness. In the United States, adult weight in both sexes decreases as social class increases. About 75% of American women feel fat, but estimates of actual obesity in women range from 30% to 25%. Although men have been less severely afflicted by the drive for thinness, they, too, have been increasingly preoccupied with changing their body shape.

Reported cases of anorexia and bulimia nervosa for the United States, Canada, and Europe (including the United Kingdom) have increased several-fold in recent decades, through both actual higher incidence and more accurate diagnosis. An estimated 0.5–1% of young women in Western societies suffer from anorexia nervosa, 2–3% of American college women meet the criteria for bulimia nervosa, and up to 5% of young women of college age in Western societies suffer from atypical or partial syndromes. Nine times as many women as men are affected. A much higher percentage of American women—over 50%—are chronic dieters or at least intermittently are restrained eaters (stop eating before satiety).

The body normally regulates nutrient intake with exquisite sensitivity around a "set point" that maintains weight within a narrow range. The range remains stable or changes slowly over time. When not afflicted by medical or psychological disorders or by coercive sociocultural norms, people who choose to eat primarily foods low in fats and concentrated sweets, who exercise regularly, and who deal reasonably with everyday stresses tend to stay

Table 14.5–1. Possible presentations of eating disorders.

Feature	Cause
Clinical	
Weight loss	Self-starvation, purging
Amenorrhea	Acquired hypothalamic dysfunction
Abdominal pain or distention	Malnutrition and electrolyte imbalance
Loss of tooth enamel	Repeated vomiting
Esophagitis or esophageal tear	Repeated vomiting
Lanugo hair	Regression to prepubertal metabolism
Fracture from minimal trauma	Osteopenia
Laboratory and radiographic	
Metabolic alkalosis	Repeated vomiting
Hypokalemia	Vomiting; diuretic or laxative abuse
Anemia	Malnutrition
Low serum estrogen levels	Suppression of GnRH and gonadotropins
Hyperprolactinemia	Cause unknown
Osteopenia	Low estrogen effect, high plasma cortisol, low body weight, perhaps too many diet sodas

within a narrow and usually normal weight range. Twin and adoption studies support a role for genetic factors in defining this weight range. However, these built-in stable patterns of "motivated behavior" are subject to many aberrations—in the United States, more often from learned sociocultural norms than from medical or psychiatric diseases.

Eating disorders can be diagnosed by relatively specific symptoms and signs. Although the fundamental causes of eating disorders are unknown, these conditions can be more accurately identified than many medical disorders for which laboratory tests exist.

EATING DISORDERS

Anorexia Nervosa

The diagnostic criteria for anorexia nervosa (Table 14.5–2) are (1) self-induced starvation to a weight at least 15% below normal; (2) an intense, irrational fear of becoming fat; and (3) hypogonadism, manifested in women by missing three consecutive menstrual periods and in men by a decrease in sexual function and interest. Although the disorder is termed "anorexia," patients lose their appetite only after losing considerable weight. Another feature seen in many patients, although not a criterion for diagnosis, is a distortion of perception in which patients perceive that they are fatter than they really are.

In more than 95% of patients, anorexia nervosa begins with a conscious wish to lose weight through dieting, often combined with exercise and occasionally augmented by self-induced vomiting and abuse of laxatives, diuretics, or diet pills. The disorder generally takes root after

months or years of self-critical scrutiny of body size and shape. Some patients begin dieting because their friends or family members are dieting or are making comments about the patient's appearance. The peaks of onset of primary anorexia nervosa are the early and late teens (ages 14 and 18). Onset is possible as early as age 7 years and as late as the 70's. The following are risk factors for anorexia nervosa—the more risk factors, the higher the risk: (1) teenage girl; (2) sensitive, self-critical, perfectionist, persevering personality; (3) family history of depressive illness; (4) family history of obesity; (5) "enmeshed" family functioning, tending to "live in each other's pockets" without freedom to grow separately, and overreacting to each other's moods and behaviors; and (6) participation in activities requiring leanness, such as ballet, modeling, wrestling, and other sports.

Anorexia nervosa, though often concealed by layers of clothing, is a relatively public disorder. Anorexic individuals usually come to medical attention because of concern by family, friends, teachers, and sometimes coaches, rather than because the patients themselves are worried.

Two major classes of patients with anorexia nervosa have been identified: those who solely restrict their food intake (restricting subtype) and those of low weight who binge and then induce vomiting or abuse laxatives or diuretics (bulimic subtype). Patients with both subtypes organize their behaviors, social lives, thinking, and ultimately their identity around promoting and maintaining weight loss and resisting weight gain. Families are distressed by the anorexic behavior, which resists both entreaties and threats. This usually makes families feel helpless, angry, or defeated, and occasionally provokes abuse.

Table 14.5–2. Criteria for diagnosis of major eating disorders.

Anorexia nervosa
 Restricting subtype
  Self-induced starvation to ≤85% of normal weight
  Irrational fear of becoming fat
  Hypogonadism
   In women: amenorrhea for 3 months
   In men: decreased libido; impotence
  Distortion of body image*
 Bulimic subtype
  All criteria for the restricting subtype, above
  Binge eating twice/wk for about 3 months
  Purging (vomiting, laxative or diuretic abuse) or other
   compensation (fasting, overexercise) to avoid weight gain*

Bulimia nervosa[†]
 Binge eating twice/wk for about 3 months
 Purging (vomiting, laxative or diuretic abuse) or other
  compensation (fasting, overexercise) to avoid weight gain*
 Irrational fear of becoming fat
 Weight usually normal or above normal
 Distortion of body image*

---

*Found in many patients, but not a diagnostic criterion.
[†]An evolving diagnostic category, binge eating disorder, is characterized by binge episodes followed by physical and emotional distress but no purging.

The final, chronic stage of the disorder has two features. The illness becomes autonomous, resisting change, and the patient develops an identity based on the anorexia nervosa, a "sick role" that derails normal social and psychological development. The chronically low weight may also be sustained by the pathophysiologic effects of malnutrition, such as slowed gastric emptying and severe abdominal distress.

Some of the more common signs of the anorexic patient's emaciation are hypotension, bradycardia, low core temperature, decreased muscle mass, and loss of both intra-abdominal and subcutaneous body fat. Radiographic and laboratory studies may reveal osteoporosis, brain shrinking, and variable degrees of anemia and endocrine dysfunction. Gonadotropins and sex steroid concentrations are low, as can be the serum triiodthyronine (T3). The serum thyroxine (T4) is usually normal. Circulating cortisol and growth hormone concentrations are often high.

Management: Most patients meeting the full criteria for anorexia nervosa need to be treated as inpatients for several weeks to months. Patients are first stabilized medically and then started on nutritional rehabilitation. The best approach to feeding is persuading patients to accept healthy amounts of food, prescribed as medicine, with the promise that they will not be allowed to become fat. Few patients require nasogastric tubes, and parenteral hyperalimentation is fraught with potential complications. Feeding may cause abdominal distress as well as mild peripheral edema, which responds to elevation of the feet; rarely, the stomach dilates. Education and support help patients understand their illness and need for treatment.

Nutritional rehabilitation is only the prelude to definitive management. The central challenge is persuading patients to think differently about their body size and nutritional needs and to appreciate the role that their illness has come to serve in their life. Management is also directed toward identifying and treating coexisting mood, anxiety, and personality disorders, and alcohol or other substance abuse. After the patient's weight has been restored to a healthy range, intensive practice in patterns of healthy daily living consolidates the treatment gains. Treatment of persons younger than 18 years old seldom succeeds unless it includes the whole family. Aftercare usually requires 2–3 years and may involve individual, group, and family treatment.

The death rate from anorexia nervosa is as high as 18%, primarily from medical complications and suicide. Most patients who survive eventually improve, but "eventually" may be years to decades. Coexisting psychiatric conditions, especially mood disorders, personality disorders, and substance abuse, often prove to be the most difficult aspects of long-term treatment. Mortality can be reduced by prompt medical stabilization of low weight and hypokalemia and by recognition and treatment of the coexisting depressive illness found in 30–50% of patients.

Bulimia Nervosa

"Bulimia," derived from the Greek words for "ox" and "hunger," is a syndrome that includes two elements (see Table 14.5–2): (1) binge eating and (2) some attempt to compensate for the extra calories, usually self-induced vomiting, laxative or diuretic abuse, overexercise, or fasting. A specific criterion for bulimia is repeated episodes of binge eating (an average of twice a week for 3 months), during which patients feel that they cannot control their eating. Purging is not essential to the diagnosis, but 80% of patients do it.

Essentially, bulimia is an attempt at anorexia by a person whose physiology does not tolerate intensive hunger from prolonged self-starvation. The term *nervosa* has been added to bulimia to emphasize the features that it shares with anorexia nervosa, primarily the relentless pursuit of lower weight and the morbid fear of fatness. Patients with bulimia may be over, under, or at ideal body weight; most are in the normal range. A diagnosis of anorexia nervosa takes precedence over bulimia if the patient's weight is less than 85% of normal.

Like anorexia nervosa, bulimia nervosa usually begins by dieting. Dieters tend toward bulimia rather than anorexia when their hunger overcomes their attempt to restrict food and they begin binge eating. The clinical disorder emerges when a morbid fear of fatness entrenches itself and patients suffer psychological distress or medical complications after binge eating and subsequent purging, especially when binges are provoked by emotional distress rather than hunger.

Bingeing is promoted by restricting food early in the day (no breakfast, salad for lunch), so an appetite builds that may not express itself until late afternoon or evening, the most common times for bingeing. In extreme cases, patients consume 10,000–30,000 calories a day and binge throughout the day. The patient's social life becomes organized around secret binge and purge episodes, requiring carefully timed entrances and exits. In a substantial minority of patients, bulimic behavior is part of a broader pattern of abnormally impulsive behavior, including alcohol or other drug abuse, sexual promiscuity, and stealing.

Patients can develop bulimia at any age from the preteens to the 50's. The peak onset is age 18–20, a few years later than that for anorexia nervosa. Fifty percent of patients have a history of anorexia nervosa or an anorexia-like episode. Bulimia may alternate with anorexia nervosa in an irregular sequence over several decades.

Bulimia has diverse complications. Nonspecific abnormalities of gastric emptying and bowel function can cause abdominal distention that may worsen patients' distorted perception of their body size and increase their desire to purge. Repeated regurgitation of gastric secretions erodes the enamel on the lingual surfaces of teeth. Serious complications include systemic hypokalemic alkalosis, leading to cardiac arrhythmias, kidney damage, and seizures. If patients use the emetic ipecac, the emetine that it contains can cause myocardial damage similar to viral myocarditis. Most deaths among patients with bulimia are caused by arrhythmias or suicide.

Even after psychological treatment has succeeded in stopping their binge-purge behavior, patients may have persistent esophageal reflux that provokes unwanted vomiting for years.

Management: After diagnosis and initial medical assessment, many patients with bulimia nervosa can be treated as outpatients, with a goal of gradually decreasing the frequency and severity of their bingeing and purging. But some patients must have their behavior interrupted abruptly by hospitalization, especially if the problem is severe and intractable or accompanied by suicide plans or medical complications. Bulimia sufferers are usually surprised and relieved to find that eating moderate quantities of food three times a day does not make them fat, as they had feared.

After bingeing and purging is stopped and any medical complications are treated, the focus of management turns to long-term inhibition of binge-purge behavior. As in managing anorexia nervosa, the physician must recognize the commonly coexisting psychiatric conditions. Both cognitive-behavioral psychotherapy and interpersonal psychotherapy have been shown to produce significant and enduring improvements, greater than antidepressants alone, although about 50% of bulimic patients benefit from the addition of an antidepressant drug. Regular moderate exercise is helpful in both managing stress and promoting a healthy body shape and composition.

Other Disorders of Eating and Appetite

Eating disorders in some patients may not fulfill all the criteria for anorexia nervosa or bulimia. For example, patients may have lost less than 15% of body weight or have fewer than two binge-purge episodes per week for 3 months, but have other typical, albeit milder, features of the disorders.

Eating abnormalities can be manifestations or secondary complications of other medical and psychiatric conditions. For example, in many people major depressive illness causes substantial weight loss. Schizophrenia may lead to weight loss in individuals deluded by suspicions of poisoned food. Patients with dementia syndromes such as Alzheimer's disease have progressive cognitive incapacity that may prevent them from eating enough. Patients with panic disorder who develop social phobias about eating or vomiting in public may avoid food.

A number of medical conditions cause weight loss, including a few in which patients actually increase their caloric intake, such as hyperthyroidism, insulin-dependent (type I) diabetes mellitus, malabsorption, tuberculosis, and intestinal parasites. Tumors of the hypothalamus can cause appetite to decrease or increase. Impaired consciousness, cocaine or amphetamine abuse, and many medicinal drugs can cause people to lose weight. The differential diagnosis of weight loss also includes conditions like occult cancer, HIV and other infections, and major depression. But unlike patients with anorexia nervosa, most people who have lost weight because of other conditions perceive themselves to be too thin and manifest no phobic fear of fatness.

OBESITY

Most obesity is a weight problem, not an eating disorder. The exception is that about 25% of seriously obese people may suffer from a newly described "binge eating disorder" characterized by "grazing" or bingeing without any purging.

The largest contribution to obesity appears to be genetic programming. Some people become progressively and severely overweight even before adolescence, and have a family history of serious obesity. The pathophysiology in these patients, and the role that genetic factors play in more common and milder forms of obesity that develop later in life, are readily inferred but still poorly understood. When both parents are obese, a child has a 90% chance of being overweight; when one parent is obese, a 40% chance; and when neither parent is obese, only a 10% chance. A few syndromes of congenital hypothalamic hyperphagia have been described, such as the Prader-Willi syndrome, in which young children develop severe obesity, hypogonadism, and some degree of mental retardation (Chapter 10.1).

Most often, mild-to-moderate obesity is acquired later in life. In addition to a genetic predisposition, this common form of overweight is attributable principally to a "good life" of an ample, high-fat diet, with infrequent exercise and poor stress management.

The essential first step in treating patients with routine mild-to-moderate adult-onset obesity is to approach it nonjudgmentally, appreciate its multifaceted pathogenesis, and consider critically whether the patient really needs to lose any weight, or, more likely, should exercise more and eat fewer fats. Unless the extra weight is causing or worsening diabetes mellitus, hyperlipidemia, or hypertension, it is not clear that mildly to moderately obese people need to lose weight. Some authorities have shown that repeated cycles of weight loss and gain may promote cardiovascular illness as much as—or even more than—simply remaining at a mildly elevated but stable weight.

The only ways proven to treat mild-to-moderate obesity effectively and safely over the long term are to get more exercise, change eating habits by lowering the fat content of food, and manage stress directly rather than by eating. Courses of virtually all appetite-suppressing drugs, whether prescribed or over-the-counter (most nonprescription drugs contain phenylpropanolamine or caffeine), are followed by a weight rebound. Furthermore, many of these compounds can cause significant medical or psychiatric complications. Similarly, thyroid hormone preparations have no demonstrated long-term efficacy but substantial risks, especially for patients with heart disease. Particularly when a patient is motivated, as by a diagnosis of hypertension or by early disease or death in obese relatives, the physician may be able to institute effective and sustainable diet and exercise changes.

Patients with morbid obesity (more than twice desirable weight) can suffer life-threatening consequences such as cardiopulmonary failure. For these patients, more aggressive approaches can sometimes be justified. Unfortunately, behavioral techniques alone seldom work. Gastric surgery with stapling to reduce stomach size has supplanted previous intestinal bypass procedures, which led to severe complications in as many as 50% of patients. There is some hope for new appetite-suppressing drugs now under investigation, such as long-term use of fenfluramine. Convincing studies are not yet available to guide practice.

ABNORMALITIES OF BODY COMPOSITION AND RATIO

Prudent clinicians do not push overweight patients to lose weight unless they have evidence of health risks. Percent of body fat, which can be estimated based on skinfold thickness (Chapter 4.10), and distribution of fat may be more critical factors in determining medical risk than is weight alone. Risk may increase when body fat exceeds 28% in women and 22% in men.

Distribution of body fat is also important. Concentration of fat in the abdomen in men, and in the upper torso—especially around the shoulders—in women, is linked to earlier onset of coronary artery disease and non-insulin-dependent (type II) diabetes mellitus. For example, risk for cardiovascular diseases increases when the ratio of waist circumference to hip circumference exceeds 0.95 in men and 0.80 in women. However, little is known about what hormonal and other factors determine body fat distribution, how to alter it, and how much the associated cardiovascular risks can be reversed. While recent enthusiasms have surfaced for giving growth hormone or testosterone to men in their 50's to 70's, to decrease fat

and increase muscle mass, conclusive studies of enduring risks and benefits are not complete. Although women may not like a gynoid (pear) distribution of weight, it is safer in the long run than the android (apple) distribution. Convincing studies have shown exercise to be an independent health-promoting factor, especially when formerly sedentary people regularly get about 4–6 hours of moderate exercise a week. Patients are more likely to exercise when the regimen is varied, enjoyable (consider groups, head phones), and close to work or home.

SUMMARY

▶ Body weight is normally determined by genetic factors, calories consumed, and energy expended with exercise.

▶ The key feature of the major eating disorders, anorexia and bulimia nervosa, is a phobic fear of fatness that leads to self-induced starvation or bingeing and purging. Typically begun as dieting spurred by social norms and personal vulnerabilities, the conditions can become self-sustaining and life-threatening. Complications include amenorrhea, esophagitis, irritable bowel symptoms, osteopenia, and cardiac abnormalities.

▶ Since dieting is a risk factor for eating disorders, physicians should ask patients about it and discourage it.

▶ Weight loss secondary to other conditions can be distinguished from primary eating disorders by patients' recognizing that they are too thin and not having a phobic fear of normal weight.

▶ Morbid obesity increases cardiopulmonary mortality, justifying aggressive intervention. Mild-to-moderate obesity requires treatment only if it is causing or worsening other medical conditions; otherwise, more exercise and less fat consumption are generally wiser than dieting.

SUGGESTED READING

Anderson AE: Bulimia nervosa. In *Conn's Current Therapy 1995.* Rakel RE (editor). WB Saunders, 1995.

Andersen AE: *Practical Comprehensive Treatment of Anorexia Nervosa and Bulimia.* Johns Hopkins, 1985.

Bowers WA, Andersen AE: Inpatient treatment of anorexia nervosa: Review and recommendations. Harvard Rev Psychiatry 1994;2:193.

Russell GFM: Bulimia nervosa: An ominous variant of anorexia nervosa. Psychol Med 1979;9:429.

Waldholtz BD, Andersen AE: Gastrointestinal symptoms in anorexia nervosa: A prospective study. Gastroenterology 1990;98:1415.

Hysteria and Other Somatization Disorders

Paul R. McHugh, MD

Most people who seek medical or surgical attention want help with the symptoms of disease. But occasionally a troubled person comes to an internist with complaints and accompanying behaviors that merely mimic organic disease. The search to explain and treat the disorder often ends inconclusively. The physician must distinguish organic disease (products of nature's action on the human organism) from artifacts (products of a human agent imitating disease).

These artificial disorders are called hysteria, conversion disorder, Briquet's syndrome, factitious disorder, malingering, and Munchausen syndrome. Patients engage in these behaviors with the goal of achieving the "sick role"—a socially defined status that can bring such advantages as relief from responsibilities, sympathy, and caring attention from medical practitioners.

Internists and psychiatrists must cooperate in detecting illness-imitating behavior. Failures usually derive from misunderstandings over the nature of the conditions and how to manage them. This chapter addresses both concerns.

HYSTERIA

Definitions

Physicians have traditionally termed most artifactual conditions "hysteria," a behavior disturbance in which people display physical signs and symptoms, more or less unconsciously, for the advantages that the patient role brings. "More or less unconsciously" implies that hysteria merges into "malingering," which is illness-imitating behavior as conscious fraud. Even most malingering patients persuade themselves that the symptoms and signs that bring them advantages are real, so they need not feel stigmatized as fraudulent when the internist's pursuit of the symptoms fails to turn up any pathology. Hysteria is better viewed as behavior that produces a medical artifact.

It is useful to differentiate acute from chronic hysteria. Acute hysteria ("conversion disorder") is the sudden appearance of signs and symptoms, often neurologic, in a person with no previous evidence of illness. Such a patient might suddenly present with paralysis or loss of sensation in the limbs, or with impaired sensory function such as blindness or deafness. Occasionally, acute hysteria takes a psychological guise such as loss of memory, dulling of consciousness, or visual or auditory hallucinations.

Chronic hysteria is also known as "somatization disorder" and "Briquet's syndrome." Patients with chronic hysteria have lifelong complaints of vague symptoms such as pain, faintness, abdominal cramping, coughing, and shortness of breath. At one time or another, they may have complained of dysfunction in every major organ system. These persons most often implicate the gastrointestinal tract, but they also report neurologic, pulmonary, cardiac, orthopedic, and genitourinary symptoms—all vividly described though vague about causes. Again, no adequate pathologic explanation emerges during evaluation and treatment, which may include radical surgery. Patients' chronic complaining is driven not by fraudulent intent but by the habit of seeking medical attention when life seems too difficult to handle.

Since hysteria is an attempt to gain the social advantages of the patient role, patients are most likely to be recognized in medical settings. In hospitals, about 2% of patients seen by psychiatric consultants have acute or chronic hysteria. The acute form is more often seen on neurologic wards, and the chronic form on medical wards. The prevalence of hysteria remains steady; the only recent change is that patients who used to be seen on psychiatric services are now distributed among the medical services.

Evaluation

Predisposing and Precipitating Factors: Both acute and chronic hysteria are usually generated by distress. The distress can be obvious, as when a person faces danger or conflict like battle or prison, from which the symptoms of illness provide an escape. Less severe distress, as from school, family, or social challenges, can promote hysterical behavior in immature or self-conscious people. Some

Acknowledgment: Patricia B. Santora, PhD, contributed to the writing of this chapter.

people develop hysterical symptoms as a reaction to disinterest or neglect. Hysterical symptoms can also be the manifestation of some other psychiatric problem such as depression or even dementia. These conditions should be considered when illness-imitating behavior appears in previously well-functioning adults.

Some aspects of hysterical behavior and its goal of achieving the status of a "sick" person derive from personality features. Many patients have a zeal for exaggeration and drama. Karl Jaspers wrote that such people "crave to appear, both to themselves and others, as more than they are and to experience more than they are ever capable of." The congruence of this personality with life troubles prompts these people to search for a medical state that will "cry out for attention."

Symptoms and Signs: A hysterical patient can imitate almost any feature of a somatic illness. The exactness of the counterfeit depends considerably on how much the patient knows about medicine. Thus, nurses and doctors can produce more persuasive artifacts than other people.

However, the symptoms of acute hysteria are usually gross and crude. They take the form of paralyses and sensory losses that do not conform to anatomic or pathophysiologic states. The symptoms and signs usually create burdens only for caregivers, whereas patients retain capacities (eg, continence) that, if lost, would inconvenience themselves.

The symptoms of chronic hysteria are usually more vague, subjective—though vividly described—complaints like indigestion, traveling pains, generalized weakness, and faintness. The pains tend to afflict the head, neck, abdomen, and lower back. But they spread across the body in idiosyncratic ways, without regard to natural physiologic boundaries, although often in accordance with the patient's concepts of physiology.

Hysterical pain often changes according to how much medical attention the patient is seeking and receiving. Patients may vary their complaints of pain as a way to divide the medical staff, claiming that some nurses and doctors are "listening to me" and others are not.

Of the many conditions that are confused with hysteria, the ones most often mistaken are those that can cause vague, fleeting symptoms and unusual behaviors. Among these conditions are some forms of spinal cord disease and peripheral neuritis (eg, multiple sclerosis, combined system disease, viral or postviral encephalomyelitis and Guillain-Barré syndrome) and disorders that disrupt consciousness (eg, delirium in a young person). The only way to prevent a mistaken diagnosis is to do thorough, repeated physical examinations and laboratory tests for differential possibilities.

Diagnosis

It is never easy to detect a medical artifact driven by a person's search for the "sick role." Diagnosis demands careful evaluation of the patient's present and past. Evaluation should start with the standard noninvasive physical and laboratory exams given to any medical patient. The only caution at this point is to avoid procedures like fine sensory exams that might suggest to the patient a potential new domain of symptoms.

Ideally, hysteria should be diagnosed on positive rather than negative grounds. The physician should seek the significant features of hysteria, rather than settle on hysteria because the medical and laboratory exams have shown nothing. The critical positive features are the form of the manifestations, the life circumstances from which they evolved, and the habitual aspects of the patient's temperament. Not all patients have all three features, but each should be considered.

Hysterical signs and symptoms, though mimicking disease, usually do not conform to the features of natural disease. Often, the physician can prove that a patient's sensory losses extend outside neuronal distributions, that reflexes remain intact despite total sensory-motor losses in a limb, or that a blind patient has no disturbance of either pupillary reflexes or the opticokinetic nystagmus of the sighted.

Hysterical symptoms—both acute and chronic—most often emerge when a person is feeling discouraged or depressed. In depressed patients, some symptoms may have been prompted by suggestion. For example, a nurse's aide caring for a paralyzed patient may develop a similar weakness. A discouraged young student who watches a film about an amnesic person may suddenly lose memory.

A key to the diagnosis is full knowledge of the patient's temperament and past habits. By learning that the patient had many previous complaints leading to medical admissions and even major surgery that proved unrevealing, the physician may suspect that the present episode should be approached psychologically and socially rather than physically. Learning that the patient tends to overreact to difficulty might also lend weight to the opinion. Conversely, people who have passed through a significant part of their life without resorting to imitative "sick role" behavior to resolve problems are unlikely to start it without some serious illness disrupting their self-control. This means that hysteria is an unlikely explanation of new symptoms in stable middle-aged persons unless supported by evidence of a serious psychological disruption such as depression or early dementia.

Finally, even after a thorough evaluation of the patient's signs, setting, and personality, the physician may overlook some medical conditions that themselves have vague and changing symptoms and signs. This concern can lead to interminable laboratory testing of hysterical patients by internists searching for ever more esoteric conditions. The tests themselves may sustain the hysterical behavior by suggesting that much is hidden but much may be found. One way to assure caregivers that an esoteric physical illness is not hidden among vague symptoms is to hold a formal ward conference involving everyone on the treatment team. The members list all possible diagnoses—including the most esoteric—and agree that if tests for these conditions are negative, the patient will be treated as hysterical unless a new sign appears.

Management

Internists' efforts to discern a physical illness from the artifactual presentation may for some time distract their attention from the patient's psychological problems. But once empathic internists realize that they are managing a psychologically driven artifact rather than natural disease, they are in a perfect position to help hysterical patients out of situations that provoke and sustain their behavior, as well as to care for them if they do develop physical illness.

It is important to diagnose hysteria quickly to prevent long periods of medical attention that can make the behavior self-perpetuating. Although there is risk in diagnosing hysteria, there is risk in overlooking it. Medical effort is wasted on pointless evaluation, opportunities for providing psychological and social treatment are missed, and the patient remains impaired and distressed.

Treatment of hysteria rests on persuasion and countersuggestion. The doctor persuades patients that they are healthy rather than ill. Sometimes all that a patient needs is for the physician to turn attention away from the symptoms and focus on the patient's present life circumstances. Patients who have come to trust the doctor's good intentions may respond especially well to statements like, "I'm aware that you've had these symptoms, but I know now that you're recovering from them and won't be troubled much longer. This is the time for us to talk about things like what may be upsetting you at home."

Certainly, this is the best tactic to use at the start with patients with Briquet's syndrome, who otherwise will only ruminate about their symptoms. A useful maneuver with these patients, once their confidence in the doctor's good will is secure, is to discuss with them how their chronic physical complaints match the descriptions of Briquet's syndrome in medical texts. Many doctors fear that patients will sense the stigma attached to this diagnosis, but in fact many patients are appreciative on learning that the internist with whom they have developed a trusting relationship has made a diagnosis that is recognized by others. What had seemed mysterious to them is now clear, and now that they understand the rationale for their treatment program, they may be better able to cooperate with it.

Some hysterical symptoms must be handled even more directly. An underlying psychological problem cannot be treated as long as the hysterical behavior is drawing everyone's attention. For example, patients who cannot walk because of hysterical paralysis must be able to walk again before their social and psychological rehabilitation can succeed. Often, the internist can simply tell patients that they will progress each day in recovering the lost function. This expectation can be delivered along with a prescription for the patient to work toward this goal with the nurses and physiotherapists. When the internist says that the process is simply one of rehabilitation, the paralysis often dissipates.

Fear that symptoms relieved will promptly be replaced by others is exaggerated, especially if the patient is encouraged to begin a psychological and social reappraisal of the life situation that promoted the illness-imitating behavior. Advice and social guidance—given by all the members of the treatment team but particularly by the social worker, who is attuned to family matters—can help to resolve these underlying difficulties and prevent the problem from recurring. The discovery and relief of underlying illnesses such as depression also prevent relapse.

Patients with chronic hysteria (Briquet's syndrome) are best managed by an internist who understands the problem, the patient, and the nature of hysterical artifacts. At the same time, the internist must remain alert to any physical illness that the patient might develop. The physician can interrupt new hysterical symptoms, provide help for the settings and depression that might precipitate them, and spare the patient needless and prolonged treatments.

BEHAVIORAL VARIANTS

Acute and chronic hysteria should be distinguished from two other behavioral syndromes that can look similar: factitious disorder and Munchausen syndrome. Patients with these conditions make more conscious efforts to produce illness-imitating symptoms than do patients with hysteria.

A person with factitious disorder purposely alters findings in the laboratory or physical exam to imitate signs of disease. Patients may heat the thermometer so they seem to have fever, inject foreign substances under their skin to produce ulcers or a rash, or ingest chemicals to change their electrolyte balance. Patients' ingenuity in producing abnormal results rests in part on their medical knowledge. Most of these patients come from the medical and nursing professions. Their transparent behavior provokes internists far more than does hysteria. But many patients with factitious disorder truly believe that they have some disease, and they create symptoms to keep the internists searching for the real problem.

Once factitious disorder is suspected and then confirmed (eg, by discovering the medications used to derange laboratory results), management is relatively simple. The behavior needs to be directly but kindly confronted, helped by such statements as, "You must be very worried if you would go to such dangerous lengths as to change your test results." If this confrontation is private and supportive, most patients will explain their problems and fears, enabling the physician to develop a new management plan.

Munchausen syndrome describes the behavior of vagrant people who have become skillful at gaining hospital admission through some behavioral display that looks life-threatening—abnormal test results, seizures, even coma. People with Munchausen syndrome are seeking admission for the bed, food, and pleasant lodging that a hospital can provide. They are not looking for aggressive procedures such as painful operations, and may leave just before being subjected to them. These people live on the largesse of the hospital system, moving from city to city as they eventually exhaust their welcome in each place. Persons with Munchausen syndrome can at first seem a great waste of medical effort, but if the internist can view them as part of the intriguing human scene, they can be helped to find their way into more useful behaviors.

SUMMARY

▶ Hysteria is a behavior in which people more or less unconsciously imitate medical conditions. Hysteria in medical patients may begin acutely (conversion disor-der) or may be lifelong (somatization disorder, Bri-quet's syndrome). In both forms, the patient's goal is to attain the sick role and its social advantages.

▶ Hysteria is diagnosed by assessing the symptoms, the setting in which they developed, and the patient's tem-perament.

▶ Managing patients with hysteria is an exercise in prompt diagnosis, countersuggestion, and psychologi-cal rehabilitation.

▶ Malingering and Munchausen syndrome are more clearly fraudulent behaviors, but, if recognized, can also be directly handled.

SUGGESTED READING

Guze SB: The validity and significance of the clinical diagnosis of hysteria (Briquet's syndrome). Am J Psychiatry 1975;132:138.

Head H: The diagnosis of hysteria. Br Med J 1922;1:827.

Reich P, Gottfried LA: Factitious disorders in a teaching hospi-tal. Ann Intern Med 1983;99:240.

Slavney PR: *Perspectives on "Hysteria."* Johns Hopkins, 1990.

Psychological Responses to Illness

Mark L. Teitelbaum, MD

Understandable psychological responses to the meaning of illness, hospitalization, and treatment are virtually ubiquitous. Most of these responses probably remain undetected by the patient's physician. It is only those exaggerated responses that cause significant distress and suffering for the patient or family or interfere with medical care that come to the physician's attention. In order to understand and deal with such meaningful responses to illness, the physician needs to take a particular perspective with the patient. Rather than viewing the patient as a bodily organism, the physician must see the patient as a person whose moods, behaviors, thoughts, and emotions can be intuitively understood and empathized with.

"LIFE-STORY" PERSPECTIVE IN MEDICINE

Seeing the patient as a subject rather than an object is the essence of the life-story perspective in medicine. A life story is the recounting of the history in which a person's attributes, strengths and weaknesses, and the characteristic way of responding to circumstances are revealed and understood. The physician "puts him- or herself in the patient's shoes" to understand the patient's response to illness and its place in the patient's life story. This response may include denial, fear, anger, or sadness. In this way, the physician grasps the meaningful connections between the patient as a person, the events that have befallen the patient, and the patient's psychological response to those events.

For all patients, being ill, hospitalized, and treated by a physician carries conscious and unconscious meanings that determine their psychological responses to these happenings. One person may experience illness as a potential or actual loss of power and control, another as loss of independence, another as the threat of financial ruin, another as loss of beauty or sex appeal, another as lonely separation from loved ones, another as distress over being diagnosed with a hereditary disease that could be passed on to children. Yet another patient sees illness as a release from the burden of life's responsibilities. The key issue is

that there is no one formula that can predict the meaning of illness for an individual patient. Likewise, it is a mistaken notion that certain personality types respond to all illnesses in the same way or that certain illnesses have the same meaning for all patients suffering from them.

Knowing the patient as a person and using the life story to interpret the patient's response to illness, hospitalization, and treatment are crucial in two ways. First, knowledge of the patient serves as the "glue" that binds physician and patient together in a relationship. This relationship makes successful collaboration between physician and patient possible. Second, it is the vehicle for the transmission of the physician's psychotherapeutic influence.

INTERACTION OF PERSONALITY, CIRCUMSTANCE, AND EMOTION

General Issues

The psychological responses of a person to illness, hospitalization, and treatment are similar to responses provoked by any perceived threat or loss. A patient may experience denial and disbelief, fear, anger, sadness, or combinations of these. Occasionally, people respond to being sick with relief, preoccupation with illness, or dramatization of illness. The predominant psychological response—its intensity and duration—depends on the patient's personality characteristics, strengths and weaknesses, the nature, intensity, and duration of the provoking circumstances, and the personal meaning of these events to the patient. The patient's perception of the social support available and of the quality of his or her relationship to the physician also influences the patient's response.

Given sufficient intensity and duration of exposure to adverse circumstances, all human beings sooner or later experience emotional distress. No one is immune. This fact has been well documented in studies of combat fatigue, in which every soldier exposed long enough to the stresses of combat eventually experiences significant emotional disturbance. Studies of the dying also reveal that the extent of emotional disturbance is directly related to the length of time that a person is physically ill and suffering.

Kinds of Responses

Denial/Disbelief: Denial of illness is a fairly common response. Such patients are unable and unwilling to believe the information being given to them by their physician. This is often associated subjectively with a feeling of shock. Such responses can provoke behavioral noncompliance with treatment. For example, wishing to sign out of the hospital prematurely may be a sign of denial of the reality of illness.

Fear: Being afraid in situations of illness and hospitalization is extremely common. One can readily understand such a response to the realistic and symbolic threats involved in being ill. Issues of uncertainty, the possibility of pain, concern about disfigurement and loss of bodily integrity, and fear of death all may play a role.

Anger: Anger is often best understood as a defensive response to being threatened. It is important to identify the nature of the threat, using the knowledge of the patient as a person contained in the life story. Excessive anger may be inappropriately directed at the physician and medical staff and may threaten the cohesiveness of the physician-patient relationship and the ability of the staff to work with the patient. Very intense responses of anger are often seen in patients who perceive having to depend on others as a threat. Such angry responses sometimes serve to maintain interpersonal distance and a feeling of independence.

Sadness: Sadness is a response to loss, and illness commonly leads to various kinds of loss, both real and perceived. Patients lose their health, may lose a valued aspect of their appearance, a body part, the ability to work, or their independence by virtue of the fact that they are sick. When confronted with a sad patient, the physician needs to distinguish understandable sadness from the mood change seen in depressive illness.

Generally, the sad mood of a person responding to adverse events tends to be reactive; that is, it is influenced by environmental events. This sadness is unlike the persistent and pervasive mood change of depressive illness. Furthermore, a realistic self-attitude is generally preserved. The understandably sad patient rarely feels guilt-ridden and does not blame him- or herself. Sleep and appetite disturbances seen in depressive illness may appear in an understandably sad patient but are usually much less severe than in depressive illness.

Relief: Paradoxically, there are some patients who respond to being ill with a feeling of relief. These are patients who may view illness as an opportunity to escape from the burdens of life or gain some advantage, either in the form of financial compensation or emotional support. Some of these patients can be problematic for the physician when not recognized, since such a response may lead to behaviors that interfere with treatment and recovery.

Illness Preoccupation/Dramatization: Some patients respond to illness by becoming preoccupied with their medical condition, that is, by excessive worry and hypochondriacal brooding out of proportion to any realistic concerns. Still others respond with self-dramatizing behaviors that give the impression that the person is sicker than is the case. Knowing the patient as a person is crucial if the physician is to reassure appropriately in the preoccupied patient and to set limits appropriately in the self-dramatizing patient.

ROLE OF PSYCHIATRIC CONSULTATION

Psychiatric consultation should be considered for patients whose responses to illness are extreme either in intensity or in duration or whose responses are associated with behaviors that interfere with treatment. Adequate preparation of a patient for psychiatric consultation is always an important ingredient of a successful consultation. However, this is sometimes overlooked. Adequate preparation not only facilitates the consultation but probably improves the patient's acceptance of recommendations made by the consultant as well. Adequate preparation involves a candid, unrushed discussion between physician and patient of the physician's reasons for seeking consultation.

Psychiatric consultation carries a variety of meanings for patients. These meanings can be the basis for an emotional reaction that might interfere with the patient's acceptance of consultation. A patient may feel stigmatized or abandoned by his or her physician or may feel that the physician devalues the patient's suffering and believes that the illness is "all in his or her head." Sometimes a patient believes that psychiatric referral means that the physician has no hope that the patient will get better. Such reactions need to be dealt with in an open and straightforward way in order to help the patient understand the reason for consultation and to be reassured that he or she will not be abandoned by the physician, that the physician knows the patient is suffering, and that the physician is hopeful about the patient's improvement.

MANAGEMENT BY THE PHYSICIAN

The Physician-Patient Relationship and Its Therapeutic Function

By virtue of the physician's role as a socially sanctioned healer and the patient's expectations of his or her relationship with the physician, there is great potential for the physician to have a psychotherapeutic influence on the patient's thinking, emotions, and behavior. Physicians exercise this psychotherapeutic function with varying degrees of conscious intent. Some exercise it inadvertently, whereas others make a conscious effort to have a psychotherapeutic impact in their practice. Psychotherapy can be done by all physicians and should not be thought of as restricted to the domain of the psychiatrist. Using several simple psychotherapeutic principles, the physician can reduce certain kinds of suffering experienced by patients and improve their quality of life.

Principles of Psychotherapy

Psychotherapy involves the development of new understanding, in the context of a special relationship based on empathy, which leads to new, more adaptive action. New knowledge or insight occurs through the collaborative construction of the patient's life story. This is the version of the history that carries meaning for the patient and is based on "narrative" truth, not "historical" truth. What is important in the history is the patient's perception, what is coherent, and what leads to illumination rather than what is historically verifiable. Through the development of the life story, previously disavowed aspects of the self are brought to light. These are often aspects that have been rejected as unacceptable and now are recognized, accepted, and reintegrated. This reintegration into awareness constitutes insight. Such new knowledge is crucial if a person is to choose consciously rather than simply respond instinctively to circumstances. Thus, with insight comes the possibility of real freedom.

Therapeutic Relationship/Empathy: Essential for the development of new knowledge is a special kind of intimate and confiding relationship that is based on empathic understanding and empathic communication: a therapeutic relationship. Empathic understanding rests on being able to understand the patient "from within," to share the patient's feelings and perceptions, and thus to understand the patient's experience and its meaning to the patient. The physician shares empathic understanding with the patient in the form of an interpretation that meaningfully links the patient's psychological response to the interaction between the kind of person the patient is and his or her life circumstances. The accumulation of interpretations linking personality, circumstance, and psychological response builds up, enriches, and illuminates the life story.

An essential ingredient of a therapeutic relationship is emotional arousal. By virtue of the intimacy that develops between physician and patient, emotions related to the patient's earliest experiences with caretakers are aroused. Such emotional arousal not only facilitates the acquisition of new knowledge but probably is therapeutic in itself. The physician's ability to arouse and sustain a feeling of hopefulness is also a major ingredient in consolidating a therapeutic relationship.

Action/Change: Armed with fresh understanding of his or her responses and an authentic, therapeutic physician-patient relationship, the patient may be influenced by the physician to take new, more adaptive action. Of course, change is always difficult. Such change comes slowly and sometimes only after repeated conversations with the physician. The process of attempting new action involves taking multiple small steps that become an accumulation of experiences, which, if positive, enhance the patient's sense of mastery and reinforce his or her efforts to continue changing in a way that is helpful.

SUMMARY

▶ Psychological responses to illness are ubiquitous and are determined by the interaction between the personality of the patient, the nature and circumstances of the illness, and the meaning of the illness to the patient.

▶ The key to interpreting and managing these responses is knowing the patient as a person in the context of his or her life story.

▶ Anger is a response to threat and sadness a response to loss, and the specific perceived threat or loss should be identified.

▶ Management of troublesome responses to illness rests on the physician's personal influence. With new self-knowledge, a patient may be persuaded to change in the context of a therapeutic physician-patient relationship that is based on empathic understanding and communication.

SUGGESTED READING

Frank JD: *Persuasion and Healing.* Shocken Books, 1977.
Frank JD et al: *Effective Ingredients of Successful Psychotherapy.* Brunner/Mazel, 1978.
Jaspers K: *The Nature of Psychotherapy: A Critical Appraisal.* The University of Chicago Press, 1964.

McHugh PR, Slavney PR: *The Perspectives of Psychiatry.* The Johns Hopkins University Press, 1983.
Yalom ID: *Existential Psychotherapy.* Basic Books, 1980.

Section 15

Special Topics

John D. Stobo, MD, and Thomas A. Traill, FRCP, Section Editors

15.1

Preventive Medicine

Michael J. Klag, MD, MPH, Daniel E. Ford, MD, MPH, and Sidney O. Gottlieb, MD

An effective clinician not only treats diseases but tries to prevent them. About 50% of all deaths in the United States each year are preventable (Table 15.1–1). The increasing emphasis on disease prevention and health promotion stems from the growing burden of patients with chronic diseases, recognition of the behavioral basis of many diseases, increasing importance of economic issues in health care decisions, and rigorous research proving the efficacy of early interventions.

There are several important reasons to stress disease prevention. First, some diseases, such as AIDS (Chapter 10.2), have no cure at this time. Second, even if a disease is treatable, the available therapies may be less than ideal, either because they do not restore full function, as with diuretic and angiotensin converting enzyme inhibitor treatment for congestive heart failure (Chapter 1.5), or because they are very expensive, as with coronary artery bypass graft surgery (Chapter 1.3). Third, prevention may be the only approach to diseases that can be fatal very soon after the first clinical manifestation. For example, about 20% of people with coronary artery disease die outside the hospital, unaware that they had the condition (Chapters 1.2 and 1.3).

This chapter describes the principles of clinical preventive medicine, provides guidelines for the periodic health examination, and outlines the principles of how patients can change their behavior.

SUCCESSES OF PREVENTIVE MEDICINE

The principles of prevention were first applied to infectious diseases. Preventive health programs reduced or eliminated many infectious diseases in the United States (Chapter 8.1). For example, long before effective antibiotics became available, deaths from cholera and tuberculosis fell because of public health campaigns to improve sanitation and ease crowded living conditions. In 1976, through efficient case identification and widespread delivery of an effective vaccine, smallpox became the only disease ever to be eradicated from the world. Vaccination programs have reduced the incidence of polio in the United States from about 18,000 cases per year in 1954 to 1 case in 1994.

Because of these trends, life expectancy in the United States has extended from 47 years in 1900 to 75 years in 1990, and the pattern of mortality has shifted from infectious to chronic diseases. Like infectious diseases, chronic diseases can be viewed as having incubation periods (although much longer) and predisposing factors. Tobacco use and other behaviors, for example, accounted for an estimated 50% of deaths in 1990 (see Table 15.1–1).

The recognition that chronic diseases do not necessarily accompany aging but are a result of lifestyle has led to remarkable achievements in the prevention of some chronic diseases, such as cardiovascular diseases (Table 15.1–2). Between 1950 and 1990, age-adjusted death rates fell by two-thirds for stroke (Chapter 13.6) and by half for heart disease. (Clinicians may not have perceived this dramatic decline in mortality because growth and aging of the population continue to increase the absolute number of patients whom physicians treat for cardiovascular disease.)

The mortality reductions are explained by both a lower incidence of cardiovascular disease and a longer survival for patients with established disease. For example, the incidence of stroke in Olmsted County, MN, fell from 209 per 100,000 population in 1945–1949 to 135 per 100,000 in 1980–1984, and the proportion of patients with stroke who died decreased from 33% to 17%. These declines can be attributed both to better medical care of persons with risk factors for cardiovascular disease and to behavior changes by the population as a whole. For example, in 1971 only 16% of Americans with hypertension were on drug treatment; in 1990, 55% were being treated. More Americans are quitting smoking: In the 1950's, 45% of adults smoked; by the early 1990's, about 25% were smokers. This complex and dangerous behavior has been reduced through the combined effects of changes in legislation, public opinion, and physician management of patients who smoke (see "Behavior Change: Smoking Cessation" below).

In contrast to the trends for cardiovascular disease,

Table 15.1–1. Potentially preventable causes of death in the United States, 1990.

Causes	Estimated Number	% of All Deaths
Tobacco	400,000	19
Diet and activity patterns	300,000	14
Alcohol	100,000	5
Microbes	90,000	4
Toxins	60,000	3
Firearms	35,000	2
Sexual behavior	30,000	1
Motor vehicles	25,000	1
Illicit use of drugs	20,000	<1
Total	1,060,000	50

Reproduced, with permission, from McGinnis JM, Foege WH: Actual causes of death in the United States. JAMA 1993;270:2207.

death rates from cancer have stayed relatively stable since 1950 (see Table 15.1–2). However, a 50% decrease in deaths from cervical cancer between 1960 and 1990 has been attributed to the widespread introduction of Papanicolaou (Pap) smear screening (Chapter 12.4). As more women have mammography, the rate of breast cancer deaths should fall similarly (Chapter 12.3).

Injuries, suicide, and homicide are also important preventable causes of morbidity and mortality in the United States. Alcohol and drug abuse contribute to accidents and violence (Chapter 14.4). Death rates from motor vehicle

Table 15.1–2. Age, race, sex-adjusted death rates per 100,000 for selected causes of death, United States, 1950 and 1990.

	1950	1990	Rank in 1990*
All causes	840.5	520.2	—
Diseases of the heart	307.2	152.0	1
Cancer	125.3	135.0	2
Cerebrovascular diseases	88.6	27.7	3
Motor vehicle accidents and other unintentional injuries	57.5	32.5	4
Chronic obstructive pulmonary disease	4.4	19.7	5
Pneumonia and influenza	26.2	14.0	6
Diabetes mellitus	14.3	11.7	7
Suicide	11.0	11.5	8
Chronic liver disease and cirrhosis	8.5	8.6	9
HIV infection	—	9.8	10
Homicide and legal intervention	5.4	10.2	11
Nephritis, nephrotic syndrome, and nephrosis	—	4.3	12
Septicemia	—	4.1	13
Atherosclerosis	—	2.7	14

*Rank based on numbers of deaths in the United States in 1990.

From Centers for Disease Control and Prevention, National Center for Health Statistics: *Vital Statistics Rates in the United States, 1940–1960.* Public Health Service, DHEW Publication No. (PHS) 1677, 1968. *Vital Statistics of the United States, vol II, Mortality, Part A, for data years 1960–1990.* Public Health Service, US Government Printing Office.

accidents have declined, partly because people are less likely to drive while under the influence of alcohol. However, homicide continues to be a major threat to the public's health. The contrast is stark between US homicide rates and those of other countries. For example, mortality from homicide for men aged 15–24 is 46 times higher in the United States (27.3 per 100,000) than in the United Kingdom (0.6 per 100,000).

TYPES OF PREVENTIVE INTERVENTIONS

Prevention efforts are classified as primary, secondary, or tertiary. *Primary prevention* is an intervention designed to keep a disease from developing. This usually involves specific protection (eg, vaccination, use of condoms to prevent HIV infection), health promotion (eg, smoking cessation to prevent lung cancer), and chemoprophylaxis (eg, use of aspirin by asymptomatic persons to prevent myocardial infarction). Primary prevention is appropriate for diseases that can be fatal within hours of the first manifestation and for diseases that have no effective treatment. The disadvantage of primary preventive interventions is that many people who will never have the disease may be subjected to an intervention.

Secondary prevention is detection of early, asymptomatic disease, usually by screening. An example is mammography to seek localized breast cancer in asymptomatic women. Secondary prevention also includes efforts to halt or slow the progression of disease after it begins. Here an example is aggressive cholesterol-lowering therapy to prevent progression of coronary artery disease in patients who have a history of angina or myocardial infarction (Chapter 4.9). Most secondary prevention is targeted at high-risk groups; thus, it leads to more efficient use of health services than do primary prevention programs. Although the ratio of benefit to cost is high for those targeted to receive the intervention, secondary prevention programs have less impact on reducing the total number of cases in a population than do primary prevention programs.

Tertiary prevention is the prevention of disability or further deterioration after disease has become well established. An example is rehabilitation after a patient has had a stroke. Tertiary prevention is usually synonymous with "routine medical care."

HIGH-RISK VERSUS POPULATION-BASED STRATEGIES

Clinicians usually think of disease prevention as it relates to their individual patients, but prevention strategies can also be applied to whole populations. Take as one of countless possible examples the goal of preventing hypertension-related disease. Physicians might screen all their patients for hypertension, then treat to lower the blood pressure of those affected (optimal blood pressure is below 120/80 mm Hg) (Chapter 1.13). This is a strategy to prevent disease in high-risk patients. A corresponding population-based strategy might be to lower by 2 mm Hg the blood pressure of everyone in the community by reducing the amount of salt used in the processing and preparation of food. The risk of future disease would fall only slightly for each individual, but the health benefits for the entire population would be substantial because they are multiplied by the number of persons in the community. Thus, a community approach might be more effective in reducing society's total burden of blood pressure-related illness than finding and treating everyone with hypertension.

In most situations, neither the strategy of preventing disease in high-risk patients nor the population-based approach is totally effective alone, so both strategies are needed. Most comprehensive prevention programs begin by targeting high-risk patients, with a goal of increasing public and physician awareness of the problem and support for the intervention. The population-based strategy can follow soon after. Practicing physicians should combine both approaches. Although they must pay special attention to the patient at obvious high risk, they should assume that every patient has some element of risk for every disease and so should try to instill in all their patients the healthy habits of eating a low-salt, low-fat diet and getting exercise, drinking alcohol in moderation, and not smoking.

PERIODIC HEALTH EXAMINATION

Physicians get their best chance to prevent disease when they evaluate healthy patients. But repeating the basic history and physical exam every year is not productive for either patient or physician. Much more useful are periodic visits for targeted testing and prevention counseling, based on the patient's age and risk factors. Recommendations on which tests to do and when to do them used to be conflicting and confusing. Now organizations and expert groups that base guidelines on review of the scientific evidence are reaching more and more consistent conclusions. The US Preventive Services Task Force, the American College of Physicians, and the Canadian Task Force on the Periodic Health Examination have developed the most comprehensive set of prevention recommendations to date (Figure 15.1–1).

Three major criteria are used to gauge the effectiveness of prevention interventions. The first criterion addresses burden of suffering. Does a given disease cause substantial disability and mortality within the population? Screening tests are recommended for rare diseases only if the tests are very accurate and available treatment is very effective, as for phenylketonuria and several other genetic metabolic disorders. The second criterion is how accurately the screening test can identify who has the target condition (test sensitivity) and who does not (test specificity). When a screening test with low sensitivity comes

back negative, patients who have early disease may be mistakenly told that they are healthy. When a screening test with low specificity is positive, many healthy people may be incorrectly labeled as having a disease. The third criterion is that the test can detect disease at a preclinical stage and that this earlier detection leads to a better outcome for the patient.

Many available tests meet the first two criteria, but few fulfill the third. Although it would seem obvious that early detection should improve prognosis, this is not always certain. Longer survival is sometimes explained by patient self-selection, as when an unusually healthy and health-conscious population seeks screening tests. Another explanation can be "lead-time bias": The disease is detected earlier in its natural history in group A patients, who were screened, than in group B patients, who were not. So the group A patients have a longer survival after diagnosis. However, these persons derive no benefit from earlier treatment, and their survival is the same as that of group B. They gained nothing from early detection except more time to worry. Only expensive large-scale randomized clinical trials can show that earlier detection and treatment truly improve outcomes. Such trials have proved the value of early detection and control of high cholesterol and hypertension. But for many interventions, trials have not been done, so recommendations must be made without definitive proof.

One result of critical evaluation of prevention recommendations is the emergence of more complex and selective guidelines. For example, instead of recommending periodic fasting blood glucose measurements for everyone, authorities now advise testing only for persons at high risk for diabetes (Chapter 4.7), that is, the markedly obese, persons with a family history of diabetes, and women with a history of gestational diabetes. As more is learned about risk factors for disease and as molecular biology contributes more to our knowledge of genetic risks (Chapters 10.1 and 10.2), prevention guidelines are likely to become even more selective and individualized.

BEHAVIOR CHANGE: SMOKING CESSATION

Physicians have a responsibility to help their patients adopt the healthiest possible lifestyles. Several aspects of the physician-patient relationship facilitate such changes. Patients view their physicians as health experts. Patients usually come to the physician with some degree of uneasiness about their current health or a perceived threat to their future health. The visit is a "teachable moment" when patients are receptive to a health message and may be especially willing to confront their high-risk behaviors.

The following are general principles of behavior change:

1. Assess the behavior: determine what people do, why they do it, and what barriers keep them from changing it.

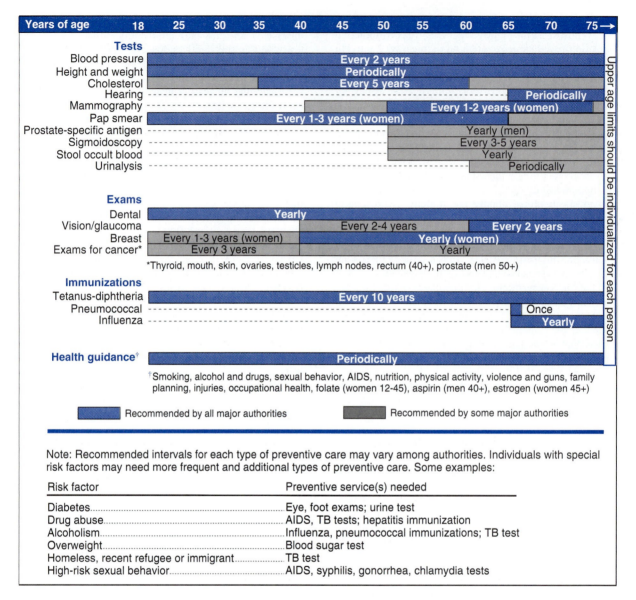

Figure 15.1–1. Summary of prevention recommendations for adults, by age. (From Adult Preventive Care Timeline [poster]. Stock No. 017-001-00502-9. US Department of Health and Human Services, Public Health Service, 1994.)

2. Determine readiness to change.
3. Set reasonable, measurable goals.
4. Use environmental cues to promote change. For example, people find it easier to cut back on drinking if they do not have beer in the refrigerator, and they are more likely to take their medicine if they keep the pill bottle next to their toothbrush.
5. Provide regular follow-up and active feedback. The physician starting a patient on a program of behavior change should schedule frequent follow-up contacts, either in person or by telephone.

Most of what we know about how physicians help patients to change their behavior comes from smoking cessation research. Many studies have shown that physicians who follow the principles are much more successful than other physicians in helping their patients to quit smoking. So although the principles of behavior change could apply equally well to improving patients' eating and drinking habits, patterns of exercise, and adherence to medication regimens, we will use smoking cessation to exemplify behavior change.

The physician should routinely ask all patients whether

they smoke. Physicians can prompt themselves to ask by keeping a checklist in the patient's chart (or putting a colored sticker indicating "smoker" on the chart) or by giving patients a questionnaire to fill out in the waiting room. The physician should ask all smokers a question such as "What do you understand to be the effects of smoking on your health?" Rather than sounding threatening, this question lets the physician learn about gaps in patients' knowledge and their concerns about their future health. Next, the physician should ask about patients' previous attempts to quit, whether they have ever managed to abstain for at least 30 days, and what has made them relapse. The physician should help patients to see unsuccessful quit attempts less as failures than as sources of information to help them do better in future attempts.

The physician's smoking cessation statement should be personal and specific, and should emphasize the benefits of change. For example, "I care about you and your health. Stopping smoking would be the best way for you to stay healthy, especially given your bronchitis. When you stop smoking, your lungs will begin to recover in a few days. You should stop smoking now, and I can help you."

For patients who have thought about quitting, the physician should then try to exact a commitment, even if minimal, to change. Patients might promise to smoke fewer cigarettes each day, limit the places where they smoke, discuss smoking cessation with a smoking spouse, or read a pamphlet about quitting. The physician should also help patients figure out ways to avoid environmental cues to smoking. Patients might hide their ash trays, get up from the dinner table rather than linger over coffee, and have paper and pencil near the telephone so they can keep their hands busy doodling during conversations.

To be most effective, the message to stop smoking must be tailored to where the smoker is in the process of behavior change. It is a waste of time to set a quit-smoking date for a patient who has not yet thought about stopping. For these patients, the physician might ask, "What is it going to take to get you to stop smoking?" Most patients will not have a ready answer. Physician: "Of course, you could wait to quit until you've had a heart attack, but both of us know that it would be better if you stop long before that." Patients might respond that they're waiting to quit until they graduate or find a job or lose weight, or they're waiting for their husband to quit first. The physician must realize that there are times in a person's life when the chances of changing a behavior are slim, for example, when the smoker is caring for a spouse with a terminal illness. Nonetheless, patients need to understand that at some point, stress can become an excuse for not trying to quit. Physician: "You will always have some stress in your life. Even if you're stressed, at some point you still need to quit. Why don't you think about this and talk with some people who have already quit? We'll talk about it again the next time you come in."

Patients who are considering quitting can take a questionnaire to learn how addicted they are to nicotine (Table 15.1–3). A score of 6 or higher means that they are more likely to suffer from the physiologic effects of nicotine withdrawal and thus are more likely to benefit from nicotine replacement therapy once they stop smoking. The higher the score and the more cigarettes smoked per day, the higher the nicotine dose should be. Nicotine replacement therapy accompanying an attempt to quit smoking doubles the probability of abstinence 6 months later.

The nicotine patch has surpassed nicotine chewing gum as the preferred method of replacement. The gum is available over-the-counter to persons over age 18; the patch and nasal spray still require a doctor's prescription.

The goal of nicotine replacement therapy is to give patients lower blood levels of nicotine than when they smoked (without the other toxins in cigarettes) and to reduce levels gradually to zero over 3–6 months. Nicotine replacement is almost certainly safer than smoking. There are several caveats: Although studies suggest that nicotine replacement can benefit smokers who have coronary artery disease, therapy in these patients should be prescribed cautiously and at low doses. Nicotine replacement should not be used by pregnant women or women who may become pregnant while on therapy.

Active follow-up improves smoking cessation rates. If patient and physician agree on a quit date, the physician's office should call the patient 1 day after that date: "Yesterday was your quit date. Did you stop smoking yesterday?"

Table 15.1–3. The Fagerstrom Tolerance Questionnaire to measure nicotine addiction.

Questions	Answers	Points*
1. How soon after you wake up do you smoke your first cigarette?	Within 30 min	1
	After 30 min	0
2. Do you find it difficult to refrain from smoking in places where it is forbidden, in church, at the library, at the movies, etc?	Yes	1
	No	0
3. Which cigarette would you hate most to give up?	The first one in the morning	1
	Any other	0
4. How many cigarettes/day do you smoke?	≤15	0
	16–25	1
	≥26	2
5. Do you smoke more frequently during the first hours after awakening than during the rest of the day?	Yes	1
	No	0
6. Do you smoke if you are so ill that you are in bed most of the day?	Yes	1
	No	0
7. What is the nicotine level of your usual brand of cigarette?	≤0.9 mg	0
	1.0–1.2 mg	1
	≥1.3 mg	2
8. Do you inhale?	Never	0
	Sometimes	1
	Always	2

*A score of 6 or higher means probable nicotine addiction.
Modified and reproduced, with permission, from Fagerstrom K-O, Schneider NG: Measuring nicotine dependence: A review of the Fagerstrom Tolerance Questionnaire. J Behav Med 1989;12:159.

If the patient quit on schedule: "Congratulations. You're off to a good start. You're going to start feeling much better off cigarettes. Are you following the plan we made?" If the patient has not quit: "We'd agreed that you would stop smoking yesterday. What happened to keep you from quitting? Let's set a new date."

The physician should schedule an appointment with the patient for the next week. This is the time to ask patients in what situations they will feel most tempted to smoke and to help them plan how they will keep from smoking in those situations. For example, "The first time you go to a bar, you have a couple of drinks, and a friend offers you a cigarette, how will you avoid smoking?" or "The next time you're home by yourself and you feel lonely and bored, what will you do instead of lighting up?" The physician's job is not to have all the answers, but to encourage patients to think ahead so that they will have a plan ready when a difficult situation arises.

Following these suggestions doubles the probability that a smoker will be abstinent 1 year after quitting. Even though the absolute success rate for quitting is only about 10% for a single attempt and most smokers have had to make several attempts, 50% of smokers in the United States have successfully quit smoking. Smokers appreciate their physician showing them genuine empathy, concern, and cautious optimism during this difficult process. With persistence and repeated attempts, physicians can help a large percentage of their smoking patients to quit.

The principles outlined here have been proven to increase success in changing behavior. Although these principles were developed for smoking cessation, they can be used to change many other unhealthy behaviors, such as obesity, sedentary lifestyle, and problem drinking.

SUMMARY

▶ Preventable lifestyle factors accounted for at least 50% of deaths in the United States in 1990.

▶ Community-based interventions have the potential to reduce society's total burden of disease more effectively than interventions targeted at individual patients.

▶ Prevention recommendations are evolving quickly and becoming increasingly complex and tailored to an individual's risk factors.

▶ Physicians should assume responsibility for helping patients adopt the healthiest possible habits. For example, physicians can best help their patients stop smoking by giving specific personal advice, getting patients to commit to change, setting a quit date, prescribing the nicotine patch, and providing active follow-up.

SUGGESTED READING

Clinician's Handbook of Preventive Services. US Department of Health and Human Services, Public Health Service, 1994. Stock No. 017-001-00496-1. Order from Superintendent of Documents, PO Box 371954, Pittsburgh, PA 15250-7954, or fax (202) 512-2250 (to be used in conjunction with the *Guide to Clinical Preventive Services* below).

Guide to Clinical Preventive Services: A Report of the US Preventive Services Task Force, 2nd ed. Williams & Wilkins, 1996. Available in bookstores or from the publisher (to be used in conjunction with the *Clinician's Handbook of Preventive Services* above).

Hayward RSA et al: Preventive care guidelines: 1991. Ann Intern Med 1991;114:758.

Rose G: Sick individuals and sick populations. Int J Epidemiol 1985;14:32.

For on-line information about prevention practice guidelines: Telnet to text.nlm.nih.gov, or dial (800) 952-4426 (login: HSTAT.FTRS).

15.2

Medical Assessment and Management of Patients Undergoing Surgery

Brent G. Petty, MD

An internist who is asked to conduct a preoperative assessment of a patient should answer four questions (Table 15.2–1). The first is: What is this patient's risk from the intended operation? The answer depends on the patient's medical condition, the nature of the surgery, the duration of anesthesia and surgery, and the skill of the surgical and anesthesiology personnel. Patients undergoing anesthesia and surgical procedures have physiologic stress that particularly affects the cardiovascular and pulmonary systems. Therefore, evaluation of patients who are to undergo surgery should be comprehensive, but should focus on these systems. The patient and the physicians involved in the patient's care need to be aware of all of the patient's important medical conditions and the impact that these conditions have on the risks of surgery and on perioperative management. For the patient, the risk issue is associated with informed consent—that is, understanding the risks of surgery in light of underlying medical conditions. An important issue in the history is when patients most recently underwent anesthesia and whether they had any problems.

The second question is: Can some timely intervention significantly reduce the patient's risk without worsening the surgical condition? Several risk factors can be ameliorated. However, whether the patient's surgical condition allows the physicians the luxury of taking the time necessary to reduce these risks depends on the nature and pace of the surgical condition. In addition, the intervention for risk reduction (eg, drug treatment) may carry some risks of its own, though usually very small.

The third question is: What prophylactic measures should be instituted? In particular, the internist should consider prevention of deep venous thrombophlebitis, pulmonary complications (especially atelectasis and pneumonia), wound infections, and endocarditis.

The fourth question is: How should the patient's regular medications be altered? All unnecessary medications that can be abruptly withdrawn should be stopped. For patients whose surgery renders them unable to take oral medications, necessary medications should be given by alternative routes (parenteral, transdermal, rectal) or substituted by another compound that can be given by an alternative route.

Two questions need never be asked. One is: Is surgery absolutely contraindicated? The answer is always "no," since even the sickest patient may undergo surgery if it is the only or most reasonable means to reverse the underlying process. The balance between the perceived risks and the benefits of the surgery determines whether to proceed. The other question that surgeons and anesthesiologists sometimes ask the internist is: Will you clear my patient for surgery? This question should also be answered "no," because the internist assesses surgical risks but cannot "clear" for surgery in the sense of ensuring a trouble-free operation.

CARDIOVASCULAR SYSTEM

Anesthesia

Anesthesia has profound effects on the circulatory system. Laryngoscopy and intubation may produce vagal effects with bradycardia, while patient manipulation and the induction of anesthesia may stimulate the sympathetic nervous system with an abrupt rise in blood pressure and potential for arrhythmias. Inhalational anesthetic agents, used during the remainder of an operation after successful induction, are negative inotropic agents and dilate the vascular bed by reducing sympathetic tone. These effects lead to a lowering of blood pressure that frequently accompanies general anesthesia. Some anesthetic agents are arrhythmogenic themselves, or they may sensitize the myocardium to the effect of circulating catecholamines. Thus, the induction and maintenance of general anesthesia have significant cardiovascular effects, initially stimulatory (hypertensive) and later depressant (hypotensive).

Table 15.2–1. Questions to be answered in perioperative consultation.

What is the patient's risk from this operation?
Can a timely intervention reduce surgical risk without worsening the surgical condition?
What prophylaxis should be instituted?
How should the patient's regular medications be altered?

Spinal anesthesia is widely assumed to be safer than general anesthesia, but little or no rigorous scientific evidence supports this assumption. Spinal anesthesia causes sympathetic ganglion blockade and may lead to serious hypotension. Overall, spinal anesthesia may present no less cardiovascular risk than general anesthesia. Although spinal anesthesia may have advantages in certain situations, the remainder of this chapter deals with the risk of general anesthesia, reflecting the greater degree of investigation into and use of general anesthesia in surgical practice.

Cardiovascular Complications

Cardiovascular complications are the leading cause of perioperative mortality. In light of the physiologic effects previously mentioned, it is not surprising that these complications take the form of ventricular arrhythmias, myocardial infarction, and congestive heart failure—any of which can be fatal. Studies comparing surgical patients' preoperative medical conditions with their outcomes have identified several risk factors for cardiovascular complications (Table 15.2–2). The most important of these risk factors are myocardial infarction within the past 6 months, preoperative heart failure (manifested by an S_3 gallop or jugular venous distention), age over 70 years, rhythm other than sinus, and reduced exercise capacity.

Table 15.2–2. Risk factors for perioperative cardiovascular complications.

Major
Myocardial infarction within past 6 months
Congestive heart failure
Age >70
Heart rhythm other than sinus
Reduced exercise capacity

Moderate
Hypoxemia
Hypokalemia
Aortic stenosis
Respiratory insufficiency (PCO_2 >50 mm Hg)
Renal failure (blood urea nitrogen >50 mg/dL or creatinine >3.0 mg/dL)
Elevated aspartate aminotransferase (AST)
Chronic liver disease
Bedridden patient
Emergency surgery
Thoracic or upper abdominal surgery

Minimal or none
Mild or moderate hypertension
Diabetes mellitus
Stable angina pectoris
Asymptomatic carotid bruits
Bifascicular conduction block

The incidence of perioperative myocardial infarction in patients with a previous myocardial infarction appears to have decreased over the past 25 years. It is not certain whether this improvement is attributable to better case selection, better case preparation, more extensive intraoperative monitoring, or improved postoperative care. Nevertheless, what both the older data showed and the more recent data confirm is that the incidence of perioperative myocardial infarction progressively falls with a longer interval between the previous infarction and surgery. The risk usually levels off at about 6 months after the previous myocardial infarction and does not fall substantially from that point, even with intervals of years since the infarction. Therefore, if a patient has had a myocardial infarction, the risk of any surgery will be less if it is delayed until at least 6 months after the infarction. Nevertheless, the incremental increase in perioperative risk at 3 months compared with 6 months after an infarction is modest; therefore, many physicians endorse proceeding with important surgery after the shorter interval. Patients with a history of myocardial infarction, regardless of when the infarction occurred, have a mortality rate of 50% if they suffer another infarction perioperatively. Many myocardial infarctions and arrhythmias occur up to several days after anesthesia.

Other Risk Factors

Less important risk factors for perioperative cardiac complications include hypoxemia, hypokalemia, aortic stenosis, respiratory insufficiency, renal failure, elevated aspartate aminotransferase (AST), signs of chronic liver disease, and a patient bedridden for noncardiac causes. Patients with valvular aortic stenosis are especially sensitive to even small increases or decreases in intravascular volume. Patients who undergo emergency operations or surgery in the thorax or upper abdomen are also at somewhat higher risk. Diastolic hypertension below 110 mm Hg does not seem to be an important risk factor, nor does diabetes mellitus, stable angina pectoris, peripheral vascular disease, or bifascicular conduction block. The ability to do moderate exercise—long a clinical measure of surgical suitability—has been confirmed in a geriatric population to be an excellent identifier of patients with low cardiovascular risk.

From this evidence, it seems reasonable to assume that surgical risk can be reduced by eliminating or decreasing the severity of identified risk factors. Measures to reduce risk may include gradual correction of congestive heart failure and electrolyte abnormalities, control of arrhythmias, and, if the surgical condition allows, delay of surgery pending recovery from myocardial infarction or acute renal failure. On the other hand, rapid reduction in blood pressure to the normal range in chronically hypertensive patients may be counterproductive, since a hasty change in intravascular volume or vascular tone may impair renal function, predispose to stroke, or increase the difficulty of managing autonomic nervous system changes (especially vasodilatation) associated with anesthesia.

Patients who are to undergo peripheral vascular surgery

have a higher incidence of coexisting coronary artery disease and perioperative myocardial infarction than many other surgical patients. Dipyridamole-thallium scans are helpful in risk stratification for patients with intermediate risk based on routine clinical assessment, but this modest benefit does not seem sufficient to justify the expense.

Occasionally, patients presenting for surgery are found to have asymptomatic carotid bruits, or noninvasive testing shows moderate carotid artery obstruction. These patients have no greater incidence of perioperative strokes than comparable patients without detectable carotid disease, so prophylactic endarterectomy is not recommended for asymptomatic surgical candidates.

RESPIRATORY SYSTEM

Several surgical factors contribute to pulmonary complications. General anesthesia decreases vital capacity, but this effect is magnified in patients undergoing thoracic or upper abdominal surgery, compared with patients having lower abdominal or extra-abdominal nonthoracic surgery. This is because upper abdominal surgery induces diaphragmatic dysfunction, leading to a restriction of lung expansion at the bases, a redirection of ventilation predominantly from the bases to the apices, and a shift to primarily "rib cage" breathing from normal abdominal breathing. Postoperative analgesics and sedatives contribute to the hypoventilation caused by general anesthesia. Not only is depth of breathing reduced with general anesthesia, but there is also decreased clearing of secretions. Since smoking also reduces sputum-clearing mechanisms, smokers are at substantially greater risk for pulmonary complications than nonsmokers. The combination of hypoventilation and reduced clearing of secretions can lead to atelectasis with ventilation-perfusion mismatches and consequent hypoxemia, respiratory failure, and pneumonia.

Various preoperative pulmonary function tests have been studied in an effort to determine which best predicts postoperative pulmonary complications. It has been shown that patients with abnormal preoperative spirometry or arterial blood gases who undergo upper abdominal surgery are at increased risk for pulmonary complications. Nevertheless, no studies have clearly delineated a minimum forced expiratory volume in the first second (FEV_1) or forced vital capacity (FVC) below which patients must not be subjected to surgery. Patients with an FEV_1 as low as 0.45 L have tolerated general anesthesia without complication. Thus, routine preoperative spirometry should not be done. On the other hand, preoperative arterial blood gases may be beneficial, not only as a predictor of postoperative complications (see Table 15.2–2), but also to establish a baseline for the patient. Such baseline arterial blood gases are not routine preoperative requirements, but may be especially helpful in patients with known or suspected pulmonary disease.

Some interventions have been shown to reduce perioperative pulmonary complications (Table 15.2–3): stopping smoking at least 2 weeks before surgery, preoperative an-

Table 15.2–3. Interventions to reduce perioperative pulmonary complications.

Smoking cessation ≥14 days before surgery
Antibiotic treatment of acute bronchitis or pneumonia
Psychological preparation for postoperative pain
Incentive spirometry before and after surgery
Effective but not excessive analgesia
Early ambulation
Prophylaxis for thromboembolism

tibiotic treatment of acute exacerbations of bronchitis and other respiratory infections, preparing the patient to anticipate postoperative pain, incentive spirometry starting before surgery and continuing afterward, effective but not excessive narcotic analgesia to control pain, and early postoperative ambulation.

ENDOCRINE SYSTEM

Several endocrinologic issues are of importance in the surgical patient. The physiologic stresses involved with surgery lead to an increase in circulating cortisol, glucagon, growth hormone, and catecholamines. The increase in catecholamines puts increased work on the cardiovascular system; elevations of cortisol, glucagon, and growth hormone interfere with glucose metabolism, potentially leading to hyperglycemia, particularly in patients with diabetes.

The dose of oral hypoglycemic agents or insulin should be reduced by 30–50% on the morning of surgery to prevent perioperative hypoglycemia. It is far better for a diabetic patient to have slightly high blood sugars for 1–2 days perioperatively than to suffer the consequences of hypoglycemia, which can be clinically silent during anesthesia or in the presence of large doses of narcotic analgesics. On the other hand, extreme postoperative hyperglycemia can lead to problems such as dehydration, delayed wound healing, and impaired leukocyte function. Frequent blood sugar determinations and supplemental short-acting insulin or intravenous dextrose can keep blood sugar levels in a desirable range in the postoperative period. With current management practices, diabetes in and of itself (not complicated by cardiac or renal disease) does not appear to increase substantially the morbidity or mortality of surgery.

Thyrotoxicosis and hypothyroidism can increase the risk of perioperative complications, particularly when thyroid dysfunction is severe or patients have coexisting heart disease. Uncontrolled hyperthyroidism may predispose surgical patients to atrial fibrillation, leading to heart failure or thromboembolism. Delirium, vomiting, and diarrhea can also complicate perioperative management of thyrotoxic patients. Ideally, thyrotoxicosis should be controlled preoperatively with antithyroid medications. Patients who require emergency surgery may be given short-term β-adrenergic blockade.

Hypothyroidism increases risks for perioperative heart failure, intraoperative hypotension, and postoperative neuropsychiatric and gastrointestinal problems, all of which are usually minor and self-limited. Another problem is that hypothyroid surgical patients are less likely to have a fever when infected. Elective operations should be postponed until euthyroidism is restored.

A marked, sustained, or refractory elevation in blood pressure at the induction of anesthesia may be a sign of pheochromocytoma, although most patients with such blood pressure increases do not, in fact, have this tumor. The cause probably relates to a sympathetic nervous system that is particularly sensitive to the normal perioperative increases in catecholamines, or an exuberant release of catecholamines by a normal adrenal medulla, not a tumor.

A common management problem is the patient undergoing general anesthesia who is receiving supraphysiologic doses of adrenocorticosteroids for therapeutic reasons, and therefore has a suppressed hypothalamic-pituitary-adrenal axis. This suppression prevents such patients from providing the usual glucocorticoid release in response to the stress of anesthesia (equivalent to 200 mg hydrocortisone); without supplementation, these patients can suffer acute adrenal insufficiency. It is important to give these patients intravenous hydrocortisone 100 mg or its equivalent, starting shortly before induction of anesthesia and continuing every 6–12 hours for 1–2 days (higher daily doses for more extensive surgery) and then returning to the usual corticosteroid dose or providing the intravenous equivalent. It is not necessary to taper the dose down to the preoperative dose. The supplement should be continued longer than 3 days only if postoperative complications arise. For minor surgery, when usual oral dosing of steroids is not interrupted, patients can continue their regular regimen.

THROMBOEMBOLISM

Thromboembolic disease can be a serious postoperative problem. The immobility required by the surgical procedure makes this a potential complication for any patient, but at particular risk are patients who are obese or elderly, have malignancies, undergo lengthy operations, are likely to have prolonged postoperative immobility of the legs (eg, patients undergoing orthopedic surgery), or have a history of thrombophlebitis.

Because of the frequency of thromboembolic disease in patients who have undergone surgery, effective but safe prophylaxis is needed. Measures should reduce the incidence of postoperative thrombophlebitis and embolism but not increase the incidence of perioperative complications, particularly bleeding. Furthermore, for such preventive measures to be widely used, they should be inexpensive and cost-effective. Measures that meet all these criteria include low-dose subcutaneous heparin (5000 U every 8–12 hours), platelet inhibitors, elastic stockings, and intermittent pneumatic leg compression systems. For reasons that are not clear, these measures may be effective in some surgical settings but not others. For example, low-dose heparin is effective in preventing thromboembolism in many surgical patients, but has not

been found to be effective in patients undergoing hip replacement. These patients appear to do best with higher-dose heparin, low molecular weight heparin, or low-dose warfarin. Some evidence exists of additive benefit when mechanical and pharmacologic measures are combined. The prophylactic measures appear to be most effective when started before surgery and should be continued until patients are ambulatory. Some studies suggest a reduction in thromboembolic complications and in graft occlusion after peripheral vascular surgery if regional anesthesia is used instead of general anesthesia.

GASTROINTESTINAL TRACT AND NUTRITION

Gastrointestinal diseases in general do not constitute serious risks for surgery. They become significant if they are severe enough to cause malnutrition, anemia, or overall debility. For example, of patients who undergo elective surgery for Crohn's disease, those with a serum albumin below 3.1 g/dL have a higher incidence of complications than those whose serum albumin is at least 3.1 g/dL. The incidence of surgical complications is also inversely correlated with serum total iron binding capacity, another measure of intravascular proteins. This relationship between serum albumin or total iron binding capacity and the incidence of surgical complications also holds for patients undergoing many other types of surgery.

For most patients undergoing elective surgery, briefly reduced caloric intake in the perioperative period is of little consequence. However, in patients already suffering from poor nutrition, such as alcoholics and patients with cancer, further restriction of calories may aggravate the underlying condition. This may delay healing, impair host defense against infection, and prolong convalescence. Some of these patients benefit from hyperalimentation before or after surgery, or both (Chapter 4.10).

Liver disease, especially chronic liver disease, appears to be an important surgical risk factor. Both nutritional and hepatic status combine in Child's classification, which is a fairly reliable indicator of prognosis for patients who are to undergo portasystemic shunts. Patients with the combination of an albumin less than 3.0 g/dL, serum bilirubin over 3.0 mg/dL, severe ascites, encephalopathy, and generalized wasting have a 50% operative mortality rate for portasystemic shunts, while patients with none of these abnormalities have a mortality rate of less than 1%. Chronic liver disease is also a risk factor for other surgical procedures. Acute viral hepatitis has been implicated as a serious perioperative risk factor. The risk of general anesthesia in patients with alcoholic hepatitis is less clear.

Obesity increases perioperative morbidity in several ways. Obese patients are more prone to wound infections or dehiscence than nonobese patients, and are more likely to develop thrombophlebitis, hypoventilation, and consequent pulmonary complications. Severe obesity also presents mechanical problems for intubation and establishment of a patent airway.

HEMATOLOGIC SYSTEM

Because oxygen delivery to tissues depends in large part on the hemoglobin concentration in blood, anemia is a particular problem in surgical patients. Furthermore, if the patient's hematocrit is low before the operation, there is less margin of safety with intraoperative bleeding. It is general practice to keep or achieve a minimum hematocrit of about 30% before surgery, usually through transfusions, except for patients undergoing minor procedures or those who have chronic, compensated anemias and potential volume contraindications to preoperative transfusion (eg, patients with chronic renal failure or aortic stenosis). This minimum hematocrit of 30% may be particularly important in patients with atherosclerotic cardiovascular disease.

Severe thrombocytopenia can interfere with hemostasis. Platelet plug and clot formation are usually normal when platelet counts exceed 70,000/μL, but at lower levels hemostasis becomes compromised; at platelet counts of 20,000/μL or less, patients face the risk of increased bleeding during surgery, bleeding from invasive cardiovascular monitoring devices, bleeding caused by invasive measures to effect regional anesthesia, and spontaneous bleeding unrelated to surgery. On the other hand, platelet function may be impaired in spite of a normal platelet count because of illness (eg, uremia) or exogenous toxins (eg, aspirin). Platelet function can be accurately assessed at the bedside by the bleeding time, but an abnormal bleeding time cannot reliably identify patients who will bleed excessively during surgery.

INFECTION

Postoperative infections are common, and several factors contribute to their development. Normal skin integrity, an extremely important barrier to invasive pathogens, is lost at the site of surgical incision, leading to a high incidence of wound infections. Invasive monitoring and support equipment also violate normal barriers to bacteria and act as portals of entry for infection. Inhalational anesthetics have an adverse effect on neutrophils, making them less active in killing bacterial invaders. There is evidence that prolonged hyperglycemia in patients with diabetes has similar and additional detrimental effects on the body's response to infection, and these patients as a group are probably more likely than comparable nondiabetic patients to develop postoperative infections.

Antibiotic prophylaxis reduces the incidence of infections in elective abdominal, gynecologic, and other surgery. Antibiotics are especially effective in reducing wound infections and urinary tract infections. Cephalosporins are popular drugs for preoperative antibiotic prophylaxis. Surgical wound infections are more common with contaminated surgery, such as that for a ruptured abdominal viscus, than with noncontaminated procedures; patients who are to undergo contaminated surgery should be started on antibiotics preoperatively. Antibiotic prophylaxis for bacterial endocarditis is indicated for patients with valvular or congenital heart disease whose operation is likely to cause bacteremia.

SUMMARY

▶ Fundamental questions regarding surgical risk, potentially beneficial interventions, prophylaxis, and medication adjustment need to be answered for all patients undergoing surgery.

▶ The most important risk factors for perioperative mortality are cardiovascular: evidence of congestive heart failure (jugular venous distention, a third heart sound), myocardial infarction within the past 6 months, and rhythm other than sinus.

▶ Perioperative pulmonary complications can be reduced by effective analgesia, early ambulation, antibiotic treatment of acute bronchitis or pneumonia, incentive spirometry, and prophylaxis for deep venous thrombophlebitis.

▶ Hypokalemia, hypoxemia, renal failure, respiratory insufficiency, and liver disease contribute only modestly to perioperative cardiac events. In contrast to widespread belief, diabetes, stable angina, and even moderate hypertension add little risk.

SUGGESTED READING

Bode RH Jr et al: Cardiac outcome after peripheral vascular surgery: Comparison of general and regional anesthesia. Anesthesiology 1996;84:3.

Christopherson R et al: Perioperative morbidity in patients randomized to epidural or general anesthesia for lower extremity vascular surgery. Anesthesiology 1993;79:422.

Gerson MC et al: Cardiac prognosis in noncardiac geriatric surgery. Ann Intern Med 1985;103(6 pt 1):832.

Kammerer WS, Gross RJ (editors): *Medical Consultation: The Internist on Surgical, Obstetric, and Psychiatric Services,* 2nd ed. Williams & Wilkins, 1990.

Preoperative pulmonary function testing. American College of Physicians. Ann Intern Med 1990;112:793.

Wong T, Detsky AS: Preoperative cardiac risk assessment for patients having peripheral vascular surgery. Ann Intern Med 1992;116:743.

15.3

Hypothermia and Hyperthermia

Keith T. Sivertson, MD

Both hypothermia and hyperthermia can cause irreversible tissue damage and death. The physician treating a patient with either condition has three concerns: (1) What must I do to restore the patient's temperature to normal? (2) What organs may have been damaged by the cold or heat? (3) Should I consider any concurrent conditions, such as alcohol intoxication or central nervous system infection, which might be preventing the patient from responding normally to changes in environmental temperature?

Both hypothermia and hyperthermia can present either as an obvious extraordinary temperature from known environmental exposure, or as shock or coma, in which the high or low temperature comes as a surprise. Temperature is an important and often overlooked vital sign in critically ill, hemodynamically unstable patients; physicians should not need to be reminded that the only way to identify hypothermia or hyperthermia is with a thermometer. Learning the cause of hypothermia or hyperthermia may require talking with the patient's family and friends and with witnesses.

TEMPERATURE REGULATION

Body temperature reflects a balance between heat production and heat loss. This balance is maintained in two ways. The first is a person's ability to recognize signals of thermal discomfort sensed by skin thermoreceptors, and avoid thermal stress by changing activity, adjusting clothing, or seeking shelter. This system breaks down when a person cannot perceive the discomfort or cannot respond to it. Thermal perception can be disrupted by any process that alters cognitive functioning, for example, use of alcohol or other drugs, head trauma, stroke, dementia, psychosis, and mental retardation. People with these conditions do not perceive discomfort or danger from heat or cold. Ability to respond is disrupted by immobility. The person understands that a hot or cold environment threatens, but is not able to take needed action.

The second way that the body balances heat production and loss is with the autonomic nervous system. The autonomic system maintains the temperature of the body's core (brain, heart, and other trunk organs) at the expense of the skin and extremities. The "thermostat" controlling heat distribution is centered in the anterior hypothalamus. Output from the hypothalamus is delivered by direct neural pathways and by catecholamine release from the adrenal medulla. The "set point" of this hypothalamic thermostat can be affected by central nervous system disease, pyrogens, or drugs such as phenothiazines or tricyclic antidepressants. When a pyrogen changes the set point, the hypothalamus defends it the same way that it defends normal temperature. Thus, fever is caused by a change in hypothalamic set point. Hyperthermia from environmental exposure is caused not by a change in set point, but by a failure of heat-dissipating mechanisms.

The skin and extremities are the primary route of adjustable heat exchange. Vasomotor responses adjust skin temperature through their ability to alter skin blood flow 20-fold or more. Heat is dissipated by peripheral vasodilation and sweating. Heat is conserved primarily by peripheral vasoconstriction, seen as skin blanching and as cold, poorly perfused extremities. Heat production can be increased by *nonshivering thermogenesis,* a rise in metabolic rate mediated by norepinephrine release. In severe cold stress, shivering can for short periods increase heat production about as much as maximum exercise.

Actual heat transfer depends on physical mechanisms of heat exchange: radiation, conduction, convection, and evaporation. *Radiation* of heat to cooler surroundings accounts for most loss of body heat. Exposure to radiant heat (eg, the sun, blast furnaces, or large engines) can increase body heat. *Conduction* by contact with a warmer or cooler object exchanges only small amounts of heat, except when the body is immersed in a liquid. Hypothermia is thought to contribute significantly to ocean drownings. Death by hyperthermia has been reported in residential hot tubs and whirlpool baths. *Convection* usually has little effect on heat loss or gain. A 2–4-mm boundary layer of still air surrounds the body. However, moving air (wind) can destroy this boundary layer and cause serious heat loss or gain. The wind-chill index, calculated from temperature and wind speed, is a way of communicating to the public the risk that exposed skin will freeze.

Evaporation of sweat from the skin or "insensible" water loss from the lungs can permit 20% of cooling at rest. When the ambient temperature is 35°C (95°F) or higher, most heat is shed by evaporation of sweat. High humidity greatly reduces the body's ability to cool itself by sweating. When the relative humidity approaches 90%, evaporation virtually stops. Sweat that does not evaporate hardly helps to dissipate heat.

COLD EXPOSURE SYNDROMES

The cold exposure syndromes are hypothermia and frostbite. *Hypothermia* is a generalized drop in body core temperature; *frostbite* is focal tissue freezing. The two phenomena can occur independently or be found in the same person.

Hypothermia

Mild hypothermia is arbitrarily defined as a core body temperature of 32–35°C (89.6–95°F), and severe hypothermia as a core temperature below 32°C. Changes with mild hypothermia result from the body's attempt to maintain a normal temperature. Below 32°C, however, the cold so severely impairs organ function that the body's protective mechanisms fail. The rate and duration of cooling affect the type and severity of derangements in a given patient. At highest risk is the patient who has been slowly cooled to a very low temperature, because that person's intravascular volume and energy stores are depleted. People can become hypothermic at surprisingly moderate temperatures if they are wet from immersion or rain. Alcohol and drug intoxication, stroke, extremes of age, and injury are common predisposing factors. (Especially after drinking heavily, some people develop severe hypoglycemia; the clinician should measure patients' glucose level.) Another potential cause of mild hypothermia is hypothyroidism. It should be excluded by measurements of the serum free T_4 and thyroid-stimulating hormone (TSH), particularly in elderly women, who have an especially high prevalence of thyroid dysfunction.

Diagnosis: In theory, hypothermia should be easy to recognize. All it takes is measuring the patient's rectal temperature with a low-reading mercury or electronic thermometer. However, hypothermia may not be the obvious diagnosis, because patients can present with a broad spectrum of symptoms ranging from confusion to cardiac arrest and apparent death.

Management: As core temperature falls, myocardial contractility, heart rate, and cardiac output decline faster than do the metabolic needs of the peripheral tissues. Respiratory rate also falls. Therefore, patients develop acidosis, often both respiratory and metabolic. This increases

myocardial irritability. Electrocardiographic (ECG) abnormalities include prolongation of PR and QT intervals and the QRS complex. The terminal vector of the QRS complex may be altered, producing the J or Osborn wave (Figure 15.3–1).

Because of patients' increased myocardial irritability, the tenets of initial care for hypothermia are to (1) avoid precipitating ventricular fibrillation; (2) prevent further cooling; (3) begin intravascular volume expansion with normal saline, adding thiamine because of the possibility of thiamine deficiency; (4) treat any hypoglycemia; and (5) gradually rewarm the patient (Table 15.3–1). The focus of treatment is the heart. The brain is relatively protected from cold—one of the reasons for using controlled hypothermia in cardiac surgery. Patients who have no spontaneous circulation are very difficult to warm. Because these patients have such a low threshold for ventricular instability and fibrillation, only essential invasive procedures should be undertaken during rewarming. In particular, a pulmonary artery or right atrial catheter should not be inserted, and the airway and the esophagus should not be manipulated unnecessarily.

Active rewarming should be started only after the hypothermic patient has been brought in from the cold. The only patients who should be quickly rewarmed are those who were quickly cooled (as from brief immersion in icy water) or are only mildly hypothermic (core temperature above 32°C [89.6°F]). Everyone else is at risk for peripheral vasodilation and resulting hypotension (rewarming shock) caused by the extremities being warmed before the core. However, some heat, in the form of warmed, humidified oxygen or trunk-only warming (warming blanket around the trunk) may be needed to prevent the patient from continuing to cool after rescue. Frostbitten extremi-

Table 15.3–1. Treatment of hypothermia.

Principle	Examples
Avoid manipulations that could trigger ventricular fibrillation	Do not catheterize the right atrium or pulmonary artery Do not unnecessarily manipulate the airway or esophagus Turn and move the patient as little as possible
Prevent further cooling	Keep the patient covered except during physical exams and essential tests such as ECGs Keep ambient temperature >22°C (71.6°F)
Slowly begin volume expansion and thiamine repletion	Give warmed 5% dextrose and normal saline, initially at 250–500 mL/hr, titrating to patient response Give thiamine, 100 mg IV
Treat hypoglycemia	Give 50–100 mL D50W IV bolus
Rewarm the patient	Use warm fluids and blankets for mild hypothermia Use active core rewarming for severe hypothermia Give warmed, humidified oxygen to all patients

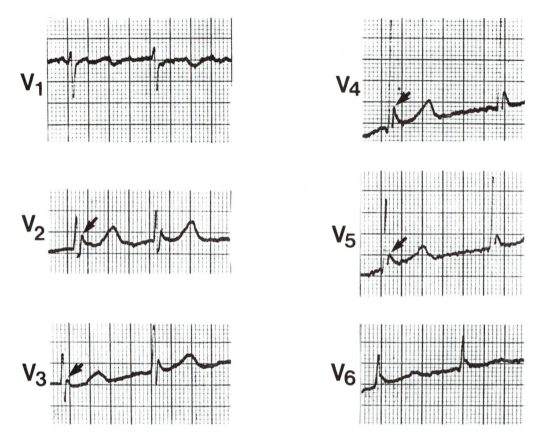

Figure 15.3–1. Hypothermia. This man was found unconscious in an unheated apartment in the wintertime. The ECG shows the characteristic Osborn ("J") waves (arrows) seen in hypothermia. The tracing also shows atrial fibrillation. (Courtesy of Abraham Genecin, MD.)

ties should not be rewarmed until the patient is brought in from the cold and hypothermia is treated. More tissue is lost from thawing and refreezing than from prolonged freezing alone.

Profoundly hypothermic patients may appear dead, but may recover completely. Cardiopulmonary resuscitation should be started in hypothermic patients who have ventricular fibrillation, asystole, or bradycardia without detectable cardiac output. If no cardiac output can be detected by a palpable carotid pulse or Doppler flow meter, chest compressions should be started, even at the risk of triggering ventricular fibrillation.

Other supportive care must be started quickly. Endotracheal intubation is indicated for patients who are not breathing or do not have a gag reflex. Ventilating with oxygen before intubation reverses hypoxemia and reduces the risk of ventricular fibrillation during intubation. An intravenous line should be started with 5% dextrose and normal saline, or with 5% dextrose and lactated Ringer's solution. Intravenous thiamine should be given because of the possibility of thiamine deficiency. If hypoglycemia is detected, 50 mL of 50% dextrose should be given intravenously. Naloxone should be given to confused or un-

conscious patients to reverse possible narcotic overdose. Other drugs should given with caution, especially to patients with a core temperature below 30°C (86°F); many drugs, such as antiarrhythmics, are typically ineffective in patients with a core temperature below 30°C. The primary treatment of ventricular tachycardia or fibrillation is not drugs but core rewarming plus cardioversion or defibrillation.

For mildly hypothermic patients (temperature above 32°C [89.6°F]), passive rewarming with blankets (allowing patients' own metabolic heat to warm them) and warm oral fluids may be adequate, and the physician should focus on finding associated illnesses or injuries. Profoundly hypothermic patients, however, will survive only with active rewarming: They should be given warmed (45°C [113°F]), humidified oxygen at a concentration of 50% or greater, and all intravenous fluids should be warmed to 45°C.

Emergency cardiopulmonary bypass through femoral arterial and venous cannulae is perhaps the method of choice for warming a patient who has profound hypothermia with poor perfusion or with an intractable cardiac arrhythmia impairing perfusion. A reasonable alternative to bypass is peritoneal dialysis with fluid heated to 45°C. Dual catheters exchange 4–6 L of fluid per hour. Dialysis also allows control of fluid balance and electrolytes.

Once started, cardiopulmonary resuscitation (CPR) must not be stopped too quickly. Cases have been reported in which patients with profound hypothermia and cardiac arrest had full neurologic recovery after more than 2 hours of CPR. These cases suggest that heroic efforts are justified in otherwise salvageable hypothermic patients.

Frostbite

Local tissue injury from cold exposure ranges from numbness with pain on warming (chilblain), to the freezing of an extremity, which when warmed develops gangrene and must be amputated (severe frostbite).

Hypothermic patients with frostbitten extremities should have their core rewarmed before the frostbitten extremities are allowed to thaw. After the core temperature is above 32–34°C (89.6–93.2°F), the frostbitten area should be warmed quickly in a water bath at 42–44°C (107.6–111.2°F). Pain is often severe, and patients may need intravenous narcotic analgesics. Vasospasm in a frostbitten extremity may persist and may require angiography, intra-arterial infusion of vasodilating drugs, and surgical sympathectomy.

HEAT EXPOSURE SYNDROMES

Preventing an abnormal elevation in body temperature depends on maintaining a balance between heat generation and dissipation. Clothing, ventilation, exercise, and water and salt repletion affect the heat load and the body's ability to regulate temperature. Everyone should avoid or limit heavy exercise in hot, humid weather. People should schedule routine water repletion before they get symptoms of heat illness. Thirst is an insensitive guide to water repletion. The very young, the very old, and persons with conditions such as cardiovascular disease are at special risk for illness from heat stress.

Heat Stroke

Heat stroke is a syndrome in which a rise in core temperature is high enough to damage cells throughout the body. The exact temperature threshold for cell damage is unknown and it differs in different people, but it is probably 42°C (107.6°F) or higher. The typical patient with heat stroke is known to have been exposed to heat and has or had both a high temperature and severe central nervous system dysfunction—delirium, coma, or seizures. The severity of the central nervous system dysfunction distinguishes heat stroke from heat exhaustion. Many patients with severe heat stroke suffer brain damage.

Heat stroke has two common presentations. One is seen most often in the very young, the elderly, and the debilitated. It tends to develop over several days during a heat wave in persons who cannot escape to cool places or drink adequate fluids. The other common presentation is exertional heat stroke. It tends to develop in healthy young persons who do heavy work or exercise in excessive heat and humidity. The onset is sudden, and dehydration is usually less severe than in patients with nonexertional heat stroke.

Simply stated, the pathophysiology of heat stroke is diffuse cellular metabolic derangement and cell death. Cell membranes tend to malfunction and release cellular enzymes into the serum. Rhabdomyolysis (dissolution of muscle) produces myoglobinuria, which can lead to acute renal failure. Coagulation times are often prolonged because of hepatic ischemia and decreased production of coagulation factors, and some patients develop disseminated intravascular coagulation. Despite an increase in cardiac output, patients may become hypotensive because of severe peripheral vasodilation and volume depletion. At core temperatures above 40°C (104°F), cardiac contractility decreases, and hypotension may result from reduced cardiac output, hypovolemia, or both.

Management: The primary treatment of heat stroke is immediate, rapid cooling (Table 15.3–2). Therapy focuses on restoring normal temperature to the brain, given the potential devastating injury and the limited ability to regenerate. Patients are undressed and sprayed with cool water while fans blow cool, dry air over them. This technique cools patients quickly and allows the staff easy access to the patients, their intravenous lines, and monitoring devices.

Supportive care is essential. Endotracheal intubation is advised for patients with inadequate ventilation or no gag reflex. All patients should receive oxygen, large-caliber intravenous access, and continuous monitoring of ECG, central venous pressure, blood pressure, and urine output with a Foley catheter. Fluid therapy must be carefully monitored to make sure that patients do not develop fluid overload, because if hypotension is primarily a result of decreased cardiac contractility, it may improve with cooling alone. Maintaining adequate urine output seems to decrease the risk of acute renal failure.

Active cooling should be stopped when core body temperature falls to 38–39°C (100.4–102.2°F). Even if pa-

Table 15.3–2. Treatment of hyperthermia.

Principle	Examples
Cool immediately and quickly	Spray cool water onto exposed patient while fans blow air over skin; this is preferable to cool water baths or a cooling blanket
Give supportive therapy	Give intravenous fluids Give supplemental oxygen Monitor ECG Monitor renal output with Foley catheter
Watch for recurrent hyperthermia	Admit to intensive care unit for continuous core temperature monitoring

tients are quickly cooled and their mental status improves, all patients with heat stroke require intensive monitoring for 2–3 days. The hyperthermia can recur 4–6 hours after cooling is stopped, and thermoregulatory mechanisms may be unstable for several weeks. Jaundice, rhabdomyolysis, and acute renal failure can be late sequelae. The severity and duration of hyperthermia govern the morbidity and mortality. Poor prognostic signs include coma for more than 10 hours, a markedly prolonged prothrombin time, and severely elevated serum liver enzymes.

Concurrent disease must be sought, especially in patients who remain comatose or whose temperature is refractory to efforts at cooling. Lumbar puncture may be needed to exclude meningitis and encephalitis. The physician should consider sepsis, head trauma, cerebrovascular accident, and severe thyrotoxicosis.

Heat Exhaustion

Heat exhaustion is a syndrome characterized by progressive dehydration over days, resulting from moderate heat exposure and inadequate fluid replacement. Most patients present with nonspecific complaints that have developed over several days. Typical symptoms are headache, irritability, anorexia, malaise, thirst, and muscle cramps. Many patients have tachycardia and tachypnea; some have orthostatic hypotension and syncope. Patients have some degree of dehydration. Impairment of central nervous system function is minimal and nonspecific. Body core temperature is usually normal or no higher than 38°C (100.4°F).

Diagnosis of heat exhaustion relies on a history of heat exposure, typical symptoms, and no concomitant disease. Treatment is rest in a cool place, and rehydration with oral or intravenous sodium chloride solution. Dehydration is indicated by an elevated blood urea nitrogen, an elevated hematocrit, or orthostatic hypotension. Young, healthy patients with serious dehydration may require 4 L or more of fluid over 6–8 hours. Older patients need slower rehydration to prevent fluid overload, and they should probably be hospitalized.

Heat Cramps

Heat cramps develop in large, heavily used muscle groups such as the calves, typically after several days of heat exposure. Although the cause is not well defined, inadequate water intake and salt depletion are most often implicated. Large amounts of water and small amounts of salt supplements are effective prophylaxis for persons at risk, for example, steel mill workers and football players. Cramps are relieved by passive stretching and by hydration with oral or intravenous sodium chloride solution.

SUMMARY

▶ Core temperature is an important and frequently overlooked vital sign in hemodynamically unstable, critically ill patients.

▶ Hypothermia protects the central nervous system, but lowers cardiac output and increases risk for ventricular fibrillation.

▶ Since profoundly hypothermic patients can recover fully after prolonged cardiopulmonary resuscitation, patients should be vigorously resuscitated.

▶ Heat stroke can cause irreversible brain injury. Treatment is immediate, rapid cooling.

▶ In patients with hypothermia or hyperthermia, the physician should seek conditions like infection and central nervous system disease that might impair the body's ability to respond to environmental exposures.

SUGGESTED READING

Auerbach PS: *Wilderness Medicine: Management of Wilderness and Environmental Emergencies,* 3rd ed. CV Mosby, 1995.

Schaller MD, Fischer AP, Perret CH: Hyperkalemia: A prognostic factor during acute severe hypothermia. JAMA 1990;264:1842.

Sterba JA: Efficacy and safety of prehospital rewarming techniques to treat accidental hypothermia. Ann Emerg Med 1991;20:896.

Shock and Multiple Organ Dysfunction Syndrome

Roy G. Brower, MD, and Henry E. Fessler, MD

Shock is the acute syndrome of organ and system dysfunction precipitated by failure of the circulation to meet the needs of metabolically active tissues. It develops within minutes or hours of an initial insult such as a severe hemorrhage. If not promptly reversed, shock progresses quickly to death. Multiple organ dysfunction syndrome (MODS) is also a syndrome of organ and system dysfunction that occurs during severe illness, but it runs a course over days to weeks rather than hours, with mechanisms that need not be directly related to circulatory failure. For example, in some patients a single process such as sepsis affects the kidney, gut, and central nervous system, leading to acute renal dysfunction, gastrointestinal bleeding, and stupor, respectively. In other patients, dysfunction of various organs and systems occurs through a progressive series of interrelated processes.

The primary purpose of this chapter is to explain a rational approach to assessing patients in shock, who represent some of our most challenging clinical problems and in whom good management can make the difference between spectacular recovery and death. The physiology of systemic blood flow is reviewed to help recognize and manage shock caused by various conditions. A secondary purpose of this chapter is to explain how multiple organ dysfunction syndrome may occur and to develop a systematic approach to managing our sickest and most complex patients.

SHOCK

An insult such as hemorrhage usually triggers compensatory autonomic cardiovascular responses including tachycardia and vasoconstriction. If these responses are adequate, organ and system function are preserved and survival requires little or no treatment. However, if the insult is severe, patients develop signs of organ and system dysfunction such as hypotension, delirium, and oliguria. These signs represent the onset of shock. Prompt intervention may be life-saving, with full recovery of organ and system function within hours or days. If treatment is inadequate, still more serious manifestations evolve, such as stupor, anuria, and cardiac and circulatory collapse.

The constellation of signs, symptoms, and laboratory abnormalities that are recognized as shock is caused by inadequate oxygen delivery via the systemic circulation to metabolically active tissues. Low blood oxygen content from anemia or hypoxemia may also contribute to poor oxygen delivery. A useful way of classifying the many potential causes of shock is to group them according to the primary circulatory problem (Table 15.4–1). According to this classification, shock is caused either by low blood flow or by poorly regulated distribution of blood flow.

Determinants of Blood Flow to Systemic Tissues

Cardiac Function: The cardiac stroke volume and therefore cardiac output are proportional to the volume of blood that fills the ventricular chambers during the preceding diastole. Since this volume correlates with atrial pressure, cardiac function may be represented by the relationship of cardiac output to atrial pressure (Figure 15.4–1A). Normally, the slope of this relationship is steep. With myocardial or valvular disease or arrhythmia, the slope is depressed.

Venous Return: The heart can pump only as much blood as it receives from the systemic circulation (ie, venous return). The characteristics of the systemic circulation that affect venous return rate are represented in the relationship of systemic venous flow to right atrial pressure, which is the pressure at the downstream end of the systemic circulation (see Figure 15.4–1B). Venous return decreases when right atrial pressure is raised because the

Table 15.4–1. Functional classification of causes of shock.

Inadequate blood flow
    Reduced blood volume (see Table 15.4–2)
        Hemorrhage
        Dehydration
        Burns
    Impaired cardiac (pump) function
        Myocardial infarction
        Acute valvular dysfunction
        Arrhythmias
    Obstruction to blood flow
        Cardiac tamponade
        Tension pneumothorax
        Pulmonary embolism

Poor distribution of cardiac output
    Sepsis
    Anaphylaxis
    Fulminant hepatic failure

pressure gradient from the systemic circulation to the right heart falls. The horizontal axis-intercept (the level of right atrial pressure when venous return is zero) is the average or mean systemic pressure. This represents the upstream pressure driving venous return and is determined by the capacitance of the systemic blood vessels and the volume of blood they contain. In a normal relaxed person, mean systemic pressure is about 7 mm Hg. The slope of the venous return-right atrial pressure relationship is inversely related to the resistance to venous flow.

Coupling of Cardiac and Venous Function: Cardiac output and venous return must be equal. If cardiac output briefly exceeds venous return, blood volume and vascular pressures in the pulmonary circulation fall, whereas blood volume and systemic vascular pressures rise. Systemic venous return then rises, whereas pulmonary venous return decreases. Within moments, cardiac output and venous return become equal again. This coupling of cardiac output and venous return can be represented graphically by combining the cardiac and venous function relationships on the same axes (see Figure 15.4–1C). The one point in common between the two relationships indicates the cardiac output-venous return and right atrial pressure in a patient whose cardiac and vascular functions were represented in Figure 15.4–1A and B.

Specific Shock Conditions

Hypovolemic Shock: Severe loss of fluid from the intravascular space may be caused by loss of blood or plasma to the environment or by sequestration into an extravascular space (Table 15.4–2). Loss of vascular volume decreases mean systemic pressure and therefore decreases the pressure gradient for venous return (Figure 15.4–2). Cardiac output and right atrial pressure are low because venous return is low.

Patients in hypovolemic shock present with arterial hypotension and low systemic venous pressures. Tachycardia and tachypnea are common, as they are in all patients

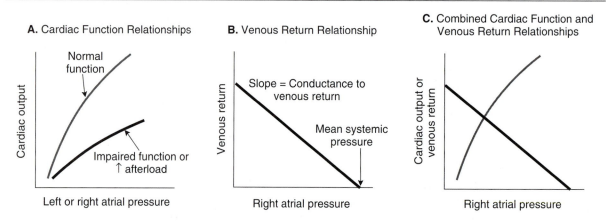

Figure 15.4–1. A: Cardiac function relationships represented as cardiac output versus atrial pressure. Atrial pressure is a convenient way to estimate preload, or ventricular end-diastolic volume. The cardiac function relationship is steep when cardiac function is normal. The relationship is depressed when cardiac function is impaired or ventricular afterload is increased. **B:** Venous return relationships. Venous return is the flow of blood back from the systemic circulation to the right heart. The horizontal axis intercept represents mean systemic pressure, which is determined by the volume of blood in the circulation and the compliance of the systemic vessels. Venous return decreases as right atrial pressure rises because the pressure gradient for venous return (mean systemic pressure – right atrial pressure) falls. The slope of the venous return relationship represents the conductance (reciprocal of resistance) to venous return, representing primarily conducting properties of venules and veins. **C:** Combined cardiac function and venous return relationships. Cardiac output and venous return must be equal. Therefore, both can be shown on the same axis. The intersection of the two relationships indicates the level of cardiac output/venous return that would occur in an individual with the cardiac function and venous function represented in panels A and B.

Table 15.4–2. Causes of hypovolemic shock.

Blood loss
  Trauma
    External bleeding
    Internal sequestration (hematoma, hemoperitoneum,
      hemothorax)
  Gastrointestinal bleeding
    Peptic ulcer, diffuse gastritis
    Diverticular bleeding

Plasma loss
  External loss
    Diarrhea (gastroenteritis, cholera)
    Dehydration (exposure, heat prostration)
    Burns
    Diabetes mellitus
    Diabetes insipidus
  Third spacing
    Severe pancreatitis
    Severe ileus, megacolon

with shock conditions. Alterations in body temperature are uncommon and suggest other processes such as infection or exposure. The pulse is characteristically weak. Reflex cutaneous vasoconstriction causes pallor and cool skin; turgor is decreased. The jugular veins are typically difficult to identify because central venous pressure, like right atrial pressure, is low. The cardiac sounds may be soft; gallop rhythms are not audible. Other physical findings and routine laboratory data may indicate the cause of hypovolemia. For example, melanotic or bloody stools and anemia suggest internal bleeding from peptic ulcer disease.

Much of our knowledge about the natural history of hypovolemic shock comes from experimental work in animals. Within minutes after bleeding, intense sympathoadrenal discharge causes peripheral vasoconstriction. This salutary response decreases systemic vascular capacitance and thus partially restores mean systemic pressure and therefore venous return. It also redistributes cardiac output to essential organs such as the heart and brain. Activation of the renin-angiotensin-aldosterone system further increases vascular tone and causes renal retention of fluid and electrolytes. Increased circulating levels of antidiuretic hormone and reduced atrial natriuretic factor contribute to the maintenance of intravascular volume.

If compensatory mechanisms are inadequate, shock develops. During the early phase of hypovolemic shock, cardiac output and arterial pressure can be returned to normal by administration of fluids. In experiments on dogs, this phase lasted about 90 minutes when more than 40% of the normal blood volume was rapidly removed. If the animals were not resuscitated with fluid within this time, shock became irreversible.

At the cellular level, the endoplasmic reticulum and mitochondria in various tissues swell, and cellular metabolic functions deteriorate. Adenosine triphosphate (ATP) production within the cell occurs predominantly by anaerobic glycolysis, resulting in progressive lactic acidosis. In the peripheral circulation, loss of spontaneous smooth muscle

tone and responsiveness to catecholamines aggravates hypotension, and venous return-cardiac output decreases. Increased vascular permeability causes further loss of intravascular fluid to the interstitial spaces. Myocardial contractility is depressed by ischemia, acidosis, and circulating myocardial depressant factors. Renal blood flow redistributes from the cortex to the medulla; tubular necrosis results in renal failure. The liver loses its ability to manufacture albumin and metabolize lactate and other metabolic substrates. Cerebral function deteriorates, resulting in stupor or coma. Pulmonary vascular permeability may increase, causing acute respiratory distress syndrome (ARDS; Chapter 2.7).

Regardless of the cause of hypovolemic shock, the mainstay of management is rapid restoration of vascular volume. Isotonic crystalloid fluids (normal saline or lactated Ringer's solution) should be used when hypovolemic shock occurs without anemia or hemorrhage. These fluids are also very useful for patients in hemorrhagic shock—whether or not blood products are used—but especially if blood is not immediately available. Fluids should be administered rapidly until blood pressure, pulse, urine output, and other clinical indicators of systemic perfusion approach normal. To ensure oxygen carrying capacity, packed red blood cells should be transfused when blood hemoglobin concentration is less than 10 g/100 mL or when bleeding is brisk.

Cardiogenic Shock: The ability of the heart to generate flow may be severely impaired by myocardial disease, valve disease, or arrhythmia (Table 15.4–3). Decreased

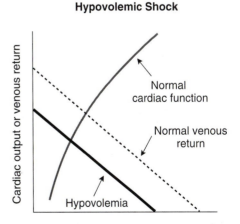

Hypovolemic Shock

Cardiac output or venous return / Right atrial pressure

Normal cardiac function
Normal venous return
Hypovolemia

Figure 15.4–2. Hypovolemic shock. The venous return relationship is shifted to the left because decreased vascular volume leads to decreased mean systemic pressure (horizontal axis intercept). The cardiac function relationship is normal. The intersection of the cardiac function and venous return relationships shifts to a lower level of cardiac output/venous return and atrial pressure.

Table 15.4–3. Causes of cardiogenic shock.

Weakening of cardiac muscle
   Myocardial infarction
   Myocarditis
Valvular dysfunction
   Acute aortic insufficiency
   Acute mitral regurgitation (rupture of papillary muscle or
     chordae)
Arrhythmias
   Tachyarrhythmias: ventricular tachycardia
   Bradyarrhythmias: nodal bradycardia
Tamponade
   Pericarditis
   Malignancy
   Cardiac rupture

systemic blood flow caused by heart disease is represented in Figure 15.4–3, where the slope of the cardiac function relationship is depressed. The venous return relationship is normal, unless there are compensatory responses by the circulation or changes in systemic vascular volume. Venous return is low because elevated right atrial pressure decreases the pressure gradient for venous return.

Patients in cardiogenic shock present with arterial hypotension and high right atrial pressure. The skin may be ashen or cyanotic, and cool from peripheral vasoconstriction. The pulse is weak. The jugular venous pressure is increased and cardiac gallop rhythms are common. Mitral or aortic murmurs may be audible; this is especially important for diagnosis and management if they are new or louder than on previous examinations. Marked dyspnea

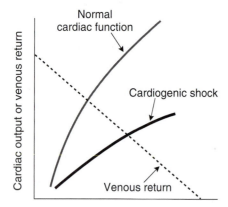

Cardiogenic Shock

Figure 15.4–3. Cardiogenic shock. The cardiac function relationship is depressed and intersects the venous return relationship at a lower level of cardiac output/venous return and higher level of atrial pressure. The same changes occur in pulmonary embolism because the right heart is unable to sustain its output with the high afterload.

occurs because high left atrial pressure causes pulmonary engorgement and edema. Auscultation of the lungs typically reveals crackles that may extend to the midthorax or even the apices. Patients may have peripheral edema if they had heart failure before shock. The chest x-ray shows pulmonary vascular congestion and edema. Cardiomegaly may not be present if the cardiac injury occurred acutely. The electrocardiogram may indicate ischemia, infarction, or arrhythmia.

Medical management of cardiogenic shock is difficult because measures to increase oxygen delivery frequently fail or have serious adverse effects. An arterial vasodilator such as nitroprusside promotes higher cardiac output, but the drug may also decrease aortic pressure and therefore coronary flow, worsening myocardial ischemia. Intravenous fluids elevate mean systemic pressure and promote venous return-cardiac output, but may also raise left atrial pressure and exacerbate pulmonary edema. Conversely, diuresis may decrease left atrial pressure and relieve pulmonary edema, but at the expense of decreasing mean systemic pressure, resulting in lower venous return and therefore cardiac output. An inotropic drug such as dobutamine may enhance myocardial function, but this may increase myocardial oxygen requirements and worsen ischemic injury or cause arrhythmias.

In patients with acute myocardial infarction, thrombolysis with streptokinase, urokinase, or tissue plasminogen activator may allow recovery of sufficient cardiac function to reverse shock (Chapter 1.3). Under some circumstances, emergency angioplasty or coronary artery bypass grafting may be life-saving. When the cause of cardiogenic shock is potentially reversible, as with angioplasty or bypass surgery, temporary improvement in cardiac output may be obtained with an intra-aortic balloon pump. When cardiogenic shock is caused by acute mitral or aortic regurgitation, a systemic vasodilator may promote forward flow and improve oxygen delivery while preparations are made for valve replacement. Shock caused by cardiac tachyarrhythmia requires immediate cardioversion.

Septic Shock:
Pathogenesis: Severe infections such as pneumonia, peritonitis, and pyelonephritis may cause septic shock. Most episodes are related to infections with gram-negative bacteria, but gram-positive organisms are increasingly implicated, as are fungi. Patients with impaired immunity, such as those with severe renal failure, alcoholism, and AIDS, are at increased risk. Despite the availability of potent antibiotics, septic shock is an increasingly common problem. About 200,000 cases occur in the United States each year, with an in-hospital mortality rate of about 50%.

In severe infections, microbial pathogens trigger a cascade of events that involve exogenous (endo- and exotoxins) and endogenous mediators (tumor necrosis factor, interleukins, platelet activating factor, leukotrienes, prostanoids), cellular elements in the blood, and vascular endothelium and smooth muscle. Diffuse vascular inflammation, intravascular coagulation, and decreased vascular smooth muscle tone lead to loss of regulation of cardiac output and its distribution.

Two phases of septic shock may be recognized. In the early phase, patients develop hypotension, tachycardia, tachypnea, and hyper- or hypothermia, with low or normal systemic venous pressure and normal or elevated cardiac output. Loss of systemic vascular tone causes hypotension (low afterload), which allows the heart to generate higher cardiac output at any level of right atrial pressure. Stress-induced endogenous catecholamines contribute further to the heart's ability to generate higher cardiac output. Vascular volume may be expanded by early infusion of intravenous fluids, raising mean systemic pressure, and increasing venous return-cardiac output (Figure 15.4–4).

During the early phase of septic shock, cardiac output is normal or high, but there are clear signs that blood flow and oxygen delivery to various organs and systems are inadequate. Besides being hypotensive, tachycardic, and tachypneic, patients are frequently oliguric and delirious or obtunded. Increased serum lactate and decreased bicarbonate concentrations indicate oxygen deprivation of metabolically active tissues. These changes imply maldistribution of flow. Vasodilatation in some vascular beds such as the skin causes high flow. In other vascular beds, there is little vasodilatation or even compensatory vaso-

constriction. Blood flow to these regions decreases. Intravascular coagulation and aggregation of platelets, polymorphonuclear leukocytes, and injured endothelial cells prevent oxygen delivery to some portions of vascular beds that may be otherwise well perfused. Vascular inflammation causes increased vascular permeability. The resulting interstitial edema impedes oxygen diffusion from capillaries to cells.

The early phase generally lasts several hours to a few days. If treatment is inadequate, cardiac output decreases despite normal or even high cardiac filling pressure. Cardiac function is depressed by circulating myocardial depressant factors, myocardial edema, ischemia, and acidosis. Sepsis-induced vasorelaxation and increased vascular permeability may lead to low mean systemic pressure and therefore low venous return. Oliguria may progress to anuria due to acute tubular necrosis. Hepatic dysfunction results in cholestasis and reduced synthesis of proteins such as albumin and clotting factors. The bowel's ability to retain enteric bacteria and their byproducts in the gut lumen may be impaired, resulting in bacteremia and further episodes of sepsis. Increased pulmonary vascular permeability to water and protein leads to ARDS. Release of vaso- and bronchoactive mediators causes maldistribution of pulmonary blood flow and ventilation, contributing to hypoxemia.

Treatment: Management of patients with septic shock involves several simultaneous measures. Isotonic fluids (normal saline or lactated Ringer's solution) should be given generously to achieve, if possible, normal or moderately increased venous return. Infusions of packed red blood cells are recommended if anemia is present. Because of the risk of precipitating pulmonary edema, intravenous fluids should be withheld when left atrial filling pressure exceeds 15–18 mm Hg. In many patients, hypotension persists despite adequate vascular filling and normal or even high cardiac output. To avoid coronary and cerebral ischemia, a vasopressor may be used to maintain systolic arterial pressure above 90 mm Hg or mean arterial pressure above 60 mm Hg. This is intended to promote myocardial and cerebral blood flow, but may worsen perfusion in other vascular beds or cause cardiac arrhythmias.

The source of infection must be identified as quickly as possible. Some sites of infection are likely to harbor gram-negative bacteria (pyelonephritis, peritonitis, cholangitis), whereas others are likely sites of gram-positive pathogens (wounds, cardiac valves, infected vascular catheters). The search for the source begins with a directed history, physical examination, and routine laboratory data. Cultures of blood and secretions from all suspected sites of infection (urine, sputum, cerebrospinal fluid, ascites, and pleural fluid) should be obtained and antibiotics begun quickly while results are pending. Antibiotics should be chosen to ensure broad-spectrum activity when the pathogen is unknown, or synergistic activity when a specific pathogen is known or suspected. Some infections require drainage (eg empyema, abscess) or surgical débridement.

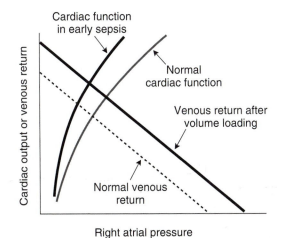

Early Septic Shock

Cardiac function in early sepsis

Normal cardiac function

Venous return after volume loading

Normal venous return

Cardiac output or venous return

Right atrial pressure

Figure 15.4–4. Early septic shock. The cardiac function relationship is steeper than normal because left ventricular afterload is lower (hypotension) and because endogenous or exogenous catecholamines stimulate increased myocardial contractility. The venous return relationship is shifted upward because of catecholamine-induced systemic vasoconstriction and iatrogenic volume expansion.

Monoclonal antibodies directed against lipid A, a component of endotoxin common among species of gram-negative bacteria, have not fulfilled early hopes that they would improve survival in patients with sepsis. Other drugs under study include interleukin receptor antagonists and anti-tumor necrosis factor antibodies. Like the anti-lipid A antibodies, these drugs are designed to interrupt the cascade of biochemical events that leads to sepsis and shock. Data are currently insufficient to show which patients benefit from these expensive new drugs.

Pulmonary Embolism (Chapter 2.8):

Pathogenesis: Embolism acutely increases pulmonary vascular resistance from mechanical obstruction of vessels and release of pulmonary vasoconstrictors. This leads to increased pressure and volume in the right heart. As right atrial pressure rises, the pressure gradient for venous return falls (see Figure 15.4–3). As in cardiogenic shock, the cardiac function relationship is depressed and intersects the venous return relationship at a lower flow and higher right atrial pressure. Hypoxemia from ventilation-perfusion mismatch and shunt contributes to poor oxygen delivery.

Clinical evaluation: Pulmonary embolism should be suspected when sudden onset of shock is associated with pleuritic chest pain and hypoxemia, especially in sedentary or postsurgical patients or in a patient with a history of venous thrombosis. Like cardiogenic shock, the clinical presentation is characterized by arterial hypotension with high central venous pressure. Tachypnea and dyspnea are marked and may be accompanied by cyanosis. The jugular veins are usually prominent. Other signs on the physical and routine laboratory examinations are subtle and variable. A loud second heart sound may be heard over the right upper sternal border, along with a right ventricular heave and gallop. There may be wheezing or coarse airway sounds from bronchoactive mediator release. Crackles may not be present initially but may develop in the first 1 or 2 days. About 50% of patients have changes in the extremities suggesting deep venous thrombosis.

The chest x-ray is often normal but may show central pulmonary vascular prominence, hyperlucency in a region deprived of flow (oligemia), regional volume loss, or a pleural-based infiltrate or effusion. The electrocardiogram usually shows nonspecific changes but may show right axis deviation and right ventricular strain. Arterial blood gas measurement usually shows hypoxemia and hypocapnia. Echocardiography may show right ventricular overload and dilatation. The suspicion of pulmonary embolism may be supported or confirmed with a perfusion scan or pulmonary angiogram, but these tests are difficult to perform when a patient is in shock.

Treatment: Management is often initiated on the basis of clinical suspicion alone. Rapid infusions of intravenous fluids increase mean systemic pressure, restoring the pressure gradient for venous return. Supplemental oxygen usually alleviates hypoxemia. Anticoagulants are given to prevent further embolism. If a large pulmonary embolus can be confirmed by perfusion scan or angiogram, thrombolytic agents such as streptokinase may be given to promote rapid dissolution of the clot and return of hemodynamic stability.

Tension Pneumothorax: Tension pneumothorax develops when a puncture in the visceral pleura functions as a valve, allowing air to be drawn into the pleural space in inspiration (or forced into it in a patient on a ventilator), but preventing it from escaping during expiration. Typical circumstances are patients who have sustained chest trauma or who have pulmonary blebs and are being mechanically ventilated; sometimes tension pneumothorax develops after inadvertent puncture with a needle, for example, while placing a central line. The resulting rise in pleural pressure compresses the heart and great veins. As right atrial pressure rises, the pressure gradient for venous return decreases. Narrowing of the venae cavae may increase the resistance to venous return, further decreasing cardiac output. Hypoxemia due to pulmonary shunt through the affected lung contributes to poor oxygen delivery.

Tension pneumothorax usually develops precipitously and causes arterial hypotension with high systemic venous pressure. Marked agitation and cyanosis are common. The affected hemithorax is hyperresonant to percussion and breath sounds are decreased. Jugular veins are distended, but the heart sounds are muffled. The trachea may be deviated to the contralateral hemithorax.

Management of tension pneumothorax must be directed toward restoring the pressure gradient for venous return. Rapid intravenous infusions of isotonic fluids help by raising mean systemic pressure. Air in the chest should be evacuated quickly, either through a chest tube or, in extreme emergencies, simply by inserting a large-bore needle between two ribs.

Cardiac Tamponade (Chapter 1.10): If fluid accumulates rapidly or in large amounts in the pericardial sac, as in pericarditis, pericardial pressure rises and compresses the heart, raising right atrial pressure. Hence, tamponade, like tension pneumothorax and pulmonary embolism, causes low venous return-cardiac output with high venous pressures. Tamponade should be suspected in a patient with shock with pulsus paradoxus (>10 mm Hg fall in systemic arterial pressure with inspiration), high jugular venous pressure with a systolic descent, and quiet heart sounds. The chest x-ray usually shows a very large cardiac silhouette, but may be normal if pericardial fluid has accumulated rapidly. The ECG may show low voltage.

As in tension pneumothorax, management of shock caused by cardiac tamponade entails restoring the pressure gradient for venous return. Isotonic fluids should be infused to increase mean systemic pressure. Right atrial pressure should be lowered by removing pericardial fluid by pericardiocentesis or a surgically created pericardial window into the pleural space.

General Approach to the Patient in Shock

Shock is an emergency. The patient in shock should be managed in a critical care unit that allows substantial commitment of time to the individual patient and provides specialized equipment for continuous monitoring and support of severe cardiovascular and respiratory disease. Expeditious assessment and treatment may make the difference between survival and death.

In many patients, a condition such as pneumonia or hemorrhage is obvious, as is the hemodynamic consequence leading to poor oxygen delivery. In others, the initial cause is less clear, and a cursory assessment may be misleading. In all patients, it is paramount to identify the pathophysiologic cause of deficient oxygen delivery. Fever and warm extremities suggest high cardiac output in sepsis. Cool extremities and thready peripheral pulses suggest low cardiac output. Look for dry mucous membranes, decreased skin turgor, soft heart sounds, flat jugular veins, low urine output, high urine specific gravity, and elevated blood urea nitrogen (BUN). If several of these are present, hypovolemia is likely.

Relative hypovolemia can also be caused by sepsis, when systemic vasodilatation causes increased vascular capacitance. In these situations, patients usually benefit from intravenous fluids. In contrast, edema of the extremities, hips, or flanks, a cardiac gallop, distended jugular veins, and basilar crackles suggest hypervolemia, and therapy is entirely different.

Assessment of central venous pressure is especially useful, either by examination of the jugular veins or by direct measurement with a central venous catheter. Low central venous pressure strongly suggests hypovolemia and warrants administration of intravenous fluids to increase venous return-cardiac output. In contrast, high central venous pressure occurs most frequently in patients with cardiac disease, in whom fluid administration is seldom beneficial. However, if other observations indicate pulmonary embolism, cardiac tamponade, or tension pneumothorax, rapid infusions of intravenous fluids may improve the hemodynamic condition and allow other lifesaving treatments.

The examination and laboratory data are frequently complicated by concurrent disease. For example, a patient with cirrhosis and gastrointestinal bleeding may have several signs of hypovolemia but also have edema and ascites, which suggest hypervolemia. The latter two findings may be from severe hypoalbuminemia and portal hypertension. A patient with pulmonary embolism may have rales, distended jugular veins, and a third heart sound, suggesting volume overload. Oliguria and high urine specific gravity may suggest hypovolemia, but are more likely secondary to low cardiac output. Because of ambiguities such as these, weigh all available information, decide which observations are most reliable or misleading, and only then formulate an assessment of the hemodynamics.

Based on the initial examination, measures to improve oxygen delivery should be started within minutes. These may include intravenous fluids (including blood products if hematocrit is less than 30% or hemoglobin is less than 10 g/100 mL), vasopressors, supplemental oxygen, and ventilatory support, when necessary. Specific measures such as antibiotics for sepsis or pericardiocentesis for tamponade should be initiated within the first hour.

Frequently, the physical examination, laboratory data, and hospital course remain ambiguous, and the cause of shock is still uncertain. Shock may be complicated by respiratory or renal failure or concurrent heart disease in patients with presumed noncardiogenic shock. In patients such as these, a flow-directed Swan-Ganz catheter may be passed from a central vein through the right heart until it wedges in a branch of the pulmonary artery. The "wedge pressure" so obtained approximates left atrial pressure. The Swan-Ganz catheter also allows periodic measurements of cardiac output by the thermodilution technique. Combined assessments of wedge pressure and cardiac output allow more precise titration of intravenous fluids, diuretics, vasopressors, and inotropic agents to promote adequate cardiac output and avoid fluid overload.

It is essential to evaluate responses to treatment frequently until the physiologic indications of inadequate oxygen delivery return to normal. Vital signs should be measured hourly if not continuously using hemodynamic monitoring equipment. Pertinent aspects of the physical examination and laboratory data should be repeated frequently during the first day to ensure that treatments have desired effects, to avoid complications of treatment, and to recognize concurrent disease at the earliest possible time.

MULTIPLE ORGAN DYSFUNCTION SYNDROME (MODS)

Therapeutic and technologic advances allow many patients to be stabilized who previously would have quickly succumbed to severe illnesses such as multilobar pneumonia or hemorrhagic shock. However, days to weeks after initial improvement, some patients develop unanticipated dysfunction of one or more organs or systems. MODS (sometimes called multisystems organ failure or multiple organs and systems failure) may manifest in various forms, predominantly in some patients as respiratory and cardiovascular failure and in others as deteriorating renal, neurologic, or hepatic function. In some patients, a disease initially confined to one organ or system may directly or indirectly cause failure in other systems. For example, mediators released during sepsis from peritonitis may cause ARDS and acute renal failure, or liver failure from acute viral hepatitis may lead to circulatory collapse and coma. In other patients, failure of various organs may be initiated by unrelated, sequential, or iatrogenic processes, such as progression of a presenting illness, nosocomial infections, drug-induced renal failure or thrombocytopenia, or even internal bleeding from an arterial puncture. An example of how MODS may evolve in one patient is shown in Figure 15.4–5.

Multiple Organ Dysfunction Syndrome
Sample Case

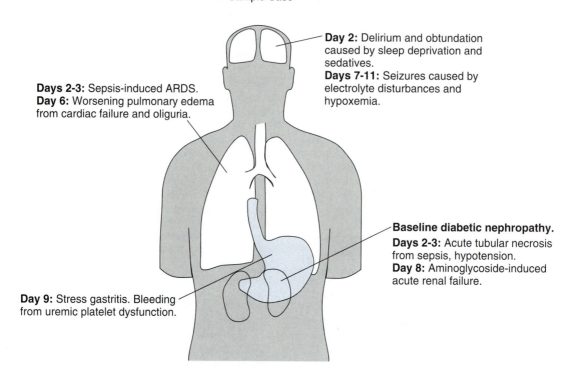

Day 2: Delirium and obtundation caused by sleep deprivation and sedatives.
Days 7-11: Seizures caused by electrolyte disturbances and hypoxemia.

Days 2-3: Sepsis-induced ARDS.
Day 6: Worsening pulmonary edema from cardiac failure and oliguria.

Baseline diabetic nephropathy.
Days 2-3: Acute tubular necrosis from sepsis, hypotension.
Day 8: Aminoglycoside-induced acute renal failure.

Day 9: Stress gastritis. Bleeding from uremic platelet dysfunction.

Figure 15.4–5. Multiple organ dysfunction syndrome case presentation. A 55-year-old man with a history of diabetes, chronic renal failure (baseline creatinine = 1.9 mg/dL), and coronary artery disease experiences septic shock from cellulitis of the left leg. He receives intravenous fluids and antibiotics, and shock resolves after 24–48 hours. However, ARDS, renal failure, obtundation and seizures, and gastrointestinal bleeding complicate his hospital course.

Pathogenesis and Clinical Manifestations

Lung Involvement: Usually an early manifestation of patients with MODS, lung involvement occurs within 72 hours of the onset of a severe illness such as sepsis. Sepsis, major trauma, and pancreatitis can cause complement activation, neutrophil and platelet margination and activation in the pulmonary vasculature, and release of endogenous mediators, lysosomal enzymes, and oxygen free radicals injure the pulmonary endothelium and increase vascular permeability to protein and fluid. Nosocomial pneumonia, aspiration pneumonitis, atelectasis, and pulmonary embolism may contribute to respiratory dysfunction. Administration of unavoidably high concentrations of inspired oxygen causes pulmonary oxygen toxicity. Some patients on mechanical ventilators experience pulmonary barotrauma. Hypoxemia contributes to oxygen deprivation and dysfunction in other tissues.

Renal Dysfunction: Also common in MODS patients, renal dysfunction has several causes. Hypotension from hemorrhage or cardiogenic shock causes decreased renal blood flow and glomerular filtration rate. Acute tubular or cortical necrosis may follow prolonged hypotensive episodes. Vasopressors used to treat hypotension frequently cause renovascular vasoconstriction, leading to ischemia and acute tubular necrosis. Aminoglycosides and other antibiotics are frequently nephrotoxic, especially in patients with episodes of hypotension, sepsis, or in whom vasopressors are used. As in the lung, sepsis-induced activation of complement, neutrophils, and platelets may cause inflammation in the renal circulation.

Regardless of the cause, renal failure presents several daunting problems that affect other organs and systems. Oliguria may cause vascular volume overload, especially in patients receiving many parenterally administered medications and nutrition. Uremia-induced immune dysfunction predisposes to nosocomial infections, and platelet dysfunction predisposes to bleeding complications. Electrolyte disorders may impair cardiovascular and neurologic function.

Myocardial Factors: Circulating myocardial depressant factors have been identified in some patients with severe illnesses such as sepsis, severe pancreatitis, and trauma. Hypotension may cause myocardial ischemia or infarction, and electrolyte abnormalities may cause life-threatening arrhythmias. Impaired cardiac output contributes to poor oxygen delivery and failure in other systems.

Neurologic Dysfunction: Neurologic dysfunction is common in critically ill patients. Delirium or obtundation are frequently attributable to sleep deprivation and the effects of failure of other organ systems, such as hypoglycemia from liver failure and inadequate cerebral perfusion from cardiac failure. Many drugs contribute to altered sensorium. Seizures may be caused by severe electrolyte disturbances, hypoxemia, and inadequate cerebral perfusion. Cerebral hemorrhage may occur in patients with coagulopathy.

Gastrointestinal Disorders: Patients with gut dysfunction may present with paralytic ileus, which prevents continued enteral nutrition. Parenteral nutrition may be used, but complications of this approach include sepsis from infected catheters and fluid and electrolyte disorders. Disuse of the bowel and hypotension or vasopressor-induced mesenteric ischemia may impair the intestinal mucosal barrier, allowing bacteria or their toxic products to enter the bloodstream, causing repeated episodes of sepsis. Stress-induced gastritis and peptic ulcer disease cause internal blood loss.

Liver Failure: Hepatic failure is a late but ominous manifestation of MODS. Impaired hepatic synthetic ability leads to hypoalbuminemia, which promotes edema formation. Hypoprothrombinemia may cause hemorrhage. Impaired hepatic clearance can contribute to lactic acidosis or accumulation of hepatically metabolized drugs.

General Approach to the Patient with MODS

A patient with MODS may sometimes be described as a "train wreck" because everything seems to be broken. It is difficult to know what problems are important, what needs immediate attention, and how to begin to put the cars back on the track.

Systems Evaluation: Successful care of complex critically ill patients begins with frequent evaluations of each of the systems and the relations among systems. Physicians and nurses must balance the overall potential benefits and risks of treatments, avoiding unnecessarily toxic therapy that may contribute to organ and system dysfunction. They must also identify dysfunction in specific systems at the earliest sign and modify treatment to minimize further damage.

Critically ill patients usually have arterial, central venous, and pulmonary arterial catheters placed for continuous or frequent monitoring of several basic or critical indicators of systems' physiologic functions, such as blood pressure, pulse and respiratory rates, right and left atrial filling pressures, cardiac output, and oxyhemoglobin saturation. These observations are complemented by frequent (about twice daily) focussed physical examinations

and reviews of key laboratory data, such as serum electrolytes, blood gases, and hematocrit. An essential tool of management and communication for each patient is a large bedside flowsheet, which integrates and displays these data so that all care-givers can understand current and recent physiologic status, trends, and responses to treatments.

One of the most daunting practical problems is organizing and digesting the vast amount of information that is accumulated about each patient. It is paramount for the clinician to develop and rigorously adhere to a comprehensive physiologic systems format in evaluating these complicated patients. Some systems may seem to be functioning (or malfunctioning) independently of others. Problems with other systems may frequently seem to be intimately intertwined. A comprehensive systems approach in thinking about the various problems allows care-givers to review and integrate all important data and observations, consider the relationships among problems, prioritize each patient's needs, and maintain a complete and rational plan of care. Verbal (rounds) and written communications (progress notes) should also be organized in a systems format, in which each physiologic system is discussed in sequence, referring to all pertinent clinical observations and laboratory data.

Treatment: Much of the current therapy for MODS is either preventive or supportive. Rapid resuscitation from shock, prompt management of infections, and attention to details of fluid, electrolyte, and nutritional status may help to prevent subsequent dysfunction of organs and systems not involved in an initial illness. New or worsening tachypnea may trigger a lung examination, chest x-ray, and arterial blood gas to identify the cause of the tachypnea, quantify the degree of dysfunction, and point toward treatment options. A decrease in urine output should prompt clinical assessment of intravascular volume, perhaps including direct measurement of right or left ventricular filling pressures.

To identify intrinsic renal disease, further evaluation should include measurement of BUN, creatinine, and a urinalysis. If there is acute renal dysfunction, sepsis, drug-induced nephrotoxicity, or another treatable or correctable cause must be sought. Once organ failure occurs, supportive measures such as dialysis and mechanical ventilation are designed to prevent additional complications while intrinsic reparative processes restore systems function. Nutritional support via enteral or parenteral routes may minimize the autocatabolism associated with the hypermetabolic state of severe illness.

Many other therapies are in stages of investigation. Some researchers advocate use of inotropic agents to increase oxygen delivery above usual normal levels to support marginally perfused tissues. Others have promoted gut sterilization with oral nonabsorbable antibiotics to prevent sepsis from bacterial translocation. The results of large multicenter trials of glucocorticoids in patients with sepsis and ARDS were disappointing, but other anti-inflammatory agents with fewer side effects may be more efficacious. Immunotherapy with agents directed against inflammatory mediators may also prove beneficial.

Prognosis: Regardless of the cause of MODS or the organs involved, failure of one or two organs persisting for 3 days or more is associated with 40% or 60% mortality rate, respectively. When three or more organs fail, mortality rate approaches 100%. About 15% of all deaths in intensive care units occur in patients with MODS. Because of these frequent deaths and the high cost of intensive care, the pathophysiology and management of MODS are the subject of much current research.

SUMMARY

▶ Shock is organ and system dysfunction caused by inadequate delivery of oxygen to metabolically active tissues. The most important determinant of oxygen delivery to an organ is blood flow.

▶ Inadequate oxygen delivery in shock can be understood by focussing on the interaction between cardiac and circulatory functions. Low cardiac output with low central venous pressure is caused by hypovolemia. Low output with high central venous pressure implies cardiogenic shock, tamponade, or pulmonary embolism. Inadequate oxygen delivery in septic shock with high cardiac output is caused by maldistribution of flow.

▶ A successful approach to shock requires rapid but precise assessment of the circulation. Initial management is directed toward restoring blood flow to oxygen-deprived tissues and reversing the process that initiated shock.

▶ Multiple organ dysfunction syndrome is similar to shock in that several organs and systems fail simultaneously or sequentially. However, the cause, pathogenesis, and natural history are different. Organ and system failures in MODS may be attributed to one or several processes. Dysfunction of an individual system may precipitate or aggravate failure in others.

SUGGESTED READING

Bone RC: Toward a theory regarding the pathogenesis of the systemic inflammatory response syndrome: What we do and do not know about cytokine regulation. Crit Care Med 1996; 24:163.

Hess ML, Warner M, Okabe E: Hemorrhagic shock. In: *Handbook of Shock and Trauma*. Altura BM et al (editors). Raven Press, 1983.

Hinshaw L: Overview of hemorrhagic shock. In: *Pathophysiology of Shock, Anoxia and Ischemia*. Cowley RA, Trump BF (editors). Williams & Wilkins, 1982.

Parrillo JE et al: Septic shock in humans. Ann Intern Med 1990; 113:227.

Pinsky MR, Matuschak GM: Multiple systems organ failure: Failure of host defense homeostasis. Crit Care Clin 1989;5:199.

Sylvester JT, Goldberg HS, Permutt S: The role of the vasculature in the regulation of cardiac output. Clin Chest Med 1983;4:111.

Skin Disease and Internal Medicine

Benjamin K. Yokel, MD, and Antoinette F. Hood, MD

About one-third of patients presenting to a primary care physician have a skin problem as either a primary or secondary complaint. Many hospitalized patients have rashes, often as a complication of therapy. Physicians must be able to recognize skin abnormalities because they may be life-threatening (eg, melanoma) or a manifestation of systemic disease (eg, systemic lupus erythematosus). These abnormalities may also be disfiguring and debilitating. Equally important, from the patient's perspective, is the fact that most skin disease can be treated effectively.

DIAGNOSIS

Clinical Evaluation

Because a complete history is crucial to the diagnosis of skin disease, in addition to asking the patient about the current problem, the physician should seek the past medical history, medication history (both prescription and over-the-counter products), family history, and histories of travel, jobs, recreation, and environmental exposures.

A complete skin examination requires checking all mucocutaneous surfaces. The patient should be fully disrobed, but draped except for the areas being examined. An accurate exam requires bright lighting, either natural or artificial. Useful equipment includes a magnifying lens, a ruler, a small flashlight, protective gloves, and glass slides to be used for diascopy (see "Diagnostic Techniques" below).

The physician should record the morphology, configuration, and distribution of all cutaneous lesions, using precise dermatologic terms. Table 15.5–1 is a glossary of some important terms, and Figure 15.5–1 illustrates many of them.

Diagnostic Techniques

The following are some of the more frequently used dermatologic diagnostic techniques:

Potassium hydroxide examination: A potassium hydroxide (KOH) exam is done to confirm or rule out superficial fungal infection. Scale is gently removed from the surface of a skin lesion and placed on a microscope slide. Potassium hydroxide 10–20% is added, a coverslip is applied, and the slide is heated. The specimen is then examined microscopically for hyphae and spores.

Diascopy: Diascopy reveals how the skin changes after blood vessels are emptied. The examiner compresses erythematous skin lesions using either two clear glass microscope slides or a clear plastic diascope. Erythema secondary to vasodilatation clears when compressed; extravasated blood (purpura) still looks red.

Wood's light examination: Pigment changes of primarily epidermal origin enhance when viewed under the Wood's (black) light, and a number of infectious organisms fluoresce.

Tzanck preparation: A Tzanck preparation is used to evaluate vesicular lesions that may be caused by herpesvirus infection. The base and roof of a fresh vesicle or bulla are exposed and gently scraped. The scrapings are placed on a glass slide, fixed, and stained with Wright or Giemsa stain. If the lesions are caused by a herpesvirus, balloon cells and multinucleate giant cells will be visible.

Scraping for mites: A drop of mineral oil is applied to skin with suspected scabies, and the lesions are scraped vigorously. The scrapings are checked under the microscope for mites, eggs, and feces.

Darkfield examination: This is the test for ulcerated genital lesions suspected of being primary syphilis. Serous exudate from a genital ulcer is applied to a glass slide and examined under the darkfield microscope for spirochetes.

Skin biopsy: Skin biopsy is a simple procedure that may help establish a diagnosis of a tumor or inflammatory disease. Tissue can be removed by any of several means: Small lesions can be shaved off with a razor blade. Lesions can be surgically excised, and the wound closed with sutures. A punch biopsy, done by a special instrument with a circular blade, re-

Table 15.5–1. Glossary: Terms used to describe skin lesions.

macule: nonpalpable area of color change <1 cm in diameter (eg, freckle).

patch: larger nonpalpable lesion (eg, café-au-lait spot).

papule: discrete, solid, raised lesion <1 cm in diameter (eg, nevus).

nodule: larger discrete, rounded, raised, solid lesion (eg, rheumatoid nodule).

cyst: circumscribed lesion containing either fluid or solid material (eg, epidermoid cyst, acne cyst).

plaque: raised, flat-topped lesion >1 cm in diameter (eg, psoriasis).

wheal: transient edematous erythematous plaque (eg, hive [urticaria]).

vesicle: fluid-filled lesion <0.5 cm in diameter (eg, varicella).

bulla: larger fluid-filled lesion (eg, bullous pemphigoid).

pustule: vesicle-like lesion filled with purulent exudate (eg, folliculitis).

erosion: area of tissue loss above the dermal-epidermal junction.

ulcer: area of tissue loss including the full thickness of epidermis, and generally some dermis as well.

fissure: thin, linear erosion or ulcer (eg, fingertip eczema).

scale: a surface change characterized by dry, whitish flakes (eg, dandruff).

crust: dried serous and serosanguineous exudate (eg, impetigo).

lichenification: accentuation of the skin markings, generally also with thickening of the skin.

atrophy: loss of substance of tissue; can involve the epidermis, dermis, or subcutaneous tissue; atrophic epidermis appears shiny and finely wrinkled, like cigarette paper.

verrucous: wart-like.

annular: arranged in a circle or ring (eg, tinea corporis).

polycyclic: arranged in multiple confluent rings.

arcuate: arranged in incomplete rings, forming arc-like patterns.

linear: arranged in a straight line or band (eg, zoster).

reticulate: arranged in a net-like pattern (eg, livedo reticularis).

morbilliform: measles-like; implies multiple widely distributed lesions that may be discrete, confluent, or both (eg, drug eruption).

moves a cylindrical plug of skin 2–6 mm in diameter. Specimens may be sent for histologic examination, culture, or other special tests.

Immunofluorescence: *Direct immunofluorescence* is used to detect the deposition of tissue-bound antibodies and complement in the skin. Characteristic deposition may be seen in certain immune-mediated bullous diseases and connective tissue disorders. Sections of skin are treated with fluorescein-conjugated antisera to human immunoglobulins (IgG, IgM, and IgA), complement, and fibrin. The sections are then examined with a special microscope adapted to detect fluorescence. *Indirect immunofluorescence* is used to detect serum autoantibodies that are directed against certain skin structures. Frozen sections of animal squamous epithelium are incubated with the patient's serum; if the serum contains skin-reacting antibodies, they attach to components of the epithelium. Then fluorescein-labeled anti-human IgG antiserum is added to identify the specific circulating antibody, and the final preparation is examined with the fluorescein microscope to localize the antibody.

PAPULOSQUAMOUS DISORDERS

Papulosquamous disorders are a heterogeneous group of skin diseases characterized by red papules, patches, and plaques, with differing amounts of scale.

Psoriasis

Psoriasis is an idiopathic inflammatory skin disorder that affects 1% of the population worldwide. Psoriasis begins at any age. Involvement can range from isolated plaques on the scalp, elbows, and knees to involvement of the whole body. The eruption can be asymptomatic or pruritic. Patients with severe disease may have fever and chills, and some develop an associated arthritis (Chapter 3.7).

Classic psoriasis appears as well-demarcated red plaques covered with thick, silvery scale and distributed over the scalp, lower back, and extensor surfaces of the extremities (see Color Plates). Many patients have palmar and plantar involvement, and a majority have nail changes—pitting, yellowish spots (oil spots), and nail dystrophy. Clinical variants include guttate psoriasis (small drop-like lesions), pustular psoriasis, inverse psoriasis (flexural distribution of lesions), and erythrodermic psoriasis (see "Exfoliative Erythroderma" below).

Limited disease can be treated topically with calcipotriene (a vitamin D derivative), corticosteroids, tar-derived preparations, or anthralin. More extensive disease may require ultraviolet light therapy or even systemic therapy with methotrexate or etretinate.

Atopic Dermatitis and Eczematous Dermatitis

Atopic dermatitis (eczema) is a common inflammatory skin disorder characterized by ill-defined red, scaly, often weepy plaques. The plaques are most pronounced in flexural areas such as the antecubital and popliteal fossae. Patients almost uniformly complain of pruritus, and many have a personal or family history of asthma or allergic rhinitis. Laboratory testing may show elevated serum IgE levels and impaired delayed-type hypersensitivity. Disease severity generally peaks in early childhood and tends to ease somewhat in later life, but this is variable. Many children with atopic dermatitis develop hand dermatitis as adults. Topical corticosteroids and emollients are the most widely used treatments, although patients with severe disease may need oral corticosteroids and ultraviolet light.

Seborrheic Dermatitis

Seborrheic dermatitis is a common condition that can present at any age. Patients typically complain of erythema and scale on the central face, eyebrows, retroauricular areas, scalp, and central chest. This disorder is especially common in patients with neurologic disorders and immunodeficiency states, including AIDS. Some dermatologists believe that seborrheic dermatitis is a hypersensitivity reaction to *Malassezia furfur* (also known as *Pityrosporum ovale*), a ubiquitous yeast. Seborrheic dermatitis responds to treatment with mild topical steroids, although topical antifungal agents may be useful as well.

Contact Dermatitis

Contact dermatitis is defined as inflammation localized to areas of skin exposed to an extrinsic agent (see Color Plates). The process may be caused by direct chemical or physical irritation of the skin (irritant contact dermatitis; eg, hand dermatitis), or it may be immune-mediated (allergic contact dermatitis; eg, poison ivy). The physician can usually obtain a history of exposure to a potential irritating or sensitizing agent, but finding the cause sometimes requires a great deal of investigation, including visits to the patient's workplace.

Other forms of eczematous dermatitis may present as red, scaly eruptions. These include *stasis dermatitis,* which can be seen on the legs and feet of patients with chronic venous insufficiency; *asteatotic eczema,* dry, scaly, fissured skin, seen in older patients; and dermatitis secondary to *nutritional deficiency,* such as pellagra or essential fatty acid deficiency.

Exfoliative Erythroderma

The condition of confluent erythema and scale involving the entire skin surface is termed exfoliative erythroderma. Many patients also have fissuring and crusting, and most report intense pruritus. Because of the massive shunting of blood to the inflamed skin, many patients have dehydration and impaired thermoregulation. Other systemic complications of exfoliative erythroderma are high-output heart failure, hypoalbuminemia secondary to the lost protein in the shed scale, and folate deficiency and anemia secondary to the accelerated keratinocyte turnover.

For nearly 50% of patients with new-onset exfoliative erythroderma, no specific cause can be found. Known causes include psoriasis, atopic dermatitis, drug reactions, cutaneous T-cell lymphoma, and occasionally other primary dermatologic disorders such as pemphigus foliaceus. The condition can also be a paraneoplastic phenomenon, especially in response to an underlying lymphoma. Rare systemic causes of erythroderma are sarcoidosis and systemic lupus erythematosus.

Management of erythroderma includes soaks and emollients to rehydrate the skin, careful attention to fluid and nutritional status, and treatment of the underlying cause.

TUMORS

Melanocytic Lesions

Melanocytic neoplasms are extremely common. Although most of these lesions are benign melanocytic nevi (moles), the incidence of malignant melanoma is rising, and every physician must be proficient at recognizing this potentially fatal tumor. Although many patients with melanoma present to their physician complaining of a changing mole, a large percentage of melanomas are detected incidentally—hence, the importance of thorough skin exams.

Most dermatologists use the ABCDE rule when screening melanocytic lesions: melanomas tend to be **a**symmetric, to have notched or irregular **b**orders, have **c**olor variation within the lesions, to have **d**iameters greater than 6 mm, and to be **e**levated above the skin surface (see Color Plates). Any patient with such a pigmented lesion should be referred to a dermatologist for further evaluation. Early melanomas tend to be macular; more advanced lesions are nodular. Patients with thin melanomas (less than 0.76 mm in microscopic thickness) have an excellent prognosis; the prognosis worsens progressively for patients with thicker melanomas. The treatment of choice for cutaneous melanoma remains surgical excision of the primary tumor.

Tumors Composed of Keratinocytes

Seborrheic keratoses represent a common benign proliferation of keratinocytes. Most patients are asymptomatic, but they may be concerned about their cosmetic appearance. Seborrheic keratoses are flesh-colored to pigmented papules or plaques. They generally have an irregular, wart-like surface and "stuck-on" appearance, as if they could be peeled off the underlying skin. Although the lesions are clinically insignificant, the sudden development of multiple seborrheic keratoses may be a marker for an underlying visceral carcinoma. Many other benign tumors, beyond the scope of this chapter, derive from keratinocytes or skin appendages (adnexal structures: eccrine sweat glands, sebaceous glands, hair, and nails).

Malignant keratinocyte-derived tumors are much more common than malignant melanomas, but fortunately tend to grow more slowly and rarely metastasize. *Basal cell carcinoma* is the most common malignancy; each year, in the United States alone, more than 500,000 people develop this tumor. Most patients with basal cell carcinoma have a fair complexion and a history of extensive sun exposure. Basal cell carcinomas appear as flesh-colored to red macules, papules, and nodules; they have a pearly or translucent surface with prominent telangiectases, rolled borders, and often depressed or ulcerated centers (see Color Plates). Although metastatic basal cell carcinoma is extremely rare, tumors can be locally invasive and aggressive, so they must be removed completely by excision, destruction, or radiation.

Squamous cell carcinomas are more aggressive than basal cell carcinomas. Many patients with squamous cell carcinomas have a history of extensive sun exposure, although the tumors can develop within areas of chronic inflammation or in skin chronically infected with human papillomavirus. Squamous cell carcinomas are especially common in immunosuppressed persons. Patients typically complain of an enlarging and ulcerating red nodule. Squamous cell carcinomas occasionally metastasize, especially from primary tumors on the lower lip and genitalia. The treatment of choice is early complete surgical excision or radiation.

Metastatic Tumors

Many internal malignancies can metastasize to the skin, particularly cancers arising in the breast, gastrointestinal tract, lung, and kidney; most patients with cutaneous

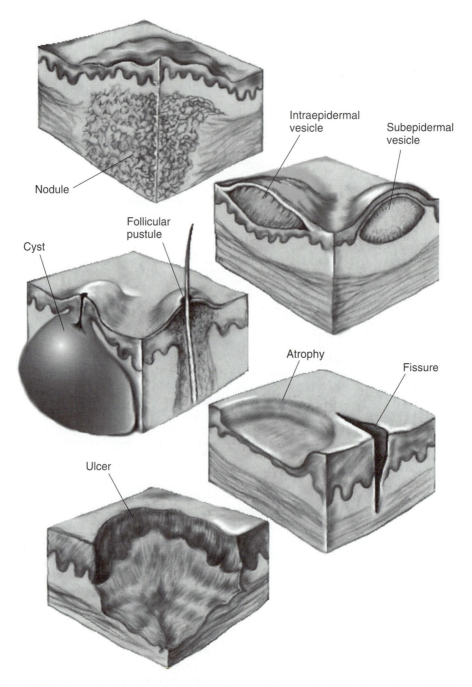

Figure 15.5–1. Types of skin lesions. (S. Elizabeth Whitmore, MD, consulted in the preparation of this figure.)

metastatic carcinoma present with multiple firm skin nodules. Patients with leukemia or lymphoma can also develop cutaneous spread of their malignancies; these patients typically present with red to plum-colored papules, plaques, and nodules. Cutaneous metastasis from sarcomas is uncommon.

Cutaneous T-Cell Lymphoma

Cutaneous T-cell lymphoma (mycosis fungoides) is a malignant proliferation of T lymphocytes arising primarily in the skin. The tumor may spread to involve lymph nodes or other organs, but its progression is generally indolent, taking years or decades. Patients present with red

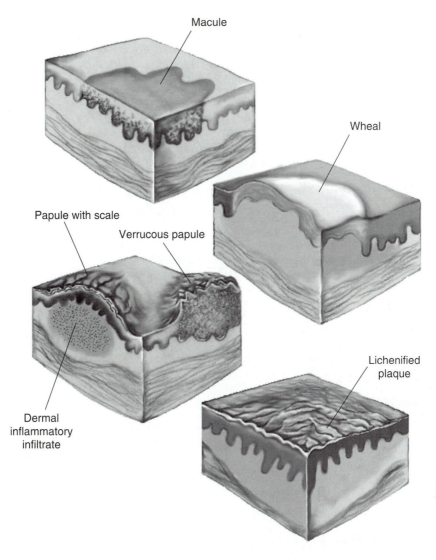

Macule

Wheal

Papule with scale

Verrucous papule

Dermal
inflammatory
infiltrate

Lichenified
plaque

Figure 15.5–1. (Continued)

to reddish-brown scaly patches and plaques; the plaques are often shaped like kidney beans. As the disease progresses, nodules and tumors form. Ultimately, the lymphoma may progress to the Sézary syndrome, a leukemic phase associated with an exfoliative erythroderma.

The diagnosis of cutaneous T-cell lymphoma is confirmed by skin biopsy that shows atypical cleaved lymphocytes invading the epidermis. Immunophenotyping of the lymphoid infiltrate may be used to confirm the histologic findings. The etiology is unknown, although infection with HTLV-1 can produce identical clinical findings.

Treatment for early cutaneous T-cell lymphoma is palliative and probably does not alter the disease's course. Ultraviolet light, topical nitrogen mustard, and electron-beam radiation may improve patients' symptoms and cos-

metic appearance. Nodules and tumors may be irradiated, and patients may need systemic chemotherapy when organs other than the skin are involved.

Miscellaneous Benign and Malignant Cutaneous Neoplasms

Lipomas are benign tumors composed of adipocytes, presenting as soft, fleshy nodules. They are of no clinical significance. *Neurofibromas* present as soft, often pedunculated (exophytic, with a stalk-like base) nodules, which tend to umbilicate or "buttonhole" when pressed. Although the lesions themselves are benign, patients with multiple neurofibromas should be evaluated for neurofibromatosis. *Epidermal inclusion cysts* arise from hair follicle epithelium, often as a result of trauma. A patient with multiple epidermal inclusion cysts should be evaluated for familial polyposis of the colon (Gardner's syndrome). Cherry *angiomas* are benign proliferations of blood vessels, appearing as bright red papules. Their frequency increases with age. *Kaposi's sarcoma* is a malignant proliferation of endothelial cells. In its classic form, this tumor is seen as purple macules, papules, plaques, and nodules on the legs of persons with chronic stasis dermatitis. Kaposi's sarcoma is now seen most often in patients infected with HIV; these patients' lesions can appear anywhere on the body (see Color Plates).

HYPERSENSITIVITY REACTIONS

Urticaria

Patients with urticaria (hives) complain of the acute onset of transient, migratory, intensely pruritic skin lesions (Chapter 10.2). The lesions are edematous red plaques, often annular or polycyclic, with central clearing (see Color Plates). Urticaria usually represents an IgE-mediated release of histamine from mast cells, but is occasionally caused by nonimmune physical stimuli. Urticaria can result from allergies to food and medication and hypersensitivity to antigens produced in response to chronic infection or a neoplasm. In most patients, no specific cause can be found.

Treatment of patients with simple urticaria should include oral antihistamines and avoidance of inciting stimuli. Patients who develop angioedema (swelling of the deeper tissues around the lips and tongue) should be watched closely for the development of laryngospasm or anaphylaxis.

Erythema Multiforme

Erythema multiforme is an uncommon inflammatory dermatosis. Although the exact etiology is unknown, the disorder can appear in association with a number of other conditions, including herpesvirus and *Mycoplasma pneumoniae* infections, and can be a drug reaction. Some patients complain of only a few isolated lesions, others of a widespread process. The characteristic lesion is a target-like annular plaque with a red border and a dusky, purpuric, or bullous center, found on the palms and soles (see Color Plates). A severe variant of erythema multiforme is *Stevens-Johnson syndrome,* in which patients develop severe erosions of mucous membranes. Although patients with erythema multiforme tend to recover spontaneously, oral steroids are often used to accelerate healing. Any underlying cause should also be treated.

A related condition that can develop as a drug reaction is *toxic epidermal necrolysis.* Affected patients present with tender, macular erythema. Later they develop multiple flaccid subepidermal bullae that rupture, leaving behind extensive areas of denuded dermis (see Color Plates). Rubbing the normal-looking skin adjacent to intact bullae often makes the epidermis separate from the dermis (Nikolsky's sign). Patients with toxic epidermal necrolysis are at great risk for fluid and electrolyte imbalances and secondary infections and should be managed as if they had severe thermal burns. The role of corticosteroids in treating toxic epidermal necrolysis is controversial.

Panniculitis

Patients with inflammation of the subcutaneous fat present with tender red nodules, usually on the legs. The most common cause is *erythema nodosum*, in which the inflammation is localized to the interlobular septa (see Color Plates). A biopsy is needed to differentiate this condition from deep forms of vasculitis. Erythema nodosum can be associated with a number of systemic disorders, including inflammatory bowel disease (Chapter 6.10), streptococcal infection, systemic fungal infection (especially coccidioidomycosis) (Chapter 8.13), and sarcoidosis (Chapter 2.5).

Vasculitis

Most patients with palpable purpuric skin lesions are found on skin biopsy to have vasculitis (Chapter 3.5; see Color Plates). Some of these patients have multiple small purpuric papules (sometimes ulcerated), which are widely distributed but concentrated on the legs and feet. Those affected probably have *leukocytoclastic vasculitis*—hypersensitivity angiitis involving the small venules (see Color Plates). Although leukocytoclastic vasculitis is often a self-limited skin disorder, it can have systemic associations. *Henoch-Schönlein purpura,* most commonly seen in children, is a form of leukocytoclastic vasculitis with abdominal pain and often with renal involvement. Leukocytoclastic vasculitis can also be associated with necrotizing angiitis involving other organs, including the central nervous system. Patients may develop small-vessel cutaneous vasculitis with such systemic inflammatory disorders as systemic lupus erythematosus (Chapter 3.2), Sjögren's syndrome (Chapter 3.4), sarcoidosis (Chapter 2.5), and cryoglobulinemia (Chapter 3.5); with an underlying neoplasm or infection; or as a drug reaction. Treatment of leukocytoclastic vasculitis is aimed at correcting identifiable causes. Isolated skin disease is treated with immunosuppressive drugs only if the patient develops severe ulceration.

Patients with vasculitis involving larger cutaneous vessels may present with nodules, bullae, and frank necrosis with ulceration. *Livedo reticularis* is a net-like pattern of macular violaceous erythema involving the legs and feet; although normal people can have this pattern, it is usually pronounced in patients with vasculitis. All patients with cutaneous lesions suggesting larger-vessel vasculitis require biopsy confirmation and thorough systemic evaluation.

LOCALIZED CUTANEOUS INFECTIONS

Some common fungal, bacterial, and viral skin infections are mentioned here. Chapter 8.12 covers skin infections in depth. Other chapters discuss the skin manifestations of infections caused by mycobacteria (tuberculosis, atypical mycobacteria) (Chapter 8.14), spirochetes (syphilis [Chapter 8.9], Lyme disease [Chapter 8.16]), rickettsiae (Rocky Mountain spotted fever) (Chapter 8.16), and parasites (pediculosis pubis, scabies) (Chapter 8.9).

Fungal Infections

Localized superficial cutaneous fungal infections (Chapter 8.13) are caused either by a group of organisms collectively known as dermatophytes or by *Candida* sp. Dermatophyte infections (tinea) can occur anywhere on the body and are named for the site of infection. For example, tinea capitis for scalp ringworm, tinea corporis for body ringworm, tinea cruris for groin infections, tinea pedis for athlete's foot. Patients may give a history of exposure to other infected people or animals; tinea pedis and tinea cruris are especially common when factors like sweating or rubber footwear increase local humidity. The classic appearance of a dermatophytosis is a red annular plaque with a scaling, occasionally pustular border. But the clinical picture is highly variable, and the ring shape is often hard to see. A KOH preparation is generally diagnostic; an occasional patient needs a fungal culture or skin biopsy. Dermatophyte infections can be treated topically with antifungal agents such as clotrimazole, or systemically with griseofulvin or ketoconazole.

Cutaneous candidiasis generally develops in intertriginous regions. It is seen most often in association with incontinence, diabetes, immunosuppression, or antibiotic treatment. The typical appearance is beefy red scaling plaques with satellite papules and pustules. Therapy should include aeration of the affected area and a topical or oral imidazole.

Tinea versicolor is a common fungal skin infection characterized by widespread scaly patches that may be red, hyperpigmented, or hypopigmented. The eruption may be pruritic or asymptomatic. It usually worsens during the warmer months. Tinea versicolor is seen most often in young and otherwise healthy adults. *Malassezia furfur* (*Pityrosporum ovale*), the causative organism, is a ubiquitous component of normal skin flora, but tinea versicolor affects only a small percentage of the population. The diagnosis is confirmed by KOH exam of a specimen of scale. The eruption generally responds to topical antifungal agents or selenium sulfide.

Many fungi can cause cutaneous infections that penetrate into the dermis and subcutaneous tissues, where they may produce localized or disseminated disease. In neutropenic patients, disseminated infections are caused by more common fungi, such as *Candida albicans*. These infections usually present as widespread red papules and nodules.

Bacterial Infections

Localized skin infection typically presents with erythematous lesions of variable morphology (Chapter 8.12). Patients with *cellulitis* develop tender, warm, indurated, often weepy red plaques in the infected area. *Erysipelas* is a superficial variant of cellulitis characterized by very superficial red plaques with sharply demarcated, palpable borders (see Color Plates). Cellulitis and erysipelas require treatment with oral or intravenous antibiotics.

Impetigo is a common infection that usually affects children. Patients present with one or several red patches covered by a honey-colored crust. Since the infection is limited to the superficial epidermis, patients can be treated topically or orally with antibiotics active against streptococci and staphylococci. Bacterial abscesses typically present as fluctuant (pus-filled), tender red nodules; these lesions require prompt surgical drainage.

Bacterial skin infection can also cause vesicles and bullae. *Bullous impetigo* is seen in children and immunosuppressed adults. Patients develop flaccid bullae filled with seropurulent fluid. The cause is *Staphylococcus aureus,* phage group 2. The organism produces a toxin that causes the skin to split at the level of the granular layer, forming blisters. The diagnosis is confirmed by bacterial culture of the blister fluid. Bullous impetigo responds promptly to oral antibiotics.

The same staphylococci occasionally release the toxin systemically, giving rise to the *staphylococcal scalded skin syndrome.* This syndrome can arise even from a very small superficial staphylococcal infection. Patients with scalded skin syndrome present with a generalized eruption of flaccid bullae, which rupture, leaving behind crusted red patches. Here, the blister fluid is sterile. Scalded skin syndrome is also treated with antibiotics.

Viral Infections

Herpes simplex infections (Chapter 8.11) present as grouped vesicles on an erythematous base (see Color Plates). Patients typically report tingling or burning sensations before the lesions appear. The infection can recur, although recurrences tend to be less severe than the initial outbreak. Although herpes simplex most commonly infects the genital and perioral regions, it can involve any part of the body. The virus is spread from person to person or from region to region by direct contact. Herpes can be spread even when there are no active lesions. Disseminated cutaneous infection, known as eczema herpeticum, is seen in patients with atopic dermatitis; infants and immunosuppressed patients can have systemic infection. Herpes simplex infections usually respond to therapy with acyclovir.

Primary herpes varicella zoster infection (Chapter 8.11) causes chickenpox—fever, malaise, and vesicular skin lesions described as "dew drops on rose petals." Patients with recurrent varicella zoster present with severe pain followed by an outbreak of vesicles and erythematous plaques in a linear, dermatomal distribution (see Color Plates). In immunosuppressed patients, the infection may spread to other organs. Zoster is treated with high-dose acyclovir or famciclovir, plus an analgesic.

Verrucae vulgaris (common warts) represent infection of keratinocytes by the human papillomavirus. Occasional lesions, especially those on mucous membranes, undergo malignant transformation. *Molluscum contagiosa* are pearly, umbilicated, flesh-colored papules caused by a poxvirus infection. These lesions are found most often in children, but are also common in immunosuppressed adults.

AUTOIMMUNE BLISTERING DISORDERS AND PORPHYRIA

A number of autoimmune disorders can produce bullae. *Bullous pemphigoid* is an uncommon dermatosis of older people. Patients present with multiple tense subepidermal bullae, especially in flexural areas. Immunofluorescence exam of the skin around the lesion reveals IgG and C3 deposits along the dermal-epidermal junction. Many patients have circulating autoantibodies directed against the basement membrane zone.

Pemphigus vulgaris is another antibody-mediated blistering disorder. Patients with pemphigus present with multiple flaccid intraepidermal bullae and erosions at the sites of ruptured bullae. Immunofluorescence reveals antibody deposition in the intracellular space within the epidermis.

Among the other autoimmune blistering disorders is *dermatitis herpetiformis,* which manifests as small pruritic vesicles on the extensor surfaces and may be associated with a gluten-sensitive enteropathy.

Patients with autoimmune blistering disorders are generally treated with oral corticosteroids. Some patients, especially those with pemphigus, require more aggressive immunosuppressive therapy.

Patients with abnormalities in heme biosynthesis can develop various forms of porphyria. Skin lesions are most commonly seen in *porphyria cutanea tarda,* caused by congenital or acquired deficiency in uroporphyrinogen decarboxylase. Affected patients complain of bullae and scarring in sun-exposed areas (see Color Plates). When a patient presents with porphyria cutanea tarda, the physician should consider iron overload and hepatitis C as precipitating factors. In many patients, the trigger is alcohol abuse.

Pruritus

Although pruritus can be a feature of many skin disorders, some people present with isolated pruritus. Pruritus without primary skin lesions has a limited differential diagnosis: scabies (although most patients with scabies have small linear red burrows in their digital web spaces), drug reaction, polycythemia, iron deficiency anemia, occult liver disease, occult autoimmune blistering disease, occult malignancy, and occult psychiatric illness. Pruritus is managed by correcting any underlying cause and sedating the patient with oral antihistamines.

Acne

A number of common skin disorders can present as eruptions of follicular pustules. *Acne vulgaris* is perhaps the best known and most common. The primary lesions of acne—small flesh-colored papules known as microcomedones—can evolve into either inflammatory red papules and pustules (whiteheads) or noninflammatory open and closed comedones (blackheads). Severe acne leads to cysts and scarring. Most affected persons have acne on their face, chest, and back. The condition is worsened by topical application of substances that occlude the follicular orifices. Acne may flare when the patient takes certain medications, including lithium, prednisone, and some oral contraceptives. Severe acne may also accompany Cushing's syndrome and other endocrine disorders. Typical acne vulgaris peaks during the teen years, but occasionally persists well into adulthood.

Acne rosacea is a facial eruption in adults, characterized by pustules, papules, and telangiectases usually involving the nose and central face. Patients with rosacea often complain of flushing. The condition responds well to oral tetracycline and to topical metronidazole or sulfur-containing preparations.

DISORDERS OF THE HAIR AND SCALP

Alopecia (hair loss) may be a localized condition or may be associated with underlying systemic disorders. In nonscarring alopecia, the follicular orifice is preserved; in scarring alopecia, the follicle is destroyed. Other complaints that the physician may encounter are scaling and itching of the scalp and excessive hair growth elsewhere on the body (Chapter 4.5).

Nonscarring Alopecia

Androgenic alopecia (male-pattern balding) is the most common cause of hair loss. This inherited condition, which can affect both women and men, is characterized by symmetric loss of terminal hairs from the vertex, frontal, and temporal areas of the scalp. Women with significant androgenic alopecia should be evaluated to rule out an underlying endocrine disorder. Treatment with topical minoxidil may provide minimal regrowth.

Alopecia areata presents as loss of hair from one or more discrete patches on the scalp or elsewhere. There is minimal underlying inflammation. Alopecia areata is an immune-mediated process; affected patients should be evaluated for autoimmune thyroid disease. Although alopecia areata is usually self-limited, it can progress until the patient has no hair on the scalp (alopecia totalis) or the entire body (alopecia universalis). Commonly used treatments are local and systemic steroids and ultraviolet light.

Telogen effluvium, the result of the synchronized conversion of multiple hair follicles into the telogen (resting) phase, can follow any major physiologic stress, including illness and pregnancy. Telogen effluvium is characterized by the relatively sudden onset of diffuse scalp hair loss. The loss is transient, and the hair grows back.

Diffuse, nonscarring alopecia can accompany systemic illnesses such as secondary syphilis, hypothyroidism, and systemic lupus erythematosus. A number of drugs can cause thinning of scalp hair; cytotoxic agents can cause complete alopecia because of their antimitotic effect on rapidly proliferating hair follicle cells. Nonscarring alopecia can also result from dermatophyte fungal infection of the scalp.

Scarring Alopecia

Scarring alopecia is caused by inflammation severe enough to destroy the hair follicle. A common cause of scarring alopecia is chronic cutaneous (discoid) lupus erythematosus, which generally also produces scalp atrophy, erythema, scale, and pigment alteration (see Color Plates). Scarring alopecia can also develop secondary to localized forms of scleroderma (morphea) (Chapter 3.10), severe bacterial or fungal infections, and less common inflammatory disorders such as folliculitis decalvans and lichen planopilaris.

DISORDERS OF MUCOUS MEMBRANES

Involvement of the mucous membranes is characteristic of a number of cutaneous disorders, including pemphigus vulgaris, erythema multiforme, and lichen planus. Mucosal lesions are also typical of a number of systemic disorders. Tender, self-healing oral erosions known as *aphthous ulcers* are common in healthy persons; similar but more aggressive lesions may be seen in Behçet's syndrome (Chapter 3.5), systemic lupus erythematosus (Chapter 3.2), and Crohn's disease (Chapter 6.10). Immunosuppressed patients often have *mucosal candidiasis,* which presents as whitish plaques on the tongue and buccal mucosa. Vertical linear white papules on the lateral surface of the tongue are typical of *oral hairy leukoplakia*; this condition, seen in people infected with HIV, is caused by the Epstein-Barr virus.

A number of tumors arise in the oral mucosa—most commonly, squamous cell carcinoma. Any patient with an enlarging or ulcerating nodule or a persistent whitish plaque should be referred to an oral surgeon for biopsy.

SUMMARY

▶ Skin disorders are common throughout life and account for up to 30% of all primary and secondary complaints that patients bring to physicians.

▶ Skin disease can cause not only discomfort and cosmetic distress but disability. Some skin disease is life-threatening.

▶ The general medical evaluation should include obtaining appropriate historical information about and examination of the skin.

▶ To diagnose dermatologic disease accurately, the physician must be able to recognize and differentiate normal from abnormal findings. The cornerstones of diagnosis are the morphology, configuration, and distribution of skin lesions.

▶ The skin often provides important evidence of and information about internal disease.

SUGGESTED READING

Callen JP et al (editors): *Dermatological Signs of Internal Disease,* 2nd ed. WB Saunders, 1995.

Callen JP et al: *Color Atlas of Dermatology.* WB Saunders, 1993.

Fitzpatrick TB et al (editors): *Dermatology in General Medicine,* 4th ed. McGraw-Hill, 1993.

Friedman RJ et al (editors): *Cancer of the Skin.* WB Saunders, 1991.

Penneys NS: *Skin Manifestations of AIDS.* JB Lippincott, 1990.

Index

NOTE: Page numbers in bold face type indicate a major discussion. A *t* following a page number indicates a table and an *i* following a page number indicates an illustration. Drugs are listed under their generic names. When a drug trade name is listed, the reader is referred to the generic name.